BERNE & LEVY
PRINCIPLES OF PHYSIOLOGY

BERNE & LEVY
PRINCIPLES OF PHYSIOLOGY

FOURTH EDITION

Matthew N. Levy, MD
Professor Emeritus
Physiology and Biomedical Engineering
Case Western Reserve University
Cleveland, Ohio

Bruce A. Stanton, PhD
Professor of Physiology
Dartmouth Medical School
Hanover, New Hampshire

Bruce M. Koeppen, MD, PhD
Dean, Academic Affairs and Education
Albert and Wilda Van Dusen
Professor of Academic Medicine
University of Connecticut Health Center
Farmington, Connecticut

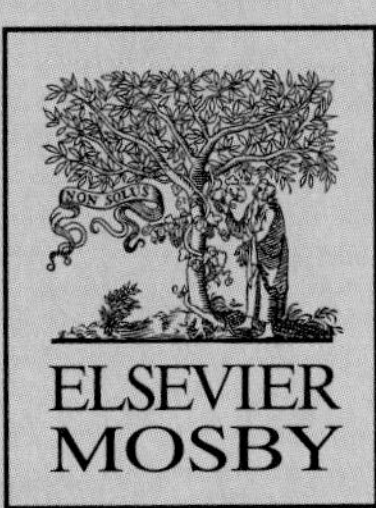

ELSEVIER
MOSBY

1600 John F. Kennedy Blvd.
Ste 1800
Philadelphia, PA 19103-2899

BERNE AND LEVY PRINCIPLES OF PHYSIOLOGY
0-323-03195-1 (Standard)
0-8089-2321-8 (International)

Library of Congress Cataloging-in-Publication Data

Berne and Levy principles of physiology/[editors] Matthew N. Levy, Bruce M. Koeppen, Bruce A. Stanton.—4th ed.
p. cm.
ISBN 0-323-03195-1
1. Human physiology. I. Levy, Matthew N., 1922— II. Berne, Robert M., 1918– III. Koeppen, Bruce M. IV. Stanton, Bruce A.
QP34.5.P744 2005
612—dc22 2004065640

Acquisitions Editor: William R. Schmitt
Developmental Editor: Andrew Hall
Design Direction: Steven Stave
Cover Designer: Steven Stave
Publishing Services Manager: Tina Rebane
Project Manager: Linda Van Pelt

Printed in China

Last digit is the print number: 9 8 7 6 5 4 3 2 1

This book is dedicated to Professor Robert M. Berne, who died October 4, 2001. Dr. Berne, together with Dr. Levy, developed the concept of this book and served as editor of the first three editions. His enthusiasm for the book and his thoughtful input were always valued, and now they are missed.

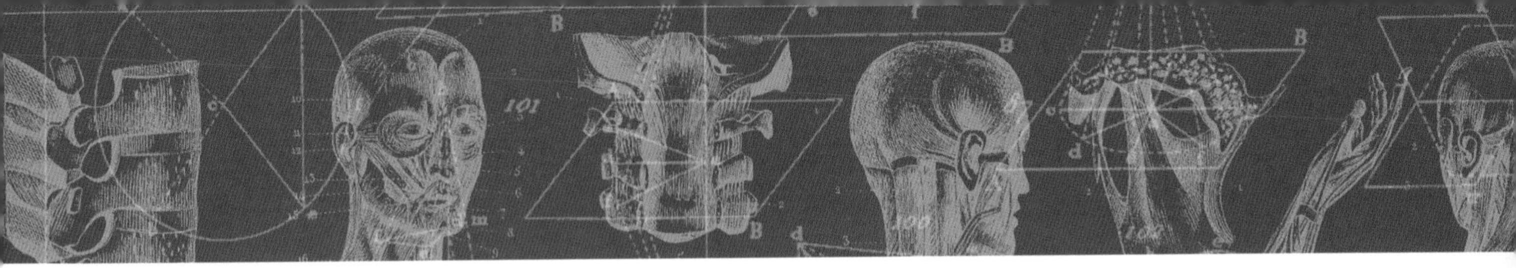

Contributors

Michelle M. Cloutier, MD
Professor of Pediatrics
University of Connecticut Health Center
Farmington, Connecticut
Director, Asthma Center
Connecticut Children's Medical Center
Hartford, Connecticut
Part Five, Respiratory System

Saul M. Genuth, MD
Professor of Medicine
Division of Clinical and Molecular Endocrinology
Case Western Reserve University
Cleveland, Ohio
Part Eight, Endocrine System

Bruce M. Koeppen, MD, PhD
Dean, Academic Affairs and Education
Albert and Wilda Van Dusen Professor of Academic Medicine
University of Connecticut Health Center
Farmington, Connecticut
Part Seven, Renal System

Howard C. Kutchai, PhD
Professor
Department of Molecular Physiology and Biological Physics
School of Medicine
University of Virginia
Charlottesville, Virginia
Part One, Cell Physiology
Part Six, Digestive System

Matthew N. Levy, MD
Professor Emeritus
Physiology and Biomedical Engineering
Case Western Reserve University
Cleveland, Ohio
Part Four, Cardiovascular System

Achilles Pappano, PhD
Professor of Pharmacology
University of Connecticut Health Center
Farmington, Connecticut
Part Four, Cardiovascular System

Bruce A. Stanton, PhD
Professor of Physiology
Dartmouth Medical School
Hanover, New Hampshire
Part Seven, Renal System

Roger S. Thrall, PhD
Professor of Medicine
Director of Pulmonary Research
University of Connecticut Health Center
Farmington, Connecticut
Director of Clinical Research
Hospital for Special Care
New Britain, Connecticut
Part Five, Respiratory System

James Watras, PhD
Associate Professor
Department of Pharmacology
University of Connecticut Health Center
Farmington, Connecticut
Part Three, Muscle

William D. Willis, Jr, MD, PhD
Professor
Neuroscience and Cell Biology
University of Texas Medical Branch
Galveston, Texas
Part Two, Nervous System

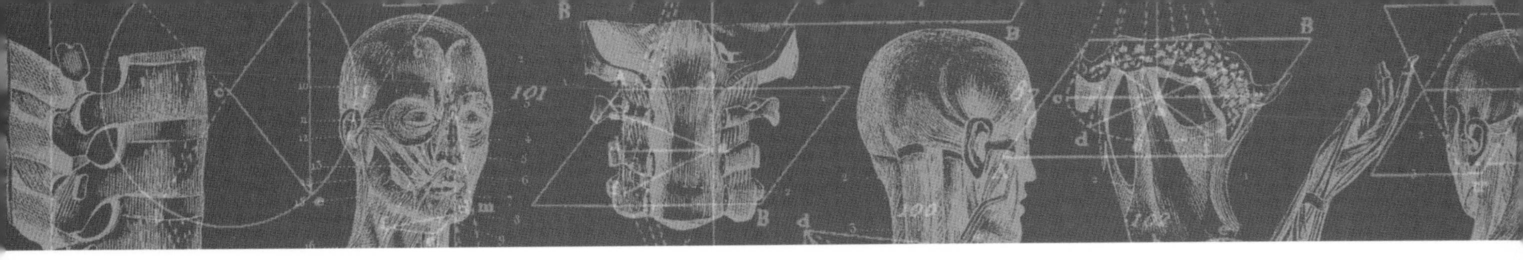

Preface

As in the previous editions of *Berne and Levy Principles of Physiology*, we have attempted in this revision to present broad concepts in a concise manner and to minimize the compilation of isolated facts. Each chapter in this edition has been revised to make the text as lucid, accurate, and current as possible. New insights from advances in molecular biology have been added, but not at the expense of providing the reader with a clear understanding of the important principles of organ physiology. We welcome to this edition new authors for the muscle, cardiovascular, and respiratory sections. The changes in these sections reflect the insight and perspective of these new authors regarding the important physiological principles at work in these organ systems.

This book has been designed to serve as an introductory text on human physiology. We believe that it will meet the learning needs of medical and dental students, other health professionals, and students in upper-level college physiology courses. To facilitate student learning, we have retained many of the popular features of earlier editions. Each chapter begins with a list of objectives. Multicolored illustrations are used to depict concepts as simply as possible. When sequential mechanisms are involved, multipanel diagrams have been designed to illustrate each step clearly. Block diagrams are used to depict the interrelationships among the various factors that may affect a specific function. Important data are accumulated in tables. The use of mathematics has been minimized, and succinct, lucid descriptions have been substituted wherever feasible. Controversial issues have been omitted to allow ample room for the explanation of important, generally accepted physiological mechanisms. We have refrained from citing the sources of the statements and assertions that appear in this text to keep nonessential details to a minimum. Throughout the book, certain sentences are set in small capital letters to emphasize important concepts, and we have used boldface to denote new terms and definitions. We have also emphasized many of the important physiological concepts by describing important clinical conditions in which such concepts are relevant. These clinical illustrations are framed in shaded boxes. Summaries are provided at the end of each chapter to highlight the key points in the chapter. Also at the end of each chapter, we have included a number of multiple-choice review questions based on illustrative clinical case studies. Answers with explanations are given at the end of the book. These questions and answers can help readers evaluate their comprehension of the material covered in the text and help in linking physiological concepts and mechanisms to clinical situations.

In Part One of this book (Cell Physiology), important physiological principles that apply across many of the organ systems are discussed. Topics include the roles of membrane transport proteins, the structure and function of ion-transporting ATPases, and signal transduction mechanisms.

Part Two (Nervous System) provides a neuroanatomical framework for the presentation of contemporary cellular neurophysiology. Substantial attention has been focused on the sensory and motor systems because of their clinical relevance. Analysis of the fundamental principles common to the various sensory systems facilitates the comprehension of the various components of each system.

In Part Three (Muscle), the basic mechanisms of contraction in skeletal, smooth, and cardiac muscles are described. The characteristics of skeletal and smooth muscle are presented in detail in this section, but the description of cardiac muscle performance is divided between Parts Three and Four.

In Part Four (Cardiovascular System), the function of the heart and vasculature is examined. Subsequently, how the various parts of the closed-loop circulatory system interact under various physiological and pathological conditions is analyzed.

Part Five (Respiratory System) emphasizes the physical principles that underlie the mechanics of breathing and the exchange of gas between the blood and the alveoli, and between the blood and the peripheral tissues. Furthermore, the neural and chemical processes that regulate respiration, the role of the lungs in immune defense, and certain nonrespiratory functions of the lungs are presented.

Part Six (Digestive System) first presents the processes of motility and secretion in the gastrointestinal tract, then explains how these functions are integrated by neural, endocrine, and paracrine mechanisms. Furthermore, the role of ion transporters in the absorption and secretion of electrolytes in the gastrointestinal tract is described.

In Part Seven (Renal System), the mechanisms by which the kidneys handle water and certain important solutes (e.g., Na^+, K^+, phosphate, and Ca^{++}) are described. The regulation of body fluid osmolality and volume and of acid-base balance is also explained.

In Part Eight (Endocrine System), similarities in the functioning of the various endocrine glands are emphasized. Major new insights into the mechanisms of hormone action, the regulation of energy storage and turnover, and the processes of reproduction are presented.

We wish to express our appreciation to all of our colleagues and students who have provided constructive criticism during the revision of this book.

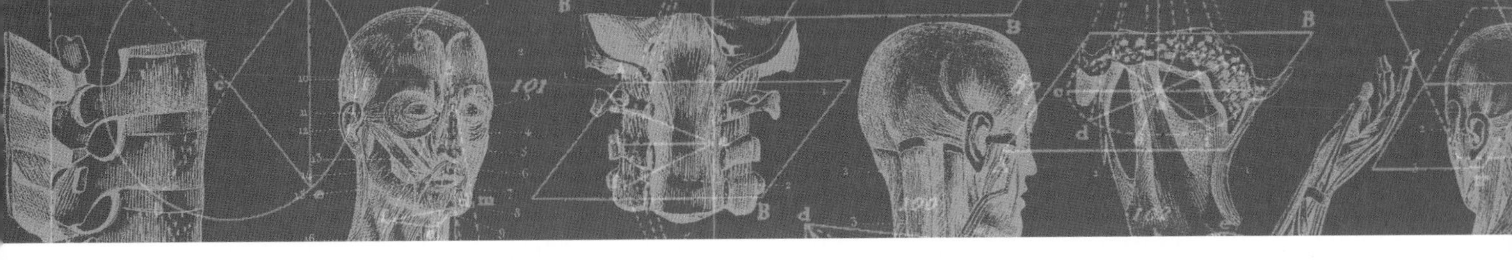

Contents

Part Seven: Renal System

Bruce M. Koeppen and Bruce A. Stanton

Part Eight: Endocrine System

Saul M. Genuth

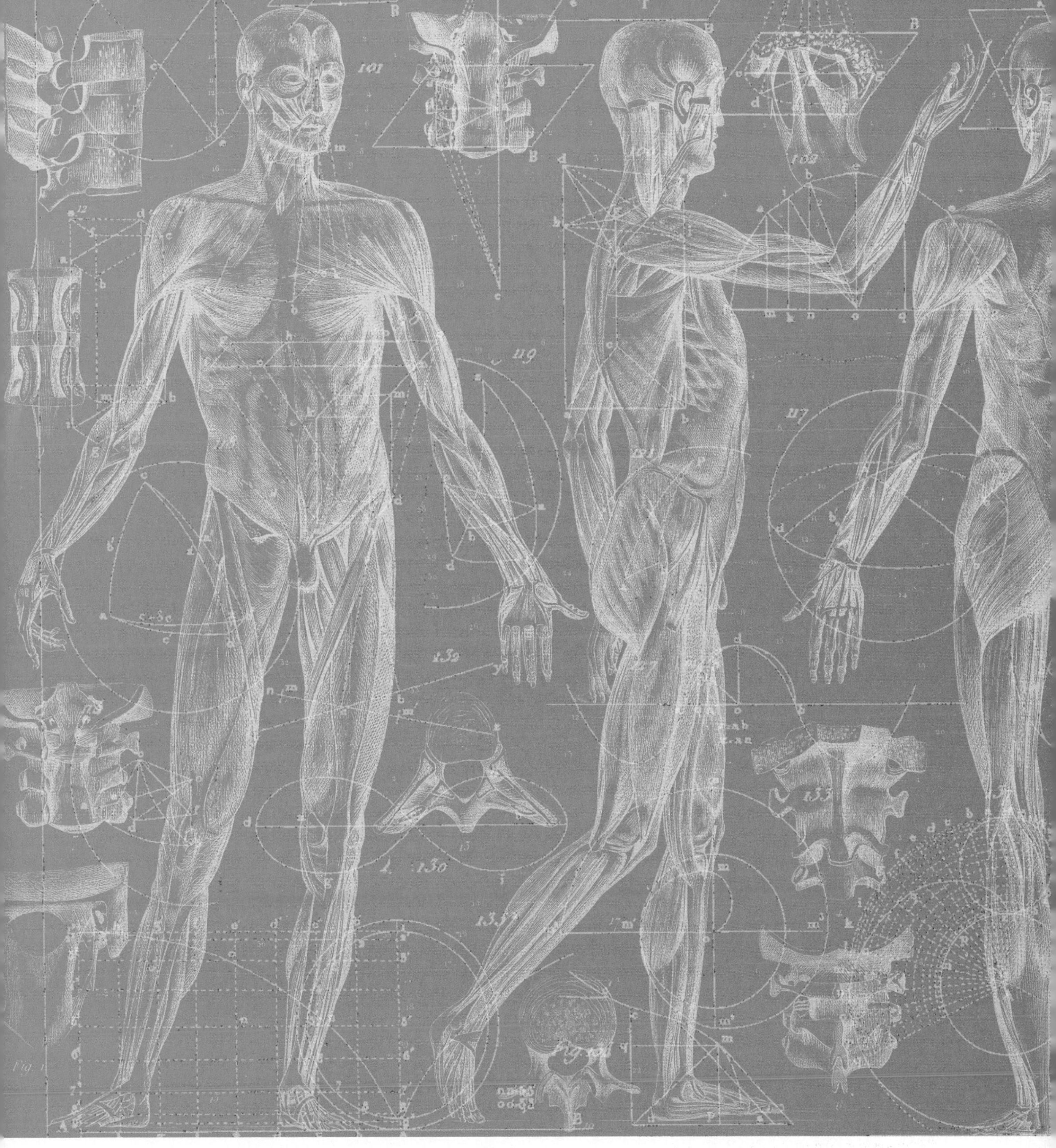

Part One: Cell Physiology

Howard C. Kutchai

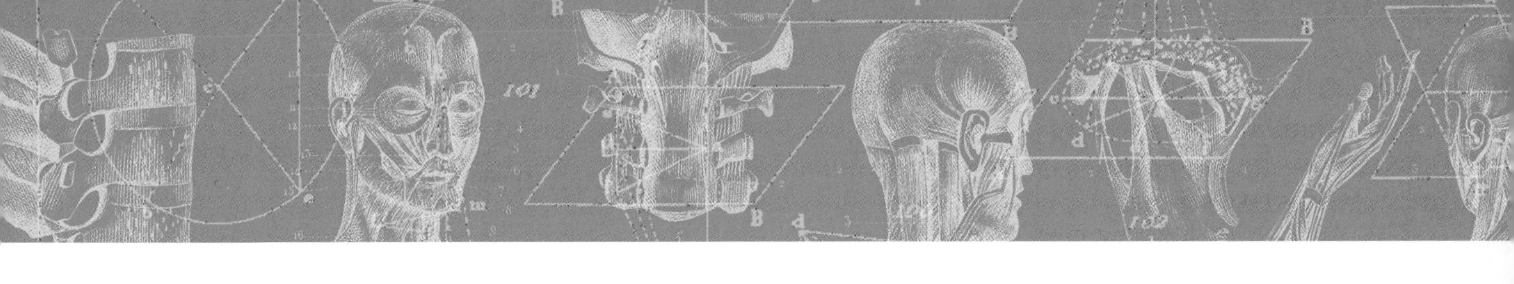

Chapter 1: Cellular Membranes and Transmembrane Transport of Solutes and Water

Objectives

- ❖ Describe the fluid mosaic model of biological membranes.
- ❖ Estimate the rate of diffusion across a membrane by Fick's first law.
- ❖ Apply van't Hoff's law to estimate the osmotic pressure of an electrolyte solution.
- ❖ Explain how the ability of a solute to cause osmotic water flow across a membrane depends on the permeability of the membrane for that solute.
- ❖ List the properties of facilitated and active transport.
- ❖ Distinguish primary from secondary active transport and define symport and antiport.
- ❖ Describe the properties of several transporters that are prominent in the lives of cells.
- ❖ Define transcellular and paracellular transport across an epithelium.

The section on cellular physiology (Chapters 1 to 5) discusses aspects of the functioning of individual cells that are later applied in the context of various organ systems. Each cell is surrounded by a plasma membrane that separates it from the extracellular milieu. Cellular organelles, such as the nucleus, mitochondria, Golgi apparatus, and endoplasmic reticulum, are bounded by membranes or contain multiple types of membranes. This chapter considers the basic structure and properties of biological membranes and some of the processes whereby molecules are transported across membranes. Chapters 2 and 3 present the basic properties of electrically excitable cells, such as neurons and muscle cells, and Chapter 4 discusses the means whereby electrical signals are communicated between cells. Chapter 5 explains the signal-transduction mechanisms whereby extracellular regulatory molecules, such as hormones, influence cellular processes.

Membranes Divide the Cell into Compartments with Specific Biochemical Functions

The plasma membrane serves as a permeability barrier that allows the cell to maintain a cytoplasmic composition far different from the composition of the extracellular fluid. The plasma membrane contains enzymes, receptors, and antigens that play central roles in the interaction of the cell with other cells and with hormones and other regulatory agents in the extracellular fluid. Plasma membrane proteins interact with proteins of the cytoskeleton and the extracellular matrix and are thereby involved in transducing signals from the cell to its surroundings and vice versa.

The membranes that enclose the various organelles divide the cell into discrete compartments and allow the localization of particular biochemical processes in specific organelles. Many vital cellular processes take place in or on the membranes of the organelles. Striking examples are the processes of electron transport and oxidative phosphorylation, which occur on, within, and across the mitochondrial inner membrane.

Most biological membranes have certain features in common. However, in keeping with the diversity of membrane functions, the composition and structure of the membranes differ from one cell to another and among the membranes of a single cell.

The lipid bilayer matrix of membranes is a barrier to the permeability of most substances

Proteins and phospholipids are the most abundant constituents of cellular membranes. A **phospholipid** molecule has a polar head group and two nonpolar, hydrophobic fatty acyl chains **(Figure 1–1, *A*)**. In an aqueous environment, phospholipids tend to form structures that allow the fatty acyl chains to be kept away from contact with water. One such structure is the **lipid bilayer** (Figure 1–1, *B*). Many phospholipids, when they are dispersed in water, spontaneously form lipid bilayers. Most of the phospholipid molecules in biological membranes have a lipid bilayer structure.

The phospholipid bilayer is responsible for certain passive permeability properties of biological membranes. Substances that are highly soluble in water typically permeate cellular membranes slowly, whereas nonpolar compounds that are more soluble in nonpolar, hydrophobic organic solvents cross cell membranes more rapidly. High concentrations of barium salts are administered by mouth or by enema to make the interior of the gastrointestinal tract opaque to x-rays and improve the contrast of diagnostic x-ray films of the gastrointestinal tract. Barium ions in this concentration would be highly toxic, but because barium is insoluble in the hydrophobic interior of membranes, it is barely absorbed from the gastrointestinal tract. Hence, the concentration of barium in the blood rises very little after the administration of barium salts.

Most membranes are a "fluid mosaic" of phospholipids and proteins

Figure 1–2 depicts the **fluid mosaic model** of membrane structure. This model is consistent with many of the properties of biological membranes. Note the bilayer structure of most of the membrane phospholipids. There are two major classes of membrane proteins: (1) **integral** or **intrinsic membrane proteins** that are embedded in the phospholipid bilayer and (2) **peripheral** or **extrinsic membrane proteins** that are associated with

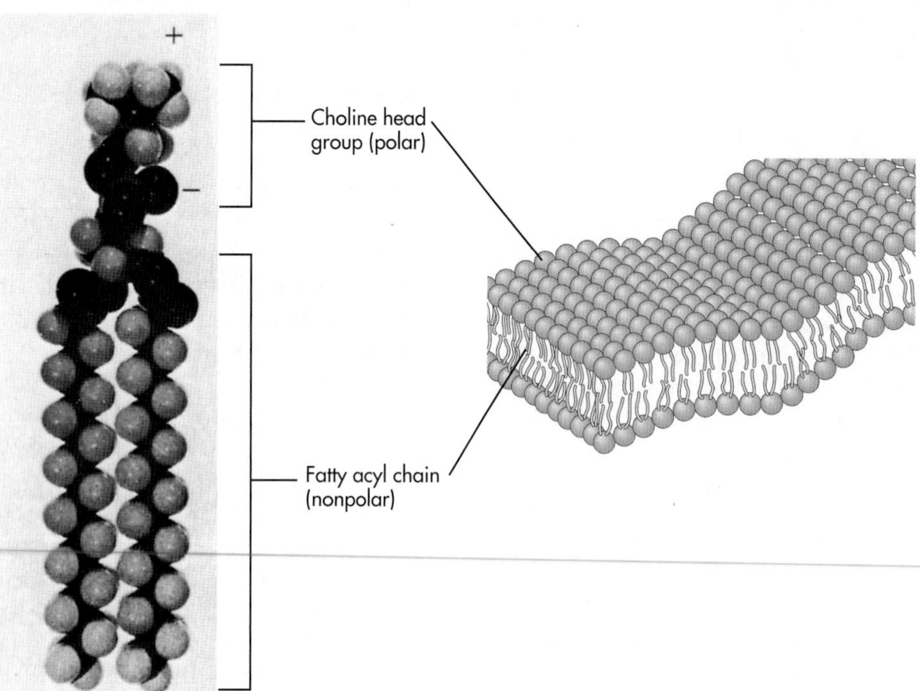

FIGURE 1–1. A, Structure of a membrane phospholipid molecule, in this case a phosphatidylcholine. B, Structure of a phospholipid bilayer. The blue spheres represent the polar head groups of the phospholipid molecules. The wavy lines represent the fatty acyl chains of the phospholipids.

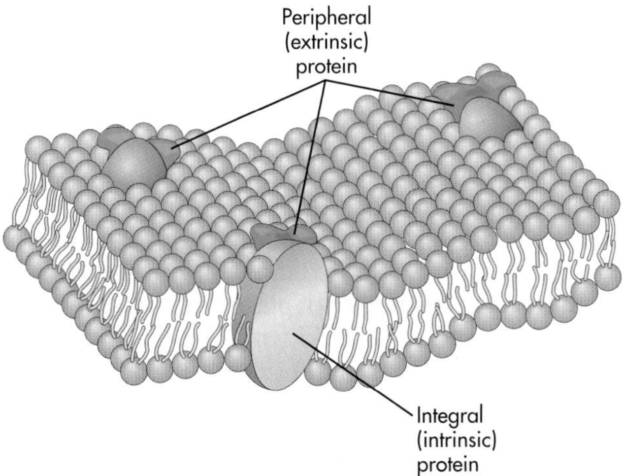

FIGURE 1–2. Fluid mosaic model of membrane structure. The integral proteins *(tan)* are embedded in the lipid bilayer matrix of the membrane, and the peripheral proteins *(green)* may be associated with the external surfaces of integral membrane proteins.

the surface of the membrane. Peripheral membrane proteins interact with the membrane predominantly by charge interactions with integral membrane proteins. The interactions of certain other proteins with the membrane are stabilized by hydrophobic "anchors" that are covalently associated with the protein and that insert into the lipid bilayer; a fatty acid linked to the protein that intercalates among the fatty acyl chains may serve this purpose. Other proteins are covalently linked to a particular class of lipid molecules—glycosylphosphatidyl inositol—that binds them to the membrane. Integral membrane proteins have still more extensive hydrophobic interactions with the interior of the membrane.

Cellular membranes are fluid structures in which many of the constituent molecules are free to diffuse in the plane of the membrane. Most lipids and proteins can move freely in the bilayer plane. The "flip-flop" of phospholipids or proteins from one phospholipid monolayer to the other occurs infrequently. A large hydrophilic moiety is unlikely to flip-flop since it must be dragged through the nonpolar interior of the lipid bilayer.

In some cases, membrane components are not free to diffuse in the plane of the membrane. Examples of this motional constraint are the sequestration of acetylcholine receptors (integral membrane proteins) at the motor end plate of skeletal muscle and the presence of different membrane proteins in the apical and basolateral plasma membranes of epithelial cells. The cytoskeleton appears to tether certain membrane proteins. The **anion antiporter,** a major protein of the human erythrocyte membrane, is bound to the **spectrin** network that undergirds the membrane via a protein called **ankyrin.**

If the motor nerve that innervates a skeletal muscle is accidentally severed, the acetylcholine receptors are no longer sequestered at the motor end plate; instead, they spread over the entire plasma membrane of the muscle cells. The entire surface of the cell then becomes excitable by acetylcholine, a phenomenon known as **denervation supersensitivity.**

Membranes Are Composed of Lipids and Proteins

Phospholipids and cholesterol are the major lipid components of membranes

Choline-containing phospholipids and amino phospholipids are the most prevalent phospholipid classes

In animal cell membranes, the most abundant phospholipids are the choline-containing phospholipids: the lecithins (phosphatidylcholines) and the sphingomyelins. Next in abundance are the amino phospholipids: phosphatidylserine and phosphatidylethanolamine. Other important phospholipids present in smaller amounts are phosphatidylglycerol, phosphatidylinositol, and cardiolipin. THE PHOSPHOLIPID BILAYER IS PRIMARILY RESPONSIBLE FOR THE PASSIVE PERMEABILITY PROPERTIES OF THE MEMBRANE.

Certain phospholipids, present in tiny proportions in the plasma membrane, play a vital role in cellular signal-transduction processes. **Phosphatidylinositol bisphosphate,** when cleaved by a receptor-activated phospholipase C, releases **inositol 1,4,5-trisphosphate (InsP3)** and **diacylglycerol.** InsP3 is released into the cytosol, where it acts on receptors in the endoplasmic reticulum to cause the release of stored Ca^{++}, an action that affects a wide variety of cellular processes (see Chapter 5). Diacylglycerol remains in the plasma membrane, where it participates, along with Ca^{++}, in activating **protein kinase C,** an important signal-transduction protein.

Cholesterol serves as a "fluidity buffer" in membranes

Cholesterol is a major constituent of plasma membranes, and its steroid nucleus lies parallel to the fatty acyl chains of membrane phospholipids. Cholesterol functions as a "fluidity buffer" in the plasma membrane. Its presence tends to keep the fluidity of the acyl chain region of the phospholipid bilayer in an intermediate range in the presence of agents that tend to fluidize biological membranes, such as alcohols and general anesthetics.

Outward-facing carbohydrate moieties of glycolipids and glycoproteins serve as receptors and antigens

Glycolipids are not abundant but have important functions. They are found mostly in plasma membranes, where their carbohydrate moieties protrude from the external surface of the membrane. The carbohydrate parts of glycolipids frequently function as receptors or antigens.

The receptor for cholera toxin (see Chapter 35) is the carbohydrate moiety of a particular glycolipid, ganglioside (GM_1). The A and B blood group antigens (see Chapter 16) are the carbohydrate moieties of other gangliosides in the human erythrocyte membrane.

Phospholipids are distributed asymmetrically between the inner and outer lipid monolayers of the membrane

In most membranes, the lipids are not distributed uniformly across the bilayer. The glycolipids of the plasma membrane are located almost exclusively in the outer monolayer. Phospholipids are also distributed asymmetrically between the inner and outer monolayers of membranes. In the red blood cell membrane, for example, the outer (extracellular) monolayer contains a higher proportion of the choline-containing phospholipids, whereas the inner monolayer contains more of the amino phospholipids.

Lipids and proteins form domains in the membrane

Phospholipids with longer and more saturated fatty acyl chains tend to associate with one another in the plane of the membrane, thereby forming domains that have a gel-like consistency, in contrast to more fluid regions of the membrane. The gel-like regions are also known as **lipid rafts.** Certain membrane proteins associate with the lipid rafts; other proteins are preferentially located in the more fluid domains of the lipid bilayer.

Membrane proteins are enzymes, transporters, and receptors

The protein composition of membranes may be simple or complex. The functionally specialized membranes of the sarcoplasmic reticulum of skeletal muscle and the discs of the rod outer segment of the retina contain only a few different proteins. In contrast, plasma membranes, which perform many functions, may have more than 100 different proteins. Membrane proteins include enzymes, transporters, and receptors for hormones and neurotransmitters.

Membrane glycoproteins mediate interactions with the extracellular matrix

Some membrane proteins are glycoproteins with covalently bound carbohydrate side chains. As with glycolipids, the carbohydrate chains of glycoproteins are located almost exclusively on the extracellular surfaces of plasma membranes. The carbohydrate moieties of membrane glycoproteins and glycolipids have important functions. The negative surface charge of cells is caused by the negatively charged sialic acid of glycolipids and glycoproteins.

Fibronectin is a large fibrous glycoprotein that helps cells attach, via cell surface glycoproteins called **integrins,** to proteins of the extracellular matrix. This linkage mediates communication between the extracellular matrix and the cell's cytoskeleton, permitting the cell to respond to alterations in its surroundings. Membrane glycoproteins are also key components of the junctional complexes that mediate the adhesion of a cell to its neighbors.

Membrane proteins have a specific orientation in the membrane

As a consequence of the way that membrane proteins are threaded across the membrane of the endoplasmic reticulum during their synthesis, the proteins have a particular orientation in the membrane. The Na^+,K^+-ATPase of the plasma membrane and the Ca^{++}-ATPase of the sarcoplasmic reticulum membrane illustrate the asymmetrical disposition of membrane proteins. In both cases, ATP is split on the cytoplasmic face of the membrane, and some of the energy liberated is used to pump ions in specific directions across the membrane. In the case of Na^+,K^+-ATPase, K^+ is pumped into the cell and Na^+ is pumped out, whereas the Ca^{++}-ATPase actively pumps Ca^{++} into the sarcoplasmic reticulum. Both of these ion-transporting ATPases are oriented in the membrane so that the part of the protein responsible for binding ATP is on the cytosolic side of the membrane.

Membranes Are Permeability Barriers

Membranes are impermeable to most water-soluble substances

Biological membranes serve as **permeability barriers.** Most of the molecules present in living systems are highly soluble in water and poorly soluble in nonpolar solvents. Such molecules are poorly soluble in the nonpolar environment in the interior of the lipid bilayer of biological membranes. Consequently, BIOLOGICAL MEMBRANES POSE A FORMIDABLE BARRIER TO THE DIFFUSION OF MOST WATER-SOLUBLE MOLECULES. For many substances, this barrier allows the maintenance of large concentration differences between the cytoplasm and the extracellular fluid.

The localization of various cellular processes in certain organelles depends on the barrier properties of cellular membranes. The spatial organization of chemical and physical processes in the cell depends on the barrier functions of cellular membranes, much as the walls in a house separate rooms with different functions. For example, the inner mitochondrial membrane is impermeable to the enzymes and substrates of the tricarboxylic cycle; thus it allows the localization of this metabolic pathway in the mitochondrial matrix. The passage of important molecules across membranes at controlled rates is central to the life of the cell. Examples are the uptake of nutrient molecules, the discharge of waste products, and the release of secreted molecules. As discussed in the next section, molecules may move from one side of a membrane to another without actually moving through the membrane itself. In other cases, molecules cross a particular membrane by passing through or among the molecules that make up the membrane.

Material may cross membranes without passing through the molecules that make up the membrane

Cells take up small samples of the extracellular medium via endocytosis

Endocytosis, a process that allows material to enter the cell without passing through the membrane (**Figure 1–3**), includes **phagocytosis** and **pinocytosis.** The uptake of particulate material is termed phagocytosis (Figure 1–3, *A*). The uptake of soluble molecules is called pinocytosis (Figure 1–3, *B*). Special regions of the plasma membrane may be involved in endocytosis. In these regions, the cytoplasmic surface of the plasma membrane is covered with a protein called **clathrin.** These clathrin-covered regions are called **coated pits,** and their endocytosis gives rise to coated vesicles. The coated pits are involved in receptor-mediated endocytosis (Figure 1–3, *C*). Proteins to be taken up are recognized and bound by specific membrane receptor proteins near the coated pits. The binding often leads to aggregation of receptor-ligand complexes, and the aggregation triggers endocytosis. Endocytosis is an active process that requires metabolic energy. Endocytosis can also occur in regions of the plasma membrane that do not contain coated pits.

Most cells cannot synthesize cholesterol, which is needed for the synthesis of new membranes, synthesis of bile acids, and synthesis of steroid hormones. Cholesterol is carried in the blood, predominantly in low-density lipoproteins (LDL). Many cells have LDL receptors in their plasma membranes. When LDL binds to these receptors, the receptor-LDL complexes migrate to coated pits, where they aggregate and are taken into the cell by receptor-mediated endocytosis. Individuals who lack LDL receptors have high levels of cholesterol-laden LDL in the blood. Consequently, such individuals tend to develop arterial disease **(atherosclerosis)** at an early age, which makes them more likely to experience heart attacks prematurely.

Certain substances are extruded from cells by exocytosis

Molecules can be ejected from cells by **exocytosis,** a process that resembles endocytosis in reverse. The release of neurotransmitters, which is considered in more detail in Chapter 4, takes place by exocytosis. Exocytosis is responsible for the release of secretory proteins by many cells. The release of pancreatic enzymes from the acinar cells of the pancreas is a well-studied example. Pancreatic enzymes play vital roles

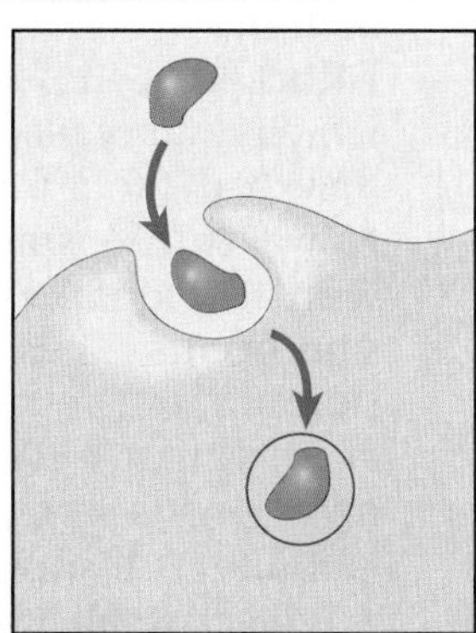

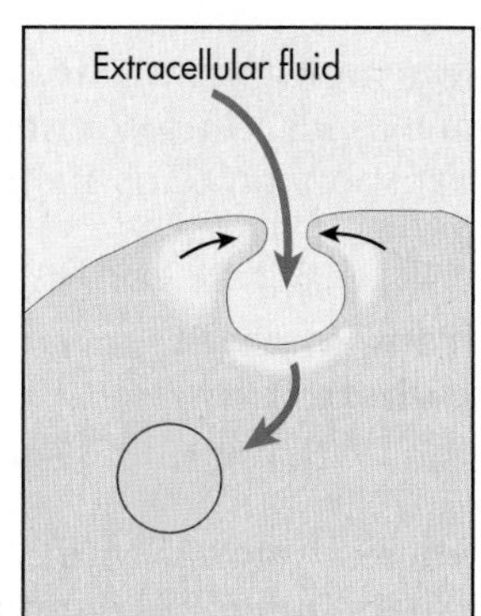

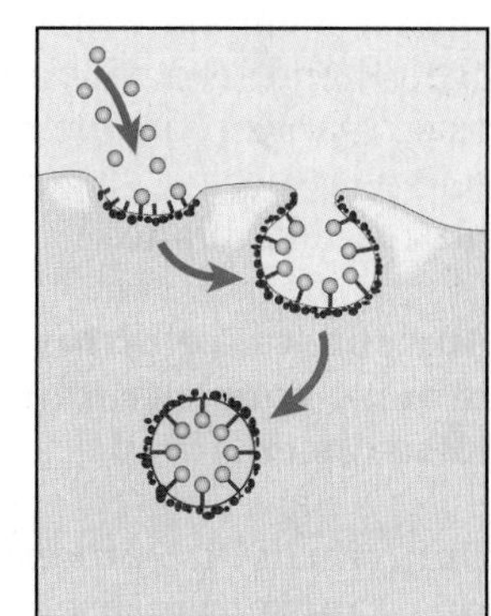

FIGURE 1–3. Endocytotic processes. A, Phagocytosis of a solid particle. B, Pinocytosis of extracellular fluid. C, Receptor-mediated endocytosis by coated pits.

in the digestion of proteins, carbohydrates, and lipids (see Chapters 34 and 35). In such cases, the proteins to be secreted are stored in secretory vesicles in the cytoplasm. A stimulus to secrete causes the secretory vesicles to fuse with the plasma membrane and to release the vesicle contents by exocytosis.

Vesicle fusion allows the mixing of vesicular contents

The contents of one type of organelle can be transferred to another type by fusion of the membranes of the organelles. In some cells, secretory products are transferred from the endoplasmic reticulum to the Golgi apparatus by the fusion of the vesicles of the endoplasmic reticulum with the membranous sacs of the Golgi apparatus. The fusion of many endocytic vesicles with lysosomes allows the endocytosed material to be digested by proteolytic enzymes in the lysosomes. The turnover of many normal cellular constituents involves their destruction in lysosomes, followed by their resynthesis.

Influenza viruses have membrane proteins that undergo a dramatic conformational change to insert a "fusion peptide" into the host cell. The fusion peptide promotes the fusion of the viral membrane with the plasma membrane of the host cell, allowing entry of the viral genome into the host cell.

The Transport of Molecules Across Membranes Occurs by Diffusion, Osmosis, and Protein-Mediated Transport Processes

The traffic of molecules across biological membranes is vital for most cellular processes. Some molecules move across biological membranes simply by diffusing among the molecules that make up the membrane, whereas the passage of other molecules involves the mediation of specific transport proteins in the membrane.

O_2 and CO_2, for example, are small molecules that are fairly soluble in nonpolar solvents. O_2 and CO_2 cross biological membranes by diffusing among membrane lipid molecules. Glucose, on the other hand, is a much larger molecule that is not very soluble in the membrane lipids. Glucose enters cells via specific glucose transport proteins in the plasma membrane.

Any substance diffuses from where it is more concentrated to where it is less concentrated

Diffusion is the process whereby atoms or molecules move because of their random thermal

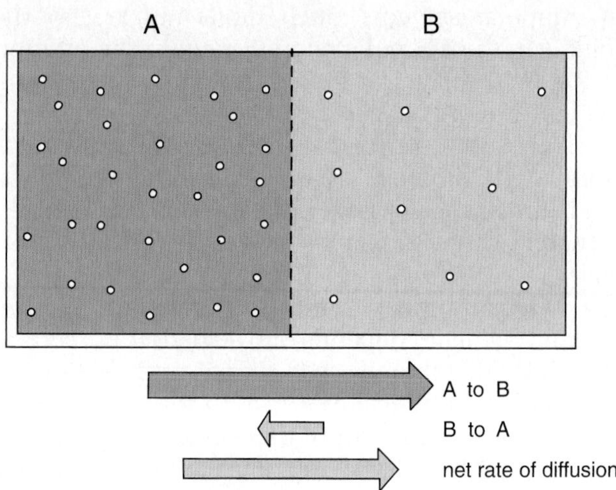

FIGURE 1–4. Chambers A and B are separated by a removable partition. Chamber A has a higher concentration of molecules than does chamber B. When the partition is removed, there will be a net diffusion of molecules from A to B.

motion; it is also called **brownian motion.** Imagine a container divided into two compartments by a removable partition **(Figure 1–4).** A much larger number of molecules of a compound are placed on side A than on side B, and then the partition is removed. Every molecule is in random thermal motion. It is equally probable that a molecule that begins on side A will move to side B in a given time and that a molecule on side B will move to side A. Because many more molecules are present on side A, the total number of molecules moving from A to B will be greater than the number moving from B to A. In this way, the number of molecules on side A decreases, whereas the number of molecules on side B increases. This process continues until the concentration of molecules on side A equals that on side B. Thereafter, the rate of diffusion of molecules from A to B equals that from B to A, and no further net movement occurs; a dynamic equilibrium exists.

Diffusion occurs rapidly over microscopic distances but slowly over macroscopic distances

Diffusion is a rapid process when the distance over which it takes place is small. A rule of thumb is that a typical molecule takes 1 msec to diffuse 1 μm. However, the time required for diffusion increases with the square of the distance over which diffusion occurs. Thus, A 10-FOLD INCREASE IN THE DIFFUSION DISTANCE MEANS THAT THE DIFFUSION PROCESS WILL REQUIRE ABOUT 100 TIMES LONGER TO REACH A GIVEN DEGREE OF COMPLETION.

Table 1–1 shows the results of calculations for a typical small water-soluble solute. A cell that is

TABLE 1–1. TIME REQUIRED FOR DIFFUSION TO OCCUR OVER VARIOUS DIFFUSION DISTANCES*

Diffusion Distance (μm)	Time Required for Diffusion
1	0.5 msec
10	50 msec
100	5 sec
1,000 (1 mm)	8.3 min
10,000 (1 cm)	14 hr

*The time required for the "average" molecule (with diffusion coefficient taken to be 1×10^{-5} cm²/sec) to diffuse the required distance was computed.

100 μm away from the nearest capillary can receive nutrients from the blood by diffusion with a time lag of only 5 seconds or so. This is sufficiently fast to satisfy the metabolic demands of many cells. However, a skeletal muscle cell that is 1 cm long cannot rely on diffusion for the intracellular transport of vital metabolites because the 14 hours required for diffusion over the 1-cm distance is too long on the time scale of cellular metabolism. Some nerve fibers are longer than 1 m. Therefore, it is no wonder that intracellular axonal transport systems are involved in transporting important molecules along nerve fibers. Because of the slowness of diffusion over macroscopic distances, it is not surprising that even small multicellular organisms have evolved circulatory systems to bring the individual cells of the organisms within a reasonable diffusion range of nutrients.

The diffusion coefficient depends on the diffusing molecule and the medium through which it is diffusing

The **diffusion coefficient (D)** is proportional to the speed with which the diffusing molecule can move in the surrounding medium. The larger the molecule and the more viscous the medium, the smaller is D. For small molecules, D is inversely proportional to the square root of MW (molecular weight). For macromolecules, D is inversely proportional to the cube root of MW. Thus, a protein that has eight times the mass of another molecule has a D only half that of the smaller molecule.

Diffusion of a substance across a membrane is described by Fick's law of diffusion

Diffusion usually leads to a state in which the concentration of the diffusing species is constant in space and time. Thus, diffusion across cellular membranes tends to equalize the concentrations on the two sides of the membrane. **Fick's first law of diffusion** states the following:

$$J = -DA\frac{\Delta c}{\Delta x} \qquad \textbf{1-1}$$

where

J = net rate of diffusion (moles or grams per second)

D = diffusion coefficient of the diffusing solute in the membrane (cm^2/sec)

A = area of the membrane (cm^2)

Δc = concentration difference across the membrane (mole/cm^3)

Δx = thickness of the membrane (cm)

Equation 1-1, Fick's law, says that the diffusion rate across a membrane is proportional to the area of the membrane and to the difference in the concentration (Δc) of the diffusing substance on the two sides of the membrane and inversely proportional to the membrane thickness (Δx). D, the diffusion coefficient, is a proportionality constant that depends on the nature of the diffusing substance and the properties of the membrane.

Membranes Are More Permeable to Lipid-Soluble Substances Than to Water-Soluble Substances

The permeability of membranes to a particular molecule is proportional to its solubility in the interior of the lipid bilayer

The more soluble a compound is in nonpolar solvents, the more permeant is that substance across biological membranes. Fat-soluble vitamins are absorbed by the epithelial cells of the small intestine by simply diffusing across their luminal plasma membranes. In contrast, water-soluble vitamins do not readily diffuse across biological membranes, so special membrane transport proteins are required for the absorption of most water-soluble vitamins (see Chapter 35).

Only rather small water-soluble molecules can diffuse rapidly across membranes

Very small uncharged, water-soluble molecules pass through cell membranes more rapidly than predicted from their lipid solubilities. For example, water permeates cell membranes about 100 times more rapidly than predicted from its molecular radius and its lipid solubility. There are two reasons for the unusually high permeability to water. Water and certain very small water-soluble molecules can pass between adjacent phospholipid molecules

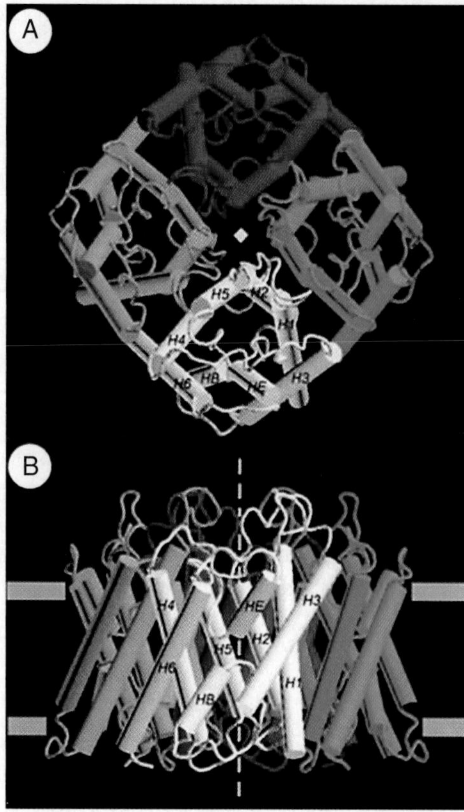

FIGURE 1–5. Structure of human aquaporin 1 (AQP1), a water channel protein. The protein is a tetramer of identical subunits. A, The tetramer viewed from above. Each monomer has a water-conducting pore through it. B, Side view of the protein. (Reproduced from Murata K et al: *Nature* 407:599, 2000.)

without actually dissolving in the region occupied by the fatty acid side chains. Moreover, the plasma membranes of many cells contain membrane proteins called **aquaporins** that form channels permitting a high rate of water flow across the membrane **(Figure 1–5).** At least seven isoforms of aquaporin are present in the kidney. Mutations in these water channels may result in defects in the ability of the kidney to produce urine that is more concentrated than body fluids (see Chapter 38).

The permeability of membranes to uncharged, water-soluble molecules decreases as the size of the molecules increases. Most membranes permit significant diffusion only of water-soluble molecules whose MWs are less than about 200. Because of their net charges, ions are relatively insoluble in membrane lipids, so membranes are impermeable to most ions. Ions diffuse across membranes mainly through protein **ion channels** that span the membrane. Certain ion channels allow only cations to pass; others are selective for anions. Some ion channels are highly specific with respect to the ions allowed to pass, whereas others allow all ions with charge of the same sign that are below a certain size to pass. Some ion channels are controlled by the voltage difference across the membrane, and others are controlled by neurotransmitters or other regulatory molecules (see Chapters 3 and 4).

Although certain water-soluble molecules such as sugars and amino acids are essential for cell survival, they do not cross plasma membranes appreciably by simple diffusion. Plasma membranes have specific proteins that allow the transfer of vital molecules into or out of the cell. The characteristics of membrane **protein-mediated transport** are discussed later in this chapter.

Water Flows by Osmosis When There Is a Solute Concentration Difference Across a Membrane

Osmosis is defined as the flow of water across a semipermeable membrane from a compartment in which the solute concentration is lower to one in which the solute concentration is greater. A SEMIPERMEABLE MEMBRANE IS A MEMBRANE PERMEABLE TO WATER BUT IMPERMEABLE TO SOLUTES. Plasma membranes and other cellular membranes are semipermeable membranes. OSMOSIS TAKES PLACE BECAUSE THE PRESENCE OF SOLUTE DECREASES THE CHEMICAL POTENTIAL OF WATER. Water tends to flow from where its chemical potential is higher to where its chemical potential is lower. Other effects caused by the decrease in the chemical potential of water (because of the presence of solute) include reduced vapor pressure, lower freezing point, and higher boiling point of the solution compared with pure water. Because these properties, and osmotic pressure as well, depend primarily on the concentration of the solute present rather than on its chemical properties, they are called **colligative properties.**

The osmotic pressure of a solution is the pressure that must be applied to it to prevent water from entering the solution across a semipermeable membrane

In **Figure 1–6**, a semipermeable membrane separates a solution containing solute (side A) from pure water (side B). Water tends to flow from side B to side A by osmosis because the presence of solute on side A reduces the chemical potential of water in the solution. Pushing on the piston increases the chemical potential of the water in the solution of side A and slows the net rate of osmotic water flow.

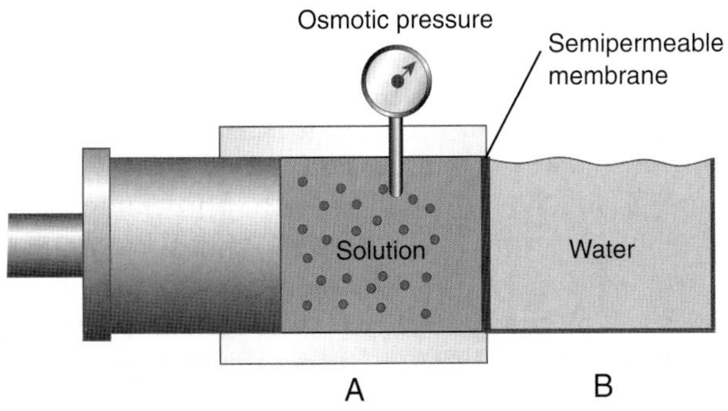

FIGURE 1–6. Osmotic pressure. When the hydrostatic pressure applied to the solution in chamber A is equal to the osmotic pressure of that solution, there is no net water flow across the membrane.

If the force on the piston is increased gradually, a pressure is eventually reached at which net water flow stops. The application of still more pressure causes water to flow in the opposite direction. The pressure on side A that is just sufficient to keep pure water from entering is called the **osmotic pressure** of the solution on side A.

THE OSMOTIC PRESSURE OF A SOLUTION DEPENDS ON THE CONCENTRATION OF SOLUTE PARTICLES IN SOLUTION. Thus, the degree of ionization of the solute must be taken into account. A 1 M solution of glucose, a 0.5 M solution of NaCl, and a 0.333 M solution of $CaCl_2$ have *approximately* the same osmotic pressure. (Actually, their osmotic pressures differ somewhat because of the deviations of real solutions from ideal behavior.) One form of **van't Hoff's law** for the calculation of osmotic pressure is

$$\pi = RT(\Phi ic) \quad \textbf{1-2}$$

where

π = osmotic pressure

R = ideal gas constant

T = absolute temperature

Φ = osmotic coefficient

i = number of ions formed by the dissociation of a solute molecule

c = molar concentration of the solute (moles of solute per liter of solution)

The osmotic coefficient (Φ) accounts for the deviation of the solution from the ideal. It depends on the particular compound, its concentration, and the temperature. The value of Φ is less than 1 for electrolytes of physiological importance (e.g., NaCl, KCl, $NaHCO_3$, $CaCl_2$), and for all solutes Φ approaches 1 as the solution becomes more and more dilute. The term **Φic** can be regarded as the **osmotically effective concentration,** and Φic, called the **osmolarity** of the solution, is expressed in osmoles/liter. When the concentration is expressed as molality *m* (moles/kg water), then **Φim** is the **osmolality** of the solution. Sometimes, a less precise estimate of osmotic pressure is computed by assuming that Φ is equal to 1.

The osmotic pressure of a solution can be estimated from its freezing point

As noted, the osmotic pressure of a solution can be obtained by determining the pressure required to prevent water from entering the solution across a semipermeable membrane (Figure 1–6). More often, however, the osmotic pressure is estimated from another colligative property, such as depression of the freezing point. The relationship that describes the osmolarity (Φic) of a solution in terms of the depression of the freezing point of water by the solute is

$$\Phi ic = \Delta T_f/1.86 \quad \textbf{1-3}$$

where ΔT_f is the freezing point depression in degrees centigrade. When the freezing point depression of a multicomponent solution is determined, the effective osmolarity (in osmoles per liter) of the solution as a whole can be obtained.

If the total osmotic pressures of two solutions (as measured by their freezing point depressions or by the osmotic pressures they develop across a semipermeable membrane) are equal, the solutions are said to be **isoosmotic** (or **isosmotic**). If solution A has a greater osmotic pressure than solution B, A is said to be **hyperosmotic** with respect to B. If solution A has less total osmotic pressure than solution B, A is said to be **hypoosmotic** to B.

Cells swell or shrink in response to changes in the solute content of extracellular fluid

The plasma membranes of most of the body's cells are relatively impermeable to many of the solutes of the extracellular fluid but are highly permeable to water. Therefore, when the osmotic pressure of the extracellular fluid is increased, water leaves the cells by osmosis, and the cells shrink until the intracellular and extracellular osmotic pressures are equal. Conversely, if the osmotic pressure of the extracellular fluid is decreased, water enters the cells. The cells swell until the intracellular and extracellular osmotic pressures are equal.

Red blood cells are often used to illustrate the osmotic properties of cells. Within a certain range of external solute concentrations, the red cell

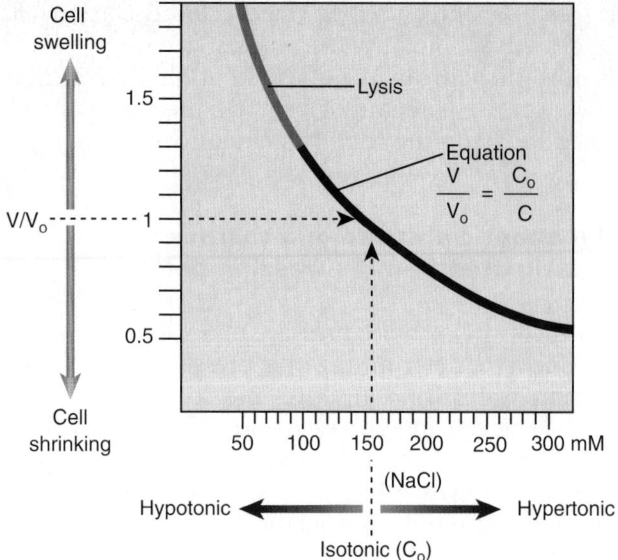

FIGURE 1–7. Osmotic behavior of human red blood cells in NaCl solutions. At 154 mM NaCl (isotonic), the red cell has a normal volume. (As explained in Equation 1-4, 154 mM NaCl has an effective osmotic concentration of 286 milliosmolar.) Red cells shrink in more concentrated (hypertonic) solutions and swell in more dilute (hypotonic) solutions. V_o and C_o are the red cell volume and intracellular solute concentration, respectively, for the red cell in blood or in an isotonic solution. V and C are, respectively, the cell volume and intracellular solute concentration in a solution that is not isotonic.

behaves like an osmometer because its volume is inversely related to the solute concentration in the extracellular medium. In **Figure 1–7**, the red cell volume, as a fraction of its normal volume in plasma, is shown as a function of the concentration of NaCl solution in which the red cells are suspended. At an NaCl concentration of 154 mM (this equals 286 milliosmolar, see Equation 1-4), the volume of the cells is the same as their volume in plasma; this concentration of NaCl is said to be **isotonic** to the red cell.

Isotonic NaCl solution (also known as **isotonic saline**) is used for intravenous rehydration or for the administration of medications. Isotonic saline is given to patients because, being isotonic, it does not cause any changes in cell volume.

A concentration of NaCl greater than 154 mM is called **hypertonic** (cells shrink), and a solution less concentrated than 154 mM is termed **hypotonic** (cells swell). When red cells have swollen to about 1.4 times their original volume, some cells lyse (burst). At this volume, the properties of the red cell membrane abruptly change; hemoglobin leaks out of the cell, and the membrane becomes transiently permeable to other large molecules as well.

The erythrocyte's intracellular substances producing an osmotic pressure that just balances the osmotic pressure of the extracellular fluid include hemoglobin, K^+, Na^+, Cl^-, organic phosphates, and glycolytic intermediates. Regardless of the chemical nature of its contents, the red cell behaves as though it is filled with a solution of impermeant molecules with an osmotically effective concentration of 286 milliosmolar, which is the same as the osmolarity of isotonic saline, as follows:

$$\begin{aligned}\Phi_{NaCl} i_{NaCl} C_{NaCl} &= 0.93 \times 2 \times 0.154 \text{ M} \\ &= 0.286 \text{ osmolar} \\ &= 286 \text{ milliosmolar}\end{aligned} \qquad \textbf{1-4}$$

The more permeable a membrane is to a particular solute, the smaller the osmotic water flow that can be caused by that solute

When a difference in hydrostatic pressure (ΔP) causes water flow across a membrane, the rate of water flow ($\dot{V}_w$) is as follows:

$$\dot{V}_w = L\Delta P \qquad \textbf{1-5}$$

where L is a constant of proportionality called the **hydraulic conductivity,** which is related to the permeability of the membrane to water.

THE OSMOTIC FLOW OF WATER ACROSS A MEMBRANE IS DIRECTLY PROPORTIONAL TO THE OSMOTIC PRESSURE DIFFERENCE ($\Delta\pi$) BETWEEN THE SOLUTIONS ON THE TWO SIDES OF THE MEMBRANE:

$$\dot{V}_w = L\Delta\pi \qquad \textbf{1-6}$$

Equation 1-6 holds only for osmosis caused by impermeant solutes. Permeant solutes cause less osmotic flow. THE GREATER THE PERMEABILITY OF A SOLUTE, THE SMALLER THE OSMOTIC FLOW IT CAUSES. **Table 1–2** shows the osmotic water flows induced across a porous membrane by solutes of different molecular sizes. The solutions have identical freezing points, so the total osmotic pressures are the same. The larger the solute molecule, the more impermeable the membrane to the solute, and the greater the osmotic water flow it causes.

Knowing the reflection coefficient of a membrane for a particular solute allows prediction of how much osmotic flow that solute can cause across that membrane

Equation 1-6 can be rewritten to take solute permeability into account by including the **reflection coefficient (σ),** as follows:

TABLE 1–2. OSMOTIC WATER FLOW ACROSS A POROUS DIALYSIS MEMBRANE CAUSED BY VARIOUS SOLUTES

Gradient Producing the Water Flow	Net Volume Flow (μL/min)*	Solute Radius (Å)	Reflection Coefficient (σ)
D_2O	0.06	1.9	0.0024
Urea	0.6	2.7	0.024
Glucose	5.1	4.4	0.205
Sucrose	9.2	5.3	0.368
Raffinose	11	6.1	0.440
Inulin	19	12	0.760
Bovine serum albumin	25.5	37	1.02
Hydrostatic pressure	25		

*Flow is expressed as microliters per minute caused by a 1 M concentration difference of solute across the membrane. The flows are compared with the flow caused by a theoretically equivalent hydrostatic pressure.
Data from Durbin RP: *J Gen Physiol* 44:315, 1960.

$$\dot{V}_w = \sigma L \Delta\pi \quad \text{1-7}$$

σ is a dimensionless number that ranges from 1 for completely impermeant solutes to 0 for extremely permeant solutes. σ is a property of a particular solute and a particular membrane and represents the osmotic water flow induced by the solute as a fraction of the theoretical maximum osmotic water flow (Table 1–2). The more permeant a substance across a particular membrane, the smaller the σ of the membrane for that substance, and the smaller the osmotic water flow the substance can cause.

The mechanism by which the kidney produces urine more concentrated than extracellular fluid (see Chapter 38) involves various parts of the nephron that have different values of σ for each important solute, such as NaCl and urea. The osmotic water flows induced by NaCl and urea in a particular segment of the nephron depend on the values of σ for the epithelium in that segment to these solutes.

Transporters Are Responsible for Moving Important Substances Across Membranes

Certain substances enter or leave cells by way of specific transporters or channels that are intrinsic proteins of the plasma membrane. Transport via such transporters or channels is called **protein-mediated transport** or simply **mediated transport.** Specific ions or molecules may cross the membranes of the mitochondrion, the endoplasmic reticulum, and other organelles by mediated transport. Mediated transport systems include **active transport** and **facilitated transport,** which have several properties in common. The principal distinction between these two processes is that ACTIVE TRANSPORT REQUIRES ENERGY AND IS CAPABLE OF "PUMPING" A SUBSTANCE AGAINST A CHEMICAL OR ELECTROCHEMICAL GRADIENT, BUT FACILITATED TRANSPORT ONLY MEDIATES THE TRANSPORT OF A SUBSTANCE DOWN ITS CHEMICAL OR ELECTROCHEMICAL GRADIENT (see Chapter 2).

Protein-mediated transport has some of the properties of enzyme catalysis

- A substance moved by a transporter is moved more rapidly than molecules that have a similar MW and lipid solubility but that cross the membrane by simple diffusion **(Figure 1–8).**

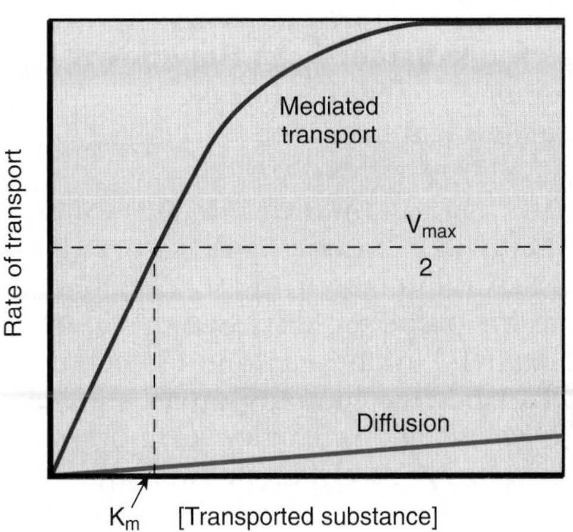

FIGURE 1–8. Movement via a transport protein shows saturation kinetics. As the concentration of the transported substance increases, the rate of its transport approaches a maximum value, the V_{max} for the transporter. The concentration of the transported substance required for the transport rate to be half-maximal is termed the K_m of the transporter. Movement of the substrate by the transporter is much faster than by simple diffusion.

- The transport rate shows **saturation kinetics:** as the concentration of the transported compound is increased, the rate of transport at first increases, but eventually a concentration is reached after which the transport rate increases no further. At this point, the transport system is said to be SATURATED WITH THE TRANSPORTED COMPOUND.
- The transporter has **chemical specificity:** only molecules with the requisite chemical structure are transported. The specificity of most transporters is not absolute, and in general, it is broader than the specificity of most enzymes. The lock-and-key relationship between an enzyme and its substrate applies to transport proteins as well.
- Structurally related molecules may compete for transport. Typically, one transport substrate decreases the transport rate of a second substrate by competing for binding to the transporter. The competition is analogous to competitive inhibition of an enzyme.
- Transport may be inhibited by compounds not structurally related to transport substrates. An inhibitor may bind to the transporter in a way that decreases the affinity of the protein for the normal transport substrate. The compound **phloretin** does not resemble a sugar molecule, yet it strongly inhibits red cell sugar transport. Active transporters, which require some link to metabolism, may be inhibited by metabolic inhibitors. The rate of Na^+ transport out of cells by Na^+,K^+-ATPase is decreased by substances that interfere with ATP generation.

Facilitated transport enhances the rate at which a substance can flow down its chemical concentration or electrochemical gradient

SOMETIMES CALLED **FACILITATED DIFFUSION,** FACILITATED TRANSPORT OCCURS VIA A TRANSPORTER THAT IS NOT LINKED TO METABOLIC ENERGY. Facilitated transport has the properties discussed previously, except that metabolic inhibitors do not generally depress it. Because facilitated transporters are not linked to energy metabolism, they cannot move substances against concentration gradients. Facilitated transporters act to equalize concentrations of transported substances on the two sides of the membrane.

Monosaccharides enter muscle cells via facilitated transporters. Glucose, galactose, arabinose, and 3-*O*-methylglucose compete for the same transporter. The rate of transport shows saturation kinetics. The nonphysiological stereoisomer L-glucose enters the cells very slowly, and nontransported sugars, such as mannitol and sorbose, enter muscle cells very slowly if at all. Phloretin inhibits sugar uptake, and insulin stimulates it.

A major action of the hormone **insulin** is to stimulate the facilitated transport of glucose across the plasma membranes of muscle and fat cells. People with **type 1 diabetes** secrete insulin at markedly subnormal rates (see Chapter 43). In this disease, the rate of glucose uptake by muscle and adipose cells is so slow that the ability of these tissues to use glucose as a metabolic fuel is markedly impaired.

An active transporter can transport a substance from where its concentration is lower to where it is higher: this requires energy

Active transport processes have most of the properties of facilitated transport. In addition, active transporters can concentrate their substrates against concentration or electrochemical potential gradients. This requires energy; hence, active transport must be linked to energy metabolism in some way. Active transporters may use ATP directly, or they may be linked more indirectly to metabolism. Because of their dependence on metabolism, any substance that interferes with energy metabolism may inhibit active transporters.

A primary active transport process has a direct link to metabolic energy

An active transporter linked directly to cellular metabolism (i.e., by using ATP to power the transport) is called a **primary active transporter.** In the cytoplasm of most animal cells, the concentration of Na^+ is much less and the concentration of K^+ is much greater than their extracellular concentrations. These concentration gradients are brought about by the action of Na^+,K^+-ATPase, an integral protein in the plasma membranes of all cells. Na^+,K^+-ATPase uses the energy of ATP to pump Na^+ out of the cell and K^+ into the cell. Na^+,K^+-ATPase transports three Na^+ ions out of the cell and two K^+ ions into the cell for each molecule of ATP hydrolyzed. Because Na^+,K^+-ATPase uses the energy in the terminal phosphate bond of ATP to power the transport cycle, it is said to be a primary active transporter. A transporter powered by some other high-energy metabolic intermediate or linked directly to a primary metabolic reaction would also be classified as a primary active transporter.

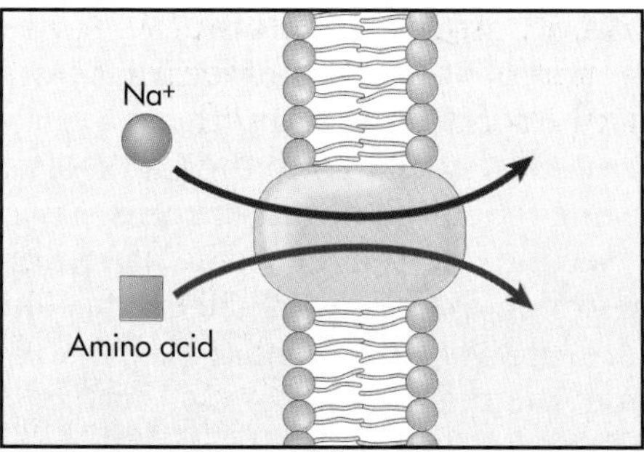

FIGURE 1–9. Many cells take up neutral amino acids via secondary active transport. The transport protein binds both Na^+ and the amino acid. Na^+ is transported down its electrochemical gradient, and the transport protein uses the energy released by Na^+ flux to transport the amino acid against a concentration gradient.

A secondary active transporter derives energy from the concentration gradient of another substance that is actively transported

The previous section emphasized that energy is required to create a concentration gradient for a transported substance. ONCE CREATED, A CONCENTRATION GRADIENT REPRESENTS A STORE OF CHEMICAL POTENTIAL ENERGY THAT CAN BE HARNESSED TO DO WORK (see Chapter 2). In most cell types, the concentration gradient of Na^+ created by Na^+,K^+-ATPase is used to actively transport other solutes into the cell. Many cells take up neutral, hydrophilic amino acids by membrane transport proteins that link the inward transport of Na^+ down its electrochemical potential gradient to the inward transport of amino acids against their concentration gradients **(Figure 1–9)**. The energy for the transport of the amino acid is provided not directly by ATP or another high-energy metabolite but indirectly from the gradient of Na^+ that is itself actively transported. Hence, the amino acid is said to be transported by **secondary active transport.** In the secondary active transport of amino acids, both the rate of amino acid transport and the extent to which the amino acid is accumulated depend on the electrochemical potential difference of Na^+ across the membrane. Certain other secondary active transporters, such as the transporter that mediates the absorption of small peptides from the small intestine (see Chapter 35), are powered by a transmembrane electrochemical potential gradient of H^+.

Membrane transport proteins may be classified according to the mechanism whereby they mediate transport across the membrane (Table 1–3)

Perhaps the simplest transport mechanism is exemplified by **pore** proteins like aquaporin (Figure 1–5). The water channel is apparently always open and available to water molecules from either side of the membrane. By contrast, **transporters,** like the glucose transporters or the Na^+,K^+-ATPase, bind a transported substrate from one side of the membrane and then must undergo a conformational change before releasing the substrate to the other side of the membrane **(Figure 1–10, *A*)**. Because protein conformational changes occur relatively slowly, transporters have the slowest rates of substrate transport (Table 1–3). Ions are transported across membranes by ion channel proteins. **Channels** (Figure 1–10, *B*), like pores, have a water-filled transport pathway that traverses the membrane and is simultaneously available from both sides of the membrane, but channels are usually **gated,** which means that the channel alternates between an open (rapidly conducting) and a closed (slowly conducting) state (Figure 1–10, *B*).

TABLE 1–3. PROPERTIES OF MEMBRANE TRANSPORT PROTEINS

Class of Membrane Transport Protein	Transport Mechanism	Accessibility of Permeation Pathway	Typical Rates of Transport
Pores (e.g., aquaporin, pore proteins in outer mitochondrial membrane)	Diffusion of substrate through the channel	Accessible from both sides of the membrane at all times	As high as 10^9/sec
Channels (gated) (e.g., voltage-gated Na^+ channels, cyclic nucleotide–gated ion channels, mechanosensitive channels)	Diffusion of substrate through open channel Very low rate of diffusion through closed channel	Open channel accessible from both sides of membrane simultaneously In closed channel, accessibility depends on location of the gating structure	When open: 10^6 to 10^8/sec
Transporters (carriers) (e.g., glucose and amino acid transporters, Na^+,K^+-ATPase)	Binding of substrate from one side, conformational change of protein, then release of substrate to other side of membrane	Accessible from only one side of the membrane at a time	10^2 to 10^5/sec

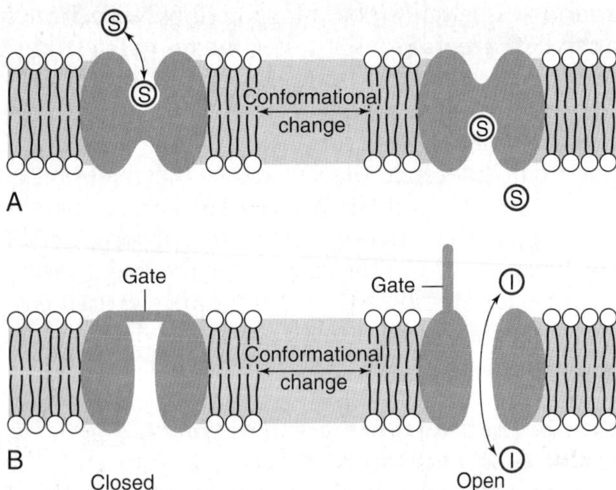

FIGURE 1–10. Transporters function differently from ion channels. A, A transporter binds the transported substance (S) on one side of the membrane and, after a conformational change, releases S at the other side of the membrane. B, An ion channel is either "open" or "closed," depending on the position of its "gate." When the channel is open, the conducted ion (I) can enter the channel from either side of the membrane and be rapidly conducted across the membrane.

Most transporters have numerous α helices that traverse the membrane. From one side of the membrane, the transported substrate binds to a site on the transporter that lies among its transmembrane helices. A rearrangement of the transmembrane helices then occurs so that the bound substrate has access to the other side of the membrane (Figure 1–10, *A*).

Cells depend on a number of membrane transport proteins

Ca^{++} is transported across membranes by Ca^{++}-ATPases and by $3Na^{+}$-$1Ca^{++}$ antiporters

Under most circumstances, the concentration of Ca^{++} in the cytosol of cells is maintained at low levels, below 10^{-7} M, whereas the concentration of Ca^{++} in extracellular fluids is on the order of 10^{-3} M. Plasma membranes contain Ca^{++}-ATPase that helps maintain the large gradient of Ca^{++} across the plasma membrane. The plasma membrane Ca^{++}-ATPase shares important properties with the Ca^{++}-ATPase of the sarcoplasmic reticulum (see Chapter 12) and the Na^{+},K^{+}-ATPase of plasma membranes. These proteins carry out the primary active transport of ions across membranes, and they capture the energy of the terminal phosphate bond of ATP to accomplish this task.

In addition, most cells store Ca^{++} in the endoplasmic reticulum or other intracellular storage vesicles. Ca^{++} is concentrated in these vesicles by a Ca^{++}-ATPase closely related to the Ca^{++}-ATPase of the sarcoplasmic reticulum of muscle cells. Because Ca^{++} is a key second messenger (see Chapter 5), many hormones or agonists elevate the intracellular level of Ca^{++} by opening Ca^{++} channels in the plasma membrane, the membranes of Ca^{++} storage vesicles, or both sites.

Certain electrically excitable cells, such as those of the heart, have an additional mechanism for controlling the level of intracellular Ca^{++}. A **$3Na^{+}$-$1Ca^{++}$ antiporter** in the plasma membrane uses the energy in the Na^{+} gradient to extrude Ca^{++} from the cell. Three Na^{+} enter the cell for every one Ca^{++} extruded. In heart cells, the rapid, transient decreases in intracellular Ca^{++} early in diastole are mediated by the $3Na^{+}$-$1Ca^{++}$ antiporter, whereas the resting level of intracellular Ca^{++} is set mainly by the Ca^{++}-ATPases of the plasma membrane and sarcoplasmic reticulum (see Chapters 13 and 18).

Glucose is transported into muscle and fat cells by facilitated transporters

Glucose is a primary fuel for most of the cells of the body, but glucose diffuses across plasma membranes very slowly. The plasma membranes of many cell types contain several different sugar transporters that mediate the facilitated transport of glucose and related monosaccharides. Red blood cells, adipocytes, and muscle cells (skeletal, cardiac, smooth) all possess glucose transporters of the GLUT family. The uptake of glucose in these cell types depends neither on the electrochemical potential difference of Na^{+} across the plasma membrane nor on cellular metabolism in any direct way. In adipocytes and muscle cells, the transport of glucose across the plasma membrane is increased by insulin (see Chapter 43), which causes more glucose transport proteins to be inserted into the plasma membrane. The source of the newly inserted protein is a preformed pool of transporters in vesicles in the cytoplasm of the cell, so that this response to insulin can occur rapidly.

Amino acids are taken up into cells via several different types of amino acid transporters

Most of the cells in the body synthesize proteins and therefore require amino acids. The synthesis of proteins is required for the turnover of cells and tissues and in processes such as wound healing. Several different amino acid transporters are present in plasma membranes. The amino acid transporters include three distinct classes of transporters for neutral, basic, and acidic amino acids (see Chapter 35). Amino acid transporters overlap significantly in substrate specificities, and the distribution of the different transport proteins varies from one cell type to another. Some of these transporters are secondary active transporters powered by the concentration gradient of Na^+ **(Na^+–amino acid symporters).** Others are Na^+-independent facilitated transporters.

You will encounter numerous transporters in your study of physiology

Among the other transporters you will learn about are

- H^+,K^+-ATPases that extrude H^+ from gastric parietal cells in exchange for K^+;
- anion antiporters that, for example, exchange Cl^- for HCO_3^- across the membrane of the red blood cell;
- Na^+-H^+ antiporters that secrete H^+ from cells into their surroundings;
- an oligopeptide-H^+ symporter that absorbs small peptides from the small intestine;
- Na^+-HCO_3^- symporters;
- Na^+-Cl^- symporters;
- K^+-Cl^- symporters;
- and many other transporters.

The steady-state concentrations of ions in the cytosol represent the net result of the actions of ion pumps and transmembrane fluxes of ions via symporters and antiporters

When an ion is in the **steady state,** its concentrations in the cytosol and in the extracellular fluid are constant in time. As examples, consider the concentrations of Na^+. Na^+ is pumped out of the cytosol against its electrochemical potential difference by the Na^+,K^+-ATPase. Na^+ then "leaks" back into the cytosol, down its electrochemical potential gradient, via the Na^+-dependent symporters and antiporters and via nonspecific cation channels. In the steady state, the rate at which Na^+ is extruded from the cell by the Na^+,K^+-ATPase is just equal to the sum of the rates that Na^+ enters the cytosol by all the Na^+ entry pathways. The cytosolic concentrations of all the other ions are similarly the result of the processes that mediate their entry into and their exit from the cytosol. The steady-state concentrations of cations and anions in the cytosol are different from their concentrations in the extracellular fluid that surrounds the cells **(Table 1–4).**

TABLE 1–4. CONCENTRATIONS OF IONS IN THE CYTOSOL OF A TYPICAL CELL AND IN THE EXTRACELLULAR FLUID THAT SURROUNDS IT

Ion	Cytosolic Concentration	Concentration in Extracellular Fluid
K^+	140 mM	4 mM
Na^+	15 mM	145 mM
Ca^{++}	$\approx 10^{-7}$ M	$\approx 10^{-3}$ M
Cl^-	20 mM	120 mM
HCO_3^-	14 mM	24 mM

Epithelial cells are polarized: the apical and basolateral plasma membranes contain different transport proteins

Epithelial cells are polarized with respect to their transport properties. That is, the transporters of the plasma membrane facing one side of the epithelial cell layer are different from the transporters of the membrane facing the other side.

The epithelial cells of the small intestine (see Chapter 35) and the proximal tubule of the kidney (see Chapter 37) are good examples of this polarity. The transporters in the brush border plasma membrane that faces the lumen of the small bowel or the renal tubule differ from the transporters of the basolateral plasma membrane of the cell **(Figure 1–11).** The tight junctions that join the epithelial cells side to side prevent mixing of the proteins of the luminal and basolateral plasma membranes. The brush border plasma membranes of these epithelia contain few Na^+,K^+-ATPase molecules, which reside mainly in the basolateral plasma membrane. Glucose (and galactose) and neutral amino acids enter these epithelial cells at the brush border via Na^+-monosaccharide symporters (secondary active transporters). However, these substances leave the cells at the basolateral membrane primarily by facilitated transporters.

The tight junctions that join epithelial cells are somewhat leaky to water and small water-soluble molecules and ions. The tightness of the tight junctions varies among epithelia. There are thus two types of pathways for transport across the epithelia: **transcellular pathways** (through the cells) and **paracellular pathways** (in between the cells) (Figure 1–11).

Neurons are also polarized cells. The axons of neurons contain proteins not present in the dendrites and vice versa. The polarity of the neuron subserves the different, highly specialized functions of the axons and the dendrites (see Chapter 6).

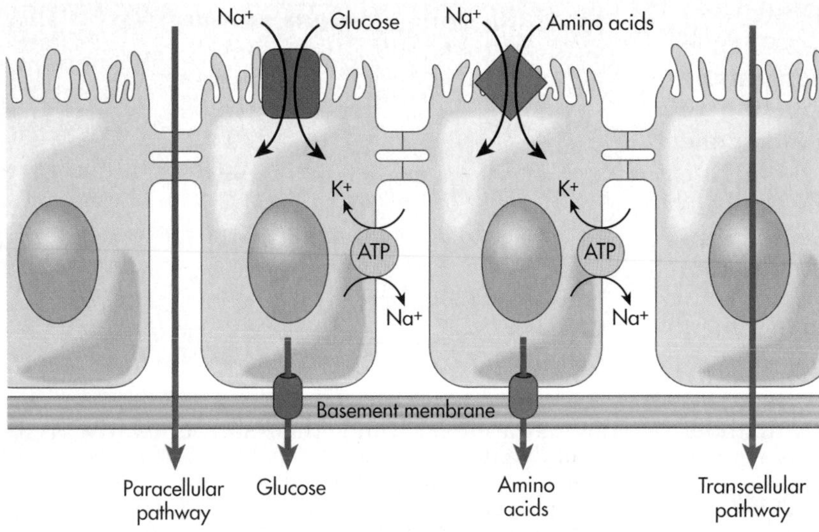

FIGURE 1–11. Epithelial transport processes that occur in the small intestine and renal tubules. Epithelia are polarized such that the transporters on one side of the cell differ from those on the other side. Glucose and neutral amino acids enter the epithelial cell at the brush border via Na^+-powered secondary active transport but leave the cell across the basolateral membrane by facilitated transport.

Summary

- Biological membranes are phospholipid bilayers with integral membrane proteins embedded in the bilayer and peripheral membrane proteins associated with the surfaces of the membrane.
- Membranes serve as permeability barriers that separate the cell from the extracellular milieu and divide the cell into biochemically specialized compartments.
- Endocytosis and exocytosis permit material to enter or to leave the cell without passing through the membrane.
- Diffusion is an effective biological transport process on the microscopic scale of distances.
- Only very small water-soluble molecules can diffuse across biological membranes at appreciable rates. Lipid-soluble molecules permeate membranes more readily. The more soluble a lipid-soluble compound is in the interior of the lipid bilayer core of the membrane, the more permeable is the compound.
- Gradients of solutes across membranes cause the flow of water by osmosis.
- The osmotic water flow caused by a particular solute depends on the permeability of the membrane to that species; the greater the permeability, the smaller the osmotic water flow.
- Membrane transporter proteins are classified as pores, channels, and transporters.
- Aquaporin is a pore protein that makes plasma membranes highly permeable to water.
- Ion channels permit specific ions to cross a membrane at high rates. Ion channels are said to be gated since they alternate between open and closed states.
- A transporter binds the molecule to be transported from one side of the membrane, then undergoes a conformational change that permits the release of the transported substrate at the other side of the membrane.
- Transporters promote the movement of various classes of molecules across the membrane. Facilitated transporters allow the transported substance to equilibrate across the membrane. Active transporters can pump the transported substrates against chemical or electrochemical potential gradients. Active transport requires a link to metabolism.
- Primary active transporters have a direct link to metabolism, frequently by consuming ATP.
- Secondary active transporters use the gradient of another substance, frequently Na^+, to power the transport of substances such as sugars and amino acids.

- Cell membranes contain a large number of different transporters. Some, like the glucose transporter of muscle cells, transport a single molecule (glucose). Symporters, like the Na^+–amino acid antiporters, use the energy of the Na^+ gradient to actively take up amino acids. Antiporters, like Na^+-H^+ antiporters, use the energy of the Na^+ gradient to actively extrude H^+ from the cell. Another class of antiporters exchanges certain anions across plasma membranes.

Bibliography

Abramson J et al: The lactose permease of *Escherichia coli:* overall structure, the sugar-binding site and the alternating access model for transport, *FEBS Lett* 555:96, 2003.

Agre P, Kozono D: Aquaporin water channels: molecular mechanisms for human diseases, *FEBS Lett* 555:72, 2003.

Alper SL et al: The AE gene family of Cl^-/HCO_3^- exchangers, *J Nephrol* 15(suppl 5):S41, 2002.

Bers DM, Barry WH, Despa S: Intracellular Na^+ regulation in cardiac myocytes, *Cardiovasc Res* 57:871, 2003.

Broer S: Adaptation of plasma membrane amino acid transport mechanisms to physiological demands, *Eur J Physiol* 444:457, 2002.

Brown GK: Glucose transporters: structure, function and consequences of deficiency, *J Inherit Metab Dis* 23:237, 2000.

Bryant NJ, Govers R, James DE: Regulated transport of the glucose transporter GLUT4, *Nature Rev Mol Cell Biol* 3:267, 2002.

Clausen T: The sodium pump keeps us going, *Ann N Y Acad Sci* 986:595, 2003.

Dohm GL: Invited review: regulation of skeletal muscle GLUT-4 expression by exercise, *J Appl Physiol* 93:782, 2002.

Hayashi H, Szaszi K, Grinstein S: Multiple modes of regulation of Na^+/H^+ exchangers, *Ann N Y Acad Sci* 976:248, 2002.

Jung H: The sodium/substrate symporter family: structural and functional features, *FEBS Lett* 529:73, 2002.

Khan AH, Pessin JE: Insulin regulation of glucose uptake: a complex interplay of intracellular signalling pathways, *Diabetologia* 45:1475, 2002.

Minokoshi Y, Kahn CR, Kahn BB: Tissue-specific ablation of the GLUT4 glucose transporter or the insulin receptor challenges assumptions about insulin action and glucose homeostasis, *J Biol Chem* 278:33609, 2003.

Putney LK, Denker SP, Barber DL: The changing face of the Na^+/H^+ exchanger, NHE1: structure, regulation, and cellular actions, *Annu Rev Pharmacol Toxicol* 42:527, 2002.

Rakowski RF, Sagar S: Found: Na^+ and K^+ binding sites of the sodium pump, *News Physiol Sci* 18:164, 2003.

Scheiner-Bobis G: The sodium pump. Its molecular properties and mechanics of ion transport, *Eur J Biochem* 269:2424, 2002.

Sterling D, Casey JR: Bicarbonate transport proteins, *Biochem Cell Biol* 80:483, 2002.

Tsunoda SP et al: Aquaporin-1, nothing but a water channel, *J Biol Chem* 279:11364, 2004.

Wood IS, Trayhurn P: Glucose transporters (GLUT and SGLT): expanded families of sugar transport proteins, *Br J Nutr* 89:3, 2003.

Self-Assessment

1. Which of the following statements about diffusion is true?

A. The rate of diffusion is inversely proportional to the diffusion coefficient.

B. The time required for the average molecule to diffuse a given distance is proportional to the square of distance.

C. Diffusion is rapid on a scale of centimeters.

D. No human cells are small enough for diffusion to suffice for intracellular transport.

2. Which of the following statements about diffusion of substance X across a typical plasma membrane is true?

A. The smaller the molecular weight (MW) of X, the slower its diffusion.

B. The more soluble is X in nonpolar (hydrophobic) solvents, the more rapidly X diffuses across membranes.

C. If X is water, its rate of diffusion across membranes is low.

D. If X is water soluble and has MW = 400, its diffusion across membranes will be fast.

3. Which of the following statements about osmosis is true?

A. An ideal semipermeable membrane is permeable to H_2O but impermeable to some solutes.

B. Water flows from where osmotic pressure is lower to where osmotic pressure is higher.

C. The more concentrated the solution, the more accurate is van't Hoff's law.

D. The osmotic pressure of a solution is proportional to its boiling point depression.

4. Which of the following is characteristic of transporters?

A. Transport via a transporter is slower than by diffusion.
B. Chemical specificity
C. Spontaneous alternation between rapidly and slowly transporting states
D. Transport rate is linearly dependent on concentration of the transport substrate.

5. Which of the following is a primary active transporter?

A. Na^+,K^+-ATPase
B. The Na^+-glucose symporter
C. The Na^+-H^+ antiporter
D. The $3Na^+$-$1Ca^{++}$ antiporter

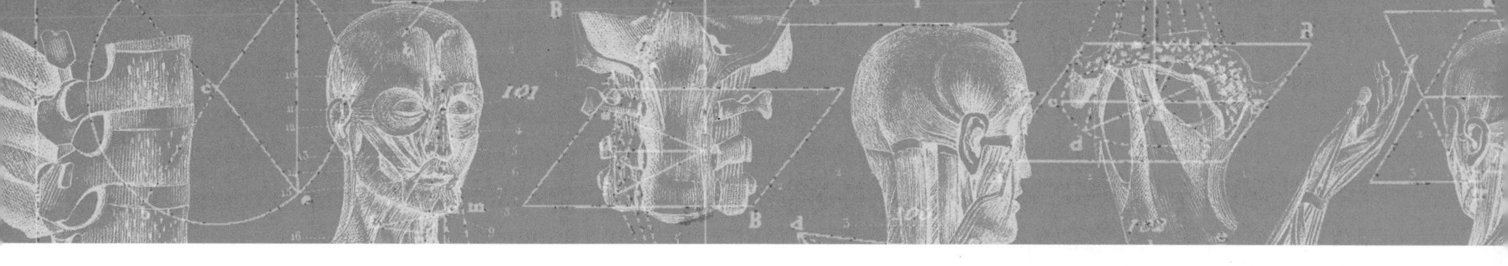

Chapter 2: Ionic Equilibria and Resting Membrane Potentials

Objectives

- Define the electrochemical potential difference ($\Delta\mu$) of an ion across a membrane and state that $\Delta\mu$ expresses the tendency for the ion to flow as a consequence of its concentration difference and the electrical potential difference across the membrane.
- Use the Nernst equation to determine whether an ion is in equilibrium across a membrane. If the ion is not in equilibrium, decide in which direction the ion will tend to flow spontaneously.
- Explain the importance of the Gibbs-Donnan equation and explain the circumstances under which it applies.
- Compute the equilibrium transmembrane electrical potential difference across a membrane that is permeable to only one ionic species.
- Estimate a cell's resting membrane potential by the chord conductance equation.

Cells have an electrical potential difference (voltage difference), called the **resting membrane potential,** across their plasma membranes. THE CYTOPLASM IS USUALLY ELECTRICALLY NEGATIVE RELATIVE TO THE EXTRACELLULAR FLUID. The resting membrane potential is necessary for the electrical excitability of neurons (see Chapters 2 to 4 and 6 to 11), skeletal muscle (see Chapter 12), smooth muscle (see Chapter 14), and the heart (see Chapters 13 and 17). This chapter discusses the basic physical chemical principles of ionic equilibria and the processes that generate the resting membrane potential in all the cells of the body. In this text, we deal with resting membrane potentials (often called simply resting potentials) in electrically excitable cells, such as nerve and muscle cells. However, resting potentials are important in cells that are not usually classified as electrically excitable, such as epithelial cells and lymphocytes.

An Ion at Equilibrium Has No Net Force Acting on It

The difference in potential energy of an ion across a membrane depends on its concentration difference and the electrical potential difference across the membrane

A membrane separates aqueous solutions in two chambers (A and B). The ion X^+ is at a higher concentration on side A than on side B (**Figure 2–1**). If no electrical potential difference exists between A and B, X^+ tends to diffuse from A to B, just as if it were an uncharged molecule. If, however, A is electrically negative with respect to B, the situation is more complex. The tendency of X^+ to diffuse from A to B because of the concentration difference

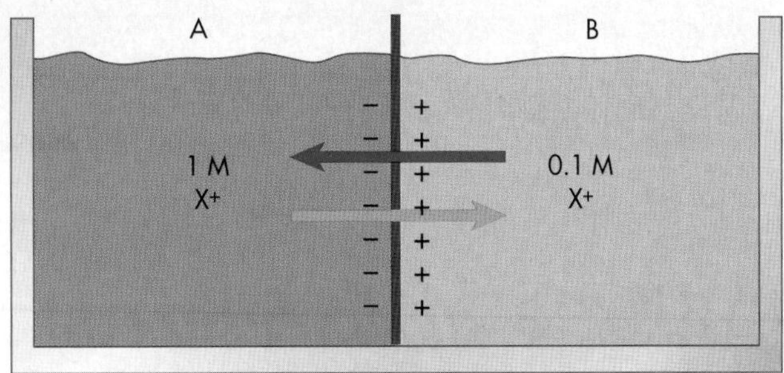

FIGURE 2–1. X^+ is present at 1 M in chamber A and at 0.1 M in chamber B. A concentration force for X^+ tends to cause X^+ to flow from A to B. However, chamber A is electrically negative with respect to chamber B, so an electrical force tends to cause X^+ to flow from B to A. The red arrow indicates the electrical gradient; the yellow arrow indicates the concentration gradient.

remains, but now X^+ also tends to move in the opposite direction (from B to A) because of the electrical potential difference across the membrane. The direction of net X^+ movement depends on whether the effect of the concentration difference or the effect of the electrical potential difference is larger. By comparing the two tendencies—concentration and electrical—one can predict the direction of net X^+ movement.

The quantity that allows a comparison of the relative contributions of ionic concentration differences and electrical potential differences across a membrane is called the **electrochemical potential difference ($\Delta\mu$)** of an ion. The electrochemical potential difference of X^+ across the membrane is defined as follows:

$$\Delta\mu(X) = \mu_A(X) - \mu_B(X) = RT\ln\frac{[X]_A}{[X]_B} + zF(E_A - E_B) \quad \textbf{2-1}$$

where

$\Delta\mu$ = electrochemical potential difference of the ion between sides A and B of the membrane

R = ideal gas constant

T = absolute temperature

$\ln\frac{[X]_A}{[X]_B}$ = natural logarithm of concentration ratio of X^+ on the two sides of the membrane

z = charge number of the ion (e.g., +2 for Ca^{++}, −1 for Cl^-)

F = Faraday's number

$E_A - E_B$ = electrical potential difference across the membrane

THE FIRST TERM ON THE RIGHT-HAND SIDE OF EQUATION 2-1 (THE LOGARITHM) EXPRESSES THE TENDENCY FOR X^+ IONS TO MOVE FROM A TO B BECAUSE OF THE CONCENTRATION DIFFERENCE, AND THE SECOND TERM, $zF(E_A - E_B)$, EXPRESSES THE TENDENCY FOR THE IONS TO MOVE FROM A TO B BECAUSE OF THE ELECTRICAL POTENTIAL DIFFERENCE. The first term represents the potential energy difference between a mole of X^+ ions on side A and a mole of X^+ ions on side B as a result of the concentration difference. The second term represents the potential energy difference between a mole of X^+ ions on side A and a mole of X^+ ions on side B caused by the electrical potential difference between A and B. Thus, $\Delta\mu(X)$ describes the difference that exists in potential energy between a mole of X^+ ions on side A and a mole of X^+ ions on side B. $\Delta\mu(X)$ is proportional to the energy possessed by the average X^+ ion on side A minus the average energy of an X^+ ion on side B. $\Delta\mu$ results from both concentration and electrical potential differences, hence the name **electrochemical potential difference.** The unit of electrochemical potential, and of both terms on the right-hand side of Equation 2-1, is energy per mole.

The X^+ ions will tend to move spontaneously from higher to lower electrochemical potential. The term $\Delta\mu$ has been defined as the electrochemical potential of the ion on side A minus that on side B. If $\Delta\mu$ is positive, the ions tend to move from A to B; if $\Delta\mu$ is zero, there is no net tendency for the ions to move at all; and if $\Delta\mu$ is negative, the ions tend to move from B to A.

If μ_A is greater than μ_B, then ions will tend to flow spontaneously from A to B. For ions to flow from B to A, work must be done. Specifically, $\mu_A - \mu_B$ is the minimal amount of work that must be done to cause 1 mole of ions to flow from B to A. When ions flow from A to B, on the other hand, energy is released. In fact, this energy can be harnessed to perform work. The maximal amount of work that can be done by 1 mole of ions flowing from A to B is $\mu_A - \mu_B$. THE ELECTROCHEMICAL POTENTIAL DIFFERENCE OF AN ION ACROSS A MEMBRANE THUS REPRESENTS POTENTIAL ENERGY THAT CAN BE USED TO PERFORM WORK.

What sort of work can be done by the electrochemical potential energy stored in an ion gradient? Chapter 1 mentions that the electrochemical potential of the Na^+ gradient is used to power the secondary active transport of sugars and amino acids. In mitochondria, the action of the electron transport enzymes creates an electrochemical potential difference of H^+ across the mitochondrial inner membrane. The H^+ ions flow back into the mitochondrial matrix via the ATP synthase enzyme complex in the mitochondrial inner membrane. The ATP synthase uses the energy released by the H^+ ions to drive the synthesis of ATP. Drugs that increase the permeability of the mitochondrial inner membrane to H^+, such as the poison dinitrophenol, collapse the H^+ gradient and prevent the synthesis of ATP.

An ion in equilibrium across a membrane satisfies the Nernst equation

In Equation 2-1, $\Delta\mu$ may be thought of as the net force on the ion; the logarithmic term is the force caused by the concentration difference, and $zF(E_A - E_B)$ is the force caused by the electrical potential difference. When the two forces are equal and opposite, $\Delta\mu$ equals zero, and there is no net force on the ion. When there is no net force on the ion, no net movement of the ion occurs, and the ion is said to be in **electrochemical equilibrium** across the membrane. At equilibrium, $\Delta\mu$ equals zero. From Equation 2-1, therefore, at equilibrium

$$\Delta\mu = RT\ln\frac{[X]_A}{[X]_B} + zF(E_A - E_B) = 0 \qquad 2\text{-}2$$

Solving for $E_A - E_B$, one obtains

$$E_A - E_B = -\frac{RT}{zF}\ln\frac{[X]_A}{[B]_B} \qquad 2\text{-}3$$

Equation 2-3 is called the **Nernst equation.** The condition of equilibrium was assumed in its derivation, and the Nernst equation is satisfied only for ions in equilibrium. It allows the computation of the electrical potential difference, $E_A - E_B$, required to produce an electrical force that is just equal and opposite to the concentration force. That electrical force equals

$$-\frac{RT}{zF}\ln\frac{[X]_A}{[B]_B} = \frac{RT}{zF}\ln\frac{[X]_B}{[B]_A}$$

The Nernst equation can be used to determine whether an ion is in equilibrium across a membrane

It is often convenient to convert the Nernst equation to a form involving the logarithm to the base 10 (log) rather than natural logarithms (ln). The formula for this conversion is ln(x) = 2.303 log(x). Because biological electrical potentials are usually expressed in millivolts (mV), the units of R may be selected so that RT/F comes out in millivolts. At 29.2°C, the quantity 2.303 RT/F is equal to 60 mV. Because this quantity is proportional to the absolute temperature, it changes by approximately 1/300 (0.33%) for each centigrade degree. Thus, the value of 60 mV for 2.303 RT/F holds approximately for most experimental conditions in biology (using 60 mV, instead of the exact value, at 37°C results in an error of about 2.6%). Thus, a useful form of the Nernst equation follows:

$$E_A - E_B = \frac{-60\text{ mV}}{z}\log\frac{[X]_A}{[X]_B} = \frac{60\text{ mV}}{z}\log\frac{[X]_B}{[X]_A} \qquad 2\text{-}4$$

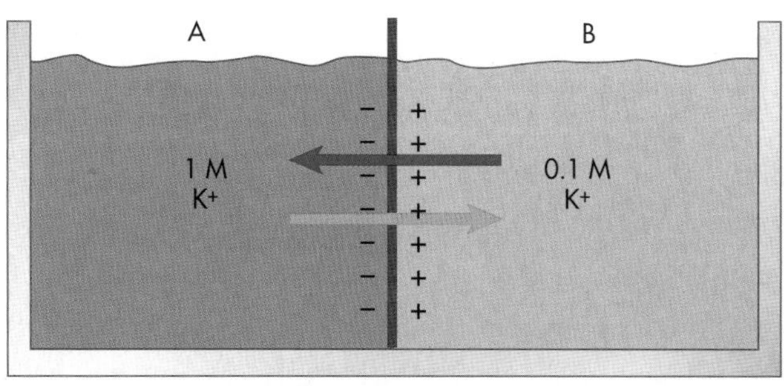

FIGURE 2–2. A membrane separates chambers containing K^+ at different concentrations. At an electrical potential difference ($E_A - E_B$) of –60 mV, K^+ is in electrochemical equilibrium across the membrane. The red arrow indicates the electrical gradient; the yellow arrow indicates the concentration gradient.

Examples of uses of the Nernst equation

Example 1. In **Figure 2–2**, K^+ is 10 times more concentrated on side A than on side B. The following is a calculation of the electrical potential difference that must exist between the chambers for K^+ to be in equilibrium across the membrane. Because K^+ should be in equilibrium, the Nernst equation holds

$$\begin{aligned} E_A - E_B &= \frac{-60\text{ mV}}{1}\log\frac{[K^+]_A}{[K^+]_B} \\ &= -(60\text{ mV})\log\frac{0.1}{0.01} \\ &= -(60\text{ mV})\log(10) = -60\text{ mV} \end{aligned} \qquad 2\text{-}5$$

The Nernst equation reveals that at equilibrium, A must be –60 mV relative to B. We know that this polarity is correct because K^+ tends to move from B to A driven by this electrical potential difference, which counteracts the tendency for it to move from A to B as a result of the concentration difference.

This example shows that AN ELECTRICAL POTENTIAL DIFFERENCE OF ABOUT 60 mV IS REQUIRED TO BALANCE A 10-FOLD CONCENTRATION DIFFERENCE OF A UNIVALENT ION. This is a useful rule of thumb.

Example 2. In **Figure 2–3,** the Nernst equation can aid in the determination of whether HCO_3^- is in equilibrium. If HCO_3^- is not in equilibrium, the equation allows the direction of net flow of HCO_3^- to be predicted.

The Nernst equation computes the electrical potential difference, $E_A - E_B$, that just balances the concentration difference of HCO_3^- across the membrane, as follows:

$$\begin{aligned} E_A - E_B &= \frac{-60\text{ mV}}{-1}\log\frac{[HCO_3^-]_A}{[HCO_3^-]_B} \\ &= +(60\text{ mV})\log\frac{1}{0.1} \\ &= +60\text{ mV}\log(10) = +60\text{ mV} \end{aligned} \qquad 2\text{-}6$$

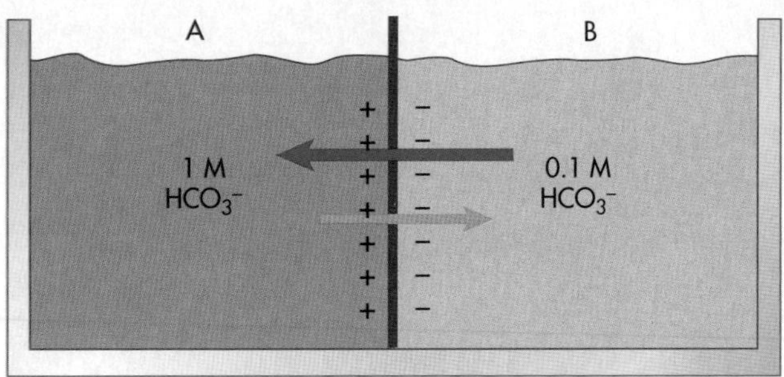

FIGURE 2–3. A membrane separates chambers containing different HCO_3^- concentrations. $E_A - E_B = +100$ mV. HCO_3^- is not in electrochemical equilibrium. If $E_A - E_B$ were +60 mV, HCO_3^- would be in equilibrium. $E_A - E_B$ (+100 mV) is stronger than it needs to be (+60 mV) to just balance the tendency for HCO_3^- to move from A to B because of its concentration difference. Thus, a net movement of HCO_3^- from B to A occurs. The red arrow indicates the electrical gradient; the yellow arrow indicates the concentration gradient.

Thus, a potential difference of +60 mV between A and B would just balance the tendency of HCO_3^- to move from A to B because of its concentration difference. However, $E_A - E_B$ is actually +100 mV. Therefore, the electrical force is in the right direction to balance the concentration force, but it is 40 mV larger than it needs to be to just balance the concentration force. Because the electrical force on HCO_3^- is larger than the concentration force, the electrical force determines the direction of net HCO_3^- movement. Net HCO_3^- flow will occur spontaneously from B to A.

In summary, the Nernst equation can be used to predict the direction that ions tend to flow, as follows:

1. If the potential difference measured across a membrane is equal to the potential difference calculated from the Nernst equation for a particular ion, then that ion is **in electrochemical equilibrium** across the membrane, and no net flow of that ion will occur across the membrane.
2. If the measured electrical potential is of the same sign as that calculated from the Nernst equation for a particular ion but larger in magnitude than the calculated value, then the electrical force is larger than the concentration force, and net movement of that particular ion tends to occur in the direction determined by the electrical force.
3. When the measured electrical potential difference is of the same sign as the potential calculated from the Nernst equation for a particular ion but numerically less, then the concentration force is larger than the electrical force, and net movement of that ion tends to occur in the direction determined by the concentration difference.
4. If the measured electrical potential difference across the membrane is of the opposite sign to that predicted by the Nernst equation for a particular ion, then the electrical and concentration forces are in the same direction. Thus, that ion cannot be in equilibrium, and it tends to flow in the direction determined by both electrical and concentration forces.

When an Ionic Species Cannot Permeate the Membrane, a Gibbs-Donnan Equilibrium May Occur

Certain properties of cells are due to the presence of impermeant anions in the cytosol

Cytoplasm typically contains proteins, organic polyphosphates, nucleic acids, and other ionized substances that cannot permeate the plasma membrane. The majority of these impermeant intracellular ions are negatively charged at physiological pH. The presence in cells of impermeant anions affects the distribution of permeant cations and anions across the plasma membrane and, as a consequence, affects the steady-state concentrations of permeant ions in the cytosol and influences the resting membrane potential. The steady-state properties of this mixture of permeant and impermeant ions are described by the **Gibbs-Donnan equilibrium.**

As a model of a cell with impermeant anions, consider a membrane separating a solution of KCl from a solution of KY, where Y^- is an anion to which the membrane is completely impermeable **(Figure 2–4, *top*)**. The membrane is permeable to water, K^+, and Cl^-. Suppose that initially chamber A contains a 0.1 M solution of KY and that chamber B contains an equal volume of 0.1 M KCl. Because $[Cl^-]_B$ exceeds $[Cl^-]_A$, there will be a net flow of Cl^- from B to A. Negatively charged Cl^- ions flowing from B to A will create an electrical potential difference (chamber A negative) that causes K^+ also to flow from B to A. Given enough time, K^+ and Cl^- come to equilibrium. At equilibrium, both $\Delta\mu(K^+)$ and $\Delta\mu(Cl^-)$ must equal zero. Setting the equation for $\Delta\mu(K^+)$ equal to that for $\Delta\mu(Cl^-)$, the following equation can be obtained:

$$[K^+]_A[Cl^-]_A = [K^+]_B[Cl^-]_B \qquad 2\text{-}7$$

Equation 2-7 is called the **Donnan relation** or the **Gibbs-Donnan equation,** and it holds for any pair of univalent cation and anion in equilibrium between the two chambers. If other univalent ions that could attain an equilibrium distribution were present, the same reasoning and an equation similar to Equation 2-7 would apply to each cation-anion pair among them.

For this model situation, application of the Gibbs-Donnan equation results in the final

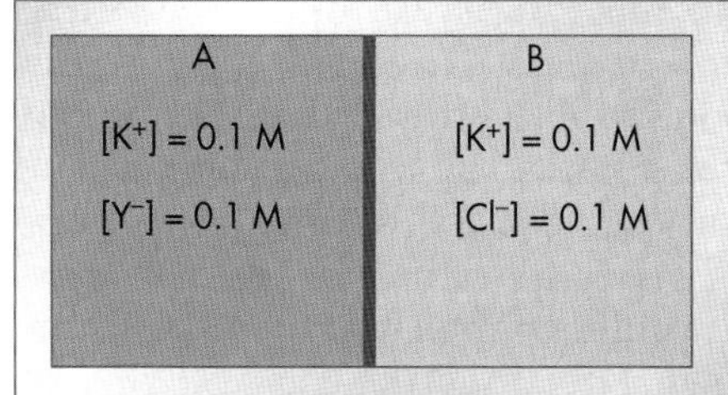

Membrane permeable to K^+ and Cl^- but impermeable to Y^-

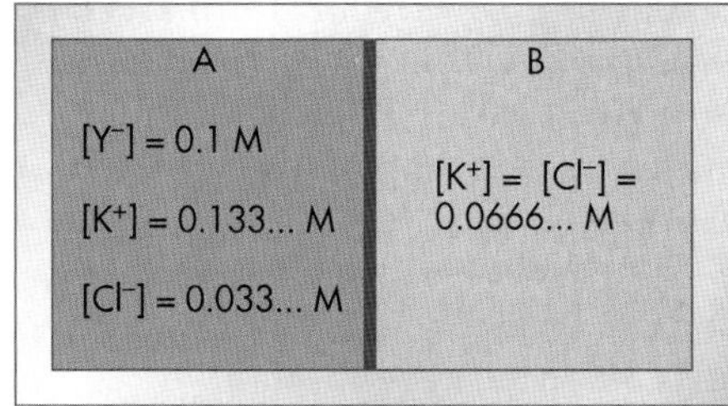

FIGURE 2–4. ***Top,*** **Initial concentrations. Before a Gibbs-Donnan equilibrium is established, a membrane separates two aqueous compartments. The membrane is permeable to water, K^+, and Cl^- but is impermeable to Y^-.** ***Bottom,*** **Equilibrium concentrations. Ion concentrations after a Gibbs-Donnan equilibrium has been attained.**

concentrations shown in Figure 2–4, *bottom*. In this Gibbs-Donnan equilibrium, K^+ and Cl^- (but not Y^-) are in electrochemical equilibrium. This means that both K^+ and Cl^- must satisfy the Nernst equation, so the equilibrium transmembrane electrical potential difference can be computed from the Nernst equation for either K^+ or Cl^-. Applying the Nernst equation to either K^+ or Cl^- results in

$$E_A - E_B = -60 \text{ mV} \log(2) = -18 \text{ mV}$$

The presence of the impermeant Y^- anions results in a negative electrical potential in the chamber that contains them. In this way, the impermeant anions in the cytoplasm of a typical cell contribute on the order of −10 mV to the resting membrane potential of the cytoplasm relative to the extracellular fluid.

Only the permeant ions (K^+ and Cl^- in this example) attain equilibrium. The impermeant anion, Y^-, cannot reach an equilibrium distribution. It may not be evident that water also does not achieve equilibrium, unless provision is made for that to occur. The sum of the concentrations of K^+ and Cl^- ions in chamber A in the preceding example exceeds that in chamber B. This is a general property of Gibbs-Donnan equilibria. When the impermeant Y^- is also taken into account, the total concentration of osmotically active ions is considerably greater in A than in B. Water tends to flow by osmosis from B to A until the total osmotic pressure of the two solutions is equal. However, ions then flow to set up a new Gibbs-Donnan equilibrium, and this requires that there be more osmotically active ions on the side with Y^-. All the water from B ends up in A unless water is restrained from moving.

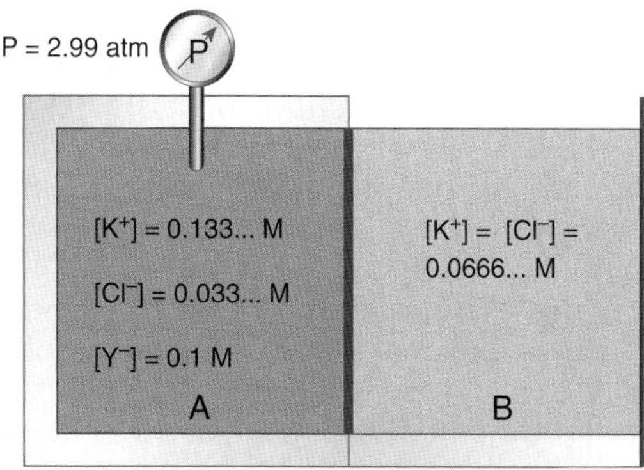

FIGURE 2–5. A hydrostatic pressure (P) of 2.99 atm is required to prevent water from flowing from B to A in the Gibbs-Donnan equilibrium in Figure 2–4. This 2.99 atm is equal to the osmotic pressure in chamber A minus that in chamber B.

This can be done by enclosing the solution in chamber A in a rigid container **(Figure 2–5)**. As fluid then flows from B to A, pressure builds up in A, and this pressure opposes further osmotic water flow. The pressure in A at equilibrium is equal to the difference between the osmotic pressures of the solutions in A and B. The rigid cell wall of plant cells allows turgor pressure to build up in the cell and to partly compensate for the osmotic effects of the Gibbs-Donnan equilibrium. Left to its own devices, the Gibbs-Donnan equilibrium results in an osmotic pressure in the cytoplasm that is in excess of that in the extracellular fluid. Since water would thus enter cells, this poses a threat to the maintenance of the normal cellular volume. Animal cells do not have rigid cell walls and have thus evolved other ways that involve ion transport processes to deal with the osmotic consequences of the Gibbs-Donnan equilibrium.

Ion transport processes are required for the regulation of cell volume

Why does the osmotic imbalance just discussed not cause animal cells to swell and finally burst? One reason is that cells actively pump Na^+ out of the cytoplasm to the extracellular fluid. The extrusion of Na^+ decreases the osmotic pressure of the cytoplasm and increases that of the extracellular fluid. The pumping of Na^+ is done by the Na^+ pump (i.e., Na^+,K^+-ATPase) in the plasma membrane. The

Na^+,K^+-ATPase splits an ATP and uses some of the energy released to extrude three Na^+ ions from the cytoplasm and to pump two K^+ ions into the cell. Whereas K^+ is only slightly removed from an equilibrium distribution, because of pumping by the Na^+,K^+-ATPase, Na^+ is far from an equilibrium distribution.

When the ATP production of a cell is compromised (e.g., in the presence of metabolic inhibitors or low O_2 levels) or when the Na^+,K^+-ATPase is specifically inhibited, Na^+ enters the cell more rapidly than it can be pumped out. As a result, the cell swells.

The plasma membranes of red blood cells from patients with **hereditary spherocytosis** are about three times more permeable to Na^+ than are red blood cells from normal individuals. The level of Na^+,K^+-ATPase in the erythrocyte membranes of such patients is also substantially elevated. When these red cells have sufficient glucose to maintain normal ATP levels, they extrude Na^+ as rapidly as it diffuses into the cell cytosol, and the red cell volume is maintained. However, when such erythrocytes are delayed in the venous sinuses of the spleen, where glucose and ATP are present at low levels, the intracellular ATP concentrations fall; Na^+ cannot be pumped out by Na^+,K^+-ATPase as rapidly as it enters, and the red cells swell. The swollen erythrocytes are prone to destruction by the spleen; consequently, patients with hereditary spherocytosis become anemic.

Every Cell Has a Resting Membrane Potential

The cytosol of a cell at rest is electronegative relative to the extracellular fluid

Communication between nerve cells depends on an electrical disturbance called an **action potential** that is propagated in the plasma membrane of the nerve cell. In striated muscle, an action potential propagates rapidly over the entire cell surface and allows the cell to contract synchronously (see Chapter 12). The action potential in nerve and muscle cells and the ionic mechanisms that account for its properties are discussed in Chapter 3. All cells that can produce action potentials have sizable resting membrane potentials (cytoplasm negative) across their plasma membranes. Inexcitable cells (e.g., epithelial cells) also have negative resting membrane potentials.

The resting membrane potential of a skeletal muscle cell is about −90 mV. By convention, membrane potential differences are expressed as the voltage in the cytoplasm minus the voltage in the extracellular fluid. A negative value denotes that the cytoplasm is electrically negative relative to the extracellular fluid. The resting membrane potential is necessary for the cell to fire an action potential.

Actively transported ions are not in electrochemical equilibrium across the plasma membrane. It is shown later that the flow of ions across the plasma membrane, down their electrochemical potential gradients, is directly responsible for generating much of the resting membrane potential. An understanding of how an ion's electrochemical potential gradient can give rise to a transmembrane difference in electrical potential can be gained by first considering a model system known as a **concentration cell.**

A concentration gradient of a permeant ionic species across a membrane produces an electrical potential difference across the membrane

In **Figure 2–6**, the membrane that separates chambers A and B is permeable to cations but not to

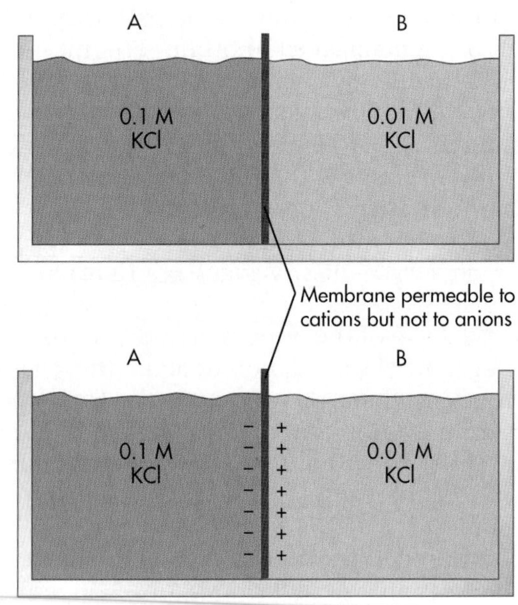

FIGURE 2–6. *Top,* Initial concentrations. A membrane that is permeable to cations but not to anions separates KCl solutions of different concentrations. *Bottom,* Equilibrium concentrations. Electrochemical equilibrium has been established. The flow of an infinitesimal amount of K^+ generated an electrical potential difference across the membrane that is equal to the equilibrium potential for K^+.

anions. Initially, no electrical potential difference exists across the membrane. K^+ flows from A to B because of the concentration force acting on it. Cl^- has the same force on it but cannot flow because the membrane is impermeable to anions. The flow of K^+ from A to B transfers a net positive charge to B and leaves a slight excess of negative charges behind on A. A thus becomes electrically negative to B (Figure 2–6, *bottom*). This electrical force is oppositely directed to the concentration force on K^+. The more K^+ that flows, the larger the opposing electrical force. Net K^+ flow stops when the electrical force just balances the concentration force, which occurs when the electrical potential difference is equal to the equilibrium (Nernst) potential for K^+:

$$E_A - E_B = \frac{-60\ \text{mV}}{+1}\log\frac{[K^+]_A}{[K^+]_B} = -(60\ \text{mV})\log\frac{0.1}{0.01}$$
$$= -60\ \text{mV}$$

Only a very small amount of K^+ flows from A to B before equilibrium is reached. This is because the separation of positive and negative charges requires a large amount of work. The electrical potential difference that builds up to oppose further K^+ movement is a manifestation of that work.

THE K^+ CONCENTRATION DIFFERENCE IN THIS EXAMPLE ACTS LIKE A BATTERY. In the example shown in Figure 2–6, by flowing down its electrochemical potential difference, K^+ creates a membrane potential that just balances the concentration difference of K^+ across the membrane. In this example, the 10-fold concentration difference of K^+ across the membrane functions as a battery that tends to bring the membrane potential to –60 mV. The natural tendency for any ion that can flow is to seek equilibrium; thus, K^+ tends to flow until its equilibrium potential difference is established. As explained later, when more than one type of ion can permeate a membrane, each ion "strives" to make the transmembrane potential difference equal to its equilibrium potential. The more permeant an ion, the greater its ability to force the electrical potential difference toward its equilibrium potential.

Gradients of ion concentrations across the plasma membrane help generate the resting membrane potential

In most tissues, a number of ions are not in equilibrium between the extracellular fluid and the cytoplasm. **Figure 2–7** gives approximate concentrations of Na^+, K^+, and Cl^- in the extracellular fluid and in the cytoplasm of human skeletal muscle. The resting membrane potential of a typical skeletal muscle cell is about –90 mV. Cl^- is close to being

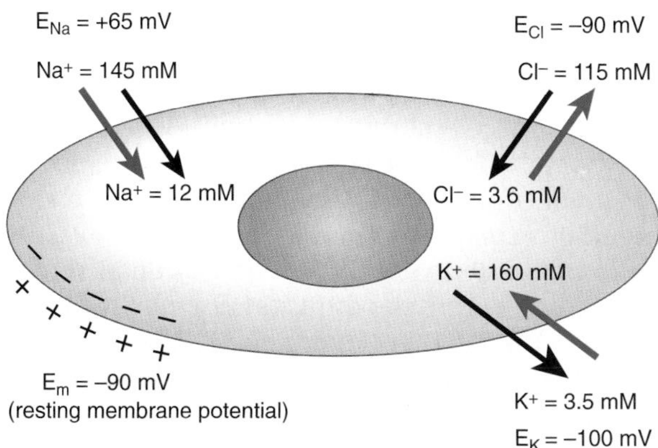

FIGURE 2–7. Approximate concentrations of Na^+, K^+, and Cl^- in the cytoplasm of a human skeletal muscle cell and in the surrounding extracellular fluid. The equilibrium potentials of the ions are indicated. The concentration forces on the ions are indicated by black arrows and the electrical forces by red arrows.

in equilibrium across the plasma membrane of skeletal muscle cells. This is known because chloride's equilibrium potential (E_{Cl}), as calculated from the Nernst equation, is about equal to the measured transmembrane potential difference (Figure 2–7). K^+ has a concentration force that tends to make it flow out of the cell. The electrical force on K^+ is oppositely directed to the concentration force. If the $E_{in} - E_{out}$ in skeletal muscle were –100 mV, the value of E_K, electrical and concentration forces on K^+, would exactly balance. Because $E_{in} - E_{out}$ is only –90 mV, the concentration force on K^+ is greater than the electrical force. Therefore, K^+ has a net tendency to flow out of the cell. Both the concentration and the electrical forces on Na^+ tend to cause it to flow into the cell. Na^+ is the ion farthest from an equilibrium distribution. The larger the difference between the measured membrane potential and the equilibrium potential for an ion, the larger the net force tending to make that ion flow.

The Na^+,K^+-ATPase contributes directly to generation of the resting membrane potential

The Na^+-K^+ pump is responsible for the high intracellular $[K^+]$ and the low intracellular $[Na^+]$. Because the pump moves a larger number of Na^+ ions out than K^+ ions in (three Na^+ to two K^+), it causes a net transfer of positive charge out of the cell and thus contributes to the resting membrane potential. Because it brings about net movement of charge across the membrane, the pump is termed **electrogenic.** In some cells, the Na^+,K^+-ATPase is directly responsible for a large fraction of the resting membrane potential. In certain smooth muscle cells, for example, the electrogenic effect of the Na^+,K^+-ATPase is responsible for more than 20 mV of the resting membrane potential. By contrast, in many vertebrate nerve and skeletal muscle cells, the direct contribution of the pump to the resting potential is small, less than 5 mV. Thus, the resting membrane potential in nerve and skeletal muscle results mainly from the diffusion of ions down their electrochemical potential gradients. The ionic gradients are maintained by the Na^+,K^+-ATPase.

Cardiac glycosides, such as **digitalis,** can increase the heart's strength of contraction (see Chapter 18). These compounds inhibit the Na^+,K^+-ATPase. Consequently, the intracellular level of Na^+ in cardiac cells is elevated. Each contraction of the heart is initiated by an increase in the cytosolic concentration of Ca^{++} (see Chapters 13 and 18). For cardiac muscle to relax, Ca^{++} must be removed from the cytosol, which is accomplished by its being pumped into the sarcoplasmic reticulum by a Ca^{++}-ATPase in the sarcoplasmic reticulum membrane and out across the plasma membrane by plasma membrane Ca^{++}-ATPase and by $3Na^+$-$1Ca^{++}$ antiporters (see Chapter 1). In the presence of cardiac glycosides, because of the elevated cytosolic [Na^+], the $3Na^+$-$1Ca^{++}$ antiporter is not as effective in extruding Ca^{++} from the cell. Consequently, Ca^{++}-ATPase can accumulate more Ca^{++} in the sarcoplasmic reticulum, so more Ca^{++} is released from the sarcoplasmic reticulum to power the next cardiac contraction, which is stronger than normal because of the higher peak level of Ca^{++} in the cytosol.

The diffusion of ions down their electrochemical potential gradients contributes to generation of the resting membrane potential

The earlier discussion of concentration cells shows how an ion gradient can act as a battery. WHEN A NUMBER OF IONS ARE DISTRIBUTED ACROSS A MEMBRANE, ALL BEING REMOVED FROM ELECTROCHEMICAL EQUILIBRIUM, EACH ION TENDS TO FORCE THE TRANSMEMBRANE POTENTIAL TOWARD ITS OWN EQUILIBRIUM POTENTIAL AS CALCULATED FROM THE NERNST EQUATION. THE MORE PERMEABLE THE MEMBRANE TO A PARTICULAR ION, THE GREATER STRENGTH THAT ION WILL HAVE IN FORCING THE MEMBRANE POTENTIAL TOWARD ITS EQUILIBRIUM POTENTIAL. In skeletal muscle (Figure 2–7), the Na^+ concentration difference can be regarded as a battery that tries to make $E_{in} - E_{out}$ equal to +65 mV. The K^+ concentration difference resembles a battery that attempts to make $E_{in} - E_{out}$ equal to –100 mV. The Cl^- concentration difference resembles a battery trying to make $E_{in} - E_{out}$ equal to –90 mV.

The chord conductance equation describes the contributions of permeant ions to the resting membrane potential

The way in which the interplay of ion gradients creates the resting membrane potential (E_m) is illustrated by a simple mathematical model. For the distribution of K^+, Na^+, and Cl^- across the plasma membrane of a cell, the following equation predicts the transmembrane potential difference across the membrane:

$$E_m = \frac{g_K}{\sum g} E_K + \frac{g_{Na}}{\sum g} E_{Na} + \frac{g_{Cl}}{\sum g} E_{Cl} \qquad \textbf{2-8}$$

where

g = the conductance of the membrane to the ion indicated by the subscript

$\Sigma g = (g_K + g_{Na} + g_{Cl})$

E = the equilibrium potentials of the ion denoted by the subscript

Conductance is the reciprocal of resistance ($g = 1/R$). The more permeable the membrane to a particular ion, the greater the conductance of the membrane to that ion.

Equation 2-8 is called the **chord conductance equation.** It states that THE MEMBRANE POTENTIAL IS A WEIGHTED AVERAGE OF THE EQUILIBRIUM POTENTIALS OF ALL THE IONS TO WHICH THE MEMBRANE IS PERMEABLE, in this case K^+, Na^+, and Cl^-. The weighting factor for each ion is the fraction of the total ionic conductance of the membrane (the sum of the individual ionic conductances) that results from the conductance of the ion in question. The sum of the weighting factors for the ions must equal 1, so if one weighting factor grows larger, the others must become smaller. The chord conductance equation shows that THE GREATER THE CONDUCTANCE OF THE MEMBRANE TO A PARTICULAR ION, THE GREATER THE ABILITY OF THAT ION TO BRING THE MEMBRANE POTENTIAL TOWARD THE EQUILIBRIUM POTENTIAL OF THAT ION.

For the skeletal muscle fiber discussed earlier, $E_{in} - E_{out} = -90$ mV. The membrane potential is much closer to E_K (–100 mV) than to E_{Na} (+65 mV) because in the resting cell, g_K is much larger than g_{Na}. The chord conductance equation predicts that in resting muscle, g_K is about 10 times larger than g_{Na}. This has been confirmed by ion flux measurements with radioactive tracers. In other types of excitable cells, the relationship between g_K and g_{Na} may be somewhat different. Other ions also may play a role in generating the resting membrane potential. Resting membrane potentials vary from approximately –10 mV in human erythrocytes to around –40 mV in some types of smooth muscle and up to –90 mV or more in vertebrate skeletal muscle and cardiac ventricular cells.

K^+ has the largest resting conductance and thus has the largest influence on the resting membrane potential. For this reason, changes that occur in $[K^+]$ in a patient's extracellular fluid affect the resting membrane potentials of all cells. An increase in extracellular K^+ partially depolarizes cells (decreases the magnitude of the resting membrane potential), whereas a decrease in the level of extracellular K^+ hyperpolarizes cells (increases the magnitude of the resting membrane potential). Either a depolarization or a hyperpolarization of cardiac cells (see Chapter 17) may lead to cardiac arrhythmias, some of which are life-threatening. **Hypokalemia** (low serum K^+ levels) may result from long-term use of diuretics. **Hyperkalemia** (elevated serum K^+ level) occurs in acute renal failure and in a disorder called **primary hyperkalemic periodic paralysis,** which is characterized by episodes of muscle weakness and flaccid paralysis.

Summary

- An ion tends to flow across a membrane if there is a concentration difference of that ion or an electrical potential difference across the membrane.
- The electrochemical potential difference ($\Delta\mu$) of an ion across a membrane includes the contributions of both the concentration difference and the electrical potential difference to the tendency of the ion to flow across the membrane.
- The electrochemical potential difference of an ion across a membrane represents a difference of chemical potential energy. This potential energy difference can be harnessed to do work (e.g., to actively transport another species or to produce ATP).
- An ion that is distributed in equilibrium across a membrane satisfies the Nernst equation, which can be used to tell whether an ion is in equilibrium or to compute what the electrical potential difference across the membrane must be for a particular ion to be in equilibrium.
- The presence in cells of impermeant anions affects the distribution of permeant cations and anions across the plasma membrane and, as a consequence, affects the steady-state concentrations of permeant ions in the cytosol and influences the resting membrane potential.
- All cells have a negative resting membrane potential; that is, the cytoplasm is electrically negative relative to the extracellular fluid.
- The diffusion of ions across the plasma membrane and down their electrochemical potential gradients contributes to the resting membrane potential.
- The flow of each ion across the plasma membrane tends to bring the resting membrane potential toward the equilibrium potential for that ion. The more permeable the membrane is to a particular ion, the greater the ability of that ion to bring the membrane potential toward its equilibrium potential.
- Three processes contribute to generation of the resting membrane potential: ionic diffusion as just described (major), the electrogenic effect of Na^+,K^+-ATPase (variable in importance), and the Gibbs-Donnan equilibrium (minor in excitable cells).

Bibliography

Aidley DJ: *The physiology of excitable cells,* ed 4, Cambridge, 1998, Cambridge University Press.

Hille B: *Ion channels of excitable membranes,* ed 3, Sunderland, Mass, 2001, Sinauer Associates.

Hodgkin AL: *The conduction of the nervous impulse,* Springfield, Ill, 1964, Charles C Thomas.

Kandel ER, Schwartz JH, Jessell TM: *Principles of neural science,* ed 4, New York, 2000, Elsevier Science.

Katz B: *Nerve, muscle, and synapse,* New York, 1966, McGraw-Hill.

Nadeau SE et al: *Medical neuroscience,* New York, 2004, Elsevier.

Nicholls JG et al: *From neuron to brain,* ed 4, Sunderland, Mass, 2001, Sinauer Associates.

Purves D et al: *Neuroscience,* ed 2, Sunderland, Mass, 2001, Sinauer Associates.

Sperelakis N, ed: *Cell physiology source book,* ed 3, New York, 2001, Elsevier.

Self-Assessment

1. With reference to the situation diagrammed below, which statement is true?

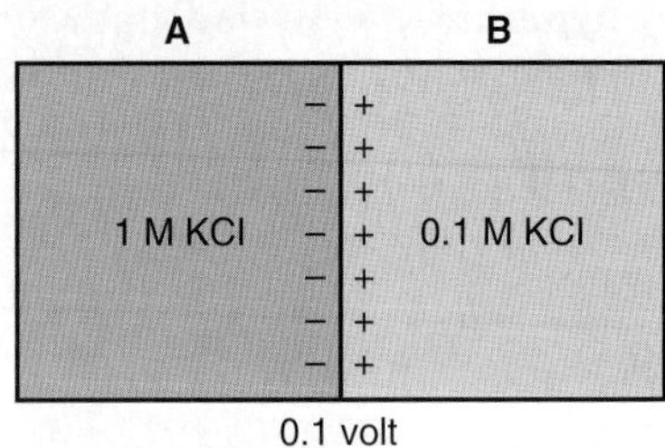

A. Cl^- is in equilibrium.
B. K^+ is in equilibrium.
C. There is a net tendency for K^+ to diffuse from B to A.
D. Work is required to cause K^+ to flow from B to A.

2. Li^+ and Cl^- are in Gibbs-Donnan equilibrium across the membrane of an erythrocyte. The impermeant ions in the cell have a predominantly negative charge. Which statement is true?

A. The concentration of Li^+ in the cell will be less than that in the extracellular fluid.
B. The concentration of Cl^- in the extracellular fluid will be less than that in the cell.
C. The sum of $[Li^+]$ and $[Cl^-]$ is greater in the cell than in the extracellular fluid.
D. The product of $[Li^+]$ and $[Cl^-]$ is greater in the cell than in the extracellular fluid.

3. In the "concentration cell" depicted below, the membrane is permeable to Cl^- but completely impermeable to K^+. Which statement is true?

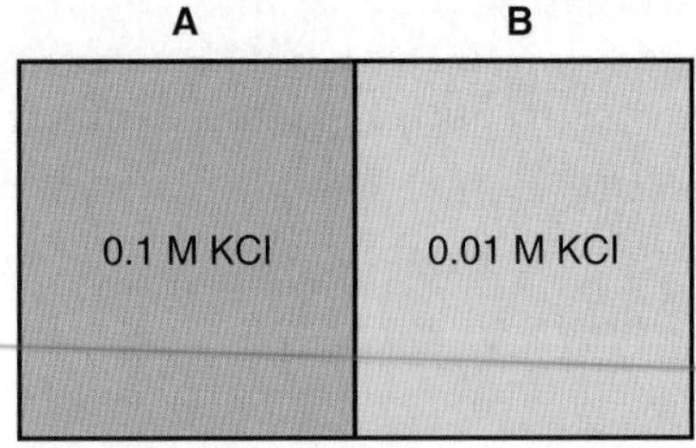

A. K^+ will diffuse from A to B.
B. A potential difference $E_A - E_B$ of +60 mV will develop.
C. Absolutely no Cl^- will flow from A to B.
D. Both K^+ and Cl^- will attain equilibrium.

4. The diagram below depicts a hypothetical skeletal muscle cell. The resting membrane potential (E_m) is −90 mV. E_{Na} = +64.8 mV. E_K = −92.6 mV. E_{Cl} = −92.1 mV. Which statement is true?

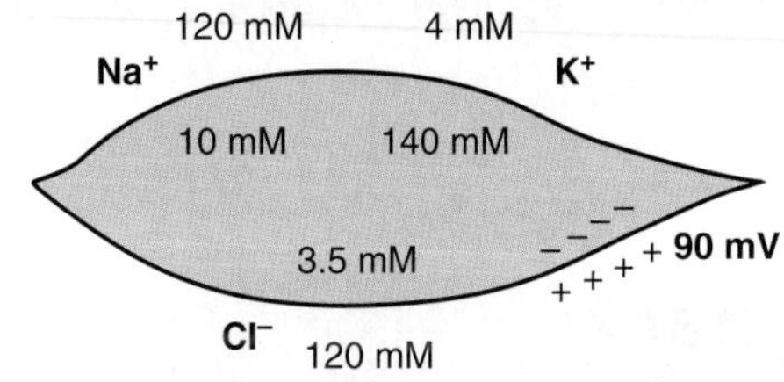

A. Cl^- will tend to flow into the cell.
B. K^+ will tend to flow into the cell.
C. Na^+ will tend to flow out of the cell.
D. K^+ is the ion closest to equilibrium.

5. For a cell with the intracellular and extracellular ion concentrations depicted in the figure in the preceding question, which statement is *not* true?

A. If the conductances (g's) for Na^+, K^+, and Cl^- are equal, then E_m = −30 mV.
B. If $g_{Cl} = g_{Na} = 0$, but g_K is significant, then E_m = −92.6 mV.
C. If $g_{Cl} = g_K = 0$, but g_{Na} is significant, then E_m = +50 mV.
D. If g_{Cl} is 0 and $g_{Na} = g_K$, then E_m = 0.

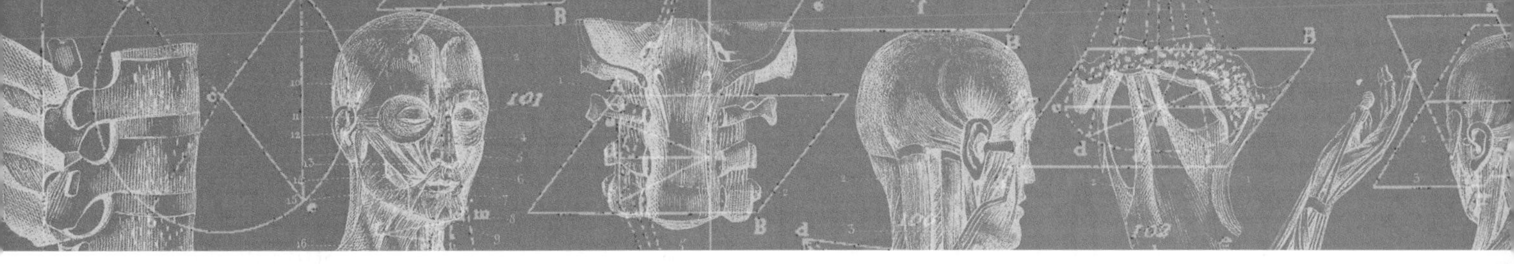

Chapter 3: Generation and Conduction of Action Potentials

Objectives

- Describe in terms of the chord conductance equation how the changes in the conductances to Na^+ and K^+ account for the form of the action potential.
- Define the absolute and relative refractory periods and accommodation and explain these phenomena in terms of the voltage-dependent properties of Na^+ and K^+ channels.
- Explain electrotonic conduction in terms of local circuit currents.
- Describe the local response and define the length constant and explain its determinants.
- Explain why an axon with large diameter conducts faster than a smaller axon.
- Discuss how myelination of an axon greatly increases its conduction velocity.

An action potential is a rapid change in the membrane potential that is propagated along the length of the cell. Action potentials are the basis for most communication between neurons (see Chapters 4 and 6 to 11). Action potentials elicit the contraction of skeletal muscle cells and permit contraction to occur nearly synchronously along the length of the cell (see Chapters 4 and 12). Action potentials in cardiac muscle cells spread from one cell to another via gap junctions, causing contractions of the ventricle to occur in a coordinated manner that permits the effective pumping of blood (see Chapters 13, 17, and 18).

Action Potentials Have Different Forms in Different Tissues

An **action potential** is a rapid change in the membrane potential followed by a return to the resting membrane potential **(Figure 3–1)**. The size and shape of action potentials differ considerably from one excitable tissue to another. An action potential is propagated with the same shape and size along the whole length of a nerve or muscle cell. Voltage-dependent ion channel proteins in the plasma membrane are responsible for action potentials. Action potentials in different cell types have different forms (Figure 3–1) because these cells have different kinds of voltage-dependent ion channels.

The Membrane Potential of a Cell Can Be Measured by Penetrating Its Plasma Membrane with a Microelectrode

Knowledge of the ionic mechanisms of action potentials was first obtained from experiments on the squid giant axon. The large diameter (up to 0.5 mm) of the squid giant axon makes it a convenient model for electrophysiological research with intracellular electrodes. The frog sartorius muscle is another useful preparation. The information learned from the squid axon and sartorius muscle applies in large part to mammalian neurons and skeletal muscle, respectively.

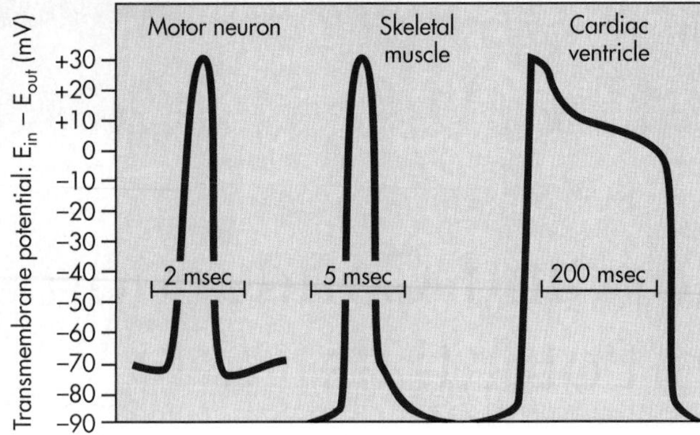

FIGURE 3–1. Action potentials from three vertebrate cell types. Note the different time scales. (Redrawn from Flickinger CJ et al: *Medical cell biology,* Philadelphia, 1979, WB Saunders.)

If the plasma membrane of a single muscle cell of a frog sartorius muscle is penetrated by a microelectrode (tip diameter < 0.5 μm), a potential difference (a voltage) is observed between the microelectrode whose tip is inside the cell and an extracellular electrode. The internal electrode is about –90 mV with respect to the external electrode. This 90-mV potential difference is the **resting membrane potential** of the muscle cell. In the absence of perturbing influences, the resting membrane potential remains at –90 mV.

Subthreshold changes in membrane potential are conducted with decrement

If a pulse of current flows across a cell's plasma membrane, the membrane potential changes. Current pulses are **depolarizing** or **hyperpolarizing,** depending on the direction of current flow. The terms depolarizing and hyperpolarizing may be confusing. A change in the membrane potential from –90 to –70 mV is a depolarization because it is a decrease in the potential difference, or polarization, across the cell membrane. If the membrane potential changes from –90 to –100 mV, the polarization of the membrane has increased; this is hyperpolarization. The larger the current passed, the larger the perturbation of the membrane potential.

When subthreshold current pulses are passed, the size of the potential change observed depends on the distance of the recording electrode from the point of current passage (**Figure 3–2,** ***A***). THE CLOSER THE RECORDING ELECTRODE TO THE SITE OF CURRENT PASSAGE, THE LARGER THE POTENTIAL CHANGE OBSERVED. The size of the potential change decreases expo-

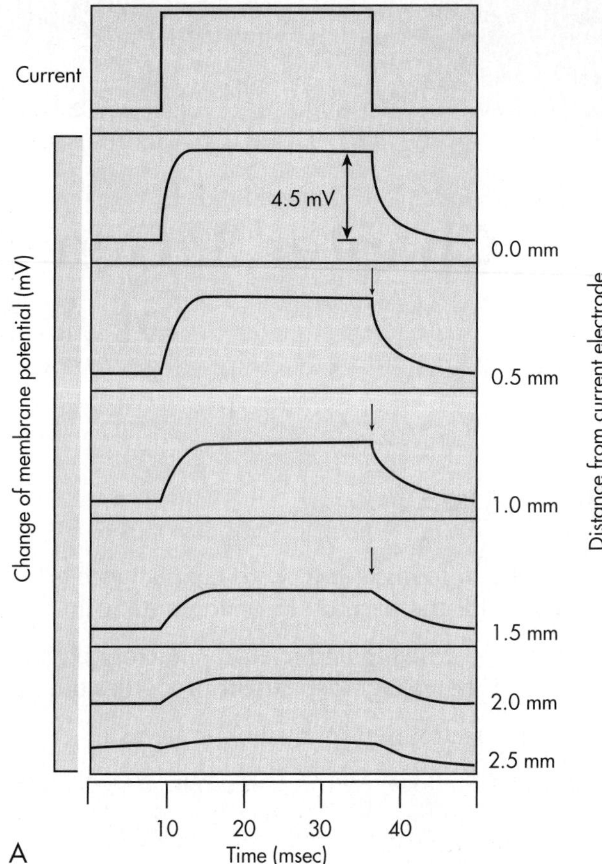

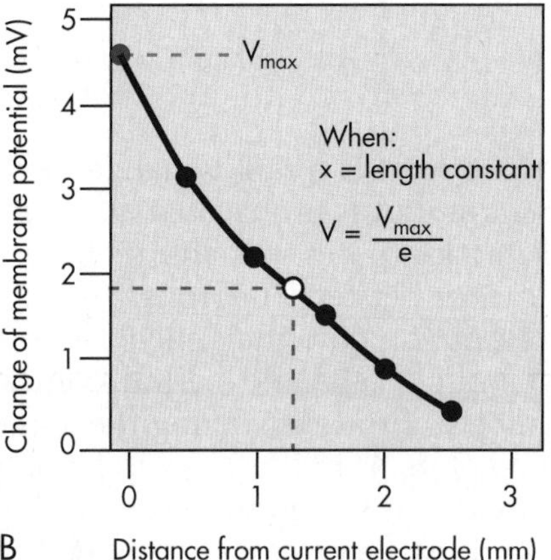

FIGURE 3–2. **A,** Responses of an axon of a shore crab to a subthreshold rectangular pulse of current recorded extracellularly by an electrode located different distances from the current-passing electrode. As the recording electrode is moved farther from the point of stimulation, the response of the membrane potential is slower and smaller. **B,** The maximum change in membrane potential from **A** is plotted versus distance from the point of current passage. The distance over which the response falls to 1/e (37%) of the maximal response (V_{max}) is the length constant. (**A** redrawn from Hodgkin AL, Rushton WAH: *Proc R Soc Biol* 133:97, 1946.)

nentially with distance from the site of current passage (Figure 3–2, *B*). The response is said to be **conducted with decrement.** The distance over which the potential change decreases to 1/e (37%) of its maximum value is called the **length constant** or space constant (*e* is the base of natural logarithms and is equal to 2.7182). A LENGTH CONSTANT OF 1 TO 2 MM IS TYPICAL FOR MAMMALIAN NERVE OR MUSCLE CELLS. Because these potential changes are observed primarily near the site of current passage and the changes are not propagated along the length of the cell (as are action potentials), they are called **local responses.**

An action potential remains the same size and shape as it spreads across the membrane

If progressively larger depolarizing current pulses are applied, a condition is reached at which a different sort of response, the action potential, occurs **(Figure 3–3).** AN ACTION POTENTIAL IS TRIGGERED WHEN THE DEPOLARIZATION IS SUFFICIENT FOR THE MEMBRANE POTENTIAL TO REACH A THRESHOLD VALUE. The action potential differs from the local response in two important ways:

- It is a much larger response, with the polarity of the membrane potential reversing (i.e., the cell interior becoming positive with respect to the exterior).
- The action potential is ***propagated without decrement*** down the entire length of the nerve or muscle cell.

THE SIZE AND SHAPE OF AN ACTION POTENTIAL REMAIN THE SAME AS THE POTENTIAL TRAVELS ALONG THE CELL.

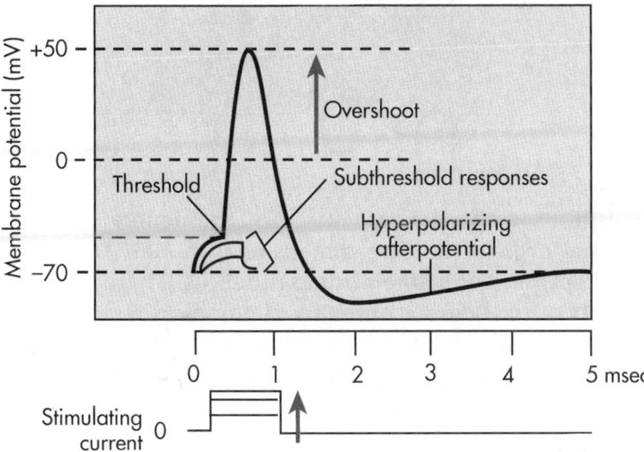

FIGURE 3–3. Responses of the membrane potential of a squid giant axon to increasing pulses of depolarizing current. When the cell is depolarized to threshold, it fires an action potential.

Unlike the local response, the action potential does not decrease in size with distance. When a stimulus larger than the threshold stimulus is applied, the size and shape of the action potential do not change. Either a stimulus fails to elicit an action potential (a subthreshold stimulus) or it produces a full-sized action potential. For this reason, the action potential is called an **all-or-none response.**

Action Potentials Involve the Flow of Ions Across the Plasma Membrane

Action potentials in neurons have a characteristic form

The form of an action potential of a squid giant axon is shown in Figure 3–3. Action potentials in many mammalian neurons have a similar shape. Once the membrane is depolarized to the threshold, an explosive depolarization occurs and completely depolarizes the membrane and even overshoots so that the membrane becomes polarized in the reverse direction. The peak of the action potential reaches about +50 mV. The membrane potential then returns toward the resting membrane potential almost as rapidly as it was depolarized. After repolarization, a transient hyperpolarization occurs that is known as the **hyperpolarizing afterpotential.** It persists for about 4 msec.

The neuronal action potential is caused by changes in the conductance of the membrane to Na^+ and K^+

In Chapter 2, the resting membrane potential was seen to be a weighted average of the equilibrium potentials for ions such as Na^+, K^+, and Cl^-. The weighting factor for each ion is the fraction that its conductance contributes to the total ionic conductance of the membrane (the chord conductance equation, Equation 2-8). In squid giant axon, the resting membrane potential (E_m) is about –70 mV. E_K is about –100 mV in squid axon; hence, an increase in the conductance to K^+ (g_K) would hyperpolarize the membrane, and a decrease in g_K would tend to depolarize the membrane. E_{Cl} is about –70 mV, so an increase in the conductance to Cl^- (g_{Cl}) would stabilize E_m at –70 mV. An increase in the conductance to Na^+ (g_{Na}) of sufficient magnitude would cause depolarization and reversal of the membrane polarity because E_{Na} is about +65 mV in squid giant axon.

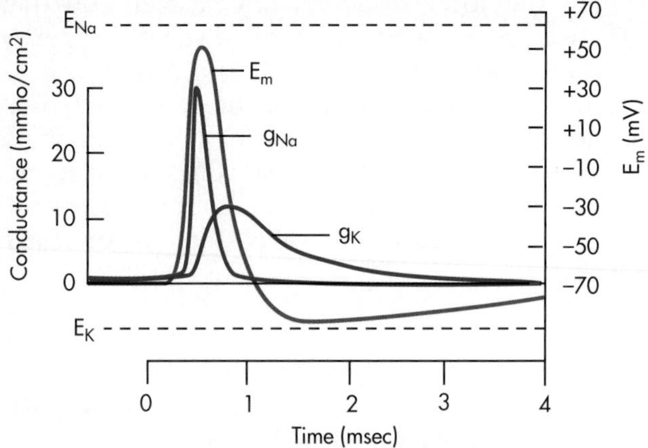

FIGURE 3–4. The action potential E_m of a squid giant axon is shown on the same time scale as the associated changes in g_{Na} and g_K. (Redrawn from Hodgkin AL, Huxley AF: *J Physiol* 117:500, 1952.)

In the 1950s, Hodgkin and Huxley showed that the action potential of squid giant axon is caused by successive increases in conductance to Na^+ and K^+. They found that g_{Na} increases rapidly during the early part of the action potential **(Figure 3–4).** g_{Na} reaches a peak about the same time as the peak of the action potential; then it decreases rapidly. g_K increases more slowly, reaches a peak at about the middle of the repolarization phase, and then returns more slowly to resting levels.

As described in Chapter 2, the chord conductance equation shows that the membrane potential is a result of the opposing tendencies of the K^+ gradient to bring E_m toward the equilibrium potential for K^+ and the Na^+ gradient to bring E_m toward the equilibrium potential for Na^+. Increasing the conductance of either ion increases its ability to pull E_m toward its equilibrium potential. The rapid increase in g_{Na} during the early part of the action potential causes the membrane potential to move toward the equilibrium potential for Na^+ (+65 mV). The peak of the action potential reaches only about +50 mV because g_{Na} quickly decreases toward resting levels and because g_K increases to oppose the depolarization. The rapid return of the membrane potential toward the resting potential is caused by the rapid decrease in g_{Na} and the continued increase in g_K. These conductance changes decrease the size of the Na^+ term in the chord conductance equation and increase the size of the K^+ term. During the hyperpolarizing afterpotential, when the membrane potential is actually more negative (more polarized) than the resting potential, g_{Na} returns to baseline levels, but g_K remains elevated above resting levels. E_m is pulled closer to the K^+ equilibrium potential (−100 mV) as long as g_K remains elevated.

Na^+ and K^+ channels open and close in response to changes in the membrane potential

Hodgkin and Huxley proposed that the ion currents pass through separate Na^+ and K^+ channels, each with distinct characteristics, in the plasma membrane. Subsequent research has supported this interpretation and has determined some of the properties of proteins that form the ion channels. The amino acid sequences of several K^+ and Na^+ channels have been determined, and knowledge of the structure of ion channels is rapidly expanding **(Figure 3–5).** Although the three-dimensional structure of the Na^+ channel remains to be determined, its intramembrane domain is known to consist of a number of α helices that span the membrane and surround the ion channel. The Na^+ channel has

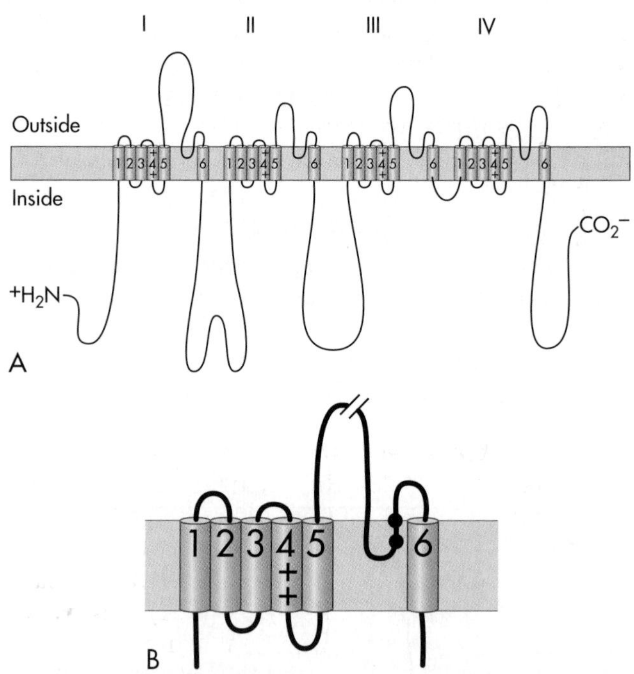

FIGURE 3–5. Model of the voltage-dependent Na^+ channel protein. A, Two-dimensional model. The cylinders represent transmembrane α helices. There are four repeats of six-cylinder domains of homologous α helices. The intracellular loop connecting domains III and IV functions as the inactivation gate; after depolarization, with a slight delay, this loop apparently swings up into the mouth of the channel to block ion conduction. B, Domain IV. The part of the extracellular loop that connects helices 5 and 6 and that dips into the membrane helps form the selectivity filter of the channel. The residues indicated by solid circles are key determinants of the ionic selectivity of the channel. (B redrawn from Catterall W: *J Bioenerg Biomembr* 28:219, 1996.)

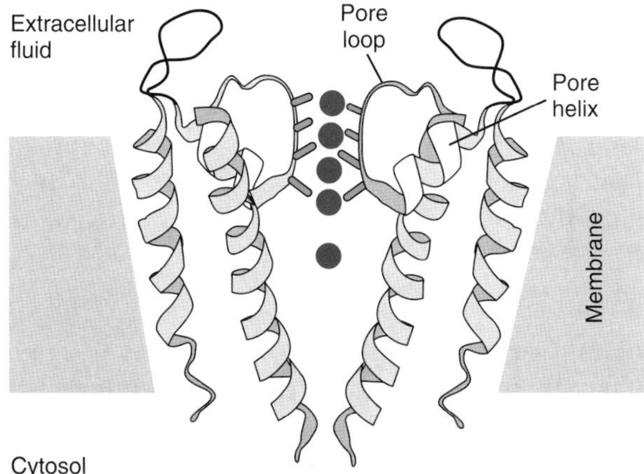

FIGURE 3–6. A representation of the structure of a K^+ channel from *Streptomyces lividans*, a fungus-like bacterium. The channel consists of four subunits; only two of the subunits are shown. Each subunit of the channel has two transmembrane α helices. The selectivity filter is formed by the pore loops of each of the four subunits. The carbonyl oxygens (greenish protrusions) coordinate with K^+ ions (red balls) and thereby cause K^+ to shed most of its waters of hydration, allowing it to pass through the pore. Shown are four positions within the selectivity filter where K^+ may be coordinated. The bottom red ball represents a K^+ ion in the central cavity of the ion channel. The amino acid sequence in the pore domain of this protein is nearly identical with the sequences of the homologous region of all known vertebrate voltage-gated K^+ channels. (From Morais-Cabral JH, Zhou Y, MacKinnon R: *Nature* 414:23, 2001.)

both an **activation gate** and an **inactivation gate** that account for the changes in g_{Na} during an action potential. Groups of charged amino acid residues that form these gates have been tentatively identified. To enter the channel's narrowest part, known as the **selectivity filter,** K^+ and Na^+, it is believed, must shed most of their waters of hydration. To strip K^+ and Na^+ of their associated water molecules, negative amino acid residues that line the pore of the channel must have a particular geometric shape; the precise geometry differs for K^+ and for Na^+ **(Figure 3–6).** This requirement is believed to confer the specificity of ion channels.

Tetrodotoxin (TTX), one of the most potent poisons known, is a specific blocker of the Na^+ channel. It binds to the extracellular side of this channel. **Tetraethylammonium** (TEA^+) blocks the K^+ channel. TEA^+ enters the K^+ channel from the cytoplasmic side and blocks the channel because it cannot pass through the channel.

The ovaries of certain species of puffer fish, also known as **blowfish,** contain TTX. Raw puffer fish is a highly prized dish in Japan. Connoisseurs of puffer fish enjoy the tingling numbness of the lips that is caused by minuscule quantities of TTX present in the flesh. Sushi chefs who are trained to remove the ovaries safely are licensed by the government to prepare this dish. Nevertheless, several people die each year from eating improperly prepared puffer fish. **Saxitoxin** is another blocker of Na^+ channels. Saxitoxin is produced by reddish dinoflagellates that are responsible for the so-called red tide. Shellfish eat the dinoflagellates, and saxitoxin becomes concentrated in their tissues. A person who eats these shellfish may experience life-threatening paralysis about 30 minutes after the meal.

An ion channel has an open state and a closed state

It is possible to study the behavior of individual ion channels. One way to do this is to incorporate either purified ion channel proteins or bits of membrane into planar lipid bilayers that separate two aqueous compartments. Electrodes placed in the aqueous compartments can then be used to monitor or impose currents and voltages across the membrane. Under some conditions, only one or a few ion channels of a particular type may be present in the planar membrane. The ion channels spontaneously oscillate between an open state, in which ions move through the channel, and a closed state.

Another way to study individual ion channels is by using a so-called **patch electrode.** A fire-polished microelectrode is placed against the surface of a cell, and suction is applied to the electrode to form a high-resistance seal around the tip of the electrode **(Figure 3–7, *A*).** The sealed patch electrode can then be used to monitor the activity of whatever channels happen to be trapped inside the seal. Sometimes, the patch trapped inside the electrode contains more than one functional ion channel (Figure 3–7, *B*).

During an action potential, there is a rapid influx of Na^+. The time course of this inward Na^+ current resembles that of the change in the Na^+ conductance shown in Figure 3–4. In contrast, the behavior of each Na^+ channel is random, like the behavior of the channels shown in Figure 3–7, *B*. The probability of each Na^+ channel's being in the open state is increased when the membrane is depolarized to threshold, and then the probability of being open decreases (channel inactivation). The macroscopic Na^+ current is the average current through thousands of Na^+ channels. The "average channel" opens (activates) promptly in response to depolarization; then after a short delay, the channel closes (inactivates) even though the applied depolarization is maintained.

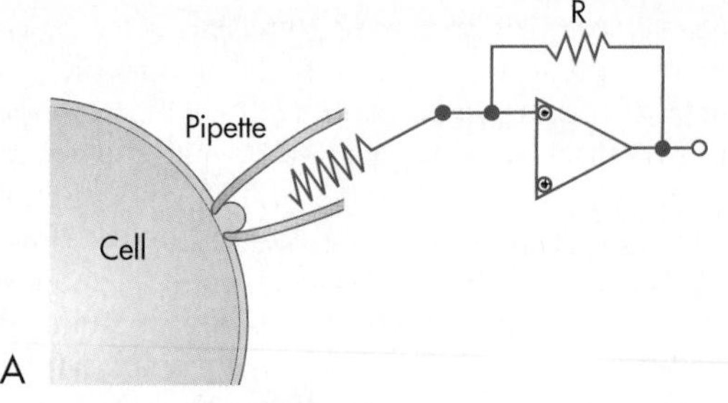

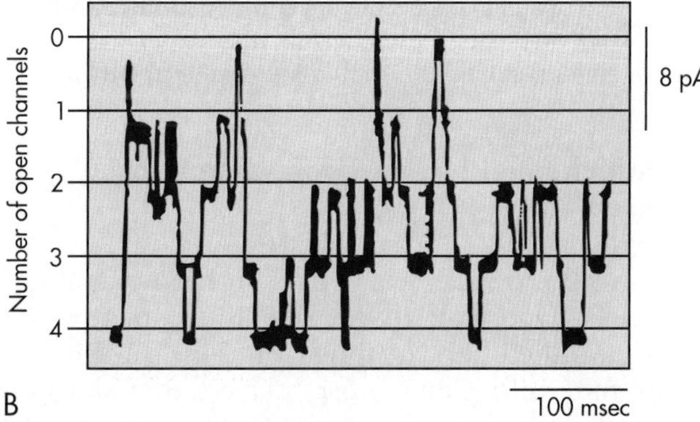

FIGURE 3–7. A, Patch electrode and circuitry required to record the ionic currents that flow through the small number of ion channels isolated in the electrode patch. B, Current recording from a patch electrode on the plasma membrane of a skeletal muscle cell. The five current levels show that this particular patch contains four different ion channels, each opening and closing independently of the others. (A redrawn from Sigworth FJ, Neher E: *Nature* 287:447, 1980; B redrawn from Hammill OP et al: *Pflugers Arch* 391:85, 1981.)

Action potentials in cardiac muscle cells have a shape different from that of nerve and muscle action potentials because different voltage-gated ion channels are present in cardiac cells

An action potential in a cardiac ventricular cell is shown in Figure 3–1. The initial rapid depolarization and overshoot are caused by the rapid entry of Na^+ through channels that are similar to the Na^+ channels of nerve and skeletal muscle. After the initial depolarization and overshoot, the cardiac ventricular action potential has a plateau phase. The plateau is caused by slow channels that are distinct from fast Na^+ channels. Slow channels open and close more slowly than fast Na^+ channels do. The slow channels belong to a particular class of Ca^{++} channels called **L-type Ca^{++} channels** (for long lasting). The Ca^{++} that enters the cell via the L-type Ca^{++} channels during the plateau phase helps initiate contraction of the ventricular cell and stimulates release of more Ca^{++} from the sarcoplasmic reticulum of the heart cell. The repolarization of the ventricular cell is brought about by the closing of the L-type Ca^{++} channels and by a much delayed opening of the K^+ channels. The ionic mechanisms of cardiac action potentials are discussed in more detail in Chapter 17.

Under Certain Circumstances, It Is More Difficult to Elicit an Action Potential

The voltage inactivation of Na^+ channels is responsible for refractory periods and accommodation

If a neuron or skeletal muscle cell is partially depolarized (e.g., by increasing the concentration of K^+ in the extracellular fluid), its action potential has a slower rate of rise and a smaller overshoot than the action potential of the normally polarized cell. This is a result of a smaller electrical force driving Na^+ into the depolarized cell and voltage inactivation of some of the Na^+ channels. The increase in g_{Na} in response to a depolarization is self-inactivating; that is, the inactivation gates close soon after the activation gates open. Once the Na^+ channels are inactivated, the membrane must be repolarized toward the normal resting membrane potential before the channels can be reopened. As the membrane potential is restored toward normal resting levels, more and more of the Na^+ channels again become capable of being activated.

The explosive depolarizing phase of the action potential may be compared to a chemical explosion. A chemical explosion requires a critical mass of material; the spike of the action potential can be generated only if a critical number of Na^+ channels are recruited. WHEN A CELL IS PARTLY DEPOLARIZED, THE POOL OF ACTIVABLE Na^+ CHANNELS IS REDUCED; consequently, a stimulus may not be able to recruit a sufficient number of Na^+ channels to generate an action potential. Voltage inactivation of Na^+ channels partially accounts for important properties of excitable cells, such as refractory periods and accommodation.

During the first part of an action potential, it is impossible to elicit another action potential

During much of the action potential, the membrane is completely refractory to further stimulation. This means that no matter how strongly the cell is stimulated, it is unable to fire a second action

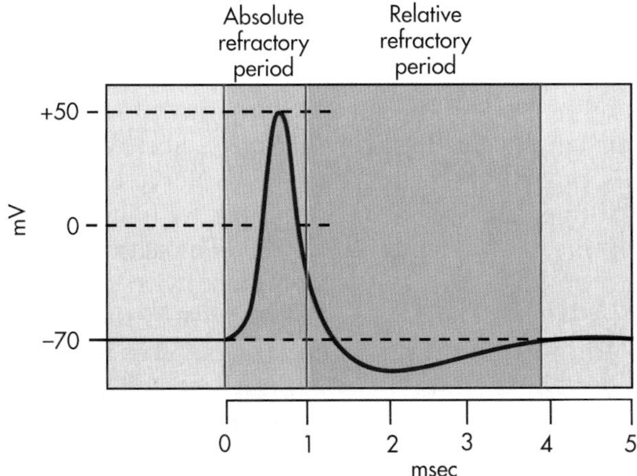

FIGURE 3–8. Action potential of a nerve, illustrating the associated absolute and relative refractory periods.

potential. This unresponsive state is called the **absolute refractory period** (Figure 3–8). The cell is refractory because a large number of its Na^+ channels are voltage inactivated and cannot be reopened until the membrane is repolarized.

During the latter part of the action potential, the cell is able to fire a second action potential, but a stronger-than-normal stimulus is required. This is the **relative refractory period.** Early in the relative refractory period, before the membrane potential has returned to the resting potential level, some Na^+ channels are voltage inactivated; hence, a stronger-than-normal stimulus is required to open the critical number of Na^+ channels needed to trigger an action potential. Throughout the relative refractory period, the conductance to K^+ is elevated, which opposes depolarization of the membrane. This also contributes to the refractoriness.

A cell that is depolarized too slowly may fail to fire an action potential

When a nerve or muscle cell is depolarized slowly, the normal threshold may be passed without an action potential being fired; this is called **accommodation.** Na^+ and K^+ channels are both involved in accommodation. During slow depolarization, some of the Na^+ channels that are opened by depolarization have enough time to become voltage inactivated before the threshold potential is attained. If depolarization is slow enough, the critical number of open Na^+ channels required to trigger the action potential may never be attained. In addition, K^+ channels open in response to the depolarization. The increased g_K tends to repolarize the membrane, making it still more refractory to depolarization.

In an inherited disorder called **primary hyperkalemic periodic paralysis,** patients suffer episodes of painful spontaneous contractures of muscles followed by periods of paralysis of the affected muscles. These symptoms are accompanied by elevated levels of K^+ in the plasma and extracellular fluid. The elevation of extracellular K^+ contributes to depolarization of skeletal muscle cells. Initially, the depolarization brings muscle cells closer to threshold, so spontaneous action potentials and contractions are more likely. As depolarization of the cells becomes more marked, the cells accommodate because of voltage-inactivated Na^+ channels. Thus, they become unable to fire action potentials and are unable to contract in response to action potentials in their motor axons.

Conduction of Action Potentials Involves Ionic Currents

Local circuit currents are responsible for the conduction of action potentials and subthreshold responses

Action potentials and subthreshold responses are conducted along a nerve or muscle cell by local current flows **(Figure 3–9).** This mechanism of

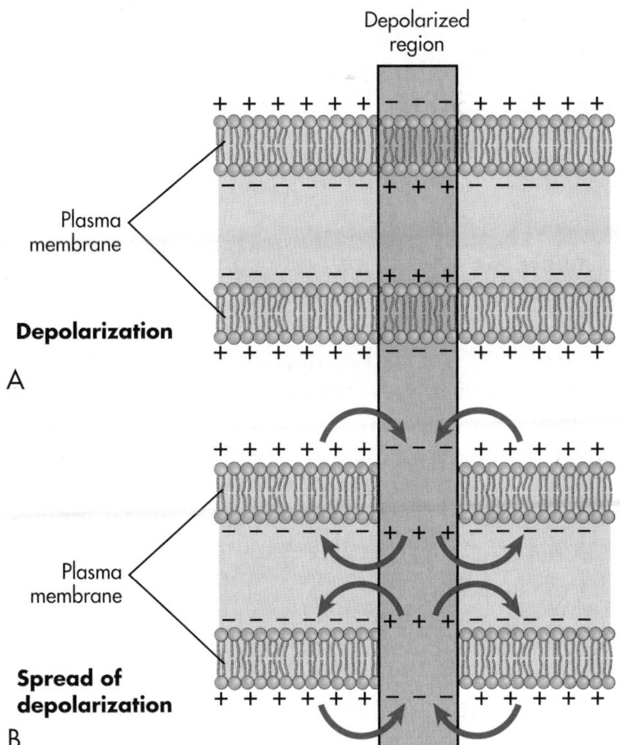

FIGURE 3–9. Mechanism of electrotonic spread of depolarization. A, Reversal of membrane polarity that occurs with local depolarization. B, Local currents that flow to depolarize adjacent areas of the membrane and allow conduction of the depolarization.

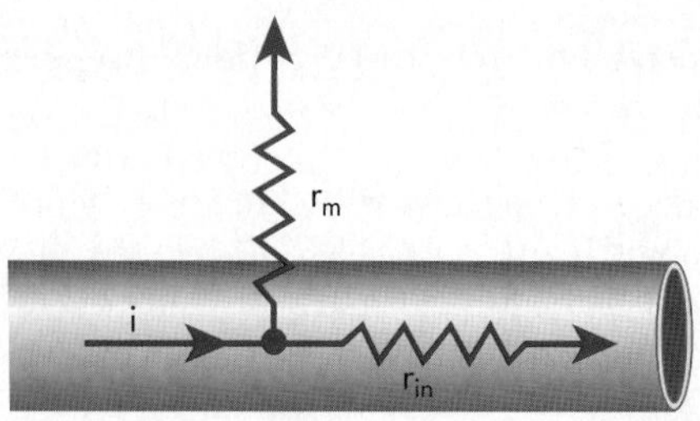

FIGURE 3–10. An axon or a muscle cell resembles an electrical cable. Currents (i) that flow across the membrane resistance (r_m) are lost from the cable. Currents that flow through the longitudinal resistance (r_{in}) carry the electrical signal along the cable. The larger the ratio r_m/r_{in}, the more efficient the signal transmission along the cell.

conduction is known as **electrotonic conduction.** Figure 3–9, *A,* shows the membrane of an axon or muscle cell that has been depolarized in a small region. In this region, the external surface of the membrane is negative relative to the adjacent membrane, and the internal face of the depolarized membrane is positively charged relative to neighboring internal areas. The potential differences cause **local circuit currents** to flow (Figure 3–9, *B*), which depolarize the membrane adjacent to the initial site of depolarization. These newly depolarized areas then cause current flows that depolarize other segments of the membrane still farther removed from the initial site of depolarization. The same factors that govern the velocity of electrotonic conduction also determine the speed of action potential propagation.

A nerve or muscle cell has some of the properties of an electrical cable

In a perfect cable, the insulation surrounding the core conductor prevents all loss of current to the surrounding medium, so a signal is transmitted along the cable with undiminished strength (**Figure 3–10**). The plasma membrane of an unmyelinated nerve or muscle cell serves as the insulation, the cytoplasm being the core conductor. The membrane has a high resistance (r_m), but (partly because of its thinness) the plasma membrane is not a perfect insulator. The resistance to current flow in the cytoplasm along the long axis of the cell is r_{in}. The higher the ratio of r_m to r_{in}, the less current lost across the plasma membrane, the better the cell can function as a cable, and the longer the distance that a signal can be transmitted electrotonically without significant decrement. r_m/r_{in} determines the **length constant** of a cell; the length constant is equal to $(r_m/r_{in})^{1/2}$.

An action potential does not diminish in size because it is self-reinforcing

Many nerve and muscle cells are much longer than their length constants (1 to 2 mm). Skeletal muscle cells can be as long as 1 to 2 cm. Nerve axons can be longer than 1 m. Conduction with decrement will not work for such long cells. The action potential conducts an electrical impulse with undiminished strength along the full length of these cells. To do this, the action potential reinforces itself as it is conducted along the cell. Thus, the action potential may be said to be **propagated** as well as conducted. The conduction of the action potential occurs via local circuit currents by the electrotonic mechanism depicted in Figure 3–9. When the areas on either side of the depolarized region reach threshold, these areas also fire action potentials, which locally reverses the polarity of the membrane potential. By local current flow, the areas of the cell adjacent to these areas are next brought to threshold, and these areas in turn fire action potentials. A cycle of depolarization occurs by local current flow followed by generation of an action potential in a restricted region that then is conducted along the length of the cell, with "new" action potentials being generated as they spread. In this way, the action potentials are regenerated as they spread, and the action potential propagates over long distances, keeping the same size and shape.

BECAUSE THE SHAPE AND SIZE OF THE ACTION POTENTIAL ARE USUALLY INVARIANT, ONLY VARIATIONS IN THE FREQUENCY OF THE ACTION POTENTIALS CAN BE USED IN THE CODE FOR INFORMATION TRANSMISSION ALONG AXONS. The maximum frequency is limited by the duration of the absolute refractory period (≈1 msec) to about 1000 impulses/sec in large mammalian nerves.

The conduction velocity is determined by the resistance and capacitance of the cell

The speed of electrotonic conduction of an action potential or a local response along a nerve or muscle cell is determined by the electrical properties of the cytoplasm and of the plasma membrane that surrounds the cell. The following discussion focuses on the mechanism of electrotonic conduction, but it applies equally well to the mechanism of propagation of the action potential.

CELLS THAT ARE LARGER IN DIAMETER HAVE A GREATER CONDUCTION VELOCITY. This is caused principally by the decrease in resistance to conduction in the cytoplasm along the length of the cell as the radius (and hence the cross-sectional area) of the cell increases.

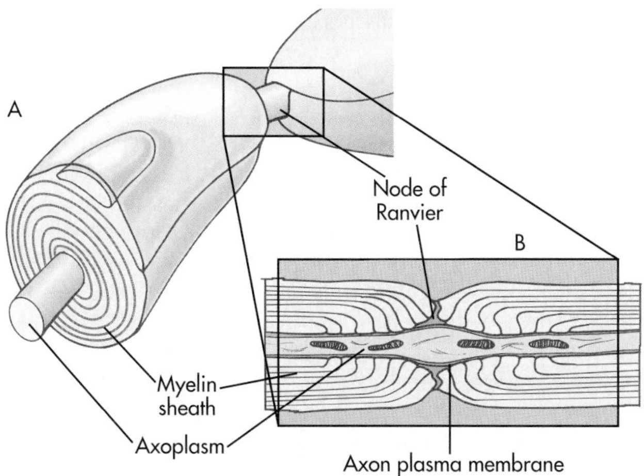

FIGURE 3–11. Myelin sheath. A, Drawing of Schwann cells wrapping around an axon to form a myelin sheath. B, Drawing of a cross section through a myelinated axon near a node of Ranvier.

Myelination results in a dramatic increase in conduction velocity

In vertebrates, certain nerve cells are coated with **myelin;** such cells are said to be **myelinated.** Myelin is formed from multiple wrappings of the plasma membranes of **Schwann cells** that wind themselves around the nerve axon **(Figure 3–11).** The myelin sheath consists of several to more than 100 layers of plasma membrane. Gaps that occur in the sheath every 1 to 2 mm are known as **nodes of Ranvier.** These nodes are about 1 μm wide and are the lateral spaces between adjacent Schwann cells along the axon. MYELIN ALTERS THE ELECTRICAL PROPERTIES OF THE NERVE FIBER AND RESULTS IN A GREAT INCREASE IN THE CONDUCTION VELOCITY OF THE FIBER.

A squid giant axon with a 500-μm diameter has a conduction velocity of 25 m/sec and is unmyelinated. If conduction velocity were directly proportional to fiber radius, a human nerve fiber with a 10-μm diameter would conduct at 0.5 m/sec. With this conduction velocity, a reflex withdrawal of the foot from a hot coal would take about 4 seconds. Even though human nerve fibers are much smaller in diameter than squid giant axons, human reflexes are much faster than this. The myelin sheath that surrounds certain vertebrate nerve fibers results in a much greater conduction velocity than that of unmyelinated fibers of similar diameters. A 10-μm myelinated fiber has a conduction velocity of about 50 m/sec, which is twice that of the 500-μm squid giant axon. The high conduction velocity permits reflexes that are fast enough to allow humans to avoid dangerous stimuli. A myelinated axon has a greater conduction velocity than an unmyelinated fiber that is 100 times larger in diameter **(Figure 3–12).** The myelin sheath increases the velocity of action potential conduction by increasing the length constant of the axon, decreasing the capacitance of the axon, and restricting the generation of action potentials to the nodes of Ranvier.

Myelination greatly alters the electrical properties of the axon. The many wrappings of membrane around the axon increase the effective membrane resistance so that r_m/r_{in} (Figure 3–10) and thus the length constant is much greater. Less of the conducted signal is lost through the electrical insulation of the myelin sheath; hence, the amplitude of a conducted signal declines less with distance along the axon. The myelin-wrapped membrane has a much smaller electrical capacitance than the naked axonal membrane. Therefore, the local currents can more rapidly depolarize the membrane as a signal is conducted. For this reason, the conduction velocity is greatly increased by myelination. BECAUSE OF THE INCREASE IN LENGTH CONSTANT AND CONDUCTION VELOCITY, AN ACTION POTENTIAL IS CONDUCTED WITH LITTLE DECREMENT AND AT GREAT SPEED FROM ONE NODE OF RANVIER TO THE NEXT.

The resistance to the flow of ions across the many layers of Schwann cell membrane that make up the myelin sheath is so high that the ionic currents are effectively localized to the short stretches of plasma membrane that occur at the nodes of Ranvier. The ion channels that participate in the action potential are also especially concentrated at the nodes of

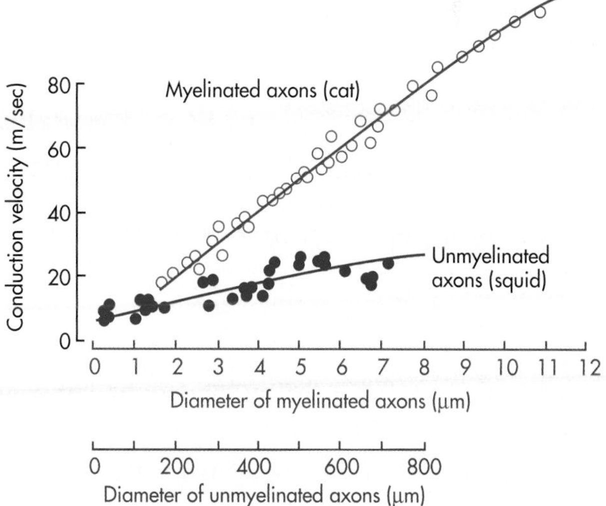

FIGURE 3–12. Conduction velocities of myelinated and unmyelinated axons as functions of axon diameter. Myelinated axons are from cat saphenous nerve at 38°C. Unmyelinated axons are from squid at 20°C to 22°C. Note that myelinated axons have greater conduction velocities than unmyelinated axons 100 times larger in diameter. (Data for myelinated axons from Gasser HS, Grundfest H: *Am J Physiol* 127:393, 1939. Data for unmyelinated axons from Pumphrey RJ, Young JZ: *J Exp Biol* 15:453, 1938.)

Ranvier. For these reasons, the action potential is regenerated only at the nodes of Ranvier (1 to 2 mm apart) rather than at each place along the fiber, as is the case in an unmyelinated fiber. The action potential is rapidly conducted from one node to the next (in about 20 μsec) and "pauses" to be regenerated at each node. The action potential appears to "jump" from one node of Ranvier to the next, a process called **saltatory conduction.**

Myelinated axons are also more efficient metabolically than unmyelinated axons are. The Na^+, K^+-ATPase extrudes the Na^+ that enters and reaccumulates the K^+ that leaves the cell during action potentials. In myelinated axons, ionic currents are restricted to the small fraction of the membrane surface at the nodes of Ranvier. For this reason, far fewer Na^+ and K^+ ions traverse a unit area of fiber membrane, and much less ion pumping is required to maintain Na^+ and K^+ gradients.

In some diseases known as **demyelinating disorders,** the myelin sheath deteriorates. In **multiple sclerosis,** scattered progressive demyelination of axons in the central nervous system results in loss of motor control. The neuropathy common in severe cases of **diabetes mellitus** is due to demyelination of peripheral axons. When myelin is lost, the length constant, which is dramatically increased by myelination, becomes much shorter. Hence, when the action potential is electrotonically conducted from one node of Ranvier to the next, it loses amplitude. If demyelination is sufficiently severe, the action potential may arrive at the next node of Ranvier with insufficient strength to fire an action potential. The axon then fails to propagate action potentials.

Summary

- ❖ Different cell types have differently shaped action potentials because their populations of voltage-dependent ion channels differ.
- ❖ The action potential in a squid giant axon and in many mammalian nerve and skeletal muscle cells is generated by the rapid activation and subsequent voltage inactivation of voltage-dependent Na^+ channels and the delayed opening and closing of voltage-dependent K^+ channels.
- ❖ Ion channels are integral membrane proteins that have ion-selective pores.
- ❖ An ion channel typically has two states, high conductance (open) and low conductance (closed). The channel oscillates randomly between the open and closed states. For a voltage-dependent channel, the fraction of time the channel spends in the open state is a function of the transmembrane potential difference.
- ❖ Cardiac muscle cells have L-type Ca^{++} channels that open and close slowly and are responsible for the long duration of the action potential in these cell types.
- ❖ The voltage inactivation of Na^+ channels is an important factor in the absolute and relative refractory periods and in the accommodation of an excitable cell to a slowly rising stimulus.
- ❖ Local circuit currents produce electrotonic conduction. This is the mechanism by which both subthreshold signals and action potentials are conducted along the length of a cell.
- ❖ A subthreshold signal is conducted with decrement. It dies away to 37% of its maximal strength over a distance of 1 length constant. The length constant is equal to $(r_m/r_{in})^{1/2}$. A typical value for the length constant is 1 to 2 mm.
- ❖ The action potential is propagated, rather than merely conducted; it is regenerated as it moves along the cell. In this way, an action potential remains the same size and shape as it is conducted.
- ❖ The velocity of conduction is determined by the electrical properties of the cell. A large-diameter cell has a faster conduction velocity.
- ❖ Myelination dramatically increases the conduction velocity of a nerve axon. Because of myelination, an action potential is conducted rapidly and with little decrement from one node of Ranvier to the next.
- ❖ Action potentials are regenerated only at the nodes of Ranvier; the internodal membrane cannot fire an action potential. The action potential "jumps" from node to node; this is saltatory conduction.

Bibliography

Bezanilla F, Perozo E: The voltage sensor and the gate in ion channels, *Adv Protein Chem* 63:211, 2003.

Catterall WA, Goldin AL, Waxman SG: International Union of Pharmacology. XXXIX. Compendium of voltage-gated ion channels: sodium channels, *Pharmacol Rev* 55:575, 2003.

Hille B: *Ionic channels of excitable membranes,* ed 3, Sunderland, Mass, 2001, Sinauer Associates.

Hodgkin AL: *The conduction of the nervous impulse,* Springfield, Ill, 1964, Charles C Thomas.

Katz B: *Nerve, muscle, and synapse,* New York, 1966, McGraw-Hill.

Keynes RD, Aidley DJ: *Nerve and muscle,* ed 3, Cambridge, 2001, Cambridge University Press.

Levitan IB, Kaczmarek LK: *The neuron: cell and molecular biology,* ed 3, New York, 2001, Oxford University Press.

MacKinnon R: Potassium channels, *FEBS Lett* 555:62, 2003.

Perozo E: New structural perspectives on K^+ channel gating, *Structure* 10:1027, 2002.

Yellen G: The voltage-gated potassium channels and their relatives, *Nature* 419:35, 2002.

Yu FH, Catterall WA: Overview of the voltage-gated sodium channel family, *Genome Biol* 4:207, 2003.

Self-Assessment

1. **Which of the following statements about the action potential in squid giant axon is correct?**
   A. The rising phase of the action potential is due to a rapid increase in the conductance to K^+.
   B. The peak of the action potential just reaches the equilibrium potential for Na^+.
   C. The repolarizing phase is due to closing of K^+ channels.
   D. The hyperpolarizing afterpotential is due to the prolonged increased conductance to K^+.

2. **Which of the following statements about ion channels is correct?**
   A. Voltage-gated Na^+ channels show both activation and inactivation in response to depolarization of the membrane.
   B. K^+ channels in neurons open more rapidly than do Na^+ channels after a depolarization.
   C. The plateau phase of the cardiac action potential is due predominantly to Na^+ channels that open and close rapidly.
   D. Most Na^+ channels open and close in unison.

3. **Which of the following statements is correct?**
   A. The absolute refractory period is due primarily to voltage activation of K^+ channels.
   B. If a neuron is depolarized very slowly, it may reach threshold without firing an action potential.
   C. Early in the relative refractory period, the cell cannot fire an action potential regardless of how strong the stimulus is.
   D. During the early part of the relative refractory period, elevated conductance to K^+ is the only cause of refractoriness.

4. **Which of the following statements about conduction mechanisms is true?**
   A. A subthreshold depolarization will sometimes cause an action potential.
   B. An action potential will be conducted by electrotonic conduction.
   C. The length constant is the length over which an electrotonically conducted signal loses 90% of its strength.
   D. Decreasing the membrane resistance will increase the length constant.

5. **Which of the following statements is true?**
   A. Myelination causes decreased membrane resistance.
   B. Saltatory conduction results in increased use of cell energy.
   C. Action potentials in myelinated axons are regenerated only at the nodes of Ranvier.
   D. The length constant of a myelinated fiber is less than that of an unmyelinated fiber of the same diameter.

Chapter 4: Synaptic Transmission

Objectives

- ❖ Explain how gap junctions mediate electrical conduction between cells.
- ❖ Describe the sequence of events at a generalized chemical synapse.
- ❖ Contrast the synthesis, secretion, and recycling of small-molecule neurotransmitters with neuropeptides.
- ❖ Discuss the sequence of events at a neuromuscular junction.
- ❖ Explain how miniature end plate potentials reveal information about the quantal nature of transmitter release.
- ❖ Explain how integration can occur at a postsynaptic neuron.
- ❖ Contrast facilitation, posttetanic potentiation, synaptic fatigue, and long-term potentiation.
- ❖ Explain the criteria for establishing that a particular substance is a neurotransmitter at a particular synapse.

This chapter as well as Chapter 5 deals with communication among cells. This chapter discusses communication among electrically excitable cells. Chapter 5 presents, in a more general context, the mechanisms whereby a regulatory molecule released by one cell can influence the activities of a target cell. A **synapse** is a site at which an electrical response is transmitted from one cell to another. At an **electrical synapse,** two excitable cells communicate directly by the passage of current between them via **gap junctions.** At a **chemical synapse,** an action potential in the presynaptic cell causes an electrical response in the postsynaptic cell via the action of a **neurotransmitter** substance released by the presynaptic cell.

At Electrical Synapses, Gap Junctions Permit Ions to Flow from One Cell to Another

AT AN ELECTRICAL SYNAPSE, A CHANGE IN THE MEMBRANE POTENTIAL OF ONE CELL IS TRANSMITTED TO ANOTHER CELL BY THE DIRECT FLOW OF CURRENT. Because current flows directly between two cells that make an electrical synapse, there is essentially no synaptic delay. Electrical synapses usually allow conduction in both directions. In this respect, electrical synapses differ from chemical synapses, which are unidirectional (see later discussion). Certain electrical synapses conduct more readily in one direction than in another; this property is called **rectification.**

Cells that form electrical synapses are joined by **gap junctions.** Gap junctions are plaque-like structures in which the plasma membranes of the coupled cells are very close (<3 nm). Freeze-fracture electron micrographs of gap junctions show regular arrays of intramembrane protein particles. The intramembrane particles consist of six subunits surrounding a central channel that is accessible to water, ions, and molecules as large as 1500 MW **(Figure 4–1, *A*)**. The hexagonal array is called a **connexon.** Each of the six subunits is a single protein (one polypeptide chain) called **connexin** (≈25,000 MW). At the gap junction, the connexons of the coupled cells are aligned to form **connexon channels,** which allow the passage of ions and water-soluble molecules from one cell to another.

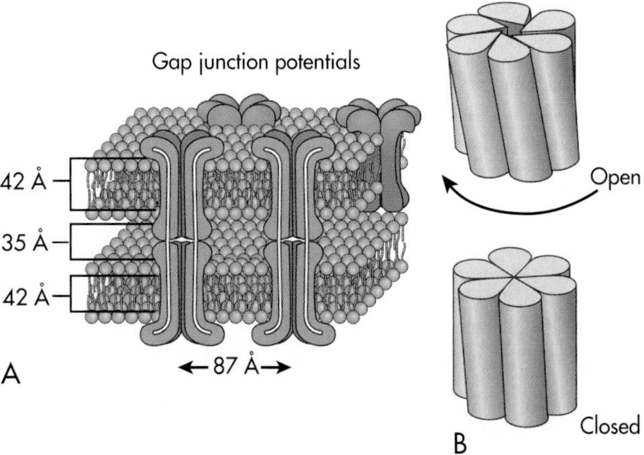

FIGURE 4–1. **A**, Structure of gap junction channels. **B**, Opening and closing of a gap junction channel. (**A** redrawn from Makowski L et al: *J Cell Biol* 74:629, 1977; **B** redrawn from Unwin PNT, Zampighi G: *Nature* 283:45, 1980.)

Connexon channels are not open continuously; they open and close (Figure 4–1, *B*) randomly, as do the voltage-gated ion channels discussed in Chapter 3. The probability of connexon channels being open may be changed by elevated intracellular Ca^{++} or H^+ in one of the cells or in response to depolarization of one or both of the cells.

Electrical synapses are widespread in the peripheral nervous system and the central nervous system (CNS) of invertebrates and vertebrates. Some neurons in the brain receive input by both electrical and chemical synapses. Electrical synapses are particularly useful in reflex pathways in which rapid transmission between cells (little synaptic delay) is necessary or when the synchronous response of a number of cells is required. AMONG THE MANY NON-NEURONAL CELLS COUPLED BY GAP JUNCTIONS ARE HEPATOCYTES, MYOCARDIAL CELLS, INTESTINAL SMOOTH MUSCLE CELLS, AND EPITHELIAL CELLS OF THE LENS.

At a Chemical Synapse, a Neurotransmitter Substance Released by the Presynaptic Cell Evokes an Electrical Response in the Postsynaptic Cell

There are several types of chemical synapses. Most share the following properties.

- The nerve ending of the presynaptic cell contains vesicles with neurotransmitter or neuromodulator substances **(Figure 4–2)**. Vesicles that contain "classic" small-molecule neurotransmitters, such as acetylcholine or norepinephrine, are small (≈50 nm in diameter), and many of the vesicles are docked near specialized release sites called **active zones** on the intracellular aspect of the presynaptic membrane. Vesicles that contain **neuropeptides** are larger and are distributed throughout the nerve terminal. Many nerve terminals contain both small

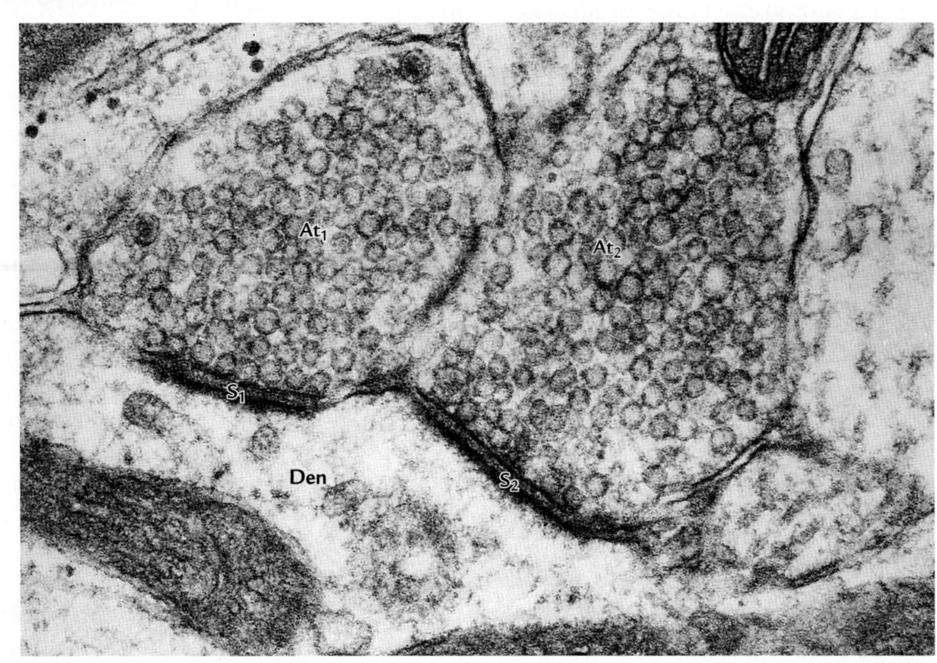

FIGURE 4–2. Synapses (S_1 and S_2) in the cerebral cortex. Two axon terminals (At_1 and At_2) synapse with a dendrite (Den) of a stellate cell. The axon terminals are packed with synaptic vesicles. (From Peters A, Palay SL, Webster H deF: *The fine structure of the nervous system,* Philadelphia, 1976, WB Saunders.)

vesicles with small-molecule transmitters and larger vesicles with neuropeptides.

- An action potential in the presynaptic neuron opens voltage-gated Ca^{++} channels that are concentrated near the active zones in the nerve terminal. The influx of Ca^{++} into the nerve terminal raises the intracellular [Ca^{++}]; this is the trigger for the release of neurotransmitter via exocytosis into the **synaptic cleft,** the narrow (20 to 40 nm in width) space that separates the presynaptic and postsynaptic cells.
- The neurotransmitter substance diffuses across the synaptic cleft to bind to specific **neurotransmitter receptor** proteins in the postsynaptic membrane. THE BINDING OF THE NEUROTRANSMITTER TO ITS RECEPTOR RESULTS IN A TRANSIENT CHANGE IN THE CONDUCTANCE OF THE POSTSYNAPTIC MEMBRANE TO ONE OR MORE IONS AND THEREBY CAUSES A TRANSIENT CHANGE IN THE MEMBRANE POTENTIAL OF THE POSTSYNAPTIC CELL. A transient depolarization of the postsynaptic cell is an **excitatory postsynaptic potential (EPSP);** a transient hyperpolarization of the postsynaptic cell is an **inhibitory postsynaptic potential (IPSP).**
- THE RECEPTOR PROTEINS FOR MANY NEUROTRANSMITTERS ARE LIGAND-GATED ION CHANNELS. Binding of the neurotransmitter to its receptor alters the probability of the ion channel's being open. In other cases, the neurotransmitter receptor is the first protein in a signal-transduction cascade that alters the probability of an ion channel's being open.
- In some instances, the neuroeffector substances, both nonpeptides and neuropeptides, function as **neuromodulators** rather than as neurotransmitters. A neuromodulator usually binds to a receptor protein in the plasma membrane of the postsynaptic cell or the presynaptic nerve terminal to initiate a signal-transduction cascade that influences the response of the postsynaptic cell to a neurotransmitter or alters the amount of neurotransmitter released by the presynaptic cell.
- The action of most nonpeptide neurotransmitters is terminated when they are actively transported back into the presynaptic nerve ending by Na^+-powered secondary active transport. The action of neuropeptides is terminated by proteolysis or by diffusion away from the postsynaptic membrane.
- Transmission at chemical synapses is one-way. An action potential in the postsynaptic cell does not cause an electrical response of the presynaptic cell. The time that elapses between an action potential in the presynaptic nerve terminal and the postsynaptic potential it evokes, typically about 0.5 msec, is called a **synaptic delay.**
- The presynaptic nerve terminal contains the enzymes for synthesis of small-molecule transmitters from simple precursors. The nerve terminal is the site of synthesis of nonpeptide neurotransmitters. In contrast, neuropeptides are synthesized in the rough endoplasmic reticulum of the cell body **(soma)** of the presynaptic neuron, and the peptide-loaded vesicles reach the nerve terminal via axonal transport.
- After a vesicle containing a nonpeptide neurotransmitter fuses with the plasma membrane, its components are recycled as coated vesicles via endocytosis. The coated vesicles fuse with early endosomes, from which new synaptic vesicles bud. The nascent neurotransmitter vesicle membrane contains an ATPase that pumps H^+ ions into the vesicle interior and a neurotransmitter transporter that couples the downhill efflux of H^+ from the vesicles to the active accumulation of neurotransmitter into the vesicle. In contrast, neuropeptide-containing vesicles are not recycled; the membrane containing the components of these vesicles is degraded.

The Neuromuscular Junction Is a Chemical Synapse

The synapses between the axons of motor neurons and skeletal muscle fibers are called **neuromuscular junctions, myoneural junctions,** or **motor end plates.** Neuromuscular junctions were the first vertebrate synapses to be well characterized, and knowledge of them aids in the comprehension of other chemical synapses.

Near the neuromuscular junction, the motor nerve loses its myelin sheath and divides into fine terminal branches, which lie in **synaptic troughs** on the surfaces of the muscle cells **(Figure 4–3).** The plasma membrane of the muscle cell lining the synaptic trough is thrown into numerous **junctional folds.** The axon terminals contain many 40-nm-diameter **synaptic vesicles** that contain **acetylcholine,** the neurotransmitter at this synapse. Many of the synaptic vesicles in the nerve terminals are docked at active zones on the prejunctional membrane; active zones are concentrated opposite the mouths of the junctional folds. **Acetylcholine receptor** protein molecules are concentrated near the crests of the junctional folds. The axon terminal and the muscle cell are separated by the **junctional cleft,** which contains a carbohydrate-rich amorphous material. When acetylcholine is released, it diffuses across the cleft to bind to acetylcholine receptors on the postjunctional membrane.

The enzyme **choline *O*-acetyltransferase** in the motor nerve terminal catalyzes the condensa-

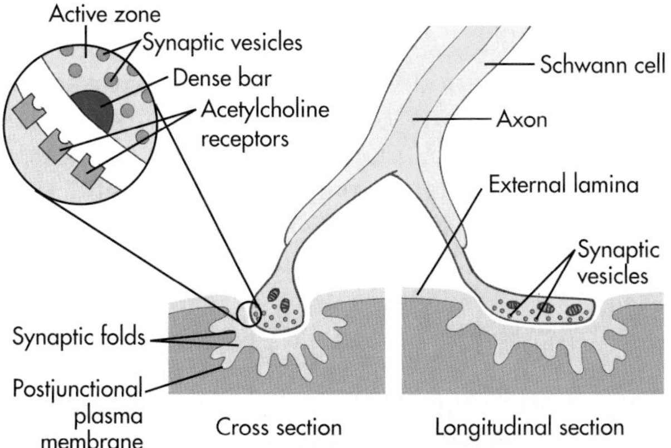

FIGURE 4–3. Structure of the neuromuscular junction in skeletal muscle. Docked vesicles are concentrated at active zones.

tion of acetyl coenzyme A (acetyl CoA) and choline to form acetylcholine. Acetyl CoA is produced by the neuron, as it is by most cells. CHOLINE CANNOT BE SYNTHESIZED BY THE MOTOR NEURON IN ADEQUATE AMOUNTS; IT IS ACTIVELY TRANSPORTED INTO THE MOTOR NEURON TERMINALS FROM THE EXTRACELLULAR FLUID by an Na^+-coupled secondary active transporter in the nerve terminal membrane that can accumulate choline against a large electrochemical potential gradient.

Acetylcholine receptors are ligand-gated channels that conduct both Na^+ and K^+

The binding of acetylcholine to an acetylcholine receptor causes a transient opening of its ion channel that increases the conductance of the postjunctional membrane to Na^+ and K^+. Because the driving force on Na^+ is much greater than that on K^+ (see Chapters 2 and 3), the inward current of Na^+ predominates, causing a transient depolarization of the end plate region. The transient depolarization is called the **end plate potential (EPP) (Figure 4–4).**

The EPP is transient because the action of acetylcholine is ended by the hydrolysis of acetylcholine to form choline and acetate

The hydrolysis of acetylcholine is catalyzed by the enzyme **acetylcholinesterase,** which is present in high concentration on the postjunctional membrane. Much of the choline liberated in the synaptic cleft is taken back up into the motor nerve terminal by an Na^+-powered secondary active transporter in the prejunctional plasma membrane.

Drugs that inhibit acetylcholinesterase are called **anticholinesterases.** In the presence of an anticholinesterase, the EPP is both larger in magnitude and longer in duration. Anticholinesterases are useful in treating disorders in which the function of neuromuscular junctions is impaired, such as **myasthenia gravis. Hemicholiniums** are medications that block the plasma membrane choline transport system and inhibit choline uptake. Prolonged treatment with hemicholiniums depletes the store of transmitter and ultimately decreases the acetylcholine content of the vesicles.

The EPP elicits an action potential in the muscle cell plasma membrane

The EPP depolarizes the postjunctional membrane by 15 to 20 mV. BECAUSE THE POSTJUNCTIONAL MEMBRANE LACKS ADEQUATE NUMBERS OF VOLTAGE-GATED Na^+ AND K^+ CHANNELS, IT DOES NOT FIRE AN ACTION POTENTIAL. Local circuit currents (see Chapter 3) depolarize the muscle cell plasma membrane on either side of the neuromuscular junction to threshold, and action potentials are generated that propagate from near the neuromuscular junction to both ends of the muscle cell to cause the muscle cell to contract (see Chapter 12). Under normal

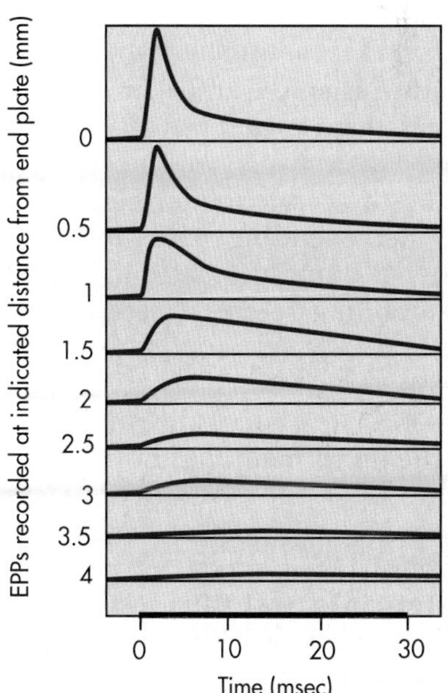

FIGURE 4–4. End plate potentials (EPPs) in a frog sartorius muscle. The preparation was treated with curare to bring the EPP just below threshold for eliciting an action potential. The EPP, recorded at increasing distances from the neuromuscular junction, decreases in amplitude and rate of rise. (Redrawn from Fatt P, Katz B: *J Physiol* 115:320, 1951.)

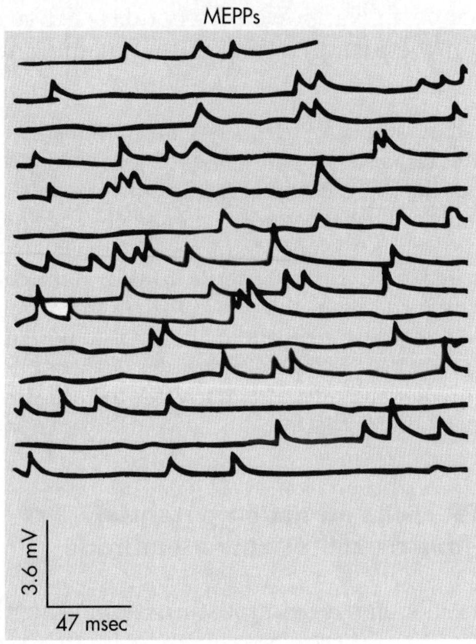

FIGURE 4–5. Spontaneous miniature end plate potentials (MEPPs) recorded at a neuromuscular junction in a fiber of frog extensor digitorum longus muscle. (Redrawn from Fatt P, Katz B: *Nature* 166:597, 1950.)

circumstances, a single action potential in the motor neuron causes a single action potential and a single twitch in each of the muscle cells innervated by that motor neuron (see Chapter 12).

Acetylcholine is released in small packets called quanta

The amount of acetylcholine released by the prejunctional nerve ending does not vary continuously; rather the amount varies in steps, with each step corresponding to the release of one synaptic vesicle. THE AMOUNT OF ACETYLCHOLINE CONTAINED IN ONE VESICLE CORRESPONDS TO A **QUANTUM** OF ACETYLCHOLINE.

Even if the motor neuron is not stimulated, small depolarizations of the postjunctional muscle cell occur spontaneously. These small spontaneous depolarizations are known as **miniature end plate potentials (MEPPs)** (Figure 4–5). They occur at random times with a frequency that averages about one per second. Each MEPP depolarizes the postjunctional membrane by only about 0.4 mV on average, not nearly enough to trigger an action potential in the adjacent muscle plasma membrane. The MEPP has the same time course as an EPP that is evoked by an action potential in the nerve terminal. The MEPP is similar to the EPP in its responses to most medications. The EPP and MEPP are both prolonged by drugs that inhibit acetylcholinesterase, and both are similarly depressed by compounds that compete with acetylcholine for binding to the receptor protein. The frequency of MEPPs may vary, but their amplitudes are within a relatively narrow range (Figure 4–5). A MEPP IS CAUSED BY THE SPONTANEOUS RELEASE OF ONE QUANTUM OF ACETYLCHOLINE INTO THE JUNCTIONAL CLEFT.

Acetylcholine receptor proteins are concentrated on the crests of the junctional folds

There are 10^7 to 10^8 acetylcholine receptor proteins per motor end plate. The acetylcholine receptor protein is an integral membrane protein that spans the hydrophobic lipid matrix of the postjunctional membrane. The acetylcholine receptor of the neuromuscular junction consists of five subunits that surround a central ion channel **(Figure 4–6).** Two of the subunits (α subunits) are identical, so there are four different polypeptide chains (i.e., α, β, δ, γ). Each α subunit contains a binding site for acetylcholine; both α subunits must bind acetylcholine to open the ion channel.

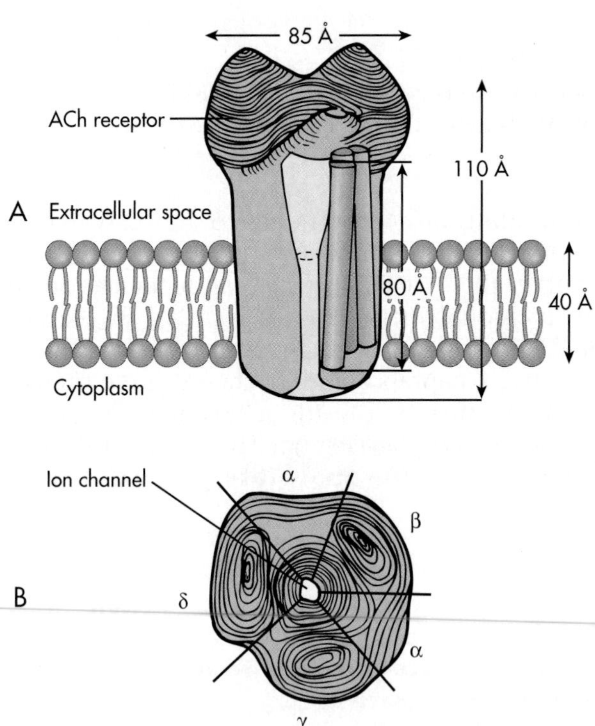

FIGURE 4–6. Structure of a nicotinic acetylcholine (ACh) receptor protein from *Torpedo*, an electric fish. A, Viewed from the side. B, Viewed looking down on the acetylcholine receptor from the extracellular surface. (Redrawn from Kistler J et al: *Biophys J* 37:371, 1982.)

So-called α **toxins** in cobra venoms are responsible for paralyzing the snake's prey. α Toxins bind to the acetylcholine binding site on the α subunits of the **acetylcholine** receptor protein and prevent acetylcholine from acting. Poison arrows whose tips are dipped in **curare,** an α toxin extracted from certain plants, are used by some South American Indians to paralyze their prey. **Succinylcholine,** which binds to the α subunit but cannot open the ion channel, is used as a paralytic agent in some surgical and medical procedures.

Acetylcholine receptor proteins are highly concentrated in the postjunctional membrane, and few acetylcholine receptors are located elsewhere on the muscle plasma membrane. The mechanisms responsible for localizing the acetylcholine receptors in the postjunctional membrane are not completely understood, but it is clear that the motor neuron plays a role. When the motor axon is damaged, acetylcholine receptors spread out over the surface of the muscle cell. When this occurs, the muscle cell becomes sensitive to acetylcholine over the entire surface of the cell. This phenomenon is called **denervation supersensitivity.**

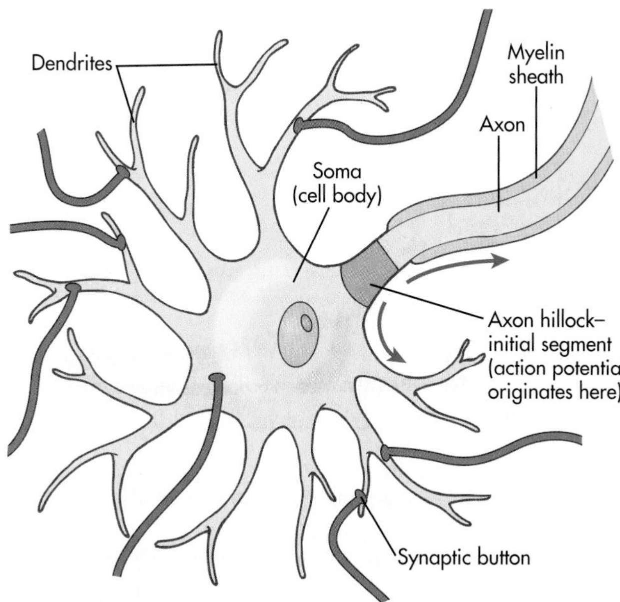

FIGURE 4–7. Spinal motor neuron with multiple synapses *(green)* on both soma and dendrites. There are about 10,000 synapses on a typical spinal motor neuron, 2000 on the soma and 8000 on the dendrites. The axon hillock–initial segment has the lowest threshold; as a result, action potentials tend to originate there.

Chemical Synapses Between Neurons Share Many of the Properties of Neuromuscular Junctions

A presynaptic cell may make synapses with the dendrites, the soma, or the axon of a postsynaptic neuron. Synapses of a presynaptic axon with a dendrite of another cell, **axodendritic synapses,** are the most numerous synapses in the CNS. Synapses are particularly common on **dendritic spines,** protuberances on the dendrites that have a highly specialized structure and function. However, **axosomatic synapses,** synapses of axons with the cell body, or soma, of a postsynaptic neuron, and **axoaxonal synapses,** synapses of an axon with the axon of a postsynaptic neuron, also occur.

A postsynaptic cell may receive one or many presynaptic inputs

Each skeletal muscle cell has only one neuromuscular junction. A single action potential in the motor neuron elicits a single action potential in the muscle cell. The neuromuscular junction is a **one-to-one synapse.**

Certain neurons receive a single synaptic input; in some cases, a single action potential in the presynaptic neuron evokes a burst of action potentials in the postsynaptic cell. This is a **one-to-many synapse.**

The most common situation is for a postsynaptic cell to receive many inputs, a **many-to-one** synaptic arrangement. In such cases, one action potential in a presynaptic cell is not typically sufficient to make the postsynaptic cell fire an action potential. The nearly simultaneous arrival of presynaptic action potentials in several input neurons that synapse on the postsynaptic cell is necessary to depolarize the postsynaptic cell to threshold.

Integration occurs at postsynaptic cells with multiple synaptic inputs

The spinal motor neuron has a many-to-one synaptic organization. About 10,000 presynaptic axons synapse on each spinal motor neuron **(Figure 4–7)**, about 8000 on dendrites and about 2000 on the soma of the motor neuron. Some of these are excitatory inputs that cause a transient depolarization, an **EPSP,** of the postsynaptic cell **(Figure 4–8)**. Other inputs cause a transient hyperpolarization, an **IPSP**. An EPSP brings the membrane potential of the postsynaptic cell closer to its threshold; an IPSP moves the membrane potential farther away from threshold. An EPSP depolarizes the postsynaptic cell by 1 to 2 mV; an IPSP hyperpolarizes it by about the same amount. The postsynaptic cell **integrates** its

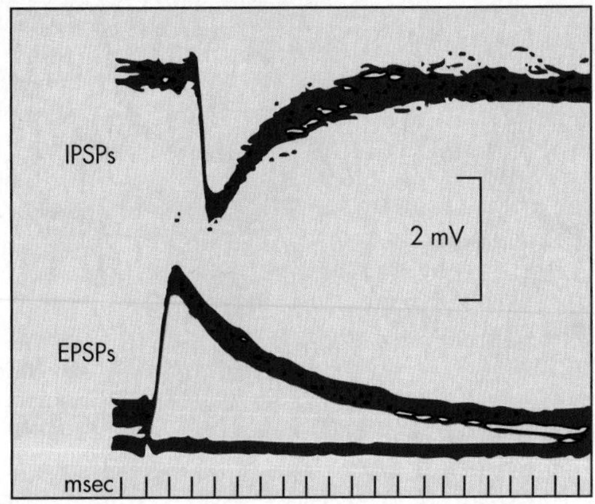

FIGURE 4–8. Inhibitory postsynaptic potentials (IPSPs) and excitatory postsynaptic potentials (EPSPs) recorded with a microelectrode in a cat spinal motor neuron in response to stimulation of appropriate peripheral afferent fibers. A total of 40 traces are superimposed. (Redrawn from Curtis DR, Eccles JC: *J Physiol* 145:529, 1959.)

many synaptic inputs. IF THE MOMENTARY SUM OF THE INPUTS DEPOLARIZES THE POSTSYNAPTIC CELL TO ITS THRESHOLD, IT FIRES AN ACTION POTENTIAL. THIS IS INTEGRATION AT THE LEVEL OF A SINGLE POSTSYNAPTIC NEURON.

Postsynaptic potentials in spinal motor neurons are caused by the opening of specific transmitter-gated ion channels

An EPSP (Figure 4–8) in a spinal motor neuron is caused by a transient increase of the conductance of the postsynaptic membrane to both Na^+ and K^+ in response to the neurotransmitter. At the cell's resting potential, the driving force for Na^+ to enter the cell is much greater than the force for K^+ to leave. Hence, in response to the neurotransmitter, a net inward flow of Na^+ ions predominates, and this depolarizes the postsynaptic cell.

An IPSP (Figure 4–8) in a cat spinal motor neuron is caused by a transient increase in the Cl^- conductance of the postsynaptic membrane in response to the binding of the inhibitory transmitter. At rest, the net tendency is for Cl^- to enter the cell. The transmitter-induced increase in Cl^- conductance allows this ion to enter the postsynaptic cell and hyperpolarize it.

The part of the membrane of the postsynaptic neuron that forms the synapse is specialized for chemical rather than for electrical sensitivity. ACTION POTENTIALS ARE NOT PRODUCED AT THE SYNAPSE. The change in membrane potential that occurs at the synapse, whether it is depolarization or hyperpolarization, is conducted electrotonically over the membrane of the postsynaptic neuron. The part of the neuron where its axon originates is called the **axon hillock;** the part of the axon very near to the neuronal cell body is called the **initial segment.** In many neurons, the **axon hillock–initial segment** region of the cell has a lower threshold than the rest of the plasma membrane of the postsynaptic cell (Figure 4–7). An action potential is generated at this site if the sum of all the inputs to the cell exceeds threshold. Once the action potential has been generated, it is conducted back over the surface of the soma and dendrites of the postsynaptic cell and propagated along its axon.

Summation of synaptic inputs occurs by spatial and temporal summation

Spatial summation occurs when two separate inputs arrive almost simultaneously **(Figure 4–9, *A* and *B*)**. The two postsynaptic potentials are added

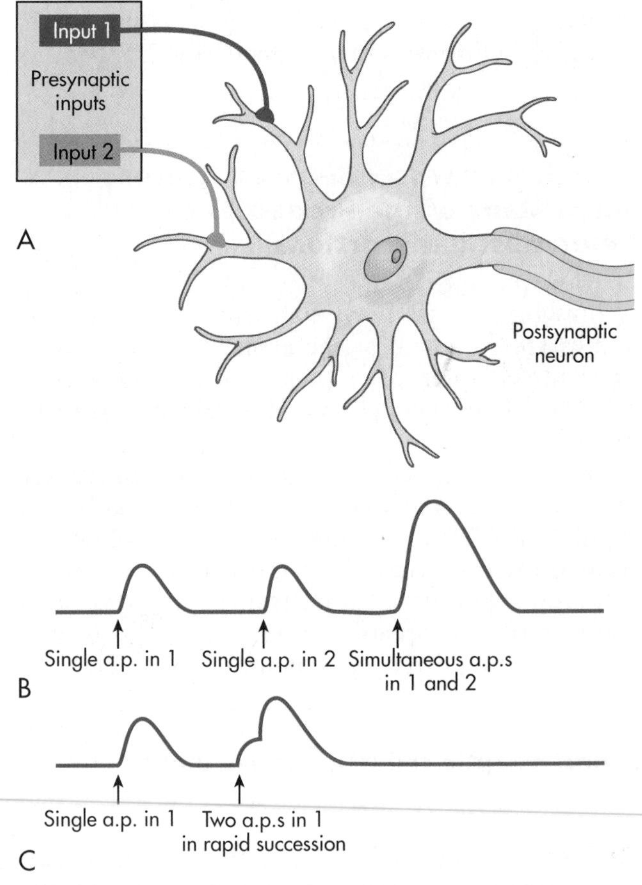

FIGURE 4–9. A, Spatial and temporal summation at a postsynaptic neuron with two synaptic inputs (1 and 2). B, Spatial summation. The postsynaptic potentials in response to single action potentials (a.p.) in inputs 1 and 2 occurring separately and simultaneously. C, Temporal summation. The postsynaptic response to two impulses in rapid succession in the same input.

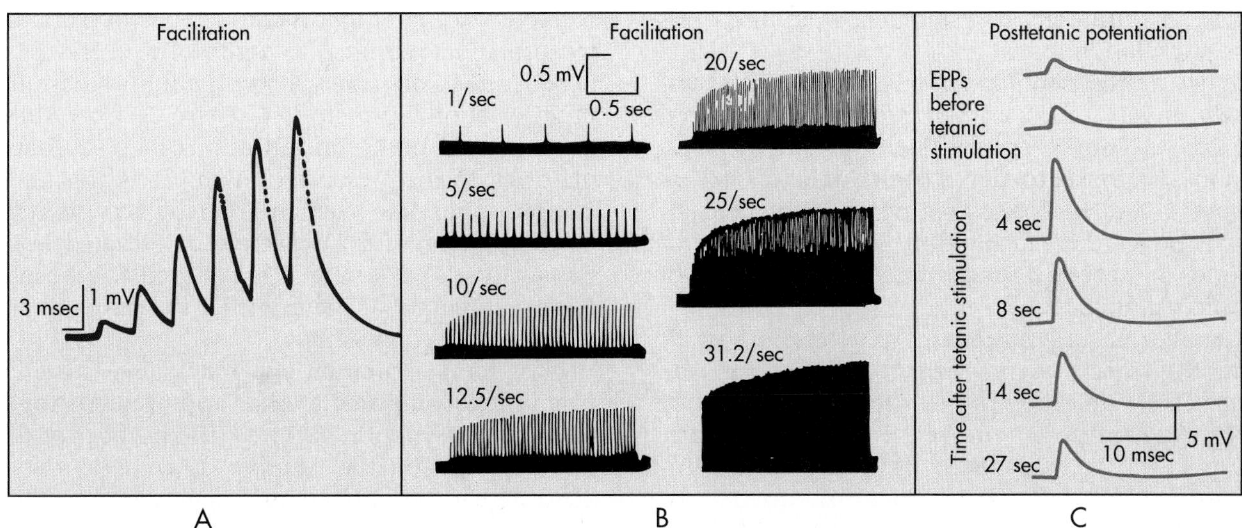

FIGURE 4–10. A, Facilitation at a neuromuscular junction. EPPs at a neuromuscular junction in toad sartorius muscle were elicited by successive action potentials in the motor axon. B, EPPs at a frog neuromuscular junction elicited by repeatedly stimulating the motor axon at different frequencies. Note that the degree of facilitation increases with the increasing frequency of stimulation. C, Posttetanic potentiation at a frog neuromuscular junction. The top two traces indicate control EPPs in response to single action potentials in the motor axon. Subsequent traces indicate EPPs in response to single action potentials after tetanic stimulation of the motor neuron. The time interval between the end of tetanic stimulation and the single action potential is shown on each trace. (A redrawn from Belnave RJ, Gage PW: *J Physiol* 266:435, 1977; B redrawn from Magelby KL: *J Physiol* 234:327, 1973; C redrawn from Weinrich D: *J Physiol* 212:431, 1971.)

so that two simultaneous excitatory inputs depolarize the postsynaptic cell about twice as much as either input alone. However, if an EPSP and an IPSP occur simultaneously, they tend to cancel each other. Even postsynaptic potentials from synapses at opposite ends of the postsynaptic cell body sum in this way. The postsynaptic potentials (EPSPs and IPSPs) sum with little decrement because cellular dimensions (<100 μm) are much smaller than the length constant (≈1 to 2 mm) for electrotonic conduction. In contrast, synaptic potentials that originate in fine dendritic branches decrease in magnitude as they are conducted to the cell body; the finer the dendrite, the greater the decrement.

Temporal summation occurs when two or more action potentials in a single presynaptic neuron occur in rapid succession so that the resulting postsynaptic potentials overlap in time (Figure 4–9, *A* and *C*). A train of impulses in a single presynaptic neuron can change the potential of the postsynaptic cell in a stepwise manner, each step caused by one of the presynaptic impulses.

Synaptic inputs to a presynaptic axon can influence the amount of transmitter it releases

The strength of individual synaptic inputs to a particular postsynaptic cell may be modulated by stimulatory or inhibitory effects on particular presynaptic axons that modulate the amount of transmitter released. **Presynaptic inhibition** and **presynaptic facilitation** are effected by means of axoaxonal synapses between modulatory neurons and presynaptic axons. Presynaptic inhibition may occur when the transmitter released at the axoaxonal synapse results in increased Cl^- conductance in the nerve terminal of the axon being modulated. The increased Cl^- conductance results in a shorter and smaller action potential, so less Ca^{++} enters the nerve terminal, and less transmitter is released. Presynaptic facilitation may occur when the transmitter released by the modulatory neuron onto the axon being modulated results in diminished voltage-gated K^+ conductance. Thus, the action potential is prolonged, which allows a greater influx of Ca^{++} and the release of more transmitter.

Repetitive stimulation can modulate the amount of transmitter released by a presynaptic neuron

When a presynaptic axon is stimulated repeatedly, the postsynaptic response may grow with each stimulation. This phenomenon is called **facilitation (Figure 4–10, *A*)**. As shown in Figure 4–10, *B*, the extent of facilitation depends on the frequency of presynaptic impulses. Facilitation dies away rapidly, within tens to hundreds of milliseconds after stimulation stops.

When a presynaptic neuron is stimulated **tetanically** (many stimuli at high frequency) for several seconds, a longer enhancement of postsynaptic response **(posttetanic potentiation)** occurs (Figure 4–10, *C*). Posttetanic potentiation persists much longer than facilitation; it lasts for tens of seconds to several minutes after the cessation of tetanic stimulation.

Facilitation and posttetanic potentiation result from the effects of repeated stimulation on the presynaptic neuron. These phenomena do not involve a change in the sensitivity of the postsynaptic cell to transmitter. With repeated stimulation, an increased number of quanta of transmitter are released, partly because repetitive stimulation leads to increased levels of intracellular Ca^{++}.

When a synapse is repetitively stimulated for a long time, a point is reached at which each successive presynaptic stimulation elicits smaller postsynaptic responses. This phenomenon is called **synaptic fatigue** (neuromuscular depression at the neuromuscular junction). The postsynaptic cell at a fatigued synapse responds normally to transmitter applied from a micropipette; thus, the defect is presynaptic. In some cases, a decrease in **quantal content** (the amount of transmitter per synaptic vesicle) contributes to synaptic fatigue. A fatigued synapse typically recovers in a few seconds.

Long-term potentiation and long-term depression involve changes in postsynaptic neurons

Repetitive high-frequency stimulation of certain synapses in the brain increases the efficacy of transmission at those synapses, a reaction that can persist for days to weeks. This phenomenon is called **long-term potentiation,** and it is probably involved in learning and memory. Repetitive low-frequency stimulation of the same synapse may lead to **long-term depression,** a persistent decrease in synaptic efficacy. In contrast with the modulatory mechanisms that result from changes in the presynaptic nerve terminal (discussed in the previous section), LONG-TERM POTENTIATION AND INHIBITION APPEAR TO INVOLVE PRIMARILY CHANGES IN THE POSTSYNAPTIC NEURON.

Ca^{++} entry into the postsynaptic region is an early required step in initiation of the changes that result in long-term enhancement of the response of the postsynaptic cell to neurotransmitter. Ca^{++} entry occurs through *N*-methyl-D-aspartate (NMDA) receptors (see later discussion), a class of glutamate receptors that permits Ca^{++} influx. The entry of Ca^{++} is believed to activate Ca^{++}–calmodulin kinase II, a multifunctional protein kinase (see Chapter 5) that is present in high concentrations in postsynaptic densities. In the presence of high $[Ca^{++}]$, this kinase can phosphorylate itself and thereby become active whether or not Ca^{++} is present at elevated levels. Ca^{++}–calmodulin kinase II is believed to phosphorylate proteins that are essential for the induction of long-term potentiation.

Long-term potentiation may also have an anatomical component. After appropriate stimulation of a presynaptic pathway, the number of dendritic spines and the number of synapses on the dendrites of the postsynaptic neurons may rapidly increase.

Whether changes in the presynaptic nerve terminal also contribute to long-term potentiation remains unresolved. The postsynaptic neuron may release a signal—nitric oxide **(NO)** has been suggested—that enhances transmitter release by the presynaptic nerve terminal, thereby contributing to long-term potentiation.

Many Compounds Serve as Neurotransmitters and Neuromodulators

Table 4–1 lists some of the substances that serve as neurotransmitters and neuromodulators. It is often difficult to prove that a substance is a neurotransmitter at a particular synapse. The candidate compound must satisfy the following criteria before it is accepted as a mediator of transmission at a particular synapse.

- The presynaptic neurons must contain the compound and must be able to synthesize it.
- The compound must be released by the presynaptic neurons in response to appropriate stimulation.
- The microapplication of the compound to the postsynaptic membrane must mimic the effects of stimulation of the presynaptic neuron.
- The effects of presynaptic stimulation and of microapplication of the compound should be altered in the same way by drugs.

Some neurotransmitters and neuromodulators have rapid and transient effects on the postsynaptic cell; others have effects that are much slower in onset and may last for minutes or even hours. Most but not all known neurotransmitters and neuromodulators fall into the major chemical classes of amines, amino acids, and oligopeptides.

TABLE 4–1. SELECTED NEUROTRANSMITTERS AND NEUROMODULATORS

Compound	Site of Action of Neurons
Acetylcholine	Neuromuscular junction, autonomic endings, autonomic ganglia, sweat glands, brain, retina, gastrointestinal tract
Biogenic amines	
Epinephrine	Brain, spinal cord
Norepinephrine	Sympathetic endings, brain, spinal cord, gastrointestinal tract
Dopamine	Brain, sympathetic ganglia, retina
Serotonin	Brain, spinal cord, retina, gastrointestinal tract
Histamine	Brain, gastrointestinal tract
Amino acids	
GABA	Brain, retina
Glutamate	Brain
Aspartate	Spinal cord, brain?
Glycine	Spinal cord, brain, retina
Purines/purine nucleotides	
Adenosine	Brain
ATP	Autonomic ganglia, brain
Gas	
Nitric oxide	Brain, spinal cord, gastrointestinal tract
Peptides	
Activins	Brain
Angiotensin II	Brain, spinal cord
Atrial natriuretic peptide	Brain
Calcitonin gene–related peptide	Spinal cord, brain
Cholecystokinin	Brain, retina, gastrointestinal tract
Corticotropin-releasing hormone	Brain
Dynorphins	Brain, gastrointestinal tract
β-Endorphins	Brain, retina, gastrointestinal tract
Endothelins	Brain, pituitary gland
Enkephalins	Brain, retina, gastrointestinal tract
FMRF amide	Brain
Galanin	Brain, spinal cord
Gastrin	Brain
Gastrin-releasing peptide	Brain
Gonadotropin-releasing hormone	Brain, autonomic ganglia, retina
Inhibins	Brain
Motilin	Brain, pituitary gland
Neuropeptide Y	Brain, autonomic nervous system
Neurotensin	Brain, retina
Oxytocin	Pituitary gland, brain, spinal cord
Secretin	Brain, gastrointestinal tract
Somatostatin	Brain, retina, gastrointestinal tract
Substance P	Brain, spinal cord, gastrointestinal tract
Vasoactive intestinal polypeptide	Autonomic nervous system, spinal cord, brain, retina, gastrointestinal tract

Acetylcholine mediates transmission between motor neurons and skeletal muscle cells and in the autonomic nervous system and the central nervous system

As discussed previously, acetylcholine is the transmitter used by all motor axons that arise from the spinal cord. Acetylcholine also plays a central role in the autonomic nervous system; it is the transmitter for all autonomic preganglionic neurons and also for postganglionic parasympathetic fibers. Betz cells of the motor cortex use acetylcholine as their transmitter. Acetylcholine is apparently an important neurotransmitter in the basal ganglia, which are involved in the control of movement. In addition, acetylcholine may be the transmitter in many other central neural pathways.

Deficits in pathways involving acetylcholine **(cholinergic pathways)** in the brain have been implicated in some forms of **senile dementia** (such as **Alzheimer's disease**). Treatment with long-lasting anticholinesterases that penetrate the blood-brain barrier may improve cognitive function in some individuals suffering from senile dementia.

Several amines serve as neurotransmitters

Dopamine, norepinephrine, and epinephrine are **catecholamines,** and they share a common biosynthetic pathway that starts with the amino acid tyrosine. Tyrosine is converted to L-dopa by tyrosine hydroxylase. L-Dopa is converted to dopamine by a specific decarboxylase. In dopaminergic neurons, the pathway stops here. Noradrenergic neurons have another enzyme, dopamine β-hydroxylase, that converts dopamine to norepinephrine. Norepinephrine is the primary transmitter for postganglionic sympathetic neurons. Chromaffin cells in the adrenal medulla add a methyl group to norepinephrine to produce the hormone epinephrine.

Neurons that contain high levels of dopamine are prominent in the midbrain regions known as the **substantia nigra** and the **ventral tegmentum.** Some of the axons of these neurons terminate in the **corpus striatum,** where they participate in controlling complex movements. Degeneration of dopaminergic synapses in the corpus striatum occurs in **Parkinson's disease** and may be a major cause of the muscle tremors and rigidity that characterize this condition. Treatment with **L-dopa,** the precursor of dopamine, may improve motor control, but only temporarily.

In contrast, hyperactivity of dopaminergic synapses may be involved in some forms of **psychosis. Chlorpromazine** and related antipsychotic drugs inhibit the dopamine receptors on postsynaptic membranes and thus diminish the effects of dopamine released from presynaptic nerve terminals.

Neurons that contain **serotonin (5-hydroxytryptamine)** are present in high concentrations in certain nuclei in the brainstem. Serotonergic neurons may be involved in temperature regulation, sensory perception, onset of sleep, and control of mood. Serotonergic neurons have been implicated in aggressive behavior in certain animal species. Fourteen different subtypes of serotonin receptors have been discovered in humans, suggesting that many functions are regulated by this compound. Thirteen distinct isoforms of the serotonin receptor are G protein–coupled receptors (see Chapter 5), and another type of serotonin receptor is a ligand-gated ion channel.

Amino acid transmitters are the most common inhibitory and excitatory neurotransmitters in the central nervous system

Glycine, the simplest amino acid, is an inhibitory neurotransmitter released by certain interneurons in the spinal cord and brainstem. **γ-Aminobutyric acid (GABA)** is not incorporated into proteins, nor is it present in all cells, as are the other naturally occurring amino acids. GABA IS PRODUCED FROM GLUTAMATE BY A SPECIFIC DECARBOXYLASE PRESENT ONLY IN CERTAIN NEURONS IN THE CNS. Among the cells that contain GABA are some neurons in the basal ganglia, cerebellar Purkinje cells, and certain spinal interneurons. In all known cases, GABA functions as an inhibitory transmitter. GABA may be the neurotransmitter at as many as one fourth of the synapses in the brain.

Glutamate and **aspartate,** dicarboxylic amino acids, strongly excite many neurons. GLUTAMATE IS THE MOST COMMON EXCITATORY NEUROTRANSMITTER IN THE BRAIN. There are five classes of **excitatory amino acid receptors** (see later discussion).

Nitric oxide is an important neurotransmitter and neuromodulator

NO mediates transmission between inhibitory motor neurons of the enteric nervous system and gastrointestinal smooth muscle cells (see Chapter 33). It also functions as a neurotransmitter and neuromodulator in the CNS. NO differs from other neuroactive compounds because it is a gas and because it is neither packaged into synaptic vesicles nor released by exocytosis. NO is highly permeant and simply diffuses from its site of production to neighboring cells. **NO synthase,** the enzyme that catalyzes the production of NO, is stimulated by an increase in cytosolic Ca^{++}.

The receptor for NO is soluble guanylyl cyclase in the target cell (see Chapter 5). NO potently stimulates this enzyme and thereby leads to an elevation of cGMP in the target cell. The elevated levels of cGMP can then influence multiple cellular processes, including certain ion channels.

Purine nucleotides and nucleosides are neurotransmitters and neuromodulators

ATP and adenosine function as neurotransmitters and neuromodulators in the central, autonomic, and peripheral nervous systems.

Many neuropeptides are neurotransmitters and neuromodulators

Certain cells release peptides that act at very low concentrations to excite or to inhibit neurons.

Many of these so-called **neuroactive peptides,** or **neuropeptides,** ranging from 2 to 40 amino acids long, have been identified (Table 4–1).

Although there are some exceptions, neuropeptides typically affect their target neurons at lower concentrations than do the classic neurotransmitters discussed previously, and the effects of neuropeptides frequently are slower to occur and more persistent. A number of neuropeptides are more familiar as hormones. A hormone is a substance that is released into the blood and that reaches its target cells via the circulation. A number of neuropeptides act as true transmitters at particular synapses and as neuromodulators at other synapses. **Table 4–2** lists some of the differences between nonpeptide neurotransmitters and peptide neurotransmitters.

In many instances, neuropeptides coexist with classic transmitters in the same nerve terminals. The classic transmitters are present in the presynaptic nerve terminal in small vesicles clustered near active zones; the neuropeptides are present in larger vesicles distributed throughout the nerve terminal. It appears that low-frequency stimulation of the presynaptic neuron preferentially releases the nonpeptide transmitter, whereas the neuropeptide is released in response to high-frequency stimulation.

Neuropeptides are synthesized in the neuronal cell body. Secretory vesicles containing the neuropeptide are released from the mature face of the Golgi complex and are then transported by **fast axonal transport** to the axon terminal. Some neuropeptides are synthesized as preprohormones (see also Chapter 41). Cleavage of a signal sequence converts a preprohormone to a prohormone. Proteolytic cleavage of the prohormone may then release one or more active peptides. In some cases, one prohormone may contain several active peptide sequences.

Opioid peptides modulate pain pathways and are important neuromodulators in the central nervous system and gastrointestinal tract

Opiates are drugs derived from the juice of the opium poppy. Compounds that are not derived from the opium poppy but that exert direct effects by binding to opiate receptors are called **opioids.** Opioids are operationally defined as direct-acting compounds whose effects are stereospecifically antagonized by **naloxone,** a morphine derivative. Opiates and opioids are useful therapeutically as powerful **analgesics** (pain relievers). They exert this effect by binding to specific opiate receptors.

The three major classes of endogenous opioid peptides in mammals are **enkephalins, endorphins,** and **dynorphins.** Enkephalins are the simplest opioids; they are pentapeptides (met-enkephalin is Tyr-Gly-Gly-Phe-Met, and leu-enkephalin is Tyr-Gly-Gly-Phe-Leu). Dynorphin and the endorphins are somewhat longer peptides that contain one or the other of the enkephalin sequences at their N termini.

Opioid peptides are widely distributed in neurons of the CNS and intrinsic neurons of the gastrointestinal tract. The endorphins are discretely localized in particular structures of the CNS, whereas the enkephalins and dynorphins are more widely distributed. Opioids also inhibit cerebral neurons that are involved in the perception of pain.

Substance P is a transmitter in the pain pathways and gastrointestinal tract

Most of the known neuropeptides are not opioids. **Substance P,** a peptide of 11 amino acids, is present in specific neurons in the brain, primary sensory neurons, and plexus neurons in the wall of the gastrointestinal tract. Substance P was the first so-called **gut-brain peptide** to be discovered. Enteric neurons contain many of the neuropeptides,

TABLE 4–2. DISTINCTION BETWEEN NONPEPTIDE AND PEPTIDE NEUROTRANSMITTERS

Nonpeptide Neurotransmitters	Peptide Neurotransmitters
Synthesized and packaged in presynaptic nerve terminal	Synthesized and packaged in soma of presynaptic neuron; transported to nerve terminal by axonal transport
Nonpeptide synthesized in active form	Active peptide formed by cleavage from much larger peptide that contains multiple neuropeptides or hormones
Present in small synaptic vesicles clustered near active zones	Present in large, clear synaptic vesicles distributed throughout nerve terminal
Action terminated by active reuptake into presynaptic nerve terminal	Action terminated by proteolysis or peptide diffusing away
Neurotransmitters and vesicle constituents recycled	Neuropeptide and vesicle constituents degraded
Released into synaptic cleft	May be released some distance from target neuron
Action typically has short latency and short duration (milliseconds)	Action may have long latency and may persist for many seconds

including substance P, that are found in the brain and spinal column (see Chapter 33). Substance P is the transmitter at synapses that primary sensory neurons (their cell bodies are in the dorsal root ganglia) make with spinal interneurons in the dorsal horn of the spinal column. Enkephalins decrease the release of substance P at these synapses and thereby inhibit the pain sensation at the first synapse in the pathway.

Vasoactive intestinal polypeptide, secretin, glucagon, and gastric inhibitory peptide are members of a family of neuropeptides

Vasoactive intestinal polypeptide (VIP) was first discovered as a gastrointestinal hormone, but it is now known to be a neuropeptide as well. VIP is widely distributed in the CNS and the intrinsic neurons of the gastrointestinal tract. In certain neurons in the brain, VIP is present in synaptic vesicles. VIP may function as an inhibitory transmitter to vascular and nonvascular smooth muscle and as an excitatory transmitter to glandular epithelial cells.

Secretin, glucagon, and **gastric inhibitory polypeptide** are peptides whose functions as gastrointestinal hormones have been well characterized. These peptides have also been found in particular neurons in the CNS, but their functions in neurons remain undetermined.

Cholecystokinin is a member of a group of neuropeptides that includes gastrin and cerulein

These peptides have similar C-terminal sequences. Cholecystokinin is a well-known gastrointestinal hormone that elicits contraction of the gallbladder and has other roles in the gastrointestinal tract (see Chapters 33 and 34). One form of cholecystokinin is present in particular neurons of the CNS.

Neurotransmitter Receptors Are Ligand-Gated Ion Channels or Signal-Transduction Proteins

Some neurotransmitter receptors, such as the acetylcholine receptor of the neuromuscular junction, are ligand-gated ion channels. Other neurotransmitters influence the function of ion channels more indirectly.

Two major classes of acetylcholine receptors are nicotinic and muscarinic acetylcholine receptors

The acetylcholine receptor at the neuromuscular junction (Figure 4–6) is a **nicotinic acetylcholine receptor;** it can be stimulated by **nicotine.** Other receptors for acetylcholine, such as those on heart cells, smooth muscle cells, and many brain neurons, are stimulated not by nicotine but by **muscarine.** They are called **muscarinic acetylcholine receptors.** Subtypes of nicotinic and muscarinic receptors are classified by their sensitivities to agonist and antagonist drugs.

MUSCARINIC ACETYLCHOLINE RECEPTORS ARE NOT ION CHANNELS. Muscarinic receptors are seven-transmembrane helix receptor proteins that are linked to heterotrimeric GTP-binding proteins. Binding of acetylcholine to M_2 muscarinic receptors in the heart's sinoatrial node activates G_i protein, which increases the probability of opening of K^+ channels (see Chapter 5). This tends to hyperpolarize the pacemaker cells of the sinoatrial node and thereby decreases the heart rate (see Chapter 17). There are five major subtypes of muscarinic receptors.

γ-Aminobutyric acid and glycine receptors mediate neurotransmission at most inhibitory synapses in the central nervous system

Glycine-mediated inhibitory synapses predominate in the spinal cord, and GABAergic synapses are the most numerous synapses in the brain. Most GABA and glycine receptors, and most other neurotransmitter receptors, belong to the superfamily of ligand-gated ion channels. They are heteropentamers, like acetylcholine receptors, and their subunits have significant sequence homology and structural similarities with the subunits of nicotinic acetylcholine receptors. Even though there may be five distinct subunits, only one or two subunit isoforms are typically required to form a functional ion channel. Different cell types in the CNS may have different receptor subtypes that consist of different combinations of subunit isoforms.

Most GABA and glycine receptors are ligand-gated Cl^- channels that mediate Cl^- influx into neurons. The Cl^- current hyperpolarizes and thus inhibits the neurons. The major classes of GABA receptors are called $GABA_A$ and $GABA_B$. The $GABA_A$ receptor is a GABA-mediated Cl^- channel. The $GABA_B$ receptor is not an ion channel itself, but it acts via protein kinase C to increase the K^+ conductance and to decrease the Ca^{++} conductance of the postsynaptic cell.

TABLE 4–3. DIFFERENT CLASSES OF EXCITATORY AMINO ACID RECEPTORS

Receptor Class	Properties
AMPA	Is widely distributed in CNS; is channel selective for Na^+ and K^+; was known as quisqualate receptor
N-methyl-D-aspartate (NMDA)	Is widely distributed in CNS; is channel selective for Ca^{++}, Na^+, and K^+; is blocked by Mg^{++} (block relieved by depolarization)
Kainate	Is present in specific areas of CNS
L-2-Amino-4-phosphonobutyrate	Is not widely distributed; may function as presynaptic glutamate receptor that inhibits glutamate release
Metabotropic	Is not an ion channel; mobilizes inositol 1,4,5-trisphosphate; increases intracellular Ca^{++} levels

General **anesthetics** prolong the open time of $GABA_A$ receptor Cl^- channels and thus prolong the inhibition of the postsynaptic neurons at GABAergic synapses. $GABA_A$ receptors may be a principal target of general anesthetics. $GABA_A$ receptors are also the targets of two major classes of medications, **benzodiazepines** and **barbiturates.** Benzodiazepines (such as **diazepam**) are widely used antianxiety and relaxant drugs. Barbiturates are used as sedatives and anticonvulsants. Both of these classes of drugs bind to distinct sites on $GABA_A$ receptors and enhance the opening of the receptors' Cl^- channels in response to GABA.

Excitatory amino acid receptors have glutamate as their most important ligand

Glutamate is the major neurotransmitter that mediates synaptic excitation in the CNS. Glutamate receptors are also known as **excitatory amino acid (EAA) receptors.** At present, five subtypes of EAA receptors are recognized **(Table 4–3).** The subtypes are classified principally on the synthetic amino acid analogues that bind tightly and specifically to them. Four of the subtypes are ligand-gated ion channels, and the fifth is a receptor (called the **metabotropic EAA receptor**) that is indirectly linked to an ion channel.

AMPA and **NMDA** receptors are widely distributed in the CNS. Stimulation of AMPA receptors by glutamate or another agonist elicits an EPSP caused by the flow of Na^+ and K^+. Stimulated NMDA receptors permit the flow of Ca^{++} as well as of Na^+ and K^+. NMDA receptors are blocked by extracellular Mg^{++} at physiological levels. The Mg^{++} block is relieved when the cell is depolarized. Thus, the first physiological response to glutamate is depolarization of the postsynaptic cell by glutamate acting on AMPA receptors. This depolarization relieves the Mg^{++} block of NMDA receptors, which then respond by permitting a Ca^{++} influx and further depolarization of the postsynaptic cell. NMDA receptors are also regulated by glycine, which binds to the receptor to enhance current flow in response to glutamate. The role of NMDA receptors in long-term potentiation was discussed previously.

Summary

- Direct electrical transmission between neighboring cells is mediated by gap junctions.
- At a chemical synapse, an action potential in the presynaptic nerve terminal causes a Ca^{++} influx, which initiates the chain of events culminating in the release of neurotransmitter.
- Neurotransmitter diffuses across the synaptic cleft and binds to neurotransmitter receptor proteins on the postsynaptic membrane, which results in a transient change in the conductance of the postsynaptic membrane to one or more ions.
- At the neuromuscular junction, acetylcholine released by the prejunctional nerve terminal binds to acetylcholine receptors in the postjunctional membrane to open ion channels conductive to Na^+ and K^+. The resulting ion flow across the postjunctional membrane causes a depolarization, called an end plate potential (EPP).
- The EPP is terminated by the hydrolysis of acetylcholine by the enzyme acetylcholinesterase. When acetylcholine is hydrolyzed, much of the choline liberated in the synaptic cleft is actively transported back into the nerve terminal.

- The release of acetylcholine is quantal. A quantum corresponds to the amount of acetylcholine in a single presynaptic vesicle.
- An action potential in an excitatory input to a spinal motor neuron causes an EPSP that depolarizes the motor neuron and brings it closer to threshold.
- An action potential in an inhibitory input causes an IPSP that hyperpolarizes the motor neuron.
- The efficacy of synaptic transmission depends on the timing and frequency of action potentials in the presynaptic neuron.
- Facilitation and posttetanic potentiation are due to increased release of neurotransmitter in response to previous multiple stimulations of a presynaptic neuron.
- Long-term potentiation involves biochemical changes that enhance the responsiveness of the postsynaptic neuron to neurotransmitter.
- Acetylcholine, biogenic amines, glutamate, glycine, and GABA are important neurotransmitters in the CNS.
- Glycine and GABA are the major transmitters at inhibitory synapses in the CNS.
- Glutamate is the major excitatory neurotransmitter in the CNS. There are five classes of EAA receptors.
- Many neuroactive peptides function as neuromodulators or neurotransmitters in the CNS.

Bibliography

Amara SB, Fonana AC: Excitatory amino acid transporters: keeping up with glutamate, *Neurochem Int* 41:313, 2002.

Boehning D, Snyder SH: Novel neural modulators, *Annu Rev Neurosci* 26:105, 2003.

Dajas-Bailador F, Wonnacott S: Nicotinic acetylcholine receptors and the regulation of neuronal signaling, *Trends Pharmacol Sci* 25:317, 2004.

Gerber SH, Sudhof TC: Molecular determinants of regulated exocytosis, *Diabetes* 51(suppl 1):S3, 2002.

Hille B: *Ion channels of excitable membranes,* ed 3, Sunderland, Mass, 2001, Sinauer Associates.

Hokfelt T, Pernow B, Wahren J: Substance P: a pioneer amongst neuropeptides, *J Intern Med* 249:27, 2001.

Jahn R, Lang T, Sudhof TC: Membrane fusion, *Cell* 112:519, 2003.

Jingami H, Nakanishi S, Morikawa K: Structure of the metabotropic glutamate receptor, *Curr Opin Neurobiol* 13:271, 2003.

Kaczmarek LK: How to make a relationship last: release sites with different levels of commitment, *Neuron* 40:7, 2003.

Kandel ER, Schwartz JH, Jessell TM: *Principles of neural science,* ed 4, New York, 2000, Elsevier Science.

Kandel ER: The molecular biology of memory storage: a dialogue between genes and synapses, *Science* 294:1030, 2001.

Katz B: *Nerve, muscle, and synapse,* New York, 1966, McGraw-Hill.

Keynes RD, Aidley DJ: *Nerve and muscle,* ed 3, Cambridge, 2001, Cambridge University Press.

LaDoux J: Structural plasticity and memory, *Nat Rev Neurosci* 5:45, 2004.

Levitan IB, Kaczmarek LK: *The neuron: cell and molecular biology,* ed 3, New York, 2001, Oxford University Press.

Lynch MA: Long-term potentiation and memory, *Physiol Rev* 84:87, 2004.

Montgomery JM, Madison DV: The grass roots of synapse suppression, *Neuron* 29:567, 2001.

Nadeau SE et al: *Medical neuroscience,* New York, 2004, Elsevier.

Nakase T, Nauss CC: Gap junctions and neurological disorders of the central nervous system, *Biochim Biophys Acta* 1662:149, 2004.

Nicholls JG et al: *From neuron to brain,* ed 4, Sunderland, Mass, 2001, Sinauer Associates.

Nitric oxide and memory, *Neuroscientist* 10:153, 2004.

Peracchia C: Chemical gating of gap junction channels; roles of calcium, pH and calmodulin, *Biochim Biophys Acta* 1662:61, 2004.

Phillips WD, Froehner SC: GABARAP and $GABA_A$ receptor clustering, *Neuron* 33:4, 2002.

Popescu G, Auerbach A: The NMDA receptor gating machine: lessons from single channels, *Neuroscientist* 10:192, 2004.

Purves D et al: *Neuroscience,* ed 2, Sunderland, Mass, 2001, Sinauer Associates.

Stevens CF: Neurotransmitter release at central synapses, *Neuron* 40:381, 2003.

Steward O, Schuman RM: Compartmentalized synthesis and degradation of proteins in neurons, *Neuron* 40:347, 2003.

Torres GE, Gainetdinov RV, Caron MG: Plasma membrane monoamine transporters: structure, regulation and function, *Nat Rev Neurosci* 4:13, 2003.

von Zastrow M: Opioid receptor regulation, *Neuromolecular Med* 5:51, 2004.

Self-Assessment

1. **Which of the following is an event in neuromuscular transmission?**
   A. Opening of voltage-gated Mg^{++} channels in the nerve terminal
   B. Binding of ACh (acetylcholine) to membrane lipids
   C. Generation of an action potential by the ACh receptor protein
   D. Reuptake of choline by the prejunctional nerve terminal

2. **Which statement about the end plate potential (EPP) is true?**
   A. The EPP is caused by increased g_{Na} and g_K of the postjunctional membrane.
   B. In the presence of an inhibitor of cholinesterase, the EPP will be the same amplitude as in the absence of the inhibitor.
   C. In health, the EPP is sometimes too small to elicit an action potential.
   D. In myasthenia gravis, EPPs may be larger in amplitude.

3. **Which statement about the acetylcholine receptor (AChR) is true?**
   A. ACh is bound to the δ subunit of AChR.
   B. AChR is a voltage-gated ion channel.
   C. AChRs are highly concentrated in the postjunctional membrane.
   D. AChRs are absent in myasthenia gravis.

4. **Which statement about synaptic transmission is true?**
   A. An IPSP is a transient depolarization of a postsynaptic cell.
   B. Two presynaptic stimuli in rapid succession may elicit a larger postsynaptic response than does a single presynaptic stimulus.
   C. IPSPs are caused by increased Na^+ conductance of the postsynaptic cell.
   D. EPSPs are caused by increased Cl^- conductance of the postsynaptic cell.

5. **Which statement about neurotransmitters is true?**
   A. Nitric oxide acts during a long time.
   B. GABA is the most common excitatory transmitter in the brain.
   C. Glutamate is an important inhibitory transmitter.
   D. Many neuropeptides are present in the brain and in the gastrointestinal system.

Chapter 5: Membrane Receptors, Second Messengers, and Signal-Transduction Pathways

Objectives

- List the components of a generalized signal-transduction pathway (agonist, receptor, second messenger, effector, biological response).
- List the components of a generalized G protein–mediated signal-transduction pathway.
- Describe the roles of protein kinases and protein phosphatases in signal transduction.
- List the major second messengers.
- Identify the major classes of second messenger–dependent protein kinases.
- Describe the general functions of receptor tyrosine kinases and receptor-associated tyrosine kinases.
- List the major classes of protein phosphatases.

This chapter discusses the signal-transduction pathways whereby regulatory molecules, such as hormones, influence intracellular processes. Basic cellular processes are regulated by a host of substances. Some regulatory substances, such as steroid and thyroid hormones (see Chapters 41, 46, and 47), enter the cell and bind to receptors that are transcription factors activated by binding the hormone. In this way, the hormone influences the transcription of certain genes. Other regulatory substances **(agonists)** exert their influences from outside the cell. Their actions are initiated when agonists bind to **receptor proteins** in the plasma membrane, thereby initiating a sequence of events called a **signal-transduction pathway** that brings about the final actions of the agonist. Agonists that act on membrane receptors and their signal-transduction pathways are the principal topic of this chapter.

A Signal-Transduction Pathway Links the Binding of a Regulatory Substance to Its Receptor with Its Intracellular Effect

An extracellular agonist's first action is to bind to the extracellular domain of specific protein receptors in the plasma membrane of the target cells. The neurotransmitters discussed in Chapter 4 and their receptors are examples of extracellular agonists. For the neurotransmitters discussed so far, the receptor is a ligand-gated ion channel, and the response of the cell is a ligand-induced ion current. The ligand-gated ion channel is both the receptor and the **effector** for the action of the neurotransmitter.

For most agonists, however, a more complex series of events links the binding of the agonist to its membrane receptor with its final effects on cellular function. Extracellular agonists exert their effects on cells via signal-transduction pathways, whereby the binding of an agonist to its plasma membrane receptor elicits an intracellular response by altering the activities of particular cellular proteins. A comprehensive discussion of this subject is beyond the scope of this book. Therefore, only certain signal-transduction pathways, especially those relevant to topics discussed in subsequent chapters, are described.

The extracellular agonists considered may be classified as **endocrine, paracrine,** or **autocrine.** Endocrine regulatory substances **(hormones)** are released by endocrine cells, and they reach their target cells, which may be far from the endocrine cells, via the bloodstream. **Paracrine** agonists are released by cells sufficiently close that the agonist can reach the target cells by diffusion. Neurotransmitters and many neuromodulators (see Chapter 4) are paracrine agonists. Paracrine agonists are secreted by one cell type and act on cells of a different type. However, some cells release regulators that act on that cell itself or on its neighbors of the same cell type. This is called **autocrine regulation.**

Protein kinases and protein phosphatases: phosphorylation of proteins is a common element of signal-transduction pathways

One or more steps in a signal-transduction pathway frequently involve the phosphorylation of particular proteins that play central roles in eliciting cellular responses. When these proteins are phosphorylated, their activities may be enhanced or suppressed. **Protein kinases** in the cell are responsible for phosphorylating particular proteins, and **protein phosphatases** catalyze the removal of phosphates from proteins. THE STATE OF PHOSPHORYLATION OF AN EFFECTOR PROTEIN DEPENDS ON THE BALANCE OF THE ACTIVITIES OF THE KINASE THAT PHOSPHORYLATES IT AND THE PHOSPHATASE THAT DEPHOSPHORYLATES IT.

A signal-transduction pathway may alter the activity of a protein kinase in response to the binding of an agonist to an extracellular site on its membrane receptor. The major classes of agonist-activated protein kinases are shown in **Figure 5–1.**

The binding of an agonist to its receptor on the cell surface frequently begins a sequence of events that leads to a change in the intracellular concentration of a **second messenger** substance, which may act to increase the activity of a protein kinase. Second messengers that regulate the activities of protein kinases include **cAMP, cGMP, Ca^{++}, inositol 1,4,5-trisphosphate (InsP3),** and **diacylglycerol.**

Cells contain protein kinases whose activities are enhanced by cAMP and cGMP. These kinases are called **cAMP-dependent protein kinases** and **cGMP-dependent protein kinases,** respectively.

The activities of **calmodulin-dependent protein kinases** are enhanced when they bind a protein called **calmodulin.** Calmodulin (MW,

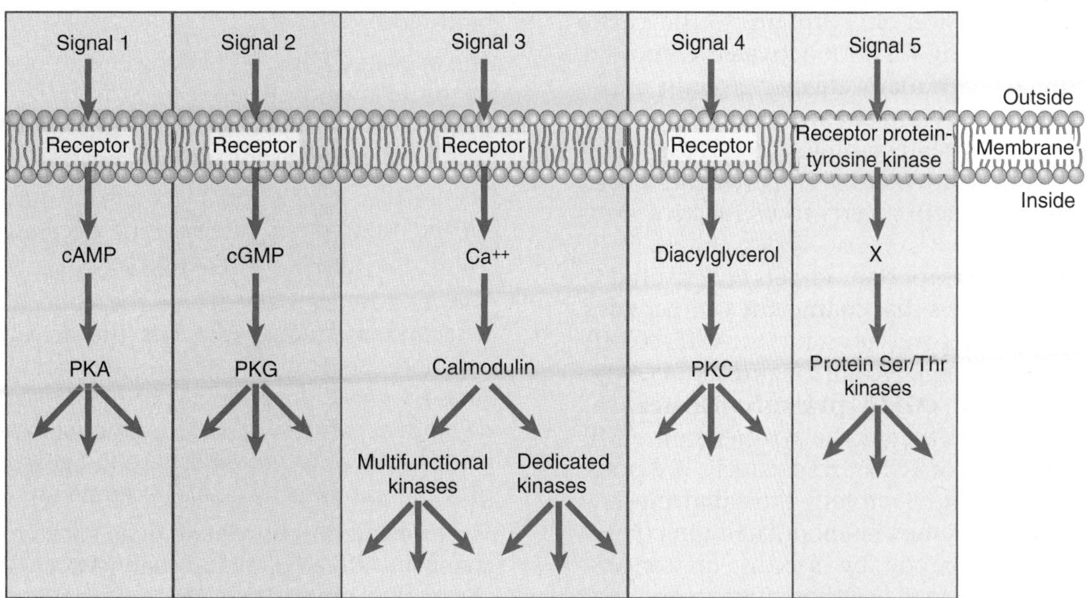

FIGURE 5–1. Signal-transduction pathways of mammalian cells involving protein kinases. PKA, cAMP-dependent protein kinase; PKC, protein kinase C; PKG, cGMP-dependent protein kinase; X, signaling pathways described later, whereby activation of a membrane receptor that phosphorylates proteins on tyrosine residues results in the activation of one or more protein kinases in the cell that phosphorylate serine or threonine residues. (Modified from Cohen P: *Trends Biochem Sci* 17:408, 1992.)

16,700) is present in all cells. Calmodulin binds four Ca^{++} ions, and the complex of Ca^{++} and calmodulin regulates a host of other intracellular proteins, many of which are not kinases.

Protein kinases of the **protein kinase C** family are activated by Ca^{++}, diacylglycerol, certain membrane phospholipids, and some breakdown products of membrane phospholipids.

Insulin and certain **growth factors** bind to membrane receptors that are themselves protein kinases that phosphorylate protein substrates on tyrosine residues. (The other protein kinases described phosphorylate proteins on serine or threonine residues.) The binding of a growth factor stimulates the **protein-tyrosine kinase** activity of the receptor.

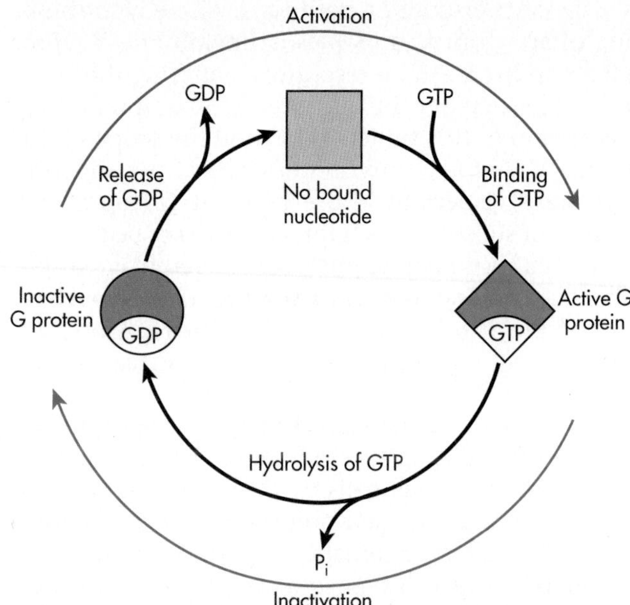

FIGURE 5–2. Activity cycle of a GTP-binding protein (G protein). The inactive form of the G protein *(blue circle)* binds GDP. The release of GDP and the binding of GTP cause the G protein to become activated *(green diamond)*. The hydrolysis of bound GTP causes the G protein to become inactivated *(blue circle)*. Pi, inorganic phosphate.

G proteins are molecular switches in signal-transduction pathways

Many hormones and other agonists alter cellular processes by signal-transduction pathways involving **heterotrimeric GTP-binding proteins,** also called simply **G proteins.** Another class of GTP-binding proteins, monomeric (or small) GTP-binding proteins, is discussed later. A G protein is a molecular switch **(Figure 5–2)** that can exist in two states. In its activated ("on") state, a G protein has a high affinity for GTP. The inactivated ("off") G protein preferentially binds GDP. When certain membrane receptors have agonist molecules bound to them, they interact with specific G proteins to promote the conversion of G proteins to their activated state by binding GTP. An activated G protein can then interact with many effector proteins, most notably enzymes or ion channels, to alter their activities. The activated G protein has GTPase activity, so eventually the bound GTP is hydrolyzed to GDP, and the G protein reverts to its inactive state (Figure 5–2).

Among the most important targets of activated G proteins are molecules that change the cellular concentrations of the second messengers cAMP, cGMP, Ca^{++}, InsP3, and diacylglycerol **(Figure 5–3). Adenylyl cyclase** and **cGMP phosphodiesterase,** the enzymes responsible for the synthesis of cAMP and the breakdown of cGMP, respectively, are powerfully modulated by G protein–mediated mechanisms. Ca^{++} channels may be modulated directly by G proteins or indirectly by second messenger–dependent protein kinases. Other effectors that are modulated by G proteins include certain K^+ channels and phospholipases C, A_2, and D.

In general, a G protein–protein kinase–mediated signal-transduction pathway involves the following events (Figure 5–3):

- A hormone or other agonist binds to its plasma membrane receptor.
- The ligand-bearing receptor interacts with a G protein and activates it; the activated G protein binds GTP.
- The activated G protein interacts with one or more of the following effectors to activate or to inhibit them: adenylyl cyclase; cGMP phosphodiesterase; Ca^{++} or K^+ channels; or phospholipases C, A_2, or D.
- The cellular level of one or more of the following second messengers increases or decreases: cAMP, cGMP, Ca^{++}, InsP3, or diacylglycerol.
- The increase or decrease of the concentration of a second messenger changes the activity of one or more second messenger–dependent protein kinases: cAMP-dependent protein kinase, cGMP-dependent protein kinase, calmodulin-dependent protein kinase, or protein kinase C. Second messengers can also directly activate certain ion channels.
- The level of phosphorylation of an enzyme or an ion channel is altered or an ion channel activity changes because of interaction with an activated G protein and causes the final cellular response.

AT EACH LEVEL OF THE SIGNAL-TRANSDUCTION CASCADE, AMPLIFICATION CAN OCCUR, SO ONE AGONIST-BEARING RECEPTOR CAN RESULT IN THE ACTIVATION OF HUNDREDS OF EFFECTORS.

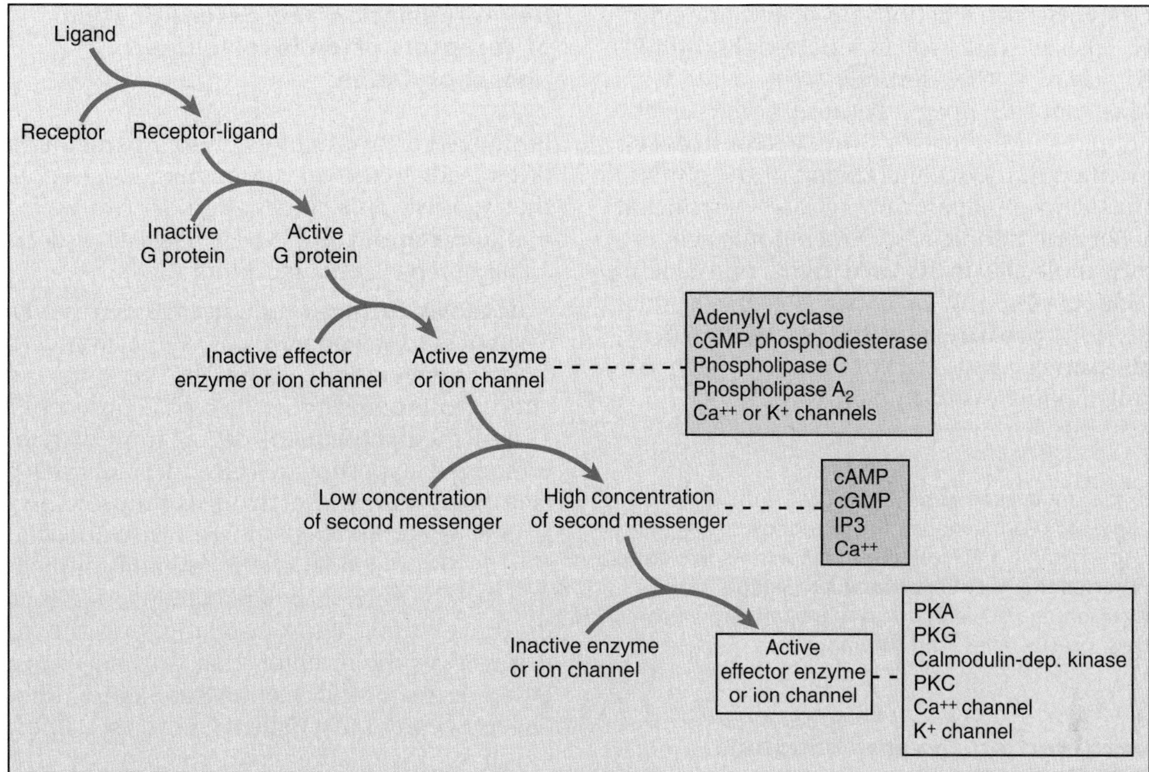

FIGURE 5–3. Signal-transduction cascade by which an extracellular ligand such as a peptide hormone can bind to its receptor to activate a G protein and, via the cascade, lead to the activation or inactivation of an ion channel, a protein kinase, or a phospholipase. The three shaded boxes to the right contain the major members of the categories to which the boxes are linked by the horizontal dashed lines.

Membrane inositol phospholipids are intermediates in certain signal-transduction pathways

Another class of extracellular agonists binds to receptors that activate a G protein called $\mathbf{G_q}$. Activated G_q stimulates the β isoform of **phospholipase C.** Phospholipase Cβ cleaves phosphatidylinositol 4,5-bisphosphate (a phospholipid present in minute quantities in the plasma membrane) into inositol 1,4,5-trisphosphate **(InsP3)** and **diacylglycerol (Figure 5–4)**, both of which are second messengers. InsP3 binds to specific ligand-gated Ca^{++} channels in the endoplasmic reticulum to release Ca^{++}, thereby increasing cytosolic [Ca^{++}]. Diacylglycerol, together with Ca^{++}, activates protein kinase C. Ca^{++} causes cytosolic protein kinase C to be bound to the plasma membrane, thus promoting its activation by diacylglycerol and certain other membrane phospholipids, notably phosphatidyl serine. Among the substrates of protein kinase C are certain proteins involved in the control of gene transcription and cellular proliferation.

The enzymes **phospholipase A_2** and **phospholipase D** are also activated by some agonists via G protein–independent pathways. Certain prod-

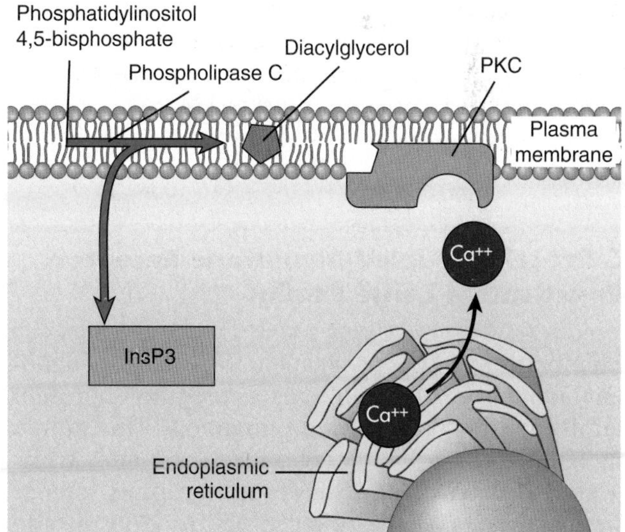

FIGURE 5–4. Signal-transduction pathway activated by the hydrolysis of inositol phospholipids of the plasma membrane. Activation of G_q by an agonist stimulates the hydrolysis of phosphatidylinositol 4,5-bisphosphate to form InsP3 and diacylglycerol. InsP3 releases Ca^{++} from the endoplasmic reticulum. Binding of Ca^{++} to PKC promotes the translocation of PKC to the plasma membrane, where diacylglycerol, together with Ca^{++}, activates PKC.

ucts of these enzymes' actions on membrane phospholipids also activate protein kinase C. Phospholipase A_2 cleaves the second fatty acid from membrane phospholipids. Because some of the phospholipids are species with **arachidonic acid** esterified to the second carbon of the glycerol backbone, phospholipase A_2 releases significant amounts of arachidonic acid. Arachidonic acid is a regulatory molecule in its own right, and arachidonic acid is also the precursor for the cellular synthesis of **prostaglandins, prostacyclins, thromboxanes,** and **leukotrienes,** which are important modulators of inflammation.

> One of the antiinflammatory actions of corticosteroids (see Chapter 47) is inhibition of the phospholipase A_2 that releases arachidonic acid from phospholipids. Aspirin and other nonsteroidal antiinflammatory agents inhibit the conversion of arachidonic acid to inflammatory prostaglandins, prostacyclins, and thromboxanes.

Signal-transduction cascades initiated by growth factors involve protein-tyrosine kinases

Proteins with intrinsic **protein-tyrosine kinase** activity make up another family of membrane receptors not linked to G proteins. When these receptors bind agonist, their tyrosine kinase activity is stimulated, and they phosphorylate specific effector proteins on particular tyrosine residues. The receptor for the hormone insulin and receptors for many growth factors are tyrosine kinases.

G Protein–Coupled Membrane Receptors Constitute a Large Family

Membrane receptors that mediate agonist-dependent activation of G proteins constitute a protein family with more than 500 members. This family includes α- and β-adrenergic receptors, muscarinic acetylcholine receptors, serotonin receptors, adenosine receptors, olfactory receptors, rhodopsin, and receptors for most peptide hormones. The members of the G protein–coupled receptor family have seven transmembrane α helices, each made up of 22 to 28 predominantly hydrophobic amino acids. After a receptor binds an agonist, the receptor undergoes a conformational change that enables the receptor to interact with and activate a specific type of G protein.

Down-regulation and desensitization of receptors often involve their phosphorylation

Prolonged exposure of a cell to a particular agonist often leads to the cell's becoming less responsive to that agonist. This comes about in two ways:

- **down-regulation**, which refers to a decrease in the number of the receptors;
- **desensitization**, which means a decreased responsiveness to the agonist.

Down-regulation occurs by receptor-mediated endocytosis of receptors via coated pits (see Chapter 1) and their subsequent degradation in lysosomes. Prolonged exposure of cells to epidermal growth factor and many other agonists for protein-tyrosine kinase receptors elicits down-regulation via endocytosis and degradation. G protein–coupled receptors may be phosphorylated when cAMP is elevated in the cytosol. Phosphorylation of the receptor desensitizes the receptor, that is to say, phosphorylation decreases the receptor's ability to influence its effector protein (e.g., adenylyl cyclase). Phosphorylation of the β-adrenergic receptor by a specific protein kinase permits the receptor to associate with a regulatory protein called **β-arrestin**. The binding of β-arrestin both desensitizes the β-adrenergic receptor and promotes its internalization via coated pits. There is a family of arrestins, each specific for down-regulating a particular class of G protein–coupled receptors.

G proteins are either heterotrimeric or monomeric

Heterotrimeric G proteins have three different subunits

A heterotrimeric G protein has three subunits: α (40,000 to 45,000 Da), β (≈37,000 Da), and γ (8,000 to 10,000 Da). At least 22 different genes encode α subunits, at least 5 genes encode β subunits, and about 12 genes encode γ subunits in mammals. The β and γ subunits are tightly associated with each other. Some heterotrimeric G proteins and the signal-transduction pathways they mediate are listed in **Table 5–1.**

The α subunit is frequently the "business end" of the heterotrimeric G protein **(Figure 5–5).** The inactive G protein exists primarily as the αβγ heterotrimer, with GDP in the nucleotide binding site of the α subunit. The interaction of the heterotrimeric G protein with a ligand-bearing receptor causes a conformational change in the α subunit to the active form, which has a higher affinity for GTP and a lower affinity for the βγ pair.

TABLE 5–1. SELECTED MAMMALIAN HETEROTRIMERIC G PROTEINS CLASSIFIED ON THE BASIS OF THEIR α SUBUNITS*

G Protein	Activated by Receptors for	Effectors	Signaling Pathways
G_s	Epinephrine, norepinephrine, histamine, glucagon, adrenocorticotropic hormone, luteinizing hormone, follicle-stimulating hormone, thyroid-stimulating hormone, others	Adenylyl cyclase Ca^{++} channels	↑ cAMP ↑ Ca^{++} influx
G_{olf}	Odorants	Adenylyl cyclase	↑ AMP (olfaction)
G_{t1} (rods)	Photons	cGMP phosphodiesterase	↓ cGMP (vision)
G_{t2} (cones)	Photons	cGMP phosphodiesterase	↓ cGMP (color vision)
G_{i1}, G_{i2}, G_{i3}	Norepinephrine, prostaglandins, opiates, angiotensin, many peptides	Adenylyl cyclase Phospholipase C Phospholipase A_2 K^+ channels	↓ cAMP ↑ InsP3, diacylglycerol, Ca^{++}
G_q	Acetylcholine, epinephrine	Phospholipase Cβ	Membrane polarization ↑ InsP3, diacylglycerol, Ca^{++}

*There is more than one isoform of each class of α subunit; more than 20 distinct α subunits have been identified.

The activated α subunit releases GDP, binds GTP, and then dissociates from βγ. The dissociated α subunit then interacts with the next protein in the signal-transduction pathway. In some cases, however, the βγ dimer is responsible for all or some of the receptor-mediated response.

Regulation of adenylyl cyclase was the first G protein–mediated regulatory pathway to be discovered

cAMP was the first of the second messengers to be discovered, and the regulation of adenylyl cyclase, the enzyme that produces cAMP, is the prototype for G protein–mediated signal-transduction pathways. Adenylyl cyclase is subject to both positive and negative control by G protein–mediated pathways (Figure 5–5). The binding of a stimulatory ligand, such as epinephrine acting through β-adrenergic receptors, results in the activation of heterotrimeric G proteins with α subunits of the type called α_s (*s* for stimulatory). Activation of the G_s-type G protein by the agonist-bearing receptor causes its α_s subunit to bind GTP and then to dissociate from βγ. The α_s subunit then interacts with adenylyl cyclase to activate it.

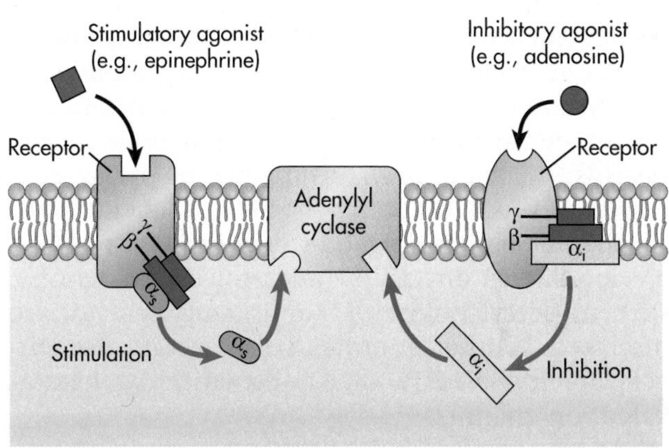

FIGURE 5–5. Receptors for agonists that stimulate adenylyl cyclase activate G_s, whose α_s subunit *(green)* dissociates from βγ and then interacts with adenylyl cyclase to stimulate it. Receptors for agonists that inhibit adenylyl cyclase activate G_i, whose α_i subunit *(yellow)* inhibits adenylyl cyclase.

Patients suffering from **cholera** experience profound diarrhea. A patient with cholera may produce up to 20 L/day of watery stool. Such patients are likely to die unless they are promptly and adequately rehydrated. Cholera is caused by **cholera toxin** that is produced by the bacterium *Vibrio cholerae.* Cholera toxin catalyzes the transfer of ADP-ribose to α_s, thereby locking α_s in the activated state. Consequently, adenylyl cyclase is persistently stimulated and thereby elevates the level of cAMP in intestinal epithelial cells. The elevated cAMP levels cause the secretion of Cl^-, Na^+, and water into the intestinal lumen by the cells in the crypts of Lieberkühn and diminished absorption of salts and water by intestinal epithelial cells near the tips of the intestinal villi. These responses cause the massive diarrhea associated with cholera.

Other regulatory substances, such as epinephrine acting at α_2 receptors and adenosine acting on A_1 receptors, inhibit adenylyl cyclase by activating G_i-type G proteins, which have α subunits of a different type, called α_i (*i* for inhibitory). Binding of the inhibitory ligand to its receptor activates the G_i-type G protein and causes its α_i subunit to dissociate from the βγ dimers. The activated α_i binds to and inhibits adenylyl cyclase. In addition, the βγ dimers may bind to free α_s subunits and thus diminish the stimulation of adenylyl cyclase by stimulatory agonists.

Certain ion channels are directly modulated by G proteins

Some ion channels are directly modulated by G proteins without the involvement of a second messenger. The binding of acetylcholine to muscarinic receptors in the heart and in certain neurons leads to the activation of a specific class of K^+ channels. Acetylcholine binding to the muscarinic receptor leads to the activation of a G protein of the G_i subclass. The activated α_i subunit then dissociates from the βγ dimer. The βγ dimer directly interacts with a particular class of K^+ channels to increase their probability of opening. The action of acetylcholine on muscarinic receptors to increase K^+ conductance of the pacemaker cells in the sinoatrial node of the heart is the major mechanism whereby parasympathetic nerves slow the heart rate (see Chapter 19). In Chapter 4, several ligand-gated ion channels that are modulated directly by an extracellular agonist, such as acetylcholine or γ-aminobutyric acid, are discussed. Neither G proteins nor second messengers are involved in direct regulation of ligand-gated ion channels.

Certain ion channels are directly modulated by a second messenger

IN SOME CASES, A SECOND MESSENGER ACTS DIRECTLY ON AN ION CHANNEL TO PRODUCE A RESPONSE. Some cells have K^+ channels that are directly activated by Ca^{++}. When intracellular Ca^{++} levels rise, **Ca^{++}-activated K^+ channels** are stimulated, which leads to repolarization or hyperpolarization of the cell.

Vision (see Chapter 8) depends on cGMP-gated ion channels. In the dark, the level of cGMP in rod photoreceptors is high. Consequently, the **cGMP-activated Na^+ channels** in the rod plasma membrane are open, and Na^+ entry maintains the rod cells in a depolarized state. **Rhodopsin** is a member of the family of G protein–coupled receptors. When rhodopsin is activated by light, it interacts with and activates a heterotrimeric G protein called **transducin (G_t).** Activated G_t interacts with cGMP phosphodiesterase to greatly increase its activity, causing a rapid decrease in the intracellular cGMP concentration. As a consequence, the cGMP-activated Na^+ channels close, and the photoreceptor cell becomes hyperpolarized. The subsequent neural processing of this signal that leads to vision is described in Chapter 8.

Olfaction (see Chapter 8) involves cAMP-gated ion channels. Humans can distinguish a large number of different odorants. Many of the odorants interact with G protein–coupled receptors in the plasma membrane of olfactory receptor cells. The odorant-bearing receptor activates **G_{olf},** a heterotrimeric G protein. Activated G_{olf} in turn stimulates adenylyl cyclase to produce cAMP. Elevated cAMP levels activate **cAMP-gated Na^+ channels** in the plasma membrane of the olfactory receptor cell. Na^+ inflow leads to depolarization of the receptor, which may trigger an action potential in the axon of the olfactory receptor.

Monomeric GTP-binding proteins regulate several cellular processes

Cells contain another family of GTP-binding proteins called **monomeric GTP-binding proteins;** they are also known as **low-molecular-weight G proteins** or **small G proteins** (MW, 20,000 to 35,000). **Table 5–2** lists the major subfamilies of monomeric GTP-binding proteins and some of their properties. The Ras-like and Rho-like monomeric GTP-binding proteins are involved in the signal-transduction pathways that link growth factor receptor tyrosine kinases to their intracellular effects. Among the processes regulated by pathways

TABLE 5–2. SUBFAMILIES OF MONOMERIC GTP-BINDING PROTEINS AND SOME OF THE INTRACELLULAR PROCESSES THEY REGULATE

Subfamily	Cellular Effects
Ras-like proteins	Control growth and differentiation
Rho-like proteins (including Rac)	Control polymerization of actin filaments and their assembly into particular structures such as focal adhesions
Rab-like proteins	Control vesicle trafficking by helping target vesicles to particular membranes
ARF-like proteins	Regulate the assembly and disassembly of vesicle coat proteins and thereby control vesicle traffic

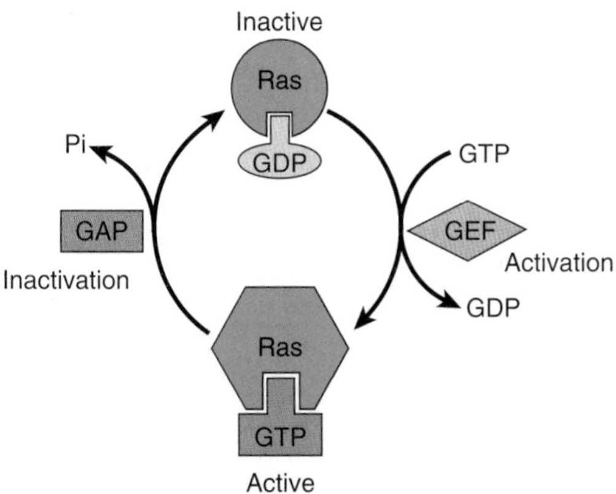

FIGURE 5–6. Activity cycle of Ras, a monomeric GTP-binding protein. The activation of Ras is enhanced by a guanine nucleotide exchange factor (GEF). The inactivation of Ras is promoted by a GTPase-activating protein (GAP). Pi, inorganic phosphate.

involving monomeric GTP-binding proteins are polypeptide chain elongation in protein synthesis, proliferation and differentiation of cells, neoplastic transformation of cells, control of the actin cytoskeleton and links between the cytoskeleton and the extracellular matrix, transport of vesicles among different organelles, and exocytotic secretion. Like their heterotrimeric cousins, monomeric GTP-binding proteins operate via the cycle of activation and inactivation shown in Figure 5–2. However, the activation and inactivation of the monomolecular GTP-binding proteins involve additional regulatory proteins that do not operate on the heterotrimeric G proteins (**Figure 5–6**). The activation of monomeric GTP-binding proteins is enhanced by **guanine nucleotide exchange factors (GEFs),** and inactivation is promoted by **GTPase-activating proteins (GAPs).** The activation and inactivation of monomeric GTP-binding proteins can occur via upstream signals that influence the activity of GEFs or GAPs, rather than by direct effects on the monomeric G protein.

A Second Messenger–Dependent Protein Kinase Is Modulated by the Cellular Level of a Second Messenger

cAMP-dependent protein kinase (PKA) participates in regulating important metabolic pathways

cAMP was first identified as a second messenger in investigations of the mechanisms involved in the hormonal control of glycogen synthesis and breakdown (see Chapters 42 and 43). The phosphorylation of rate-determining enzymes in these metabolic pathways by cAMP-dependent protein kinases is responsible for the hormonal regulation of glycogen metabolism.

In the absence of cAMP, PKA is composed of four subunits, two regulatory subunits and two catalytic subunits. The presence of the regulatory subunits greatly inhibits the enzymatic activity of the complex. In the presence of micromolar levels of cAMP, each regulatory subunit binds two molecules of cAMP. The binding of cAMP causes the regulatory subunits to dissociate from the catalytic subunits, and in this way the catalytic subunits become activated. The active catalytic subunit phosphorylates target proteins on particular serine and threonine residues.

Comparison of the amino acid sequence of PKA with representatives of the other classes of protein kinases shows that in spite of vast differences in their regulatory properties, the different classes of protein kinases share a common core with high amino acid homology (**Figure 5–7**). The core structure includes the ATP-binding domain and the enzyme's active center, where phosphate from ATP is transferred to the acceptor protein. The three-dimensional structures of the core regions of the different protein kinases also have many features in common. Regions of the kinases outside the catalytic core may participate in the regulation of kinase activity.

Calmodulin-dependent protein kinases are activated by the complex of Ca^{++} with calmodulin

A host of vital cellular processes, including the release of neurotransmitters, the secretion of hormones, and muscle contraction, are regulated by the cytosolic level of Ca^{++}. One way that Ca^{++} exerts control is by binding to calmodulin. The complex of Ca^{++} and calmodulin can then influence the activity of many different proteins, among them a group of protein kinases known as **calmodulin-dependent protein kinases** (**Figure 5–8**). Dedicated calmodulin-dependent protein kinases, such as myosin light-chain kinase and phosphorylase kinase, have only one cellular substrate. Multifunctional calmodulin-dependent protein kinases phosphorylate more than one substrate protein.

Myosin light-chain kinase plays a central role in regulating the contraction of smooth muscle (see Chapter 14). Elevation of cytosolic [Ca^{++}] in a smooth muscle cell stimulates the activity of myosin light-chain kinase; the resulting phosphorylation of the regulatory light chains of myosin allows the contraction of smooth muscle cells to proceed.

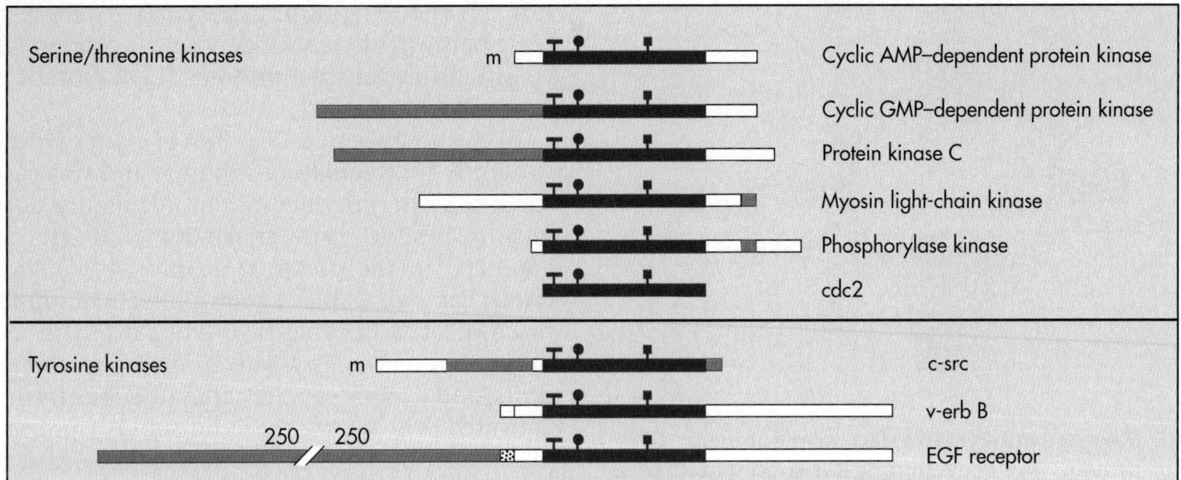

FIGURE 5–7. Protein kinase family. All known protein kinases share a common catalytic core *(blue)* that contains ATP- and peptide-binding domains and an active site where phosphoryl transfer occurs. Conserved residues are aligned with lysine 72 *(blue circles)*, aspartate 184 *(blue squares)*, and the glycine-rich loop *(blue rectangles)* of the catalytic subunit of cAMP-dependent protein kinase. Regions important for regulation are orange. The membrane-spanning segment of the epidermal growth factor (EGF) receptor is stippled. Sites of myristoylation are indicated by *m*. A covalently attached myristic acid residue helps anchor the protein kinase in the plasma membrane. (Modified from Taylor S et al: *Annu Rev Cell Biol* 8:429, 1992.)

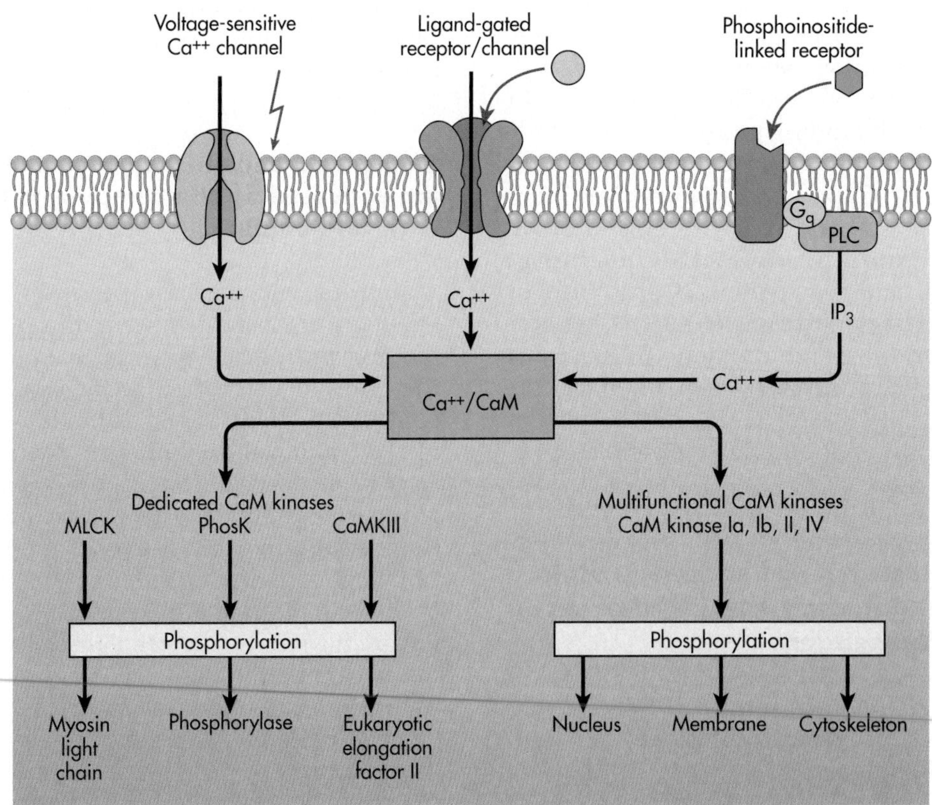

FIGURE 5–8. Dedicated calmodulin-dependent protein kinases phosphorylate specific effector proteins. Multifunctional calmodulin-dependent protein kinases phosphorylate multiple proteins of the nucleus or cytoskeleton or membrane proteins. CaM, calmodulin; CaMKIII, calmodulin-dependent kinase III; MLCK, myosin light-chain kinase; PhosK, phosphorylase kinase; PLC, phospholipase C. (Modified from Schulman H: *Curr Opin Cell Biol* 5:247, 1993.)

TABLE 5–3. PROPERTIES OF MAMMALIAN ISOZYMES OF PROTEIN KINASE C

Group	Subspecies	Apparent Molecular Mass (Da)	Activators	Tissue Expression
cPKC	α	76,799	Ca^{++}, DAG, PS, FFA, LysoPC	Universal
	βI	76,790	Ca^{++}, DAG, PS, FFA, LysoPC	Some tissues
	βII	76,933	Ca^{++}, DAG, PS, FFA, LysoPC	Many tissues
	γ	78,366	Ca^{++}, DAG, PS, FFA, LysoPC	Brain only
nPKC	δ	77,517	DAG, PS	Universal
	ε	83,474	DAG, PS, FFA	Brain, muscle
	η(L)	77,972	?	Lung, skin, heart lymphocytes, glia
	θ	81,571	?	Skeletal muscle, lymphocytes
aPKC	ζ	67,740	PS, FFA	Universal
	λ	67,200	?	Ovary, testis, others

DAG, diacylglycerol; PS, phosphatidylserine; FFA, *cis*-unsaturated fatty acids; LysoPC, lysophosphatidylcholine.

Calmodulin-dependent protein kinase II is among the most abundant proteins in the nervous system. This kinase participates in the mechanism by which an increase in Ca^{++} in a nerve terminal causes the exocytotic release of neurotransmitter (see Chapter 4).

Protein kinase C (PKC) is activated by Ca^{++} and membrane lipids

The primary action of certain lipophilic tumor-promoting substances, most notably the phorbol esters, is direct activation of **PKC.** This powerfully stimulates cell division in many cell types and converts normal cells with controlled growth properties into transformed cells (tumor cells) that grow uncontrollably.

In an unstimulated cell, much of the PKC is present in the cytosol and is inactive. When cytosolic levels of Ca^{++} rise, Ca^{++} binds to PKC. The binding of Ca^{++} causes PKC to bind to the inner surface of the plasma membrane, where it can be activated by the diacylglycerol produced by the hydrolysis of phosphatidylinositol 4,5-bisphosphate. Other membrane phospholipids, notably phosphatidyl serine, and some of their breakdown products (free fatty acids and lysophosphatidyl choline) can also activate PKC. About 10 different isoforms of PKC have been discovered (**Table 5–3**).

Tyrosine Kinases Play Key Roles in the Control of Cellular Proliferation

Receptors for certain growth factors are tyrosine kinases

The receptors for certain peptide hormones and growth factors are proteins with glycosylated extracellular domains, a single transmembrane sequence, and an intracellular domain with protein-tyrosine kinase activity. Members of this superfamily of peptide receptors include the receptors for insulin and related growth factors, epidermal growth factor, nerve growth factor, platelet-derived growth factor, colony-stimulating factor, fibroblast growth factor, and hepatocyte growth factor. The binding of hormone or growth factor to its receptor triggers multiple cellular responses, including Ca^{++} influx, increased Na^+-H^+ antiport activity, stimulation of the uptake of sugars and amino acids, and stimulation of phospholipase Cβ to hydrolyze phosphatidylinositol 4,5-bisphosphate.

The known protein-tyrosine kinase receptors fall into eight subfamilies. The binding of ligand to the receptor results in dimerization of the receptor-ligand complexes. The dimerization enhances binding affinity and activates the protein-tyrosine kinase activity. Each monomer in a dimer phosphorylates the other monomer on multiple tyrosine residues. In subclass II receptors, the insulin receptor family, the unliganded receptor exists as a disulfide-linked dimer, and binding of insulin results in a conformational change of both "monomers." This conformational change enhances insulin binding and activates the receptor's tyrosine kinase activity, which leads to enhanced autophosphorylation of the receptor's cytoplasmic domains.

Protein-tyrosine kinases that are "out of control" play a central role in cell transformation and cancer. In some cell types, a mutation of a growth factor receptor renders the receptor active in phosphorylating tyrosines regardless of the presence or absence of the growth factor. Other tumor cells secrete a growth factor and overexpress its receptor. This leads to abnormally high rates of protein-tyrosine kinase activity and to uncontrolled cell division.

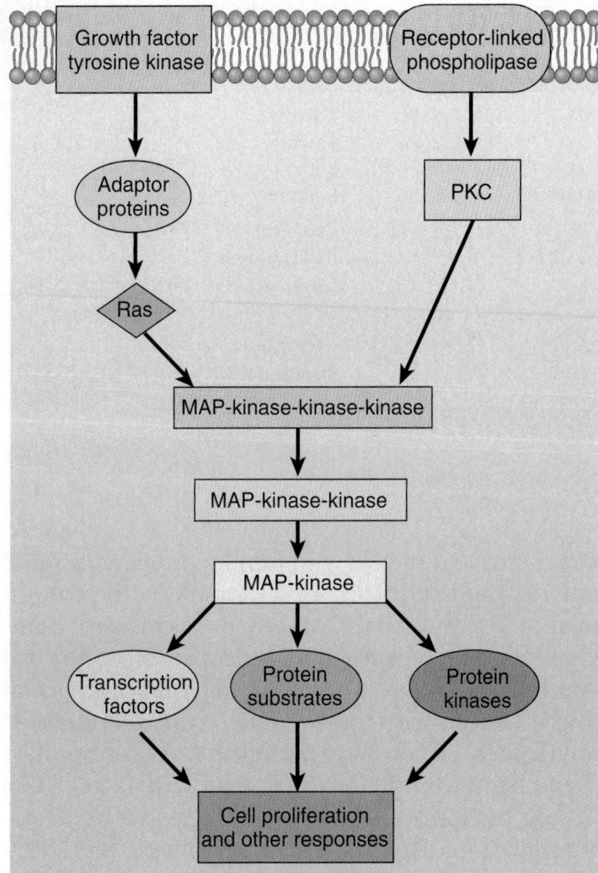

FIGURE 5–9. The MAP kinase cascade is involved in the cell-proliferation responses elicited by agonists that stimulate protein kinase C and by growth factors that activate membrane protein-tyrosine kinase receptors. MAP-kinase-kinase-kinase can be activated either by activated Ras or by PKC. The cascade results in the phosphorylation and activation of MAP kinase, which in turn phosphorylates transcription factors, protein substrates, and other protein kinases important in eliciting proliferation and other cellular responses.

Monomeric GTP-binding proteins of the Ras family (Table 5–2) are involved in coupling the binding of mitogenic ligands and their protein-tyrosine kinase receptors to the resulting intracellular effects on cell proliferation. When Ras is inactive, cells cannot respond to the growth factors that operate via receptor tyrosine kinases.

Mutations in Ras may produce overactive forms of Ras that constitutively activate the downstream effectors normally active only in the presence of growth factors. In such cases, cell growth may be uncontrolled, even in the absence of growth factors. Approximately 30% of human cancers involve mutations of Ras.

The activation of Ras by an activated receptor tyrosine kinase in turn activates a signal-transduction pathway, which ultimately turns on the transcription of certain key genes that promote cell growth. The **mitogen-activated protein (MAP) kinase cascade** (**Figure 5–9**) is involved in the responses to activated Ras. Protein kinase C also activates the MAP kinase cascade. The MAP kinase cascade is an important point of convergence for multiple effectors that promote cellular proliferation.

Certain other growth factor receptors form complexes with intracellular tyrosine kinases

The receptors for **growth hormone, prolactin,** and **erythropoietin** (as well as receptors for interferon and many cytokines) are not themselves protein kinases. However, on activation, these receptors form signaling complexes with intracellular tyrosine kinases that bring about their intracellular effects (**Figure 5–10**). The binding of hormone

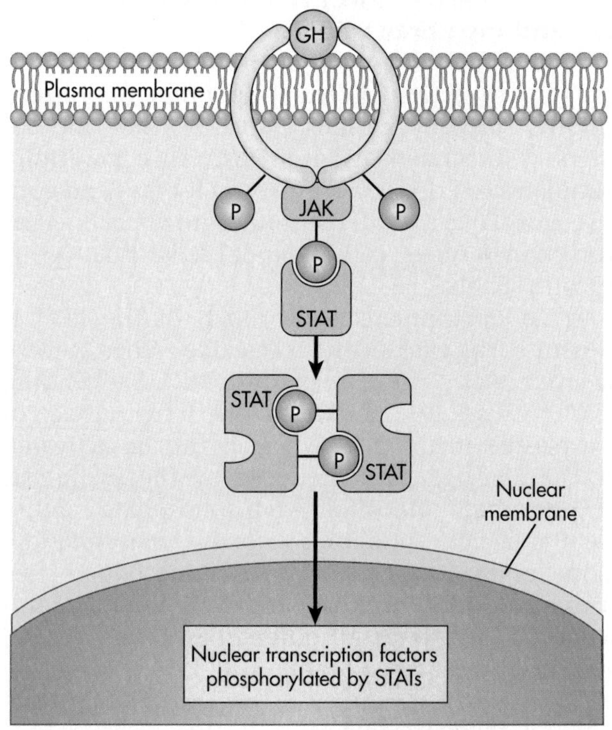

FIGURE 5–10. Receptors for growth hormone (GH) have no intrinsic tyrosine kinase activity. The receptor dimerizes in response to GH binding. The dimeric receptor binds one or more JAK tyrosine kinases, which phosphorylate themselves and the receptor. STAT tyrosine kinases bind to the complex and are phosphorylated. The phosphorylated STATs dissociate as dimers that are translocated to the nucleus, where they phosphorylate key transcription factors. P, phosphate.

TABLE 5–4. PROPERTIES OF SUBTYPES OF SERINE/THREONINE PROTEIN PHOSPHATASES

Subtype	PP-1	PP-2A	PP-2B	PP-2C
Preferred subunit of phosphorylase kinase	β Subunit	α Subunit	α Subunit	α Subunit
Inhibition by interleukin-1 and interleukin-2	Yes	No	No	No
Absolute requirement for divalent cations	No	No	Yes (Ca^{++})	Yes (Mg^{++})
Stimulation by calmodulin	No	No	Yes	No
Inhibition by okadaic acid	Yes (20 nM)	Yes (0.2 nM)	Yes (5 μM)	No
Phosphorylase phosphatase activity	High	High	Very low	Very low

induces dimerization of the hormone receptor. The receptor dimer binds one or more members of the **Janus family** of tyrosine kinases **(JAKs)**. The JAKs then cross-phosphorylate one another and also phosphorylate the receptor. Members of the **signal transducers and activators of transcription (STAT) family** bind to phosphotyrosine domains on the complex of receptor and JAK proteins. The STAT proteins are phosphorylated by the JAKs and then dissociate from the signaling complex. The phosphorylated STAT proteins form dimers that move to the nucleus to activate the transcription of certain genes.

Protein Phosphatases Undo the Work of Protein Kinases

The extent of phosphorylation of a regulated protein depends on the activities of the protein kinase that phosphorylates the protein and the protein phosphatase that dephosphorylates it. In addition to the different types of protein kinases discussed, all cells also contain protein phosphatases whose task is to reverse the effects of protein phosphorylation. Protein phosphatases are classified as **protein-serine/threonine phosphatases** or **protein-tyrosine phosphatases.**

Serine/threonine protein phosphatases are subject to complex regulation

The serine/threonine protein phosphatases are a large family of structurally related molecules. They are classified as type 1 **(PP-1)** or type 2 **(PP-2).** The type is based on which subunit of phosphorylase kinase they prefer to dephosphorylate **(Table 5–4).** PP-2 is further subclassified into PP-2A, PP-2B, and PP-2C on the basis of regulation by Ca^{++} and Mg^{++} and susceptibility to being inhibited by okadaic acid, a complex fatty acid produced by marine dinoflagellates. PP-2B is also called **calcineurin,** and it is especially abundant in certain regions of the brain.

There are a large number of different protein-tyrosine phosphatases

Protein-tyrosine phosphatases are not structurally homologous to serine/threonine protein phosphatases. **Figure 5–11** depicts four of the more than 65 known protein-tyrosine phosphatases. Whereas two are small cytosolic proteins, two others are larger transmembrane proteins. Some of the transmembrane protein-tyrosine phosphatases are receptors whose phosphatase activity is modulated by extracellular ligands.

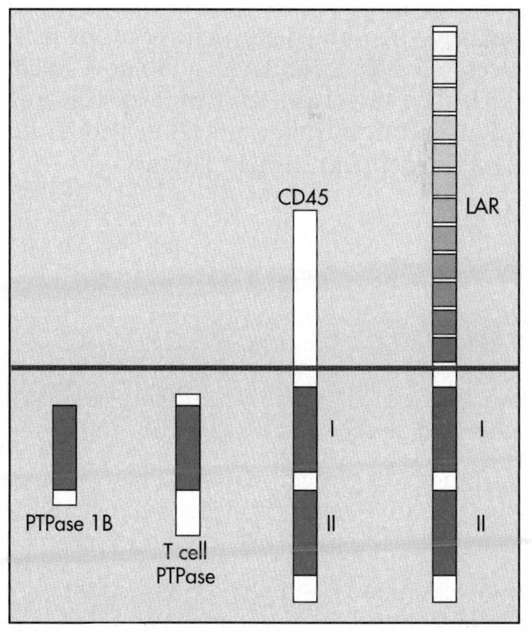

FIGURE 5–11. Four of more than 65 known protein-tyrosine phosphatases (PTPases). PTPase 1B from human placenta and PTPase from human T cells are small cytosolic PTPases. CD45 (leukocyte common antigen) and LAR (leukocyte common antigen–related protein) are transmembrane PTPases. The orange cytosolic segments of each protein are their PTPase catalytic domains. (Modified from Tonks NK, Charbonneau H: *Trends Biochem Sci* 14:497, 1989.)

Atrial Natriuretic Peptide Receptors Have Guanylyl Cyclase Activity

Atrial natriuretic peptide (ANP) is released by cells in the atrium of the heart in response to an elevation of atrial pressure. This hormone increases the excretion of NaCl and water by the kidney (see Chapter 38) and diminishes the constriction of certain blood vessels. The membrane receptors for ANP themselves possess guanylyl cyclase activity that is stimulated when ANP is bound to the receptor. No second messenger is required to activate guanylyl cyclase. ANP receptors have an extracellular ANP-binding domain, a single transmembrane helix, and an intracellular guanylyl cyclase domain. The binding of ANP stimulates the guanylyl cyclase activity and elevates intracellular levels of the second messenger cGMP.

Nitric Oxide Is a Short-Lived Paracrine Mediator

Nitric oxide (NO) is a paracrine mediator that is released by endothelial cells and certain neurons. NO is rapidly oxidized, so its biological lifetime is only several seconds. For this reason, NO affects only cells in the immediate vicinity of the cell that produces it. NO stimulates a soluble guanylyl cyclase in the target cell and thereby elevates the intracellular concentration of cGMP, thus stimulating cGMP-dependent protein kinase.

The production of NO is catalyzed by **NO synthase,** a Ca^{++}-calmodulin–dependent enzyme that accelerates the conversion of arginine to citrulline plus NO. An increase in cytosolic Ca^{++} levels is often the stimulus for the enhanced formation and release of NO. NO is a neurotransmitter that is released by nerve terminals of certain neurons in the central nervous system (see Chapter 4) and by some neurons of the enteric nervous system (see Chapter 33). NO is released by endothelial cells in response to agonists such as acetylcholine. NO released by endothelial cells acts on nearby vascular smooth muscle cells to cause vasodilation (see Chapter 23).

Signal Transduction Components Are Localized Within the Cell

If kinases, phosphatases, and the proteins that regulate them were all free to diffuse in the cytoplasm, it would be difficult to achieve the temporal and spatial specificity of particular agonist-initiated responses. cAMP-stimulated protein kinases, for example, are bound to particular intracellular proteins by members of a family of **A kinase anchoring proteins (AKAPs)**. Serine/threonine protein phosphatases are commonly anchored to particular subcellular structures via targeting subunits that are associated with the catalytic phosphatase subunit. The specific localization of kinases and phosphatases permits the coordination of the myriad cellular processes regulated by signal-transduction pathways.

Summary

- Heterotrimeric GTP-binding proteins serve as intermediaries between a receptor that has been activated by binding an agonist and enzymes and ion channels whose activity is modulated in response to agonist binding.
- A GTP-binding protein is activated by interacting with an agonist-bearing receptor. It then changes the activity of an enzyme or an ion channel and thereby alters the intracellular concentration of a second messenger, such as cAMP, cGMP, Ca^{++}, InsP3, or diacylglycerol.
- An increased level of a second messenger may increase the activity of a second messenger–dependent protein kinase: cAMP-dependent protein kinase, cGMP-dependent protein kinase, calmodulin-dependent protein kinase, or protein kinase C.
- Myriad cellular processes are regulated via the phosphorylation of enzymes and ion channels.
- Certain membrane receptors for hormones and growth factors are protein-tyrosine kinases or are associated with tyrosine kinases activated by binding of the agonist.
- Monomeric GTP-binding proteins are intermediaries between the binding of growth factors to their protein-tyrosine kinase receptors and the downstream effects on cellular proliferation.

- The small G proteins also regulate the function of the actin cytoskeleton and intracellular vesicular trafficking.
- Protein phosphatases, themselves subject to complex regulation by agonists and second messengers, reverse the effects of protein phosphorylation.

Bibliography

Bayer KU, Schulman H: Regulation of signal transduction by protein targeting: the case for CaMKII, *Biochem Biophys Res Commun* 289:917, 2001.

Cohen P: Protein kinases—the major drug targets of the twenty-first century? *Nat Rev Drug Discov* 1:309, 2002.

Cohen P: The regulation of protein function by multisite phosphorylation—a 25 year update, *Trends Biochem Sci* 25:596, 2000.

Etienne-Manneville S, Hall A: Rho GTPases in cell biology, *Nature* 420:629, 2002.

Hudmon A, Schulman H: Structure-function of the multifunctional Ca^{2+}/calmodulin-dependent protein kinase II, *Biochem J* 364:593, 2002.

Kohout TA, Lefkowitz RJ: Regulation of G protein–coupled receptor kinases and arrestins during receptor desensitization, *Mol Pharmacol* 63:9, 2003.

Krumenacker JS, Hanafy KA, Murad F: Regulation of nitric oxide and soluble guanylyl cyclase, *Brain Res Bull* 62:505, 2004.

Meng EC, Bourne HR: Receptor activation: what does the rhodopsin structure tell us? *Trends Pharmacol Sci* 22:587, 2001.

Nishizuka Y: Discovery and prospect of protein kinase C research: epilogue, *J Biochem* 133:155, 2003.

Pierce KL, Luttrell LM, Lefkowitz RJ: New mechanisms in heptahelical receptor signaling to mitogen activated protein kinase cascades, *Oncogene* 20:1532, 2001.

Pierce KL, Premont RT, Lefkowitz RJ: Seven-transmembrane receptors, *Nat Rev Mol Cell Biol* 3:639, 2002.

Schmidt A, Hall A: Guanine nucleotide exchange factors for Rho GTPases: turning on the switch, *Genes Dev* 16:1587, 2002.

Spiegel AM, Weinstein LS: Inherited diseases involving G proteins and G protein–coupled receptors, *Annu Rev Med* 55:27, 2004.

Tonks NK, Neel BG: Combinatorial control of the specificity of protein tyrosine phosphatases, *Curr Opin Cell Biol* 13:182, 2001.

Self-Assessment

1. **Which statement about heterotrimeric G proteins is true?**
   A. Activation involves binding GDP.
   B. Interaction with an agonist-bearing receptor promotes inactivation of a G protein.
   C. Activation is reversed when GTP is bound.
   D. On activation, the α subunit tends to separate from βγ.

2. **Which statement about inositol phospholipid–linked signaling is true?**
   A. Agonists that activate G_q increase the activity of phospholipase Cβ.
   B. Cleavage of phosphatidylinositol bisphosphate produces InsP3 and fatty acids.
   C. Protein kinase C is stimulated in the cytoplasm by diacylglycerol.
   D. InsP3 causes uptake of Ca^{++} by the endoplasmic reticulum.

3. **Which statement about regulation of ion channels is true?**
   A. Acetylcholine binding to muscarinic receptors leads to opening of Na^+ channels.
   B. The action of acetylcholine on K^+ channels is mediated by βγ subunits.
   C. cAMP-activated Na^+ channels in rod cells are opened by light.
   D. cGMP-activated K^+ channels in olfactory cells are opened by odorants.

4. **Which statement about protein kinases is true?**
   A. Protein kinase A is activated when a regulatory subunit is bound.
   B. Calmodulin-dependent protein kinases are activated by calmodulin in the absence of Ca^{++}.
   C. Some isoforms of protein kinase C are activated by cholesterol.
   D. Activation of myosin light-chain kinase promotes contraction of smooth muscle.

5. **Which statement about signal transduction involving protein-tyrosine kinases is true?**
   A. Protein-tyrosine kinases have seven transmembrane α helices.
   B. Heterotrimeric G proteins couple binding of growth factors to cellular responses.
   C. The MAP kinase cascade is involved in numerous pathways initiated by receptor protein-tyrosine kinases.
   D. The normal form of Ras promotes uncontrolled growth of cells.

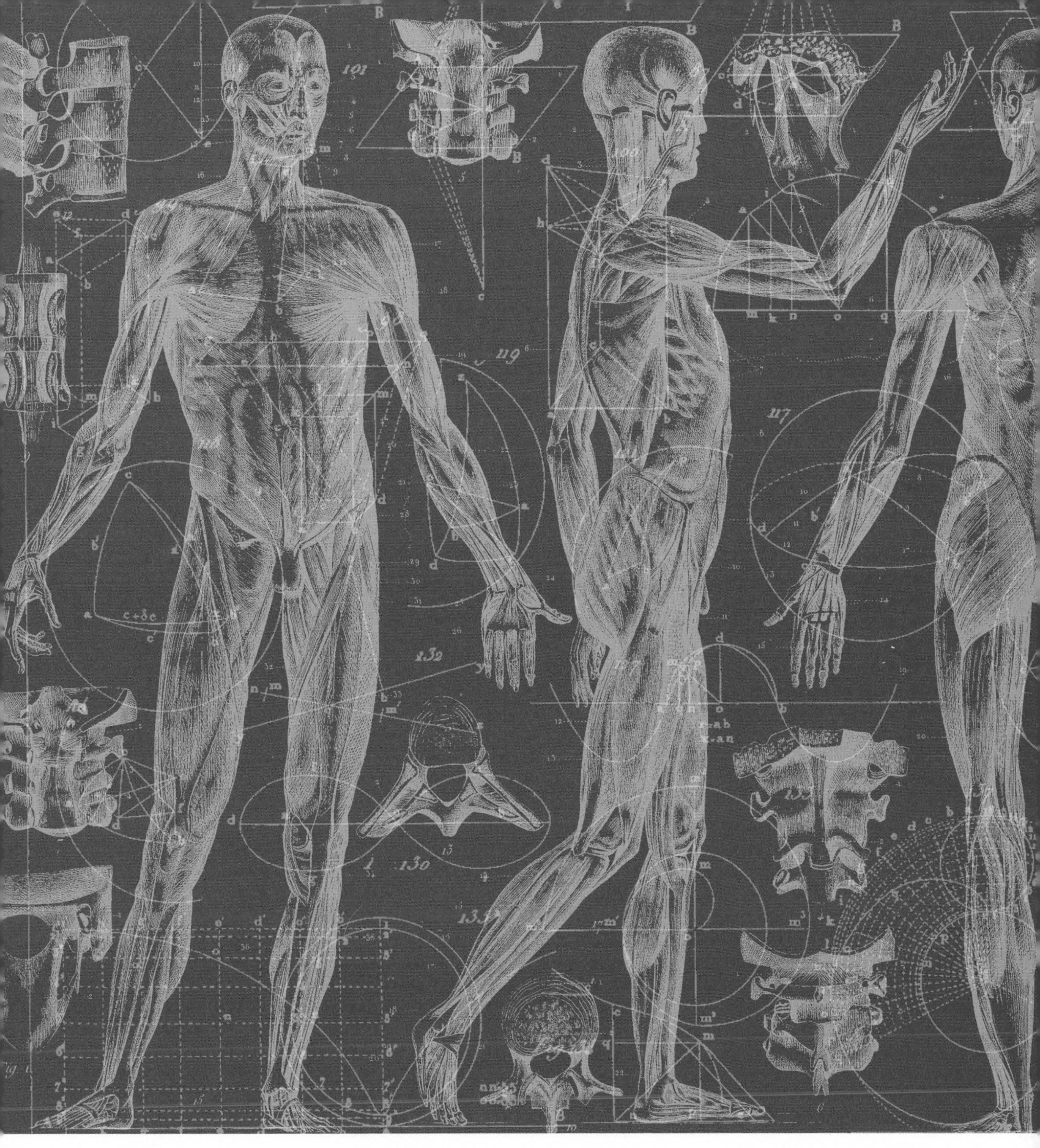

Part Two: Nervous System

William D. Willis, Jr.

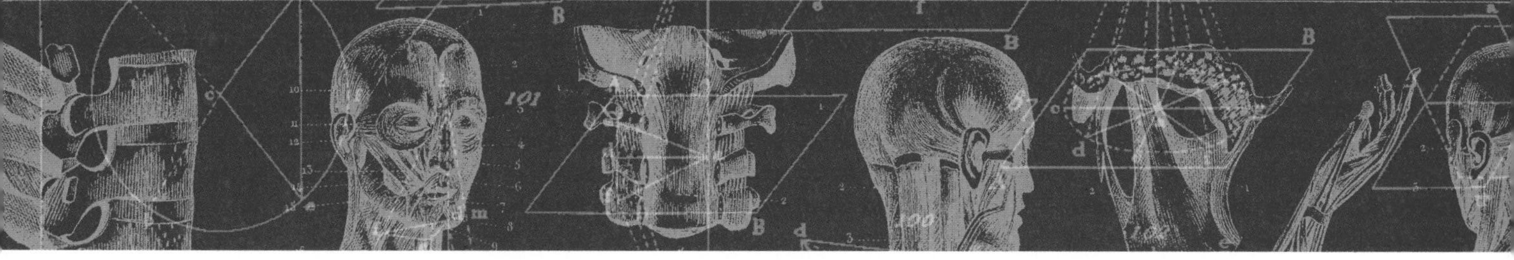

Chapter 6: Cellular Organization

Objectives

- ❖ Explain the cellular composition of the nervous system.
- ❖ Describe the organization of the peripheral and central nervous system, the environment of neurons, and the structure of neurons.
- ❖ Discuss the functional properties of neurons and the ways that information is distributed and chemical substances are transported in nervous tissue.
- ❖ Discuss the pathological responses of nervous tissue and some representative diseases that result from disorders of neural function.

The nervous system is responsible for most of the functions that characterize higher organisms. In humans, it is the source of conscious awareness, sensation, voluntary movement, thought, memory and learning, prediction, emotion, and other forms of cognitive behavior. On a simpler level, the nervous system mediates reflex activity and controls autonomic and endocrine responses. Elements of the nervous system are distributed throughout the body and influence all other systems.

The nervous system is a communication network that allows an organism to interact in appropriate ways with the environment. This system has **sensory components** that detect environmental events, **integrative components** that process sensory data and information stored in memory, and **motor components** that generate movements and other activity. The nervous system can be divided into peripheral and central parts, each with a number of further subdivisions.

The Nervous System Consists of a Complex Aggregate of Cells

The nervous system consists of a highly complex aggregation of cells, part of which is a communication network and another part a supportive matrix. THE COMMUNICATION NETWORK IS FORMED BY **NEURONS,** WHICH ARE THE FUNCTIONAL CELLULAR UNITS OF THE NERVOUS SYSTEM. The human brain contains approximately 10^{12} neurons. Neurons are specialized for receiving information, making decisions, and transmitting signals to other neurons or to effector cells such as muscle or gland cells. This specialization depends on different types of extensions of the cell body, or **soma,** of a neuron. Most neurons have several **dendrites** and an **axon.** Different types of neurons have consistent forms that relate to their functional properties (**Figure 6–1**). The dendrites receive contacts called **synapses** from other neurons, and the axon forms synapses with other neurons or effector cells. Information is transmitted in a neuron by conduction of an electrical signal, the nerve impulse or **action potential** from a trigger zone on the initial segment of the axon, along the axon to the synaptic endings. A chemical **neurotransmitter** is then released and signals information to the next cell. **Synaptic transmission** can have an excitatory or an inhibitory effect.

THE SUPPORTIVE CELLS OF THE NERVOUS SYSTEM INCLUDE THE **NEUROGLIA** ("NERVE GLUE"). The human brain has 10 times as many neuroglia as neurons. Different types of neuroglia are shown in **Figure 6–2**. Some neuroglia, called **astrocytes** because of their star-shaped appearance in stained histological sections, help maintain an appropriate local

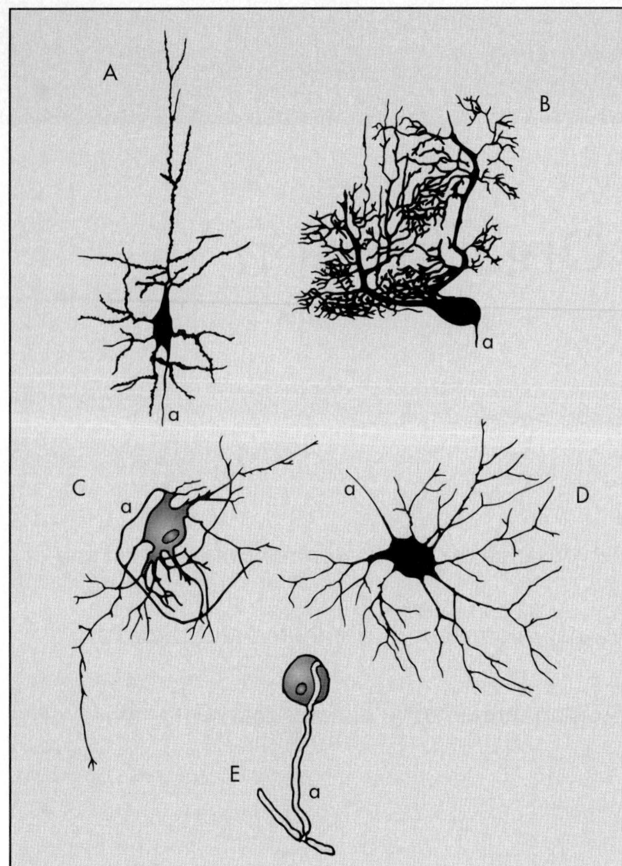

FIGURE 6–1. Various forms of neurons. **A,** Pyramidal cell from the cerebral cortex. **B,** Cerebellar Purkinje cell. **C,** Sympathetic postganglionic neuron. **D,** Spinal cord motor neuron. **E,** Dorsal root ganglion cell. a, axon. (Redrawn from Willis WD Jr, Grossman RG: *Medical neurobiology: neuroanatomical and neurophysiological principles basic to clinical neuroscience,* ed 3, St. Louis, 1981, Mosby.)

environment for neurons. Others, named **oligodendroglia** because they have a limited number of processes, ensheathe axons to increase the speed of propagation of nerve impulses (see Chapter 3). **Microglia** are phagocytes that remove the products of cellular damage from the central nervous system. They are probably derived from the circulation. **Ependymal cells** form an epithelium that separates the central nervous system from the ventricles, a series of cavities within the brain; these cavities contain cerebrospinal fluid (CSF).

The nervous system is also richly supplied with blood vessels.

The Nervous System Consists of a Peripheral and a Central Division

The nervous system can be divided into a **peripheral nervous system (PNS)** and a **central nervous system (CNS).**

The peripheral nervous system is an interface between the central nervous system and the environment

The PNS provides an interface between the CNS and the environment, including both the external world and the body apart from the nervous system. The PNS includes sensory and motor components. The sensory component detects environmental signals and is formed by **sensory receptor organs** and **primary afferent neurons.** Motor components command effector organs to perform muscular or glandular activity and include the axons of **somatic motor neurons** as well as **autonomic preganglionic and postganglionic neurons** and their axons. Autonomic neurons can be further subdivided into **sympathetic, parasympathetic,**

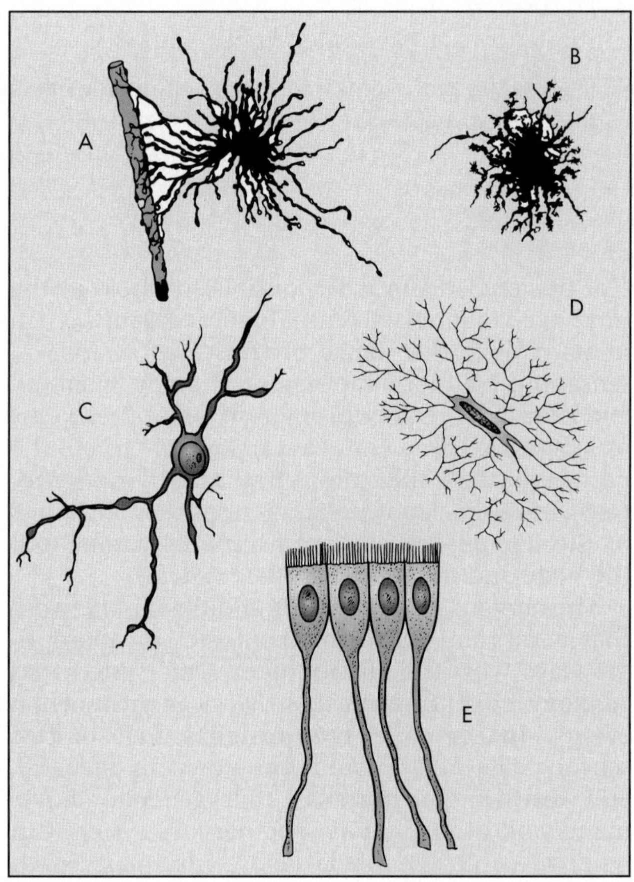

FIGURE 6–2. Different types of neuroglial cells of the central nervous system. **A,** Fibrous astrocyte; note the glial foot processes in association with a capillary. **B,** Protoplasmic astrocyte. **C,** Oligodendrocyte; each of the processes is responsible for the production of one or more myelin sheath internodes around central axons. **D,** Microglial cell. **E,** Ependymal cells. (Redrawn from Willis WD Jr, Grossman RG: *Medical neurobiology: neuroanatomical and neurophysiological principles basic to clinical neuroscience,* ed 3, St. Louis, 1981, Mosby.)

and **enteric neurons.** Somatic motor axons cause contractions of skeletal muscle fibers. Autonomic motor axons excite or inhibit cardiac muscle, smooth muscle, or glands. The sympathetic nervous system prepares the organism for emergency action, whereas the parasympathetic nervous system promotes more routine activities such as digestion. The sympathetic and parasympathetic nervous systems ordinarily work together in regulating visceral function.

The central nervous system includes the spinal cord and brain

The CNS includes the **spinal cord** and **brain** (**Figure 6–3**). The brain can be subdivided into the following regions on the basis of embryological development: myelencephalon, metencephalon, mesencephalon, diencephalon, and telencephalon.

In the adult brain, the myelencephalon becomes the **medulla;** the metencephalon, the **pons** and **cerebellum;** the mesencephalon, the **midbrain;** the diencephalon, the **thalamus, hypothalamus, and subthalamus;** and the telencephalon, the **basal ganglia** and various lobes of the **cerebral cortex.** The diencephalon and basal ganglia are hidden from view in Figure 6–3.

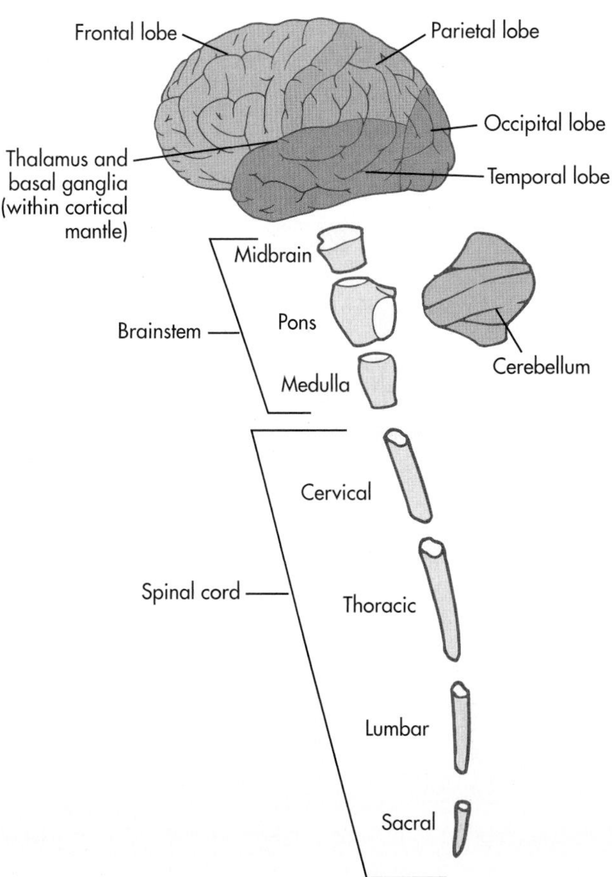

FIGURE 6–3. Exploded view showing the major components of the central nervous system. Also shown are four of the major divisions of the cerebral cortex: the frontal, parietal, occipital, and temporal lobes.

The Local Environment of Neurons Is Controlled

The local environment of most neurons is controlled so that neurons are normally protected from extreme variations in the composition of the extracellular fluid that bathes them. This control is provided by the regulation of the circulation of the CNS (see Chapter 25), the presence of a blood-brain barrier, the buffering function of astrocytes, and the exchange of substances with CSF. Substances are exchanged freely between the extracellular fluid of the CNS and the CSF. However, the entry of substances from the blood into the CNS is controlled by secretory processes in the choroid plexuses, which form CSF, and by the blood-brain barrier (**Figure 6–4**).

The fluid compartments of the cranium are the brain, blood, and cerebrospinal fluid

The cranial cavity contains the brain, blood, and CSF. The human brain weighs about 1350 g, of which approximately 15%, or 200 mL, is extracellular fluid. The intracranial blood volume is about 100 mL, half of it extracellular fluid, and the cranial CSF volume is another 100 mL. Thus, the extracellular fluid space in the cranial cavity totals approximately 350 mL.

The blood-brain barrier restricts the movement of substances into the brain

The movement of large molecules and highly charged ions from the blood into the brain and spinal cord is severely restricted by the **blood-brain barrier** (Figure 6–4). The restriction is at least partly caused by tight junctions between the capillary endothelial cells of the CNS. Astrocytes may also help limit the movement of certain substances. For example, astrocytes can take up K^+ and thus regulate the concentration of K^+ in the extracellular space. Some substances are removed from the CNS by transport mechanisms. For example, penicillin is transported from CSF across the epithelium of the choroid plexuses and into the blood.

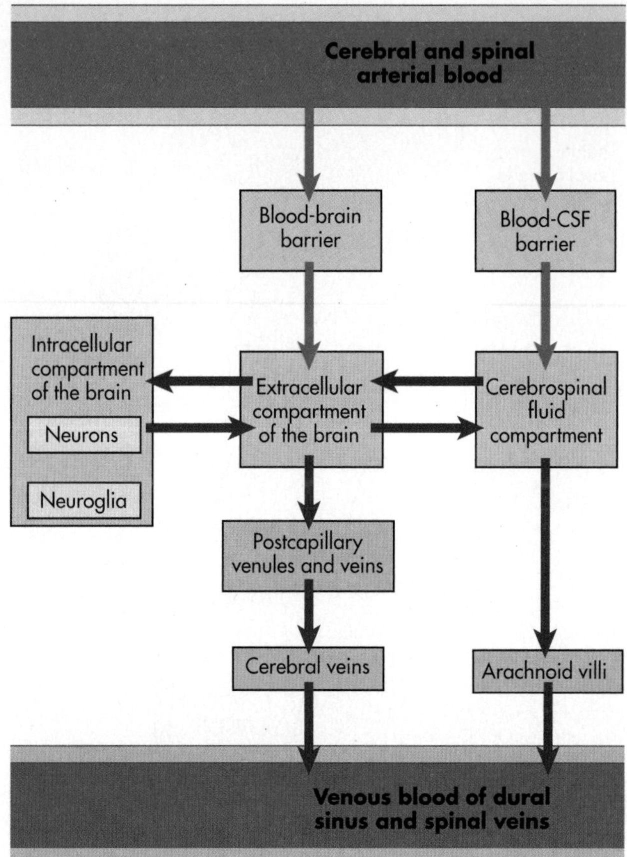

FIGURE 6–4. Structural and functional relationships involved in the blood-brain and blood-CSF barriers. Substances entering the neurons and neuroglial cells (i.e., intracellular compartment) must pass through the cell membrane. Arrows indicate the direction of fluid flow under normal conditions.

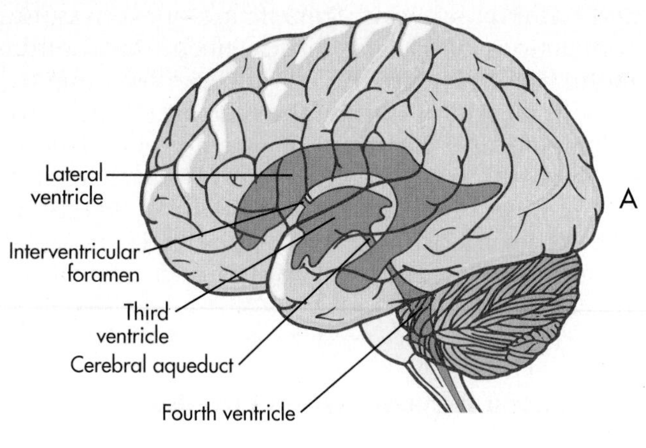

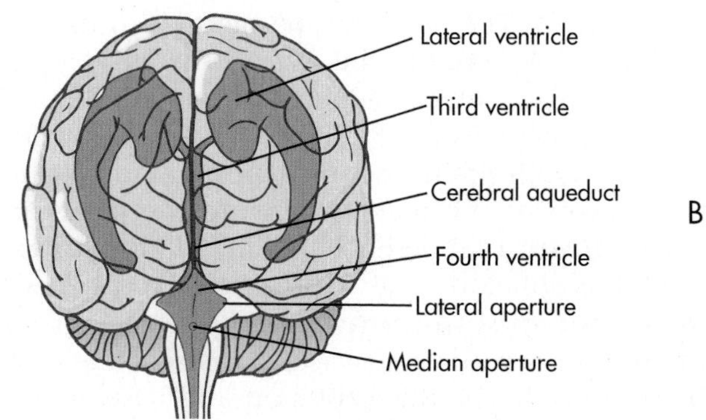

FIGURE 6–5. Ventricular system in situ as seen from the side (A) and front (B).

Cerebrospinal fluid influences the environment of neurons

The extracellular fluid within the CNS communicates directly with the CSF. THUS, THE COMPOSITION OF CSF INDICATES THE COMPOSITION OF THE EXTRACELLULAR ENVIRONMENT OF NEURONS IN THE BRAIN AND SPINAL CORD. The main constituents of CSF in the lumbar cistern (from which CSF can readily be removed by lumbar puncture) are shown in **Table 6–1**. For comparison, the concentrations of the same constituents in the blood are also given. CSF has lower concentrations of K^+, glucose, and protein but greater concentrations of Na^+ and Cl^- than in blood. Furthermore, CSF contains practically no blood cells. The increased concentrations of Na^+ and Cl^- allow CSF to be isotonic to blood, despite the much lower concentration of protein in the CSF.

CSF is formed largely by the **choroid plexuses,** which are capillary loops covered by specialized ependymal cells that are located in the ventricular system of the brain. The **ventricular system** includes the two **lateral ventricles** in the telencephalon, the **third ventricle** of the diencephalon, and the **fourth ventricle** of the metencephalon and myelencephalon. Each lateral ventricle connects to the third ventricle via an **interventricular foramen,** and the third ventricle connects with the fourth through the **cerebral aqueduct.** Choroid plexuses are found in the lateral ventricles, third ventricle, and fourth ventricle (**Figure 6–5**).

TABLE 6–1. CONSTITUENTS OF CSF AND BLOOD

Constituent	Lumbar CSF	Blood
Na^+ (mEq/L)	148	136–145
K^+ (mEq/L)	2.9	3.5–5
Cl^- (mEq/L)	120–130	100–106
Glucose (mg/dL)	50–75	70–100
Protein (mg/dL)	15–45	$6–8 \times 10^3$
pH	7.3	7.4

CSF ESCAPES FROM THE FOURTH VENTRICLE THROUGH OPENINGS IN ITS CONNECTIVE TISSUE ROOF (Figure 6–5). These openings are the unpaired **median aperture** and the paired **lateral apertures.** After leaving the ventricular system, CSF circulates through the subarachnoid spaces surrounding the brain and spinal cord. Much of the CSF is removed by bulk flow through the valvular **arachnoid villi** into the dural venous sinuses.

The volume of CSF within the cerebral ventricles is approximately 35 mL, and that in the subarachnoid spaces of the brain and spinal cord is about 100 mL. CSF is produced at a rate of about 0.35 mL/min, which allows the CSF to be turned over approximately four times daily.

The pressure in the CSF column of adults is about 12.0 to 18.0 cm H_2O when a person is recumbent. The rate at which CSF is formed is relatively independent of the pressure in the ventricles and subarachnoid space and of the systemic blood pressure. However, the absorption rate of CSF is a direct function of CSF pressure.

Obstruction of the circulation of CSF leads to increased CSF pressure and hydrocephalus. In **hydrocephalus,** the ventricles become distended. In young children, the intracranial volume may be increased because the cranial sutures are not closed, so the head can enlarge. However, if the increase continues, brain substance may be lost. In adults, an increase in the ventricular size compromises the flow of blood and causes the loss of brain tissue. When the obstruction is within the ventricular system or in the roof of the fourth ventricle, the condition is called a **noncommunicating hydrocephalus.** If the obstruction is in the subarachnoid space or arachnoid villi, it is known as a **communicating hydrocephalus.**

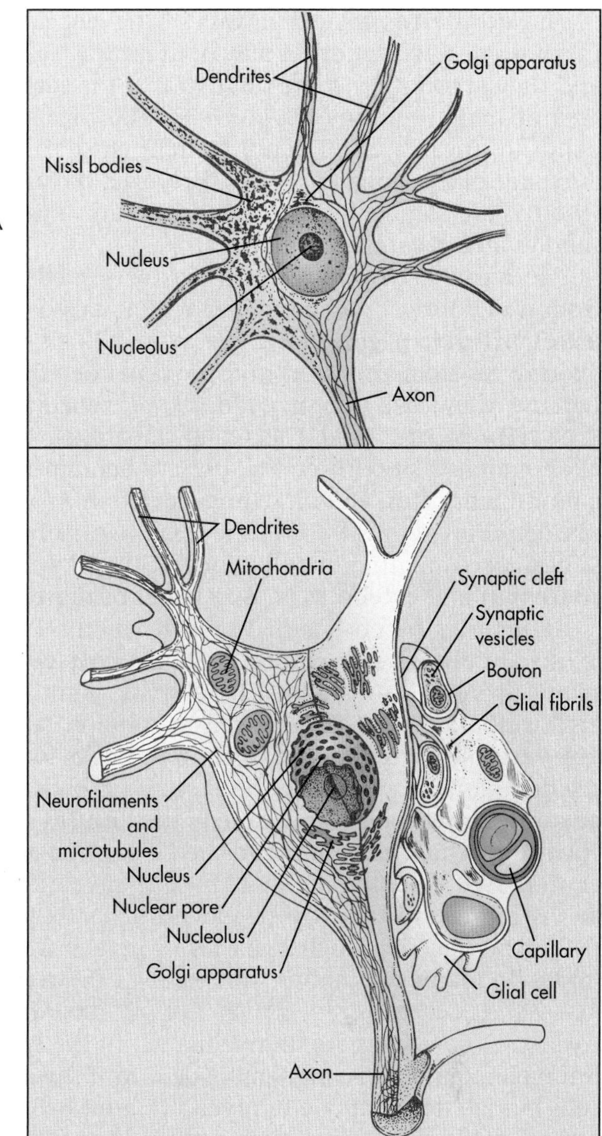

FIGURE 6–6. Organelles of neurons. A, Organelles typical of a neuron shown as they are seen with the light microscope. The left side of the neuron includes structures seen with a Nissl stain, whereas the right side includes structures seen with a heavy metal stain. B, Structures visible with an electron microscope. (Redrawn from Willis WD Jr, Grossman RG: *Medical neurobiology: neuroanatomical and neurophysiological principles basic to clinical neuroscience,* ed 3, St. Louis, 1981, Mosby.)

The Microscopic Anatomy of the Neuron Is Complex

Most neurons have a cell body or soma, one or more dendrites, and an axon. The **cell body** (Figure 6–6) contains the nucleus and nucleolus of the neuron. It possesses a well-developed biosynthetic apparatus for the manufacture of membrane constituents, synthetic enzymes, and other chemical substances needed for the specialized functions of the nerve cell. The neuronal biosynthetic apparatus includes **Nissl bodies,** which are stacks of **rough endoplasmic reticulum,** the organelle that is responsible for protein synthesis. The soma also contains a prominent **Golgi apparatus,** which packages materials into vesicles for transport to other parts of the cell, and numerous mitochondria and cytoskeletal elements, including neurofilaments and microtubules. **Neurofilaments** are thin, rod-like structures, whereas **microtubules** are larger, cylinder-like structures. **Lipofuscin** is a pigment formed from incompletely degraded membrane components, and it accumulates in some neurons. A few groups of neurons in the brainstem contain melanin pigment.

The **dendrites** are extensions of the cell body. In some neurons, dendrites may be as long as 1 mm, and they account for more than 90% of the surface area of many neurons (Figure 6–6). The proximal dendrites (near the cell body) contain Nissl bodies and parts of the Golgi apparatus. However, the main cytoplasmic organelles in dendrites are microtubules and neurofilaments.

The **axon** arises from the soma (or sometimes from a dendrite) in a specialized region called the **axon hillock** (Figure 6–6). The axon hillock and axon differ from the soma and proximal dendrites because they lack rough endoplasmic reticulum, **free ribosomes,** and the Golgi apparatus. The axon contains smooth endoplasmic reticulum and a prominent cytoskeleton. Axons may be short and, like dendrites, terminate near the soma **(Golgi type 1 neurons),** or they may be long **(Golgi type 2 neurons)** and extend as far as a meter or more.

Axons may be ensheathed or bare. In the PNS, axons are always surrounded by **Schwann cells.** Many axons are surrounded by a spiral, multilayered wrapping of a Schwann cell membrane called a **myelin sheath.** A series of Schwann cells forms a series of internodes along the axon. Gaps between adjacent internodes are called the **nodes of Ranvier,** which are the sites of nerve impulse generation (see Chapter 3). In the CNS, myelinated axons are ensheathed by oligodendroglia **(Figure 6–7).** One oligodendroglial cell forms myelin internodes on many CNS axons. THE PRESENCE OF MYELIN ALLOWS NERVE IMPULSES TO BE CONDUCTED MORE RAPIDLY. Other axons are unmyelinated. In the PNS, unmyelinated axons are embedded in Schwann cells but are not wrapped in myelin **(Figure 6–8).** A group of such axons and the accompanying Schwann cells are called a **bundle of Remak.** In the CNS, unmyelinated axons are bare. Unmyelinated axons conduct action potentials slowly.

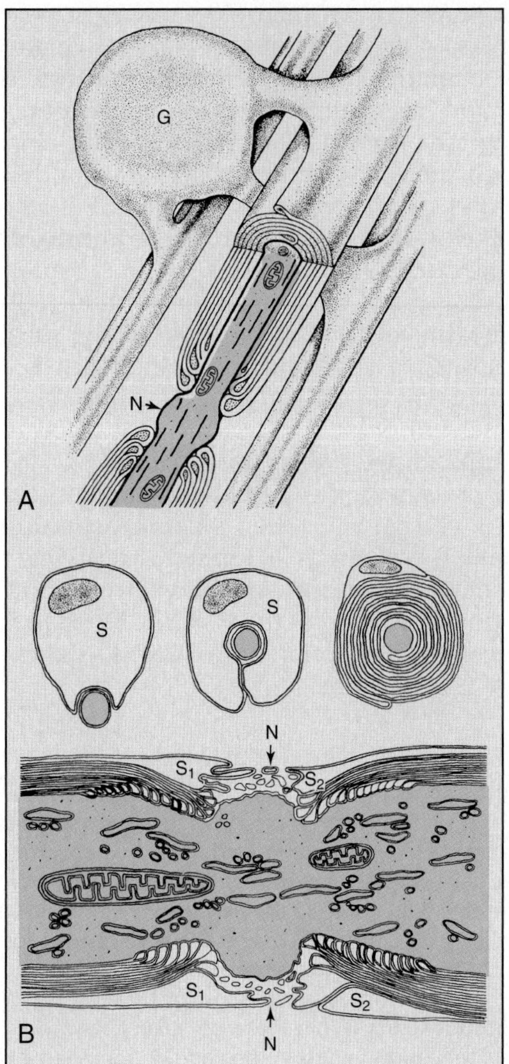

FIGURE 6–7. A, Myelin sheath in the CNS. Each oligodendroglial process forms an internode for one axon. One oligodendroglial cell can myelinate internodes on as many as 40 or 50 separate axons. G, oligodendrocyte; N, node of Ranvier. B, Myelin sheath in the PNS. S, S_1, S_2, Schwann cells. (A from Berne R, Levy MN, Koeppen BM, Stanton BA: *Physiology*, ed 5, Philadelphia, 2004, Elsevier; B redrawn from Patton HD: *Introduction to basic neurology*, Philadelphia, 1976, WB Saunders.)

In some diseases of the nervous system, myelin may be lost over one or more internodes of many axons without interruption of the axons. In such cases, conduction of nerve impulses may be slowed or blocked, and the function of the affected axons is therefore abnormal. Such demyelination occurs in the PNS in the **Guillain-Barré syndrome** and diphtheria. An important demyelinating disease of the CNS is **multiple sclerosis.**

The Nervous System Performs Several Important Functions

Functions of the nervous system include **sensory detection, information processing, learning and memory,** and **behavior.**

Learning and memory permit behavior to change appropriately in response to environmental challenges on the basis of past experience. Other systems, such as the endocrine and immune systems, share these functions, but the nervous system is specialized for them.

Excitability is a cellular property that enables neurons to perform their functions. It is manifested by electrical events such as **nerve impulses** (or **action potentials**), **receptor potentials,** and

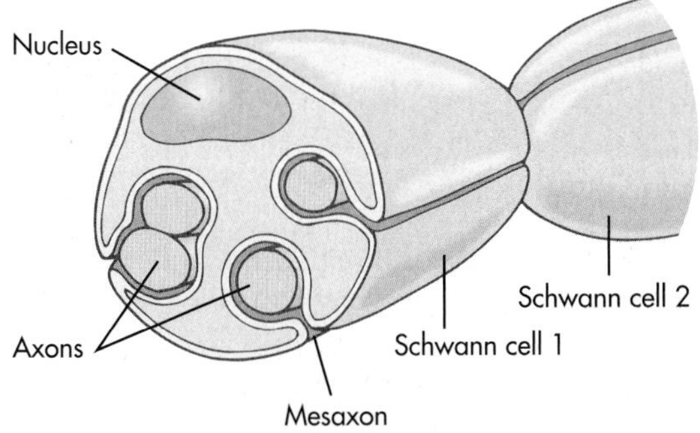

FIGURE 6–8. Three-dimensional view of a bundle of Remak. The cut face of the bundle is shown to the left. The mesaxon is a membrane indentation of the Schwann cell. To the right, the junction of the Remak bundle with an adjacent Schwann cell is depicted.

synaptic potentials (see Chapters 3 and 4). Chemical events often accompany these electrical ones.

Sensory detection is accomplished by special nerve cells called **sensory receptors.** Various forms of energy, including mechanical events that impinge on the body wall, chemicals, temperature gradients, light, sound, and, in some animals, electrical fields, are sensed.

Information processing in neural circuits depends on intercellular communication, which is accomplished by nerve cells as they respond to and generate chemical signals. The mechanisms involved require both electrical and chemical changes. Learning and memory require special forms of information processing and mechanisms for the storage and retrieval of the information.

Behavior may be covert, as in cognition or memory, but it is often readily observable as a motor act, such as a movement or an autonomic response. In humans, a particularly important set of behaviors are those involved in language.

Information Is Transmitted as a Series of Nerve Impulses

A major role of axons is to transmit information from the region of the cell body and dendrites of a neuron to the synapses on other neurons or effector cells. The information is generally transmitted as a series of **nerve impulses.**

The speed of transmission of information depends partly on the conduction velocity of the axon. Conduction velocity in turn depends on the diameter of the axon and whether the axon is unmyelinated or myelinated. Unmyelinated axons are generally less than 1 μm in diameter and conduct at speeds less than 2.5 m/sec. About 1 second would be required for a signal in an unmyelinated axon that supplies a sensory receptor in a person's foot to reach the spinal cord if the axonal conduction velocity were 1 m/sec. Myelinated axons have diameters of 1 to 20 μm and conduct at speeds of 3 to 120 m/sec. A spinal motor neuron with an axon that conducts at 100 m/sec would be able to trigger the contraction of a toe muscle in about 10 msec.

In the CNS, certain neurons that lack axons (e.g., **amacrine cells** of the retina) signal information by electrical current flow rather than by the generation of action potentials. This current flow produces a **local potential,** which decays over a short distance (millimeters to hundreds of micrometers, depending on the length constant of the neuron involved). Local potentials differ from action potentials in that they do not propagate and therefore cannot spread over long distances. In contrast, action potentials can propagate over long distances along axons (see also Chapter 3).

Signaling by local potentials is also characteristic of sensory receptors, which produce **receptor potentials** (see Chapter 7), and of communication between nerve cells by **synaptic potentials** (see Chapter 4).

Neurons encode information

Information conveyed by axons may be coded in several ways. Sets of neurons may be dedicated to a general function, such as a particular sensory modality. For example, the visual pathway includes the retina, optic nerve and tract, lateral geniculate nucleus of the thalamus, and visual parts of the cerebral cortex (see Chapter 8). The normal means of activating the visual system is by light striking the retina, leading to axonal and synaptic transmission of visual information to higher levels in the visual pathway. However, mechanical or electrical stimulation of the visual system also produces a visual response, although a distorted one. Thus, neurons of the visual system can be regarded as a **labeled line** that, when activated, causes a visual sensation. A LABELED LINE CONSISTS OF A SET OF NEURONS, INCLUDING SENSORY RECEPTORS AND CNS PROCESSING CIRCUITS, THAT TOGETHER ARE RESPONSIBLE FOR SIGNALING A PARTICULAR TYPE OF SENSATION. A labeled line is usually activated by sensory stimulation. However, it may also be activated artificially. For example, one can cause a person to see flashes of light by pressing on the eye or by stimulating the cerebral cortex with electrical shocks. Other sensory systems provide further examples of labeled lines.

Information is also coded by the nervous system through **spatial maps.** The body surface may be mapped by an array of neurons in the somatic sensory or motor systems. This type of map is termed a **somatotopic map** (or in humans, a **homunculus** [see Chapters 7 and 9]). In the visual system, there are **retinotopic maps**. In the auditory system, the frequency of sounds is represented in **tonotopic maps** (see Chapter 8).

A third method for coding information is by **patterns of nerve impulses.** Axons transmit a sequence of nerve impulses that results in synaptic transmission of information to a new set of neurons. The information communicated is coded in terms of the structure of the nerve impulse trains. Several different types of nerve impulse codes have been proposed. A common code is likely to depend on the mean discharge frequency. For example, the intensity of a sensory stimulus may be signaled by the mean firing rate of the sensory neuron. Other candidate codes depend on the time of firing, temporal pattern, and duration of bursts of discharges.

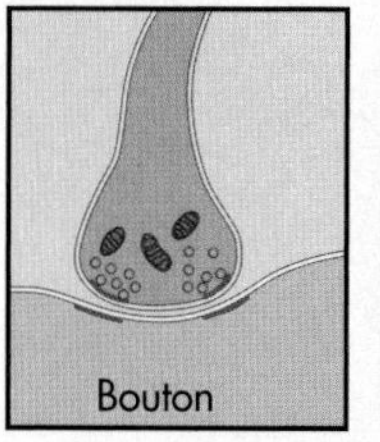

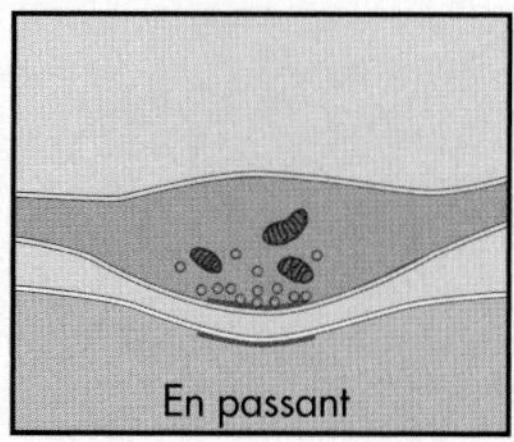

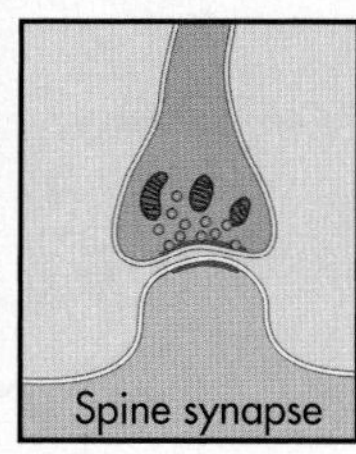

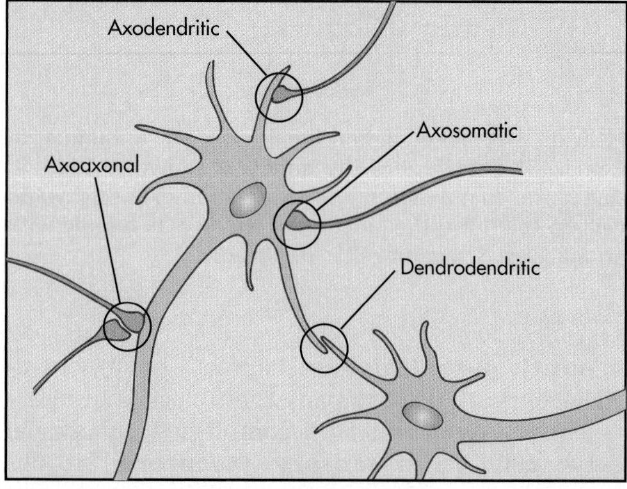

FIGURE 6–9. The drawings of electron micrographs at the top show a synaptic bouton at the termination of an axon, an en passant synapse made by an axon that continues past the synapse, and a spine synapse on a dendritic spine. The drawing at the bottom illustrates axodendritic, axosomatic, axoaxonal, and dendrodendritic synapses.

Synaptic Transmission Allows Neurons to Communicate

Neurons communicate with one another at specialized junctions called **synapses** (see Chapter 4). Synapses are typically formed between the terminals of the axon of one neuron and the dendrites of another **(Figure 6–9)**; these are called **axodendritic synapses.** However, several other types of synapses, including **axosomatic, axoaxonal,** and **dendrodendritic** (Figure 6–9), occur. The synapse between a motor neuron and a skeletal muscle fiber is called an **end plate** or **neuromuscular junction.**

Axonal Transport Moves Substances Within Neurons

Many axons are too long to allow the effective movement of substances from the soma to the synaptic endings simply by diffusion. Certain membrane and cytoplasmic components that originate in the biosynthetic apparatus of the soma and proximal dendrites must be distributed along the processes, especially to the presynaptic elements of synapses, to replenish secreted or inactivated materials. A special transport mechanism, called **axonal transport,** accomplishes this distribution.

There are several types of axonal transport. Certain membrane-bound organelles and mitochondria are transported relatively rapidly by **fast axonal transport.** Substances (e.g., proteins) that are dissolved in cytoplasm are moved by **slow axonal transport.** Fast axonal transport proceeds as rapidly as 400 mm/day, whereas slow axonal transport occurs at about 1 mm/day. This means that synaptic vesicles can travel from a motor neuron in the spinal cord to a neuromuscular junction in a person's foot in about 2½ days, whereas the transport of many soluble proteins over the same distance would take nearly 3 years.

AXONAL TRANSPORT REQUIRES METABOLIC ENERGY AND INVOLVES Ca^{++} IONS. Microtubules in the cytoskeleton provide a system of guide wires along which membrane-bound organelles move during fast axonal transport. These organelles attach to transport filaments, which are moved along the microtubules through a link similar to that between the thick and thin filaments of skeletal muscle fibers. A MOTOR PROTEIN CALLED KINESIN FORMS THIS LINK. Ca^{++} ions trigger the movement of the organelles along the microtubules.

Axonal transport occurs in both directions. Transport from the soma toward the axonal termi-

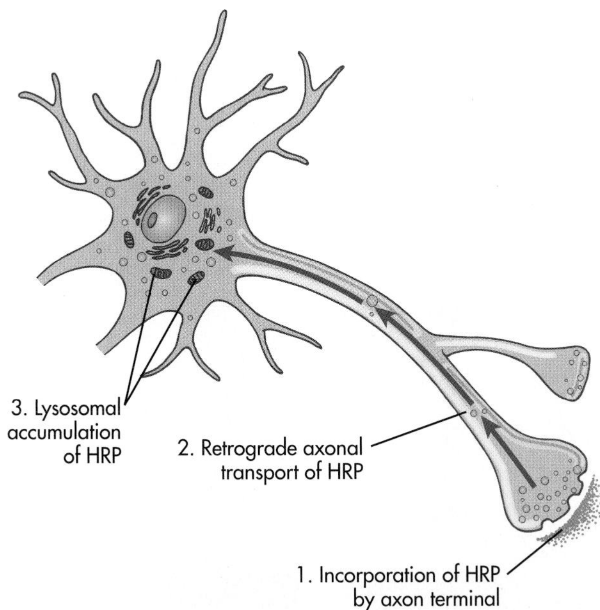

FIGURE 6–10. Endocytotic incorporation (1), retrograde axonal transport (2), and lysosomal accumulation (3) of horseradish peroxidase (HRP) in a neuron.

nals is called **anterograde axonal transport.** This process allows the replenishment of synaptic vesicles and enzymes responsible for neurotransmitter synthesis in synaptic terminals. Transport in the opposite direction is **retrograde axonal transport** (Figure 6–10). Retrograde axonal transport is rapid, although the speed is only about half that of fast anterograde transport. A DIFFERENT MOTOR PROTEIN KNOWN AS DYNEIN IS RESPONSIBLE FOR RETROGRADE TRANSPORT. This process returns synaptic vesicle membrane to the soma for lysosomal degradation. Marker substances, such as the enzyme horseradish peroxidase, can be transported anterogradely or retrogradely and can be used in experiments to trace neural pathways.

Axonal transport is important in pathological processes. Primary afferent neurons and motor neurons link the CNS with the periphery and thus form a protoplasmic bridge that crosses the blood-brain barrier. Certain viruses, such as the rabies virus and poliovirus, and toxins, such as tetanus toxin, can enter the CNS from the periphery if they are taken up and transported in the axons of these neurons.

Neurons and Neuroglia React to Injury

Injury to nervous tissue elicits responses by neurons and neuroglia. Severe injury causes cell death. Once a neuron is lost, it cannot be replaced because neurons are postmitotic cells; that is, they are fully differentiated and no longer undergo cell division. Most neurons complete their differentiation before birth, although neuroglial cells continue to divide even in adulthood. Thus, most tumors of the CNS originate from neuroglial precursor cells rather than from neurons.

The axonal reaction is a pathological response to axonal injury

When an axon is transected, the soma of the neuron may show the **axonal reaction.** Nissl bodies normally stain well with basic aniline dyes, which attach to the ribonucleic acid of the ribosomes **(Figure 6–11, *A*)**. During the axonal reaction, the cisterns of the rough endoplasmic reticulum become distended with the products of protein synthesis. The ribosomes become disorganized; thus, the Nissl bodies are stained weakly by basic aniline dyes. This alteration in staining is termed **chromatolysis** (Figure 6–11, *C* and *D*). The soma may also become swollen and rounded, and the nucleus may assume an eccentric position in the cytoplasm. THESE MORPHOLOGICAL CHANGES REFLECT THE CYTOLOGICAL PROCESSES THAT ACCOMPANY PROTEIN SYNTHESIS. The damaged neuron is repairing itself.

Wallerian degeneration is the response to interruption of an axon

If a nerve fiber is cut, the axon distal to the transection dies (Figure 6–11, *B* and *C*). Within a few days, the axon and all of the synaptic endings formed by the axon disintegrate. If the axon was myelinated, the myelin sheath becomes fragmented and is eventually phagocytosed and removed. However, the Schwann cells that formed the myelin sheath remain viable. This sequence of events was originally described by Waller and is thus called **wallerian degeneration.**

If the axons that provide the sole or predominant synaptic input to a neuron or an effector cell are interrupted, the postsynaptic cell may undergo degeneration and even death. The best known example of this is the atrophy of skeletal muscle fibers after their innervation by motor neurons is interrupted.

In neuroanatomical investigations, these pathological changes have been useful for tracing neural pathways. For example, retrograde chromatolysis has been used to reveal groups of neurons

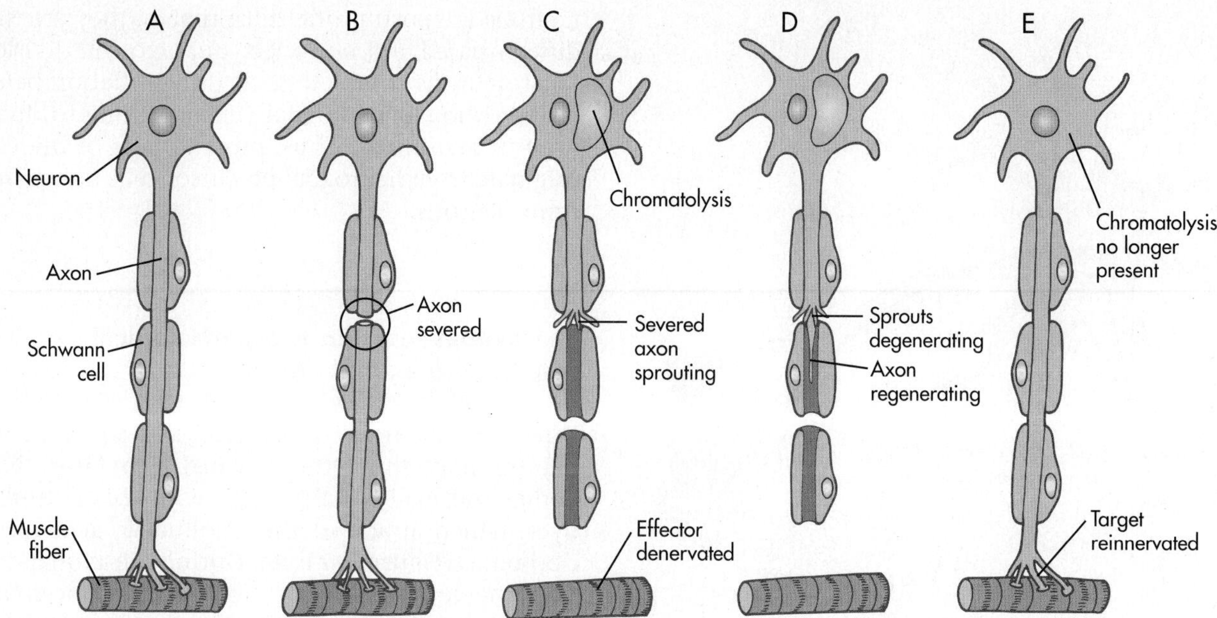

FIGURE 6–11. **A,** Normal motor neuron innervating a skeletal muscle fiber. **B,** The motor axon has been severed, and the motor neuron is beginning to undergo chromatolysis. **C,** The chromatolysis is associated eventually with sprouting. **D,** One of the sprouts is associated with regeneration of the axon. The excess sprouts degenerate. **E,** When the target cell is reinnervated, chromatolysis is no longer present. (Redrawn from Willis WD Jr, Grossman RG: *Medical neurobiology: neuroanatomical and neurophysiological principles basic to clinical neuroscience,* ed 3, St. Louis, 1981, Mosby.)

whose axons have been deliberately interrupted. The projection target of axons can be determined by following the course of interrupted axons undergoing wallerian degeneration. Synaptic targets can also be mapped if neurons undergo **transneuronal degeneration** after an axon bundle is transected.

Regeneration can occur in the peripheral nervous system, but it is unsatisfactory in the central nervous system

Many neurons can regenerate a new axon if the axon is lost through injury. The proximal stump of the damaged axon develops sprouts (Figure 6–11, *C*). In the PNS, these sprouts elongate and grow along the path of the original nerve if this route is available. The Schwann cells in the distal stump of the nerve not only survive the wallerian degeneration but also proliferate and form rows along the course previously taken by the axons. Growth cones of the sprouting axons find their way along the rows of Schwann cells and may eventually reinnervate the original peripheral target structures (Figure 6–11, *D* and *E*). The Schwann cells then remyelinate the axons. The rate of regeneration is limited by the rate of slow axonal transport to about 1 mm/day.

Nerve growth factor and other growth factors play an important role in the growth of sensory, somatic motor, and autonomic axons in peripheral nerves during development, in their maintenance, and in their regeneration after injury.

Transection of axons in the CNS also results in wallerian degeneration followed by sprouting. Proper guidance for the sprouts is generally lacking, however, because the oligodendroglia do not form a path along which the sprouts can grow. One reason the oligodendroglia do not form a path comparable to the path formed by Schwann cells is that a single oligodendroglial cell myelinates many central axons, whereas a given Schwann cell provides myelin for only a single axon in the PNS. Alternatively, different chemical signals, such as different growth factors or growth-inhibiting factors, may affect the peripheral and central attempts at regeneration differently. Another obstacle is the formation of glial scars in the CNS by astrocytes.

Summary

- The general functions of the nervous system include sensory detection, information processing, and behavior.
- The functional cellular unit of the nervous system is the neuron.
- Nervous tissue contains not only neurons but also supporting cells or neuroglia (Schwann cells in the PNS; astrocytes, oligodendroglia, microglia, and ependymal cells in the CNS) and blood vessels.
- The nervous system is subdivided into the PNS (sensory, somatic motor, and autonomic neurons) and the CNS (spinal cord and brain).
- The extracellular environment of neurons in the CNS is highly regulated. CSF is secreted by the choroid plexuses. The blood-brain barrier restricts the entry of substances into the brain.
- The parts of neurons include the cell body, dendrites, and axon. Axons may be myelinated or unmyelinated.
- Information is conducted along axons by nerve impulses, whose conduction velocity depends on the presence or absence of myelin and the diameter of the axon. The largest myelinated axons have the fastest conduction velocities.
- Several coding mechanisms are used by neurons to convey information in neural networks. These include labeled lines, spatial maps, and patterns of nerve impulses.
- Information is transmitted from neuron to neuron or from neuron to effector organ by means of synaptic transmission.
- Materials are moved along axons by axonal transport. The movements can be rapid or slow and away from or toward the cell body.
- Neurons respond to damage either by cell death or by less drastic changes, such as the axonal reaction (chromatolysis) and wallerian degeneration. Viable axons in the PNS may subsequently regenerate.

Bibliography

Cajal SR: *Histology of the nervous system,* New York, 1995, Oxford University Press.

Goldberg JL, Barres BA: The relationship between neuronal survival and regeneration, *Annu Rev Neurosci* 23:579, 2000.

Goldstein LSB, Yang ZH: Microtubule-based transport systems in neurons: the roles of kinesins and dyneins, *Annu Rev Neurosci* 23:39, 2000.

González-Scarano F, Baltuch G: Microglia as mediators of inflammation and degenerative diseases, *Annu Rev Neurosci* 22:219, 1999.

Graham DI, Lantos PL, eds: *Greenfield's neuropathology,* London, 1997, Arnold.

Huang EJ, Reichardt LF: Neurotrophins: roles in neuronal development and function, *Annu Rev Neurosci* 24:677, 2001.

Kandel ER, Schwartz JH, Jessell TM, eds: *Principles of neural science,* ed 4, New York, 2000, McGraw-Hill.

Kettenmann H, Ranson BR, eds: *Neuroglia,* New York, 1995, Oxford University Press.

Nicholls JG, Martin AR, Wallace BG: *From neuron to brain,* ed 3, Sunderland, Mass, 1992, Sinauer Associates.

Paxinos G, Mai JK, eds: *The human nervous system,* ed 2, Amsterdam, 2004, Elsevier Academic Press.

Case Studies

Case 6–1

A 59-year-old man became depressed during several years after a business failure. He became confused and had memory lapses. His family was concerned that he might be developing Alzheimer's disease. He experienced progressively greater difficulty in walking. On examination, he did not know the date and had difficulty with mental arithmetic. His gait was unsteady, and he tended to fall. He had signs of interruption of the voluntary motor pathways. The results of blood chemical analysis were normal. However, in the CSF, the protein level was elevated, and the white blood cell count was high, but the glucose level was low. A magnetic resonance scan showed a massively dilated ventricular system. A microbe screening demonstrated cryptococci in the CSF.

1. **What is the most likely reason for the patient's changed mental state and motor difficulties?**
   A. Alzheimer's disease
   B. Brain tumor
   C. Encephalitis
   D. Hydrocephalus
   E. Hypoglycemia

2. **If all of the ventricles are dilated, where is the most likely site of the obstruction?**
   A. Arachnoid villi
   B. Cerebral aqueduct
   C. Interventricular foramen
   D. Roof of the fourth ventricle
   E. Third ventricle

Case 6–2

An 18-year-old woman was well until 3 years ago, when she suddenly lost sight in her right eye. Her vision then gradually improved. Then 2 years ago, she developed a hearing loss in her right ear lasting 3 weeks. A month later, she experienced numbness and tingling in her right leg, which improved during 2 weeks. A neurological examination revealed no significant abnormalities. However, 2 months later, she developed blurred vision and on examination had weakness of adduction of the left eye and nystagmus. Some 6 months ago, she became weak in the left leg. Currently, she is experiencing normal eye movements but a left-sided weakness, a left-sided facial weakness, and hyperactive phasic stretch reflexes in the left arm and leg; Babinski's sign was elicited on the left. The results of blood and spinal fluid chemical analysis were normal.

1. **Which nervous system cell type is most likely to be affected in this patient?**
   A. Astrocyte
   B. Motor neuron
   C. Oligodendroglial cell
   D. Pyramidal cell
   E. Schwann cell

2. **What is the basic defect caused by disrupted function of this cell type?**
   A. Abnormal axonal transport
   B. Blockade or slowed conduction velocity of axons
   C. Chromatolysis
   D. Failure of synaptic transmission
   E. Wallerian degeneration

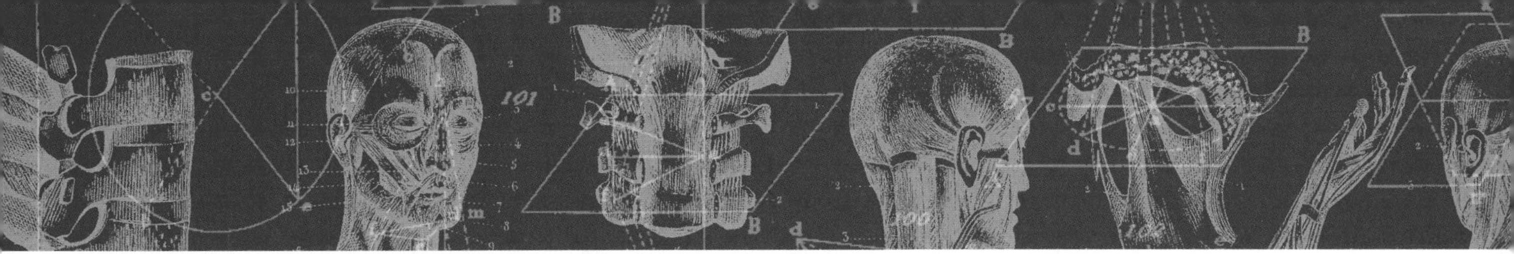

Chapter 7: General Sensory System

Objectives

- ❖ Describe the basic principles of sensory physiology.
- ❖ Discuss the organization of the somatovisceral sensory system.
- ❖ Explain how pathways that descend from the brain can modulate sensory transmission.

The nervous system can be regarded as a complex of several subsystems with different functional roles. These subsystems interact, however, and their activity leads to unified behavior. Some neural subsystems are concerned with sensory function. This chapter considers the general sensory system, or **somatovisceral sensory system,** which analyzes sensory events relating to the mechanical, thermal, or chemical stimulation of the body and face. Chapter 8 describes the special sensory systems.

The somatovisceral sensory system involves **sensory receptors,** which respond to various stimuli by the process of **sensory transduction.** The sensory receptors then provide sensory information about these stimuli to the central nervous system (CNS). Sensory information is encoded in various ways, and this encoded information is then transmitted through sensory pathways that ascend in the spinal cord white matter to brain areas that process the information in ways that eventually lead to sensory perception. One of these ascending pathways is known as the **dorsal column–medial lemniscus** pathway. This pathway is largely responsible for the sensations of flutter-vibration and touch-pressure as well as for proprioception. Another pathway is the **spinothalamic tract,** which is largely responsible for pain and temperature sensations. Components of the **trigeminothalamic tract** have similar roles in mediating sensations arising from the face and oral, nasal, and cranial cavities. Neural pathways also descend from the brain to control transmission in the ascending somatosensory pathways. The **endogenous analgesia system** is an example of this type of pathway.

There Are Several Principles of Sensory Physiology

Transduction allows sensory receptors to respond to stimuli

Useful features of environmental events are detected by **sensory receptors,** which then provide information about the events to the CNS. The interaction of an environmental event with a sensory receptor is called a **stimulus.** The effect of the stimulus on the sensory receptor may lead to a **response,** such as an increase in neural activity. The process that enables a sensory receptor to respond usefully to a stimulus is called **sensory transduction.**

ENVIRONMENTAL EVENTS THAT LEAD TO SENSORY TRANSDUCTION CAN INVOLVE MECHANICAL, THERMAL, CHEMICAL, AND OTHER FORMS OF ENERGY, DEPENDING ON THE SENSORY APPARATUS. Although humans cannot sense electrical or magnetic fields, other animals, such as fish, can respond to such stimuli.

The manner in which sensory transduction is accomplished varies with the receptor type. For example, a **chemoreceptor** may respond when a molecule of a chemical stimulant reacts with a receptor molecule in the surface membrane of the chemoreceptor. The reaction may open ion channels and induce the influx of ionic current. For example, many nociceptors contain transient receptor potential vanilloid 1 (TRPV1) receptors on their surface membranes. TRPV1 receptors can be activated by capsaicin (the active ingredient of chili peppers), noxious heat, or lowered pH. A cation channel is opened, allowing the influx of Ca^{++} and movements of Na^+ and K^+ across the nociceptor membrane, resulting in depolarization and activation of a number of signal-transduction pathways. On the other hand, mechanically sensitive ion channels in the surface membrane of a **mechanoreceptor** are opened in response to the application of a mechanical force along the membrane. Ion channels in the outer segment of a **photoreceptor** are open in the dark but closed when photons are absorbed by pigment on the disc membrane. The signal for closure of the ion channels in photoreceptors is transmitted by second-messenger molecules. Thus, the details of sensory transduction vary with receptor type, but often, transduction depends on changes in ionic current through ion channels in response to the activation of receptor molecules. Receptor molecules and ion channels are sometimes directly coupled, but in other cases, they are coupled indirectly through second-messenger cascades.

Sensory transduction generally induces a **receptor potential** in the peripheral terminal of a primary afferent sensory neuron. A receptor potential is usually a depolarizing event that results from inward current flow, and it may bring the membrane potential of the sensory receptor toward or past the threshold needed to trigger a nerve impulse. For example, in **Figure 7–1**, *A,* a mechanical stimulus distorts the ending of a mechanoreceptor and causes inward current flow at the terminal and longitudinal and outward current flow along the axon. The outward current produces a depolarization, the receptor potential, which may exceed threshold for an action potential. In this case, the action potential is generated at a trigger zone in the first node of Ranvier of the afferent fiber. However, in photoreceptors, the cessation of inward current flow during phototransduction leads to a hyperpolarization of the receptor.

In some sensory receptor organs, the peripheral terminal of a primary afferent fiber contacts a separate, peripherally located sensory cell. For example, in the cochlea, primary afferent fibers contact hair cells. Sensory transduction in such sense organs is made more complex by this arrangement. In the cochlea, a receptor potential is produced in the hair cells in response to sound. The receptor potential is a depolarization of the hair cell's membrane, and the depolarization liberates an excitatory neurotransmitter onto the primary afferent terminal. The resulting inward current depolarizes the primary afferent fiber terminal and produces a **generator potential.** This depolarization brings the membrane potential of the primary afferent fiber toward or beyond threshold for firing nerve impulses.

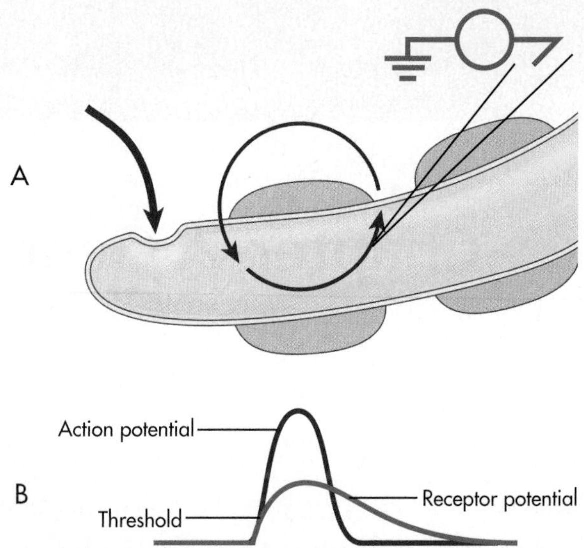

FIGURE 7–1. A, The terminal region of a myelinated mechanoreceptor afferent fiber is shown as if cut in longitudinal section. The surface membrane is indicated by a light yellow line, the axoplasm by the orange area, and the myelin internodes by the light blue areas. The current flow produced by stimulation of the mechanoreceptor at the site indicated by the large arrow is shown by the smaller arrows. The tip of an intracellular microelectrode has been placed in the axon, as indicated. B, The receptor potential produced by the current *(red line)* and an action potential that may be triggered by the receptor potential if it exceeds threshold *(blue line)* are shown.

Sensory receptors have the property of **adaptation** to maintained stimuli. A long-lasting stimulus may produce a prolonged repetitive discharge, or it may result in a brief response (one or a few discharges), depending on whether the sensory receptor is slowly or rapidly adapting. The adaptation rates differ because a prolonged stimulus may produce either a maintained or a transient receptor potential in the sensory receptor. The functional implication of the adaptation rate is that different temporal features of a stimulus can be analyzed by receptors that have different adaptation rates. For example, during an indentation of the skin, a slowly adapting receptor may respond repetitively at a rate proportional to the amount of indentation (**Figure 7–2,** ***A***). Such a response can signal skin position. On the other hand, rapidly adapting receptors in the skin respond best to transient mechanical stimuli. The information signaled may reflect stimulus velocity (Figure 7–2, *B*) or acceleration (Figure 7–2, *C*) rather than the amount of skin indentation.

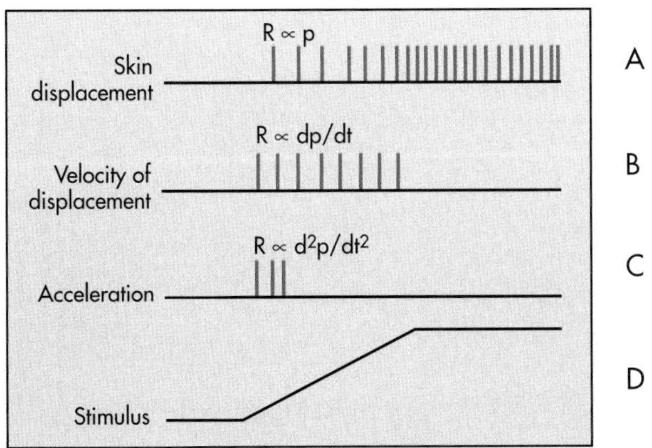

FIGURE 7–2. Responses of slowly and rapidly adapting mechanoreceptors to displacement of the skin. The discharges of the primary afferent fibers supplying the receptors in response to the ramp and hold stimulus (D) are termed the responses (R). A, R is proportional to skin position (p). The receptor is slowly adapting and signals skin displacement. B, R is a function of the velocity of displacement (dp/dt). C, R is a function of acceleration (d^2p/dt^2). The receptors in B and C are rapidly adapting, but they signal different dynamic features of the stimulus.

The stimulation of receptive fields affects the discharges of sensory neurons

The relationship between the location of a stimulus and the activation of particular sensory neurons is a major theme in sensory physiology. The **receptive field** of a sensory neuron is the region that, when it is stimulated, affects the discharge of the neuron. For example, a sensory receptor might be activated by the indentation of only a small area of skin. That area is the **excitatory receptive field** of the sensory receptor. A sensory neuron in the CNS might be excited by the stimulation of a receptive field several times as large as that of a primary afferent neuron. The receptive fields of sensory neurons in the CNS are typically larger than the receptive fields of sensory receptors because the central neurons receive information from many sensory receptors, each with a slightly different receptive field. The location of the receptive field is determined by the location of the sensory-transduction apparatus responsible for signaling information about the stimulus to the sensory neuron.

In general, the receptive fields of sensory receptors are excitatory. However, a sensory neuron in the CNS can have either an excitatory or an **inhibitory receptive field** (Figure 7–3). Inhibition results from data processing in sensory neural circuits and is mediated by inhibitory interneurons.

Sensory coding depends on nerve impulses in sensory neurons

Sensory neurons encode stimuli. In the process of sensory transduction, one or more aspects of the stimulus must be encoded in a way that can be interpreted by the CNS. The **encoded information** is an abstraction based on the responses of sensory receptors to the stimulus and on information processing within the sensory pathway. SOME OF THE ASPECTS OF STIMULI THAT ARE ENCODED INCLUDE MODALITY, SPATIAL LOCATION, THRESHOLD, INTENSITY, FREQUENCY, AND DURATION. Other aspects encoded are presented in reference to particular sensory systems (see Chapter 8).

A **sensory modality** is a readily identified class of sensation. For example, maintained mechanical stimuli applied to the skin result in a sensation of **touch-pressure,** and transient mechanical stimuli may evoke a sensation of **flutter-vibration.** Other cutaneous modalities include **cold, warm,** and **pain. Vision, audition, position sense, taste,** and **smell** are examples of noncutaneous modalities. In most sensory systems, the encoding of sensory modality is by labeled-line sensory channels (see Chapter 6). A **labeled-line sensory channel** consists of a set of neurons devoted to a particular sensory modality.

Stimulus location is often signaled by the activation of the particular population of sensory neurons whose receptive fields are affected by the stimulus (**Figure 7–4,** ***A***). In some cases, an inhibitory receptive field or a contrasting border between an excitatory and an inhibitory receptive field can have localizing value. The resolution of two different adjacent stimuli may depend on the excitation of partially separated populations of

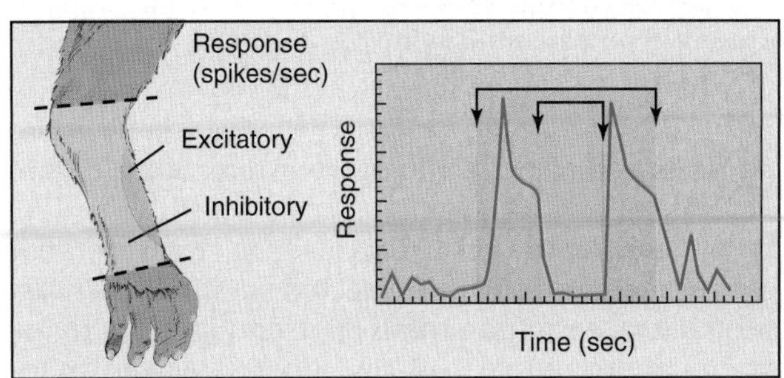

FIGURE 7–3. Excitatory and inhibitory receptive fields of a central somatosensory neuron located in the primary somatosensory cerebral cortex. The excitatory receptive field is on the forearm and is surrounded by an inhibitory receptive field. The graph shows the response to an excitatory stimulus and the inhibition of that response by a stimulus applied in the inhibitory field.

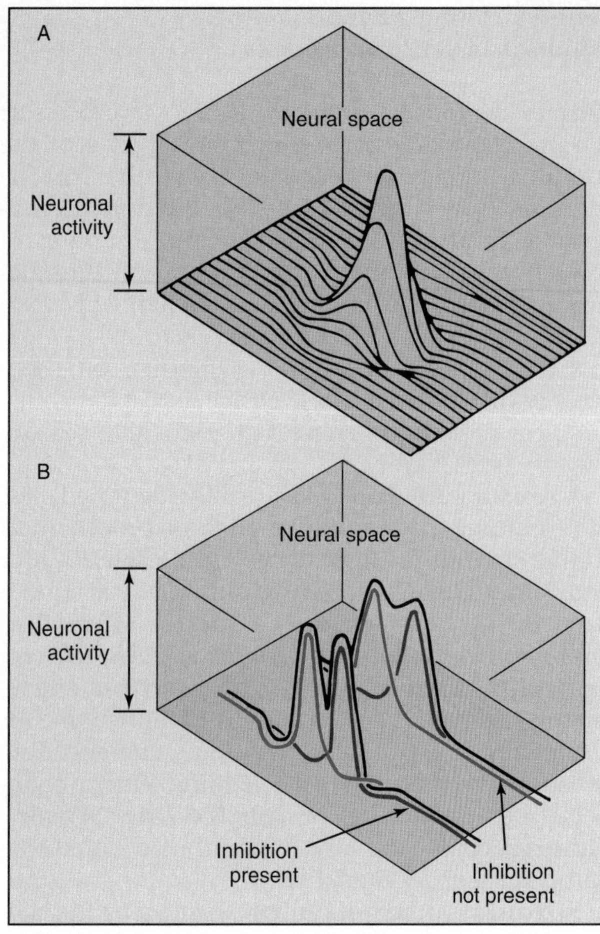

FIGURE 7–4. Activity of a large population of neurons distributed in neural space (e.g., in the cerebral cortex). **A,** The activity of the neurons in response to a stimulus applied to a single point on the skin is plotted on the vertical axis. Note that an excitatory peak is surrounded by an inhibitory trough; these are determined by the excitatory and inhibitory receptive fields of sensory neurons in the central somatosensory pathways. **B,** Neural activity in response to the stimulation of two adjacent points on the skin. Note that the sum of the activity *(black line)* is separated better into two peaks when inhibition is present than when it is not.

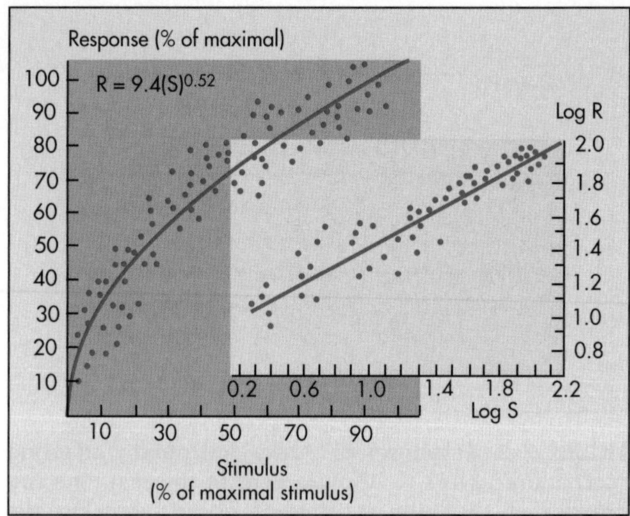

FIGURE 7–5. Stimulus-response function for a slowly adapting mechanoreceptor. The rate of discharge is plotted against stimulus strength (normalized to maximal). The plots are on linear and log-log scales. The stimulus-response function is response (R) = $9.4(S)^{0.52}$.

neurons and also on inhibitory interactions (Figure 7–4, *B*).

A **threshold stimulus** is the weakest that can be detected. To be detected, a stimulus must produce receptor potentials large enough to activate one or more primary afferent fibers. Weaker intensities of stimulation can produce subthreshold receptor potentials; however, such stimuli would not excite central sensory neurons. Furthermore, the number of primary afferent fibers that need to be excited for sensory detection depends on the requirements for spatial and temporal summation in the sensory pathway (see Chapter 4). Thus, a stimulus at threshold for detection may be much greater than threshold for activation of the most responsive primary afferent fibers. Conversely, a stimulus that excites some primary afferent fibers may not lead to perception of that stimulus.

Stimulus intensity may be encoded by the mean frequency of the discharge of sensory neurons. The relationship between stimulus intensity and response can be plotted as a stimulus-response function. For many sensory neurons, the stimulus-response function approximates an exponential curve (**Figure 7–5**). The general equation for such a curve follows:

$$\text{Response} = \text{Stimulus}^{n} \times \text{Constant}$$

The exponent *n* can be less than, equal to, or greater than 1. Many mechanoreceptors have stimulus-response functions with fractional exponents (Figure 7–5). Thermoreceptors have linear stimulus-response curves. Nociceptors may have linear or positively accelerating stimulus-response functions; that is, the exponent for these curves is 1 or more.

Another way in which stimulus intensity is encoded is by the number of sensory receptors activated. A stimulus that is threshold for perception may activate just one or a few primary afferent fibers, whereas a strong stimulus may excite many similar receptors. Central neurons that receive input from a particular class of sensory receptors would be more powerfully activated as more primary afferents are caused to discharge, and a greater activity in central sensory neurons will result in the perception of a stronger stimulus.

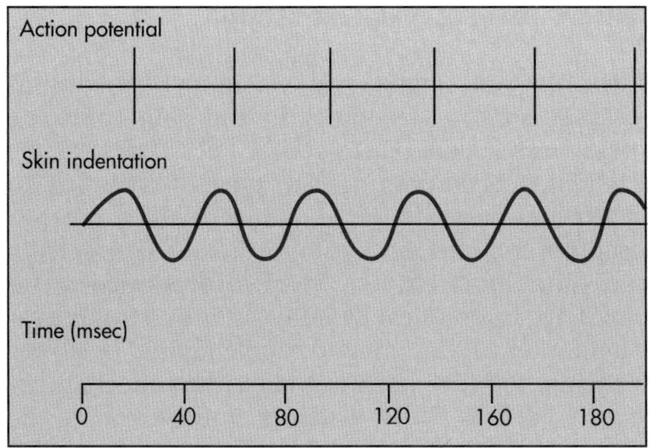

FIGURE 7–6. Coding for the frequency of stimulation: discharge of a rapidly adapting cutaneous mechanoreceptor in phase with a sinusoidal stimulus. *Top,* Action potential. *Center,* Stimulus. *Bottom,* Time in milliseconds.

Stimuli of different intensities may activate different sets of receptors. For example, a weak mechanical stimulus applied to the skin might activate only mechanoreceptors, whereas a strong mechanical stimulus might activate both mechanoreceptors and nociceptors. In this case, the sensation evoked by the stronger stimulus would be more intense, and the quality would be different.

Stimulus frequency can be encoded by the intervals between the discharges of sensory neurons. The interspike intervals sometimes correspond exactly to the intervals between stimuli **(Figure 7–6)**, but in other cases, a given neuron may discharge at intervals that are multiples of the interstimulus interval.

Stimulus duration may be encoded in slowly adapting sensory neurons by the duration of the enhanced firing. In rapidly adapting neurons, the beginning and end of a stimulus may be signaled by transient discharges.

Sensory pathways conduct sensory information to sensory-processing areas of the brain

A **sensory pathway** can be viewed as a set of neurons arranged in series **(Figure 7–7)**. First-, second-, third-, and higher-order neurons serve as sequential elements in a particular sensory pathway. However, several parallel sensory pathways often transmit similar sensory information.

The **first-order neuron** in a sensory pathway is the primary afferent neuron. The peripheral endings of this neuron form a sensory receptor (or receive input from an accessory sensory cell, such as a hair cell), and thus the neuron responds to a stimulus and transmits encoded information to the CNS. The primary afferent neuron often has its soma in a dorsal root or cranial nerve ganglion.

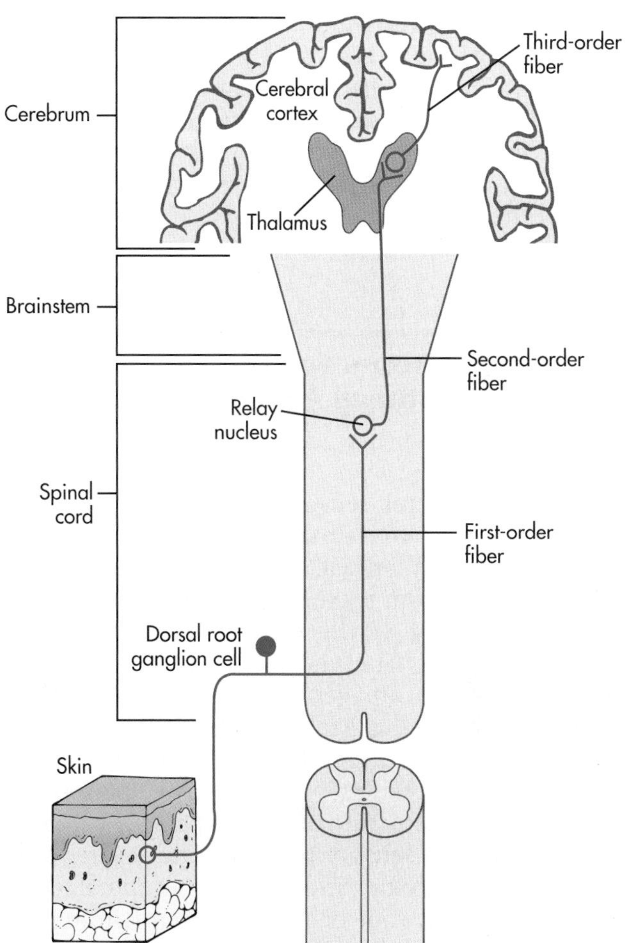

FIGURE 7–7. General arrangement of sensory pathways showing first-, second-, and third-order neurons. Note that the axon of the second-order neuron crosses the midline, so sensory information from one side of the body is transmitted to the opposite side of the brain.

The **second-order neuron** is likely to be located in the spinal cord or brainstem. It receives information from first-order neurons and transmits information to the thalamus. The information may be transformed at the level of the second-order neuron by local neural processing circuits. The ascending axons of second-order neurons typically cross the midline; thus, sensory information that originates on one side of the body reaches the contralateral thalamus.

The **third-order neuron** is generally located in a sensory nucleus of the thalamus. Again, local circuits may transform information from second-order neurons before the signals are transmitted to the cerebral cortex.

Fourth-order neurons in the appropriate sensory-receiving areas of the cerebral cortex and

higher-order neurons in the same and other cerebral cortical areas process the information further. There may also be interactions between the cerebral cortex and subcortical structures. At some undetermined site, the sensory information results in sensory perception, which is a conscious awareness of the stimulus.

The Somatovisceral Sensory System Responds to Stimuli Applied to the Body or to Viscera

The somatovisceral sensory system includes primary afferent neurons that form sensory receptor organs in the skin, muscle, joints, and viscera. Information arising from these sensory receptors reaches the CNS by way of the axons of the first-order sensory neurons. The cell bodies of the primary afferent neurons are generally in dorsal root or cranial nerve ganglia. Each ganglion cell gives off a branch or **neurite** that bifurcates into a peripheral process and a central process. The peripheral process has the structure of an axon and terminates peripherally as a sensory receptor. The central process is also an axon and enters the spinal cord through a dorsal root or the brainstem through a cranial nerve. The central process typically gives rise to numerous collateral branches that end synaptically on several second-order neurons.

The processing of somatovisceral sensory information involves a number of CNS structures, including the spinal cord, brainstem, thalamus, and cerebral cortex. The ascending pathways arise from second-order sensory neurons that are located in the spinal cord and brainstem and that generally project to the contralateral thalamus. The most important ascending somatovisceral pathways that carry information from the body are the **dorsal column–medial lemniscus pathway** and the **spinothalamic tract.** The main somatovisceral projection that represents the face is the trigeminothalamic tract. The organization of these pathways is described in the following sections. Ancillary somatovisceral pathways include the spinocervicothalamic pathway, the postsynaptic dorsal column pathway, the dorsal spinocerebellar tract, the spinoreticular tract, and the spinomesencephalic tract.

The somatovisceral sensory system can be regarded as a general sensory system. The sensory modalities mediated by the somatovisceral sensory system include touch-pressure, flutter-vibration, position sense, joint movement, thermal sense, pain, and visceral distention.

Sensory receptors detect stimuli

The somatovisceral sensory system includes various types of sensory receptors in the skin, muscles, joints, and viscera. **Cutaneous receptors** can be subdivided according to the type of stimulus to which they respond. The major types of cutaneous receptors include mechanoreceptors, thermoreceptors, and nociceptors. **Mechanoreceptors** respond to mechanical stimuli such as stroking or indentation of the skin and can be rapidly or slowly adapting. Rapidly adapting cutaneous mechanoreceptors include **hair follicle receptors** in the hairy skin, **Meissner's corpuscles** in the nonhairy (glabrous) skin, and **pacinian corpuscles** in subcutaneous tissue (**Figure 7–8,** ***A***). Hair follicle receptors and Meissner's corpuscles respond best to stimuli repeated at rates of about 30 to 40 Hz, and they contribute to the sensation of flutter. In contrast, pacinian corpuscles prefer stimuli repeated at approximately 250 Hz. They are responsible for vibratory sensation. Slowly adapting cutaneous mechanoreceptors include **Merkel cell endings** and **Ruffini's corpuscles** (Figure 7–8, *B*). Merkel cell endings have punctate receptive fields, whereas Ruffini's corpuscles have large receptive fields and can be activated by stretching or indentation of the skin. Merkel cell endings contribute to touch-pressure sensation. Ruffini's corpuscles probably contribute both to touch-pressure sensation and to position sense, at least with respect to distal joints such as those in the fingers. The axons of all of these receptor types are myelinated, so they conduct relatively rapidly, which permits signals transmitted from these receptors to be perceived soon after the stimulus occurs.

The two types of **thermoreceptors** in the skin are **cold receptors** and **warm receptors.** Both are slowly adapting, although they also discharge phasically when skin temperature changes rapidly. These are among the few receptor types that discharge spontaneously under normal circumstances. Cold receptors are supplied by small myelinated axons, whereas warm receptors are supplied by unmyelinated axons.

Nociceptors respond to stimuli that threaten to produce damage or actually do so. There are two major classes of cutaneous nociceptors: the **A-δ mechanical nociceptors** and the **C polymodal nociceptors.** A-δ mechanical nociceptors are supplied by finely myelinated (or A-δ) axons, whereas C polymodal nociceptors are supplied by unmyelinated (or C) fibers. The A-δ mechanical nociceptors respond to strong mechanical stimuli, such as pricking the skin with a needle or crushing the skin with forceps. Many do not respond to noxious thermal or chemical stimuli unless they have previously been

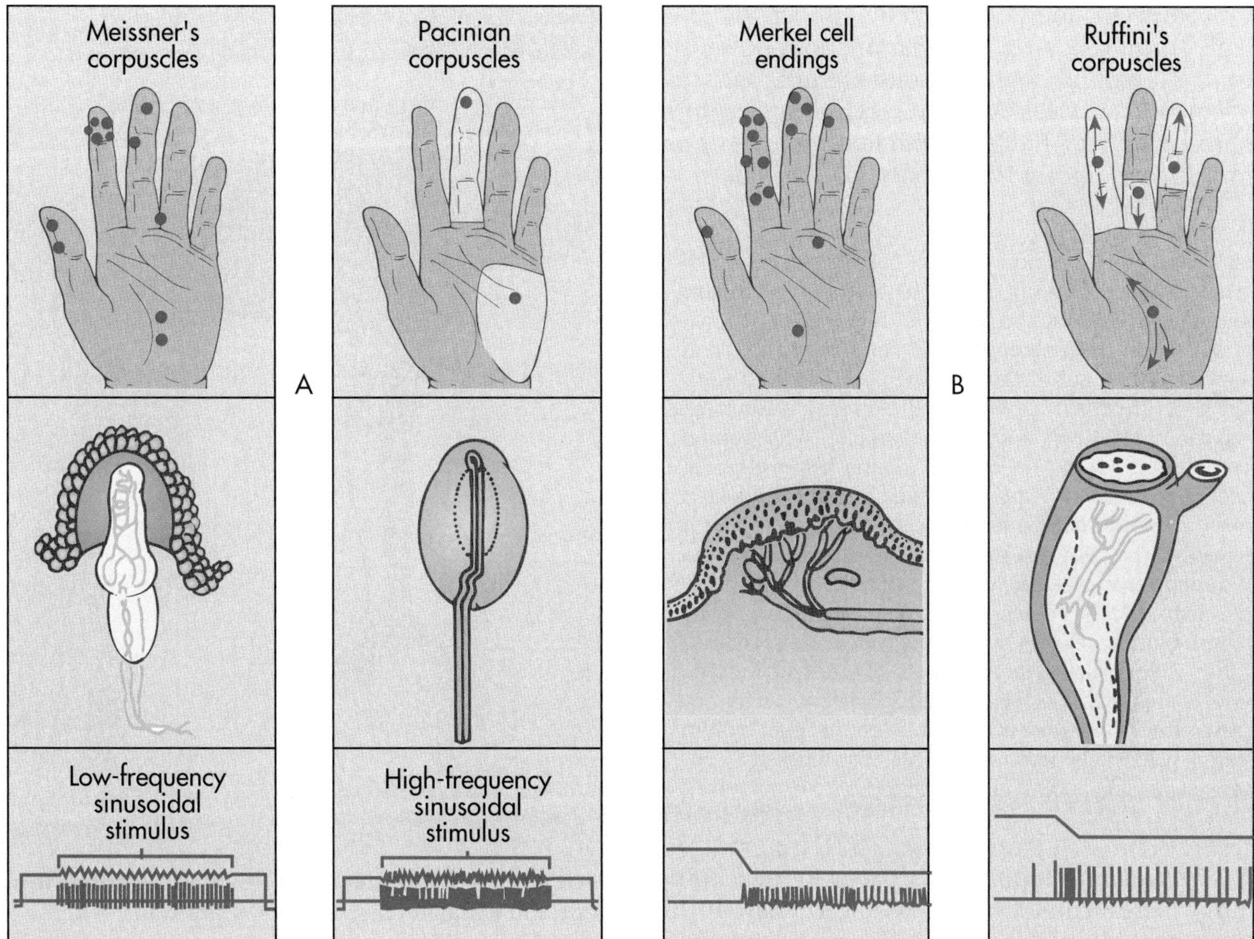

FIGURE 7–8. The receptive fields of several types of cutaneous mechanoreceptors are shown in the top row. Many more receptors are present than are indicated. Their density is greater on the more distal parts of the fingers. Red dots indicate the centers of the receptive fields, and yellow shading indicates the extent of the receptive fields. A, Rapidly adapting mechanoreceptors: Meissner's corpuscles and pacinian corpuscles. B, Slowly adapting mechanoreceptors: Merkel cell endings and Ruffini's corpuscles. The red arrows on the receptive fields of Ruffini's corpuscles show the directions of skin stretch that activated the afferent fibers. The second row of drawings shows the morphological structures of the receptors; the third row shows the responses to sinusoidal stimuli (A) or to step indentations of the skin (B).

sensitized. However, some A-δ nociceptors, termed mechano-heat nociceptors, respond to strong mechanical and thermal stimuli. C polymodal nociceptors respond to several types of noxious stimuli, including mechanical, thermal, and chemical.

Skeletal muscle also contains several types of sensory receptors. These are chiefly mechanoreceptors and nociceptors, although some muscle receptors possess thermosensitivity or chemosensitivity. The best-studied muscle receptors are the stretch receptors, which include **muscle spindles** and **Golgi tendon organs.** Although these play an important role in proprioception, they are also important in motor control. Therefore, their structure and function are discussed in Chapter 9.

Other sensory receptors in muscle include nociceptors that respond to pressure applied to the muscle and to the release of metabolites, especially during **ischemia** (inadequate blood flow). Muscle nociceptors are supplied by medium-sized and small myelinated (group II and III) axons or by unmyelinated (group IV) afferent fibers.

Joints are associated with several types of sensory receptors, including rapidly and slowly adapting mechanoreceptors and nociceptors. The rapidly adapting mechanoreceptors are pacinian corpuscles, which respond to mechanical transients, including vibration. The slowly adapting joint receptors are Ruffini's corpuscles, which respond best to movements of a joint to extremes of flexion or extension; these endings signal pressure or torque applied to the joint. Joint mechanoreceptors are innervated by medium-sized (group II) afferent fibers. Joint nociceptors are activated by probing of a joint capsule or by hyperextension or hyperflexion, although many articular nociceptors fail to respond to joint movements under normal conditions. If sensitized by inflammation, however, they can respond to innocuous stimuli, such as movements or weak pressure. Joint nociceptors are innervated by finely myelinated (group III) or unmyelinated (group IV) primary afferent fibers.

Arthritis is a common painful condition caused by inflammation of one or more joints. The nociceptors become sensitized by the release of a number of chemical substances from nerve endings, mast cells, and blood elements. These substances include neuropeptides (substance P, calcitonin gene–related peptide), histamine, bradykinin, serotonin, and prostaglandins. The sensitized nerve endings cause the joint to develop **hyperalgesia,** a condition in which the threshold for pain is lowered and the amount of pain produced by a given stimulus is increased. The joint also becomes swollen. This is caused by **neurogenic edema,** which is the collection of edema fluid that follows an increase in capillary permeability caused by the release of the neuropeptide substance P from joint nociceptors. Another peptide, calcitonin gene–related peptide, causes **vasodilation,** which increases the temperature of the joint. Arthritic pain is often treated successfully with substances that block the synthesis of prostaglandins, such as acetylsalicylic acid.

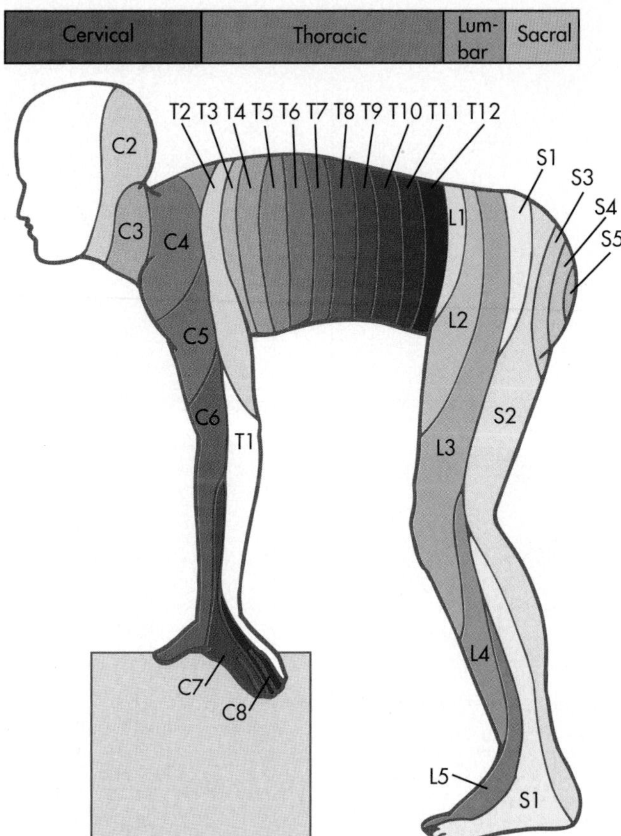

FIGURE 7–9. Dermatomes represented on a drawing of a person assuming a quadrupedal position.

Viscera are also supplied with sensory receptors. Most of these are involved in reflexes and have little to do with sensory experience. However, some visceral mechanoreceptors are responsible for the sensation of distention, and visceral nociceptors produce visceral pain. Pacinian corpuscles are present in the mesentery and in the capsules of visceral organs, such as the pancreas; these presumably signal mechanical transients. Whether visceral pain can result from overactivity of the mechanoreceptor afferents that respond to visceral distention is still controversial. Some viscera, however, clearly contain specific nociceptors.

Dermatomes, myotomes, and sclerotomes form embryonic segments of the body

Primary afferent fibers in the adult are distributed systematically, as determined during embryological development. The mammalian embryo becomes segmented, and each body segment is called a **somite.** A somite is innervated by an adjacent segment of the spinal cord or, in the case of a somite of the head, by a cranial nerve. The portion of a somite destined to form skin is called a **dermatome.** Similarly, the part of a somite that forms muscle is a **myotome,** and the part that forms bone is a **sclerotome.** Viscera are also supplied by particular segments of the spinal cord or particular cranial nerves.

Many dermatomes become distorted during development, chiefly because of the way the upper and lower extremities are formed and because humans maintain an upright posture. However, the sequence of dermatomes can readily be understood if they are pictured on the body in a quadrupedal position **(Figure 7–9).**

Although a dermatome receives its densest innervation from the corresponding spinal cord segment, it is also innervated by several adjacent spinal segments. Thus, transection of a dorsal root produces little sensory loss in the corresponding dermatome. Anesthesia of any given dermatome requires interruption of several successive dorsal roots.

Spinal roots and the spinal cord contribute to sensory pathways

Axons of the peripheral nervous system enter or leave the CNS through the spinal roots (or through cranial nerves). The dorsal root on one side of a given spinal segment is composed entirely of the central processes of **dorsal root ganglion cells.**

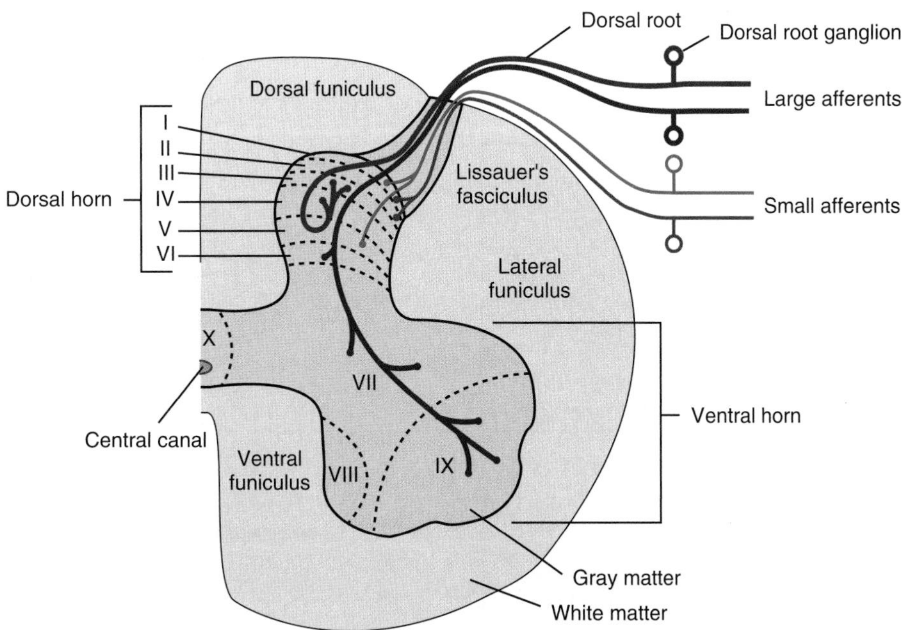

FIGURE 7–10. Distribution of large and small primary afferent fibers in the spinal cord. The gray matter on one side of the spinal cord is outlined, and the boundaries between the laminae are shown. Laminae I to VI form the dorsal horn; parts of laminae VI and VII make up the intermediate region; and part of lamina VII, plus laminae VIII and IX, forms the ventral horn. Lamina X is the gray matter surrounding the central canal. Terminals of two large primary afferent fibers are shown. One, from a hair follicle receptor *(purple)*, synapses in laminae III to V. The other, from a muscle spindle *(blue)*, synapses in laminae VI, VII, and IX. Terminals from two fine afferent fibers are also shown. The small myelinated fiber (A-δ) from a cutaneous nociceptor *(red)* ends in laminae I and V; the unmyelinated (C) afferent fiber *(green)* synapses in laminae I and II.

The **ventral root** consists chiefly of motor axons, including α motor axons, γ motor axons, and, at certain segmental levels, autonomic preganglionic axons. Ventral roots also contain many primary afferent fibers, whose role is still unclear.

The spinal cord can be subdivided into gray matter and white matter **(Figure 7–10)**. The gray matter includes the cell bodies and dendrites of the intrinsic neurons of the spinal cord. There, synaptic connections are made by primary afferent fibers, by interneurons, and by pathways descending from the brain. The **gray matter** is subdivided into the **dorsal horn,** the **intermediate region,** and the **ventral horn.** The neurons of the gray matter form layers, or **laminae.**

The gray matter of the spinal cord is surrounded by **white matter** (Figure 7–10). The white matter between the dorsal midline of the spinal cord and the entry line of the dorsal roots is called the **dorsal funiculus.** The white matter between the dorsal root entry line and the ventral root is the **lateral funiculus.** The white matter found between the ventral root exit line and the ventral midline is the **ventral funiculus. Lissauer's fasciculus** is a zone of fine nerve fibers that caps the dorsal horn. The white matter contains axons that belong to primary afferent fibers, spinal cord interneurons, and long ascending and descending pathways that connect the spinal cord and brain.

The trigeminal nerve transmits sensory information from the face and cranial cavities

The arrangement for primary afferent fibers that supply the face is comparable to that for fibers supplying the body. Peripheral processes of neurons in the **trigeminal ganglion** pass through the ophthalmic, maxillary, and mandibular divisions of the trigeminal nerve to innervate dermatome-like regions of the face **(Figure 7–11, *A*)**. The trigeminal nerve also innervates the oral and nasal cavities and the dura mater.

The large myelinated fibers that supply the mechanoreceptors of the skin and structures of the oral and nasal cavities synapse in the **principal sensory nucleus** of the trigeminal nerve (Figure 7–11, *B*). Small myelinated and unmyelinated nociceptive and thermoreceptive primary afferent fibers of the trigeminal nerve terminate in the nerve's **spinal nucleus** (Figure 7–11, *C*). Primary afferent fibers from stretch receptors have their cell bodies in the **mesencephalic nucleus** of the trigeminal

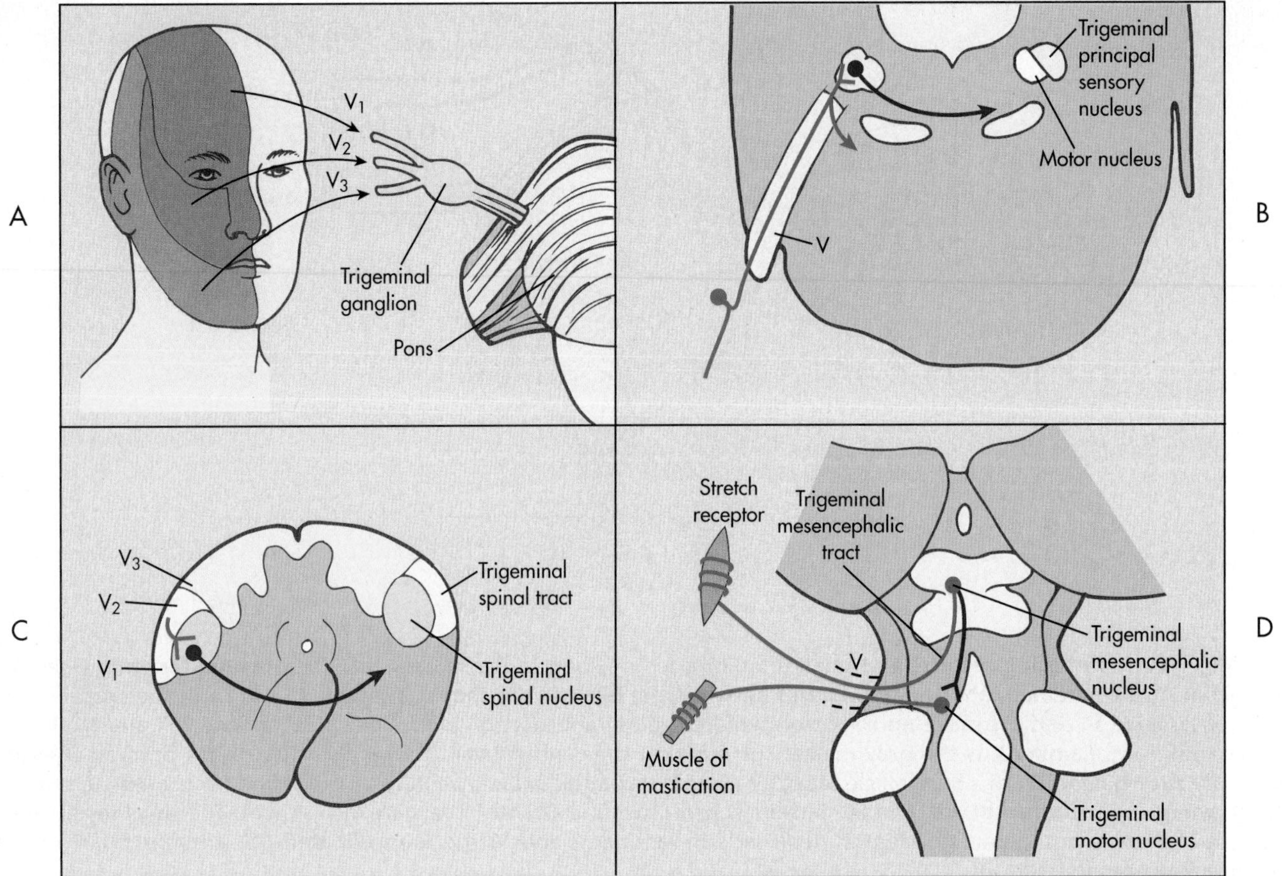

FIGURE 7–11. A, Dermatome-like areas of distribution of the ophthalmic (V_1), maxillary (V_2), and mandibular (V_3) divisions of the trigeminal nerve. B, Synaptic terminals of large myelinated primary afferent fibers of the trigeminal nerve in the main sensory nucleus and crossing of the trigeminothalamic tract. C, Descending branches of fine myelinated and unmyelinated primary afferent axons of the trigeminal nerve synapsing in the spinal nucleus and the projection of second-order neurons crossing in the trigeminothalamic tract. D, Location of cell bodies of primary afferent proprioceptive neurons of the trigeminal nerve in the mesencephalic nucleus. Synaptic connections of collaterals of these neurons are made with motor neurons in the trigeminal motor nucleus.

nerve (Figure 7–11, *D*). This arrangement is exceptional because all other primary afferent cell bodies in the somatovisceral system are in peripheral ganglia. The central processes of the proprioceptors synapse in the **motor nucleus** of the trigeminal nerve.

The dorsal column–medial lemniscus pathway includes the fasciculus gracilis and fasciculus cuneatus

The ascending branches of many large myelinated nerve fibers travel rostrally in the dorsal column to the medulla (see a standard textbook of neuroanatomy). The dorsal column can be subdivided into two smaller components, the **fasciculus gracilis** and the **fasciculus cuneatus.** Axons that innervate sensory receptors of the lower extremity and the lower trunk (T7 segment and caudally) ascend in the gracile fasciculus, whereas fibers from receptors of the upper extremity and upper trunk ascend in the cuneate fasciculus (T6 segment and rostrally). These axons are the first-order neurons of the dorsal column–medial lemniscus pathway. The second-order neurons are in the nucleus gracilis and nucleus cuneatus, which are collections of neurons in the caudal medulla. These nuclei are often called collectively the **dorsal column nuclei.** Axons of the fasciculus gracilis synapse in the nucleus gracilis, and axons of the fasciculus cuneatus synapse in the nucleus cuneatus.

Many neurons in the dorsal column nuclei respond in much the same way as the primary afferent fibers that synapse on them. Some behave like rapidly adapting receptors, responding to hair movement or to mechanical transients applied to the glabrous skin. Others discharge at high frequencies when vibratory stimuli are applied to their receptive fields and thus resemble pacinian corpuscles. Still other neurons in the dorsal column nuclei have slowly adapting responses to cutaneous stimuli. In the cuneate nucleus, many neurons are activated by muscle stretch. The main differences between the responses of dorsal column neurons and those of the primary afferent fibers are that

- dorsal column neurons have larger receptive fields because more than one primary afferent fiber synapses on a given dorsal column neuron;
- they sometimes respond to more than one class of sensory receptors because of the convergence of several different types of primary afferent fibers on the second-order neurons; and
- they often have inhibitory receptive fields mediated through interneuronal circuits in the dorsal column nuclei.

The dorsal column nuclei project to the contralateral thalamus by way of the **medial lemniscus.** The medial lemniscus terminates in the **ventral posterolateral (VPL) nucleus** of the thalamus. Neurons in the VPL nucleus in turn project to the **primary (SI)** and **secondary (SII) somatosensory cortex.**

Some projections of trigeminal nuclei are comparable to the dorsal column–medial lemniscus pathway

Large myelinated primary afferent fibers that supply mechanoreceptors in the skin of the face synapse in the principal sensory nucleus of the trigeminal nerve. Second-order neurons in the principal sensory nucleus project to the contralateral thalamus by way of the **trigeminothalamic tract** (Figure 7–11, *B*). Some neurons project ipsilaterally. The projections are to the **ventral posteromedial (VPM) thalamic nucleus.** Third-order neurons of the VPM nucleus project to the SI and SII somatosensory cortex. This pathway of the trigeminal system is equivalent for the face to the dorsal column–medial lemniscus pathway for the body.

Other somatovisceral sensory pathways are included in the dorsal spinal cord

Three other pathways that carry somatovisceral sensory information ascend in the dorsal part of the spinal cord on the same side as the afferent input: the spinocervical tract, the postsynaptic dorsal column pathway, and the dorsal spinocerebellar tract.

The cells of origin of the **spinocervical tract** receive input largely from cutaneous mechanoreceptors, although some of these cells are also activated by cutaneous nociceptors. The cells of origin of the **postsynaptic dorsal column pathway** receive information similar to that reaching spinocervical tract neurons. In addition, some of these neurons are activated by nociceptors in visceral organs. The information conveyed by these neurons is eventually conveyed to the VPL nucleus of the thalamus.

The **dorsal spinocerebellar tract** responds to input from muscle and joint receptors of the lower extremity. The main destination of the tract is the cerebellum, but it also provides proprioceptive information from the leg to the contralateral VPL nucleus of the thalamus after a relay in the medulla. Proprioceptive information from the arm is signaled by the dorsal column pathway.

Sensory functions of the dorsal spinal cord pathways are mostly mechanoreceptive

THE SENSORY QUALITIES MEDIATED BY THE ASCENDING PATHWAYS IN THE DORSAL PART OF THE SPINAL CORD INCLUDE FLUTTER-VIBRATION, TOUCH-PRESSURE, JOINT MOVEMENT, POSITION SENSE, AND VISCERAL DISTENTION. Each of these qualities of sensation depends on activity in a set of sensory neurons that collectively form a labeled-line sensory channel. A sensory channel may involve several parallel ascending pathways, and it includes particular afferent neurons and sensory-processing mechanisms at the levels of the spinal cord, brainstem, thalamus, and cerebrum.

Flutter-vibration is a complex sensation. **Flutter** refers to recognition of repetitive events that have low-frequency components. The sensory receptors that detect flutter include hair follicles and Meissner's corpuscles. Ascending sensory tracts that convey information needed for flutter sensation include the dorsal column–medial lemniscus pathway, the spinocervical tract, and the postsynaptic dorsal column pathway. High-frequency vibration is detected primarily by pacinian corpuscles. Branches of pacinian corpuscle afferents ascend in the dorsal column, and some postsynaptic dorsal column neurons respond to activation of pacinian corpuscles.

Touch-pressure sensation involves the recognition of skin indentation by Merkel cell endings and Ruffini's corpuscles. The ascending pathways that convey information from these receptors include the dorsal column–medial lemniscus and the postsynaptic dorsal column pathways.

Proprioception, the senses of joint movement and joint position, is complex and depends on sensory information that arises from muscle, joint, and cutaneous receptors. For some proximal joints, such as the knee, the most important information is derived from stretch receptors in the muscles that move the joint. In distal joints, however, such as those of the digits, Ruffini's corpuscles in the skin and nail beds and joint receptors also contribute.

Visceral pain depends on the activation of visceral nociceptors. It has been shown that visceral pain signals are conveyed in large part by postsynaptic dorsal column neurons.

The thalamus and cerebral cortex are responsible for higher processing of tactile and proprioceptive information

The medial lemniscus synapses in the VPL nucleus of the thalamus, as described earlier. The responses of many neurons in the VPL nucleus resemble those of the first- and second-order neurons of the dorsal column–medial lemniscus pathway. The responses may be dominated by a particular type of receptor, and the receptive fields may be small, although larger than that of a primary afferent fiber. Thalamic neurons often have inhibitory receptive fields. A notable difference between neurons in the VPL nucleus and neurons at lower levels of the dorsal column–medial lemniscus pathway is that the excitability of the thalamic neurons depends on the stage of the sleep-wake cycle and on the presence or absence of anesthesia.

The SI receiving area of the cerebral cortex is in the postcentral gyrus of the parietal lobe. Within any particular area of the SI cortex, all of the neurons along a line perpendicular to the cortical surface have similar response properties and receptive fields. The SI cortex is thus said to have a **columnar organization.** A comparable columnar organization has also been demonstrated for other primary sensory-receiving areas, including the primary visual and auditory cortices.

The location of cortical columns in the SI region is related systematically to the location of the receptive fields on the body surface. This relationship is called a **somatotopic map** because the body surface is mapped in the SI cortex. The lower extremity is represented in the medial aspect of the postcentral gyrus, whereas the upper extremity is mapped on the dorsolateral aspect of the postcentral gyrus, and the face is mapped dorsal to the lateral fissure (**Figure 7–12**). This somatotopic map for humans is called a **homunculus,** meaning "a little man." The somatotopic organization of the SI cortex is a means for encoding stimulus location. The somatotopic organization at the cortical level reflects the same type of organization at lower levels of the somatovisceral sensory system, including the dorsal column nuclei and the VPL and VPM nuclei of the thalamus.

Besides being responsible for the initial processing of somatovisceral sensory information, the SI cortex also begins higher-order processing, such as **feature extraction,** the recognition of special features of a stimulus. For example, certain neurons in area 1 respond preferentially to a stimulus moving in one direction across the receptive field but not in the opposite direction (**Figure 7–13**). This response pattern is the result of the organization of inhibitory circuits in the cortex. Such neurons might contribute to the perceptual ability to recognize the direction of an applied stimulus.

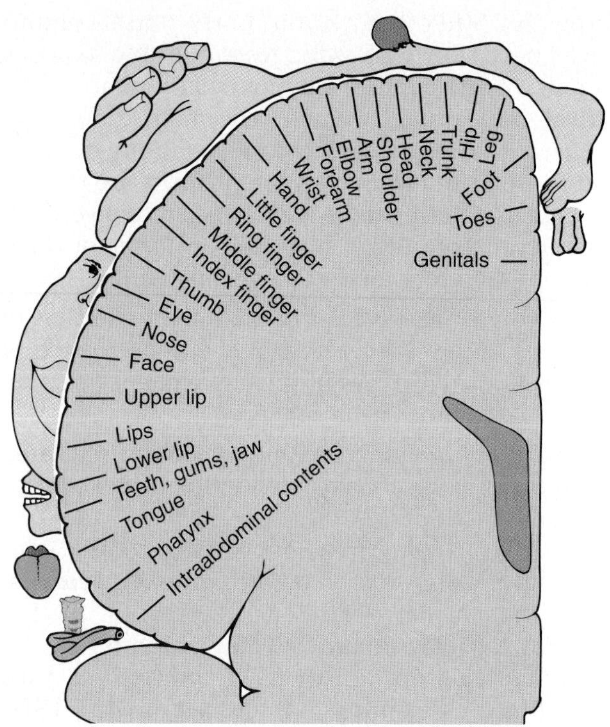

FIGURE 7–12. Sensory homunculus of the primary somatosensory cortex. One cerebral hemisphere is drawn as if it were sectioned in the coronal plane. The sizes of the different parts of the homunculus indicate the proportionate amounts of cortex dedicated to different parts of the body and head.

The spinothalamic tract is responsible for somatic pain and temperature sensations

The **spinothalamic tract** originates from spinal cord neurons that project mainly to the contralateral thalamus. The place where the axon of a spinothalamic tract cell crosses is within the same segment as the cell body, and the axon ascends in the lateral or ventral funiculus. The spinothalamic tract terminates in several nuclei of the thalamus, including the VPL nucleus and several nuclei of the medial thalamus. Imaging studies have shown that several regions of the cerebral cortex receive

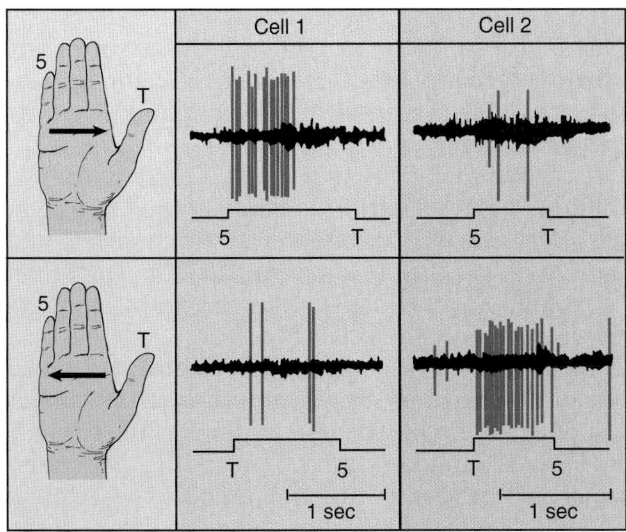

FIGURE 7–13. Feature extraction by cortical neurons. The responses of two cortical neurons to stimuli moved across the palm are shown. Cell 1 was excited strongly by movement of the stimulus toward the thumb (T) but only weakly by movements in the opposite direction. Cell 2 showed the converse behavior.

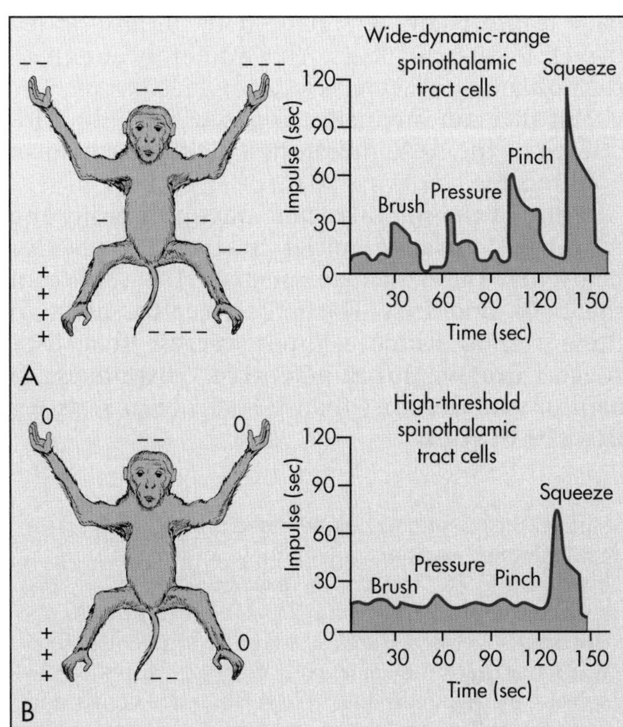

FIGURE 7–14. **A**, Responses of a wide-dynamic-range spinothalamic tract cell. **B**, Responses of a high-threshold spinothalamic tract cell. The figures at left indicate the excitatory *(plus signs)* and inhibitory *(minus signs)* receptive fields. The graphs at right show the responses to graded intensities of mechanical stimulation in the receptive field.

nociceptive input from these thalamic nuclei, including the SI and SII (primary and secondary somatosensory cortices), the anterior cingulate gyrus, and the insular cortex.

The cells of origin of the spinothalamic tract are found chiefly in spinal cord laminae I and V. Effective stimuli include noxious mechanical, thermal, and chemical stimuli. Some spinothalamic neurons are excited by activity in cold or warm thermoreceptors or sensitive mechanoreceptors.

Spinothalamic tract cells often receive a convergent excitatory input from several classes of sensory receptors. For example, a given spinothalamic tract neuron may be activated weakly by tactile stimuli but more powerfully by noxious stimuli **(Figure 7–14)**. Such neurons are called **wide-dynamic-range** cells because they are activated by stimuli that have a wide range of intensities. Wide-dynamic-range neurons mainly signal noxious events, the weak response to tactile stimuli perhaps being ignored by higher centers. However, in pathological conditions, these neurons may be activated sufficiently by normally innocuous stimuli to evoke a sensation of pain. This would explain some pain states in which activation of mechanoreceptors causes pain. This condition is called **mechanical allodynia.** Other spinothalamic tract cells are activated only by noxious stimuli. Such neurons are often called **nociceptive-specific cells** or high-threshold cells (Figure 7–14).

An example of a pathological state in which **allodynia** is prominent is **central pain,** which can result from damage to the CNS. For example, a lesion involving the VPL nucleus may result in a central pain syndrome called **thalamic pain.** The quality of the pain is typically burning, although it can be sharp. Pain is often evoked by weak stimulation, such as contact of the clothing with the skin. Patients with thalamic pain often prefer moistened clothing to dry clothing and sometimes wear a wet cotton glove on the affected side.

Spinothalamic tract cells often have inhibitory receptive fields. Inhibition may result from weak mechanical stimuli, but the most effective inhibitory stimuli are usually noxious ones. The nociceptive inhibitory receptive fields may be very large and include most of the body and face (Figure 7–14).

The **gate control theory of pain** explains how innocuous stimuli may inhibit the responses of dorsal horn neurons that transmit information about painful stimuli to the brain. In this theory, pain transmission is prevented by innocuous inputs mediated by large myelinated afferent fibers, whereas pain transmission is enhanced by inputs carried over fine afferent fibers. The inhibitory interneurons of lamina II serve as a gating mechanism. The circuit diagram originally proposed has been criticized, but the basic notion of a gating mechanism is still viable.

Many of the spinothalamic tract cells projecting to medial thalamic nuclei have large receptive fields that often include much of the surface of the body and face. The large receptive fields of these spinothalamic neurons suggest that they trigger **motivational-affective responses** to painful stimuli rather than participate in **sensory discrimination.**

Various therapeutic techniques have been developed for the treatment of pain. Some of these involve the surgical interruption of nociceptive pathways, such as the spinothalamic tract. For example, an **anterolateral cordotomy** involves a surgical lesion in the ventrolateral white matter of the spinal cord at a level rostral to the spinal cord segments that receive the pain signals and in the white matter on the opposite side (because the spinothalamic tract crosses within the spinal cord). After such a lesion, pain and temperature sensations are lost on the opposite side of the body, below the level of the lesion. Cordotomies can be effective, at least for a few months. However, pain may recur, so cordotomies are of limited value when survival time is extended. In cases of chronic pain, other modalities of treatment, such as **transcutaneous electrical nerve stimulation (TENS)** or stimulation of the dorsal funiculus with an implanted electrode, are often tried. These approaches are based on the gate theory of pain and depend on inhibitory processing of nociceptive signals in the CNS.

Some projections of trigeminal nuclei are comparable to the spinothalamic tract

Nociceptors and thermoreceptors of the face enter the brainstem with the trigeminal nerve and synapse in the spinal nucleus of the trigeminal nerve (Figure 7–11, C). Second-order neurons of the spinal nucleus project to the contralateral VPM thalamic nucleus and medial thalamus through the trigeminothalamic tract. Third-order thalamic neurons in turn project to the face area of the somatosensory cortex. This pathway for the face is equivalent to that involving the spinothalamic tract for the body. PAIN IN THE TRIGEMINAL DISTRIBUTION IS OF PARTICULAR IMPORTANCE BECAUSE IT INCLUDES BOTH TOOTH PAIN AND HEADACHES.

Other somatovisceral sensory pathways in the ventral spinal cord accompany the spinothalamic tract

Two other pathways, the spinoreticular tract and the spinomesencephalic tract, transmit somatovisceral sensory information and ascend in the ventral part of the spinal cord. The cells of origin of the **spinoreticular tract** are often difficult to activate, but when receptive fields are found, these are generally large, sometimes bilateral, and the effective stimuli include noxious ones. The reticular formation is located within the core of the brainstem, and it is involved in attentional mechanisms and arousal. Ascending fibers from the reticular formation extend to the medial thalamus and from there to wide areas of the cerebral cortex.

Many cells of the **spinomesencephalic tract** respond to noxious stimuli, and the receptive fields are generally small. The terminations of the tract are in several midbrain nuclei, including the **periaqueductal gray** (the area around the cerebral aqueduct), which is an important component of the endogenous analgesia system (see later discussion in this chapter). Information from the midbrain is also relayed to the **limbic system.** This may provide one pathway by which noxious stimuli can trigger emotional responses. Motivational-affective responses may also result from activation of the periaqueductal gray and midbrain reticular formation. The midbrain reticular formation is an important part of the arousal system, and stimulation in the periaqueductal gray causes vocalization and aversive behavior.

Sensory functions of the ventral spinal cord pathways include pain reactions

The most important sensory modalities mediated by ventral spinal cord pathways are pain and thermal sensations. Thermal sense depends on input from cold and warm receptors to spinothalamic tract neurons. Pain resulting from the stimulation of nociceptors is mediated partly by spinothalamic tract cells and partly by the spinoreticular and spinomesencephalic tracts. The sensory-discriminative component of pain is processed in the SI and SII regions of the somatosensory cortex. This component of pain allows judgments about the location, intensity, and duration of a painful stimulus. Pain is also characterized by motivational-affective responses.

THE MOTIVATIONAL-AFFECTIVE RESPONSES TO PAINFUL STIMULI INCLUDE ATTENTION AND AROUSAL, SOMATIC AND AUTONOMIC REFLEXES, ENDOCRINE RESPONSES, AND EMOTIONAL CHANGES. These collectively account for the unpleasant nature of painful stimuli. The motivational-affective responses depend on several ascending pathways, including the component of the spinothalamic tract that projects to the medial thalamus, the spinoreticular tract, and the spinomesencephalic tract. As indicated previously, these pathways have access to attentional, orientational, and arousal systems as well as to the limbic system.

Cortical regions involved in the motivational-affective responses to painful stimuli include the anterior cingulate gyrus and the insula, as demonstrated by imaging studies.

Pain that originates from the skin is generally well localized, presumably because spinothalamic tract cells have relatively discrete cutaneous receptive fields. Also, the ascending system through which they signal is somatotopically organized. However, pain that originates from deep structures, including muscle and viscera, is poorly localized and is often mistakenly attributed to superficial structures **(referred pain).**

Angina pectoris is a type of visceral pain that results from ischemia (inadequate blood flow) to the heart. The pain is often referred to the inner aspect of the left arm, although other regions of referral, such as the jaw, abdomen, or back, are not uncommon. The ischemia, generally caused by arteriosclerotic narrowing of one or more coronary arteries, releases algesic chemicals that sensitize visceral nociceptors supplying the heart. The nociceptors activate spinothalamic tract neurons in the left upper thoracic spinal cord. These neurons are also excited by sensory receptors supplying the left upper trunk and the T1 dermatome, which courses along the inner aspect of the arm (Figure 7–9). Presumably, activation of visceral nociceptors in the heart results in the excitation of spinothalamic neurons that also signal pain originating from the body wall. This in turn leads to a misinterpretation of the source of the pain. This concept is the basis of the **convergence-projection theory** of referred pain.

Centrifugal control of somatovisceral sensation allows the brain to control sensory information

SENSORY EXPERIENCE IS NOT JUST THE PASSIVE DETECTION OF ENVIRONMENTAL EVENTS; INSTEAD, IT MORE OFTEN DEPENDS ON EXPLORATION OF THE ENVIRONMENT. Tactile cues are sought by moving the hand over a surface. Visual cues result from scanning visual targets with the eyes. Thus, sensory information is often received as a result of activity in the motor system. Furthermore, sensory transmission in pathways to the sensory centers of the brain is regulated by descending control systems. This allows the brain to control its input by filtering the incoming sensory messages. Important information can be processed and unimportant information ignored.

The tactile and proprioceptive somatosensory pathways are regulated by descending pathways. However, of particular interest are the descending control systems that regulate the transmission of nociceptive information. These systems presumably reduce excessive pain under certain circumstances.

Soldiers on the battlefield, athletes in competition, accident victims, and others facing stressful circumstances often feel little or no pain at the time a wound occurs or a bone is broken. Later, however, pain may be severe. Although the descending regulatory pathways that control pain are part of the more general centrifugal system that modulates all forms of sensation, the pain-control system is so important that it is distinguished as a special **endogenous analgesia system.**

Several descending pathways contribute to the endogenous analgesia system. The activity of these descending pathways inhibits spinothalamic tract neurons. The **raphe nuclei,** which are at the midline of the medulla, and the **periaqueductal gray,** which is near the midline in the midbrain, give rise to direct and indirect projections to the medullary and spinal dorsal horns, and these pathways inhibit nociceptive neurons, including trigeminothalamic and spinothalamic tract cells **(Figure 7–15,** ***A*****).**

The endogenous analgesia system can be subdivided into pathways that release one of the **endogenous opioids** and those that do not. The endogenous opioid substances are neuropeptides that activate one or more of the several forms of opiate receptors. Some of the endogenous opioids are the **enkephalins, dynorphin, β-endorphin,** and the recently discovered **endomorphins.** Opioid analgesia can generally be antagonized with the narcotic antagonist **naloxone.** Therefore, naloxone is used as a test of whether analgesia is mediated through an opioid mechanism.

Opiates typically inhibit neural activity in the nociceptive pathways. Two sites of action have been proposed for opiate inhibition, presynaptic and postsynaptic (Figure 7–15, *B*). The presynaptic action of opiates on nociceptive afferent terminals is thought to prevent the release of excitatory transmitters, such as the neuropeptide **substance P.** The postsynaptic action produces an inhibitory postsynaptic potential, reducing cAMP levels as well. How can an inhibitory neurotransmitter activate descending pathways? One hypothesis is that the descending analgesia system is under tonic inhibitory control by inhibitory interneurons in both the midbrain and the medulla. The action of opiates would inhibit the inhibitory interneurons and thereby disinhibit the descending analgesia pathways. However, evidence indicates that another opioid action can be postsynaptic excitation.

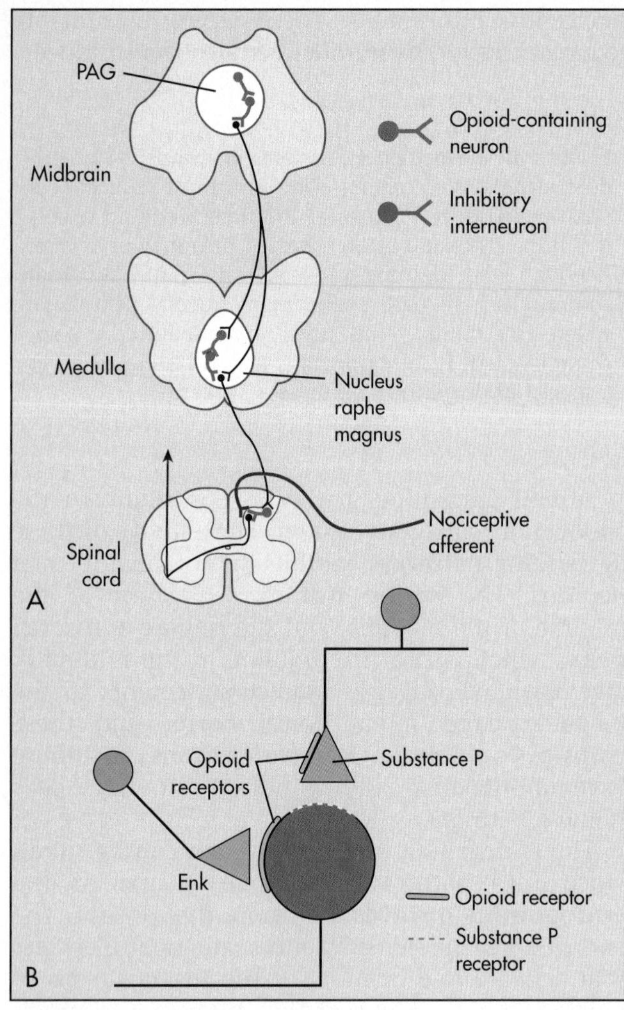

FIGURE 7–15. A, Neurons that play a role in the endogenous analgesia system. The periaqueductal gray (PAG) activates the raphe-spinal pathway, which in turn inhibits spinothalamic tract cells. Interneurons containing opioid neurotransmitters are at each level. B, Possible presynaptic and postsynaptic sites of action of enkephalin (Enk). The presynaptic action prevents the release of substance P from nociceptors, and the postsynaptic action is inhibition of nociceptive neurons.

Opiate receptors are found in the brain and spinal cord. At the spinal level, opiate receptors are located not only on the dorsal horn neurons but also on the terminals of nociceptors within the dorsal horn. Because of the presence of these opiate receptors, pain can sometimes be treated by the application of morphine to the spinal cord. This is done by the use of a **morphine pump** connected to a catheter introduced into the epidural space. The morphine can diffuse across the meninges and enter the spinal cord dorsal horn. The advantage of this route of delivery of morphine is that the morphine has a direct action on pain-processing circuits without seriously affecting thought processes, as may happen with systemically administered morphine. However, there is still a danger that morphine given by a morphine pump can depress respiration if the drug spreads rostrally in the cerebrospinal fluid.

The dose of morphine applied by the pump can be controlled by the patient **(patient-controlled analgesia).** The total dose of morphine that successfully minimizes pain is less when it is regulated by the patient than when it is regulated by the health care team.

Some endogenous analgesia pathways operate by neurotransmitters other than opioids and thus are unaffected by naloxone. One way of engaging a nonopioid analgesia pathway is through any of several types of stress. The analgesia so produced is called **stress-induced analgesia.**

Many neurons in the raphe nuclei release **serotonin** as a neurotransmitter. Serotonin is able to inhibit nociceptive neurons and presumably plays an important role in the endogenous analgesia system. Other brainstem neurons release catecholamines, such as **norepinephrine.** Catecholamines also inhibit nociceptive neurons, and therefore catecholaminergic neurons contribute to the endogenous analgesia system. Many other substances also undoubtedly participate in the analgesia system. Furthermore, there is evidence that endogenous opiate antagonists exist that can prevent opiate analgesia.

Summary

- Sensory receptors respond to stimuli by various transduction mechanisms. The specific mechanism depends on the type of receptor.
- Transduction causes a receptor potential, which is usually a depolarization that may cause the sensory receptor's primary afferent fiber to discharge.
- In some sensory receptors, the primary afferent fiber develops a generator potential in response to the release of synaptic transmitter from a separate sensory receptor cell.

- The responses of sensory receptors can be rapidly or slowly adapting, depending on the type of information to be signaled.
- A sensory receptor has a receptive field, which is the region that, when it is stimulated, affects the discharge of the neuron. Central sensory neurons may have both excitatory and inhibitory receptive fields.
- Sensory information is encoded so that modality, spatial location, threshold, intensity, frequency, and duration are all recognized.
- Somatovisceral sensory receptors include mechanoreceptors, thermoreceptors, and nociceptors.
- Cutaneous sensory receptors include a number of types of mechanoreceptors—hair follicle receptors, Meissner's corpuscles, pacinian corpuscles, Merkel cell endings, and Ruffini's corpuscles. The skin also contains cold and warm thermoreceptors and several kinds of nociceptors.
- Skeletal muscle contains stretch receptors as well as nociceptors. Joints and viscera are also supplied with mechanoreceptors and nociceptors.
- The dorsal column–medial lemniscus pathway mediates the sensations of flutter-vibration, touch-pressure, and proprioception. The path is somatotopically organized. The cortical representation of the body forms a sensory homunculus.
- The spinothalamic tract mediates pain and temperature sensations. The motivational-affective part of the pain response involves nonsomatotopic connections with the medial thalamus. Visceral pain is often referred to somatic structures.
- The somatovisceral sensory pathways, including the spinothalamic tract, are controlled by pathways that descend from the brain. The endogenous analgesia system regulates pain by releasing endogenous opioid substances and certain monoamines, such as serotonin and norepinephrine, as neurotransmitters in the spinal cord dorsal horn.

Bibliography

Belmonte C, Cervero F: *Neurobiology of nociceptors,* Oxford, 1996, Oxford University Press.

Casey KL, Bushnell MC: *Pain imaging,* Seattle, 2000, IASP Press.

Caterina MJ, Julius D: The vanilloid receptor: a molecular gateway to the pain pathway, *Annu Rev Neurosci* 24:487, 2001.

Gebhart GF, ed: *Visceral pain,* Seattle, 1995, IASP Press.

Hamill OP, Martinac B: Molecular basis of mechanotransduction in living cells, *Physiol Rev* 81:685, 2001.

Hansson PT et al: *Neuropathic pain: pathophysiology and treatment,* Seattle, 2001, IASP Press.

Mason P: Contributions of the medullary raphe and ventromedial reticular region to pain modulation and other homeostatic functions, *Annu Rev Neurosci* 24:737, 2001.

Mountcastle VB: *Perceptual neuroscience: the cerebral cortex,* Cambridge, Mass, 1998, Harvard University Press.

Penfield W, Jasper H: *Epilepsy and the functional anatomy of the human brain,* Boston, 1954, Little, Brown.

Romo R, Salinas E: Touch and go: decision-making mechanisms in somatosensation, *Annu Rev Neurosci* 24:107, 2001.

Steriade M, Jones EG, McCormick DSA: *Thalamus, vol 1, Organization and function,* Amsterdam, 1997, Elsevier.

Steriade M, Jones EG, McCormick DSA: *Thalamus, vol 2, Experimental and clinical aspects,* Amsterdam, 1997, Elsevier.

Willis WD, Coggeshall RE: *Sensory mechanisms of the spinal cord,* ed 3, New York, 2004, Kluwer Academic/Plenum Publishers.

Willis WD, Westlund KN: Pain system. In Paxinos G, Mai JK, eds: *The human nervous system,* ed 2, Amsterdam, 2004, Elsevier Academic Press.

Case Studies

Case 7–1

A 74-year-old woman awakens with a feeling of numbness on the left side of her body. She also has difficulty moving her left arm and leg. Her physician finds that she cannot distinguish between a coin and a paper clip when these are placed in her left hand while her eyes are closed. Her ability to recognize that two separate points on the skin are stimulated simultaneously is much poorer on her left than on her right side. She fails to recognize the vibration of a tuning fork placed against her left wrist or ankle. Pinpricks feel duller on the left than on the right side. Several weeks after the initial incident, she begins to feel burning pain on the left side, and even gentle contact of objects with the skin of her left arm or leg causes additional pain.

1. **What is the most likely location of the lesion that produces her symptoms?**
   A. Central part of the right medulla
   B. Cerebral cortex around the right central sulcus
   C. Peripheral nerves of the left arm and leg
   D. Posterior thalamus and adjacent internal capsule on the right
   E. Right half of the spinal cord above C5

2. **The patient's ability to feel pinpricks is diminished, but she can perceive spontaneous pain and allodynia for what reason?**
   A. Her lesion has damaged the brainstem reticular formation pathways that project to the medial thalamus.
   B. The pain symptoms are imaginary and do not reflect changes in the nervous system.
   C. Spinothalamic input to the VPL nucleus is largely interrupted, but there are plastic changes in denervated cortical circuits.
   D. Nociceptive primary afferent fibers have been destroyed in peripheral nerves, but mechanoreceptive afferents become nociceptive.
   E. Spinal cord nociceptive neurons such as spinothalamic tract cells stop signaling pinprick sensations but discharge spontaneously and in response to touch.

Case 7–2

Cancer of the descending colon develops in a 46-year-old man. As the disease progresses, he has severe pelvic pain. Morphine is administered systemically to counteract the pain. However, unless the dose is so high that he becomes somnolent, he obtains insufficient pain relief. An alternative method for pain control in this patient is clearly desirable. The therapy chosen is a morphine pump to infuse morphine epidurally through a catheter placed over the lumbosacral spinal cord.

1. **This approach is likely to be successful because of which reason?**
   A. Morphine will reach the periaqueductal gray in the cerebrospinal fluid via the cerebral aqueduct.
   B. There are opiate receptors in the spinal cord dorsal horn, and activation of these will reduce nociceptive transmission.
   C. The morphine would act on the cancer cells in the pelvic region, preventing these cells from inducing pain.
   D. Nociceptors in the meninges are responsible for the pain, and morphine would block their activity.
   E. When morphine reaches the spinal cord, it will cause the release of substance P from the terminals of nociceptors in the dorsal horn.

2. **Morphine is more likely than a local anesthetic to succeed in this case because of which reason?**
   A. Morphine is unlikely to cause respiratory depression.
   B. Local anesthetic infusion may cause itching sensations.
   C. Tolerance will develop to the local anesthetic.
   D. Morphine will block all types of sensation.
   E. Morphine will block pain preferentially.

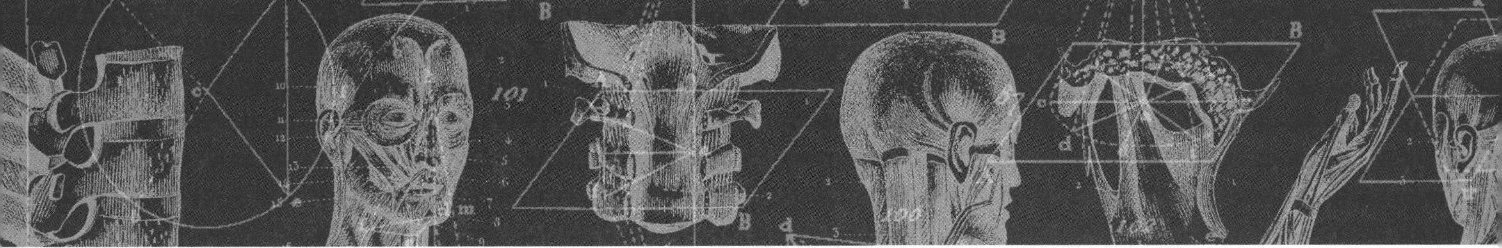

Chapter 8: Special Senses

Objectives

- ❖ Describe the visual system, including the eye and the central visual pathways.
- ❖ Explain the auditory system, including the cochlea and the central auditory pathways.
- ❖ Describe the vestibular system, including the labyrinth and the central vestibular pathways.
- ❖ Explain the chemical senses, including taste and smell.

In the evolution of the nervous system, an important trend has been **encephalization,** in which special sensory organs developed in the heads of animals and appropriate neural systems developed in the brains. These special sensory systems, which include the **visual, auditory, gustatory,** and **olfactory systems,** allowed the animal to detect and analyze light, sound, and chemical signals in the environment. In addition, the **vestibular system** evolved to signal the position of the head.

The Visual System Detects and Interprets Photic Stimuli

In vertebrates, effective photic stimuli are electromagnetic waves of lengths between 400 and 700 nm, which make up **visible light.** Light enters the eye and impinges on **photoreceptors** in a specialized sensory epithelium, the **retina.** The photoreceptors are the **rods** and **cones.** RODS HAVE LOW THRESHOLDS FOR DETECTING LIGHT, AND THEIR **PHOTOPIGMENT** BLEACHES IN STRONG LIGHT. THUS, RODS OPERATE BEST UNDER CONDITIONS OF REDUCED LIGHTING **(SCOTOPIC VISION).** However, rods neither provide well-defined visual images nor contribute to color vision. CONES, IN CONTRAST, ARE NOT AS SENSITIVE TO LIGHT BUT OPERATE BEST UNDER DAYLIGHT CONDITIONS **(PHOTOPIC VISION).** CONES ARE RESPONSIBLE FOR HIGH VISUAL ACUITY AND COLOR VISION.

The structure of the eye is complex

The wall of the eye is formed of three concentric layers **(Figure 8–1).** The outer layer is the fibrous coat, which includes the transparent **cornea** with its epithelium, the **conjunctiva,** and the opaque **sclera.** The middle layer is the vascular coat, which includes the **iris** and **choroid.** The iris contains both radially and circularly oriented smooth muscle fibers, which constitute the **pupillary dilator** and **sphincter** muscles; the iris forms a diaphragm to control the size of the **pupil.** THE DILATOR IS ACTIVATED BY THE SYMPATHETIC NERVOUS SYSTEM AND THE SPHINCTER BY THE PARASYMPATHETIC NERVOUS SYSTEM (see Chapter 10). The choroid is rich in blood vessels that supply the outer layers of the retina. The inner retinal layers are nourished by tributaries of the central artery and veins of the retina; these vessels enter the eye through the optic nerve.

The inner layer of the eye is the neural coat, the **retina** (Figure 8–1). The functional part of the retina covers the entire posterior eye except for the **blind spot,** which is the optic nerve head. Visual acuity is highest in the central part of the retina, the **macula lutea,** especially in the fovea. The **fovea** is a pitlike depression in the middle of the macula where visual targets are focused; it is the **fixation point,** or point at which light rays are focused when the eyes are directed at a visual target of interest.

Besides the retina, the eye contains a **lens** to focus light on the retina, **pigment** to reduce light

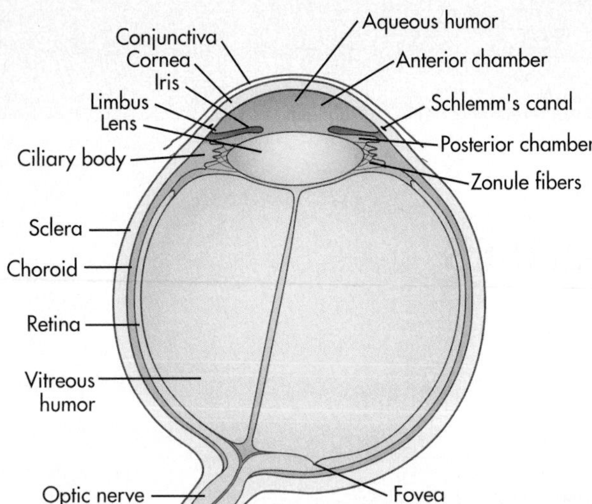

FIGURE 8–1. Right eye as viewed from above.

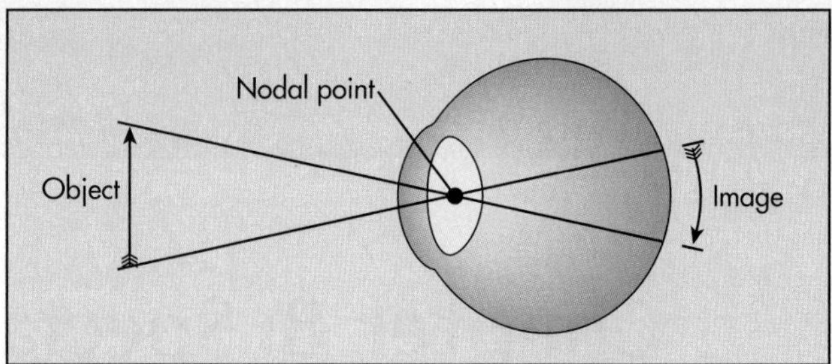

FIGURE 8–2. Image formation in the eye. The image is reversed as rays of light pass through the nodal point of the lens.

scatter, and fluids called **aqueous humor** and **vitreous humor** that help maintain the shape of the eye. Externally attached **extraocular muscles** aim the eye toward an appropriate visual target.

The lens is held in place behind the iris by the **suspensory ligaments** (or **zonule fibers**), which attach to the wall of the eye at the **ciliary body** (Figure 8–1). WHEN THE CILIARY MUSCLES ARE RELAXED, THE TENSION EXERTED BY THE SUSPENSORY LIGAMENTS TENDS TO FLATTEN THE LENS. WHEN THE CILIARY MUSCLES CONTRACT, TENSION ON THE SUSPENSORY LIGAMENTS IS REDUCED, ALLOWING THE LENS TO ASSUME A MORE SPHERICAL SHAPE BECAUSE OF ITS ELASTIC PROPERTIES. Contraction of the ciliary muscle causes relaxation of the suspensory ligaments because the ciliary muscle encircles the eye and serves as a sphincter that reduces the diameter of the eye. The ciliary muscles are activated by the parasympathetic nervous system via the oculomotor nerve.

Light scattering within the eye is minimized by pigment. The choroid contains an abundance of pigment. In addition, the outermost layer of the retina is a pigment-containing epithelium. Besides light absorption, the pigment cells of the **retinal pigment layer** are involved in the turnover of photoreceptor outer segments and the regeneration of **rhodopsin,** the photopigment found in the rods.

The space around the iris is filled with aqueous humor, which is a clear fluid resembling cerebrospinal fluid. The aqueous humor is actively secreted by the **ciliary processes,** which form an epithelium that is posterior to the iris and protrudes into a space called the **posterior chamber** (Figure 8–1). The aqueous humor circulates through the posterior chamber, out the pupil, and into the anterior chamber. It is then reabsorbed into **Schlemm's canal** and returned to the venous circulation.

Imbalance in the secretion and reabsorption of aqueous humor can increase the pressure in the eye, a condition that threatens the viability of the retina. This malady is known as **glaucoma.** Reabsorption can be increased surgically, and secretion can be reduced by medication therapy. Cholinergic medications, such as pilocarpine, which constrict the pupil, are helpful because they reduce the resistance to drainage of the aqueous humor.

The space behind the lens contains a gelatinous material, the **vitreous humor.** The vitreous humor turns over very slowly, so it does not contribute actively to glaucoma.

The extraocular muscles insert on the sclera from their origins on the bony orbit. Details concerning the organization and operation of the eye movement control system are described in Chapter 9.

Physical properties of the eye are termed physiological optics

The eye is often compared to a camera. Both devices capture images by using a lens system to focus light on a photosensitive surface. The quality of the image is enhanced by use of a diaphragm to reduce the effect of spherical aberrations of the lens and to increase depth of field. The diaphragm also controls the amount of entering light.

Like a camera, the eye produces an inverted image of an object **(Figure 8–2)**. The inversion is caused by the crossing of light rays from the object at a nodal point within the lens. The image is inverted both from side to side and from above downward.

The ability of a lens to bend light is called its **refractive power.** The unit of refractive power is the **diopter.** For an image to be in focus on the retina, light coming from any point on the object and passing through the cornea and lens must be refracted just enough so that it falls on a corresponding point on the retina. THE CORNEA IS THE

MAIN REFRACTIVE SURFACE OF THE EYE. It has a refractive power of 43 diopters. HOWEVER, THE LENS IS CRUCIAL FOR FOCUSING IMAGES ON THE RETINA because its refractive power can vary from 13 to 26 diopters. THE REFRACTIVE POWER OF THE LENS IS ALTERED BY CHANGES IN THE SHAPE OF THE LENS THROUGH RELAXATION OR CONTRACTION OF THE CILIARY MUSCLES. **Accommodation** is the process by which contraction of the ciliary muscle causes the lens to become more rounded. The result of accommodation is that images of nearby objects are brought into focus on the retina.

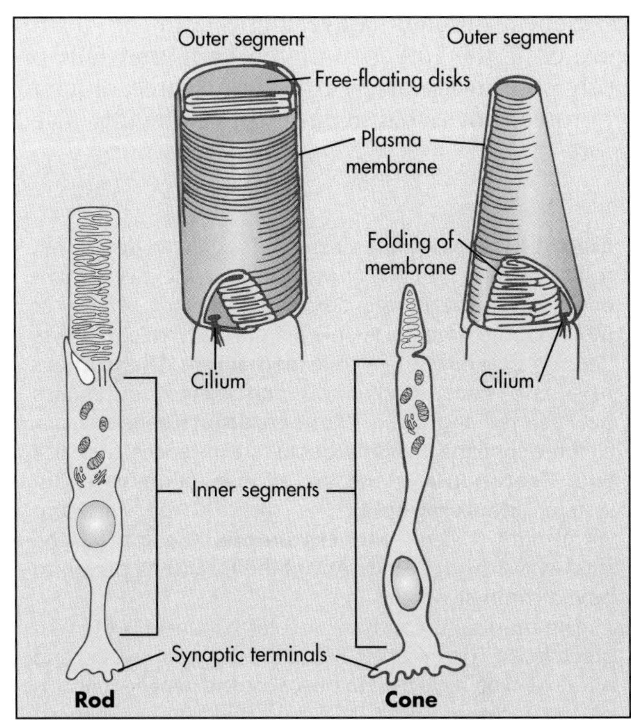

FIGURE 8–3. Structure of rods and cones. The inner and outer segments and the synaptic terminals are shown, as are details of the membranous discs in the outer segments.

During aging, the lens loses its elasticity. This loss reduces the ability of the eye to accommodate. This visual disturbance is called **presbyopia.** Other common defects in focusing ability are myopia, hypertropia, and astigmatism. In **myopia** (nearsightedness), images are focused in front of the retina because the eye is disproportionately long for the refractive system. In **hypermetropia** (farsightedness), images are focused behind the retina because the eye is short relative to the refractive system. **Astigmatism** is the result of asymmetrical focusing, usually because the cornea lacks radial symmetry.

The outermost retinal layers contain the pigment epithelium

The pigment cells capture stray light. They also phagocytose photoreceptor membrane shed from the outer segments of the rods and cones. Substances that move between the photoreceptors and the blood vessels within the choroid must pass through the pigment cell layer. Interactions between pigment cells and photoreceptor cells are important in visual function.

Individual photoreceptor cells can be subdivided into three regions: the **outer segment,** the **inner segment,** and the **synaptic terminal** (Figure 8–3). The outer segment contains a stack of **membranous discs** that are rich in photopigment. The inner segment connects with the outer segment by way of a modified cilium. The inner segment of the photoreceptor cell contains the nucleus, mitochondria, and other organelles. The synaptic ending contacts one or more **bipolar cells.**

THE ROD IS SO SENSITIVE TO LIGHT THAT IT CAN RESPOND TO A SINGLE PHOTON. The greater sensitivity of rods than cones is partly caused by the long outer segments of rods. Consequently, rods contain more photopigment, which is arranged in a monomolecular layer on each outer-segment disc. The pigment is **rhodopsin,** which is composed of a chromophore, retinal, and a protein, opsin. **Retinal** is the aldehyde form of **vitamin A.** In the dark, retinal is bound to opsin in the 11-*cis*-retinal form. Absorption of light causes a change to the all-*trans*-retinal form, which no longer binds to opsin. Before the photopigment can be regenerated, all-*trans*-retinal must be transported to the pigment cell layer, reduced, isomerized, and esterified.

Cones also contain 11-*cis*-retinal attached to an opsin. However, three different **cone opsins** are found in three different types of cones, each sensitive to a different part of the visible light spectrum. ONE CONE TYPE RESPONDS BEST TO BLUE LIGHT (420 nm), ANOTHER TO GREEN (531 nm), AND THE THIRD TO RED (558 nm). The presence of three types of cones gives the retina a mechanism for **trichromatic color vision.** Light causes a series of changes in the photopigment of cones; these changes resemble the sequence in rods, but the reactions and the recovery are quicker.

Color vision requires at least two photopigments. A single pigment absorbs light over much of the spectrum but absorbs best at a particular **wavelength.** The amount of light absorbed depends on its wavelength and **intensity.** The light of one wavelength and a given intensity could produce the same effect on a particular photoreceptor as another light of a different wavelength and intensity. Therefore, the signal is ambiguous because intensity can substitute for wavelength. However, with at least two different photoreceptors that have different pigments, different wavelengths can be distinguished if the intensity of the light that falls on both photoreceptors is the same. Three different photoreceptor types reduce the ambiguity even more.

Color blindness is often based on a genetic defect that results in the loss of one or more of the cone mechanisms or in a change in the absorption spectra of one or more photopigments. People are normally **trichromats** because they have three cone mechanisms. **Dichromats** have two cone mechanisms and cannot distinguish between red and green. **Monochromats** generally lack all three cone mechanisms, but in rare instances, they lack two. **Protanopia** is the loss of the long-wavelength system; **deuteranopia,** the loss of the medium-wavelength system; and **tritanopia,** the loss of the short-wavelength system. Any of these causes a person to be a dichromat.

The most common type of color blindness is the red-green form. This occurs in 8% of the male population and is a sex-linked recessive trait because the genetic defect is on the X chromosome. The main difficulty experienced by people with red-green color blindness occurs when there is a serious need to distinguish these colors, such as at traffic lights.

CONES ARE MOST CONCENTRATED IN THE FOVEA, WHERE ALL OF THE PHOTORECEPTORS ARE CONES **(Figure 8–4).** This is the region of the retina that provides the greatest visual acuity. In the fovea, the retina is thinned to just the four outer layers; thus, the image there is of the highest quality. Rods are most concentrated in the parafoveal region.

NO PHOTORECEPTORS EXIST IN THE OPTIC DISC (Figure 8–4), which is where the ganglion cell axons collect to leave the eye as the **optic nerve.** The optic disc is therefore a **blind spot.** The optic disc is in the medial retina. Therefore, the part of the visual field that would be imaged on the blind spot is on the temporal side of the field of vision of that eye. The blind spot is not noticed in binocular vision since the region of the visual field that fails to be seen by the blind spot in one eye is seen by the opposite eye because the light falls on the temporal side of that retina.

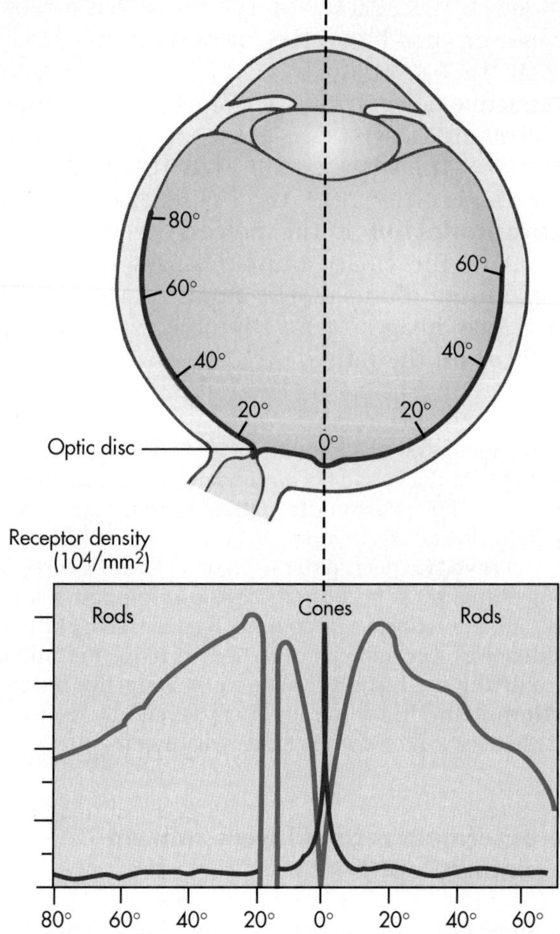

FIGURE 8–4. Density of cones and rods in different parts of the retina.

Information processing takes place in the retina

The most direct route for information flow through the retina is from **photoreceptors** to **bipolar cells** and then to **ganglion cells.** The ganglion cells provide the output of the retina to the **thalamus.**

The neural pathways in the retina can be subdivided into **rod pathways** and **cone pathways.** Convergence from photoreceptors onto bipolar cells is greater in the rod than in the cone pathways. This convergence enhances the sensitivity of the rod pathways. Cone pathways display much less convergence, in keeping with their role in visual acuity.

Because the photoreceptor cells and many of the retinal interneurons have short processes, action potentials are not required for transmitting information to the next cell in the circuit. Instead, local potentials alter neurotransmitter release, which in turn provides for information transfer. In darkness, photoreceptor cells have open Na^+ channels, which result in a **dark current** and consequently a tonic release of neurotransmitter onto bipolar cells and **horizontal cells** (**Figure 8–5**). When light is absorbed by photopigment in the outer segments of the photoreceptors, the Na^+ channels are closed, leading to a hyperpolarization of the photoreceptor cells and a decrease in the release of transmitter, which is probably glutamate.

This information processing involves an amplification mechanism that depends on a second-messenger system. cGMP maintains the Na^+ channels in an open configuration (Figure 8–5). Light activates a G protein called **transducin** in the photoreceptor membrane. Transducin in turn activates a phosphodiesterase, which hydrolyzes cGMP. Low-

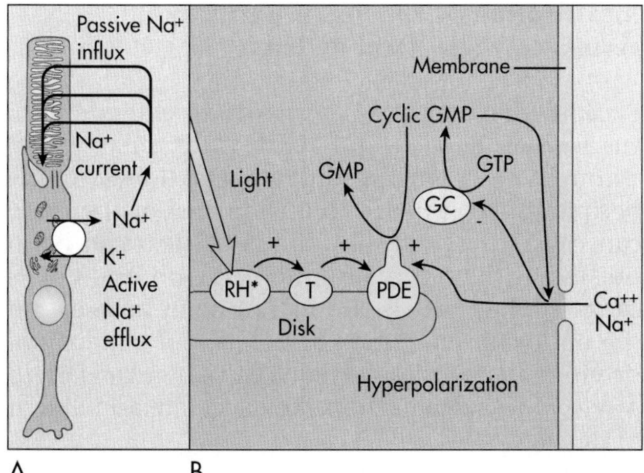

FIGURE 8–5. A, Dark current in a photoreceptor caused by passive influx of Na^+, which is returned to the extracellular space by pumping. Light closes the Na^+ channels and thus reduces the dark current. B, Second-messenger system underlying phototransduction. When light reacts with rhodopsin (RH), G protein transducin (T) is activated. This in turn activates phosphodiesterase (PDE), which breaks down cGMP into GMP. The dark current depends on cGMP, and thus a fall in cGMP concentration reduces the dark current, which causes hyperpolarization of the photoreceptor. GC, guanylyl cyclase.

ering of the cGMP concentration causes the Na^+ channels to close and the membrane to hyperpolarize.

The **receptive field** of a photoreceptor is generally a small circular area that is coextensive with the area of the retina occupied by the photoreceptor. Bipolar cells are of two types, **on-center** and **off-center** (**Figure 8–6**). An on-center bipolar cell is depolarized when light shines in the center of its receptive field and hyperpolarized when light shines in an annulus around the center of the receptive field. An off-center bipolar cell behaves in the converse manner. The different responses to stimulation of the center of the receptive field depend on differences in the receptors that respond to glutamate released from the synaptic endings of the photoreceptors on the bipolar cells. Interneuronal pathways involving horizontal cells determine the responses to stimulation of the area surrounding the center of the receptive field.

Ganglion cells, like bipolar cells, may have center-surround antagonistic receptive fields (Figure 8–6), or like amacrine cells, they may have large receptive fields. The type of receptive field presumably reflects the dominant input. Ganglion cells in primates can be classified as P cells, M cells, or W cells. Both P and M cells have center-surround receptive fields controlled by bipolar cells. P cells have smaller receptive fields than those of M cells, respond more tonically to stimuli, have slower axons, sum multiple responses in a linear fashion, and distinguish between colors. They are responsible for high visual acuity and color vision, and they project to the parvocellular layers of the lateral geniculate nucleus. M cells respond to complex stimuli in an unpredictable fashion and are insensitive to wavelength. They are motion detectors and project to the magnocellular layers of the lateral geniculate nucleus. W cells often have large, diffuse receptive fields. They signal the intensity of ambient light and are probably controlled by amacrine cells. One projection target of W cells is the superior colliculus.

Central visual projections begin in the retina

The **optic nerves** from the two eyes converge at the optic chiasm (**Figure 8–7**). Some of the optic nerve fibers decussate in the chiasm and join the optic

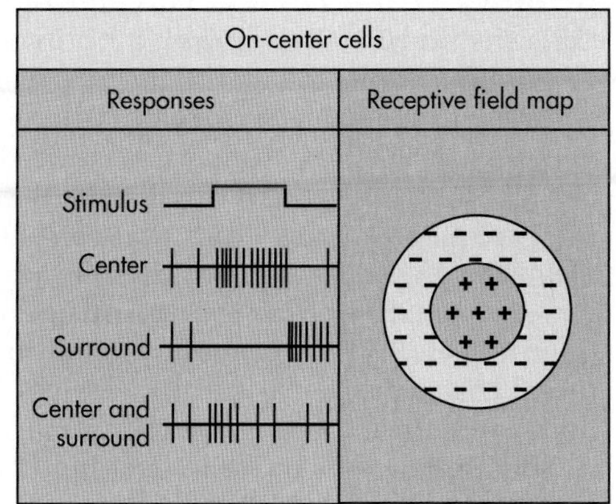

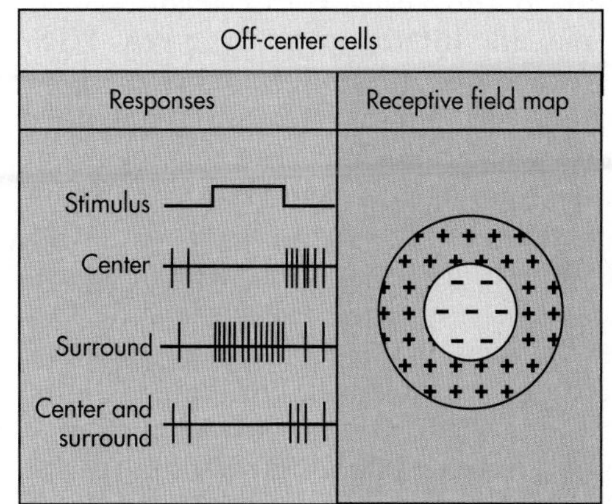

FIGURE 8–6. Center-surround receptive field organization of retinal ganglion cells. *Left,* Responses to light stimuli on the center or in a surrounding annulus for on- and off-center ganglion cells. The effect of stimulating the entire field is also shown. *Right,* Receptive fields. Plus signs indicate excitation, and minus signs indicate inhibition.

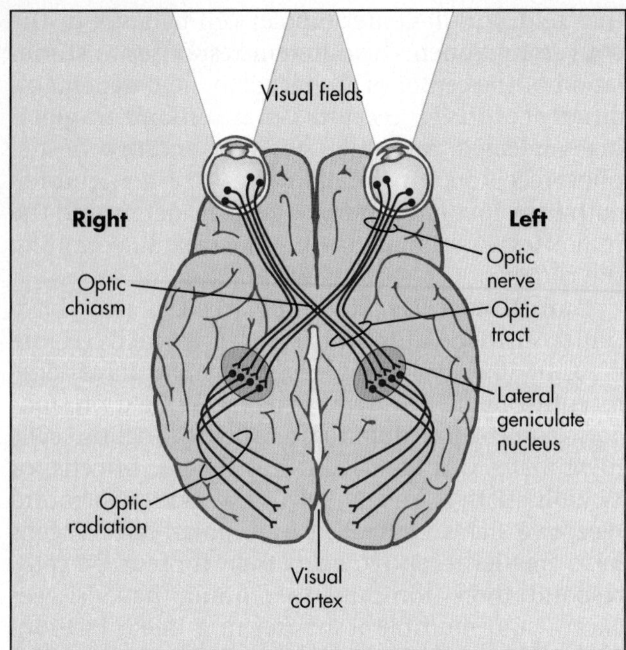

FIGURE 8–7. Main visual pathway as viewed from the base of the brain.

tract, and some continue posteriorly in the optic tract on the same side as the eye of origin. The fibers that cross originate from the **nasal hemiretinas** of the two eyes. The uncrossed fibers originate from the **temporal hemiretinas.** Because of this arrangement, each optic tract contains both uncrossed and crossed fibers. The optic tract fibers synapse in the lateral geniculate nucleus (Figure 8–7).

The lateral geniculate nucleus relays visual information to the cerebral cortex

Most neurons in the **lateral geniculate nucleus (LGN)** project to the visual cortex (Figure 8–7); however, some are interneurons. A given LGN neuron receives a dominant input from one or a few retinal ganglion cells, and the responses resemble those of the ganglion cells. Thus, the LGN neurons can be classified as P or M cells, and they have on- or off-center receptive fields. However, LGN neurons are subject to input from regions other than the retinas. These other regions include the visual cortex, several brainstem nuclei, and the reticular nucleus of the thalamus. Inhibitory actions that originate from the brainstem or thalamic reticular nucleus can prevent visual signals from reaching the cortex or can reduce these signals. In effect, the LGN serves as a filter for visual information before it accesses the visual cortex.

Interruption of the visual pathway results in visual field deficits

Because the central visual pathway extends from the base of the brain just above the pituitary gland through the temporal and parietal lobes to the occipital lobe, damage to a wide area of the brain can cause loss of vision. The visual loss can be in one eye if the retina or optic nerve on one side is involved, but the visual loss can be in both eyes if the optic chiasm, optic tract, LGN, optic radiation, or visual cortex is involved. The particular pattern of visual loss depends on the exact site and extent of damage.

A visual field defect is described in terms of the part of the visual world that a patient is unable to see. Each eye has a visual field that can be subdivided into a temporal and a nasal visual hemifield. The hemifield can be further subdivided into an upper and a lower quadrant.

Loss of vision in one eye is simply **blindness** in that eye or a **scotoma** (partial blindness in one visual field). A lesion affecting the optic chiasm causes loss of vision in the temporal fields of both eyes, a condition called **bitemporal hemianopia.** This can happen, for example, because of a pituitary tumor. Destruction of an optic tract causes loss of vision in the contralateral half of the visual field of each eye, or **contralateral homonymous hemianopia.** A similar visual field deficit results from destruction of an LGN, the entire optic radiation, or the primary visual cortex on one side. Macular vision may be spared in cortical lesions, perhaps because of the large size of the macular representation or because of collateral circulation in the case of a vascular lesion.

The striate cortex is the primary visual receiving area

The optic radiation ends chiefly in layer IV of the **primary visual cortex.** This area of cortex contains the **stripe of Gennari**, a horizontal layer of myelinated axons that can be seen grossly and that gives rise to the name **striate cortex** for this region of cortex. Projections from the magnocellular (large-celled) and parvocellular (small-celled) layers of the LGN are separate, and axons that carry information from the two eyes end in alternating patches of cortex called **ocular dominance columns** (**Figure 8–8, *B***). Recordings from neurons in area 17 reveal that a given cell usually receives input from both eyes, although one eye is dominant.

The retina is mapped onto the striate cortex **(retinotopic map).** The macular region is represented at and for a distance anterior to the occipital pole. The remainder of the retina is represented

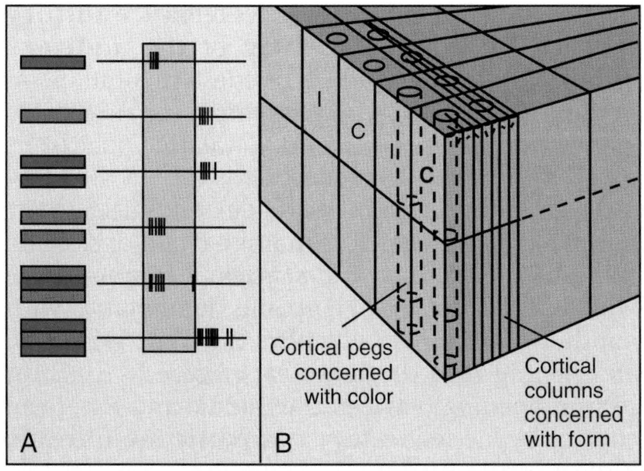

FIGURE 8–8. A, Responses of a simple cell in the striate cortex to various combinations of red and green bars. The cell responded best to a red bar flanked by two green bars. B, Diagram of the columns in the visual cortex. Ocular dominance columns are indicated by I (ipsilateral eye) and C (contralateral eye), orientation columns by the short bars at various angles. The cortical pegs contain neurons that have double-opponent color fields.

still more anteriorly along the medial aspect of the occipital lobe. The macular representation occupies more cortical volume than does the representation of the rest of the retina because of the requirements for visual acuity.

Most neurons in the striate cortex respond best to elongated stimuli. A rectangular visual target or an edge evokes a more vigorous response than a small spot does. The orientation of the stimulus is an important factor. Neurons in a region of striate cortex perpendicular to the cortical surface all respond best to elongated stimuli having the same orientation (Figure 8–8, *B*). These neurons form **orientation columns.**

The processing of visual information depends on many cortical areas

The striate or primary visual cortex receives visual information from the LGN and begins analysis of that information. The striate cortex connects with many other cortical areas, known as the **extrastriate visual cortex,** that participate in the further processing of visual information. These cortical areas are interconnected with other nuclei of the thalamus.

Stereopsis is binocular depth perception. It depends on slight differences in the images in the two eyes such that a given cortical neuron has its receptive field at points on the two retinas that are slightly out of correspondence. This provides the brain with a signal that can be used to judge differences in the distances of objects.

Color vision depends on the discrimination of wavelengths of light. Retinal ganglion cells and LGN neurons may respond selectively to one wavelength and be inhibited by another. These cells are called **spectral opponent neurons.** An example would be a neuron excited by a red light shone in the center of its receptive field and by a green light shone in the surrounding part of the field (Figure 8–8, *A*). Spectral opponent cells belong to the P cell category. Neurons in the cortex discriminate wavelength and brightness; thus, they permit the perception of true color. Such neurons are concentrated in **cortical pegs,** which are sets of neurons within the ocular dominance columns (Figure 8–8, *B*).

The superior colliculus mediates orienting reflexes

The **superior colliculus** is a layered midbrain structure that serves as a visual center and coordination center for orientation reflexes occurring in response to visual, auditory, and somatic stimuli. The dorsal three layers are involved in visual processing, whereas the deeper four layers also process other sensory input.

Retinal ganglion cells project to the upper layers of the superior colliculus. The ganglion cells include both M and W cells. The superior colliculus also receives a projection from the cerebral cortex. The cortical neurons involved in this projection are activated by M cells. Thus, the visual input to the superior colliculus is concerned with motion detection and light intensity. The output of the upper layers of the superior colliculus influences visual processing in the cortex. Experiments in animals suggest that the superior colliculus is important in determining the location of objects in visual space, whereas the cortex determines what the objects are. The deep layers of the superior colliculus are considered with the motor system (see Chapter 9).

The Auditory System Is Designed to Analyze Sound

Audition is important not only for the recognition of environmental cues but also for communication, especially language in humans.

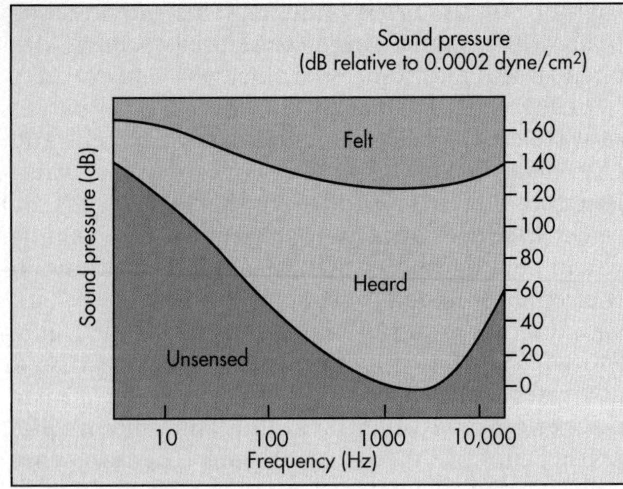

FIGURE 8–9. Sound levels for human hearing as a function of frequency. Below the range for hearing, sound is not sensed; above the hearing range, it is detected by both the auditory and the somatosensory systems.

Sound is produced by pressure waves in the air

Sound is produced by alternating waves of pressure in the air. Sound waves are composed of the sum of a set of sinusoidal waves of the appropriate amplitudes, frequencies, and phases. Thus, sound can be regarded as a mixture of pure tones. THE HUMAN ACOUSTIC SYSTEM ACTS AS A FILTER THAT IS SENSITIVE TO PURE TONES WITHIN A RANGE OF FREQUENCIES FROM APPROXIMATELY 20 TO 15,000 Hz. Threshold varies with frequency. Sound intensity is measured in **decibels (dB),** which are expressed in terms of a reference level of sound pressure (P_r), often 0.0002 dyne/cm^2, which is the threshold for hearing. The formula for sound intensity follows:

$$\text{Sound pressure (decibels)} = 20 \log(P/P_r)$$

where P is pressure.

THE EAR IS MOST SENSITIVE TO TONES FROM 1000 TO 3000 Hz. At these frequencies, threshold is by definition zero. Threshold is higher at frequencies less than 1000 Hz and greater than 3000 Hz **(Figure 8–9).** For example, threshold at 100 Hz is approximately 40 dB. Speech has an intensity of about 65 dB. Damage to the acoustic apparatus can be produced by sounds that exceed 100 dB, and discomfort results from sound pressures that exceed 120 dB.

Structures of the external, middle, and inner ear contribute to hearing

The ear can be subdivided into the **external ear, middle ear,** and **inner ear.** The external ear includes the **pinna** and the **external auditory meatus,** which leads by way of the **auditory canal** to the outer surface of the tympanic membrane **(Figure 8–10, *A*).** The auditory canal contains glands that secrete **cerumen,** a wax that guards the ear from invasion by insects.

The middle ear is a cavity that extends deep to the tympanic membrane. It contains a chain of ossicles, the **malleus, incus,** and **stapes** (Figure 8–10, *A*), which connect the tympanic membrane with another membrane that covers the **oval window,** an opening into the inner ear (Figure 8–10, *B*). A second opening between the middle and inner ear, covered by the **secondary tympanic membrane,** is the **round window.** The middle ear contains two muscles, the **tensor tympani** and the **stapedius;** the tensor tympani attaches to the malleus, and the stapedius attaches to the stapes. Contraction of the middle ear muscles dampens movements of the ossicular chain. The eustachian tube provides an opening from the middle ear to the nasopharynx.

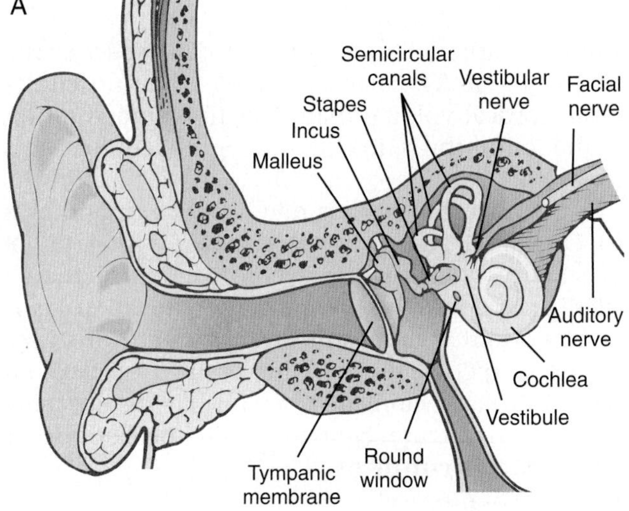

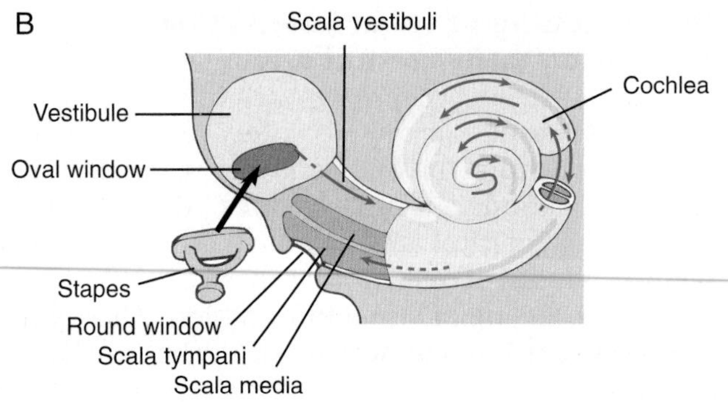

FIGURE 8–10. Structure of the cochlea. A, Components of the ear, including the membranous labyrinth. B, Cochlea in more detail. The arrows indicate the path of fluid movement that would result from movement of the stapes into the oval window.

This permits pressure differences between the environment and the middle ear to be equalized.

The inner ear is a cavity within the temporal bone and contains the **cochlea** (Figure 8–10, *A*) and **vestibular apparatus.** The cochlea is the organ of hearing and is formed by elements of both the **bony labyrinth** and the **membranous labyrinth.** The space in the bony labyrinth just inside the oval window is the **vestibule.**

The cochlea is a coiled structure formed by the division of the bony labyrinth into two compartments. The partition between the compartments is formed by a component of the membranous labyrinth; this component is called the **cochlear duct,** or **scala media.** The portion of the bony labyrinth in continuity with the vestibule is the **scala vestibuli.** This extends along the $2^1/_2$ turns of the human cochlea to the end of the cochlear duct. At this point, the scala vestibuli connects with the **scala tympani** by way of a space called the **helicotrema.** The scala tympani spirals back to the bony interface with the middle ear and ends at the **secondary tympanic membrane** that covers the **round window.** The base of the cochlea is near the oval and round windows (Figure 8–10, *B*), and the apex is at the helicotrema. The bony core of the cochlea is the **modiolus.**

The cochlear duct is a tube and is part of the membranous labyrinth **(Figure 8–11,** ***A*****).** The **basilar membrane** forms the base of the cochlear duct and can be regarded as the main partition between the scala vestibuli and scala tympani. The basilar membrane is narrowest near the base of the cochlea and widest near the helicotrema. The basilar membrane is attached internally to a ledge, the **spiral lamina,** that arises from the modiolus. Externally, the basilar membrane is anchored to the wall of the cochlea by the **spiral ligament.** Contained within the spiral ligament is a vascular structure, the **stria vascularis.** The roof over the

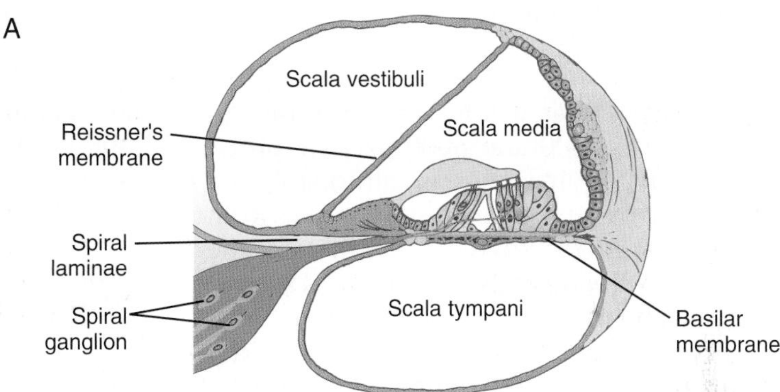

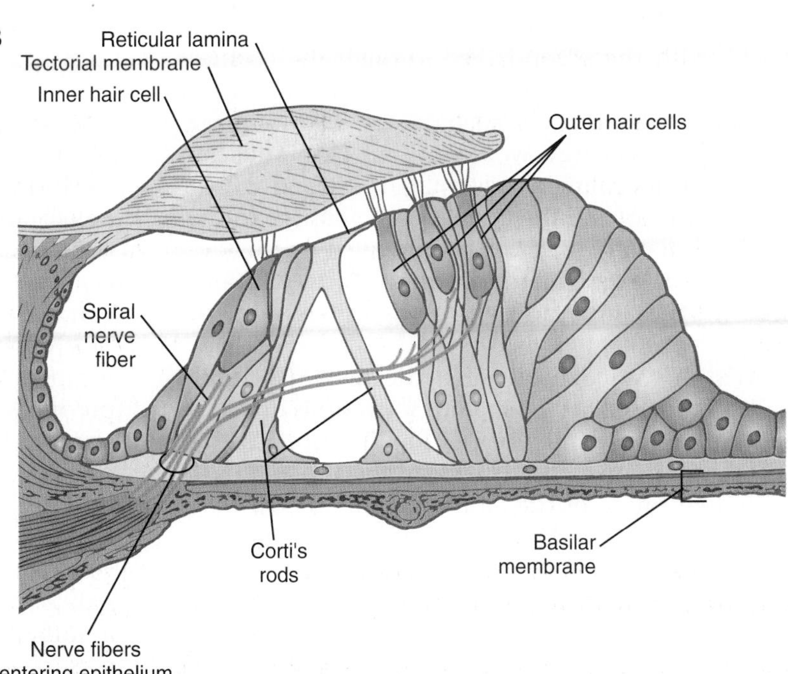

FIGURE 8–11. A, Organ of Corti within the cochlear duct (scala media). B, Enlargement of the organ of Corti.

cochlear duct is formed by **Reissner's membrane.** The cochlear duct contains **endolymph,** a fluid with high [K^+]; the endolymph is secreted by the stria vascularis. The bony labyrinth contains **perilymph,** which resembles cerebrospinal fluid.

The **organ of Corti** is the sense organ for hearing (Figure 8–11, *B*). It lies within the cochlear duct along the basilar membrane. The organ of Corti consists of **hair cells,** the **tectorial membrane,** a stiff framework, and several types of supportive cells. The **stereocilia** of the hair cells contact the tectorial membrane. The hair cells are innervated by primary afferent fibers and efferent fibers of the cochlear nerve. The cell bodies of the primary afferent fibers are in the **spiral ganglion,** which is contained in the modiolus. The spiral ganglion cells are bipolar neurons whose peripheral processes reach the hair cells through the spiral lamina. The central processes join the **cochlear nerve,** which projects into the brainstem.

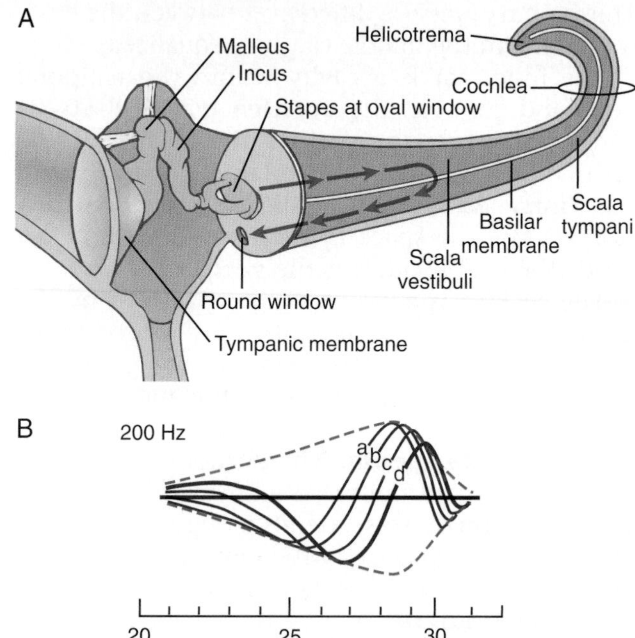

FIGURE 8–12. A, Impedance-matching arrangement of the ear. The tympanic membrane and ossicular chain oscillate in response to sound waves in the air. The movements of the stapes in the oval window produce comparable oscillations of the fluid columns within the cochlea. The distance along the basilar membrane at which the oscillation is maximal depends on the frequency of the sound. The largest displacements of the basilar membrane are near the base of the cochlea for high frequencies and near the apex for low frequencies. B, Traveling wave produced by a 200-Hz sound at four different times (*a* to *d*). The dashed line is the envelope of the peaks of the successive positions of the wave, showing a maximal deflection of the basilar membrane about 29 mm from the stapes.

Sound transduction depends on the organ of Corti

The external ear acts as a filter that is tuned to frequencies between 800 and 6000 Hz. The pinna serves little function in humans, although it is important in many animals. Pressure waves that reach the tympanic membrane cause it and the ossicular chain to vibrate at the frequency of sound. The ossicular chain in turn oscillates the oval window and the fluids within the cochlea. The round window completes the hydraulic pathway.

The middle ear mechanism serves as an **impedance-matching device** to couple airborne sound waves with those conducted through the cochlear fluids **(Figure 8–12, *A*)**. If sound waves were to be conducted directly from air to the oval window, most of the energy would be reflected and lost. With the mechanical advantage provided by the ratio of the area of the tympanic membrane to that of the oval window, plus that provided by the lever action of the ossicular chain, only 10 to 15 dB are lost in the impedance-matching process of the ear.

Within the cochlear duct, the maximal amplitude of the oscillations extends for various distances along the basilar membrane; the distance depends on the frequency of the sound (Figure 8–12, *B*). Although much of the basilar membrane oscillates in a **traveling wave** in response to a particular frequency of sound, high frequencies result in movements that are largest in the basal part of the cochlea, whereas low frequencies induce movements that are largest near the apex of the cochlea.

As the basilar membrane oscillates, the stereocilia of the hair cells in the organ of Corti are subjected to shear forces at their junctions with the tectorial membrane **(Figure 8–13)**. When the stereocilia are bent in a direction toward the longest cilia, a hair cell becomes depolarized because of an increased conductance of the apical membrane to cations. This depolarization is a **receptor potential,** and it causes the release of an excitatory transmitter that produces a **generator potential** in the primary afferent fibers synapsing on the hair cells. As the oscillations of the basilar membrane move in the opposite direction, the membrane of the hair cell is hyperpolarized, and less transmitter is released. The generator potential in the primary afferent terminals is thus an oscillatory one, and if its amplitude is sufficient during the depolarizing phases, it triggers action potentials in primary afferent nerve fibers.

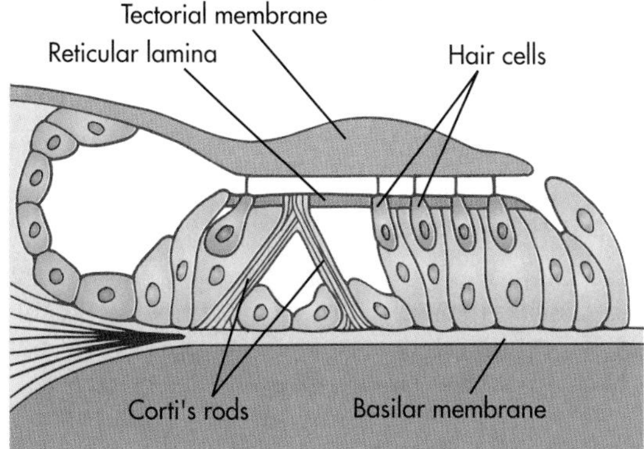

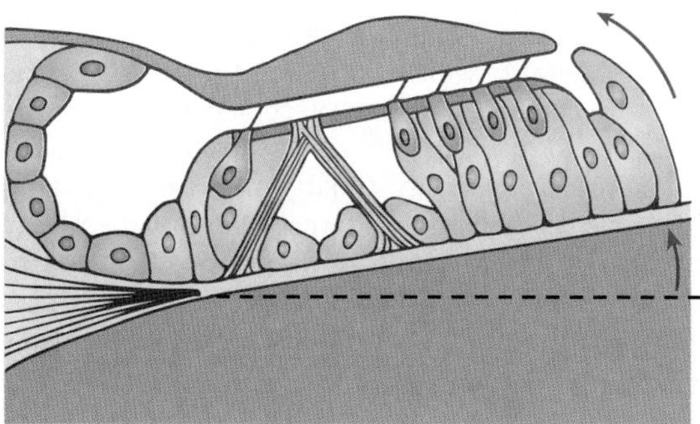

FIGURE 8–13. Transduction in the organ of Corti. An upward movement of the basilar membrane causes the development of shear forces between the stereocilia of the hair cells and the tectorial membrane, resulting in displacement of the cilia *(arrow).*

The difference in potential between the endolymph and the intracellular fluid of the hair cells is unusually high. This potential difference is an important factor in the sensitivity of the auditory system. If the potential in the perilymph is considered the reference potential, the endolymph has a positive steady potential of about 85 mV. This is called the **endocochlear potential** and is the result of electrogenic pumping by the stria vascularis. The resting potential of the hair cells is approximately 85 mV with reference to the endolymph. Because of the positive potential in the endolymph, however, the transmembrane potential across the apical membrane of the hair cells can be as great as 170 mV. This increases the ionic driving forces across the transducer membrane.

An oscillatory potential called the **cochlear microphonic potential** can be recorded from the bony labyrinth of the cochlea. This potential results from the current flow associated with the activity of the hair cells in response to sound. The cochlear microphonic potential has the frequency of the sound stimulus, and its amplitude is graded with the sound intensity.

Cochlear nerve fibers that innervate hair cells at different points along the length of the organ of Corti are tuned to different frequencies of sound. The tuning properties of the primary afferent fibers can be demonstrated by constructing tuning curves that relate the threshold for activation of the fiber to the frequencies of sound stimuli **(Figure 8–14)**. The frequency that activates the fiber at the lowest intensity is called the **characteristic frequency** of the fiber. Cochlear nerve fibers that innervate the organ of Corti near the base of the cochlea have high characteristic frequencies, whereas those innervating the apex have low characteristic frequencies. The organ of Corti is thus organized **tonotopically.**

For the lower part of the frequency range detected by the cochlea (<4000 Hz), the discharges of a given cochlear nerve fiber show **phase locking.** That is, they occur consistently at a particular phase of the sound oscillation. The discharges of a population of afferent nerve fibers

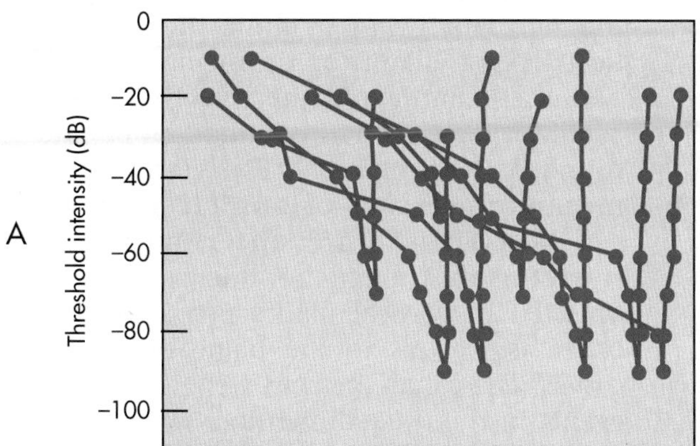

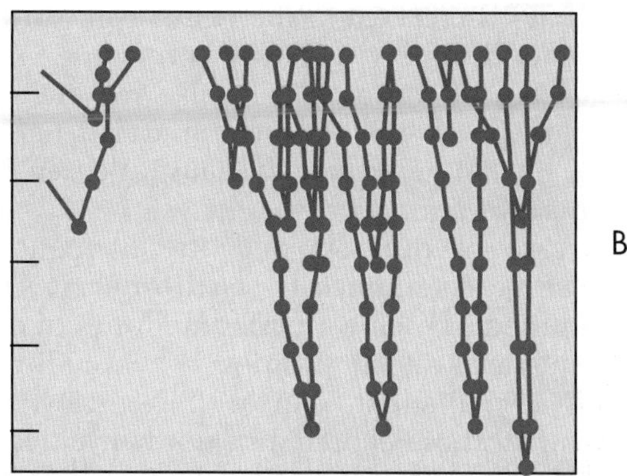

FIGURE 8–14. Tuning curves for neurons in the auditory pathway. A, Tuning curves for excitation of 7 neurons in the cochlear nerve. B, Tuning curves for 12 neurons in the inferior colliculus.

could signal the stimulus frequency. This is **volley coding of acoustic signals.** However, cochlear afferent fibers with higher characteristic frequencies do not show phase locking. Coding in these depends on **place coding;** the afferent fibers that innervate regions near the base of the cochlea signal frequencies that depend on the site innervated. **Intensity coding** depends on the number of discharges evoked by sounds of different intensities and presumably also on the number of neurons that discharge.

The central auditory pathway is responsible for sound localization and analysis of sound frequency

The **superior olivary complex** is concerned with **sound localization.** Neurons in the medial superior olivary nuclei compare the arrival times of sound in the two ears, whereas neurons in the lateral superior olivary nuclei compare differences in the intensity of sounds that reach the two ears. A sound originating from a source located to the left reaches the left ear first, and the head provides an acoustic shield that lowers the intensity of the sound reaching the right ear. By means of these **binaural cues,** signals from the superior olivary nuclei allow the central auditory pathways to judge the location of the sound source.

Binaural processing occurs also in the cerebral cortex, as shown by the presence of **summation** and **suppression columns** in the auditory cortex. The responses of the neurons in these columns depend on whether sounds are introduced into the left or right ear or both ears. In summation columns, neurons respond better when sounds reach both ears rather than only one. Neurons of suppression columns respond better to sound in one ear than to simultaneous sound in both.

Frequency analysis within the central auditory pathways is reflected in the **tonotopic maps** characteristic of many auditory structures. The tonotopic map of the cochlea is also reflected in tonotopic maps in the cochlear nuclei, inferior colliculus, medial geniculate nucleus, and several regions of the auditory cortex.

The degree of deafness and the frequencies affected can be determined by **audiometry.** The patient is tested in each ear with pure tones of different frequencies and intensities. When auditory thresholds for different sample frequencies are compared with those expected in normal subjects, hearing deficits can be described in terms of decibel losses for a certain range of frequencies or for the entire frequency spectrum.

> The bilateral organization of the central auditory pathway is the reason that neurological lesions of the brainstem at levels rostral to the cochlear nuclei do not produce unilateral deafness (although large unilateral lesions of the auditory cortex do interfere with the localization of sounds in space). Unilateral deafness implies a defect in the sound-conduction system (e.g., tympanic membrane, ossicle chain) or in the initial stages of the auditory pathway (i.e., organ of Corti, cochlear nerve, cochlear nuclei). These conditions are called **conduction deafness** and **sensorineural deafness,** respectively.
>
> The type of deafness can be assessed by Weber's test and the Rinne test. For **Weber's test,** a vibrating tuning fork is placed on the forehead. Normally, the sound is not localized to either ear. In conduction deafness, the sound is localized to the deaf ear; in sensorineural deafness, the sound is localized to the normal ear. For the **Rinne test,** the base of the tuning fork is placed against the mastoid process. In normal subjects, when the sound disappears, it can be heard again if the tuning fork is moved to a position in the air near the external auditory meatus (**air conduction** is better than **bone conduction**). In conduction deafness, bone conduction is better that air conduction, so sound is not restored when the tuning fork is moved.

The Vestibular System Is Part of the Membranous Labyrinth of the Inner Ear

The sensory role of the vestibular system is a form of proprioception. THE VESTIBULAR APPARATUS DETECTS HEAD MOVEMENTS AND THE POSITION OF THE HEAD IN SPACE. To accomplish this, it uses two sets of sensory epithelia to transduce angular and linear accelerations of the head.

The vestibular apparatus includes the semicircular ducts and otolith organs

The **vestibular apparatus** is contained within the bony labyrinth, but unlike the cochlea, its function depends mainly on the membranous labyrinth. The vestibular apparatus is connected with the cochlear duct, contains endolymph, and is surrounded by perilymph. The vestibular apparatus includes three pairs of **semicircular canals** on each side (Figure 8–15): **anterior, posterior,** and **horizontal.** The anterior and posterior canals are oriented in vertical planes perpendicular to each other as well as to the plane of the horizontal canals. The canals are thus well positioned to sense events in the three dimensions of space. The superior canal on one side is parallel to the posterior canal on the other side; the horizontal canals are in the same plane.

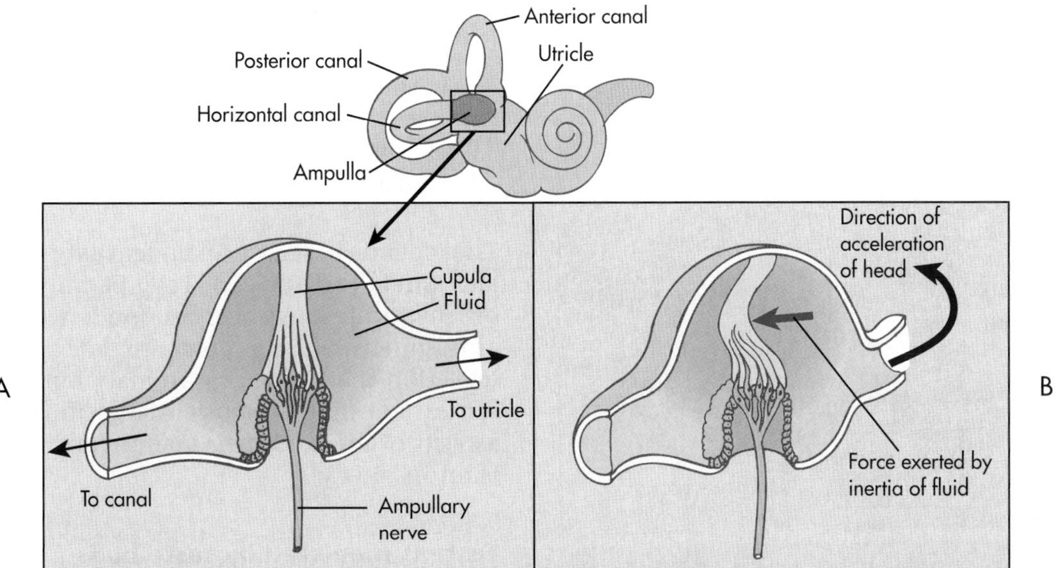

FIGURE 8–15. A, Relationship of the cupula to the ampulla when the head is stationary. B, Displacement of the cupula when the head is rotated.

Each of the semicircular canals has a dilation called an **ampulla** (Figure 8–15). Within the ampulla is a sensory epithelium known as an **ampullary crest.** The apical surface of each of the hair cells of the sensory epithelium has both **stereocilia** and a single **kinocilium** (unlike cochlear hair cells, which lack kinocilia). The arrangement of the kinocilium with respect to the stereocilia gives a **functional polarity** to the vestibular hair cells. The cilia are all oriented in the same way relative to the axis of the semicircular duct. The cilia contact a gelatinous mass, the **cupula,** which extends across the ampulla and occludes it completely (Figure 8–15, *A*). Pressure shifts in the endolymph produced by angular accelerations of the head distort the cupula (Figure 8–15, *B*) and bend the cilia of the ampullary crest.

The semicircular canals connect with the **utricle,** one of the otolith organs. The sensory epithelium of the utricle is the **utricular macula,** which is oriented horizontally along the floor of the utricle. The **otolithic membrane** is a gelatinous mass that contains numerous **otoliths** formed from crystals of calcium carbonate. The hair cells of the macula are oriented in relation to a groove called the **striola,** along the length of the macula. For example, the kinocilia in the utricle are on the striolar side of the hair cells. The **saccule** is a separate part of the membranous labyrinth, and the **saccular macula** is oriented vertically. Linear accelerations of the head shift the otolithic membranes with respect to the hair cells. This shift results in bending of the cilia and sensory transduction. Angular accelerations do not substantially affect the otolithic membranes because the otolithic membranes do not protrude into the endolymph.

Vestibular transduction depends on neuroepithelia-containing hair cells

When the stereocilia on the vestibular hair cells are bent toward the kinocilium, the hair cell is depolarized because of an increased conductance of the hair cell membrane to cations **(Figure 8–16).** Bending of the cilia in the opposite direction leads to hyperpolarization. When vestibular hair cells are depolarized, they release more neurotransmitter (probably an excitatory amino acid such as glutamate), and when they are hyperpolarized, they release less. The neurotransmitter excites primary afferent fibers that end on the hair cells. In the absence of overt stimuli, vestibular primary afferent fibers are spontaneously active (Figure 8–16). The activity either increases or decreases, depending on the direction in which the cilia are bent.

In the ampullary crest of the horizontal semicircular duct, the kinocilia are arranged so that they are on the utricular side of the ampulla (Figure 8–16). If the head is rotated to the left, inertial forces shift the endolymph relatively to the right in both of the horizontal canals. In the left ear, this means that the stereocilia of the hair cells of the left horizontal canal bend toward the kinocilium (toward the utricle) and that the discharges of the primary afferent fibers supplying the left ampullary crest increase. Conversely, the stereocilia in the crest of the right horizontal duct bend away from

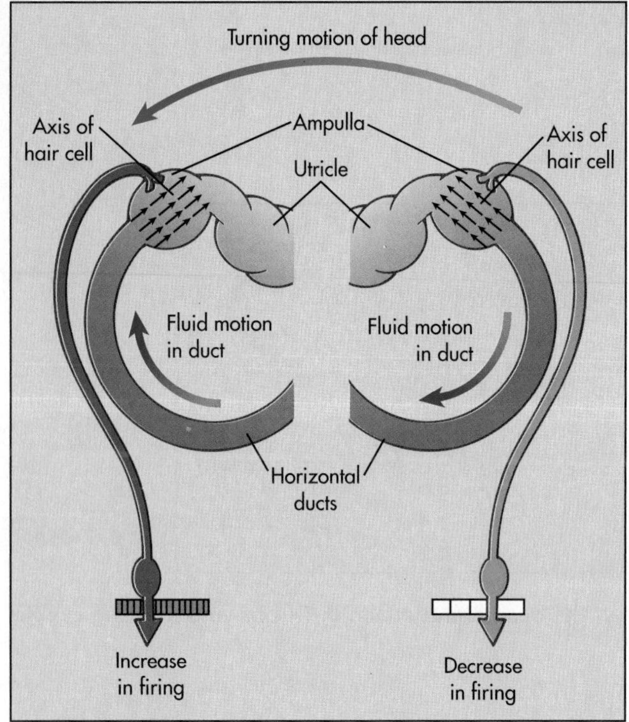

FIGURE 8–16. Effect of head movement on the hair cells in the ampullae of the horizontal semicircular ducts. The functional polarity of the hair cells is indicated by small arrows.

their kinocilia (away from the utricle), and thus the discharges of the primary afferent fibers of this crest are reduced.

The orientation of the kinocilia in the utricular macula is toward the striola. The orientation in the saccular macula is away from the striola. That is, hair cells on the two sides of the striola are functionally polarized in opposite directions. The changes in the discharges of vestibular afferents from a macula produced by linear acceleration of the head differ for different hair cells. The pattern of input to the central nervous system is analyzed and interpreted by the central vestibular pathways in terms of head position.

Central vestibular processing and vestibular sensation involve ascending and descending pathways

Primary afferent fibers from the vestibular apparatus reach the brainstem by way of the **vestibular nerve** (cranial nerve VIII). Most of the afferents terminate in the **vestibular nuclei.** The vestibular nuclei connect with the **cerebellum** and **reticular formation,** the **oculomotor nuclei,** and the **spinal cord.** These connections are important for vestibular control of eye and head movements and posture. A pathway to the cerebral cortex by way of the thalamus is responsible for vestibular sensation.

The Chemical Sensory System Involves Taste and Smell

The chemical senses include **taste (gustation)** and **smell (olfaction).** They permit the detection of chemical substances in food, water, and the atmosphere. Humans are less adept at chemical detection than are many animals, but the chemical senses contribute substantially to the affective aspects of life, and their malfunction can be significant in disease.

Taste is mediated by taste buds

The human gustatory system recognizes many different taste stimuli. However, these can generally be classified as four primary taste qualities: sweet, salty, sour, and bitter.

The sensory receptors for taste are the **taste buds.** Most taste buds are on the tongue, but some are on the palate, pharynx, larynx, and upper esophagus. Taste buds occur in groups on papillae (Figure 8–17). **Fungiform papillae** are mushroom-like structures, several hundred of which are present on the anterior two thirds of the tongue. The taste buds of the fungiform papillae respond mainly to sweet and salty substances but also to sour. **Foliate papillae** are folded structures on the posterior edge of the tongue, and their taste buds respond best to sour stimuli. The taste buds on fungiform and foliate papillae are innervated by the **chorda tympani** branch of the **facial nerve. Circumvallate papillae** are large, round structures encircled by a depression; they are on the posterior tongue and respond to bitter substances. The foliate and circumvallate papillae are innervated by the **glossopharyngeal nerve.** Taste buds in the region of the epiglottis and upper esophagus are supplied by the **vagus nerve.**

A taste bud consists of a group of some 50 **gustatory receptor cells** in association with supporting cells and basal cells. The gustatory cells are continuously replaced by the differentiation of supporting cells from basal cells. The apical membranes of the gustatory cells have microvilli that protrude into a **taste pore,** where they come into contact with saliva.

Receptor molecules on the microvilli recognize chemical substances in the saliva. The gustatory cells are in synaptic contact with primary afferent nerve terminals. Gustatory signals apparently evoke a receptor potential in the gustatory cell, which

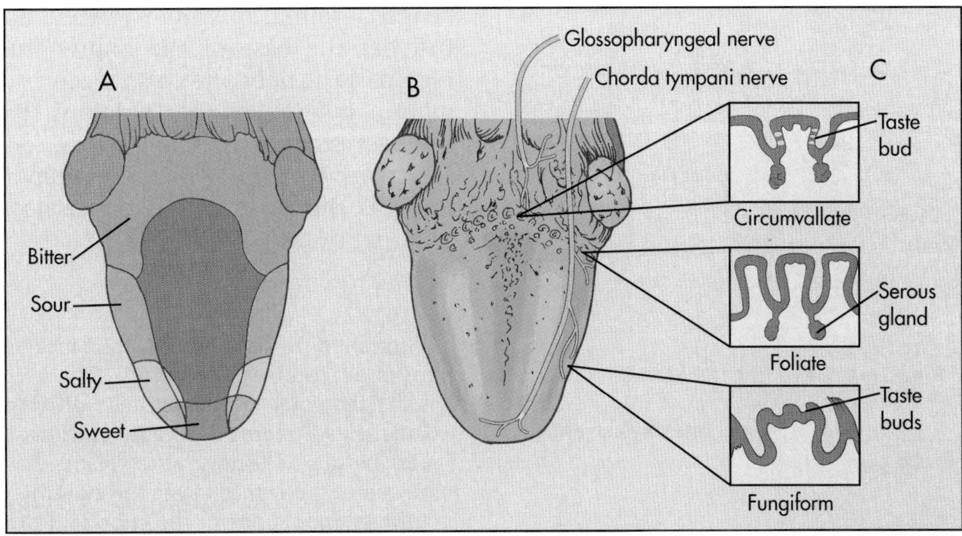

FIGURE 8–17. Peripheral sensory apparatus for gustation. A, Taste qualities associated with different regions of the tongue. B, Innervation of taste buds in the anterior two thirds and posterior one third of the tongue by the facial and glossopharyngeal nerves. C, Arrangement of the taste buds on the three types of papillae.

leads to transmitter release, generator potential, and coded pattern of nerve impulses in the primary afferent fiber. Individual gustatory cells do not appear to be completely selective for a particular primary taste. Rather, they respond best to one type of taste stimulus and less well to others. The recognition of a particular taste quality depends on the activity of a population of gustatory cells. This is a modified labeled-line system.

The primary afferent fibers from the taste buds enter the brainstem and travel caudally in the **solitary tract,** ending in the **nucleus of the solitary tract.** Ascending gustatory fibers reach a special part of the **ventral posteromedial nucleus** of the thalamus. This nucleus projects to the **postcentral gyrus,** ending adjacent to the area representing the tongue. An unusual feature of the gustatory projection is that it is ipsilateral rather than crossed.

Smell depends on the olfactory mucosa and central olfactory pathways

The human olfactory system can recognize many odors. These are difficult to classify, but there are at least seven primary odors: camphoraceous, musk, floral, peppermint, ethereal, pungent, and putrid.

The sensory receptors for olfaction are located in the **olfactory mucosa,** a specialized area of about 2.5 cm^2 in each nasal mucosa. The **olfactory receptor cells** are themselves primary afferent neurons. They have an apical process with cilia that extend into a layer of mucus, in which are dissolved chemical substances that elicit olfactory responses. The base of the olfactory receptor cells gives rise to an axon that projects centrally to end in the **olfactory bulb.** Associated with the olfactory receptor cells are supporting and basal cells that replace olfactory receptor cells as they turn over.

Olfactory transduction depends on the binding of odorants (dissolved in the mucous layer) to receptor molecules on the cilia of olfactory receptor cells. The resulting receptor potential increases the firing rate of the primary afferent fiber. The firing rate is a function of the concentration of the odorant.

The coding mechanism for odors is a modified labeled-line system similar to that for taste. Olfactory receptors respond best to a particular type of odorant and less well to others. Olfactory receptors are grouped according to sensitivity to the class of odorant and are located in different regions of the olfactory mucosa. The central nervous system is presented with a spatially coded input that partly represents odor qualities.

The central olfactory pathway is complex. An unusual feature is that the primary afferent neurons synapse directly on neurons of the telencephalon, whereas in all other sensory systems, sensory processing occurs at several lower stages before information reaches the telencephalon. The primary afferent axons from olfactory receptors are unmyelinated axons that collect into filaments of the **olfactory nerve** (Figure 8–18). The olfactory nerve bundles pass through the base of the skull and synapse in the **olfactory bulb.** The main projections of the olfactory bulb form the **olfactory**

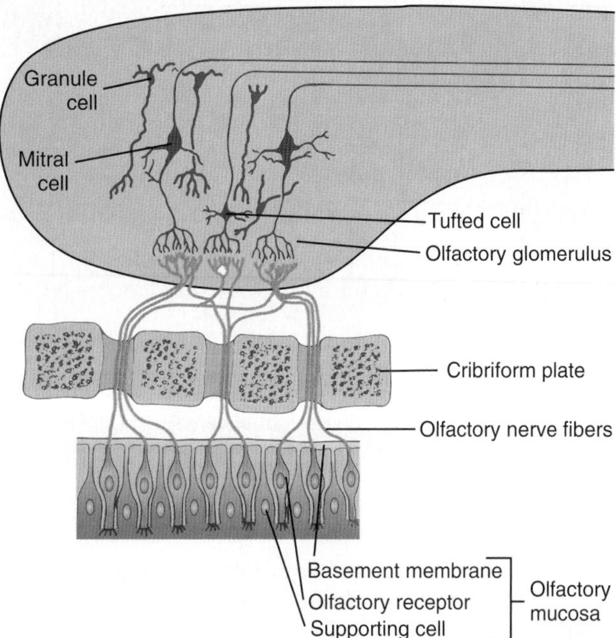

FIGURE 8–18. Initial part of the olfactory pathway, showing the olfactory receptor cells, their projection to the olfactory bulb, and their synapses in the glomeruli with projection cells known as tufted and mitral cells. Also shown are some of the granule cells, which serve as inhibitory interneurons.

tract. Terminations are made in a number of structures at the base of the brain. The orbitofrontal region of the neocortex also receives olfactory information by way of the thalamus. Presumably, the limbic system projections of the olfactory system are involved in the affective responses to odors, whereas the neocortex is concerned with the discrimination of odors.

Important disturbances in olfaction include **anosmia,** the loss of olfaction, and **uncinate fits,** seizures originating in the temporal lobe that cause **olfactory hallucinations.** Head trauma can cause anosmia on one or both sides because olfactory nerve filaments can be torn as they enter the cranial cavity through the cribriform plate of the ethmoid bone or the cribriform plate may be fractured. Unilateral anosmia can be produced by compression of an olfactory bulb or tract by a tumor, such as an **olfactory groove meningioma.** Uncinate fits are epileptic seizures that originate in a region of the temporal lobe near the olfactory cortex. These seizures begin with a **sensory aura** in which the person undergoing the seizure has an olfactory hallucination of an unpleasant odor, such as burning rubber. After this, there may be automatisms, such as movements of the lips and chewing.

Summary

- ❖ Vision depends on the detection of visible light by photoreceptors in the eye. Rods are very sensitive but do not provide high-resolution images or information about color. Cones are less sensitive but have good resolving power and allow color vision.
- ❖ Light is focused on the retina by the refractive surfaces of the eye: the cornea and the lens.
- ❖ The lens has a variable refractory power so that focus can be changed according to the distance of the object to be imaged on the retina.
- ❖ Photoreceptors release an excitatory neurotransmitter under conditions of darkness because of a membrane conductance for Na^+.
- ❖ Many photoreceptors and retinal ganglion cells have a center-surround receptive field organization. Some ganglion cells (P cells) provide signals appropriate for high visual acuity and color; other cells (M cells) have nonlinear responses that are appropriate for motion detection. Still other cells (W cells) may have diffuse receptive fields and signal brightness.
- ❖ The auditory system analyzes sound. Sound frequency determines pitch.
- ❖ Sound causes oscillatory movements of the tympanic membrane. These movements are transmitted to the oval window by a chain of ossicles.
- ❖ Oscillations of the oval window are transmitted to the fluids within the cochlea, resulting in oscillations of the basilar membrane.
- ❖ Transduction of sound occurs when movements of the basilar membrane cause the stereocilia on the hair cells of the organ of Corti to bend.

- Cochlear nerve fibers transmit signals to the cochlear nuclei in the brainstem. Ascending connections are made bilaterally in the superior olivary complex, inferior colliculus, thalamus, and cortex.
- The semicircular ducts of the vestibular apparatus detect angular accelerations of the head because of an inertial shift in the endolymph, which causes the cilia of the hair cells to bend.
- The otolith organs (utricle and saccule) detect linear accelerations of the head because of shifts in the otolithic membrane in response to changes in gravitational forces.
- The vestibular apparatus sends signals to the brainstem that are used to control eye movements and posture and to evoke vestibular sensations.
- Taste receptors are most sensitive to one of the primary tastes: sweet, salty, sour, and bitter.
- Olfactory receptor cells in the nasal mucosa signal smell.

Bibliography

Burns ME, Baylor DA: Activation, deactivation, and adaptation in vertebrate photoreceptor cells, *Annu Rev Neurosci* 24:779, 2001.

Cumming BG, DeAngelis GC: The physiology of stereopsis, *Annu Rev Neurosci* 24:203, 2001.

Dacey DM: Parallel pathways for spectral coding in primate retina, *Annu Rev Neurosci* 23:743, 2000.

Eatock RA: Adaptation in hair cells, *Annu Rev Neurosci* 23:285, 2000.

Ehret G, Romand R: *The central auditory system,* New York, 1997, Oxford University Press.

Faurion A: Physiology of the sweet taste, *Progr Sensory Physiol* 8:130, 1987.

Ferster D, Miller KD: Neural mechanisms of orientation selectivity in the visual cortex, *Annu Rev Neurosci* 23:441, 2000.

Kauer JS, White J: Imaging and coding in the olfactory system, *Annu Rev Neurosci* 24:963, 2001.

Mombaerts P: Molecular biology of odorant receptors in vertebrates, *Annu Rev Neurosci* 22:487, 1999.

Oyster C: *The human eye: structure and function,* Sunderland, Mass, 1999, Sinauer Associates.

Wandell BA: Computational neuroimaging of human visual cortex, *Annu Rev Neurosci* 22:145, 1999.

Wilson VJ, Jones GM: *Mammalian vestibular physiology,* New York, 1979, Plenum.

Case Studies

Case 8–1

A 67-year-old woman awakens with impaired vision. On examination, she cannot see objects well in the right visual field of either eye. Some vision is retained in the central regions of the visual fields, but vision is absent in both the upper and lower quadrants.

1. **What is the name for this type of visual field defect?**
   A. Bitemporal hemianopia
   B. Central scotoma
   C. Homonymous hemianopia with macular sparing
   D. Inferior homonymous quadrantanopia
   E. Superior homonymous quadrantanopia

2. **Which artery is involved?**
   A. Anterior cerebral
   B. Anterior choroidal
   C. Internal carotid
   D. Middle cerebral
   E. Posterior cerebral

3. **Which part of the visual pathway has been damaged?**
   A. LGN
   B. Occipital lobe
   C. Optic chiasm
   D. Optic tract
   E. Retina

Case 8–2

A 16-year-old boy notices that he has difficulty understanding what his English teacher is saying in class. He has been a good student, but his grades are falling. On interview by his physician, he admits an enthusiasm for loud rock music. Weber's test shows that sound does not localize to either ear. The Rinne test shows that air conduction is better than bone conduction bilaterally. Audiometry demonstrates a 40- to 60-dB loss of hearing at frequencies above 2500 Hz.

1. **What is the boy's hearing deficit called?**
   A. Bilateral conduction deafness
   B. Complete deafness
   C. Conduction deficit on the left
   D. Sensorineural deafness on both sides
   E. Sensorineural deficit on the right

2. **Which structure is most likely to be affected?**
   A. Cerebral cortex of temporal lobe
   B. Cochlear nerve
   C. Hair cells of the cochlea
   D. Ossicular chain
   E. Tympanic membranes

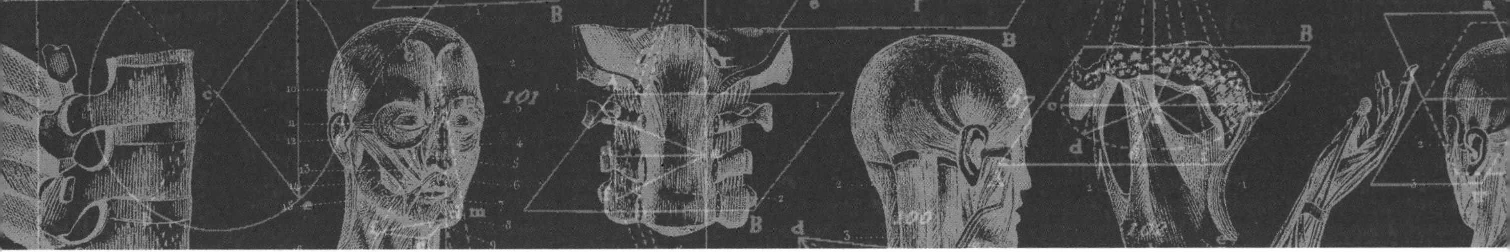

Chapter 9: Motor System

Objectives

- ❖ Describe the properties of motor units and of motor neurons.
- ❖ State the structure and function of the muscle stretch receptors (muscle spindles and Golgi tendon organs).
- ❖ Indicate the role of motor neurons and interneurons in spinal cord reflexes.
- ❖ Identify the changes in motor control that occur after transection of the spinal cord or upper brainstem.
- ❖ Describe vestibular and other postural reflexes, locomotion, and the control of eye movements.
- ❖ State the role of the cerebral cortex in motor control.
- ❖ Describe the organization of the cerebellum and the motor consequences of cerebellar disease.
- ❖ Identify disorders caused by damage to the basal ganglia and associated structures.

The term **motor system** refers to the neural pathways that control the sequence and pattern of contractions of skeletal muscles. Skeletal muscle contractions result in **posture, reflexes, rhythmic activity** (e.g., locomotion, respiration), and **voluntary movements.** A given motor act may involve several of these. Motor acts make up a substantial part of the readily observable behavior of an organism. Motor behaviors that are especially important in humans include speech and movements of the digits and eyes.

Motor control depends on sensory signals from muscle **stretch receptors** and the **reflex activity** of the spinal cord. The higher motor centers of the brain superimpose commands on spinal cord reflex activity. These centers include the **brainstem, motor cortex, cerebellum,** and **basal ganglia.** Voluntary movements are initiated by commands generated in the cerebral cortex in concert with activity in a number of cortical control systems. Motor programs are developed by these cortical areas so that muscles are contracted in a coordinated way. The cerebellum and basal ganglia help regulate activity in the motor regions of the cerebral cortex.

The Motor Units in the Spinal Cord Are Highly Organized

The motor unit is the basic element in motor control

The **motor unit** consists of an **α motor neuron,** its **motor axon,** and all the skeletal muscle fibers that it innervates (see Chapter 12). A **muscle unit** is the set of skeletal muscle fibers in a motor unit. The discharge of an α motor neuron normally results in the contraction of each of the muscle fibers that it supplies because the **end plate potential** in skeletal muscle fibers is normally suprathreshold (see Chapters 4 and 12). In mammals and other vertebrates, no inhibitory synapses exist on skeletal muscle fibers, although they do exist in many invertebrates. This means that all decisions about whether a skeletal muscle fiber will contract are normally made by the α motor neuron. Furthermore, each time an α motor neuron discharges, the entire muscle unit contracts. This means that the smallest gradation of force that can be generated by a muscle depends on the force of contraction of the weakest muscle units in that muscle.

A given skeletal muscle contains a number of motor units. The ratio of the total number of skeletal muscle fibers in a muscle to the number of α motor neurons is the **innervation ratio.** This is the number of muscle fibers in the average motor unit. The innervation ratio is large for muscles that are used for coarse movements (e.g., 2000 fibers for the gastrocnemius muscle) and small for muscles that produce finely graded movements (e.g., 3 to 6 for the eye muscles). The muscle fibers in a motor unit are distributed widely in a muscle, and they are separated by fibers belonging to other motor units. All the skeletal muscle fibers in a motor unit are of the same histochemical type. That is, the muscle fibers are all of type I, type IIb, or type IIa. The contractile properties of these muscle fiber types are summarized in **Table 9–1**. The motor units that twitch slowly and resist fatigue are classified as **S (slow)** and have type I fibers. S motor units depend on oxidative metabolism for their energy supply and have weak contractions (**Figure 9–1**). The motor units with fast twitches are **FF (fast, fatigable)** and **FR (fast, fatigue resistant).** FF motor units have type IIb fibers, use glycolytic metabolism, and have strong contractions, but they fatigue easily. FR motor units have type IIa fibers and rely on oxidative metabolism; their contractions are of intermediate force, and these motor units resist fatigue (Figure 9–1).

TABLE 9–1. MUSCLE FIBER CONTRACTILE PROPERTIES

Type	Speed	Strength	Fatigability	Motor Unit
I	Slow	Weak	Fatigue resistant	S
IIb	Fast	Strong	Fatigable	FF
IIa	Fast	Intermediate	Fatigue resistant	FR

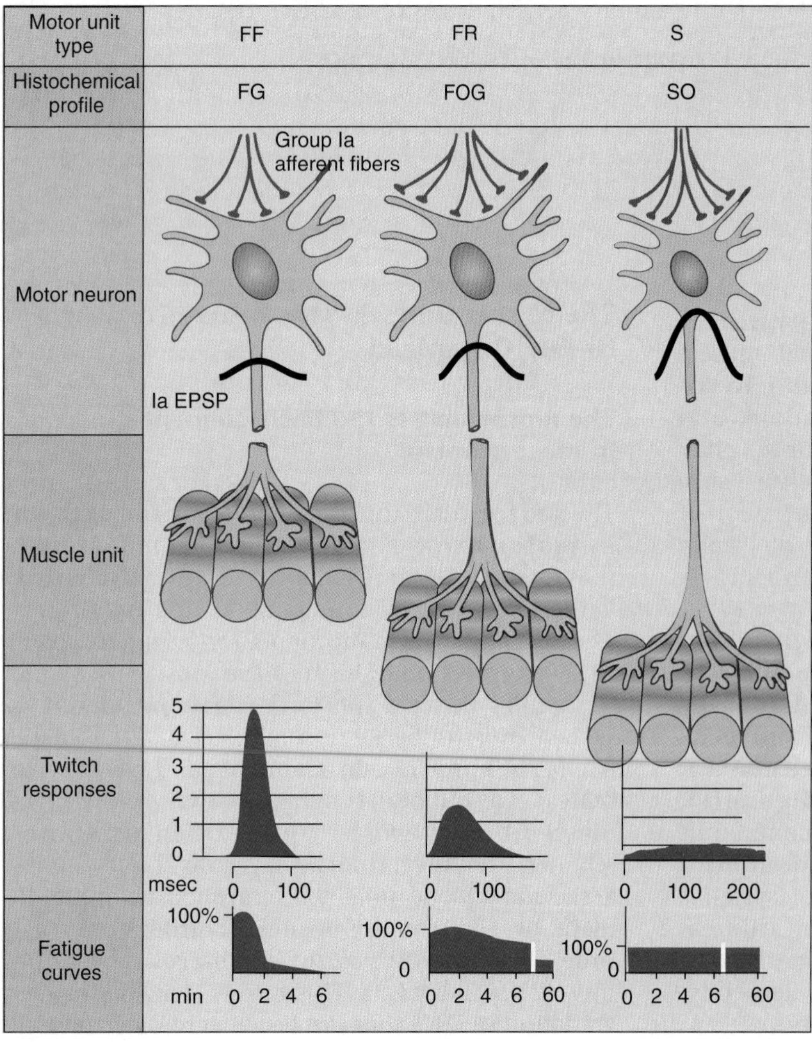

FIGURE 9–1. Summary of features of motor units in a mixed muscle (medial gastrocnemius muscle of a cat). Relative sizes are shown for motor neurons, muscle fibers, monosynaptic excitatory postsynaptic potentials (EPSP) evoked by volleys in group Ia afferent fibers, and twitch responses. FF, fast, fatigable; FG, fast, glycolytic; FOG, fast, oxidative-glycolytic; FR, fast, fatigue resistant; S, slow; SO, slow, oxidative.

α Motor neurons form the final common pathway

The only way in which the central nervous system can cause skeletal muscle fibers to contract is by evoking discharges in α motor neurons. Therefore, all motor acts depend on neural circuits that eventually impinge on α motor neurons. This is why these neurons are called the **final common pathway.**

The motor nucleus contains α motor neurons

The α motor neurons are large neurons found in lamina IX of the spinal cord ventral horn and in **cranial nerve motor nuclei** that supply skeletal muscles. Each muscle or group of synergistic muscles (i.e., those having a similar action) has its own **motor nucleus.** The α motor neurons that supply a given muscle are generally arranged as a longitudinal column of cells, often extending two or three segments in the spinal cord and several millimeters in the brainstem. The set of α motor neurons that innervates a muscle is called the **motor neuron pool** of the muscle.

The motor nuclei of different muscles or muscle groups are located in different parts of the ventral horn. That is, motor nuclei have a **somatotopic organization.** Motor nuclei that supply the axial muscles of the body are in the medial part of the ventral horn in the cervical and lumbosacral enlargements and in the most ventral part of the ventral horn in the upper cervical, thoracic, and upper lumbar segments of the spinal cord. The innervation ratio for the motor units in these muscles is large because the role of the axial muscles includes gross activities such as maintenance of posture, support for limb movements, and respiration.

Motor nuclei that innervate the limb muscles are in the lateral part of the ventral horn in the cervical and lumbosacral enlargements. The most distal muscles are supplied by motor nuclei in the dorsolateral part of the ventral horn, whereas more proximal muscles are innervated by motor nuclei in the ventrolateral ventral horn. The innervation ratios of these muscles are smaller for the distal muscles and larger for the proximal ones.

Motor neurons are large cells with several processes

The individual α motor neuron **(Figure 9–2)** is a cell with a large soma (≤70 μm in diameter). Each of the

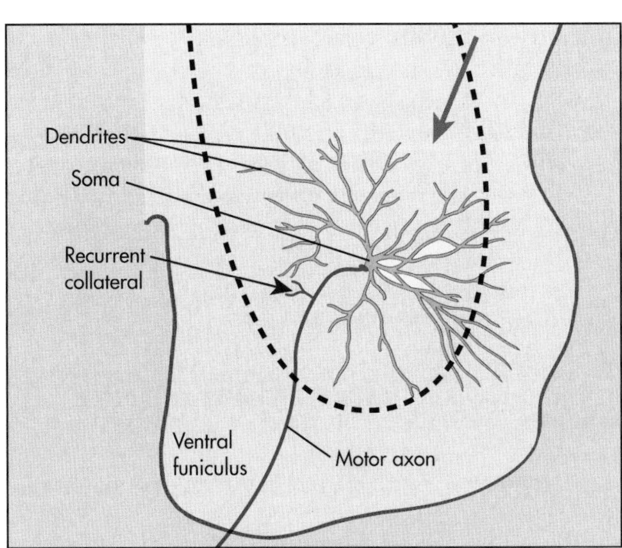

FIGURE 9–2. An α motor neuron injected intracellularly with horseradish peroxidase. The blue arrow indicates a recurrent collateral of the motor axon. The green arrow shows the direction followed by the microelectrode.

5 to 22 dendrites may be as long as 1 mm. The large myelinated axon has a diameter of 12 to 20 μm, and its conduction velocity is 72 to 120 m/sec. The axon of an α motor neuron is often called an **α motor axon.** It arises from an axon hillock on the soma or a proximal dendrite and has a short, unmyelinated **initial segment** before the myelin sheath begins. These axons collect in bundles that leave the ventral horn, pass through the ventral white matter of the spinal cord, and enter a filament of the ventral root. Just before leaving the ventral horn, some α motor axons give off **recurrent collaterals.** Recurrent collaterals typically project dorsally and synapse on interneurons, called **Renshaw cells,** in the ventral part of lamina VII (see later section).

Synaptic integration depends on postsynaptic potentials

The dendrites and soma of the α motor neuron are covered with synapses from primary afferent fibers, interneurons, and pathways that descend from the brain. Most of the synapses are from interneurons. Approximately half of the surface membrane lies beneath synaptic endings. Some of the synapses are excitatory, whereas others are inhibitory.

The part of the α motor neuron membrane with the lowest threshold is thought to be the **initial segment,** which therefore serves as a **trigger zone** for the generation of action potentials. Excitatory synaptic currents depolarize all parts of the membrane of the motor neuron, but in terms of the initiation of an action potential, the depolarization

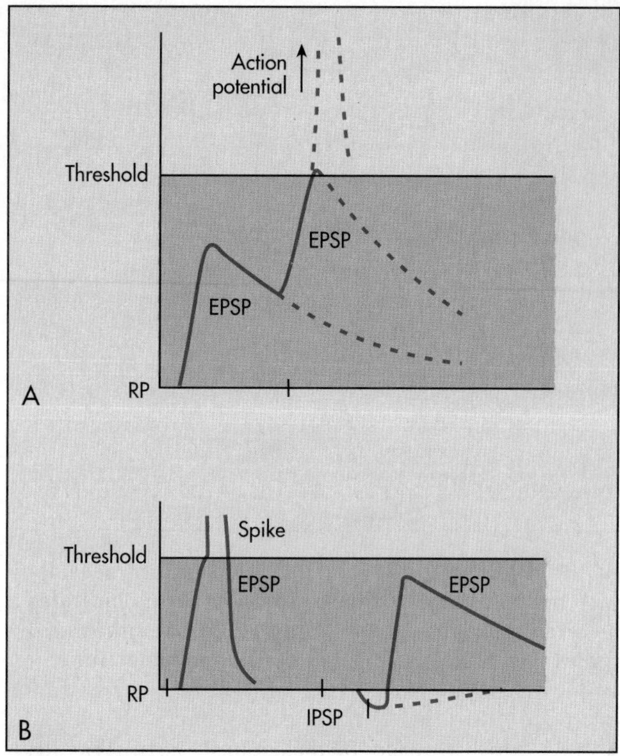

FIGURE 9–3. Synaptic integration. A, Summation of two EPSPs recorded from an α motor neuron. The second EPSP exceeds threshold, so an action potential is triggered. The two EPSPs can result from the stimulation of separate pathways (spatial summation) or the repetitive activation of a single pathway (temporal summation). B, An EPSP and the action potential it triggers are shown at the left, and the interaction between the EPSP and an inhibitory postsynaptic potential (IPSP) at the right. Note that the IPSP prevents the EPSP from triggering the spike. RP, resting potential.

of the initial segment is crucial. The **excitatory postsynaptic potentials (EPSPs)** produced by activation of more than one excitatory pathway to a motor neuron may sum **(Figure 9–3, *A*)**, and the summed EPSPs may exceed threshold for discharge **(spatial summation).** Alternatively, repetitive activation of an excitatory pathway can produce **temporal summation** (see Chapter 4). **Inhibitory postsynaptic potentials (IPSPs)** interfere with the excitatory ones and tend to prevent the discharge of an action potential (Figure 9–3, *B*). The interaction of excitatory and inhibitory synaptic currents in determining whether a neuron discharges is termed **synaptic integration.**

The location of a synapse on the membrane of a neuron such as an α motor neuron may determine the effectiveness of that particular synapse in synaptic integration. Analysis of the **passive electrical properties** of α motor neurons indicates that synaptic currents can reach the initial segment from even the most distant part of the dendritic tree. However, synaptic potentials produced by distal synapses are smaller and slower than those produced by proximal synapses. For example, if a synapse on a dendrite is one **length constant** (see Chapter 3) away from the initial segment, the size of the membrane potential change in the initial segment is only about one third (1/e) of that generated in the dendrite. Furthermore, synaptic potentials are considerably slowed.

In many neurons, inhibitory synapses, which prevent the generation of action potentials, tend to be located near the initial segment. Another arrangement is that excitatory and inhibitory synapses from neural pathways with antagonistic functions are located near each other on a given dendrite but away from the initial segment. This allows different pathways to influence the motor neuron independently. In still another arrangement, excitatory synaptic endings of one pathway receive axoaxonal synapses from another. These axoaxonal synapses cause presynaptic inhibition, which can reduce the effectiveness of a pathway to the motor neuron without altering the excitability of the motor neuron, allowing it to participate in other pathways.

Action potentials generated by α motor neurons have special features

When a motor neuron discharges in response to synaptic excitation, the potentials follow a characteristic sequence. A recording from the soma first reveals an EPSP **(Figure 9–4, *A*)**. Arising from this is a spike potential with two phases: an initial small spike, on which is superimposed a slightly delayed but larger spike. The first small spike is believed to represent the action potential generated by the initial segment; it is small in a recording from the soma because of **electrotonic decrement.** The larger spike is thought to represent invasion of the soma by the action potential. However, the spike also travels distally in the motor axon to cause a contraction of the muscle unit. The activation of a motor neuron in this fashion is called **orthodromic activation** because the sequence is in the normal, or orthograde, direction.

Under experimental conditions, an action potential may be initiated in the motor axon and conducted retrogradely to the motor neuron. This is called **antidromic activation** (Figure 9–4, *B*). A recording from the soma of the motor neuron reveals that the antidromic action potential arises directly from the resting membrane potential and has the same series of small and larger spikes as the orthodromic action potential. The missing part of

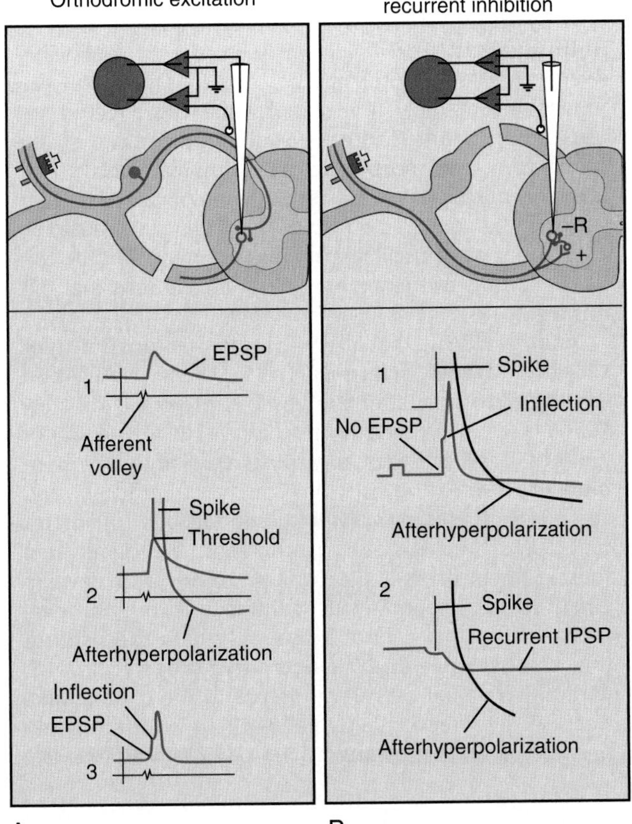

FIGURE 9–4. Orthodromic and antidromic action potentials recorded from motor neurons. A, Monosynaptic EPSP (1), a larger EPSP that reaches threshold on some trials (2), and a low-gain recording of an orthodromic action potential (3). In 3, the arrows indicate the EPSP (smaller crest) and the inflection between the initial segment and the soma-dendritic spikes (upper crest). The drawing at the top shows the recording arrangement and the interruption of the ventral root to prevent antidromic activation. B, Recordings in 1 show an antidromic action potential in a motor neuron at high gain (truncated spike) and at low gain. Note the inflection on the rising phase of the spike. Also note that the spike is succeeded by a large afterhyperpolarization. This is best seen in the high-gain record. In 2, most of the records are with the stimulus subthreshold for the motor axon, and thus the potentials recorded are IPSPs caused by the activity of Renshaw cells (R) excited by other motor axons. The drawing at the top shows the experimental arrangement. Note that the dorsal root is cut to prevent orthodromic excitation.

the potential sequence is the EPSP. After the spike, a long afterhyperpolarization occurs. This is also present in orthodromic action potentials, but it is often obscured by the EPSP.

The afterhyperpolarization is an important feature of the motor neuronal action potential because it helps determine the characteristic firing rate of the neuron. Large α motor neurons have shorter afterhyperpolarizations (≈50 msec long) than those of small α motor neurons (≈100 msec long). Therefore, large α motor neurons tend to discharge at rates of up to about 20 Hz, whereas small ones discharge at approximately 10 Hz.

Muscle fibers contract with a twitch when a motor neuron discharges once. However, repetitive discharges result in a **tetanic contraction** of the muscle (see Chapter 12). The contractile force of a tetanic contraction increases with the rate of discharge of the motor neuron up to a limit imposed by the properties of the muscle. When the tetanic contraction is submaximal, muscle force increases with each motor neuronal discharge. This condition is called an **unfused** or **incomplete tetanus.** When the tetanic contraction is maximal, the contraction becomes a **fused** or **complete tetanus.** The motor neuronal firing rate that produces a fused tetanus in the motor unit causes the greatest contractile force possible for that motor unit.

The characteristic firing rates of α motor neurons match the mechanical properties of the skeletal muscle fibers they innervate. For example, large motor neurons fire at fast rates and innervate fast-twitch muscle fibers; that is, the muscle units of large motor neurons are either the FF or the FR type (Table 9–1). Small motor neurons fire at low rates and innervate slow-twitch muscle fibers; the muscle units of small motor neurons are the S type.

The contraction of a muscle is regulated by the nervous system in two ways. The first is by altering the **firing rates** of α motor neurons. As already indicated, the effects of changing the firing rate are limited by the firing rate at which a tetanus in a given motor unit becomes fused. The second means of regulating muscle tension is by changing the number of active α motor neurons. This activation is called **recruitment.**

The recruitment of α motor neurons is orderly. Small α motor neurons are usually recruited more easily than large ones are. This may be related to differences in the membrane properties of small and large α motor neurons or reflect the synaptic organization that controls their discharges. This difference is called the **size principle.** Not only are the small α motor neurons recruited before the large ones during excitation, but also the activity of the small α motor neurons persists longer than that of the large ones during inhibition. Because the diameters of the motor axons of large α motor neurons are greater than the diameters of the axons of small α motor neurons, the action potentials recorded extracellularly from the ventral root are greater for the large than for the small α motor neurons (**Figure 9–5**). This allows evaluation

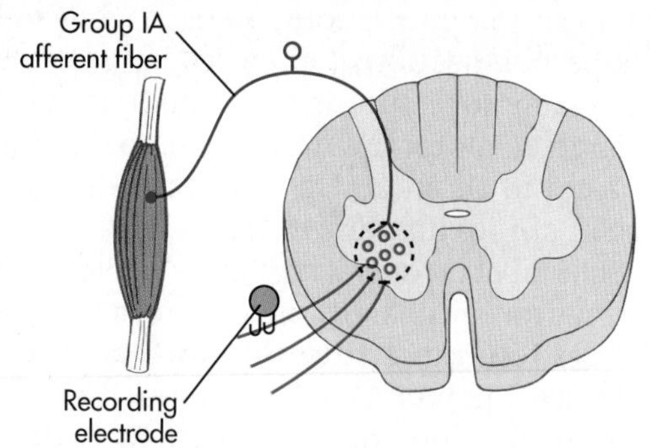

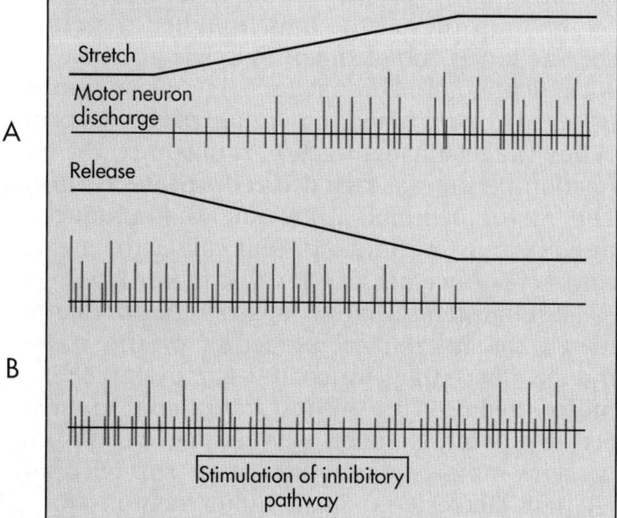

FIGURE 9–5. Size principle and motor neuron recruitment. ***Top,*** **Arrangement of the electrode during the experiment. A, Stretching the muscle activates several motor neurons. The motor axon with the smallest action potential in the ventral root filament is activated first; then progressively larger units begin to discharge. The converse sequence is seen when the muscle is released from the stretch: the large units stop firing first. B, An inhibitory input causes cessation of discharge of the larger units but not of the small unit.**

of the recruiting sequence by recordings from the ventral root.

Because of the progressive and orderly recruitment of small and then large α motor neurons, a weak activation of a motor neuronal pool discharges only the small α motor neurons. This activity produces a weak, slow contraction of slow-twitch muscle fibers. This type of muscle activity is suited to the maintenance of posture and to slow movements, such as walking. The recruitment of large α motor neurons activates powerful fast-twitch muscle fibers. The contractions of these fibers add to the initial force evoked by the slow-twitch fibers, and the resulting movements are appropriate to vigorous activity, such as running and jumping.

Several diseases of the central nervous system cause weakness by destroying α motor neurons. One of these is **poliomyelitis.** For unknown reasons, the poliovirus selectively kills α motor neurons and thus paralyzes the muscles they supply. The α motor neurons affected are usually concentrated in only a few motor nuclei of the spinal cord, but more widespread loss can occur, and cranial nerve motor nuclei are sometimes involved (bulbar polio). The denervated muscle undergoes atrophy, although some muscle fibers may be reinnervated by collateral sprouts of the axons of α motor neurons that did not die.

Another disease that affects α motor neurons is **amyotrophic lateral sclerosis (ALS),** often called **Lou Gehrig's disease** after the baseball player of the New York Yankees who died of this disease. In ALS, α motor neurons at all levels of the spinal cord and brainstem gradually die. As they die, they discharge erratically and cause **fasciculations** (visible contractions of motor units). After an α motor neuron dies, the denervated muscle fibers of its motor unit **atrophy** and develop **fibrillations** (spontaneous contractions of individual muscle fibers that cannot be seen through the skin but that can be observed by **electromyography**). In ALS, cortical pyramidal cells that give rise to the corticospinal tract (see later section) also die, resulting in further weakness of voluntary movements and pathological reflexes.

Muscle stretch receptors are important sense organs

Skeletal muscles and their tendons contain specialized sensory receptors called **stretch receptors** that discharge when the muscles are stretched. These receptors include **muscle spindles** and **Golgi tendon organs.** These receptors are involved in sensory experience and contribute to proprioception (see Chapter 7). However, they are discussed here because of their importance in motor control.

The most complex muscle receptor is the muscle spindle. Muscle spindles are composed of elongated bundles of narrow muscle fibers called **intrafusal muscle fibers** enclosed within a connective tissue capsule. The spindles are richly innervated with both sensory and motor endings. Most of the muscle spindle lies freely within the spaces between the regular or **extrafusal muscle fibers,** but its distal ends merge with the connective tissue in the muscle. This parallel arrangement is important for the operation of the muscle spindle. When the whole muscle contracts, the muscle spindle is unloaded unless the intrafusal fibers also contract.

The intrafusal muscle fibers are of two main types: **nuclear bag fibers** and **nuclear chain fibers.** Their names are based on the arrangement of their nuclei (**Figure 9–6**). Nuclear bag fibers are larger than nuclear chain fibers and have a cluster of nuclei near the midpoint (resembling a "bag" of oranges). Nuclear chain fibers have a single row of nuclei near the midpoint.

The two types of sensory endings in a muscle spindle are a **primary ending** and one or more **secondary endings** (Figure 9–6). The primary ending has spiral terminals on both nuclear bag and nuclear chain fibers, and it is innervated by a large, myelinated afferent nerve fiber called a **group Ia fiber.** Secondary endings have spraylike terminals that are chiefly on nuclear chain fibers. The secondary endings are supplied by medium-sized **group II fibers.**

The γ motor neurons provide the motor innervation of muscle spindles (Figure 9–6). The endings may be small end plates or elongated trail endings. There are two types of γ motor neurons: **dynamic γ motor neurons** innervate chiefly the nuclear bag intrafusal muscle fibers, and **static γ motor neurons** supply nuclear chain fibers.

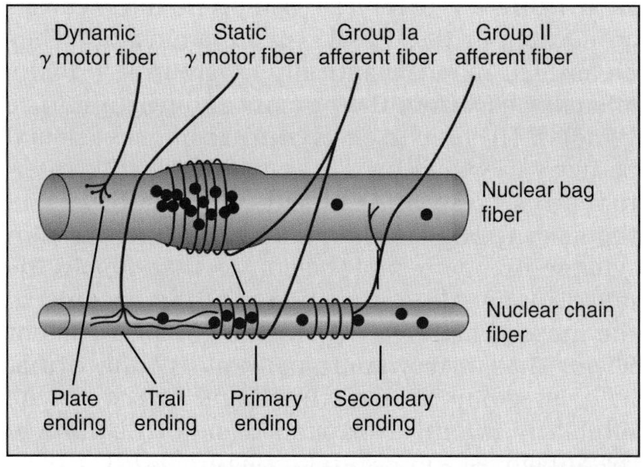

FIGURE 9–6. Innervation of nuclear bag and nuclear chain fibers of a muscle spindle.

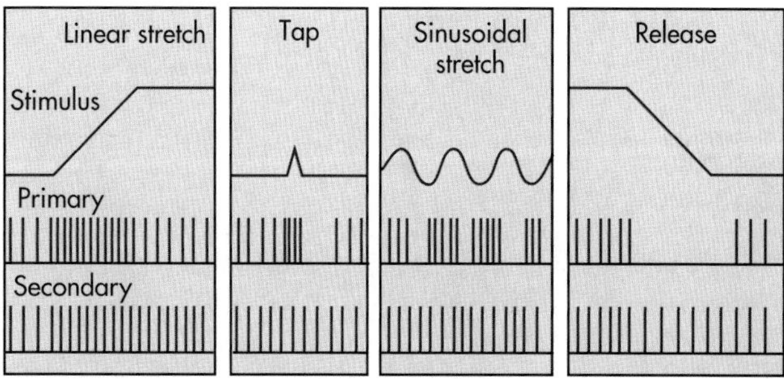

FIGURE 9–7. Responses of primary and secondary endings of a muscle spindle to linear stretch, tap, sinusoidal stretch, and release of the muscle.

Primary endings respond to maintained muscle stretch with a slowly adapting discharge that has both a dynamic and a static component **(Figure 9–7)**. The dynamic response signals the rate of stretch of muscle, and the static component signals muscle length. Secondary endings have only a static response; thus, they signal muscle length. The dynamic response probably results from the property of nuclear bag fibers of elastic rebound after an initial rapid elongation during muscle stretch.

The γ motor neurons regulate the sensitivity of muscle spindles to muscle stretch. They can also prevent the unloading effect of muscle shortening by contraction of the intrafusal muscle fibers during or just before contraction of the extrafusal muscle fibers **(Figure 9–8)**. Dynamic γ motor neurons enhance the dynamic responses of the primary endings, and static γ motor neurons increase the static responses of both primary and secondary endings. THE CENTRAL NERVOUS SYSTEM CAN THUS INDEPENDENTLY REGULATE DYNAMIC AND STATIC RESPONSES OF MUSCLE SPINDLES.

Another type of muscle stretch receptor is the **Golgi tendon organ.** These receptors are found in

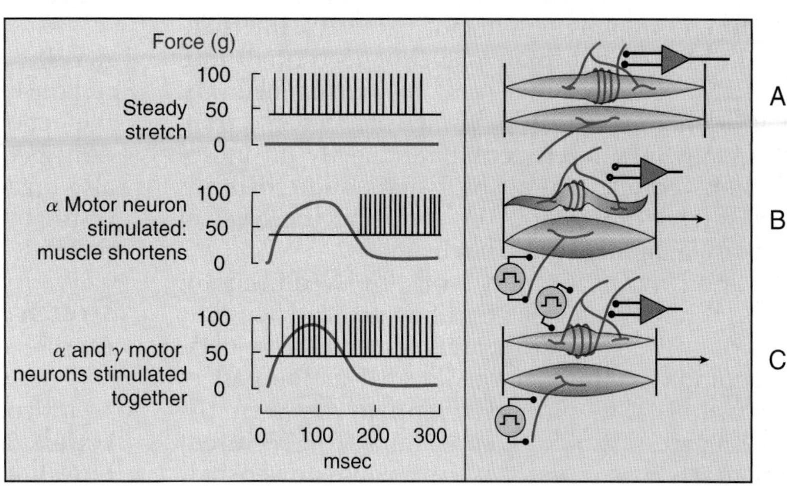

FIGURE 9–8. Effect of the activation of γ motor neurons. A, Stretch of the muscle activates an afferent fiber supplying a muscle spindle. B, The discharge stops when a muscle contraction is produced by activity in α motor neurons. C, The effect of unloading is avoided because α and γ motor neurons are coactivated.

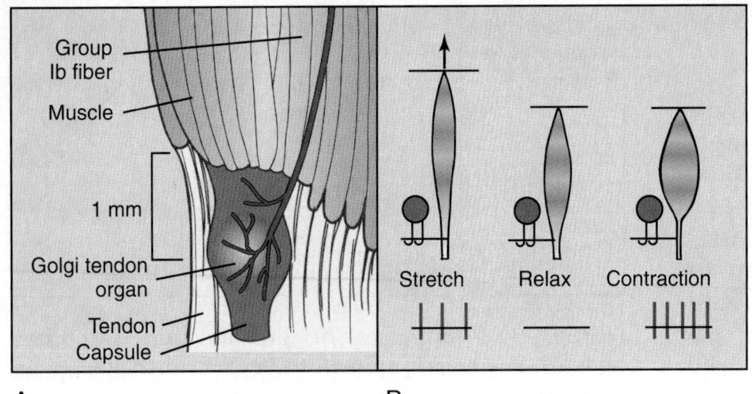

FIGURE 9–9. **A,** Structure of a Golgi tendon organ and its relationship to the tendon of a muscle. **B,** The recordings at the bottom show that a Golgi tendon organ can be activated by either muscle stretch or muscle contraction. The activity of Golgi tendon organs signals muscle tension.

tendons, in the connective tissue within skeletal muscles, and around joint capsules. Golgi tendon organs are supplied by large, myelinated primary afferent nerve fibers, called **group Ib fibers.** The terminals of group Ib fibers interdigitate with bundles of collagen fibers, an arrangement that allows the application of mechanical force to the terminals when the muscle is either contracted or stretched (**Figure 9–9**). Golgi tendon organs are therefore arranged in series with the muscle and its tendon.

Spinal cord interneurons form motor control circuits

Most of the synapses on α motor neurons originate from spinal cord interneurons. **Interneurons** are neurons interposed between primary afferent neurons and motor neurons. Interneurons whose processes are confined to the spinal cord are often called **propriospinal neurons.**

Most spinal cord interneurons are located in the dorsal horn. Many are involved in sensory processing and contribute directly or indirectly to the transmission of sensory information to the brain. Dorsal horn interneurons also influence reflex activity, often through polysynaptic pathways. Interneurons in the intermediate nucleus and ventral horn directly affect the discharge of motor neurons. Furthermore, axons in pathways that descend from the brain only rarely terminate directly on motor neurons. Instead, they usually end on interneurons and alter motor output by changing the level of activity in spinal cord neural circuits.

Various types of interneurons involved in motor control have been well characterized. The Renshaw cell has already been mentioned. **Renshaw cells** are inhibitory interneurons located in the part of lamina VII that protrudes ventrally between the lateral part of lamina IX and lamina VIII. Recurrent collaterals from α motor axons synapse on Renshaw cells. When the motor axons discharge, they release acetylcholine at the synapses on Renshaw cells and excite these cells. The Renshaw cells in turn synapse on and inhibit α motor neurons; the discharge of α motor neurons causes an inhibitory feedback via Renshaw cells. This is called **recurrent inhibition** (Figure 9–4, *B*).

Another well-studied interneuron is the **group Ia inhibitory interneuron.** These interneurons are located in the dorsal part of lamina VII. They are excited monosynaptically by group Ia primary afferent fibers from the primary endings of muscle spindles. The term **monosynaptic** implies a neural pathway in which there is only one synaptic interruption between one element of the pathway and the next. Group Ia inhibitory interneurons in turn synapse on the α motor neurons that supply the muscle or muscle group serving as the antagonist to the muscle that gives rise to the group Ia afferent fibers. Thus, a disynaptic pathway is formed that involves group Ia fibers from one muscle group, inhibitory interneurons, and α motor neurons to the antagonist muscle group (**Figure 9–10**).

Spinal cord reflexes underlie motor responses

A **reflex** is a relatively simple, stereotyped motor response to a defined sensory input. Some of the reflexes mediated by spinal cord circuits are described here. However, many other reflexes are also organized at the level of either the spinal cord or the brain (see later section).

Stretch reflexes are responses to muscle spindle input

A particularly important spinal reflex is the **stretch reflex.** Stretching a muscle causes a reflex contraction of that muscle and a reflex relaxation of the antagonist muscles. The stretch reflex has phasic

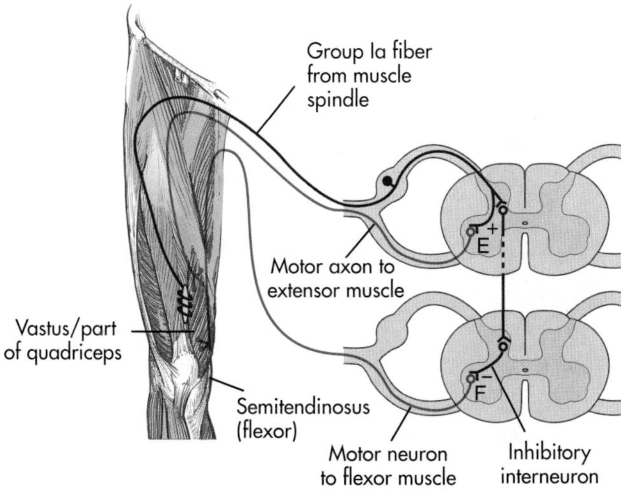

FIGURE 9–10. Reflex pathway for the stretch reflex. The illustration is for the quadriceps stretch reflex, but similar connections can be made for other muscles, including flexor muscles. A muscle spindle is shown to be supplied by a group Ia fiber that enters the spinal cord through a dorsal root and makes monosynaptic excitatory connections with an α motor neuron to the quadriceps muscle in the same segment and a group Ia inhibitory interneuron in another segment. The inhibitory interneuron synapses with an α motor neuron to the antagonistic flexor muscle, semitendinosus. E, extensor motor neuron; F, flexor motor neuron.

and tonic components. The **phasic stretch reflex** is elicited by stretching the muscle quickly. This is often done clinically by tapping the tendon of the muscle with a reflex hammer. For example, when the patellar tendon is struck, a knee jerk reflex results. The **tonic stretch reflex** results from a slower stretch of a muscle, such as occurs during passive movement of a joint by an examining physician. THE TONIC STRETCH REFLEX IS IMPORTANT IN THE MAINTENANCE OF POSTURE.

Hinge joints, such as the knee and ankle, are extended or flexed by extensor and flexor muscles, which are antagonists because they produce opposite movements of the joint. A phasic stretch reflex produced by stretching an extensor muscle results in contraction of the extensor muscle and relaxation of the flexor muscle. Conversely, a phasic stretch reflex of the flexor muscle involves a concomitant relaxation of the extensor muscle. This organization of the stretch reflex pathways is called **reciprocal innervation.**

The neural basis of a spinal reflex is the reflex arc, a circuit that includes a set of primary afferent fibers, interneurons, and α motor neurons. The reflex arc for the phasic stretch reflex of a particular muscle includes (1) the group Ia afferent fibers from primary endings of muscle spindles located within that muscle, (2) the monosynaptic excitatory connections of these afferents with α motor neurons that innervate the muscle, and (3) a disynaptic inhibitory pathway involving group Ia inhibitory interneurons that synapse with α motor neurons innervating the antagonistic muscles (Figure 9–10).

The reflex arc for the tonic stretch reflex involves the same connections described for the phasic stretch reflex. However, group II afferent fibers from secondary endings of muscle spindles also contribute because they make monosynaptic excitatory connections with the α motor neurons that supply the muscle containing the muscle spindles.

The sensitivity of the primary and secondary endings of muscle spindles is controlled by dynamic and static γ motor neurons. The activation of these neurons can result in a sufficiently strong excitatory input in group Ia afferent fibers to discharge the α motor neurons. However, the group Ia fibers in humans discharge after contractions of skeletal muscle. This pattern of discharge indicates that γ motor neurons do activate muscle spindles during voluntary movements but at about the same time as the activation of α motor neurons. Presumably, the shortening of the muscle spindles prevents unloading. Thus, voluntary and other movements depend on the coactivation of α and γ motor neurons.

In neurological examinations, a reflex hammer is commonly used to elicit **phasic stretch reflexes.** The limb to be examined is placed in a position that allows relaxation of the joint operated on by the muscle tested. The tendon of each muscle tested is struck briskly with the reflex hammer, and the subsequent contraction of the muscle is observed (or felt). Responses on the two sides are compared. The fact that tendons are struck gave rise to a misleading terminology for the stretch reflex *(deep tendon reflex);* this terminology should be avoided. The sensory receptors responsible for the phasic stretch reflex are muscle spindles within the muscle and not receptors in the tendon. Muscles that are often tested include the biceps brachii, the quadriceps, and the triceps surae. When phasic stretch reflexes appear to be reduced, it is sometimes possible to enhance them by **Jendrassik's maneuver,** in which the subject interlocks the fingers of the two hands and pulls the hands apart against resistance. **Tonic stretch reflexes** are examined by flexing and extending joints.

In pathological conditions, the stretch reflexes may be either diminished or hyperactive. Causes of decreased stretch reflexes include the death of motor neurons as a result of motor neuron disease (e.g., poliomyelitis, ALS) and the interruption of peripheral nerves or spinal roots (such as occurs in peripheral neuropathy or after a herniated disk). Increased stretch reflexes are seen in diseases that affect the descending motor pathways, such as cerebrovascular accidents (strokes) that interrupt the internal capsule.

The inverse myotatic reflex depends on input from Golgi tendon organs

An important reflex whose afferent limb is group Ib afferent fibers from Golgi tendon organs is sometimes called the **inverse myotatic reflex.** Group Ib afferent fibers from extensor muscles synapse monosynaptically on inhibitory interneurons **(Figure 9–11)**. The inhibitory interneurons in turn synapse on the α motor neurons that supply the same and other extensor muscles in the limb. Flexor muscles are relatively unaffected by this pathway. This pathway is activated by increases in muscle force, which can be produced by either stretch or contraction of the muscle, rather than by stretch alone. Therefore, the word *myotatic* (which refers to muscle stretch) is probably inappropriate.

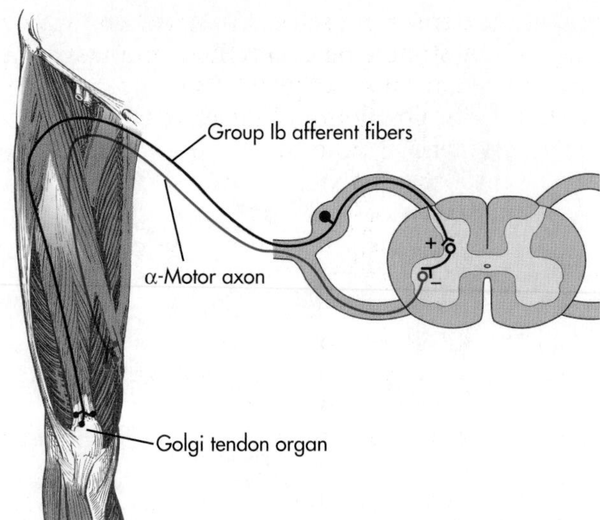

FIGURE 9–11. Pathway for the inverse myotatic reflex produced by Golgi tendon organs. A Golgi tendon organ is shown in the patellar tendon. Its group Ib afferent fiber enters the spinal cord through a dorsal root to terminate on an inhibitory interneuron that synapses on a motor neuron to the quadriceps muscle.

Reflexes may form negative-feedback loops

The stretch and the group Ib (inverse myotatic) reflexes are examples of negative-feedback loops. In a **negative-feedback loop,** the output of the system is compared with the desired output **(Figure 9–12)**. Any difference (error) is fed back to the input so that a corrective action can be made. The variable regulated by a negative-feedback system is the **controlled variable.** In the stretch reflex, the controlled variable is the muscle length; in the group Ib pathway, it is muscle force.

An example of how these negative-feedback loops might operate is the muscle behavior in a soldier at attention. The knees tend to flex because of gravitational forces. If slight flexion occurs,

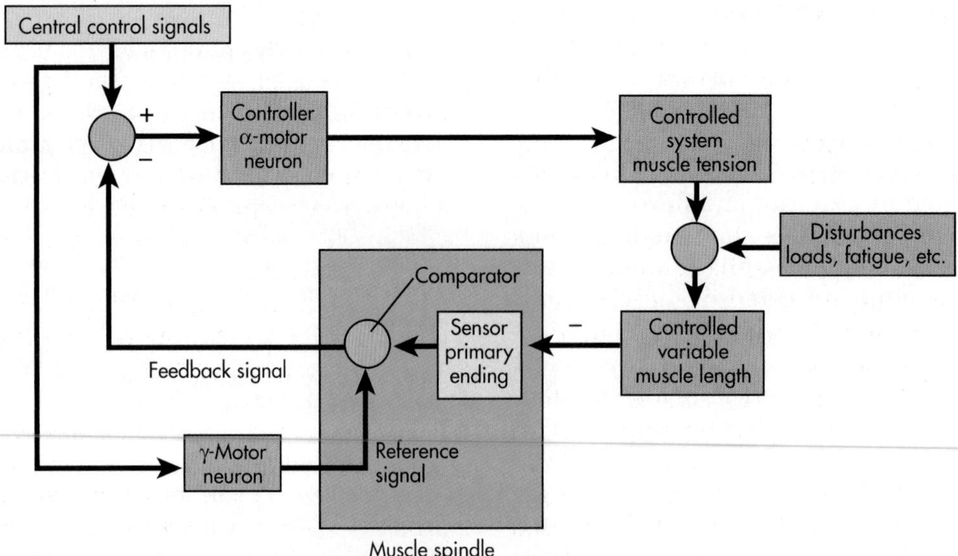

FIGURE 9–12. Operation of the stretch reflex as a negative-feedback system that regulates muscle length. Length is determined by the level of muscle tension, which depends on activity in α motor neurons. Muscle length is detected by the muscle spindle, which has its sensitivity set by γ motor neurons. If the muscle length is increased, such as by a changed load, feedback conveyed by the primary endings increases the discharges of α motor neurons, which reduces muscle length through further contraction of the muscle.

the knee extensor muscles are stretched, which activates the stretch reflex in these muscles. The result is restoration of knee extension. In terms of muscle length, gravitational forces tend to stretch the knee extensors; the stretch reflex acts as a negative-feedback mechanism to control muscle length, keeping it constant. On the other hand, if the knee extensor muscles begin to fatigue, the force that they exert on the patellar tendon decreases, causing the knee to flex. However, a reduction in the tension in the patellar tendon reduces the activity of Golgi tendon organs in the tendon. Decreased activity in group Ib afferent fibers reduces the inverse myotatic reflex (which inhibits α motor neurons to the knee extensor muscles), which allows the knee extensor muscles to contract more vigorously. Thus, a reduction in tension in the patellar tendon causes a negative feedback, which restores the tension toward its original level.

Reflexes control muscle stiffness

The concurrent regulation of muscle length and muscle force makes it possible to control muscle stiffness. Muscle has mechanical properties that resemble those of a spring. When a spring is slack, it exerts no force. When the spring is lengthened beyond a threshold point, known as the **set point** (or resting length), each increment of stretch is associated with the development of an increment of force. The relationship between length and force in an ideal spring is linear, and the slope of the length-force curve is the stiffness of the spring:

$$\text{Stiffness} = \text{Change in force} \div \text{Change in length}$$

The stiffness of different springs varies, being greater if more force is produced for a given increment of stretch.

Muscles also have characteristic **length-force relationships** (see Chapter 12). These are determined with the muscle relaxed or activated by nerve stimulation, and the curves that represent these relationships can be highly nonlinear. If a muscle is passively stretched, the muscle develops force as it is stretched beyond the set point (resting length). When the nerve to the muscle is stimulated, the length-force curve shifts, now having a lower set point and a greater slope. The increased slope indicates that contraction has increased the stiffness of the muscle. It is the interplay between length and force that regulates muscle stiffness and that sets joint position.

In a joint whose position is controlled by sets of agonist and antagonist muscles, a particular joint angle **(equilibrium point)** can actually be attained in several ways. Because the extensor and flexor muscles are reciprocally innervated, neural circuitry is available to cause one muscle to be activated and the antagonist to be relaxed. The combination of these two events determines the equilibrium point of the joint. Another possibility is **co-contraction** of the agonist and antagonist muscles. Although this mechanism requires more energy than the one using reciprocal innervation, co-contraction can provide stability in case of unanticipated changes in load because the stiffness of the joint is increased. One typically uses co-contraction to perform a new task until the task is learned, when co-contraction is replaced by the strategy of relaxing the antagonist.

Flexion reflexes have several roles

Other important reflexes, such as the flexion reflex, also operate at the spinal cord level. In the flexion reflex, the **physiological flexor muscles** of one or more joints in a limb contract and the **physiological extensor muscles** relax. THE PHYSIOLOGICAL FLEXOR MUSCLES ARE THOSE THAT TEND TO WITHDRAW THE LIMB FROM A NOXIOUS STIMULUS. The flexion reflex has several uses. The **flexor withdrawal reflex** consists of a defensive removal of a limb from a threatening or damaging stimulus. For example, if one steps on a nail, the foot is withdrawn reflexly by flexion of the ankle, knee, and hip. This reflex takes precedence over other reflexes. It may be accompanied by a **crossed extensor reflex,** which involves the contraction of the extensor muscles and the relaxation of the flexor muscles of the contralateral limb. The crossed extension serves as a postural adjustment to compensate for the loss of the antigravitational support by the limb that flexes. In quadrupeds, the converse pattern can occur in the other pair of limbs. The flexion reflex is also involved in locomotion and in the scratch reflex.

The flexion reflex is initiated by the flexion reflex afferent fibers, which supply high-threshold muscle and joint receptors, many cutaneous receptors, and nociceptors. It seems likely that the lower threshold receptors help modulate locomotion and that the nociceptors are crucial for evoking the flexor withdrawal reflex. The flexion reflex pathway from primary afferent fibers to the α motor neurons is polysynaptic and involves both excitatory and inhibitory interneurons (**Figure 9–13**). There are both uncrossed and crossed components of the pathway. The α motor neurons involved are those appropriate to the reflex movements already described.

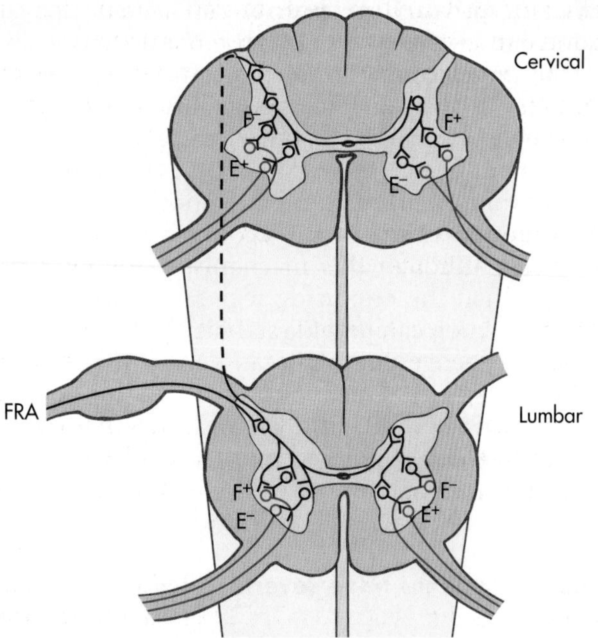

FIGURE 9–13. Flexion reflex pathway. The receptive field of flexion reflex afferents (FRA) on the lower extremity is not shown. The activation of these afferents leads to input over the dorsal roots of the lumbar enlargement. Via polysynaptic connections, flexor motor neurons (F) of the lower extremity on the side stimulated are activated and extensor motor neurons (E) inhibited, resulting in flexion of the lower extremity. Crossed connections activate extensor motor neurons and inhibit flexor motor neurons to the opposite lower extremity, the crossed extensor reflex. A reverse pattern of reflex activity may be produced in the upper extremities.

Descending Motor Pathways Have a Complex Organization

The descending motor pathways have traditionally been divided into pyramidal and extrapyramidal components. The **pyramidal system** includes the corticospinal and corticobulbar tracts; *pyramidal* refers to the presence of at least part of these tracts in the medullary pyramid. THE PYRAMIDAL SYSTEM IS THE MAIN PATHWAY THAT MEDIATES VOLUNTARY MOVEMENTS OF THE DISTAL PARTS OF THE EXTREMITIES AS WELL AS MIMETIC MOVEMENTS OF THE FACE MUSCLES AND MOVEMENTS OF THE TONGUE. The **extrapyramidal system** originally referred to motor pathways other than the corticospinal and corticobulbar tracts. At present, however, *extrapyramidal* is most usefully applied to motor disorders associated with lesions involving the **basal ganglia,** without reference to the particular motor pathways affected.

A helpful classification of descending motor pathways is based on their site of termination in the spinal cord. One set of pathways ends on motor neurons in the lateral part of lamina IX or on the interneurons that project to them **(Figure 9–14).** THIS LATERAL SYSTEM OF DESCENDING PATHWAYS CONTROLS THE MUSCLES OF THE DISTAL PART OF THE LIMBS. THESE MUSCLES SUBSERVE FINE MOVEMENTS USED IN MANIPULATION AND OTHER PRECISE ACTIONS, ESPECIALLY OF THE DIGITS. A parallel control system ends in the brainstem and regulates the part of the facial motor nucleus that supplies the muscles of the lower part of the face as well as the hypoglossal nucleus, which innervates the tongue.

The other set of pathways ends on motor neurons in the medial part of lamina IX or on interneurons that project to them (Figure 9–14). THIS MEDIAL SYSTEM OF DESCENDING PATHWAYS CONTROLS AXIAL AND GIRDLE MUSCLES AS WELL AS MOST CRANIAL NERVE MOTOR NUCLEI. THE MUSCLES OF THE BODY THAT ARE REGULATED BY THE MEDIAL SYSTEM CONTRIBUTE TO POSTURE, BALANCE, AND LOCOMOTION. Muscles in the head are involved in activities such

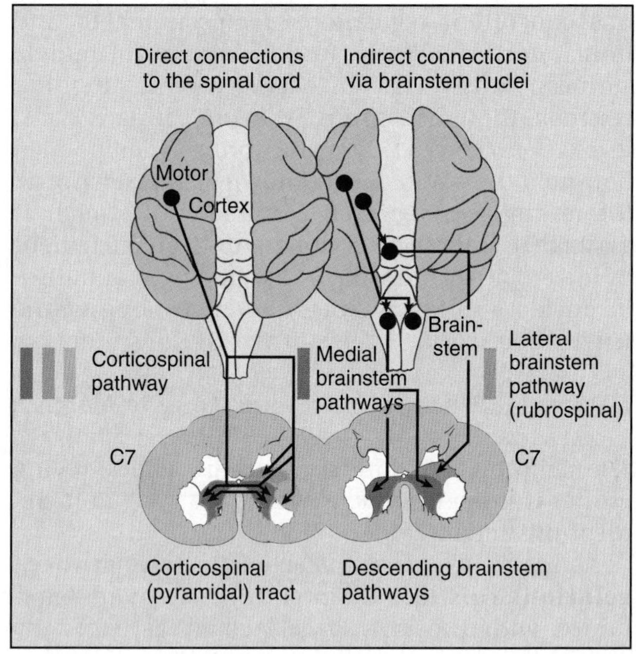

FIGURE 9–14. Lateral and medial motor control systems. Descending motor pathways in the lateral funiculus include the lateral corticospinal tract *(left)* and rubrospinal tract *(right)*. The lateral corticospinal tract projects directly to motor neurons innervating distal muscles as well as to interneurons controlling these motor neurons. The rubrospinal tract projects onto lateral interneurons. Medial pathways include the ventral corticospinal tract *(left)* and several pathways from the medial brainstem *(right)*. These pathways end in the medial ventral horn and control motor neurons to axial and proximal muscles.

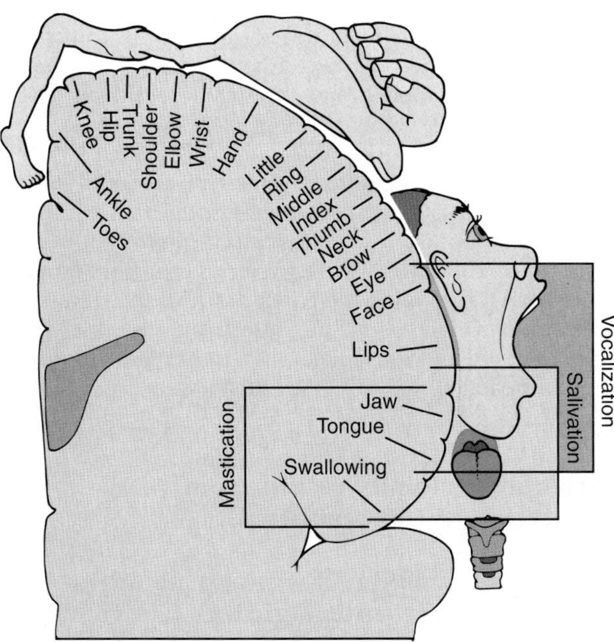

FIGURE 9–15. Somatotopic organization (homunculus) of the motor cortex.

as closure of the eyelids, chewing, swallowing, and phonation.

The lateral system has a somatotopic organization

The lateral system includes two pathways from the brain to the spinal cord (Figure 9–14): the lateral corticospinal tract and the rubrospinal tract. In addition, the part of the corticobulbar tract that controls the lower face and the tongue can be considered part of the lateral system.

The motor cortex has a somatotopic organization **(Figure 9–15)** resembling that of the somatosensory cortex (see Chapter 7). The cells of origin of the component of the **lateral corticospinal tract** controlling the upper extremity are in the dorsolateral precentral gyrus (arm representation), whereas neurons controlling the lower extremity are in the vertex and medial part of the precentral gyrus (leg area). **Corticobulbar tract** neurons that control the lower face and tongue are in the lateral precentral gyrus, just dorsal to the lateral fissure. These neurons project contralaterally to spinal cord motor nuclei or to the hypoglossal nucleus and part of the facial motor nucleus. Many of the terminations of the corticospinal tract are on interneurons, but some are directly on motor neurons, allowing a direct influence on the cerebral cortex on motor neurons that supply distal muscles, such as those controlling hand and digit movements.

The **rubrospinal tract** originates in the red nucleus. This tract appears to be much less significant in humans than in other animals.

The medial system can exert bilateral control

The **ventral corticospinal tract** projects bilaterally to influence motor neurons on both sides of the body. This is an important arrangement because the axial muscles on both sides often function together. Much of the **corticobulbar tract** belongs to the medial system and provides a bilateral innervation of many cranial nerve motor nuclei.

The **tectospinal tract** originates from the deep layers of the superior colliculus and helps control head movements. The **lateral** and **medial vestibulospinal tracts** originate from vestibular nuclei and help control posture and head movements, respectively. The **pontine** and **medullary reticulospinal tracts** arise from the reticular formation; they influence posture and control sensory transmission. The descending projections of monoaminergic nuclei in the brainstem form an additional modulatory system.

The Brainstem Controls Posture and Movement

A hierarchic organization of the motor system can be demonstrated by the effects of lesions at different levels of the neuraxis. A lesion can result in a particular effect by either

- abolishing functions subserved by a structure whose influence is removed by the lesion or
- allowing an action to appear through removal of an inhibitory influence.

The latter responses are called **release phenomena.** Lesions that are particularly instructive include spinal cord transection and decerebration.

Spinal cord transection produces characteristic deficits

Spinal cord transection at a cervical level caudal to the phrenic nucleus (thus sparing respiration) results in severe motor loss as well as in a complete loss of sensation from the body at dermatomal levels below that of the transection. The most

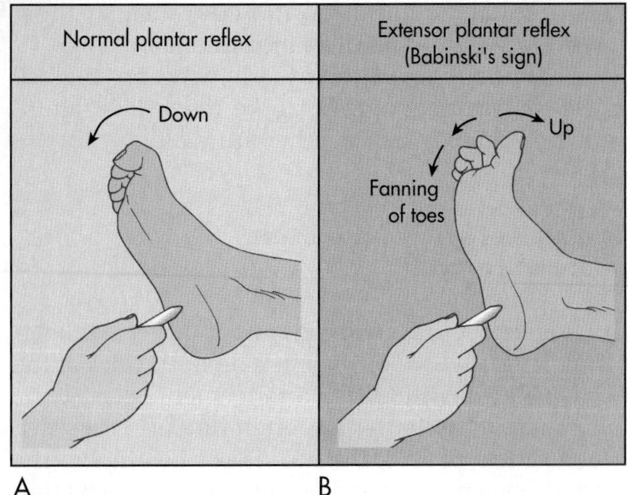

FIGURE 9–16. Babinski's sign. A, The normal response to stroking the plantar surface of the foot. B, Babinski's sign (extensor plantar reflex) in a person with interruption of the corticospinal tract.

important change is the loss of voluntary movements. IMMEDIATELY AFTER TRANSECTION, A PERIOD OF SPINAL SHOCK FOLLOWS IN WHICH REFLEXES ARE ABSENT. This presumably results from the loss of the excitatory actions of pathways descending from the brain. After a time, up to months, **hyperactive stretch** and **flexion reflexes** develop. Hyperactive stretch reflexes may result in **clonus,** alternating contractions of extensor and then flexor muscles. **Mass reflexes** are associated with hyperactive flexion reflexes and are characterized by flexion of one or both limbs and evacuation of the bladder and bowel. These changes may reflect the loss of descending inhibition and also rearrangements in spinal cord circuits, possibly because of the sprouting of primary afferent fibers and the formation of new synaptic connections within the spinal cord. Other release phenomena include the appearance of pathological reflexes, such as **Babinski's sign (Figure 9–16),** which follows interruption of the lateral corticospinal tract. Although locomotion is not regained in humans, a capability for locomotion reappears in experimental animals after spinal transection. This can be attributed to activation of a **locomotor pattern generator** within the neural circuitry of the spinal cord. A PATTERN GENERATOR IS A NEURAL CIRCUIT THAT CONTROLS A SPECIFIC TYPE OF MOTOR BEHAVIOR, OFTEN A RHYTHMIC BEHAVIOR SUCH AS LOCOMOTION OR RESPIRATION. In animals with chronic spinal transections, locomotion can be triggered by afferent signals rather than by pathways descending from the brain. It is hoped that a way will be found to activate the spinal cord locomotor pattern generator in humans with spinal cord injury.

Spinal cord injury is unfortunately a relatively common occurrence and generally affects young adults. Frequent causes are automobile and motorcycle accidents and gunshot wounds. Although incomplete transections are more frequent than complete ones, incomplete lesions may nevertheless be disastrous. When spinal injuries affect the upper cervical spinal cord, they are often fatal because of the interruption of the respiratory control pathways that descend from the brainstem to the phrenic motor nucleus. A lesion below the phrenic nucleus may result in paralysis of all four extremities, **quadriplegia,** whereas a lesion of the thoracic spinal cord causes **paraplegia,** which is paralysis of the lower extremities.

Decerebrate rigidity results from transection of the brainstem

Transection of the brainstem at a midbrain level results in **decerebrate rigidity.** This condition develops immediately after the brainstem is transected. In experimental animals, the "rigidity" is expressed as an exaggerated extensor (antigravity) posture caused by hyperactive stretch reflexes. The term *decerebrate rigidity* is unfortunate because the condition more closely resembles spasticity than the rigidity that results from basal ganglion disease (see later discussion). Activation of γ motor neurons is thought to be important in decerebrate rigidity because the hyperactive reflexes are lost after transection of the dorsal roots in experimental animals. Dorsal rhizotomies can interrupt input from muscle spindle afferents whose activity is increased in decerebrate rigidity because of an increased excitatory drive by pathways descending from the lower brainstem. The extensor posture can also be reduced or eliminated by lesions of the vestibular nuclei.

Postural reflexes include vestibular, tonic neck, and righting reflexes

Various reflexes assist in postural adjustments that occur as the head is moved or the neck is bent. The receptors that trigger these reflexes include the **vestibular apparatus** and **stretch receptors in the neck.** The visual system also contributes to postural adjustments, but the reflexes described here are elicited in the absence of visual cues.

Angular accelerations of the head activate the sensory receptors in the semicircular ducts and elicit reflexes that cause eye, neck, and limb movements that tend to oppose changes in position. For example, if the head is turned to the left **(Figure 9–17),** the eyes are reflexly rotated to the right through a similar angle. This action is called the **vestibuloocular reflex.** The two eyes move together in the same direction and through the same

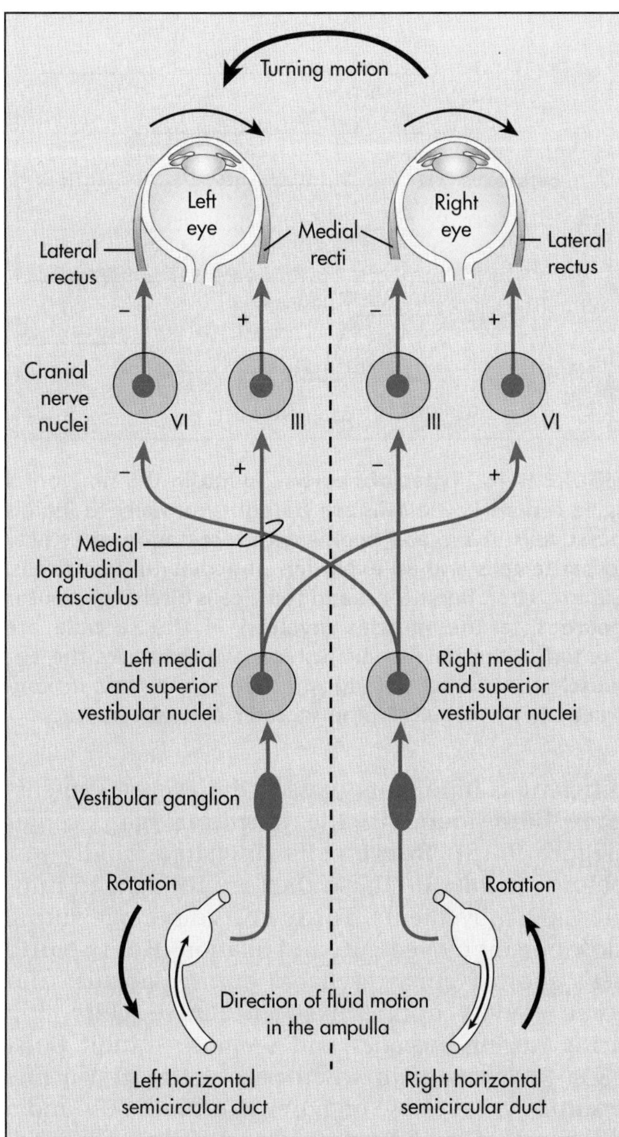

FIGURE 9–17. Neural circuit for the vestibuloocular reflex, a vestibular reflex that helps maintain a visual target despite head movement. The horizontal semicircular ducts, brainstem pathways, and eyes are viewed from above. Rotation of the head to the left is indicated by the thick black arrows. Fluid movement within the ducts is indicated by the thin black arrows. The neural activity produced by the vestibular system causes the eyes to move conjugately to the right. As the eyes reach the limit of their movement, they are quickly returned to the left.

angle, so the eye movements are said to be **conjugate.** If head rotation exceeds the range of eye movement, the eyes are quickly deflected to the left and another visual target is found. If the head continues to rotate to the left, there is an alternation of slow eye movements to the right followed by rapid eye movements to the left. These alternating slow and fast eye movements are called **nystagmus.** A similar response pattern affects the neck muscles and is called the **vestibulocollic reflex.** The same stimulus also tends to increase contractions of the extensor (antigravity) muscles on the left side of the body. This response opposes the tendency to fall to the left as the leftward head rotation continues.

The neural mechanism that underlies these reflexes depends on stimulation of sensory receptors in the semicircular ducts. In the case of rotation of the head in a plane parallel to the ground, the semicircular canals that are primarily involved are the horizontal ones (Figure 9–17). The inertia of the endolymph within the horizontal semicircular canals causes the endolymph to lag behind as the head rotates. This relative shift of the endolymph deflects the cupulae of the ampullae of the horizontal canals and bends the stereocilia of the hair cells in the ampullary crest (see Chapter 7). The hair cells of one duct depolarize and thereby increase the discharges in the vestibular afferent fibers supplying that duct. The opposite occurs in the other horizontal canal. The mismatch in input from the left and right canals to the brainstem results in reflex discharges that tend to counteract the positional changes resulting from the head rotation.

Several reflexes can be elicited by linear accelerations of the head and activation of the otolith organs. If an experimental animal is dropped, the stimulation of the utricles leads to extension of the forelimbs, the **vestibular placing reaction.** The response is in preparation for landing. If the head is tilted, the otolith organs cause the eyes to rotate in the opposite direction, the **ocular counterrolling response.** Ocular counterrolling tends to keep the visual axes aligned with the horizon.

Other postural reflexes that depend on the vestibular apparatus tend to keep the body position normal despite tilting (without bending the neck). If the neck is bent, the **tonic neck reflexes** are triggered, resulting in postural adjustments that are opposite to those evoked by vestibular stimulation. **Righting reflexes** also tend to restore the position of the head and body in space to normal; these involve the vestibular apparatus, neck stretch receptors, and mechanoreceptors in the body wall.

The spinal cord contains a pattern generator for locomotion

As described earlier, a pattern generator for locomotion is contained within the neural circuitry of the spinal cord. Actually, separate pattern generators exist for each limb. The activity of these is coupled so that the movements of the limbs are coordinated during locomotion.

The pattern generators for locomotion and for other rhythmic activities (e.g., respiration) are regarded as **biological oscillators.** Many biological oscillators operate on the basis of the reciprocal inhibition of circuits called **half-centers** that control antagonistic muscles. The details of how half-centers work and the factors that cause switching between the two half-centers vary with the particular oscillator being considered.

The locomotor pattern generator is normally activated by commands that descend from the brainstem. The midbrain locomotor center helps initiate locomotion by activating neurons in the pontomedullary reticular formation. These neurons transmit the descending commands. The locomotor pattern generator converts tonic activity in the descending pathways into rhythmic discharges of motor neurons to the muscles involved in locomotor activity. The midbrain locomotor center can be activated by voluntary commands from the motor cortex. It can also be engaged by afferent signals, as can the activity of the locomotor pattern generator in the spinal cord. These afferent signals modify the ongoing motor program so that motor performance is altered in accord with environmental demands.

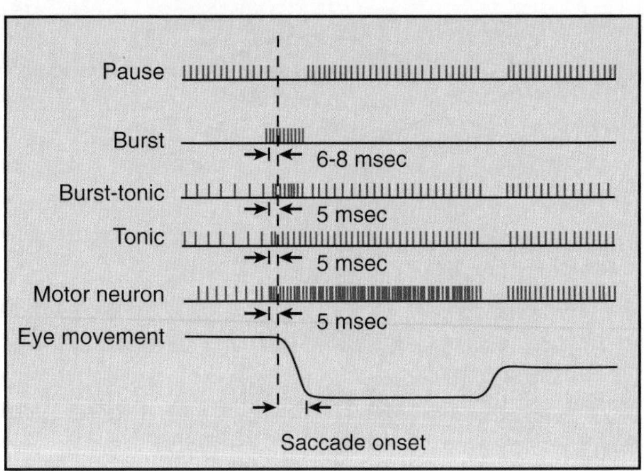

FIGURE 9–18. Types of neurons found in the horizontal gaze center. Pause cells are thought normally to inhibit burst cells. A saccade begins with a cessation of activity in pause cells and an explosion of activity in burst cells. Slightly later, burst-tonic and tonic cells discharge. Motor neurons to the muscles involved in the saccade are excited in the burst-tonic fashion, which causes the eye muscle to contract quickly and then to maintain its contraction. This results in the saccadic eye movement.

Control of eye position depends on brainstem circuits and the cerebral cortex

Movements of the eyes are generally **conjugate** (in the same direction), although sometimes they are **convergent** or **divergent** when they are targeted on nearby objects (as in reading) or on distant objects.

A rapid conjugate movement of the eyes is called a **saccade.** A saccade usually causes a visual target to be imaged on the fovea. However, saccades can be made in the dark. Once the eyes have located a visual target, fixation is maintained by **smooth pursuit movements.** Smooth pursuit movements do not take place in the dark because they require a visual target. Actually, during fixation, the eyes drift somewhat and are returned to the target by microsaccades. Without these small movements, the retina would adapt and lose sight of the target.

Misalignment of the two visual axes can cause double vision, or **diplopia.** Such misalignment, or **strabismus** (cross-eye), can result from weakness of the muscles of one eye, causing its visual axis to differ from that of the other eye. Over time, the misaligned eye may lose visual acuity, a condition called **amblyopia.**

Horizontal eye movements are organized by the **horizontal gaze center,** which is located near the abducens nucleus in the pons. There is also a **vertical gaze center** in the midbrain pretectum. Neurons with response properties corresponding to different components of saccadic eye movements have been found in the horizontal gaze center (Figure 9–18). **Burst cells** discharge rapidly just before saccades occur, so they are thought to initiate these movements. **Tonic cells** discharge during slow pursuit movements and fixation. **Burst-tonic** cells show a burst discharge during saccades and tonic activity during fixation. **Pause cells** stop firing during saccades and seem to inhibit burst cells. Saccades occur when pause cells stop firing, resulting in a release of activity in burst cells and a discharge of eye muscle motor neurons. Feedback that occurs when the eye is on target inhibits the burst cells and reactivates the pause cells.

The vestibular nuclei and the gaze centers send direct projections to the motor nuclei that supply the eye muscle (Figure 9–17). The circuit is reciprocally organized so that a signal causing an eye movement excites a set of agonistic motor neurons and inhibits the antagonistic ones. For example, neurons in the horizontal gaze center send projections to abducens motor neurons of the ipsilateral eye as well as ascending projections through the medial longitudinal fasciculus to excite motor neurons to the contralateral medial rectus muscle (**Figure 9–19**). Appropriate connections are made to inhibit the motor neurons of the antagonistic muscles.

Neurons in the deep layers of the superior colliculus and activated by visual, auditory, or somatosensory stimuli project to the horizontal gaze center (see Chapter 7). They produce saccadic eye movements that are part of an orientation response to a novel or threatening stimulus.

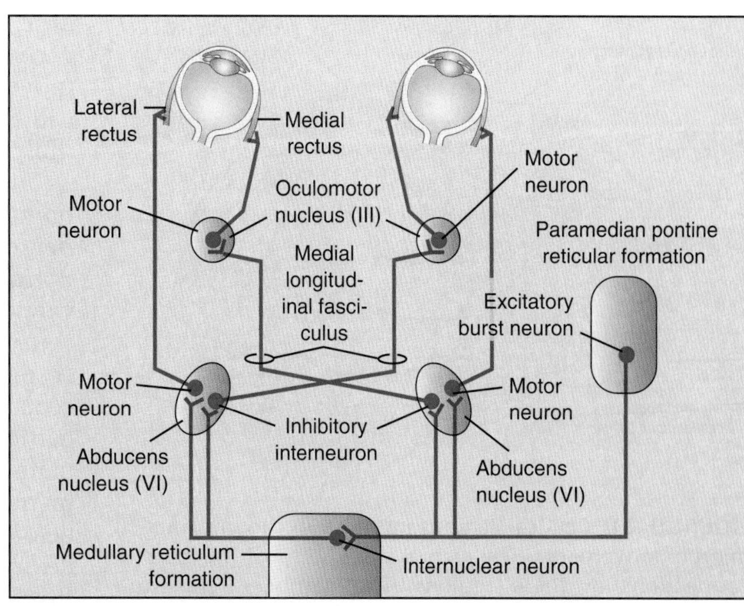

FIGURE 9–19. Organization of the horizontal gaze center. Activation of burst neurons in the right gaze center results in the direct excitation of abducens motor neurons on the right and oculomotor neurons to the medial rectus muscle on the left through an interneuronal pathway via the medial longitudinal fasciculus. Concurrently, the contralateral saccadic mechanism is inhibited by way of the reticular formation.

The **frontal eye fields** in the premotor region of the frontal lobe trigger voluntary saccadic eye movements via a projection to the contralateral horizontal gaze center. The **occipital eye fields** are involved in smooth pursuit movements, optokinetic nystagmus, and visual fixation. Adjustments for near vision include convergence, pupillary constriction, and accommodation of the lens. The occipital eye fields are connected with the superior colliculus and the pretectal region and influence the vertical and horizontal gaze centers.

The Cerebral Cortex Controls Voluntary Movement

The **corticospinal** and **corticobulbar tracts** are the most important pathways used in the initiation and execution of voluntary movements. THE LATERAL CORTICOSPINAL TRACT AND THE COMPARABLE PART OF THE CORTICOBULBAR TRACT CONTROL THE FINE MOVEMENTS PRODUCED BY THE MUSCLES OF THE CONTRALATERAL DISTAL EXTREMITIES, LOWER FACE, AND TONGUE. THE VENTRAL CORTICOSPINAL TRACT AND PART OF THE CORTICOBULBAR TRACT, AS WELL AS MORE INDIRECT PATHWAYS, PROVIDE FOR POSTURAL SUPPORT OF VOLUNTARY MOVEMENTS.

Corticospinal and corticobulbar neurons do not operate in isolation. Their discharges represent decisions based on input from many sources. The motor cortex receives projections from the **ventral lateral nucleus** of the thalamus, **postcentral gyrus, posterior parietal cortex, supplementary motor cortex,** and **premotor cortex.** The ventral lateral thalamic nucleus is part of the circuitry by which the cerebellum and basal ganglia regulate movements (see later discussion). The postcentral gyrus processes and then transmits somatosensory information to the motor cortex, which provides feedback about movements and contacts between the skin and objects being explored. The posterior parietal cortex, supplementary motor cortex, and premotor cortex help program movements.

Motor programs are developed in the sensorimotor cortex

Voluntary movements require contractions and relaxations in the proper sequence, not only of the muscles directly involved in the movements but also of the appropriate postural muscles. Therefore, a mechanism is needed for programming these complex events. The cortical areas thought to be responsible for cortical motor programs include the **posterior parietal lobe, supplementary motor cortex,** and **premotor cortex** (Figure 9–20).

The posterior parietal lobe receives somatosensory information from the postcentral gyrus and visual information from the occipital cortex. The posterior parietal cortex connects with the supplementary motor cortex and premotor cortex (Figure 9–20) and is important for processing sensory information that leads to goal-directed movements.

A lesion of the posterior parietal cortex causes deficits in visually guided movements. Humans may develop a **neglect syndrome** (especially if the lesion is in the nondominant hemisphere for language, generally the right hemisphere). In this syndrome, a patient is unable to recognize objects placed in the contralateral hand and unable to draw three-dimensional objects accurately. In fact, the patient may deny that the contralateral limbs even belong to him or her.

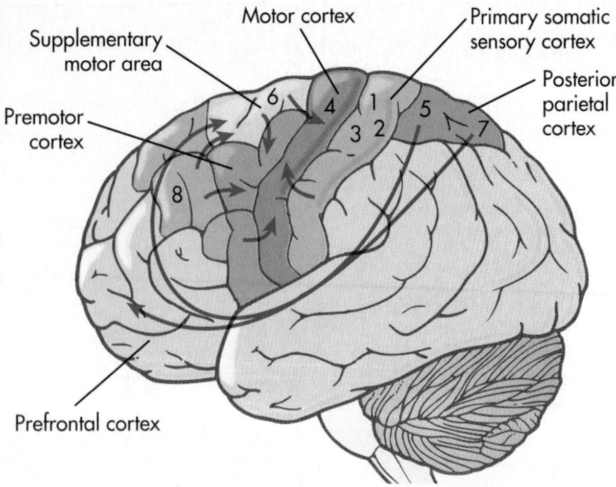

FIGURE 9–20. Cortical regions involved in the programming of movements. The arrows show some of the interconnections of these regions. The numbers refer to Brodmann's areas.

The supplementary motor cortex is concerned with complex, often bilateral movements. A lesion in the supplementary motor cortex is likely to cause deficits in orientation during movements and impairment of bilateral coordination. The premotor cortex is influenced by the cerebellum, posterior parietal lobe, and supplementary motor cortex, and it projects to the motor cortex. It is especially involved in the control of axial and proximal muscles. A lesion of the premotor cortex in humans or monkeys results in the appearance of the **grasp response,** in which touching the palm or extending the fingers elicits a grasping movement of the hand.

The motor cortex is the main motor output region

The motor cortex is recognizable microscopically by the presence of the **giant pyramidal,** or **Betz,** cells. However, many more projections of this area arise from small and medium-sized pyramidal cells than from Betz cells. The corticospinal and corticobulbar tracts originate from pyramidal cells in layer 5 of the motor cortex as well as from other cortical regions, including the premotor cortex, supplementary motor cortex, and postcentral gyrus. The somatotopic organization of the motor cortex has already been described (Figure 9–15).

The motor cortex controls both distal and proximal muscles. HOWEVER, THE CORTICOSPINAL AND CORTICOBULBAR PROJECTIONS OF THE LATERAL SYSTEM ARE ESPECIALLY IMPORTANT FOR CONTROL OF THE DISTAL MUSCLES OF THE CONTRALATERAL EXTREMITIES, LOWER FACE, AND TONGUE. A lesion that interrupts the corticospinal and corticobulbar tracts eliminates movements of distal muscles, but other pathways can still be used to activate proximal and axial muscles.

The lateral corticospinal tract makes monosynaptic excitatory connections with α motor neurons, especially those that are located in the dorsolateral part of the ventral horn and that innervate distal muscles. The same pathway also excites γ motor neurons. Thus, when the lateral corticospinal tract commands a voluntary movement, it coactivates α and γ motor neurons. In addition, the corticospinal tract influences interneurons that regulate reflex transmission. During learned movements, some pyramidal tract neurons discharge just before a particular phase of the movement (e.g., flexion or extension of a joint). The activity encodes the force exerted by the muscles involved in the movement rather than the position of the joint. Some neurons encode the rate at which force is developed, whereas others encode the steady-state force.

When the corticospinal and corticobulbar tracts are completely interrupted, the distal muscles of the contralateral upper and lower extremities and muscles of the contralateral lower face and tongue are paralyzed **(hemiplegia).** Unless the lesion is restricted to these tracts, the deficit is a **spastic paralysis.** Spasticity usually accompanies hemiplegia produced by a lesion of the internal capsule or a lesion at other levels of the nervous system because the corticoreticulospinal pathway, along with the pyramidal tract, is interrupted. Spasticity is also present in spinal cord injuries when transection at an upper cervical level causes quadriplegia or transection below the cervical enlargement causes paraplegia. Spastic paralysis is associated with an increase in muscle tone and increased phasic stretch reflexes. The latter may lead to **clonus,** such as in the ankle, in response to a brisk passive movement. Interruption of the lateral corticospinal tract at any level causes an important release response, Babinski's sign (Figure 9–16).

The Cerebellum Assists in the Regulation of Posture and Movement

The cerebellum assists in the performance of coordinated movements by receiving sensory information about the status of movements and then adjusting the activity of the various descending motor pathways to optimize performance. These functions improve with practice; thus, the cerebellum is involved in learning motor skills. Destruction of the cerebellum produces no sensory deficits; therefore, it has no essential role in sensation.

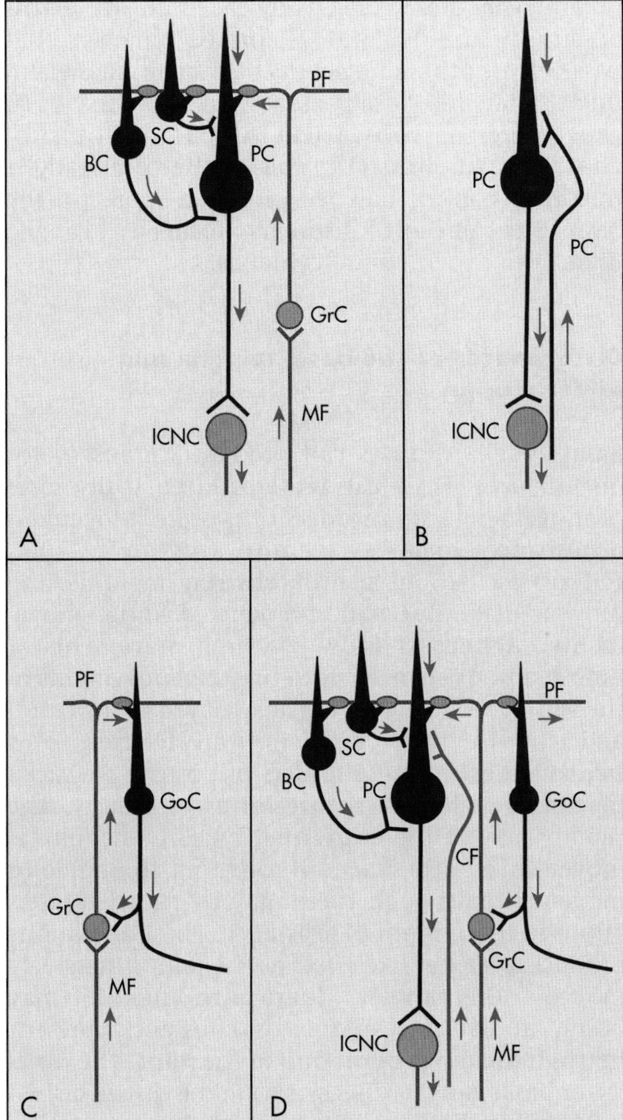

FIGURE 9–21. Excitatory and inhibitory circuits in the cerebellar cortex. Excitatory neurons are green; inhibitory neurons are blue. **A,** Connections made by mossy fibers (MF) through granule cells to Purkinje cells (PC), stellate cells (SC), and basket cells (BC). Purkinje cells inhibit neurons of the deep cerebellar nuclei. **B,** Climbing fiber (CF) input to a Purkinje cell. **C,** Excitation of a Golgi cell (GoC) by a mossy fiber through the granule cell (GrC) pathway, with inhibition of granule cells by the Golgi cell. **D,** Combination of these circuits. ICNC, deep cerebellar nuclear cell; PF, parallel fiber.

The organization of the cerebellum is consistent throughout

Afferent fibers from other parts of the central nervous system approach the cerebellum through the cerebellar white matter. Two types of afferent fibers are found: **mossy fibers** and **climbing fibers** (Figure 9–21). Mossy fibers originate from various sources, but all climbing fibers are derived from the contralateral **inferior olivary nucleus.** In the cerebellar cortex, the mossy fibers synapse in the granular layer on the dendrites of **granule cells.** There is considerable divergence because a given mossy fiber branches repeatedly and synapses on many different granule cells. An individual climbing fiber synapses at many sites on the soma and dendritic tree of one or a few **Purkinje cells.** Thus, the climbing fiber pathways show little divergence.

The granule cell axons form bundles of **parallel fibers** that synapse on the dendrites of Purkinje cells and of several classes of interneurons, including **Golgi cells, basket cells,** and **stellate cells.** Granule cells are the only excitatory interneurons in the cerebellar cortex; the other types are all inhibitory. The mossy fiber–granule cell pathway and the climbing fiber pathway are able to excite Purkinje cells; hence, they may be regarded as the excitatory circuits of the cerebellar cortex. Mossy fiber–granule cell excitation typically elicits single action potentials in a set of Purkinje cells **(simple spike response),** whereas a climbing fiber evokes a high-frequency burst of action potentials in a Purkinje cell **(complex spike).** Other pathways in the cerebellar cortex feature inhibition: Golgi cells inhibit granule cells, basket cells inhibit Purkinje cell somas, and stellate cells inhibit Purkinje cell dendrites. All of these inhibitory interneurons are activated by the mossy fiber–granule cell pathway.

A surprising observation is that although Purkinje cells are the only output neurons of the cerebellar cortex, their synaptic actions are inhibitory. This inhibition modulates the discharges of the neurons of the deep cerebellar nuclei and lateral vestibular nucleus.

The cerebellum has three functional systems

The cerebellum can be considered on phylogenetic and functional grounds to be composed of the following major components: the archicerebellum, the paleocerebellum, and the neocerebellum. The **archicerebellum** is the earliest part of the cerebellum to evolve and is related in function primarily to the vestibular system. The archicerebellum is thus often referred to as the **vestibulocerebellum.** It corresponds in the human to the flocculonodular lobe and parts of the vermis in addition to the nodule. THE ARCHICEREBELLUM HELPS CONTROL AXIAL MUSCLES AND THUS BALANCE. IT ALSO COORDINATES HEAD AND EYE MOVEMENTS. A lesion of the archicerebellum can result in a "drunken" stagger called an **ataxic gait** and in **nystagmus.**

The **paleocerebellum** receives somatotopically organized information from the spinal cord; hence, it is often called the **spinocerebellum.** The paleocerebellum regulates both movement and muscle tone. Lesions of the paleocerebellum produce deficits in coordination similar to those seen after damage to the neocerebellum.

The **neocerebellum** is the dominant component of the human cerebellum. It occupies the hemispheres of the cerebellum. The input is from wide areas of the cerebral cortex; hence, this region is sometimes called the **cerebrocerebellum.** THE NEOCEREBELLUM MODULATES THE OUTPUT OF THE MOTOR CORTEX. Because the right side of the neocerebellum controls activity in the left cortex and because the left cortex influences movements of the right limbs, the neocerebellum regulates motor activity of the same side of the body. The neocerebellum interacts with neurons of the premotor cortex in programming movements.

Lesions of the neocerebellum affect chiefly the distal limbs. The neurological signs include delayed initiation of movements, **ataxia of the limbs** (incoordination), and reduced muscle tone. The limb ataxia results in **asynergy** (lack of synergy in movements), **dysmetria** (inaccurate movements), **intention tremor** (oscillations at the end of a movement), and **dysdiadochokinesia** (irregular performance of pronation and supination movements of the forearm). Reduced muscle tone leads to **pendular phasic stretch reflexes** in the lower extremity. Bilateral lesions of the neocerebellum may result in **dysarthria** (slow, slurred speech, synonymous with "scanning speech"). These classic neocerebellar signs are often seen in **multiple sclerosis.**

The Basal Ganglia Also Regulate Posture and Movement

Like the neocerebellum, THE BASAL GANGLIA HELP REGULATE THE ACTIVITY OF THE MOTOR CORTEX. Unlike the archicerebellum and paleocerebellum, the basal ganglia exert only a minor influence on descending motor pathways other than the corticospinal and corticobulbar tracts. Judging from the effects of lesions, the role of the basal ganglia is often opposed to that of the neocerebellum.

The basal ganglia are important structures in the telencephalon

The basal ganglia include the **caudate nucleus,** the **putamen** (neostriatum), and the **globus pallidus** (paleostriatum). The caudate nucleus and putamen are often collectively called the **striatum** because of the "striations" formed by fibers that pass between these nuclei in the human. Brainstem nuclei that are closely associated with the basal ganglia are the **substantia nigra** and the **subthalamic nucleus.** The role of the basal ganglia in motor control has been inferred more on the basis of the effects of disorders of the basal ganglia than from experimental evidence.

Disturbances of the basal ganglia may affect motion

Basal ganglia diseases can produce various motor disturbances. These can be categorized as disorders of movement and disorders of posture. Movement disturbances include **tremor** (rhythmic, "pill-rolling" oscillations at rest), **chorea** (rapid flicking movements), **ballism** (violent, flailing movements), **athetosis** (slow, writhing movements of limbs), and **dystonia** (slow, twisting movements of the torso). Movements that are delayed in initiation and slow to reach completion are referred to as **bradykinesia.** The disorders of posture produced in basal ganglia disease are forms of rigidity. The rigidity may be the **cogwheel** type. As the joint is moved, resistance occurs throughout the range of movement, although there may be repeated alterations in the amount of resistance. These alterations produce a ratchet-like effect as the joint is passively moved. Alternatively, **lead-pipe** rigidity may occur, in which resistance is constantly present through the range of motion of the joint. The rigidity of basal ganglia disease should be distinguished from "decerebrate rigidity," which is more similar to spasticity (see previous discussion).

Parkinson's disease is caused by a lesion of the substantia nigra and is characterized by tremor, rigidity, and bradykinesia. The loss of dopaminergic projections to the striatum is thought to be crucial. **Hemiparkinsonism** results when one substantia nigra is affected; the manifestations are then contralateral because they are caused by inappropriate regulation of the corticospinal tract. Destruction of part of the subthalamic nucleus on one side results in **hemiballism,** which is characterized by ballistic movements on the contralateral side. **Huntington's chorea** is a genetic disorder in which there is loss of striatopallidal and striatonigral neurons containing γ-aminobutyric acid; cholinergic striatal interneurons are also lost. Loss of inhibitory input to the globus pallidus is thought to underlie the choreiform movements characteristic of the disease. The cerebral cortex also degenerates, leading to severe mental retardation. In **cerebral palsy,** athetosis often occurs because of damage of the striatum and globus pallidus.

Summary

- The basic element of motor control is the motor unit, which comprises an α motor neuron and all of the muscle fibers that it innervates.
- Motor units have a variable number of muscle fibers, depending on the coarseness or fineness of the movements made by the particular muscle.
- All of the muscle fibers of a motor unit are of the same histochemical type.
- The α motor neurons form the final common pathway for movements.
- The α motor neurons are found in motor nuclei of the spinal cord ventral horn and in cranial nerve motor nuclei. Spinal cord motor nuclei are arranged somatotopically.
- EPSPs can sum spatially or temporally, and the synaptic currents may reach threshold at the initial segment. IPSPs may prevent the threshold from being reached.
- The afterhyperpolarization in α motor neurons is often quite large and helps regulate the discharge rate.
- Repetitive firing of α motor neurons can produce an unfused or a fused tetanus of the muscle fibers that they innervate. Contractile force can therefore be increased by increasing the discharge rates of α motor neurons up to the point that a fused tetanus is produced. Contractile force can also be increased by the recruitment of additional α motor neurons.
- The recruitment of α motor neurons is orderly. Small α motor neurons are generally activated before large ones in most motor acts.
- Muscles and tendons contain stretch receptors; these include muscle spindles and Golgi tendon organs.
- The primary endings of muscle spindles signal the rate of change in muscle stretch as well as muscle length. The secondary endings signal muscle length.
- Golgi tendon organs are supplied by group Ib afferent fibers. They respond to both muscle stretch and muscle contraction and signal the tension in the tendon.
- Spinal cord reflexes are relatively simple, stereotyped responses to a defined sensory input.
- The stretch reflex involves a monosynaptic, excitatory connection between group Ia afferent fibers from muscle spindles in a muscle and the α motor neurons that supply the muscle as well as synergistic muscles; it also involves a disynaptic inhibitory connection to antagonist motor neurons.
- The inverse myotatic reflex involves a disynaptic pathway from Golgi tendon organs through inhibitory interneurons to α motor neurons of the same muscle. This reflex controls muscle tension.
- Both the stretch reflex and the inverse myotatic reflex represent negative-feedback loops. The controlled variable of the stretch reflex is muscle length, and that of the inverse myotatic reflex is muscle tension.
- The flexion reflex involves afferent fibers that supply the skin, muscle, and joints. These excite α motor neurons to flexor muscles and inhibit α motor neurons to extensor muscles in the limb.
- The lateral corticospinal tract controls muscles of the distal extremities, lower face, and tongue.
- The ventral corticospinal tract controls the proximal limb and axial muscles and thus provides for postural support.
- Spinal cord transection causes sensory loss and paralysis below the level of the lesion. Stretch and flexion reflexes become hyperactive, and pathological reflexes, such as Babinski's sign, appear.
- Transection of the upper brainstem may lead to decerebrate rigidity, in which the stretch reflexes also become exaggerated.
- Locomotion is organized by a pattern generator in the spinal cord. Locomotion can be triggered by activity in the midbrain locomotor center, and it can be modified by segmental afferent input.

- ❖ Eye position is controlled by several motor systems.
- ❖ The motor cortex issues commands that are transmitted by the corticospinal and corticobulbar tracts and that evoke voluntary movements.
- ❖ The lateral corticospinal tract and the equivalent part of the corticobulbar tract control fine movements of distal muscles of the limbs and of the lower face and tongue.
- ❖ Interruption of the lateral corticospinal tract and the corticobulbar tract on one side in the brain results in a contralateral hemiplegia. If other descending pathways, such as the inhibitory corticoreticulospinal pathway, are also interrupted, the paralysis becomes spastic with hyperactive phasic stretch reflexes.
- ❖ The cerebellum helps coordinate movements and is involved in learning motor skills.
- ❖ The output of the cerebellum influences the activity of motor pathways descending from the brainstem and corticospinal and corticobulbar tracts.
- ❖ Damage to the vestibulocerebellum can produce an ataxic (staggering) gait and nystagmus.
- ❖ Damage to the neocerebellum causes tremor and incoordination of the limbs and reduced muscle tone, resulting in pendular stretch reflexes.
- ❖ Disturbances of the basal ganglia result in disorders of movement and posture, including resting tremor, chorea, ballism, athetosis, dystonia, bradykinesia, and rigidity.

Bibliography

Cope TC, ed: *Motor neurobiology of the spinal cord,* Boca Raton, 2001, CRC Press.

Creutzfeldt OD: *Cortex cerebri: performance, structural and functional organization of the cortex*, New York, 1995, Oxford University Press.

Hunt CC: Mammalian muscle spindle: peripheral mechanisms, *Physiol Rev* 70:643, 1990.

Jami L: Golgi tendon organs in mammalian skeletal muscle: functional properties and central actions, *Physiol Rev* 72:623, 1992.

Leigh RJ, Zee DS: *The neurology of eye movements*, ed 3, New York, 1999, Oxford University Press.

Middleton FA, Strick PL: Basal ganglia and cerebellar loops: motor and cognitive circuits, *Brain Res Rev* 31:236, 2000.

Olanow CW, Tatton WG: Etiology and pathogenesis of Parkinson's disease, *Annu Rev Neurosci* 22:123, 1999.

Robinson FR, Fuchs AF: The role of the cerebellum in voluntary eye movements, *Annu Rev Neurosci* 24:981, 2001.

Shepherd GM: *The synaptic organization of the brain*, ed 4, New York, 1998, Oxford University Press.

Tanji J: Sequential organization of multiple movements: involvement of cortical motor areas, *Annu Rev Neurosci* 24:631, 2001.

Wilson VJ, Jones GM: *Mammalian vestibular physiology,* New York, 1979, Plenum.

Wise SP et al: Premotor and parietal cortex: corticocortical connectivity and combinatorial computations, *Annu Rev Neurosci* 20:25, 1997.

Case Studies

Case 9–1

A 74-year-old man suddenly found that he could not move his left arm and leg. Examination in the emergency department demonstrated weakness in the left arm and leg, especially in the distal parts of these extremities. The patient also had difficulty in using the muscles of his lower face, and the left side of his tongue was not as strong as the right side. Babinski's sign was present on the left side. In an examination 1 month later, the distribution of weakness had not changed, although the weakness was not quite as profound. The left biceps, triceps, patellar, and ankle jerk reflexes were markedly increased, and there was ankle clonus on the left. The ability of the patient to recognize tactile and vibratory stimuli was reduced on the left side of the face and body, and proprioception was impaired in the left arm and leg.

1. **Which part of the nervous system is most likely affected by the stroke?**
   A. Basal ganglia on the right
   B. Cerebellum on the left
   C. Internal capsule on the right
   D. Precentral and postcentral gyri on the right
   E. Spinal cord on the left

2. **Which of the following provides evidence indicating that the paralysis is of the spastic type?**
   A. Babinski's sign
   B. Clonus and hyperactive phasic stretch reflexes
   C. Deficits in somatic sensation
   D. Paralysis of the tongue
   E. Weakness of the arm and leg

Case 9–2

A 56-year-old woman noticed that her movements had slowed and that her hands shook when she was resting. These changes developed during several years. Her physician found that she had a pill-rolling tremor of her hands while the hands were at rest and that she initiated and executed movements slowly. Her face was not expressive. When her joints were passively bent, there was resistance to the movement, but the resistance gave way and then resumed repeatedly as the bending progressed. Phasic stretch reflexes were normal, as was muscle strength.

1. **Which structures of the central nervous system are most likely to be affected in this patient?**
   A. Basal ganglia and substantia nigra
   B. Brainstem reticular formation
   C. Deep nuclei of the cerebellum
   D. Primary motor cortex
   E. Supplementary motor cortex

2. **Relief of some symptoms may be provided by replacement therapy for which of the following?**
   A. Dopamine
   B. Epinephrine
   C. γ-Aminobutyric acid
   D. Glutamate
   E. Substance P

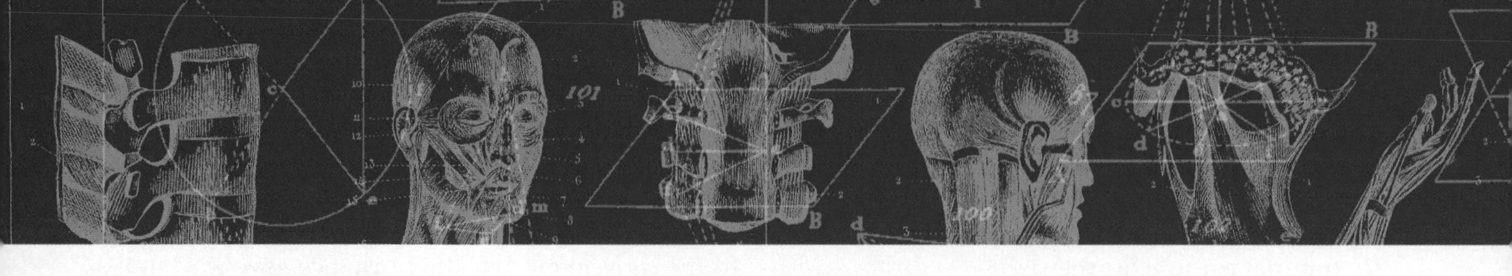

Chapter 10: Autonomic Nervous System and Its Control

Objectives

- ❖ Describe and compare the organization of the sympathetic, parasympathetic, and enteric nervous systems.
- ❖ Explain the operation and control of the autonomic nervous system and the neurotransmitters and receptors that are used.
- ❖ Discuss the relationship of the activity of the hypothalamus and limbic system to autonomic and other functions.

The autonomic nervous system is a motor system concerned with the regulation of smooth muscle, cardiac muscle, and glands. It is not directly accessible to voluntary control. Instead, it operates in an automatic fashion on the basis of **autonomic reflexes** and central control. A MAJOR FUNCTION OF THE AUTONOMIC NERVOUS SYSTEM IS **HOMEOSTASIS,** WHICH IS THE MAINTENANCE OF THE INTERNAL ENVIRONMENT IN AN OPTIMAL STATE. For instance, the autonomic nervous system in cooperation with the somatic motor system helps keep the body temperature relatively constant. Another important role is making the appropriate adjustments in smooth muscle tone, cardiac muscle activity, and glandular secretion for different behaviors. For example, the autonomic activity that can be observed during digestion is different from that seen during a sprint.

The Autonomic Nervous System Is Highly Organized

The sympathetic nervous system innervates structures in the body wall and internal viscera

The **sympathetic nervous system** is a widely distributed motor system. It reaches not only the viscera contained in the body cavities but also the skin and muscles of the body wall. It does this through a sequential pathway consisting of two types of motor neurons called **preganglionic** and **postganglionic neurons.**

The cell bodies of the sympathetic preganglionic neurons are located in the thoracic and upper lumbar spinal cord (T1 to about L2) in the **intermediolateral** and **intermediomedial cell columns** (**Figure 10–1**). The motor axons of the sympathetic preganglionic neurons leave the spinal cord in the T1 to L2 ventral roots. The motor axons are small myelinated **B fibers** or in some cases unmyelinated **C fibers.** They pass from the spinal nerves into the **white communicating rami.**

When the sympathetic preganglionic axons in a given white ramus reach the **sympathetic paravertebral ganglion** of the same segment, they may (1) synapse in that ganglion, (2) turn rostrally or caudally to synapse in a paravertebral ganglion at another segmental level, or (3) continue through a splanchnic nerve to synapse in a **prevertebral ganglion** (Figure 10–1). In this way, preganglionic axons that originate from motor neurons limited to spinal cord segments T1 to L2 are able to synapse on postganglionic neurons in the entire chain of paravertebral sympathetic ganglia (including the superior, middle, and inferior cervical sympathetic ganglia and the ganglia below L2 that do not receive white communicating rami) as well as in the prevertebral ganglia of the abdominal cavity **(Figure**

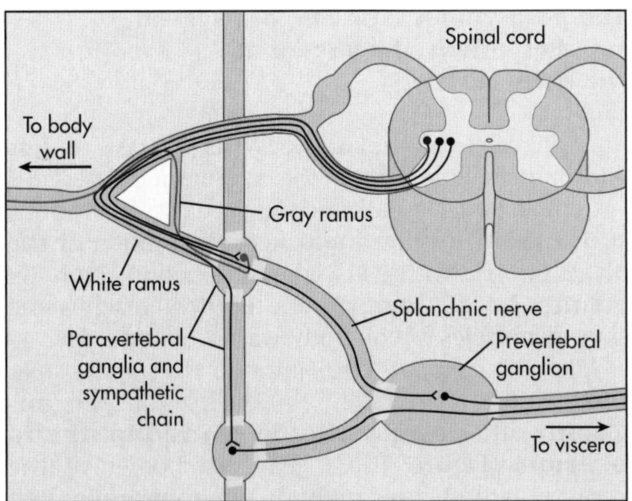

FIGURE 10–1. Distribution of sympathetic preganglionic projections to paravertebral and prevertebral ganglia.

10–2). Preganglionic axons also directly innervate the chromaffin cells of the **adrenal medulla,** which are developmentally comparable to sympathetic ganglion cells.

Sympathetic postganglionic neurons are located in the paravertebral and prevertebral ganglia. The axons are unmyelinated **C fibers** that distribute either to the body wall or to the viscera in the body cavities (Figure 10–2). If they are destined for the body wall, they pass from a paravertebral ganglion into a spinal nerve via a **gray communicating ramus.** Gray rami are found in all ganglia of the sympathetic chain and connect with the appropriate spinal nerves. Sympathetic postganglionic axons destined for viscera in the body cavities enter **splanchnic nerves** and distribute to their targets. Postganglionic axons originating in prevertebral ganglia distribute to their targets through the sympathetic plexuses near the target organs.

The sympathetic preganglionic neurons that supply the head are in the upper thoracic segments. Their axons leave the spinal cord in the white

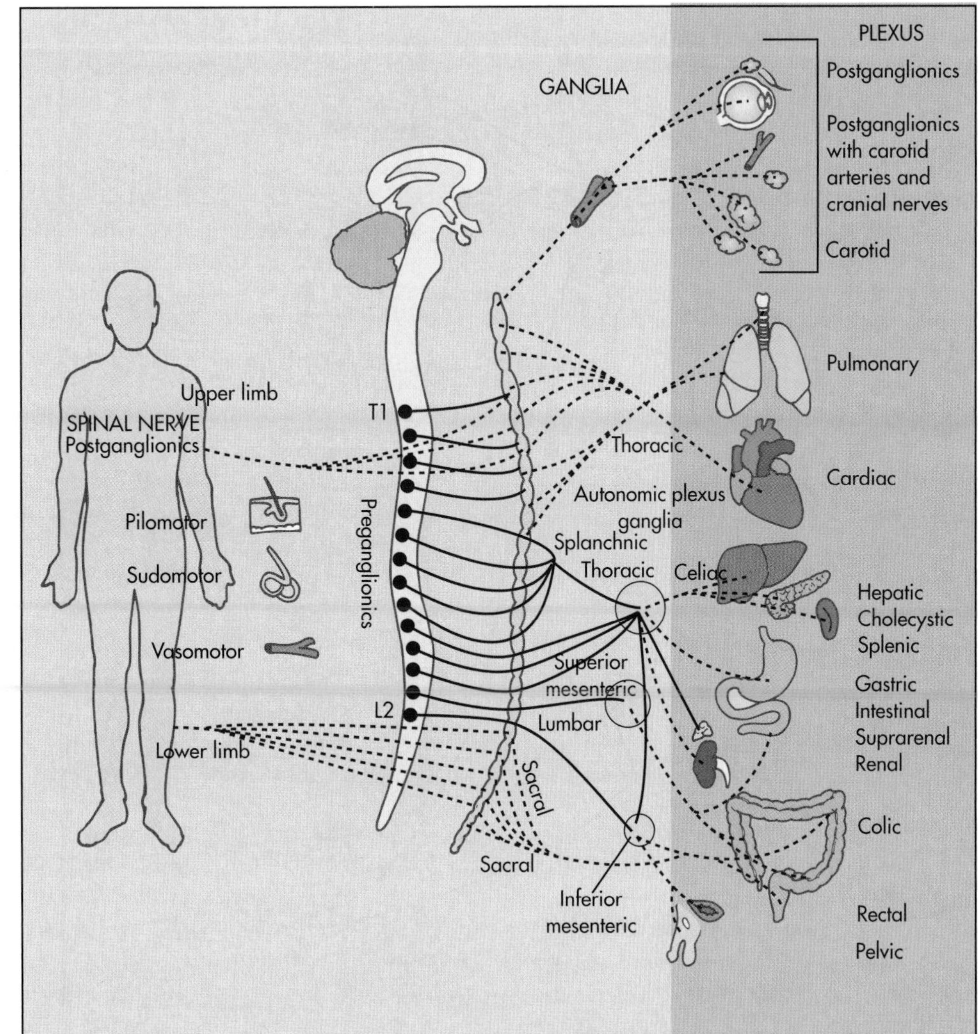

FIGURE 10–2. Sympathetic nervous system.

communicating rami at T1 and T2, enter the **sympathetic chain,** and ascend to the superior cervical sympathetic ganglion, where they synapse on sympathetic postganglionic neurons. The postganglionic axons pass into the head through a plexus around the great vessels. They synapse on smooth muscle and glands of the face, eyes, and other structures of the head.

Interruption of the sympathetic supply to the head (or of descending pathways from the hypothalamus that control sympathetic activity) results in **Horner's syndrome.** This syndrome consists of (1) **partial ptosis** (drooping of the eyelid caused by paralysis of the superior tarsal muscle of the eyelid), (2) **pupillary constriction** (because the unopposed parasympathetic supply of the iris is intact), (3) **anhidrosis of the face** (caused by interruption of the innervation of the sweat glands of the face), and (4) **enophthalmos** (retraction of the globe of the eye because innervation of the smooth muscle of the orbit has been interrupted).

The parasympathetic nervous system supplies chiefly the viscera of the body cavities

The **parasympathetic nervous system** is less widely distributed than the sympathetic nervous system. A parasympathetic supply exists for various structures in the head and neck, but much of the distribution is to the viscera contained in the body cavities. No parasympathetic outflow reaches the skin or muscles of the body wall or extremities.

Like the sympathetic outflow, the parasympathetic outflow involves a sequence of **preganglionic** and **postganglionic parasympathetic neurons** (Figure 10–3). The cell bodies of the parasympathetic preganglionic neurons are located in either the **brainstem** or **sacral spinal cord (S2 to S4).** Cranial nerve nuclei that contain preganglionic parasympathetic neurons include the **Edinger-Westphal nucleus** (cranial nerve III), **superior salivatory nucleus** (cranial nerve VII),

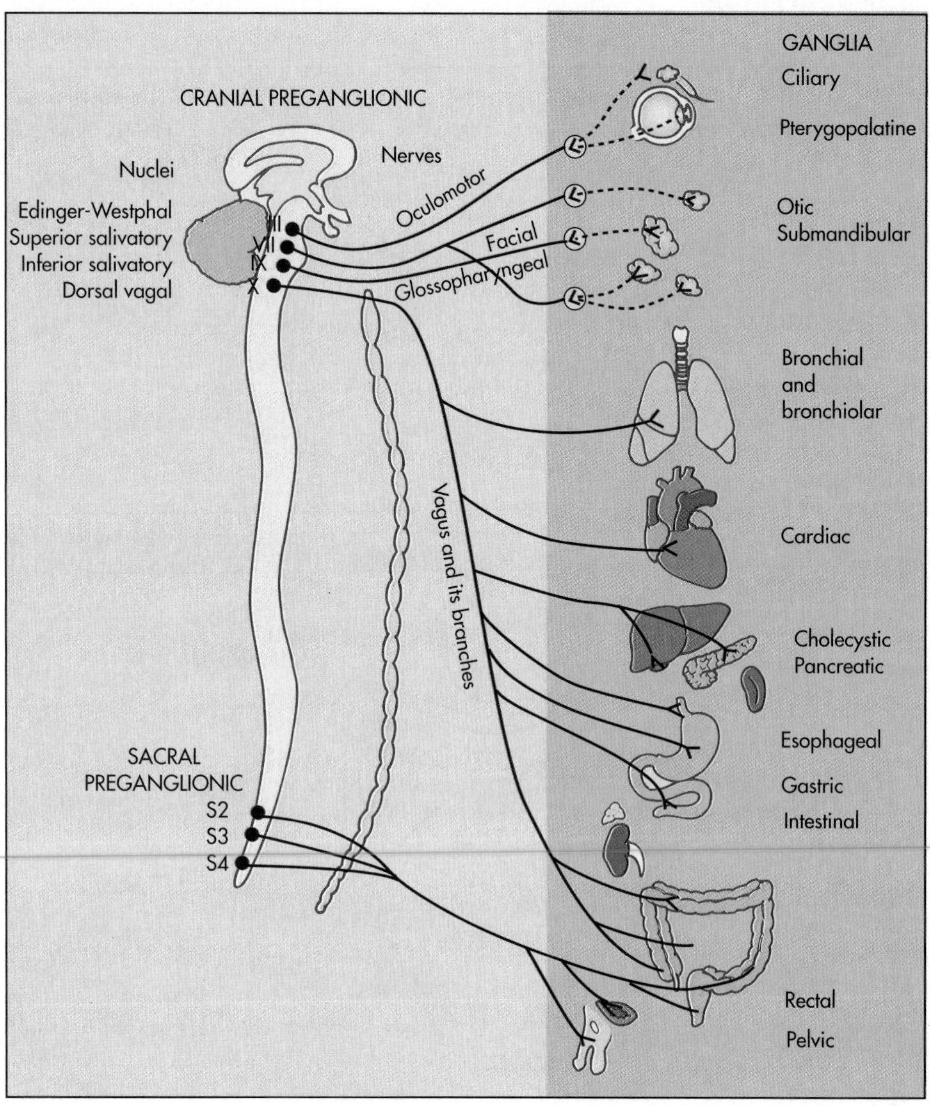

FIGURE 10–3. Parasympathetic nervous system.

inferior salivatory nucleus (cranial nerve IX), and **nucleus ambiguus** and **dorsal motor nucleus of the vagus** (cranial nerve X). Sacral parasympathetic neurons are located in the **sacral parasympathetic nucleus.** No lateral horn exists in the sacral spinal cord, but the parasympathetic nucleus is in a roughly similar position.

The cranial parasympathetic preganglionic axons leave the brainstem in the appropriate cranial nerves and synapse on ganglion cells in the appropriate **cranial parasympathetic ganglia** (Figure 10–3): **ciliary ganglion** (cranial nerve III), **sphenopalatine** and **submaxillary ganglia** (cranial nerve VII), **otic ganglion** (cranial nerve IX), and **ganglia in or near the walls of target viscera** in the thoracic and abdominal cavities (cranial nerve X). For the gastrointestinal tract, the vagal preganglionic axons synapse on neurons belonging to the **enteric nervous system** (see later discussion). The sacral parasympathetic preganglionic axons distribute to the abdominal and pelvic cavities and synapse on ganglion cells in these regions. The **splenic flexure** of the colon is the boundary between the gastrointestinal organs supplied by the vagus nerve and those supplied by the sacral parasympathetics. Parasympathetic postganglionic neurons directly innervate nearby target organs.

The parasympathetic preganglionic neurons that control pupil size are located in the **Edinger-Westphal nucleus,** which is near the midline just ventral to the cerebral aqueduct. The preganglionic axons leave the midbrain with the **oculomotor nerve** and synapse in the **ciliary ganglion,** which is in the orbit just behind the eye. Axons of the postganglionic neurons of the ciliary ganglion pass into the eye through short ciliary nerves, and some terminate on smooth muscle cells of the iris that form the **pupillary sphincter.**

When there is a large **increase in intracranial pressure,** such as happens during a **cerebral hemorrhage** or because of a **brain tumor,** the brain may shift position, causing herniation of the uncus **(uncal herniation)** in the medial temporal lobe through the tentorial notch of the dura. This may compress the oculomotor nerve and cause a sudden unilateral dilation of the pupil. A **fixed, dilated pupil** is an indicator of impending death unless the high intracranial pressure is relieved by surgery.

The enteric nervous system controls functions of the gut wall

The **enteric nervous system** is a miniature nervous system within the wall of the gastrointestinal tract (see Chapter 33). Reflex networks in this system organize gut movements that can occur even when the gut is removed from the body. Afferent neurons, interneurons, and motor neurons are included in the system. Parasympathetic and sympathetic connections to the enteric nervous system permit autonomic control. The component of the enteric nervous system in **Auerbach's myenteric plexus** controls the activity of the muscular layers, and that in **Meissner's submucosal plexus** controls the muscularis mucosae and intestinal glands.

Autonomic Functions Are Coordinated

The sympathetic nervous system actively regulates visceral function under normal circumstances. The parasympathetic nervous system often acts contrary to the sympathetic nervous system when a given organ is innervated by both systems. However, it is more appropriate to view concurrent control of organs by activity in the sympathetic and parasympathetic nervous systems as a means of coordinating visceral activity.

The preganglionic neurons of the autonomic nervous system, like α motor neurons of the somatic motor system, use **acetylcholine** as their neurotransmitter **(Figure 10–4)**. Some of the **acetylcholine receptors** on postganglionic neurons, like those of skeletal muscle, are of the nicotinic type. Nicotinic receptors are activated by low doses of nicotine and are blocked by curare. Other acetylcholine receptors on postganglionic neurons are of

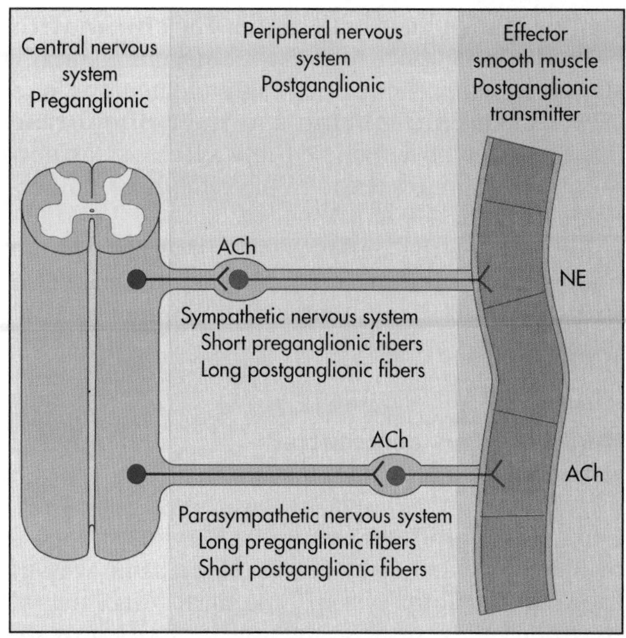

FIGURE 10–4. Transmitters of autonomic ganglia and postganglionic synapses. ACh, acetylcholine; NE, norepinephrine.

the muscarinic type. **Muscarinic receptors** are activated by **muscarine** and blocked by **atropine.**

Autonomic neurotransmission depends on cholinergic, adrenergic, and peptidergic receptors

Parasympathetic and some sympathetic postganglionic neurons also use acetylcholine as a neurotransmitter. The receptors on target organs are of the muscarinic type. The cholinergic sympathetic postganglionic axons include those that supply sweat glands (the **sudomotor fibers**) as well as **vasodilator fibers** in skin and skeletal muscle. Postganglionic parasympathetic neurons also release neuropeptides, such as **vasoactive intestinal polypeptide.**

Sympathetic postganglionic neurons generally use **norepinephrine** as their neurotransmitter (Figure 10–4), although some use acetylcholine. Receptors for norepinephrine include α- and β-**adrenergic receptors.** The α receptors are more powerfully activated by norepinephrine than by isoproterenol; the converse is true of β receptors. Phenoxybenzamine can be used to block α-adrenergic receptors, and propranolol can be used to block β-adrenergic receptors. However, selective antagonists are available for many of the subtypes of adrenergic receptors. Sympathetic postganglionic neurons also release neuropeptides, such as **neuropeptide Y,** and **ATP.**

The **adrenal medulla** is supplied by sympathetic preganglionic axons, which release acetylcholine as their neurotransmitter. The **chromaffin cells** of the adrenal medulla are developmentally similar to sympathetic postganglionic neurons, and they secrete **epinephrine** and **norepinephrine** into the circulation, where these agents act as hormones. In humans, the ratio of epinephrine to norepinephrine is 4:1.

Neurons of the enteric nervous system release not only acetylcholine and norepinephrine but also **serotonin,** ATP, and a variety of peptides as neurotransmitters and neuromodulators.

Higher centers can control autonomic function

The operation of the autonomic nervous system is regulated hierarchically in much the same way as the somatic motor system. The most direct neural control of many organs is by means of **autonomic reflexes.** However, autonomic neurons are also regulated by pathways that descend from the brainstem. In addition, autonomic function is controlled by higher autonomic centers, including the **hypothalamus** and other parts of the **limbic system.**

Autonomic reflexes are mediated by neural circuits in the spinal cord and brainstem. The afferent limbs of these reflex pathways include both visceral and somatic afferent fibers. The pathways involve interneurons that receive convergent input from visceral and somatic sensory receptors. The efferent limbs are formed by sympathetic and parasympathetic preganglionic and postganglionic neurons. The actions of the two autonomic systems are generally reciprocal.

Brainstem pathways that regulate the activity of autonomic preganglionic neurons originate from several sites, including the **reticular formation, raphe nuclei,** and **locus ceruleus complex.** These brainstem structures receive information about the visceral activities that they regulate via ascending tracts. Some autonomic functions depend strongly on these brainstem pathways. For example, **micturition** and **defecation** depend on the integrity of pathways that interconnect the sacral spinal cord and the pons.

The urinary bladder is emptied by means of the **micturition reflex,** which involves both the sympathetic and parasympathetic nervous systems and a descending control system (see also Chapter 36). As the bladder fills to near its capacity, receptors in the bladder wall are activated. Signals ascend to the **micturition center** in the pons, activating descending pathways that cause a parasympathetic contraction of the **detrusor muscle** of the bladder and relaxation of the **internal** and **external sphincters.** Simultaneously, the sympathetic system relaxes the neck of the bladder and no longer causes constriction of the internal sphincter. The bladder can thus begin to empty. The receptors in the bladder wall also respond to contraction of the bladder wall musculature and ensure complete emptying.

After spinal cord injury, the micturition reflex is disturbed by disruption of the long pathways connecting the sacral spinal cord and the micturition center in the pons. The bladder now fills excessively **(atonic neurogenic bladder)** and must be drained by catheterization. Later, a spinal reflex pathway becomes operative, but it is overactive **(spastic bladder).** However, the bladder does not empty completely, so it is predisposed to **infection,** and there is frequent **incontinence.**

Higher centers that regulate autonomic function include the hypothalamus and other components of the limbic system. Limbic structures are interconnected with nonlimbic parts of the nervous system, including the neocortex, cerebellum, and basal ganglia. The hypothalamus projects to the brainstem (e.g., to the reticular formation) and to the spinal cord. The limbic system controls motivation directly through neural pathways and indirectly through the endocrine system.

The Hypothalamus Performs a Variety of Functions

The hypothalamus (see Chapter 45) has several broadly defined functions, which include the regulation of homeostasis, motivation, and emotional behavior. These functions are mediated through hypothalamic control of autonomic and endocrine activity as well as by interactions between the hypothalamus and other parts of the limbic system.

If the hypothalamus is stimulated electrically, particular regions can be shown to relate to particular autonomic responses. For example, stimulation in the lateral and posterior hypothalamus produces responses mediated by the sympathetic nervous system. Stimulation in the anterior hypothalamus activates parasympathetic output. The responses include changes in heart rate and blood pressure. Other global functions controlled by the hypothalamus include food and water intake, emotional behavior, and regulation of the immune system.

Neuroendocrine cells of the hypothalamus regulate neuronal and endocrine functions

The neurons in some hypothalamic nuclei release peptides, either as hormones or as neuromodulator substances. Such neurons are classified as **neuroendocrine cells.** Neuroendocrine structures include the **paraventricular** and **supraoptic nuclei,** which give rise to the **hypothalamohypophysial tract** from the hypothalamus to the **posterior pituitary gland.** This tract releases the peptide hormones **oxytocin** and **vasopressin** into the circulation (see Chapter 45). The paraventricular nucleus also sends peptide-containing axons to various sites within the central nervous system, including the solitary nucleus, the dorsal motor nucleus of the vagus, and the intermediolateral cell column of the spinal cord. Oxytocin and vasopressin apparently are used both as hormones and as neuromodulators in autonomic neural circuits.

Neuroendocrine cells in a number of hypothalamic nuclei secrete hormones into the **portal system** that supplies the **anterior pituitary gland** (see Chapter 45). These hormones trigger or inhibit the release of pituitary hormones into the circulation, and they are important in endocrine regulation. As in the case of oxytocin and vasopressin, the same hypothalamic substances can be used as neuromodulatory substances at synaptic terminals within the central nervous system.

Temperature regulation is an important hypothalamic function

Homeothermic animals regulate their body temperature. WHEN THE ENVIRONMENTAL TEMPERATURE DECREASES, THE BODY ADJUSTS BY REDUCING HEAT LOSS AND INCREASING HEAT PRODUCTION. CONVERSELY, WHEN THE TEMPERATURE INCREASES, THE BODY INCREASES ITS HEAT LOSS AND REDUCES HEAT PRODUCTION.

Information about the external temperature is provided by **thermoreceptors** in the skin (and probably other organs such as muscle). Internal temperature is monitored by **central thermoreceptive neurons** in the anterior hypothalamus. The central thermoreceptors monitor the temperature of the blood. The system acts as a servomechanism with a set point at the normal body temperature. Error signals, representing deviations from the set point, lead to responses that tend to restore body temperature toward the set point. These responses are mediated by the autonomic nervous system, somatic nervous system, and endocrine system.

Cooling causes **shivering,** which consists of asynchronous muscle contractions that lead to increased heat production. There is also an increase in the activity of the thyroid gland and sympathetic nervous system, both of which tend to raise heat production metabolically. Heat loss is reduced by **cutaneous vasoconstriction** and by **piloerection.** (Piloerection is effective in animals with fur, although not in humans; in humans, the result is goose bumps.)

Warming the body has the opposite effects. The activity of the thyroid gland decreases, which leads to reduced metabolic activity and less heat production. Heat loss is increased by **sweating** and **cutaneous vasodilation.**

The hypothalamus serves as the temperature servomechanism. The heat loss responses are organized by the **heat loss center,** which is thought to be composed of neurons in the preoptic region and anterior hypothalamus. Lesions here prevent sweating and cutaneous vasodilation; this results in **hyperthermia** when the individual is placed in a warm environment. Conversely, electrical stimulation here causes cutaneous vasodilation and sweating. Neurons in the posterior hypothalamus form a **heat-production and heat-conservation center.** Lesions in the area dorsolateral to the mammillary bodies eliminate heat production and conservation, leading to **hypothermia** in a cold environment. Electrical stimulation in this region evokes shivering.

In **fever,** the set point for body temperature is elevated. An example mechanism is the release of a **pyrogen** by certain bacteria. The pyrogen changes the set point, which leads to increased heat production by shivering and to heat conservation by cutaneous vasoconstriction.

The Limbic System Includes Parts of the Telencephalon as well as the Hypothalamus

The limbic system includes the **limbic lobe** of the telencephalon as well as the **hypothalamus** and several **thalamic** and **midbrain nuclei.** The limbic components of the telencephalon include the **cingulate, parahippocampal,** and **subcallosal gyri** as well as the **hippocampal formation** (hippocampus, dentate gyrus, and subiculum) and the amygdaloid nuclei.

The functions of the limbic system include the regulation of aggressive behavior and sexuality. More generally, the limbic system appears to be concerned with motivational states, which in turn are vital for the survival of both the individual and the species.

Bilateral removal of temporal lobe structures, including the amygdaloid nuclei, results in a complex set of changes in behavior called the **Klüver-Bucy syndrome.** Animals previously wild become tame; they develop a pronounced tendency to put objects into their mouths, and they become sexually hyperactive. These changes result chiefly from damage to the amygdaloid nuclei.

The **hippocampus** appears to be important for the storage of recent memory (see also Chapter 11). MEMORIES ARE STORED IN THE FOLLOWING SEQUENCE: SHORT-TERM MEMORY, RECENT MEMORY, AND LONG-TERM MEMORY. Short-term memory is easily disrupted and is presumed to depend on ongoing neural events. Long-term memory seems to result from a permanent functional or structural change in the nervous system. Bilateral lesions of the hippocampus may not interfere with either short- or long-term memory but may prevent the process by which short-term memories are permanently stored. The process of recollection of memories may also be disrupted, resulting in **amnesia.**

Bilateral lesions of the temporal lobes that damage the hippocampus and degenerative diseases that destroy hippocampal circuits, notably **Alzheimer's disease,** can lead to deficits in the consolidation of recent memory. A patient with such disturbances may be able to remember a conversation for a short time but minutes later may repeat the same conversation as if it had never happened. However, memories of childhood events may still be relatively clear.

Summary

- Sympathetic preganglionic neurons are located in the intermediolateral (and intermediomedial) cell columns of the T1 to L2 segments of the spinal cord. Their axons leave the spinal cord through ventral roots and enter the sympathetic chain through white communicating rami.
- Sympathetic preganglionic neurons synapse on postganglionic neurons in the paravertebral or prevertebral ganglia. Postganglionic axons synapse in target organs.
- Parasympathetic preganglionic neurons are located in cranial nerve nuclei and the sacral preganglionic nucleus. Postganglionic axons synapse in target organs.
- The enteric nervous system is in the wall of the gastrointestinal tract in the myenteric and submucosal plexuses. It coordinates the movements and glandular secretions of the gut.
- The sympathetic and parasympathetic nervous systems regulate the activity of smooth muscle, cardiac muscle, and glands. These components of the autonomic nervous system often act in a reciprocal fashion.
- Preganglionic sympathetic and parasympathetic neurons release acetylcholine as their neurotransmitter. This neurotransmitter acts on nicotinic cholinergic receptors (and also on muscarinic receptors) on postganglionic neurons. Nicotinic receptors are blocked by curare.

- Parasympathetic and some sympathetic postganglionic neurons (sudomotor and vasodilator neurons) also release acetylcholine. The postsynaptic receptors on target cells in this case are muscarinic and can be blocked by atropine.
- Most sympathetic postganglionic neurons release norepinephrine, which acts on α- and β-adrenergic receptors.
- The adrenal medulla receives sympathetic preganglionic input and releases epinephrine and norepinephrine into the general circulation.
- The autonomic nervous system operates reflexly and in response to descending control systems, especially the hypothalamus and other parts of the limbic system.
- The hypothalamus regulates homeostasis, motivation, and emotional behavior through control of the autonomic nervous system, endocrine system, and somatic nervous system. Some of the functions regulated include body temperature, cardiovascular activity, appetite, water intake, and immune responses.
- The hypothalamus controls endocrine function both by the direct release of hormones in the posterior pituitary gland and by the release of peptides into the portal circulation of the anterior pituitary gland.
- The limbic system comprises not only the hypothalamus but also a number of forebrain structures, including the hippocampus, amygdaloid nuclei, and several nuclei in the midbrain. Functions of the limbic system include the regulation of aggressive behavior and sexuality. The hippocampus is involved in the storage of recently acquired memories and in memory consolidation.

Bibliography

Appenzeller O, Oribe E: *The autonomic nervous system: an introduction to basic and clinical concepts,* ed 5, Amsterdam, 1997, Elsevier.

Bannister R: *Autonomic failure: a textbook of clinical disorders of the autonomic nervous system,* New York, 1983, Oxford University Press.

Blessing WW: *The lower brainstem and bodily homeostasis,* New York, 1997, Oxford University Press.

DeGroat WC et al: Mechanisms underlying the recovery of urinary bladder function following spinal cord injury, *J Auton Nerv Syst* 30:S71, 1990.

Elfin LG, Lindh B, Hökfelt T: The chemical neuroanatomy of sympathetic ganglia, *Annu Rev Neurosci* 16:471, 1993.

Gershon M: *The second brain,* New York, 1998, Harper Collins.

LeDoux JE: Emotion circuits in the brain, *Annu Rev Neurosci* 23:155, 2000.

Loewy AD, Spyer KM: *Central regulation of autonomic functions,* New York, 1990, Oxford University Press.

Lopes da Silva FH et al: Anatomic organization and physiology of the limbic cortex, *Physiol Rev* 66:235, 1990.

Case Study

Case 10–1

A 24-year-old man was rescued from a car wreck. After his neck was stabilized by paramedics, he was taken to the emergency department. Imaging studies showed that he had a fracture of the C5 vertebra with likely damage to the spinal cord. Although he could breathe adequately, he could not move his arms or legs. Phasic stretch reflexes were absent in all extremities, and he could feel no form of stimulus to the skin below his shoulders. Babinski's sign was observed bilaterally. The systemic arterial blood pressure was 116/76 mm Hg. The urinary bladder was full, so the patient's bladder was catheterized. On follow-up examination several weeks later, the phasic stretch reflexes were hyperactive in all four extremities, and there was ankle clonus bilaterally. The basal blood pressure remained lower than normal, and plasma norepinephrine and epinephrine levels were also below normal. However, the blood pressure periodically became elevated until the bladder was emptied after stimulation of the lower abdominal wall.

1. The blood pressure increased in this patient when the bladder became distended for which of the following reasons?

A. Activity in the hypothalamospinal tract was increased by the visceral afferent input from the bladder.
B. Bladder distention was excessive because of hypotonus of the bladder wall and thus became painful.
C. Infection of the bladder resulted in a buildup of bacterial products that caused vasoconstriction.
D. Responses to plasma catecholamines were increased because of α-adrenoreceptor up-regulation after denervation.
E. Spinal autonomic reflexes were enhanced after recovery from spinal shock.

2. If this patient were placed in a cold or hot environment, which of the following would occur?

A. His body could not thermoregulate, so he would tend to become hypothermic or hyperthermic.
B. Excessive vasodilation in a hot environment would cause him to become hypothermic.
C. Exaggerated shivering in a cold environment would result in hyperthermia.
D. Peripheral and central thermoreceptors would become hyperactive, which would enhance thermoregulation.
E. Lack of hypothalamic control of sweating and shivering would balance out, so he would have no problem with thermoregulation.

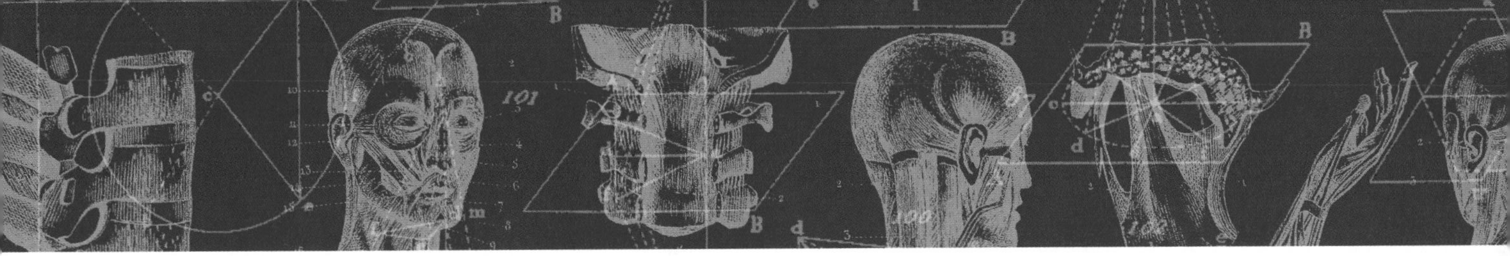

Chapter 11: Higher Functions of the Nervous System

Objectives

- ❖ Describe the electroencephalogram and evoked potentials and their relationship to states of consciousness and epilepsy.
- ❖ Explain learning and memory.
- ❖ Discuss how cerebral dominance relates to language function.

The central nervous system is responsible for the higher functions that characterize humans, including consciousness, thought, perception, learning, memory, and language. States of consciousness, including the sleep-wake cycle, are generally studied with the help of neurophysiological techniques such as the electroencephalogram and evoked potentials.

Learning and memory depend on alterations in neural functions and even in structure. The human brain is actually two brains. The left hemisphere is dominant for certain functions, including handedness and language, and the opposite hemisphere is dominant for other functions, such as spatial relations and music.

The Electroencephalogram Records the Electrical Activity of Cerebral Neurons

The higher functions of the human brain are expressed on the background of continuous thalamocortical interactions. Neurons of nearly all the nuclei of the thalamus project to the cerebral cortex, and the cerebral cortex projects back to the thalamus.

Recordings from the surface of the cerebral cortex **(electrocorticogram)** or from the scalp **(electroencephalogram [EEG])** reveal the incessant oscillations of extracellular potentials caused by membrane potential oscillations in large numbers of cortical neurons. The oscillations are produced in response to the rhythmical alterations of activity in thalamocortical circuits. On a single-neuron level, activity corresponding to the EEG consists of alternating **excitatory** and **inhibitory postsynaptic potentials.** The excitatory potentials often result in discharges of cortical neurons.

The normal EEG can be described in terms of its frequency composition. Several characteristic frequency ranges can be recognized **(Figure 11–1).** These are called **alpha waves** (8 to 13 Hz), **beta waves** (>13 Hz), **theta waves** (4 to 7 Hz), and **delta waves** (<4 Hz). Other transient waves are also seen. The dominant frequency depends on several factors, including age, state of consciousness, recording site, action of drugs, and presence of disease. During the early years of life, the EEG is dominated by low frequencies. In mature individuals at rest with the eyes closed, the EEG recorded from the posterior region of the brain shows an alpha rhythm, whereas that recorded from the anterior part of the brain has a beta rhythm. If the individual is aroused, lower voltage, higher frequency beta rhythms take the place of the lower frequency alpha waves (Figure 11–1). Slower waves of theta and delta frequencies are associated with deeper levels of sleep. **BRAIN DEATH** IS A PERSISTENT ISOELECTRICAL EEG IN THE ABSENCE OF DEPRESSANT DRUGS.

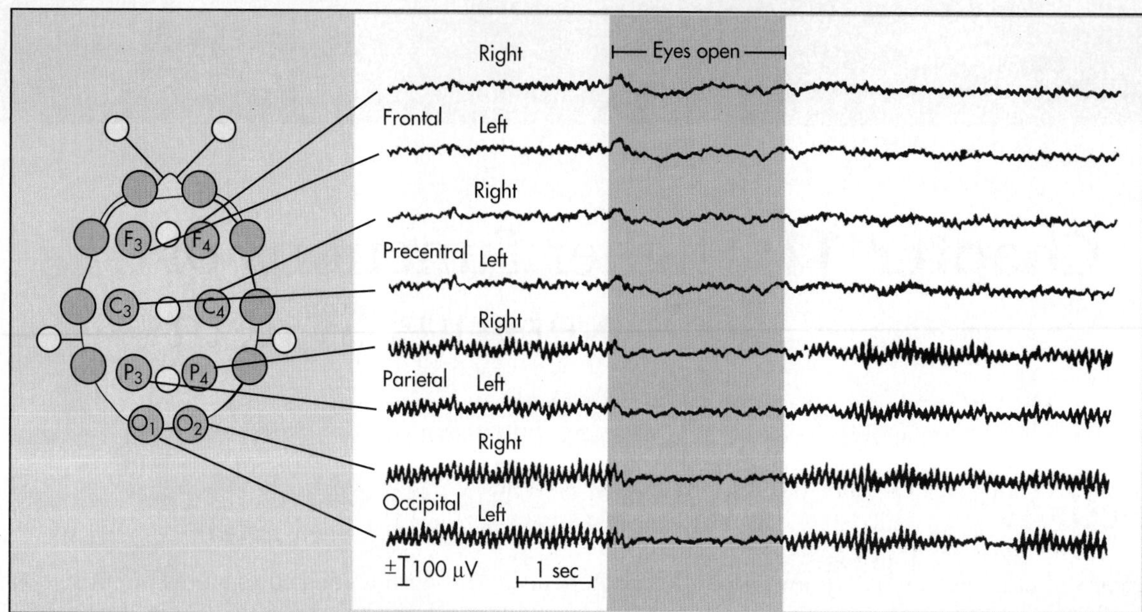

FIGURE 11–1. EEG recorded from a normal human. Recordings are from eight sites on the scalp. In the resting condition, an alpha rhythm is prominent over the parietal and occipital lobes. When the eyes are opened, the alpha rhythm is blocked and replaced by a beta rhythm.

Evoked Potentials Are Changes in Electrical Activity Induced by Activation of Neural Pathways in the Brain

The EEG represents spontaneous activity that is not linked to a particular event. Similar activity can be evoked in response to a stimulus that activates a neural pathway to the thalamus and circuits within the cerebral cortex. Such stimulus-linked activity is called a **cortical evoked potential.** Evoked potentials can easily be produced in humans by stimulating a peripheral nerve with electrical shocks, the retina with flashes of light, or the ear with an acoustic stimulus such as a click. The recorded waveform is largest over the appropriate region of the brain.

States of Consciousness Vary with the Activity in Different Regions of the Brain

Mental processes occur in the brains of conscious subjects. Consciousness is not understood, but it is required for perception, thought, and use of language. The conscious state appears to depend on an interaction between the **brainstem reticular formation** and **thalamocortical circuits.** When consciousness is depressed, the EEG becomes more synchronous and slowed in frequency. During behavioral arousal, as in response to a painful stimulus, the EEG changes to a low-voltage, high-frequency pattern (EEG arousal).

Sleep is active, not the absence of brain activity

Sleep is an alteration rather than a loss of consciousness. This is shown by the ease with which sleep is interrupted by significant environmental events such as a baby's cry. Sleep has a circadian rhythm as well as a more rapid oscillation. **Circadian rhythms** repeat at approximately daily intervals. The sleep rhythm, along with many other biological rhythms, is normally entrained by the **light-dark cycle.** When a person rapidly changes location to a different time zone, it takes days for the circadian rhythms to be re-entrained. The sleep disturbance and other disorders that result are collectively known as **jet lag.**

The various stages of sleep are characterized by different types of motor, autonomic, EEG, and psychological activity. The major distinction is between **rapid eye movement (REM) sleep** and **non-REM sleep.** When an individual falls asleep, the initial type is non-REM sleep. The EEG becomes more synchronized and slows (**Figure 11–2,** *A*). There are four levels of non-REM sleep. In the first level **(stage 1),** the person is drowsy, and the EEG shows 7- to 10-Hz rhythms. Over time, the depth of non-REM sleep increases; that is, the EEG becomes progressively slower, and the person becomes difficult to arouse. In **stage 2,** or light

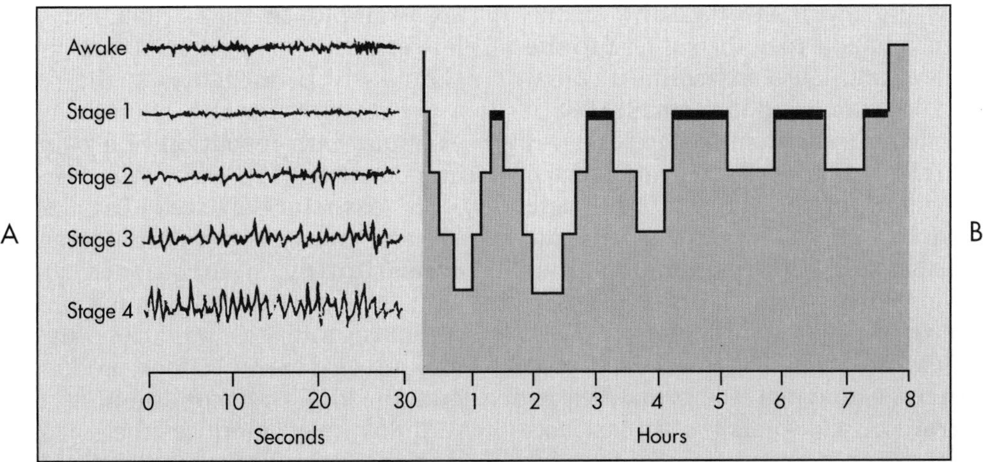

FIGURE 11–2. Stages of sleep and changes during the night. A, EEG recordings during the waking state and progressively deeper levels of non-REM sleep. The EEG in REM sleep would resemble that shown for the awake individual. B, Different sleep stages experienced during a typical night for a young adult. The bars represent periods of REM sleep.

sleep, a person is easily aroused; the dominant EEG frequencies are 3 to 7 Hz, with bursts of 12- to 14-Hz sleep spindles. During **stage 3** sleep, muscle tone and reflex activity are depressed, blood pressure falls, the heart rate slows, and the pupils constrict; the EEG shows 1- to 2-Hz high-voltage waves. **Stage 4** is the deepest level of sleep, and it is also characterized by 1- to 2-Hz EEG waves. The amount of time spent in the deepest stage of non-REM sleep decreases with age, and this stage may entirely disappear after the age of 60 years.

After about 90 minutes, sleep lightens and changes to a period of REM sleep that lasts approximately 20 minutes. During REM sleep, the EEG becomes desynchronized and has a low voltage; the pattern is similar to that seen during arousal (Figure 11–2). Tone in many muscles disappears, and reflexes are inhibited. Interrupting this tonic inhibition are phasic motor events, including rapid movements of the eyes and brief contractions of other muscles. Autonomic events include irregular respiration, reduced blood pressure interrupted by episodes of hypertension, and penile erection in males. Dreams tend to occur during REM sleep, although they can also occur in non-REM sleep. It is difficult to awaken individuals from REM sleep, but spontaneous awakening often occurs. REM sleep recurs about six times in a night. The proportion of time spent in REM sleep is greatest in the fetus and newborn, but it declines sharply during early infancy and then further with aging.

Sleep appears to be triggered by an active mechanism that involves the reticular formation and monoaminergic neurons in the brainstem. Some of the neurotransmitters associated with sleep include serotonin, norepinephrine, and acetylcholine. Several sleep-inducing peptides have been discovered as well.

Attention depends on neural mechanisms

Attention is the process by which perception is directed at particular events. It involves orientation to stimuli that are potentially significant, such as novel stimuli or stimuli likely to lead to a reward or a punishment. Repeated attention to a stimulus may result in the loss of interest in or **habituation** to the stimulus. Application of a threatening stimulus enhances attention; this process is termed **sensitization.**

Several forms of epilepsy exist

Epilepsy refers to disease states characterized by behavioral and EEG seizures. The seizures may be partial or generalized. In **partial seizures,** only part of the brain shows abnormal activity. Consciousness is retained in partial simple seizures but lost in partial complex seizures. In **generalized seizures,** large regions of the brain are involved, and consciousness is lost.

Partial seizures may originate in a damaged area of the motor cortex. Such seizures are characterized by contractions of muscles in the somatotopically appropriate region on the contralateral side and a focal EEG spike train. (An EEG spike is a synchronous wave that results from simultaneous activity in many neurons.) The seizures often spread to adjacent areas in a **march** of convulsive activity to other contralateral parts of the body. For example, the seizure may start with contractions of the fingers, but the movements may then spread to the arm, shoulder, face, and lower extremities. Partial seizures may also originate from the somatosensory cortex and produce focal sensory experiences contralaterally. Psychomotor seizures are partial seizures that originate in the limbic lobe. These are characterized by semipurposeful movements, changes in consciousness, hallucinations, and illusions. A common hallucination is an unpleasant odor **(uncinate fit).**

Generalized seizures include **grand mal** and **petit mal seizures.** Grand mal attacks may be preceded by an **aura.** Consciousness is soon lost, followed by tonic and clonic contractions of muscles on both sides of the body. Petit mal attacks are brief losses of consciousness, accompanied by a characteristic EEG pattern.

Learning and Memory Are Processes Based on Experience

Learning is a process by which behavior is modified on the basis of experience. **Memory** is the storage of information that has been learned. There are several stages of memory, including short-term memory, recent memory, and long-term memory (see Chapter 10). **Short-term memory** appears to depend on ongoing neural activity because it is easily disrupted (e.g., by anesthesia). **Recent memory** refers to the process by which information in short-term memory is transformed into long-term memory. This process seems to depend on activity transmitted by the hippocampal formation because damage to the hippocampus and related structures prevents the consolidation of short-term memory into long-term memory. **Long-term memory** apparently depends on permanent changes in widely distributed sets of neurons. The changes may include morphological and functional changes. In addition to memory stores, mechanisms must exist for accessing these stores, retrieving the information, recalling it to consciousness, comparing it to other information, and using the information for decisions.

Experiments are being performed to elucidate the mechanisms of learning and memory. Simple forms of learning have been studied in the simple nervous systems of invertebrates. Habituation and sensitization are examples of **nonassociative learning** because they do not require learning an association between two events. In habituation, a response to a particular stimulus diminishes with repetition of the stimulus. Habituation is thus the process of learning that a stimulus is unimportant. For example, an alarm clock may in time become less effective than when it was first put into use. Conversely, sensitization is the process by which a person learns that a stimulus is important. For example, with repetition of a painful stimulus, an individual quickly learns to respond.

In **associative learning,** the relationship between two different stimuli is learned. In **classic conditioning,** a conditioned stimulus is paired with an unconditioned stimulus. The unconditioned stimulus initially produces an unconditioned response; for example, food produces salivation in a hungry dog. After conditioning, the conditioned stimulus may produce the same response; for example, ringing a bell at the time food is presented ultimately causes salivation even if the food is omitted. Extinction is the opposite process; if food is not presented in association with the ringing of the bell, the dog soon no longer salivates. In **operant conditioning,** reinforcement of a response changes the probability of the response. Operant behaviors are not reflexes but rather spontaneous actions. An example of operant conditioning would be an animal's avoidance of a wire grid that induces an electrical shock when the animal happens to step on the grid. In this case, the conditioning stimulus provides **negative reinforcement.** Conversely, an example of **positive reinforcement** would be giving a porpoise a fish when it successfully jumps out of the water and through a hoop.

Habituation, sensitization, and classic conditioning have been demonstrated in invertebrate models, and the neural mechanisms that underlie both nonassociative and associative learning are being investigated. A major theme of such work is that synaptic efficacy changes during these simple forms of learning. These changes depend on the activation of second-messenger systems. Long-term changes are accompanied by structural as well as functional changes. A parallel experimental approach in mammals involves the enhancement or depression of synaptic transmission for hours to days or even longer after the activation of particular pathways in the hippocampus and cerebellum. The mechanisms that underlie **long-term potentiation** and **long-term depression** are under active study.

Cerebral Dominance Denotes the Disparate Behavior Between the Halves of the Brain

The halves of the human brain are not equivalent. IN A REAL SENSE, THE HUMAN HAS TWO BRAINS THAT COMMUNICATE WITH EACH OTHER VIA THE CEREBRAL COMMISSURES. The left hemisphere is dominant in

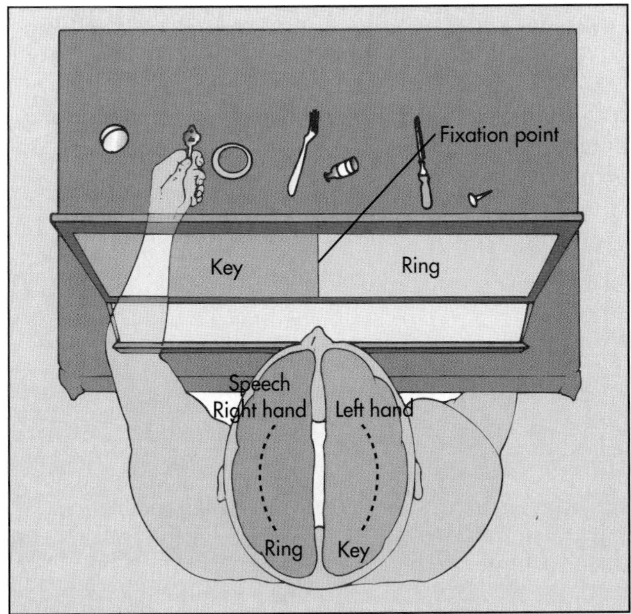

FIGURE 11–3. Technique for investigating a patient with a disconnection syndrome caused by transection of the corpus callosum. The subject is asked to look at a fixation point at the center of the screen. Pictures are projected on the screen. If the picture is in the left visual field, the image is processed in the right hemisphere (key in this instance). The subject can also reach under the screen to find objects that can be identified by tactile cues. (See also text.)

most individuals with respect to control of the preferred hand (right in most people) and language. However, the right hemisphere can be considered dominant for other functions (e.g., music, spatial relationships).

Cerebral dominance has been studied best in patients whose left and right hemispheres have been disconnected by surgical division of the corpus callosum. Visual images can be shown separately to the left and right visual fields of such individuals, and they can be asked to identify objects placed in the right or left hand **(Figure 11–3)**. If a picture of an object, such as a ring, is presented to the left hemisphere, the subject can identify the object verbally as a ring. If a picture of a key is presented to the right hemisphere, the subject cannot identify it verbally. This is because information about the key that reaches the right hemisphere does not gain access to the language centers of the left hemisphere. However, the subject can identify the picture in another way, by picking up a key with the left hand after feeling a group of objects.

Language is processing by certain cortical areas

Language depends on activity in the left hemisphere in most people. This can be demonstrated by injecting local anesthetic into the carotid circulation on the left while an individual is speaking. The anesthetic stops speech (causes **aphasia**).

Analysis of aphasia that occurs after damage to the left hemisphere of adults has revealed that several major zones are important for language. One of these is called **Broca's area,** which is located in the inferior frontal gyrus just anterior to the face representation in the motor cortex **(Figure 11–4)**. The other important region for the control of language is **Wernicke's area,** which is in the supramarginal and angular gyri of the temporal lobe and the posterior part of the superior temporal gyrus. A structural correlate of cerebral dominance for language is the greater size of the left than of the right **planum temporale** (temporal plane, the superior surface of the temporal lobe [Figure 11–4]).

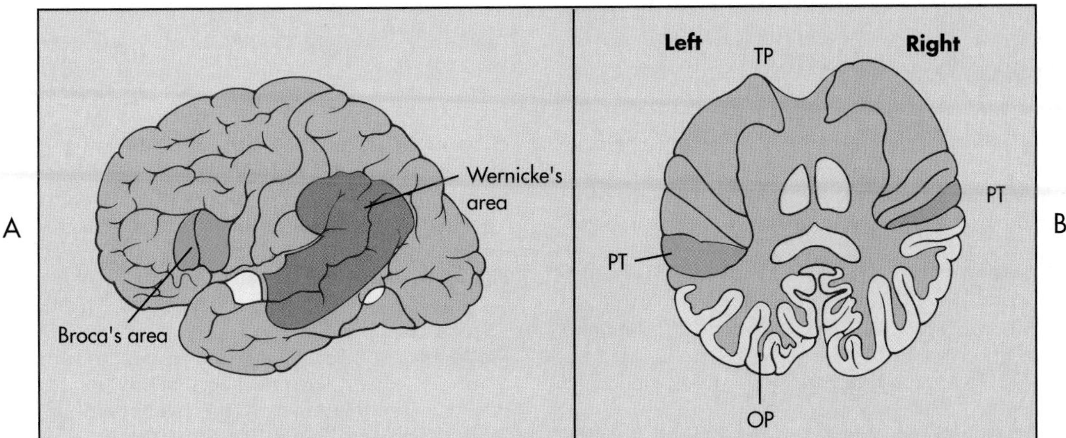

FIGURE 11–4. Areas of the cerebral cortex important for language. **A**, Broca's and Wernicke's areas. **B**, The relative size of the planum temporale (PT) on the two sides of the brain. OP, occipital pole; TP, temporal pole.

Damage to Broca's area diminishes the ability of the individual to speak and write. The person understands spoken or written words, and there is nonfluent speech. Although the lesion may also result in hemiplegia, there is not necessarily an impediment to sound production. Vocabulary is often reduced to expletives. This type of aphasia is called **expressive** or **Broca's aphasia.** Damage to Wernicke's area diminishes the comprehension of spoken or written language. However, the person has fluent speech, much of which is meaningless, with frequent **paraphasias** and **neologisms.** This type of aphasia is called **receptive** or **Wernicke's aphasia.**

Summary

- The EEG can be recorded from scalp electrodes, and it is produced by ongoing activity in thalamocortical neural circuits. It represents the summed synaptic potentials of numerous cerebral cortical neurons.
- The EEG has waves of different characteristic frequencies, which range from more than 13 Hz (beta waves) to 8 to 13 Hz (alpha waves), 4 to 7 Hz (theta waves), and less than 4 Hz (delta waves). Beta waves are observed in the aroused state and in REM sleep, alpha waves in quiet wakefulness, and delta waves in non-REM sleep.
- Events in cortical neurons can be triggered by the stimulation of sensory pathways. When recorded in a way similar to that used for the EEG, these events are called evoked potentials.
- Consciousness is a state resulting from activity of the brain. It may be impaired or lost in disease states.
- Sleep is an alteration of consciousness and occurs with a circadian rhythm. Sleep is subdivided into REM and non-REM forms.
- Learning and memory allow the modification of behavior on the basis of experience. Memory includes short-term, recent, and long-term stages. Learning can be nonassociative or associative, depending on whether conditioned and unconditioned stimuli are paired.
- The cerebral hemispheres differ in that one is dominant for some functions and the second is dominant for other functions.
- Damage to Broca's or Wernicke's area results in the loss of the ability to use language.

Bibliography

Aldrich MS: *Sleep medicine,* New York, 1999, Oxford University Press.

Alvarez PS, Zola-Morgan S, Squire LR: Damage limited to the hippocampal region produces long-standing memory impairment in monkeys, *J Neurosci* 15:3796, 1995.

Chen C, Tonegawa S: Molecular genetic analysis of synaptic plasticity, activity-dependent neuronal development, learning, and memory in the mammalian brain, *Annu Rev Neurosci* 20:157, 1997.

Engel J, Pedley TA: *Epilepsy: a comprehensive textbook,* Philadelphia, 1997, Lippincott-Raven.

Gazzaniga M: Principles of human brain organization derived from split-brain studies, *Neuron* 14:217, 1995.

Kryger MH, Roth T, Dement WC, eds: *Principles and practice of sleep medicine,* ed 2, Philadelphia, 1994, WB Saunders.

Malenka RC, Nicoll RA: Long-term potentiation: a decade of progress? *Science* 285:1870, 1999.

Martin SJ, Grimwood PD, Morris RGM: Synaptic plasticity and memory: an evaluation of the hypothesis, *Annu Rev Neurosci* 23:649, 2000.

McCarley RW: Sleep, dreams and states of consciousness. In Conn PM, ed: *Neuroscience in medicine,* Philadelphia, 1995, JB Lippincott, p 535.

McCormick DA, Bal T: Sleep and arousal: thalamocortical mechanisms, *Annu Rev Neurosci* 20:185, 1997.

Price CJ: The anatomy of language: contributions from functional imaging, *J Anat* 197:335, 2000.

Wada J, Rasmussen T: Intracarotid injection of sodium amytal for the lateralization of cerebral speech dominance: experimental and clinical observations, *J Neurosurg* 17:266, 1960.

Case Study

Case 11–1

A 78-year-old man suddenly developed a right-sided hemiplegia. He was unable to give a satisfactory history because the only words that he could speak were curse words. However, he did nod his head appropriately in response to questions.

1. **Damage to which part of the brain produced the speech disorder in this patient?**
   A. Corpus callosum
   B. Inferior frontal gyrus on the left
   C. Inferior frontal gyrus on the right
   D. Posterior part of the superior temporal gyrus on the left
   E. Posterior part of the superior temporal gyrus on the right

2. **What other neurological deficit is this patient likely to have?**
   A. Difficulty writing
   B. Intention tremor on the right
   C. Left homonymous hemianopia
   D. Loss of hearing in the left ear
   E. Babinski's sign on the left

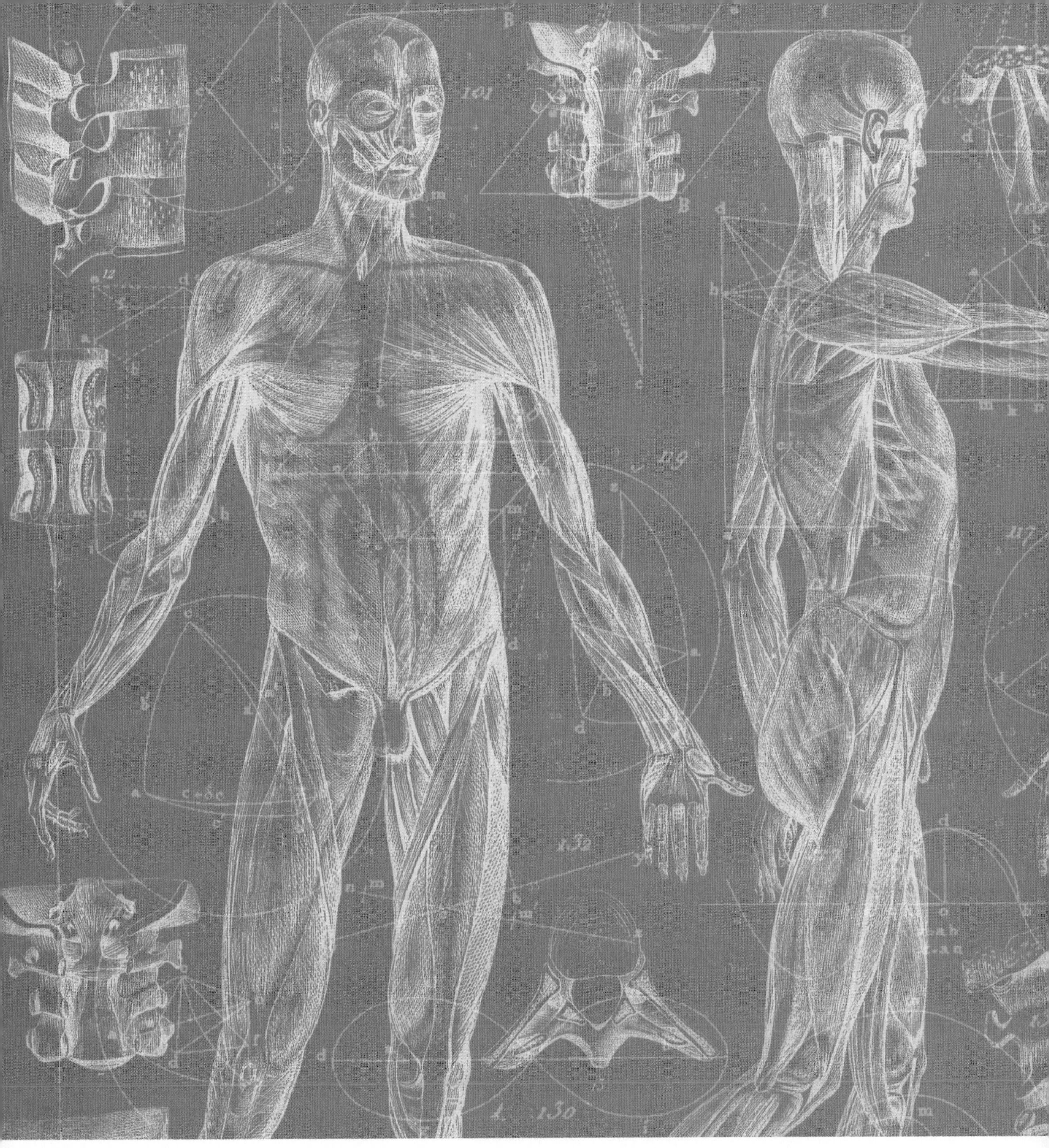

Part Three: Muscle

James Watras

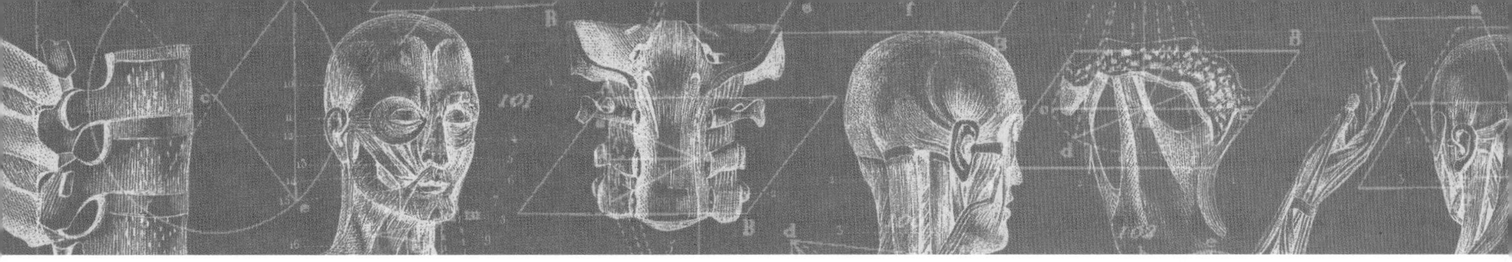

Chapter 12: Skeletal Muscle

Objectives

- ❖ Describe the organization of skeletal muscle fibers and the molecular basis of contraction.
- ❖ Identify mechanisms by which force of contraction can be increased.
- ❖ Compare skeletal muscle fiber types and their recruitment pattern.
- ❖ Describe pathophysiological conditions affecting skeletal muscle.

Different Types of Muscle Do Different Types of Work

Muscle cells are highly specialized cells for the conversion of chemical energy into mechanical energy. SPECIFICALLY, MUSCLE CELLS USE THE ENERGY IN ADENOSINE TRIPHOSPHATE (ATP) TO GENERATE FORCE OR DO WORK. As work can take many forms (such as locomotion, pumping blood, or peristalsis), several types of muscle have evolved. The three basic types of muscle are skeletal muscle, cardiac muscle, and smooth muscle. In this chapter, the function of skeletal muscle is discussed. Cardiac muscle and smooth muscle are discussed in Chapters 13 and 14, with particular emphasis on comparison and contrast of the mechanisms underlying regulation of force in the three muscle types.

As the name implies, skeletal muscle usually acts on the skeleton. Moreover, in limbs, skeletal muscle often crosses a joint, thereby allowing a lever action **(Figure 12–1)**. Skeletal muscles attach to bone by way of tendons; the proximal and distal attachments are termed origin and insertion, respectively. Also, the point of insertion is typically close to the joint. This arrangement requires that the muscle exert more force than the lifted weight, but it allows large movements after small degrees of cell shortening. Also note in Figure 12–1 that there are muscles on either side of the elbow joint, allowing opposing actions (e.g., to flex or to extend your arm against a load). Not all skeletal muscles act on the skeleton, however, as noted by the striated muscles of lips and esophagus (which participate in the voluntary acts of speaking and swallowing).

Skeletal Muscles Have a Striated Appearance due to the Highly Organized Array of Contractile Elements

Skeletal muscle is composed of numerous muscle fibers, with each muscle fiber representing a single cell. A given muscle fiber is typically 10 to 80 μm in diameter and may extend up to 25 cm in length, as in some leg muscles. Connective tissue surrounds the entire muscle and attaches the muscle to the skeleton. There are, however, connective tissue sheaths around groups of muscle fibers in the muscle, forming a fasciculus **(Figure 12–2)**, and around individual muscle fibers within the muscle. The muscle fiber, in turn, contains numerous **myofibrils,** which represent a highly organized array of contractile elements.

The myofibril has alternating regions of light and dark, with a thin line, called the **Z line,** in the middle of each light band **(Figures 12-2 and 12-3)**. These repeating bands within the myofibril are often in register with those in adjacent myofibrils and muscle fibers, yielding the appearance of striations in the muscle. Consequently, skeletal muscle is classified as a striated muscle.

The region between two adjacent Z lines in a myofibril is called a **sarcomere,** which represents the basic contractile unit in skeletal muscle. The

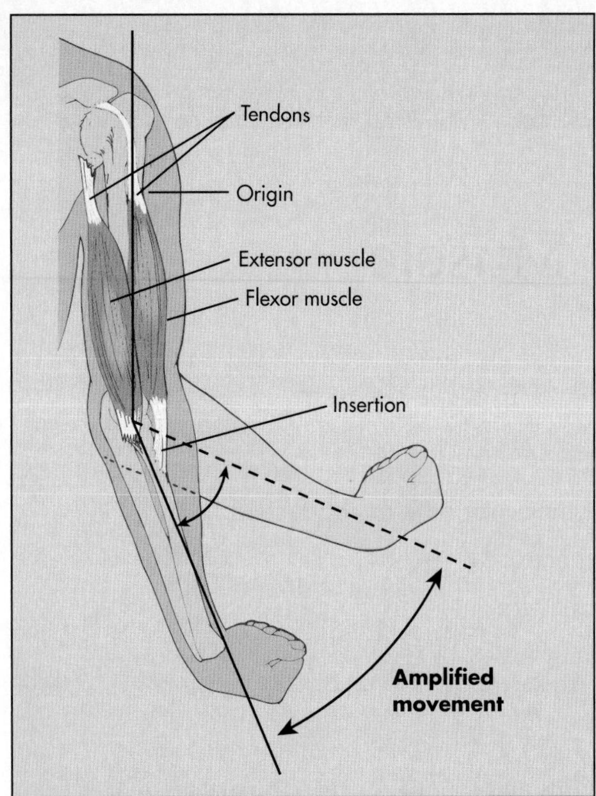

FIGURE 12–1. In limbs, skeletal muscles often span a joint, with the distal attachment (insertion) of the muscle occurring near the joint. Such an arrangement allows the limited contractions of muscle to cause large movement of the lever (arm). Also note that both sides of a joint are spanned by muscle, allowing the arm to flex or extend under load.

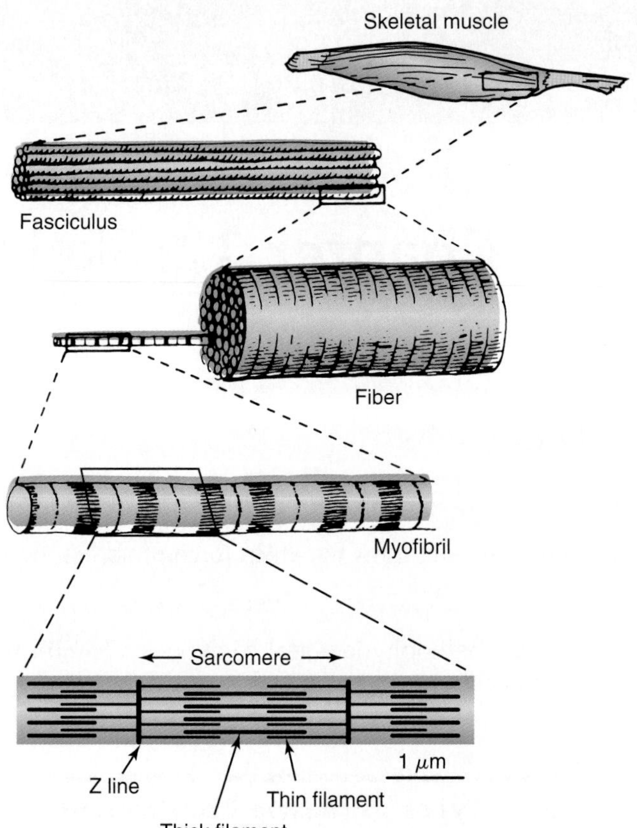

FIGURE 12–2. Skeletal muscle is composed of bundles of muscle fibers (each called a fasciculus); each muscle fiber contains numerous myofibrils. The striations are due to the arrangement of thick and thin filaments. The sarcomere represents the contractile unit in striated muscle and is bounded by Z lines. Thin filaments extend from the Z line toward the center of the sarcomere and overlap thick filaments. Contraction results from thick filaments pulling thin filaments toward the center of the sarcomere. (Redrawn from Bloom W, Fawcett DW: *A textbook of histology,* ed 10, Philadelphia, 1975, WB Saunders.)

light band **(I band)** contains actin thin filaments, extending from the Z line toward the middle of the sarcomere. The dark band **(A band)** contains **myosin thick filaments.** The darkest regions at the ends of the A band represent regions of overlap between the actin thin filaments and the myosin thick filaments. It is within this region of overlap that the force of contraction is developed, with the myosin thick filaments pulling the actin thin filaments toward the center of the sarcomere. Initiation of contraction, however, requires a rise in intracellular Ca^{++}, as discussed subsequently.

The bottom of Figure 12–3 shows myofibrils surrounded by an intracellular membrane network termed the **sarcoplasmic reticulum (SR).** The SR plays a key role in the regulation of cytosolic [Ca^{++}] and thus is critical for the initiation and termination of contraction. The entire muscle fiber is surrounded by a plasma membrane, termed **sarcolemma,** with invaginations **(T tubules)** extending deep into the muscle fiber. The sarcolemma and T tubules stimulate Ca^{++} release from the SR and thus play a key role in the initiation of contraction.

Muscular dystrophies are degenerative disorders, the most common of which is Duchenne's muscular dystrophy (DMD). DMD was first described by G.B. Duchenne and is an X-linked recessive muscle-wasting disease associated with a defect in the dystrophin gene. DMD affects 1 in 3500 male children; most are wheelchair bound by the age of 12 years, and many die of respiratory failure in adulthood. Dystrophin is a large protein that is localized on the inside surface of the plasma membrane of several cells including skeletal muscle, smooth muscle, retina, and brain. Dystrophin is thought to play a structural role in association with glycoproteins. DMD is associated with a loss in dystrophin, which may weaken the sarcolemma of skeletal muscle, leading to muscle wasting. It has also been suggested that the dystrophin-glycoprotein complex may participate in a signaling cascade, with mutations of this complex promoting apoptosis or cell death.

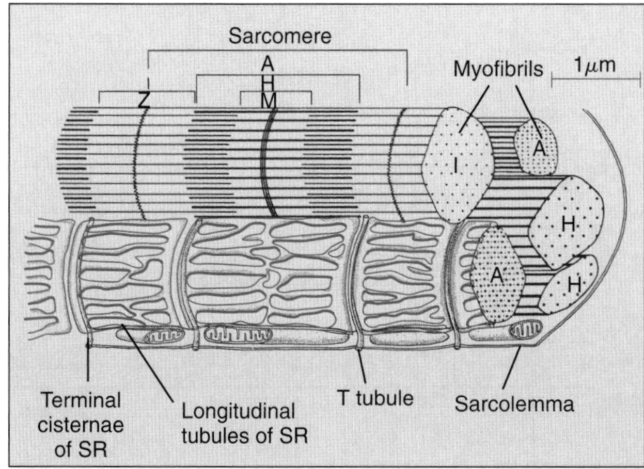

FIGURE 12–3. The myofibrils in a skeletal muscle fiber are surrounded by an internal membrane network called the sarcoplasmic reticulum (SR). T tubules represent invaginations of the sarcolemma and come close to the sarcoplasmic reticulum. T tubules allow the transmission of action potentials into the center of the muscle fiber and the activation of Ca^{++} release channels in the adjacent sarcoplasmic reticulum. (From Berne R, Levy MN, Koeppen BM, Stanton BA: *Physiology,* ed 5, Philadelphia, 2004, Elsevier.)

Contraction of Skeletal Muscle Is Controlled by the Central Nervous System

Skeletal muscle is a voluntary muscle that we consciously contract. Contraction is initiated when neurons in the motor cortex of the brain send impulses to the α **motor neurons** in the ventral horns of the spinal cord (see Chapter 9). The axon of the α motor neuron exits the spinal cord via the ventral root and synapses on skeletal muscle fibers (**Figure 12–4**). Each muscle fiber is innervated by only one α motor neuron, but a given α motor neuron can innervate many muscle fibers. A **MOTOR UNIT** REFERS TO ALL OF THE MUSCLE FIBERS INNERVATED BY A GIVEN α MOTOR NEURON. The size of the motor unit may vary from just a few muscle fibers where fine motor control is needed, as in the lateral rectus of the eye, to more than 2000 muscle fibers, as in the gastrocnemius of the leg, where high levels of force are required to maintain posture and to walk.

Acetylcholine released from the α motor neuron at the neuromuscular junction (end plate) initiates an action potential in the innervated muscle fiber (see Chapter 4). The action potential then travels along the length of the muscle fiber and down the invaginations in the sarcolemma called T tubules. As described in the next section, the action potential ultimately leads to an increase in the intracellular [Ca^{++}], which then initiates muscle contraction.

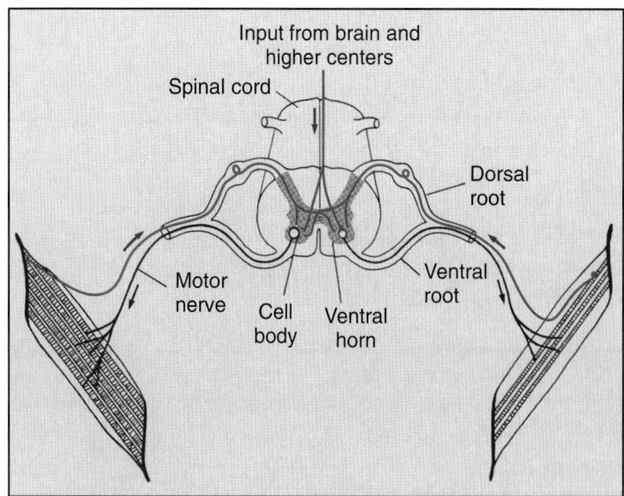

A

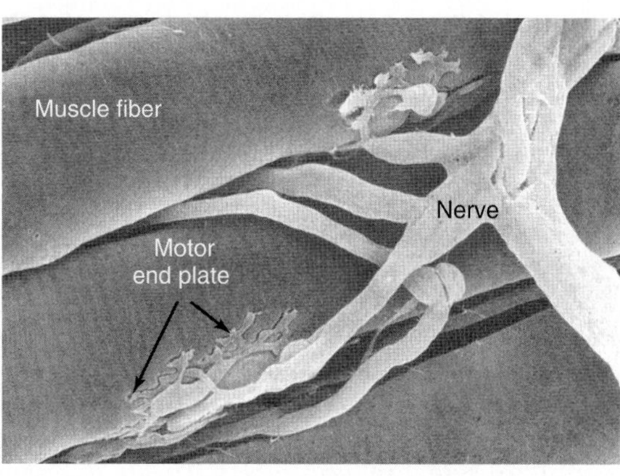

B

FIGURE 12–4. **A**, Contraction of skeletal muscle is controlled by the central nervous system. Impulses from the motor cortex of the brain pass down the spinal cord, activating α motor neurons, which in turn activate multiple muscle fibers in a given muscle. A motor unit represents all of the muscle fibers innervated by a given motor neuron. **B**, Scanning electron micrograph of skeletal muscle fibers innervated by a single α motor neuron. The site of innervation is called a motor end plate. (**A** from Berne R, Levy MN, Koeppen BM, Stanton BA: *Physiology,* ed 5, Philadelphia, 2004, Elsevier; **B** from Desaki J, Uehara Y: *J Neurocytol* 10:107, 1981.)

The Skeletal Muscle Action Potential Causes Ca^{++} Release from the SR into the Cytosol, Promoting Actin-Myosin Interaction and Hence Contraction

Before it is described how an action potential initiates SR Ca^{++} release and thus contraction, it is important to note that there is a gap (≈15 nm) between the T tubule and the SR, and there is no evidence that the SR is depolarized during an action potential. Instead, the SR Ca^{++} channel protein, also

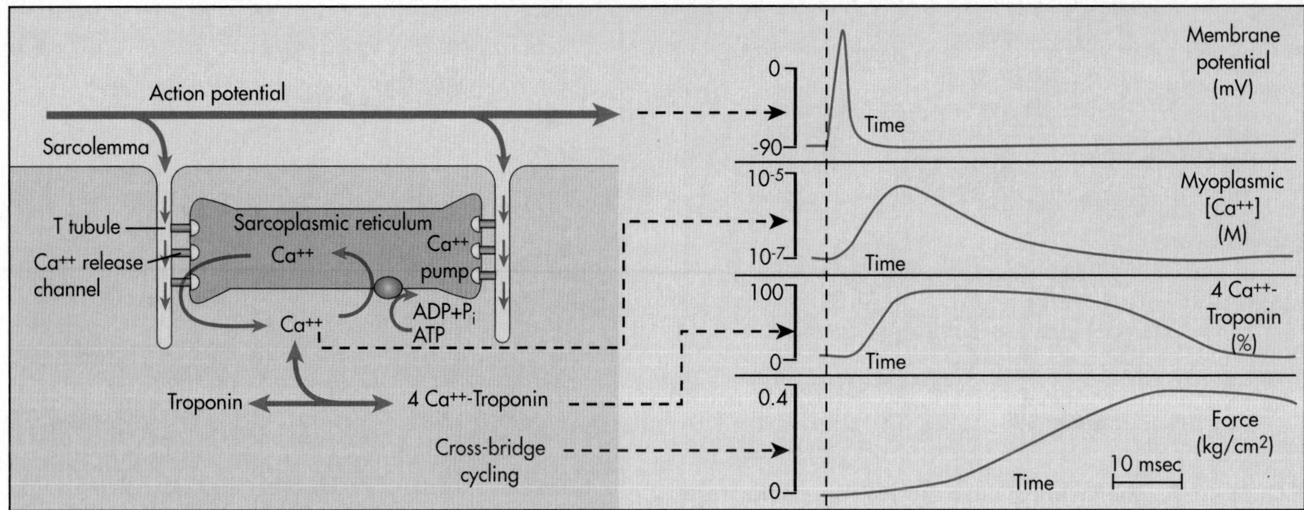

FIGURE 12–5. Activation of an α motor neuron induces an action potential in the innervated muscle fiber, which passes down the T tubules, resulting in a conformational change in the dihydropyridine receptor in the T-tubule membrane. This voltage-dependent conformational change in the dihydropyridine receptor results in opening of the closely apposed SR Ca^{++} release channel (ryanodine receptor), releasing Ca^{++} into the cytosol and thereby promoting contraction. The time course of the changes in the action potential, intracellular [Ca^{++}], Ca^{++} binding to troponin, and force generation are shown on the right. Relaxation follows as Ca^{++} is reaccumulated by the SR through the action of the SR Ca^{++} pump (SERCA).

called the **ryanodine receptor,** a large protein that extends into the gap between the SR and the T tubules, appears to abut a voltage-gated Ca^{++} channel, also called the **dihydropyridine receptor,** in the adjacent T-tubule membrane. Because skeletal muscle can contract without extracellular Ca^{++}, the voltage-gated Ca^{++} channel appears to act more as a voltage sensor, undergoing a conformational change as the action potential passes down the T tubule. This conformational change in the T-tubule voltage sensor is hypothesized to induce a conformational change in the SR Ca^{++} release channel, causing it to open. Release of Ca^{++} from the SR increases the cytosolic [Ca^{++}] from 0.1 μM to perhaps 1 μM. These interactions are depicted in **Figure 12–5,** with the rise in intracellular Ca^{++} lasting less than 80 msec. The fall in intracellular [Ca^{++}] is due to the closure of the SR Ca^{++} release channel as the action potential passes, coupled with Ca^{++} reaccumulation by the SR through the action of the **SR Ca^{++} pump (SERCA).**

Myosin Cross-Bridges in the Thick Filament Pull the Actin Thin Filaments Toward the Center of the Sarcomere, Resulting in Contraction

The action potential–dependent rise in cytosolic [Ca^{++}] initiates contraction by promoting the interaction of **myosin** with **actin.** Actin filaments extend from the Z line toward the center of the sarcomere, whereas myosin filaments are centrally located, overlapping the actin thin filaments to some extent **(Figure 12–6, *A*).** Myosin binding sites on the actin thin filaments, however, are blocked by **tropomyosin** at low cytosolic [Ca^{++}] . When the cytosolic [Ca^{++}] rises in the muscle fiber after an action potential, Ca^{++} binds to the **troponin complex.** The troponin complex that is associated with tropomyosin moves the tropomyosin into the actin groove, exposing the myosin binding sites and hence promoting contraction (Figure 12–6, *B*). A four-state model of this **cross-bridge cycling** is provided in **Figure 12–7,** where at low cytosolic [Ca^{++}], the myosin cross-bridge is energized by partial hydrolysis of ATP (state 1). As the cytosolic [Ca^{++}] rises after action potential–induced release of Ca^{++} from the SR, myosin binds to actin (state 2), followed by a ratchet action of the myosin head (state 3), which pulls the actin filament toward the center of the sarcomere and releases ADP and inorganic phosphate. Binding of ATP to the myosin head in state 3 then decreases myosin affinity for actin, resulting in myosin detachment from actin (state 4), followed by a partial hydrolysis of ATP again to energize the myosin head (state 1). If the cytosolic [Ca^{++}] is still high (i.e., greater than ≈0.2 μM), then the myosin is able to reattach to the actin filament and undergo another cross-bridge cycle to further contract the muscle. Thus, the thin filaments essentially slide past the thick filaments

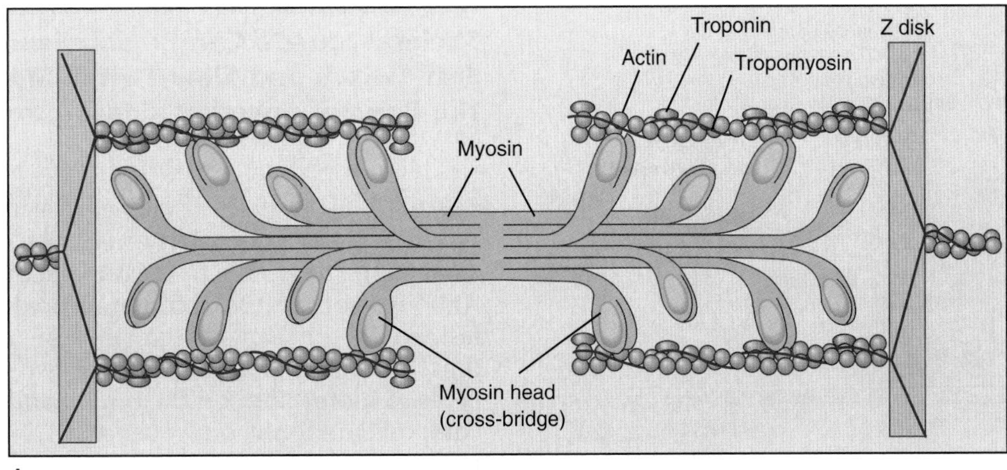

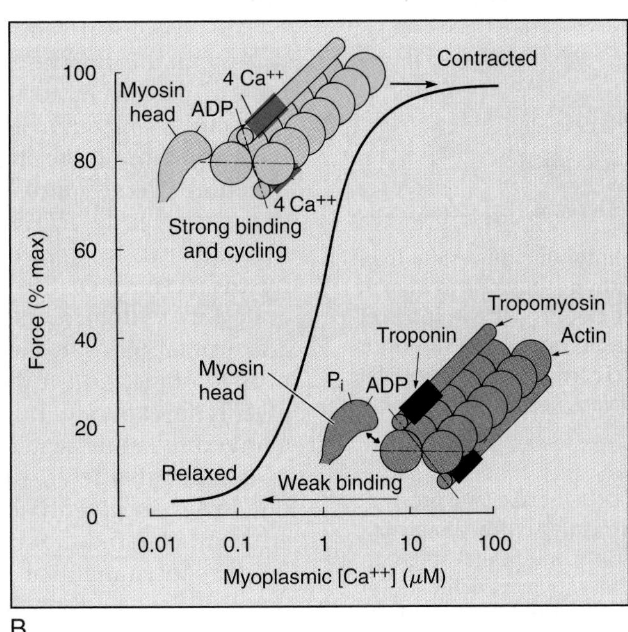

FIGURE 12–6. A, The thin filament is composed of an actin polymer, with the regulatory proteins troponin and tropomyosin. The thick filament is composed of myosin, with the heads of myosin extending as cross-bridges to the underlying actin thin filament. B, At low intracellular [Ca^{++}], tropomyosin blocks myosin binding sites on actin and thus prevents contraction. As the intracellular [Ca^{++}] is raised, Ca^{++} binds to troponin, inducing a conformational change such that tropomyosin moves into the actin groove, exposing myosin binding sites on actin. Myosin then binds to actin, pulling the actin filament toward the center of the sarcomere and hence contracting the muscle. (B from Berne R, Levy MN, Koeppen BM, Stanton BA: *Physiology,* ed 5, Philadelphia, 2004, Elsevier.)

toward the center of the sarcomere during contraction of skeletal muscle, hence the name **sliding filament theory.** AS THE INTERACTION OF MYOSIN WITH ACTIN IS CONTROLLED BY THE AVAILABILITY OF MYOSIN BINDING SITES ON ACTIN, SKELETAL MUSCLE CONTRACTION IS SAID TO BE THIN FILAMENT REGULATED. If cytosolic ATP is depleted, the cross-bridge cycle stops in state 3, termed the rigor state as in **rigor mortis** (Figure 12–7).

In the preceding discussion, Ca^{++} binding to the troponin complex induced a change in the tropomyosin such that it moved into the actin groove, thereby uncovering myosin binding sites. The troponin complex actually contains three proteins: troponin T, troponin I, and troponin C. Troponin T binds to tropomyosin. Troponin I moves tropomyosin over myosin binding sites and thus "inhibits" myosin binding to actin. Binding of four molecules of Ca^{++} to troponin C, however, removes this inhibition by moving tropomyosin into the actin groove, exposing myosin binding sites.

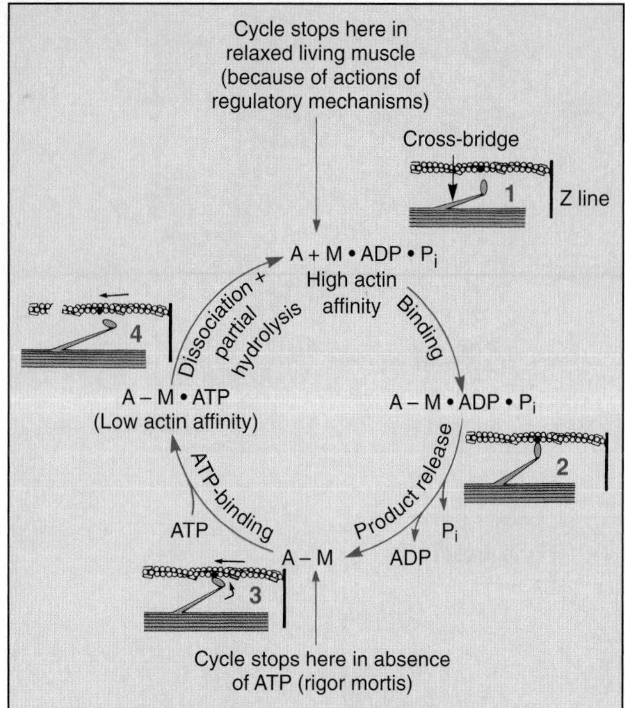

FIGURE 12–7. Contraction of skeletal muscle results from a ratchet action of myosin and is hypothesized to involve a four-step process (see text for details). If the intracellular [Ca^{++}] is still elevated, the cycle repeats, resulting in more shortening of the muscle. (From Berne R, Levy MN, Koeppen BM, Stanton BA: *Physiology,* ed 5, Philadelphia, 2004, Elsevier.)

Malignant hyperthermia, central core disease, and Brody's disease are genetic diseases associated with abnormal regulation of the intracellular [Ca^{++}] in skeletal muscle. Malignant hyperthermia is the most common of these genetic defects and may have life-threatening consequences during certain types of surgical procedures. Specifically, anesthetics such as halothane and ether or the muscle relaxant succinylcholine can stimulate Ca^{++} release from the SR, resulting in muscle rigidity, increased heart rate, hyperventilation, and hyperthermia. Malignant hyperthermia is an autosomal dominant trait, linked to a defect in the SR Ca^{++} channel (ryanodine receptor), with an incidence of 1 in 15,000 children or 1 in 50,000 adults treated with anesthetics.

Central core disease is a rare autosomal dominant trait characterized by muscle weakness and a loss of mitochondria in the core of skeletal muscle fibers. Central core disease is hypothesized to be due to a defect in the SR Ca^{++} channel (ryanodine receptor) that causes the SR to release/leak Ca^{++}, which is then accumulated by mitochondria, resulting in mitochondrial Ca^{++} overload and hence loss of mitochondria.

Brody's disease is a rare genetic disorder characterized by painless muscle cramping during exercise. Brody's disease appears to result from a defect in the SR Ca^{++} pump (SERCA) found in fast-twitch skeletal muscle. Muscle cramping is attributable to slowed Ca^{++} uptake by the SR and prolonged elevation of the intracellular [Ca^{++}].

Skeletal Muscle Can Be Subdivided into Fast-Twitch and Slow-Twitch Muscle on the Basis of Speed of Contraction

SKELETAL MUSCLE CAN BE SUBDIVIDED INTO TWO BASIC TYPES ON THE BASIS OF SPEED OF CONTRACTION **(Figure 12–8, *A*)**, **FAST TWITCH** AND **SLOW TWITCH.** Although some muscles contain a predominance of fast-twitch or slow-twitch muscle fibers, most muscles contain a mixture of the two muscle fiber types. A motor unit, on the other hand, is typically composed of only one fiber type. Thus, skeletal muscles usually contain both fast-twitch motor units and slow-twitch motor units.

The basis for this difference in contraction speed is attributable to the expression of either a "fast-twitch" myosin molecule or a "slow-twitch" myosin molecule. Although these two myosin isoforms have the same basic structure, they are products of different genes and hence differ in primary sequence and ATPase activity. Histochemical methods can be used to distinguish the fiber types by the activity of the myosin ATPase. Fast-twitch and slow-twitch fibers also differ in terms of size and metabolic profiles. In humans, fast-twitch muscle fibers tend to be of large diameter, high in glycolytic capacity, but low in oxidative capacity. Conversely, slow-twitch muscle fibers are typically of smaller diameter, higher in oxidative capacity, but lower in glycolytic capacity. This basic difference in metabolic activity is consistent with the fatigue resistance of slow-twitch muscle fibers (Figure 12–8, *B*). By comparison, fast-twitch muscle fibers are easily fatigued. Because of this difference in fiber fatigability, slow-twitch fibers tend to be recruited first during a muscle contraction, whereas fast-twitch fibers tend to be recruited last. The smaller diameter of slow-twitch muscle fibers also facilitates fatigue resistance by increasing the surface-to-volume ratio of the cell (and thus increasing diffusion and uptake of oxygen and metabolic substrates from the blood). The higher oxidative capacity of the slow-twitch muscle fibers is also manifested in their reddish color, which is due to the abundance of myoglobin, mitochondria, and high vascular supply. By comparison, fast-twitch muscles, which rely more on anaerobic metabolism, tend to be white or pale.

In addition to these differences between fast-twitch and slow-twitch fibers, other muscle proteins are also expressed in a fiber type–specific manner. These include the SR Ca^{++} pump (SERCA), the three troponin subunits, and tropomyosin. The differential expression of SERCA isoforms contributes to the differences in the speed of relaxation between fast-

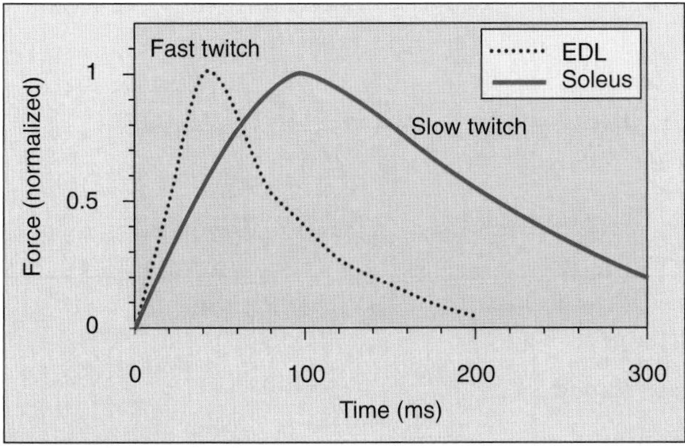

A

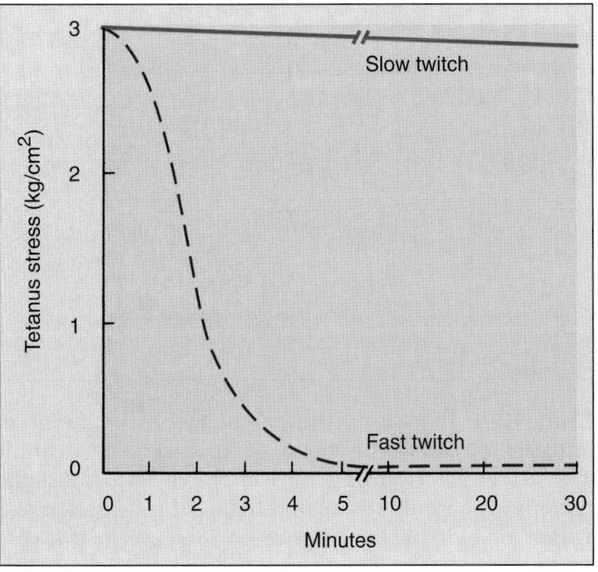

B

FIGURE 12–8. A, Skeletal muscle fibers can be classified as either fast twitch or slow twitch. The extensor digitorum longus (EDL) is a fast-twitch skeletal muscle found in the leg; a single action potential produces a rapid rise in force development (reaching peak force within 30 msec). The slow-twitch muscle soleus of the leg, on the other hand, requires more time (90 msec) to reach peak force. B, Fast-twitch muscle fibers fatigue, with a decline in tension, more quickly than slow-twitch muscle fibers during continuous stimulation. (B from Berne R, Levy MN, Koeppen BM, Stanton BA: *Physiology,* ed 5, Philadelphia, 2004, Elsevier.)

and slow-twitch muscle. The activity of SERCA is higher in fast-twitch muscle fibers, thereby leading to faster relaxation. Differential expression of troponin and tropomyosin isoforms influences the Ca^{++} dependency of contraction. Slow fibers begin to develop tension at lower Ca^{++} concentrations than do fast fibers.

An important determinant of the muscle fiber type is its innervation. This is shown by cross-innervation studies, where muscle fibers in a fast-twitch motor unit increase oxidative capacity, decrease contraction speed, and express the slow-type myosin isoform when an α motor neuron from a slow motor unit is surgically connected. Similarly, muscle fibers in a slow-twitch motor unit adopt properties associated with a fast-twitch muscle fiber, including the synthesis of a fast-twitch muscle myosin, when they are cross-innervated with an α motor neuron that typically innervates fast-twitch muscle fibers. This mutability is not due to a trophic substance from the nerve, however, but instead reflects the activity pattern of the neuron. For example, chronic electrical stimulation of an α motor neuron innervating a fast-twitch motor unit promotes the synthesis of slow-twitch myosin and increases oxidative capacity. Likewise, decreased activity of slow-twitch muscle (e.g., after immobilization) promotes atrophy and the progression to a fast-twitch phenotype, including the synthesis of fast-twitch muscle myosin. Thus, the expression of myosin isoforms appears to be activity dependent, with frequent stimulation promoting synthesis of slow-twitch myosin and disuse promoting synthesis of fast-twitch myosin. The mechanism promoting the synthesis of slow-twitch muscle myosin in a fast-twitch muscle after chronic electrical stimulation or cross-innervation is not clear, although there is evidence to suggest that it may involve a modest, chronic elevation of intracellular $[Ca^{++}]$. Efforts to change fast-twitch muscle fibers into slow-twitch muscle fibers through endurance exercise programs have been largely unsuccessful, perhaps because of the need for more frequent (chronic) stimulation of the fast-twitch muscle fibers.

The Force of Contraction of Skeletal Muscle Is Increased by Recruitment of More Motor Units and by Tetanus

Recruitment

A simple means of increasing the force of contraction of a muscle is to recruit more muscle fibers. As all of the muscle fibers within a motor unit are activated simultaneously, one recruits more muscle fibers by recruiting more motor units. As noted, there is a difference in recruitment pattern between fast-twitch and slow-twitch muscle fibers. Typically, slow-twitch muscle fibers are recruited first. This is due to differences in the α motor neurons innervating slow-twitch and fast-twitch muscle fibers. That is, α motor neurons innervating slow-twitch muscles are more easily excited because of a lower threshold. The small diameter of slow-twitch α motor neurons may contribute to this increased excitability. A motor unit typically contains either fast-twitch or slow-twitch muscle fibers, so when more force is needed, motor units containing fast-twitch muscle fibers are recruited as well. This recruitment order is consistent with their fatigue resistance, in that motor units containing oxidative, fatigue-resistant muscle fibers tend to be recruited first and thus can withstand continuous stimulation.

Slow-twitch motor units tend to be small (containing 100 to 500 muscle fibers) and thus suited for fine motor control or a gradual increase in force. Fast-twitch motor units, by contrast, tend to be large (containing 1000 to 2000 muscle fibers) and would provide large amounts of force during maximal efforts of short duration.

The process of increasing the force of contraction by recruitment of additional motor units is termed **spatial summation,** since one is "summing" forces from muscle fibers within a larger area of the muscle. This is in contrast to **temporal summation,** which is discussed next.

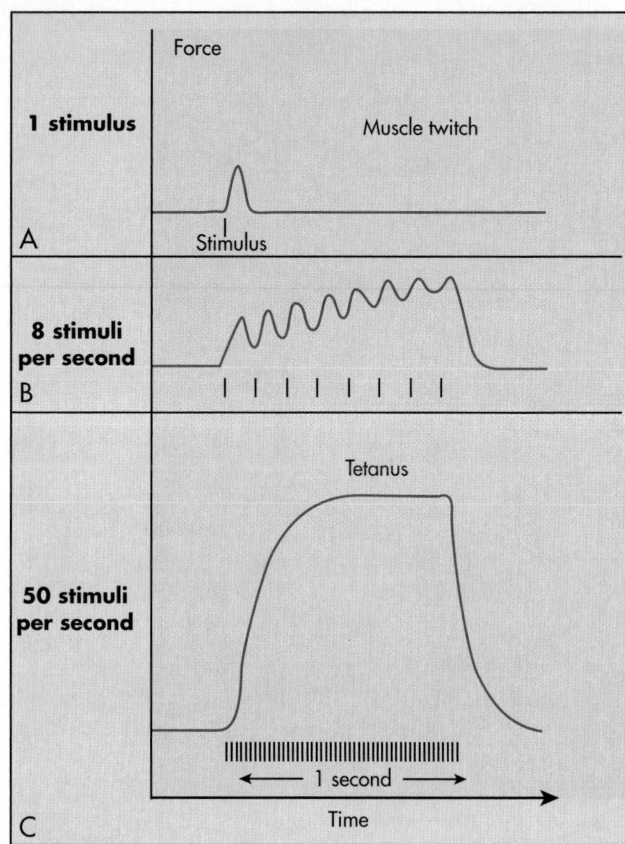

FIGURE 12–9. Increasing the frequency of stimulation of a muscle increases the force of contraction. A single action potential induces a muscle twitch (**A**), but if the muscle is repeatedly stimulated before it relaxes, there is a fusion of twitches and hence an increase in the contractile force (**B**). At high levels of stimulation, the fusion of twitches occurs quickly, resulting in a rapid rise in contractile force (**C**). The increase in force at high frequencies of stimulation is termed tetanus or tetany.

Tetanus

Tetanus refers to the ability to increase the force of contraction by repeated stimulation of skeletal muscle before it has time to relax (**Figure 12–9**). This is possible because of the brevity of the action potential (about 5 msec) compared with the duration of the twitch (20 to 100 msec). The end result is that during repeated stimulation, Ca^{++} is being released from the SR faster than it can be reaccumulated, resulting in a prolonged elevation in the intracellular [Ca^{++}]. One interpretation of the increase in force with increasing frequency of stimulation is that during an ordinary twitch after a single stimulation, the rise in intracellular [Ca^{++}] is brief, such that it falls before myosin can fully stretch the series elastic elements in the muscle fiber. The series elastic elements are thought to include connective tissue in muscle and cytoskeletal components within the muscle fiber that are stretched during muscle contraction (**Figure 12–10**). By prolongation of the intracellular Ca^{++} transient, as during repeated stimulation, there is sufficient time to fully stretch the series elastic component and thus express the full force developed by the actin-myosin interactions.

Slow fibers can be tetanized at lower frequencies of stimulation than fast fibers. This is due to the longer duration of the twitch in slow-twitch muscle compared with that of fast-twitch muscle. Tetanized fast-twitch motor units, however, develop greater force than do tetanized slow-twitch motor units because of the larger diameter of fast-twitch muscle fibers and the greater number of muscle fibers in a fast motor unit.

Muscle Spindles and Golgi Tendon Organs Modulate Force Through Reflex Arcs

The α motor neurons receive inputs from a variety of sources within the central nervous system, including reflex arcs from afferent nerve fibers in

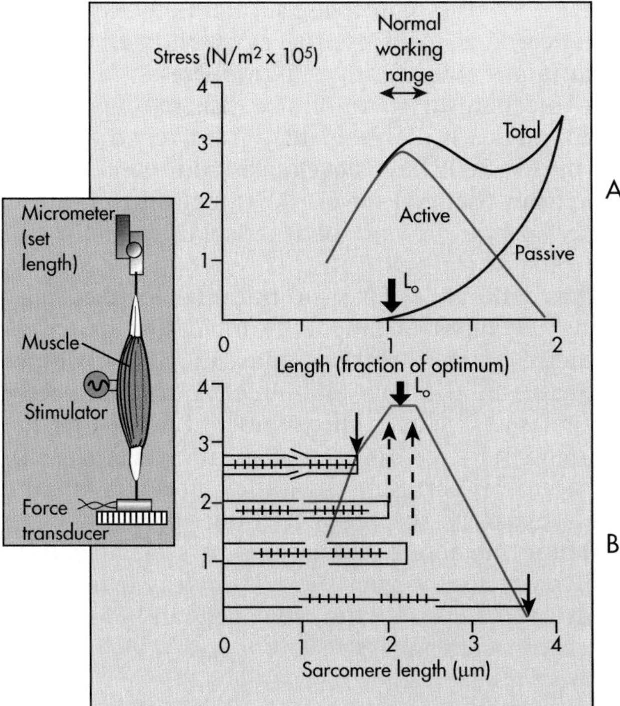

FIGURE 12–10. The force of contraction is dependent on the length of the sarcomere. The inset shows the experimental setup, with a micrometer used to adjust muscle length and a force transducer to measure isometric tension. A, The force of contraction at a given length is calculated by subtracting the passive tension from the total tetanic tension. The force of contraction is then plotted as a function of sarcomere length. Contractile force is maximal at sarcomere lengths between 2 and 2.5 μm but gradually decreases at sarcomere lengths above or below this range. B, The overlap of the thick and thin filaments at the various muscle lengths explains this length dependence of contractile force.

the skeletal muscle (see also Chapter 9). There are two basic types of afferent pathways.

The first afferent pathway is from sensors **(muscle spindles)** in specialized fibers running parallel to the skeletal muscle fibers. This afferent pathway is responsible for the stretch reflex, whereby stretch of a muscle results in a reflex stimulation of the α motor neuron innervating the stretched muscle. The second afferent pathway involves sensors **(Golgi tendon organ)** in the tendon of the muscle. The Golgi tendon organ is of low sensitivity and is activated when the force on a muscle is extremely high, resulting in an inhibition of the muscle that was stretched and stimulation of the opposing (antagonist) muscle. The Golgi tendon organ thus serves to protect the stretched or overloaded muscle from damage.

Afferent Signals from the Spindles Contribute to Skeletal Muscle Tone

The skeletal system supports the body in an erect posture with the expenditure of relatively little energy. However, even at rest, muscles normally exhibit some level of contractile activity. Isolated, (i.e., denervated) unstimulated muscles are in a relaxed state and are said to be **flaccid.** However, relaxed muscles in the body are comparatively firm. This firmness, or tone, is caused by low levels of contractile activity in some of the motor units and is driven by reflex arcs from the muscle's spindles. Interruption of the reflex arc, by sectioning the sensory afferent fibers, abolishes this resting muscle tone.

Muscles Convert the Chemical Energy in ATP into Mechanical Energy, Although the ATP Pool Must Be Continually Replenished

Muscle cells convert chemical energy of ATP into mechanical energy. Although the ATP pool in skeletal muscle is small and capable of supporting only a few contractions, the ATP pool is continually replenished during contraction such that even when the muscle fatigues, the ATP stores are only modestly decreased. This replenishment of ATP pools is accomplished in part by the creatine phosphate pool, which converts ADP into ATP, especially during intense exercise. The **creatine phosphate** pool, however, is also small (about five times the size of the ATP pool). Intense exercise is associated with the depletion of the creatine phosphate store, although this does not necessarily imply that the fatigue is caused by depletion of the creatine phosphate store. Muscle cells also contain glycogen, which can be metabolized during muscle contraction to provide glucose for oxidative phosphorylation and glycolysis, both of which will generate ATP to replenish the ATP store. Muscle cells can also take up glucose from the blood. Fatty acids represent an important source of energy for muscle cells during prolonged exercise and can be derived from the blood or from triglycerides within the muscle. The fatty acids are subjected to β-oxidation within the mitochondria, ultimately yielding ATP for muscle contraction.

When the Energy Demands of Exercise Exceed the Aerobic Capacity of the Muscle, an Oxygen Debt Is Developed

If the energy demands of exercise cannot be met by oxidative phosphorylation, an **oxygen debt** is incurred. After completion of exercise, respiration remains above the resting level to "re-pay" this oxygen debt. The extra oxygen consumption during this recovery phase is used to restore metabolite levels, such as creatine phosphate and ATP, and to metabolize the lactate generated by glycolysis.

Muscle Fatigue Is Not due to Depletion of ATP

The ability of the muscle to meet energy needs is a major determinant of the duration of the exercise. HOWEVER, FATIGUE IS NOT THE RESULT OF DEPLETION OF ENERGY SOURCES. Instead, metabolic byproducts seem to be important factors in the onset of fatigue. Fatigue may potentially occur at any of the points involved in muscle contraction, from the brain to the muscle cells, as well as in the cardiovascular and respiratory systems that maintain energy supplies (i.e., fatty acids and glucose) and oxygen delivery to the exercising muscle.

Several factors have been implicated in muscle fatigue. Decreases in force during tetany are paralleled by depletion of glycogen and creatine phosphate stores and the accumulation of lactic acid. Importantly, the decline in force/stress occurs when the ATP pool is not greatly reduced, so that the muscle fibers do not go into rigor. Evidently, some factor associated with energy metabolism can inhibit contraction (e.g., in the fast fibers), but this factor has not been clearly identified. One potential candidate is phosphate (which can inhibit SR Ca^{++} release and actin-myosin interaction). Decreases in intracellular pH due to lactate accumulation may also inhibit actin-myosin interaction.

Regardless of whether the muscle fatigues as a consequence of high-intensity exercise of short duration or prolonged exercise, the cytoplasmic ATP level does not decrease substantially. Given the reliance of all cells on the availability of ATP to maintain viability, fatigue may represent a protective mechanism to minimize risk of muscle cell injury or death. Consequently, it is likely that skeletal muscle cells have developed redundant systems to ensure that ATP levels do not drop to dangerously low levels and hence risk the viability of the cell.

An endurance exercise training regimen can delay the onset of fatigue by increasing oxidative capacity of the exercised muscles. This includes increases in the level of mitochondrial oxidative enzymes as well as in the number of mitochondria, along with increases in vascularization (i.e., density of capillaries perfusing the muscle fibers). Similarly, high-resistance exercise training programs can promote metabolic adaptations in skeletal muscle that postpone fatigue, such as increased levels of creatine phosphate and glycogen and decreased levels of lactate.

The Cross-Sectional Diameter of a Skeletal Muscle Increases by Hypertrophy

As the skeleton grows, the muscle cells lengthen. Lengthening is accomplished by formation of additional sarcomeres at the ends of the muscle cells, a process that is reversible. For example, the length of a cell decreases when terminal sarcomeres are eliminated, which can occur when a limb is immobilized with the muscle in a shortened position or when an improperly set fracture leads to a shortened limb segment. Changes in muscle length affect the velocity of shortening, and the extent of shortening, but do not influence the amount of force that can be generated by the muscle.

Skeletal muscles have a limited ability to form new fibers **(hyperplasia).** Instead, the gradual increase in strength and diameter of a muscle during growth or after an exercise regimen is achieved mainly by **hypertrophy.** Doubling of the myofibrillar diameter by addition of more sarcomeres in parallel (hypertrophy), for example, may double the amount of force generated. Muscles immobilized in a cast, by contrast, lose mass **(atrophy).** Also, space flight exposes astronauts to a microgravity environment that mechanically unloads their muscles. This unloading leads to a rapid loss of muscle mass and weakness.

The Length-Tension Relationship of Skeletal Muscle Contraction Is Consistent with the Sliding Filament Theory

To assess the length-tension relationship of skeletal muscle contraction, the skeletal muscle is stretched (or pre-contracted) to various lengths, and then the force of contraction is measured after a tetanic stimulus. The basic setup is shown in the inset to Figure 12–10, with the muscle extended between two points. The top of the muscle is attached to a micrometer (for setting muscle length), and the bottom of the muscle is attached to a force transducer (to measure force). As the muscle is not able to shorten during the contraction, this is called an **isometric contraction.**

When the skeletal muscle is stretched beyond its normal working range, the force of contraction decreases (as shown in Figure 12–10, *A*). There is also an increase in the passive tension on the skeletal muscle during these high degrees of stretch (lower curve in Figure 12–10, *A*), reflecting the elastic properties of connective tissue and cytoskeletal components within the muscle. The active force developed during the tetanic contraction is redrawn in Figure 12–10, *B,* with the abscissa representing sarcomere length. The sarcomere length of skeletal muscle at rest is approximately 2 µm, but as the muscle is stretched beyond a sarcomere length of 2.5 µm, there is a progressive decrease in the ability of the muscle to generate the force of contraction. The force of contraction also decreases when the sarcomere length is reduced below ≈2 µm. This length dependence of skeletal muscle contraction has been attributed to changes in the overlap of the thick and thin filaments. At sarcomere lengths of 2 to 2.5 µm, there appears to be optimal overlap of thick and thin filaments, with all of the myosin cross-bridges being capable of interacting with the underlying actin thin filaments in the presence of a high intracellular [Ca^{++}]. As the sarcomere is stretched beyond 2.5 µm, the actin thin filaments are pulled away from the thick filaments, such that fewer and fewer of the myosin cross-bridges overlap the actin thin filament, until at 3.7 µm, actin filaments no longer overlap the myosin thick filaments and contractile force drops to zero. At sarcomere lengths below 2 µm, on the other hand, actin filaments on opposing sides of the sarcomere collide, or disrupt actin-myosin interactions on the opposite side of the sarcomere, resulting in a decreased force of contraction. At ≈1.3 µm, the ends of the thick filaments abut the Z lines, limiting further shortening of the sarcomere. Thus, the length dependence of skeletal muscle contraction can be explained by the overlap of thick and thin filaments and therefore is consistent with the sliding filament theory of contraction.

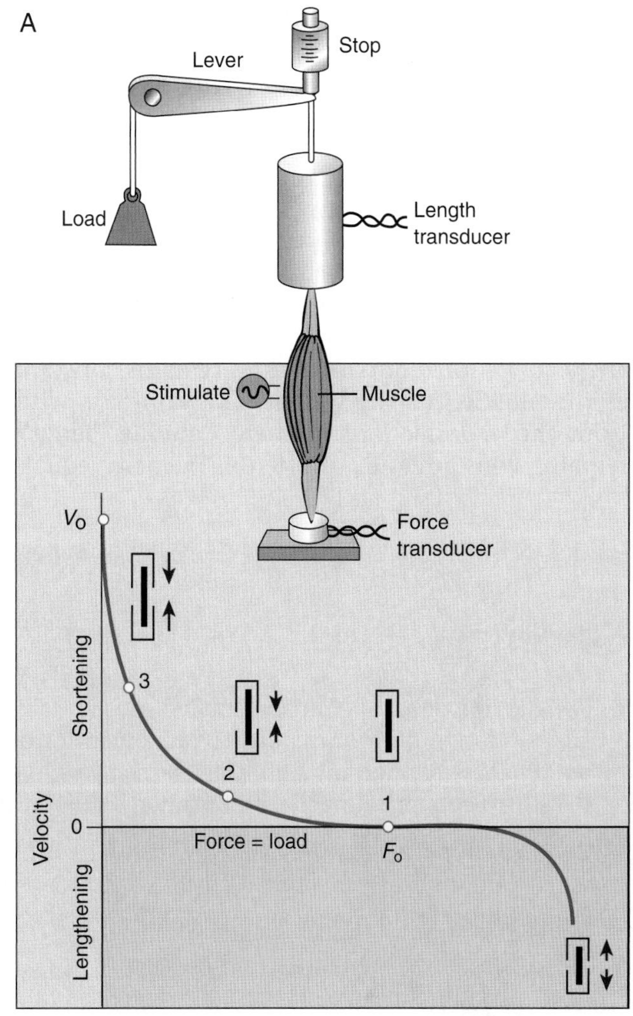

FIGURE 12–11. The velocity of muscle shortening decreases with increase in load. A, The experimental setup used to measure shortening velocity while lifting various loads. B, Load 1 (F_o) represents the maximal tetanic tension, as the muscle can only hold the load. Decreasing the load results in an exponential increase in the shortening velocity. The *y* intercept (V_o) represents the predicted velocity of shortening at zero load. F_o reflects the maximal number of actin-myosin interactions; V_o reflects the maximal rate of cross-bridge cycling.

The Speed of Muscle Shortening Decreases with an Increase in Load

The force-velocity relationship of skeletal muscle is a biophysical property of skeletal muscle that provides insights into the maximal rate of cross-bridge cycling and maximal number of cross-bridge interactions. The experimental protocol is shown in **Figure 12–11, *A*,** where the velocity of muscle shortening after tetanic stimulation is measured while lifting various loads. Load 1 (also denoted F_o in Figure 12–11, *B*) is equivalent to the maximal isometric tension of the muscle, so the muscle can hold this weight but cannot generate the force needed to lift it (i.e., shortening velocity equals zero). If the weight is decreased slightly to load 2, the muscle can lift it with measurable shortening velocity. The contraction is termed **isotonic** since the load, or force of contraction, remains constant as the muscle lifts the weight. This contrasts with isometric contractions, where muscle length remains constant (i.e., shortening velocity equals zero). Decreasing the weight further to load 3 results in an even faster velocity of shortening. Mathematical analysis of this force-velocity relationship yields an exponential fit, with the *y* intercept reflecting the predicted maximal velocity of muscle shortening (V_o) if there were no load. Thus, V_o represents the theoretical maximal rate of actin-myosin interactions, with fast-twitch muscle fibers exhibiting a significantly higher V_o than slow-twitch muscle fibers. The F_o, on the other hand, reflects the maximal number of cross-bridge interactions and increases with muscle fiber diameter. If a load in excess of F_o is imposed on the muscle, the muscle cannot even hold the load and is thus stretched (as shown in Figure 12–11, *B*).

Summary

- Skeletal muscle is a voluntary, striated muscle composed of numerous muscle cells (muscle fibers). Striations are due to the highly organized arrangement of thick and thin filaments in the skeletal muscle fibers. The sarcomere (bounded by Z lines) is the contractile unit in skeletal muscle; contraction results from myosin thick filaments pulling actin thin filaments toward the center of the sarcomere.
- Contraction of skeletal muscle is under the control of the central nervous system. Motor centers in the brain send impulses down the spinal cord to α motor neurons, which in turn innervate skeletal muscle fibers. A motor unit refers to all muscle fibers innervated by a given motor neuron.
- The α motor neuron initiates contraction of skeletal muscle by producing an action potential in the muscle fiber, which induces Ca^{++} release from the sarcoplasmic reticulum. The rise in the intracellular [Ca^{++}] exposes myosin binding sites on actin, allowing actin-myosin interaction and hence contraction. Extracellular Ca^{++} is not needed for skeletal muscle contraction.
- The force of contraction can be increased by activating more α motor neurons (recruitment) or by increasing the frequency of action potentials in the muscle fiber (tetany).
- There are two basic types of skeletal muscle fibers, distinguished on the basis of their speed of contraction (i.e., fast twitch and slow twitch). The difference in speed of contraction is attributed to the expression of different myosin isoforms. During muscle contraction, slow-twitch muscles are typically recruited first. They have higher oxidative capacity, have smaller diameter, and constitute smaller motor units than fast-twitch muscle fibers.
- The increase in skeletal muscle mass that follows strength training is due to hypertrophy.
- Muscle fatigue during exercise is not due to depletion of ATP, although accumulation of various metabolic products (e.g., lactate, inorganic phosphate, ADP) has been implicated. Endurance exercise training regimens can postpone fatigue by increasing oxidative capacity but do not change muscle fiber type.

Bibliography

Allen DG, Westerblad H: Role of phosphate and calcium stores in muscle fatigue, *J Physiol* 536(pt 3):657, 2001.

Baur CP et al: A multicenter study of 4-chloro-*m*-cresol for diagnosing malignant hyperthermia susceptibility, *Anesth Analg* 90:200, 2000.

Carroll S et al: Calcium transients in single fibers of low-frequency stimulated fast-twitch muscle of rat, *Am J Physiol* 277(pt 1):C1122, 1999.

Dirksen RT, Beam KG: Role of calcium permeation in dihydropyridine receptor function. Insights into channel gating and

excitation-contraction coupling, *J Gen Physiol* 114:393, 1999.
Gordon AM et al: Regulation of contraction in striated muscle, *Physiol Rev* 80:853, 2000.
Huxley AF: Mechanics and models of the myosin motor, *Philos Trans R Soc Lond B Biol Sci* 355:433, 2000.
Jurkat-Rott K et al: Genetics and pathogenesis of malignant hyperthermia, *Muscle Nerve* 23:4, 2000.
MacLennan DH: Ca^{2+} signalling and muscle disease, *Eur J Biochem* 267:5291, 2000.
O'Brien KF, Kunkel LM: Dystrophin and muscular dystrophy: past, present, and future, *Mol Genet Metab* 74:75, 2001.
Pette D, Staron RS: Myosin isoforms, muscle fiber types, and transitions, *Microsc Res Tech* 50:500, 2000.
Rando TA: The dystrophin-glycoprotein complex, cellular signaling, and the regulation of cell survival in the muscular dystrophies, *Muscle Nerve* 24:1575, 2001.
Sahlin K et al: Energy supply and muscle fatigue in humans, *Acta Physiol Scand* 162:261, 1998.

Case Studies

Case 12–1

A 5-year-old boy shows slow muscular development, with progressive weakness. Clinical tests showed evidence of soluble proteins characteristic of skeletal muscle cells in the serum; a muscle biopsy confirmed necrosis of both fast- and slow-type muscle fibers. DNA analysis reveals a defect in the dystrophin gene. Immunocytochemical analyses failed to detect dystrophin in the skeletal muscle biopsy specimen.

1. **What is the significance of skeletal muscle proteins in the serum?**
   A. It is diagnostic of muscular dystrophy.
   B. It implies either injury or necrosis of skeletal muscle cells.
   C. It demonstrates that these proteins are being secreted into the serum.
   D. This is a normal occurrence after exercise.
   E. It results from atrophy of the muscle cell.

2. **Duchenne's muscular dystrophy occurs only in boys. Why is it not seen in girls?**
   A. The defective gene is X-linked.
   B. Testosterone is required for the expression of the muscle wasting.
   C. Girls do not require dystrophin.
   D. Dystrophin deficiency is lethal (in utero) in girls.
   E. Estrogen protects against muscle wasting.

3. **The dystrophin deficiency characteristic of Duchenne's muscular dystrophy is likely to promote muscle wasting by which of the following mechanisms?**
   A. Impairment in skeletal muscle proliferation
   B. Impairment in muscle hypertrophy
   C. Impairment in structural integrity of skeletal muscle
   D. Inadequate oxygen delivery to the muscle
   E. Increased Ca^{++} release from the SR

Case 12–2

A patient received a muscle relaxant before surgery but soon developed massive spontaneous contractions and increased heart rate. The patient began to hyperventilate and experienced a dramatic increase in body temperature. The physician administered dantrolene, a blocker of SR Ca^{++} channels, which reversed the condition. The patient was later shown to have malignant hyperthermia.

1. **The massive contractions were likely to have been caused by which of the following?**
   A. Hyperexcitability of the α motor neurons
   B. Inhibition of acetylcholine esterase
   C. Hyperexcitability of Ca^{++} channels in the sarcolemma
   D. Hyperexcitability of Ca^{++} channels in the SR
   E. Increased Ca^{++} sensitivity of the thin filaments

2. **The rise in body temperature was primarily attributable to which of the following?**
   A. Heat produced by cross-bridge cycling
   B. Heat produced by SR Ca^{++} reaccumulation
   C. Heat produced by increased ATP production
   D. Decreased heat dissipation
   E. Heat produced by Ca^{++} influx through sarcolemma

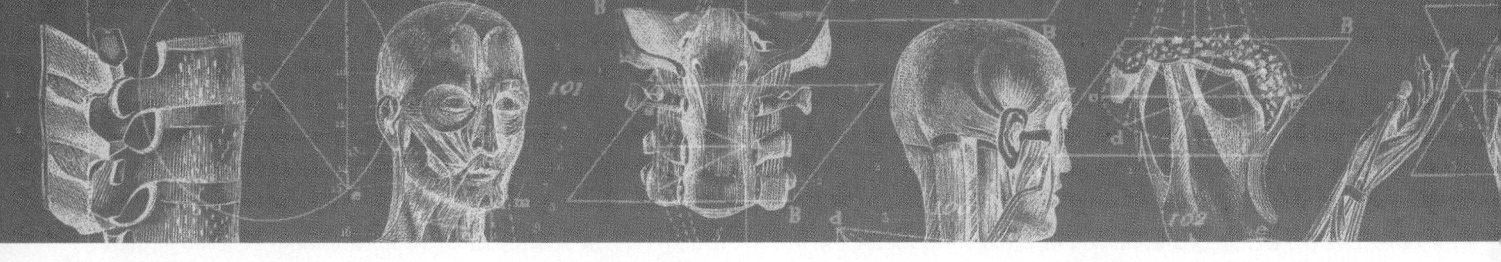

Chapter 13: Cardiac Muscle

Objectives

- ❖ Explain the organization of cardiac muscle cells and the molecular basis of contraction.
- ❖ Identify mechanisms by which force of contraction can be increased.
- ❖ Describe pathophysiological conditions affecting cardiac muscle.

Cardiac Muscle Is a Striated Muscle but Unlike Skeletal Muscle Is Involuntary

In contrast to skeletal muscle, which is voluntary and under the control of the central nervous system, the heart is an involuntary striated muscle; a built-in pacemaker allows the heart to contract rhythmically without any outside influence. Moreover, cardiac muscle cells form an **electrical syncytium** such that all of the cardiac muscle cells contract in a synchronous (wavelike) fashion, which is important for the pumping action of the heart. Differences between cardiac and skeletal muscle are also evident in terms of excitation-contraction coupling and the regulation of force, as discussed later.

Cardiac Muscle Cells Form an Electrical Syncytium

Cardiac muscle cells are much smaller than skeletal muscle cells. Typically, cardiac muscle cells measure 10 μm in diameter and approximately 100 μm in length. Cardiac cells are connected to each other through **intercalated disks,** which include a combination of mechanical junctions and electrical connections **(Figure 13–1).** The mechanical connections, which keep the cells from pulling apart when they contract, include the **fascia adherens** and **desmosomes. Gap junctions** between cardiac muscle cells, on the other hand, provide electrical connections between cells, allowing the propagation of the action potential throughout the heart, thereby permitting a synchronous contraction of the heart.

The basic organization of thick and thin filaments in cardiac muscle cells is comparable to that in skeletal muscle. Cardiac muscle is a striated muscle; the **sarcomere** represents the contractile unit. Similarly, myofibrils in the cardiac muscle cells are surrounded by the internal membrane network, the **sarcoplasmic reticulum (SR).** However, the SR in the heart is less dense than that in skeletal muscle. Terminal regions of the SR abut the **T tubule** or lie just below the **sarcolemma** (see bottom of Figure 13–1) and play a key role in the elevation of the intracellular [Ca^{++}] during an action potential. The mechanism by which the action potential initiates Ca^{++} release from the SR in heart is distinct from that in skeletal muscle (as discussed later). The heart contains an abundance of mitochondria, with up to 30% of the volume of the heart being occupied by mitochondria. The high density of mitochondria provides the heart with great oxidative capacity, more so than typically seen in skeletal muscle.

The sarcolemma of cardiac muscle also contains invaginations (T tubules), comparable to those in skeletal muscle. However, in cardiac muscle, they are oriented at the Z lines rather than at the A band–I band junction as in skeletal muscle. In cardiac muscle, connections between the T tubules and the SR also tend to be fewer and less well developed than in skeletal muscle.

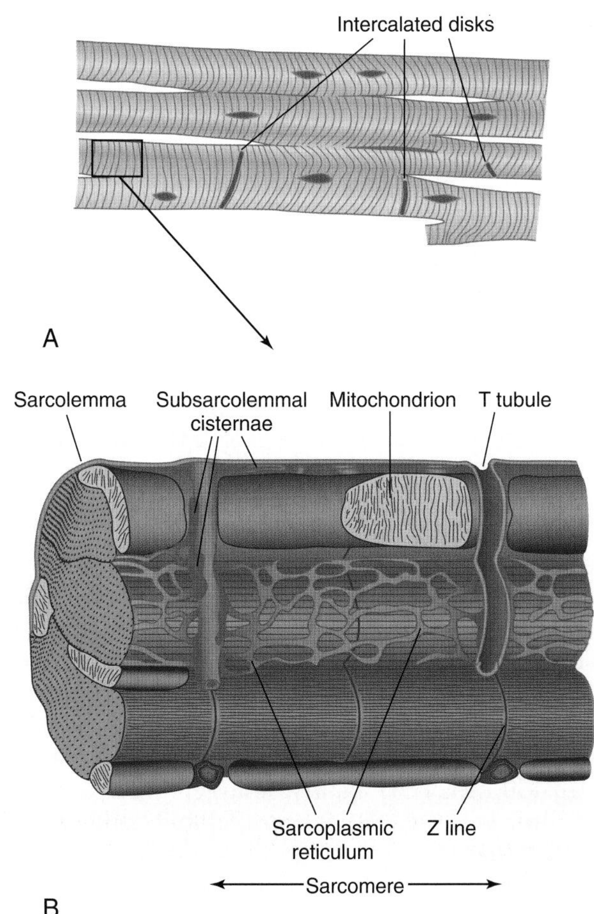

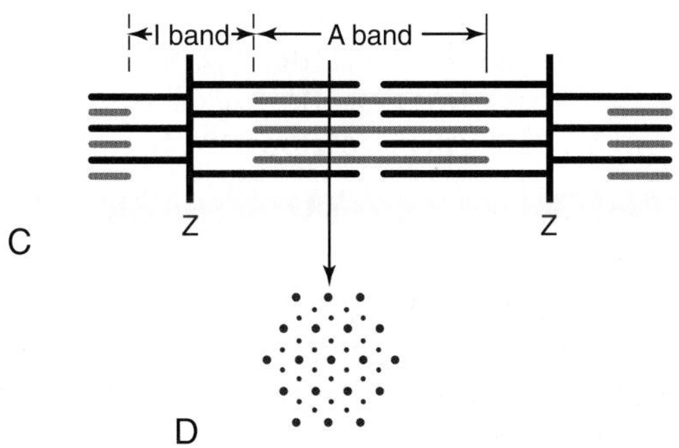

FIGURE 13–1. A, The heart is composed of a serial and parallel arrangement of cardiac muscle cells, connected in series by intercalated disks. B, Individual cardiac muscle cells are small (10 μm in diameter, 100 μm long) and composed of myofibrils, as in skeletal muscle. The cardiac muscle cell is mononucleate and has an abundance of mitochondria. Sarcoplasmic reticulum surrounds each myofibril and has enlarged regions (cisternae) that abut the sarcolemma and T tubules. The density of sarcoplasmic reticulum is considerably less than in skeletal muscle. C, The sarcomere, bounded by Z lines, is the basic contractile unit of cardiac muscle. Actin (thin) filaments extend from the Z lines toward the center of the sarcomere and overlap myosin (thick) filaments. D, Each myosin is surrounded by six thin filaments forming a hexagonal array. (B from Fawcett DW, McNutt NS: *J Cell Biol* 42:1-45, 1969.)

Familial cardiomyopathic hypertrophy occurs in approximately 0.2% of the general population but represents a leading cause of sudden death among otherwise healthy adults. It has been linked to genetic defects in a variety of proteins in cardiac sarcomeres, including myosin, troponin, tropomyosin, and myosin-binding protein C, a structural protein located in the middle of the A band of the sarcomere. Familial cardiomyopathic hypertrophy is an autosomal dominant disease, and transgenic studies indicate that expression of only a small amount of the mutated protein can result in the development of the cardiomyopathic phenotype. Moreover, mutation of a single amino acid in the myosin molecule is sufficient to produce cardiomyopathic hypertrophy. The pathogenesis of familial cardiomyopathic hypertrophy is variable, however, even within a family with a single-gene defect, in terms of both onset and severity, suggesting the presence of a modifying locus.

The Heart Can Beat on Its Own, Without Outside Influence

Cardiac muscle is an involuntary muscle, with an intrinsic pacemaker. The pacemaker represents a specialized cell (located in the **sinoatrial node** of the right atrium) that is able to undergo spontaneous depolarization and generate action potentials (see Chapter 17). The action potential is then propagated between atrial cells via gap junctions as well as through specialized conduction fibers in the atria. The action potential can pass throughout the atria within approximately 70 msec. For the action potential to reach the ventricles, it must pass through the **atrial-ventricular node,** after which the action potential passes throughout the ventricle through specialized conduction pathways (**bundle of His** and **Purkinje system**) and gap junctions in the intercalated disks **(Figure 13–2).** The action potential can pass through the entire heart within 220 msec after initiation in the sinoatrial node. As contraction of a cardiac muscle cell typically lasts 300 msec, this rapid conduction promotes a nearly synchronous contraction of the heart muscle cells. This is a very different scenario than for skeletal muscle, in which cells are grouped into motor units that are recruited independently as the force of contraction is increased.

Extracellular Ca^{++} Is Required for an Action Potential to Release Ca^{++} from the Sarcoplasmic Reticulum and thus Initiate Contraction

The action potential in cardiac muscle has a long plateau phase due to the activation of a

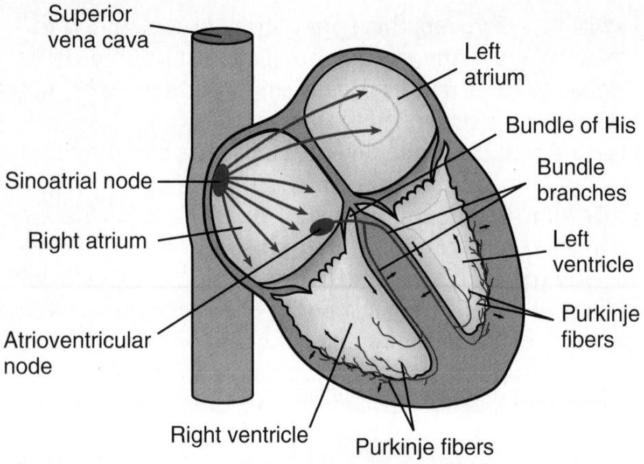

FIGURE 13–2. Contraction of the heart is initiated by a pacemaker located in a specialized region of the atria called the sinoatrial node. The pacemaker depolarizes spontaneously, initiating an action potential that travels throughout the atria by specialized conduction pathways and gap junctions. The action potential enters the ventricular myocardium through the atrioventricular node and passes throughout the ventricular muscle via conduction pathways (bundle of His and Purkinje fibers) and also by gap junctions. The action potential can pass throughout the heart quickly (within 220 msec), allowing synchronous contraction of the heart. (From Berne R, Levy MN, Koeppen BM, Stanton BA: *Physiology,* ed 5, Philadelphia, 2004, Elsevier.)

voltage-gated **L-type Ca^{++} channel.** Ca^{++} INFLUX INTO THE CELL VIA THIS CHANNEL IS CRITICAL FOR CONTRACTION OF CARDIAC MUSCLE. Thus, unlike skeletal muscle, cardiac muscle will not contract in the absence of extracellular Ca^{++}. However, the amount of Ca^{++} entering the cardiac muscle cell during an action potential is small and unable to promote actin-myosin interaction. The influx of Ca^{++} during an action potential serves as a trigger to induce Ca^{++} release from the SR, which then promotes actin-myosin interaction and hence contraction (Figure 13–3).

Contraction of Cardiac Muscle Results from Myosin Cross-Bridges in the Thick Filament Pulling the Actin Thin Filaments Toward the Center of the Sarcomere

As described for skeletal muscle, a rise in the cytosolic [Ca^{++}] in cardiac muscle initiates contraction by binding to **troponin** C, resulting in movement of **tropomyosin** such that **myosin** binding sites on the actin thin filament are exposed. The myosin cross-bridges then bind to the underlying actin, resulting in a ratchet action of the myosin head, which pulls the actin filament toward the center of the sarcomere. ATP is then needed to release myosin from the actin, followed by partial hydrolysis of ATP to energize the myosin head for another cross-bridge cycle. Thus, the four-state myosin cross-bridge cycle described for skeletal muscle applies to cardiac muscle as well (see Figure 12-7).

Relaxation of skeletal muscle simply requires the reaccumulation of Ca^{++} by the SR through the action of the **SR Ca^{++} pump (SERCA).** Although SERCA plays a key role in the decrease in the cytosolic [Ca^{++}] and hence the relaxation of cardiac muscle, the process is more complex in cardiac muscle. This is due to the fact that some "**trigger Ca^{++}**" enters the cardiac muscle cell through the sarcolemmal Ca^{++} channels during each action potential. A mechanism must therefore exist to extrude this trigger Ca^{++}; otherwise, the amount of Ca^{++} in the SR would continuously increase, resulting in Ca^{++} overload. In particular, some Ca^{++} is extruded from the cardiac muscle cell through the sarcolemmal **$3Na^+$-$1Ca^{++}$ antiporter** and a **sarcolemmal Ca^{++} pump** (Figure 13–3, *A*). Note that the extracellular [Ca^{++}] is in the millimolar range, whereas the intracellular [Ca^{++}] is submicromolar, so that the extrusion of Ca^{++} is against a large chemical gradient. Similarly, the [Na^+] is considerably higher in the extracellular media than within the cell. The antiporter uses the Na^+ gradient across the cell to power the uphill movement of Ca^{++} out of the cell. Because $3Na^+$ enter the cell in exchange for $1Ca^{++}$, the $3Na^+$-$1Ca^{++}$ antiporter is electrogenic and creates a depolarizing current. The sarcolemmal Ca^{++} pump, on the other hand, uses the energy in ATP to extrude Ca^{++} from the cell. Both extrusion mechanisms and SERCA thus contribute to the relaxation of cardiac muscle by decreasing the cytosolic [Ca^{++}].

Cardiac Muscle Cannot Increase Force of Contraction by Recruiting More Muscle Cells or Tetany

AS THE HEART REPRESENTS AN ELECTRICAL SYNCYTIUM, WITH ALL OF THE CARDIAC MUSCLE CELLS CONTRACTING DURING A SINGLE BEAT, IT IS NOT POSSIBLE TO INCREASE THE FORCE OF CONTRACTION BY RECRUITING MORE MUSCLE FIBERS AS IS THE CASE IN SKELETAL MUSCLE. Moreover, tetany of the heart would lead to death, as it would defeat the critical pumping action of the heart. The heart has therefore developed alternative strategies to increase the force of contraction. The long action potential found in cardiac muscle, which is due to activation of the voltage-gated L-type Ca^{++} channel (Figure 13–3, *B*), results in a long refractory period (Figure 13–3, *C*), which in turn prevents tetany. Modulation of L-type Ca^{++} channels

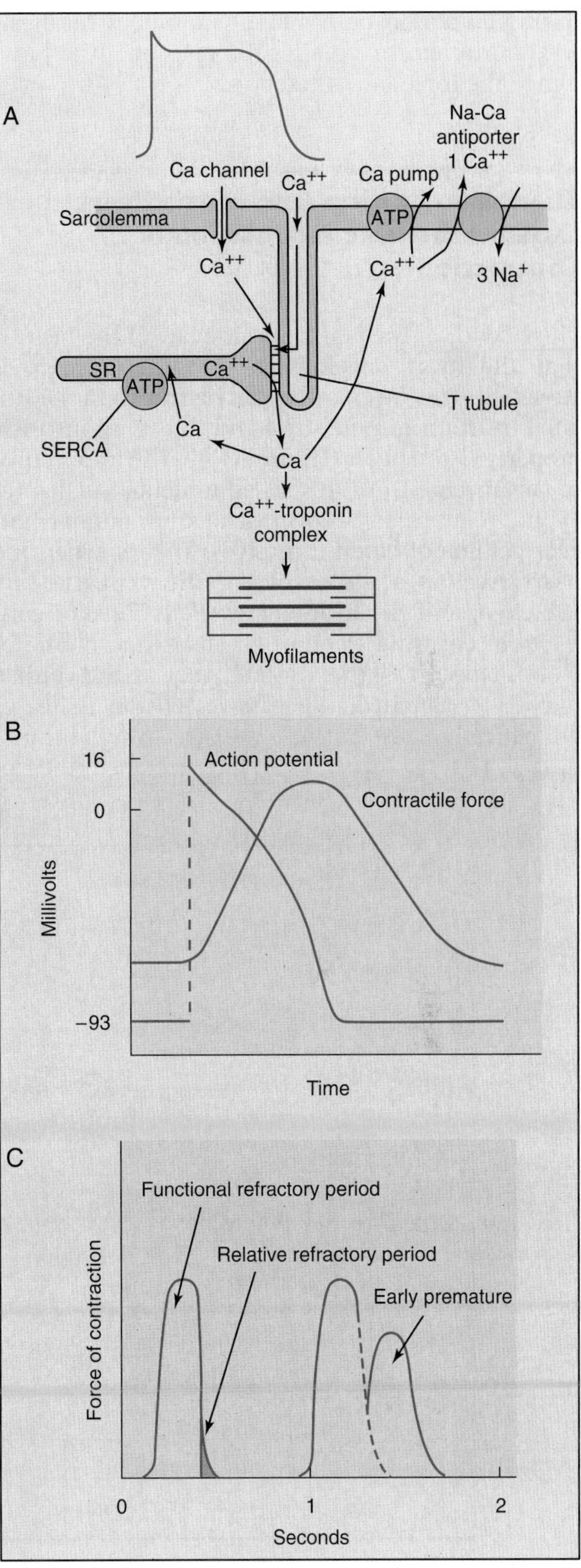

FIGURE 13–3. **A**, The action potential in cardiac muscle has a long plateau due to opening of voltage-dependent Ca^{++} channels. The influx of Ca^{++} through these channels is small but critical for the opening of SR Ca^{++} channels. Ca^{++} release from the SR then increases the intracellular $[Ca^{++}]$ sufficiently to expose myosin binding sites on actin and hence allow contraction. Relaxation occurs as the intracellular $[Ca^{++}]$ is lowered from the combined actions of Ca^{++} uptake by the SR and Ca^{++} extrusion by the sarcolemmal Ca^{++} pump and the sarcolemmal $3Na^{+}$-$1Ca^{++}$ antiporter. **B**, The long action potential in cardiac muscle (lasting ≈300 msec) overlaps the contraction, resulting in a long refractory period that decreases the likelihood of tetany. **C**, The mechanical refractory period of cardiac muscle, with a second stimulation able to induce a contraction near the end of the first contraction. (**A** and **B** from Berne R, Levy MN, Koeppen BM, Stanton BA: *Physiology*, ed 5, Philadelphia, 2004, Elsevier; **C** from Guyton AC: *Textbook of medical physiology*, ed 11, 2005, Philadelphia, Elsevier.)

during an action potential also provides the heart with a mechanism to alter the cytosolic [Ca^{++}] and hence the force of contraction.

The Frank-Starling Law of the Heart Explains Intrinsic Modulation of Contraction

The essence of the Frank-Starling law of the heart is that the heart develops more force when it is stretched. This mechanism can be shown in the isolated heart (or muscle strip) and thus is an intrinsic property of the heart **(Figure 13–4)**. The importance of this mechanism is discussed in detail in Chapter 18, but it essentially allows the heart to pump whatever volume of blood it receives. That is, when the heart receives a lot of blood, the ventricles are stretched, and the heart increases its force of contraction, ensuring ejection of this extra volume of blood. Note in Figure 13–4, *A,* that as the cardiac muscle is stretched, the passive tension increases dramatically, preventing overstretching of the heart. This resistance to being overstretched is attributable to the abundance of connective tissue in the heart.

The mechanism underlying this stretch-induced increase in force of contraction appears to involve an increase in Ca^{++} sensitivity of actin-myosin interaction (as shown in Figure 13–4, *B*), so that at submaximal Ca^{++} concentrations, more myosin molecules will interact with actin, thereby increasing force development. There is also an increase in the maximal force of contraction on stretch, suggesting that stretching of the heart can also increase the maximal number of myosin molecules that can interact with actin (Figure 13–4, *B*). The mechanism underlying the increase in maximal force of contraction is not clear, but it does not appear to be due to simple changes in overlap of thick and thin filaments.

Extrinsic Control of Contraction Occurs by Hormonal Stimulation of Adrenergic Receptors

The sympathetic nervous system is stimulated when we become excited and is said to prepare the indi-

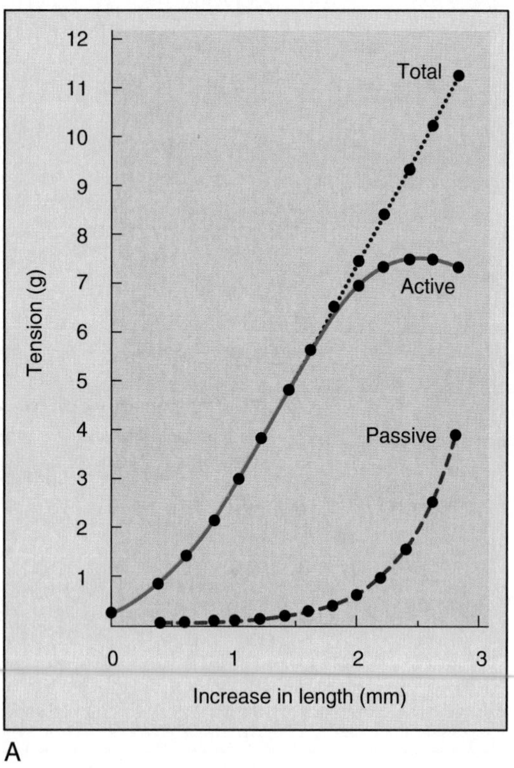

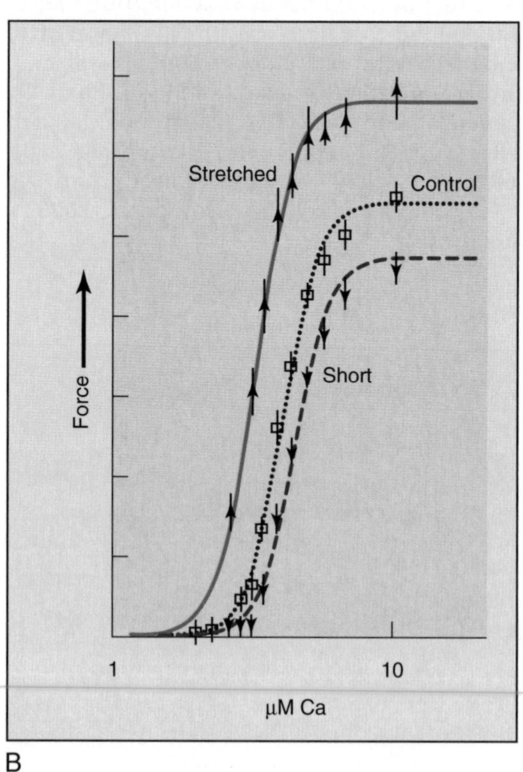

FIGURE 13–4. A, Stretching of cardiac muscle results in an increase in the force of contraction. The high passive resistance *(dashed line)* prevents overstretching of the cardiac muscle and is attributable to the abundance of connective tissue in the heart. B, The mechanism underlying this response involves a stretch-induced increase in Ca^{++} sensitivity of actin-myosin interaction, allowing more myosin molecules to bind to actin in the presence of Ca^{++}. (A redrawn from Downing SE, Sonnenblick EH: *Am J Physiol* 207:705-715, 1964. Used with permission. B from Dobest DP, Konhilas PP, DeTombe PP: *Am J Physiol* 282:H1055-1062, 2002. Used with permission.)

vidual for "fight or flight." In the case of the heart, increased levels of the adrenal medullary hormone **epinephrine** or the sympathetic neurotransmitter **norepinephrine** activate β-adrenergic receptors on the cardiac muscle cells, activating **adenylyl cyclase,** increasing **cAMP,** and thus promoting cAMP-dependent phosphorylation of numerous proteins in the cardiac muscle cells. Importantly, both voltage-gated L-type Ca^{++} channels (responsible for the trigger Ca^{++}) and a protein associated with SERCA, called **phospholamban,** are phosphorylated by **cAMP-dependent protein kinase.** The combined action of these phosphorylations increases the amount of Ca^{++} in the SR. Specifically, phosphorylation of the sarcolemmal Ca^{++} channel results in more trigger Ca^{++} entering the cell, and phosphorylation of phospholamban increases the activity of SERCA, allowing the SR to accumulate more Ca^{++} before it is extruded by the $3Na^{+}$-$1Ca^{++}$ antiporter and sarcolemmal Ca^{++} pump. The net result is that the SR releases more Ca^{++} into the cytosol during the next action potential, which promotes more actin-myosin interactions and hence greater force of contraction **(Figure 13–5).** The increased activity of SERCA after sympathetic stimulation also results in a shortened contraction because of the rapid reaccumulation of Ca^{++} by the SR. This in turn allows the heart to increase its rate of contraction. An additional consequence of the sympathetic stimulation is an increase in the heart rate due to a direct effect on the pacemaker cells (see Chapter 17).

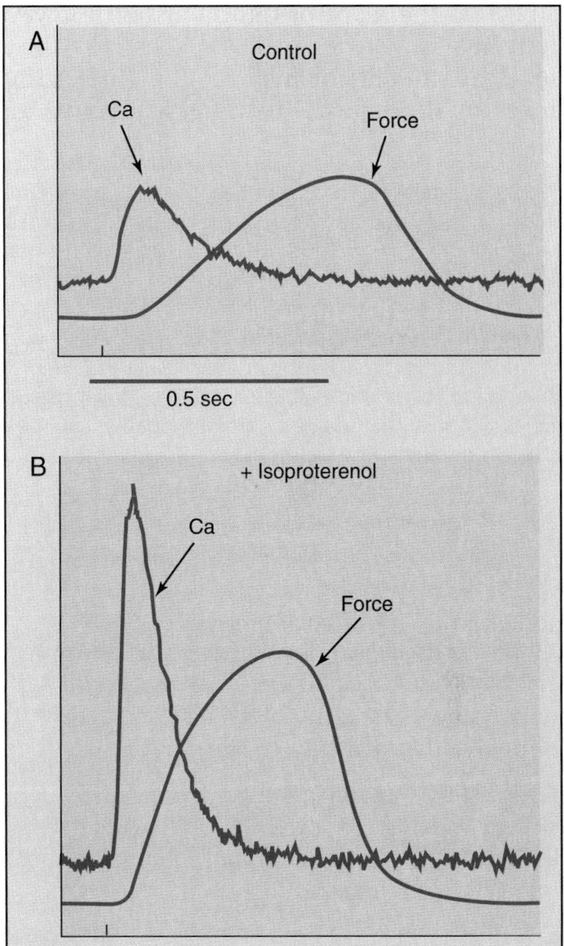

FIGURE 13–5. The force of contraction of cardiac muscle increases on stimulation of the sympathetic nervous system because of activation of β-adrenergic receptors. A, The rise in intracellular Ca^{++} and the force generation in response to a single action potential in control cardiac muscle. B, In the presence of the β-adrenergic receptor agonist isoproterenol, the action potential induces a more forceful contraction, which is also shorter in duration. The increase in force is attributable to an increase in the intracellular [Ca^{++}]. The duration of the Ca^{++} spike is also reduced, which is due in part to stimulation of SR Ca^{++} uptake. (From Morgan JP, Morgan KG: *Am J Med* 77:33–46, 1984.)

Cardiac Muscle Relies Largely on Aerobic Metabolism, Including Oxidation of Fats, to Meet Energy Demands

As in skeletal muscle, myosin uses the energy in ATP to generate force, so the ATP pool, which is small, must be continually replenished. This replenishment of ATP pools is typically accomplished by aerobic metabolism, including the oxidation of fats and carbohydrates. During times of ischemia, the **creatine phosphate** pool, which converts ADP into ATP, may decrease. As in skeletal muscle, the creatine phosphate pool is small.

When cardiac muscle is completely deprived of oxygen because of occlusion of a coronary vessel (i.e., stopped-flow ischemia), contractions quickly cease (within 30 seconds). This is not due to depletion of either ATP or creatine phosphate, because these levels decline more slowly. Even after 10 minutes of stopped-flow ischemia, when creatine phosphate levels are near zero and only 20% of the ATP remains, reperfusion can restore these energy stores as well as contractile ability. However, prolonging the stopped-flow ischemia for 20 minutes results in further drops in ATP level such that reperfusion has considerably less effect with only limited restoration of ATP and creatine phosphate levels or contractile activity.

Cardiac Hypertrophy

Cardiac muscle cells increase in size **(hypertrophy)** in response to pressure overload. The mechanisms underlying cardiac hypertrophy are complex and beyond the scope of this discussion. However, a dysregulation of cytosolic Ca^{++} has been implicated as a stimulus for hypertrophy. Interestingly, changes in the regulation of cardiac contraction also occur with severe (pathological) hypertrophy, including loss of β-adrenergic control of the force of contraction, along with loss of the response to stretch (Frank-Starling law of the heart).

High blood pressure, defects in heart valves, and weakened ventricular walls due to myocardial infarctions can all lead to heart failure, a leading cause of death. Heart failure may be seen with thickening of the walls of the ventricle or with dilated ventricles (i.e., increased volume).

Contractile defects associated with myocardial hypertrophy appear to involve defects in intracellular Ca^{++} handling, resulting in a lower contractile force and a slower relaxation. Studies suggest that dilated cardiomyopathy can be prevented in an animal model by down-regulation of a protein called phospholamban. The mechanism underlying this preventive effect of phospholamban down-regulation is thought to involve an increase in SR Ca^{++} uptake activity, since phospholamban typically inhibits SERCA. Increased activity of SERCA would facilitate relaxation of the heart because of rapid Ca^{++} uptake by the SR. In addition, the force of contraction is increased because more Ca^{++} is available for release. Increased Ca^{++} uptake by the SR may also decrease the activation of Ca^{++}-dependent phosphatases that have been implicated in the development of cardiac hypertrophy.

Summary

- Cardiac muscle is an involuntary, striated muscle. Cardiac muscle cells are connected mechanically and electrically, forming an electrical syncytium. Action potentials are initiated in the sinoatrial node and spread quickly throughout the heart, allowing synchronous contraction, a feature important for the pumping action of the heart.
- Contraction of cardiac muscle involves Ca^{++}-dependent interaction of actin and myosin filaments, as in skeletal muscle. However, unlike in skeletal muscle, an influx of extracellular Ca^{++} is required. Specifically, the influx of Ca^{++} during an action potential triggers Ca^{++} release from the SR, which then promotes actin-myosin interaction and contraction.
- Relaxation of cardiac muscle involves the reaccumulation of Ca^{++} by the SR and Ca^{++} extrusion from the cell via the $3Na^{+}$-$1Ca^{++}$ antiporter and the sarcolemmal Ca^{++} pump.
- The force of contraction of cardiac muscle is increased by stretch (Frank-Starling law of the heart) and by sympathetic stimulation. This is in contrast to skeletal muscle, which increases force by recruiting more muscle fibers or by tetany.
- Heart failure can result from pressure overload (hypertrophic cardiomyopathy), volume overload (dilated cardiomyopathy), or genetic mutations (familial hypertrophic cardiomyopathy). Typically, the contractility and rate of relaxation are reduced in these failing hearts and involve disturbances in Ca^{++} handling.

Bibliography

Chang J et al: Activation of the heat shock response: relationship to energy metabolites. A ^{31}P NMR study in rat hearts, *Am J Physiol Heart Circ Physiol* 280:H426, 2001.

Chaudhri B et al: Interaction between increased SERCA2a activity and beta-adrenoceptor stimulation in adult rabbit myocytes, *Am J Physiol Heart Circ Physiol* 283:H2450, 2002.

Dobesh DP et al: Cooperative activation in cardiac muscle: impact of sarcomere length, *Am J Physiol Heart Circ Physiol* 282:H1055, 2002.

Koch WJ et al: Functional consequences of altering myocardial adrenergic receptor signaling, *Annu Rev Physiol* 62:237, 2000.

Li L et al: Phosphorylation of phospholamban and troponin I in beta-adrenergic–induced acceleration of cardiac relaxation, *Am J Physiol Heart Circ Physiol* 278:H769, 2000.

Maass AH, Leinwand LA: Mechanisms of the pathogenesis of troponin T–based familial hypertrophic cardiomyopathy, *Trends Cardiovasc Med* 13:232, 2003.

Marx J: Heart disease. How to subdue a swelling heart, *Science* 300:1492, 2003.

McMullen JR et al: Phosphoinositide 3-kinase(p110α) plays a critical role for the induction of physiological, but not pathological, cardiac hypertrophy, *Proc Natl Acad Sci USA* 100:12355, 2003.

Neagoe C et al: Titin isoform switch in ischemic human heart disease, *Circulation* 106:1333, 2002.

Page E, Fozzard H, Solaro RJ, eds: *The heart. Handbook of physiology, section 2, cardiovascular system, vol 1,* New York, 2002, Oxford University Press.

Robbins J: Remodeling the cardiac sarcomere using transgenesis, *Annu Rev Physiol* 62:261, 2000.

Wilkins BJ et al: Calcineurin/NFAT coupling participates in pathological, but not physiological, cardiac hypertrophy, *Circ Res* 94:110, 2004.

Case Studies

Case 13–1

During a routine medical checkup, a 25-year-old man is found to have an enlarged heart. He is a professional athlete and does not have high blood pressure or high cholesterol level, and he is otherwise in good health. He mentions that his father and paternal grandfather had both died at an early age of apparent heart attacks. A few months after the medical checkup, he died suddenly of an apparent heart attack. DNA analyses indicate mutations in a gene for cardiac myosin, at a site associated with familial cardiac hypertrophy.

1. **Analysis of the heart showed that many cardiac sarcomeres were in disarray, which was probably due to which of the following?**
   A. Effects of his physical training
   B. Decreased ATP production by cardiac mitochondria
   C. Development of an arrhythmia
   D. Myocardial infarction
   E. Development of cardiac hypertrophy

Case 13–2

A 50-year-old man is frequently short of breath when performing tasks of moderate intensity. He is seen by his physician, who diagnoses exertional angina.

1. **The exertional angina is due to which of the following?**
   A. Impaired Ca^{++} handling by the cardiac muscle
   B. Altered sensitivity of the actin-myosin interactions
   C. Depletion of ATP in the cardiac muscle
   D. Myocardial energy demands exceeding energy supply
   E. Inhibition of sarcolemmal Ca^{++} channels

2. **Coronary artery arteriography is performed, and there is no obvious blockage of coronary vessels. Instead, a suitable treatment for this condition might be which of the following?**
   A. Elevation of cardiac phospholamban through DNA transfer technology
   B. Inhibition of cardiac SERCA through DNA transfer technology
   C. Creatine supplements to be taken daily
   D. β-Adrenergic agonists to be taken at times of attacks
   E. Vasodilators to be taken at times of attacks

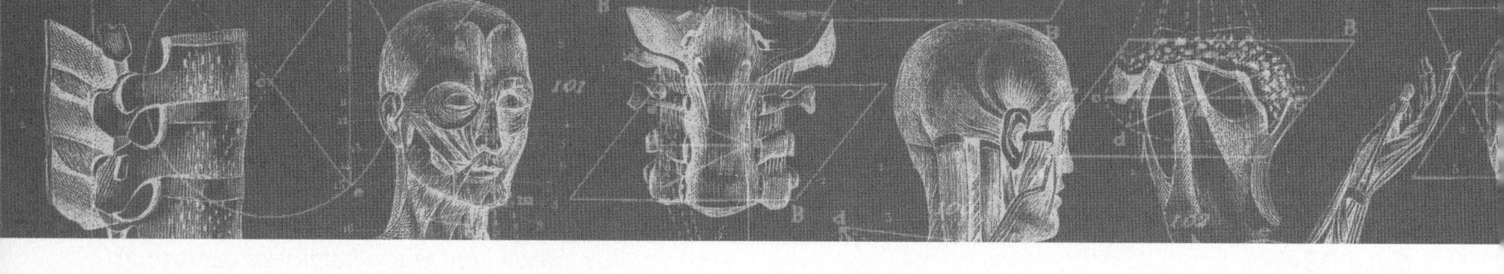

Chapter 14: Smooth Muscle

Objectives

- ❖ Explain the organization of smooth muscle cells and the molecular basis of contraction.
- ❖ Describe latch state.
- ❖ Identify mechanisms regulating the smooth muscle tone.
- ❖ Describe pathophysiological conditions affecting smooth muscle.

Smooth Muscle Is a Diverse Group: Some Types Exhibit Spontaneous, Synchronous Activity, Whereas Other Types of Smooth Muscle Act Independently

SMOOTH MUSCLE IS AN INVOLUNTARY MUSCLE THAT LACKS STRIATIONS, RESULTING IN "SMOOTH" APPEARANCE MICROSCOPICALLY. Smooth muscle has been divided into two groups, single-unit and multi-unit.

Single-unit smooth muscle, such as intestinal smooth muscle, acts like an electrical **syncytium** and undergoes wavelike contractions (e.g., peristalsis). Multi-unit smooth muscle, such as vascular smooth muscle, acts independently of its neighbors, being modulated by hormones or neurotransmitters. In actuality, these two divisions represent extremes; many smooth muscles have some degree of communication with neighboring cells. In addition to this difference in coupling, smooth muscles also show considerable structural diversity. Some smooth muscle cells exhibit a spindle-shaped appearance, whereas others may be more rectangular (see scanning electron micrographs in **Figure 14–1**).

Smooth Muscles Lack Sarcomeres but Contain the Contractile Elements Actin and Myosin

Smooth muscle cells are relatively small compared with skeletal muscle cells and approximate the size of a cardiac myocyte (approximately 10 μm in diameter and 100 μm in length). Unlike cardiac or skeletal muscle, however, smooth muscle lacks striations. Recall that the striations in skeletal and cardiac muscle are attributed to the highly organized array of sarcomeres aligned across the width of the muscle fiber. SMOOTH MUSCLE LACKS SARCOMERES (i.e., there are no Z lines). Instead, smooth muscles contain **dense bodies,** which represent the functional equivalent of a Z line **(Figure 14–2).** Actin filaments extend between the dense bodies. Myosin filaments are located in the central region between the dense bodies where they overlap with the thin filaments, analogous to the sarcomere of striated muscle. Dense bodies are present throughout the smooth muscle, with no evidence of alignment like the Z lines of skeletal muscle. The thin filaments are roughly aligned with the long axis of the smooth muscle cell. Adherent junctions between smooth muscle cells provide mechanical links and thus prevent cells from pulling apart during contraction. Gap junctions electrically couple the cells and are present to varying degrees, depending on the smooth muscle. There may also be pacemaker activity, particularly in unitary smooth muscle as in the intestine, and varying degrees of neuronal innervation (e.g., from the sympathetic and parasympathetic nervous system).

SMOOTH MUSCLE LACKS T TUBULES BUT CONTAINS NUMEROUS SMALL INVAGINATIONS OF THE SARCOLEMMA CALLED **CAVEOLAE.** The caveolae appear to serve a function similar to that of T tubules. Smooth muscles also contain sarcoplasmic reticulum (SR),

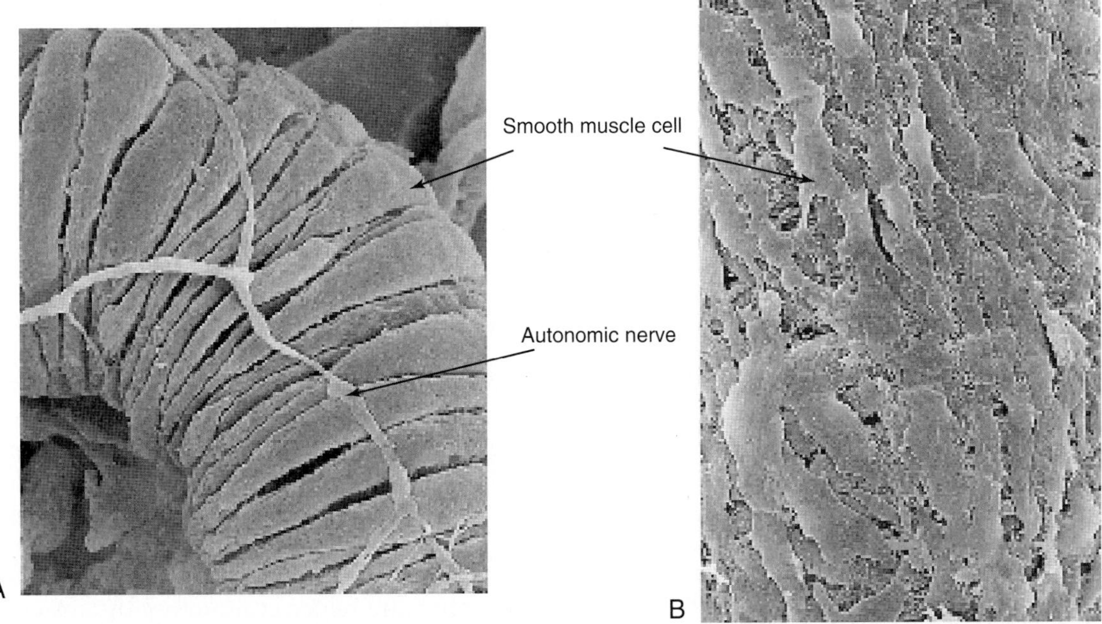

FIGURE 14–1. Scanning electron micrographs of smooth muscle in a small arteriole (**A**) and in the outer layer of the epididymis (**B**). The circumferential arrangement of smooth muscle cells shown in the arteriole facilitates vasoconstriction, which decreases blood flow to perfused tissues. In some tissues, such as the small intestine, smooth muscle cells may be arranged into a circumferential layer and a longitudinal layer to facilitate the movement of intestinal contents during peristalsis. (From Uehara Y et al. In Motta PM, ed: *Ultrastructure of smooth muscle,* Norwell, Mass, 1990, Kluwer Academic.)

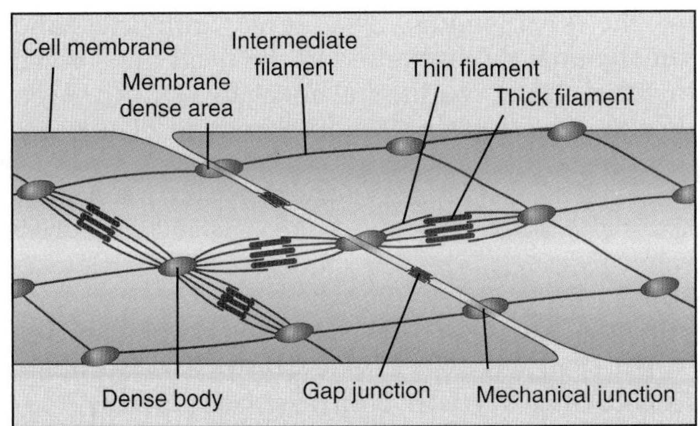

FIGURE 14–2. Smooth muscle cells are often coupled to each other through a series of mechanical and electrical connections. The mechanical connections, formed by desmosomes and fascia adherens, and electrical connections, formed by gap junctions, facilitate synchronous contractions necessary for the squeezing action of hollow organs. Although smooth muscle cells lack Z lines, there are dense bodies anchoring actin thin filaments and myosin thick filaments that extend between opposing thin filaments. These contractile units are randomly positioned, both parallel and perpendicular to the long axis of the cell, which allows the smooth muscle to exert force in several directions.

some of which is directly under the sarcolemma close to the caveolae, analogous to the arrangement of SR and T tubules in striated muscle. ALTHOUGH SMOOTH MUSCLE CONTAINS ACTIN, MYOSIN, AND TROPOMYOSIN, IT LACKS TROPONIN. Without troponin, particularly troponin I, tropomyosin does not block myosin binding sites on the actin thin filament. Consequently, smooth muscle uses a different system for regulating actin-myosin interaction, called **thick filament regulation** (as discussed later).

Numerous Factors Can Initiate Contraction of Smooth Muscle by Increasing the Cytosolic [Ca^{++}]

Numerous hormones and neurotransmitters that increase the cytosolic [Ca^{++}] induce contraction of smooth muscle. As shown in **Figure 14–3**, some of these hormones and neurotransmitters may increase the cytosolic [Ca^{++}] by depolarizing the smooth muscle membrane, thereby activating voltage-gated Ca^{++} channels that can then trigger Ca^{++}-induced Ca^{++} release via the **ryanodine receptor** from the underlying SR, comparable to

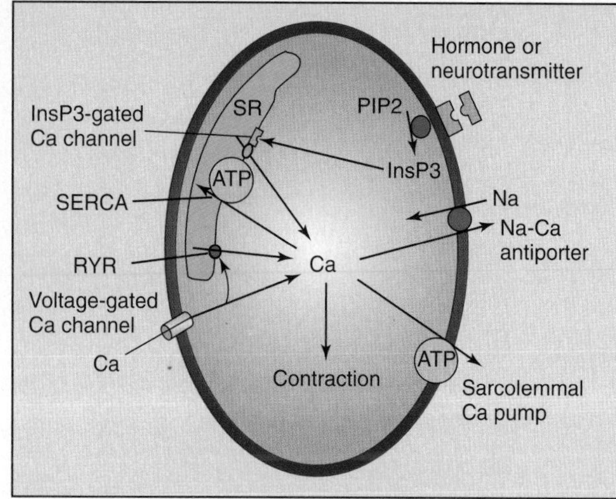

FIGURE 14–3. Contraction of smooth muscle is Ca^{++} dependent, and there are several mechanisms by which the cytosolic [Ca^{++}] can be increased. Hormones and neurotransmitters, for example, may depolarize the smooth muscle cell, activating voltage-gated Ca^{++} channels in the sarcolemma. The influx of Ca^{++} may then initiate contraction or activate the SR Ca^{++}-gated Ca^{++} channel, called the ryanodine receptor (RYR), resulting in further increase in the cytosolic [Ca^{++}]. The cytosolic [Ca^{++}] may increase in the absence of a change in membrane potential when hormones and neurotransmitters activate phospholipase C. Phospholipase C produces InsP3, which activates an InsP3-gated Ca^{++} channel in the SR. Relaxation of smooth muscle occurs when the cytosolic [Ca^{++}] falls because of Ca^{++} uptake by the SR Ca^{++} pump (SERCA) and Ca^{++} extrusion from the cell by the $3Na^+$-$1Ca^{++}$ antiporter and sarcolemmal Ca^{++} pump.

the excitation-contraction coupling in the heart. Alternatively, many hormones and neurotransmitters, such as vasopressin, angiotensin, acetylcholine (binding to muscarinic receptors), and epinephrine or norepinephrine (binding to α-adrenergic receptors), increase the intracellular [Ca^{++}] in smooth muscle without changing membrane potential, a process that is called **pharmacomechanical coupling.**

The steps involved in pharmacomechanical coupling are as follows. Hormone and neurotransmitter binding to receptors on the smooth muscle membrane activates phospholipase C, resulting in the production of inositol 1,4,5-trisphosphate (InsP3). InsP3 then diffuses to the underlying SR, opening InsP3-gated Ca^{++} channels, releasing Ca^{++} from the SR into the cytosol. The rise in the intracellular [Ca^{++}] then initiates contraction of smooth muscle, with no change in membrane potential.

Ca^{++} Promotes Actin-Myosin Interaction by Stimulating Myosin Phosphorylation

The overall structure of smooth muscle myosin is comparable to that in striated muscle, although the amino acid sequence is different. Myosin, whether it is obtained from skeletal, cardiac, or smooth muscle, is composed of four proteins, two large or "heavy" chains and two smaller or "light" chains. However, in contrast to skeletal or cardiac muscle myosin, one of the light chains in smooth muscle myosin actually inhibits binding of myosin to actin. Ca^{++}-dependent phosphorylation of this "regulatory light chain" by a **myosin light-chain kinase** allows smooth muscle myosin to interact with actin. As shown in **Figure 14–4**, the smooth muscle myosin then goes through the four-step cross-bridge cycle, pulling the dense bodies closer together and hence contracting the smooth muscle, consistent with the sliding filament theory of muscle contraction. As noted, smooth muscle lacks troponin, which in skeletal and cardiac muscle is critical for blocking myosin binding sites on actin. Thus, SMOOTH MUSCLE RELIES ON Ca^{++}-DEPENDENT MYOSIN PHOSPHORYLATION (i.e., THICK FILAMENT REGULATION) FOR MODULATING ACTIN-MYOSIN INTERACTION.

Relaxation of smooth muscle is typically accomplished by decreasing the intracellular [Ca^{++}] through Ca^{++} reaccumulation into the SR via the SR Ca^{++} pump (SERCA) and Ca^{++} extrusion from the cell by the sarcolemmal $3Na^+$-$1Ca^{++}$ antiporter and sarcolemmal Ca^{++} pump, as in the heart and shown in Figure 14–3. Additional mechanisms, however, do exist for relaxing smooth muscle. These are described in the following.

Smooth Muscle Tone Can Be Decreased by Inhibiting Myosin Light-Chain Kinase or Activating Myosin Dephosphorylation

Myosin light-chain kinase is a Ca^{++}-calmodulin–dependent enzyme, so a decrease in the cytosolic [Ca^{++}] after SR reaccumulation and extrusion from the cell represents an effective means of relaxing smooth muscle. However, regulation of smooth muscle tone is more complex, and alternative pathways for relaxing smooth muscle have been identified. In particular, cAMP CAN RELAX SMOOTH MUSCLE BY INHIBITING MYOSIN LIGHT-CHAIN KINASE EVEN IN THE PRESENCE OF ELEVATED CYTOSOLIC Ca^{++}. This inhibitory action of cAMP is used in the treatment of the bronchospasm of asthma. Another means of decreasing

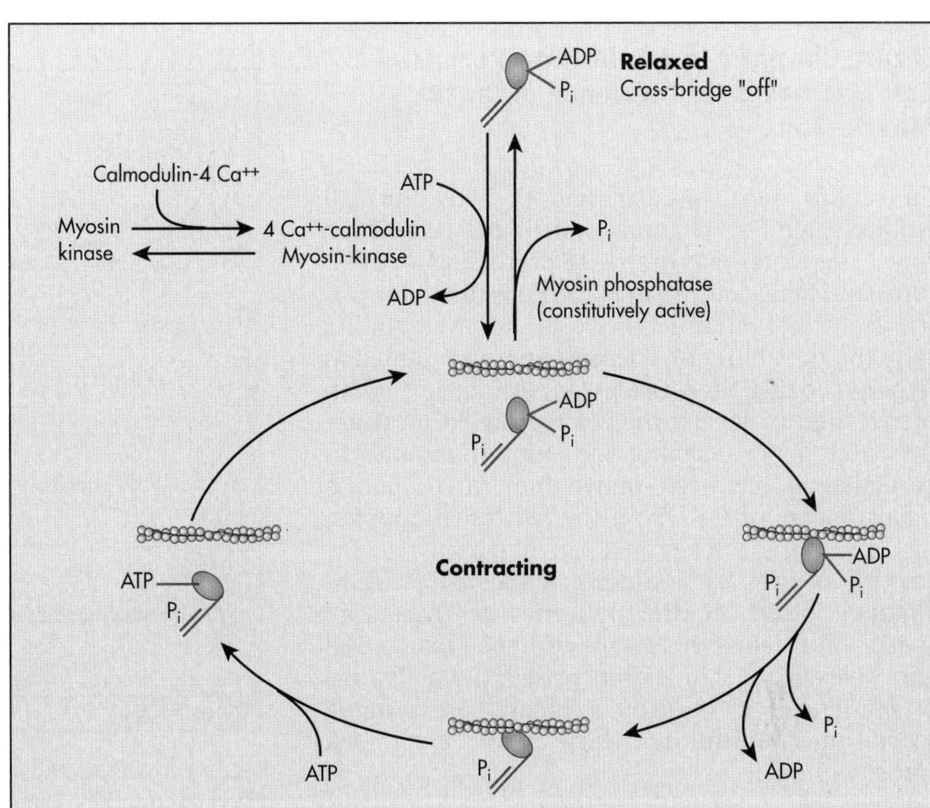

FIGURE 14–4. Contraction of smooth muscle is thick filament regulated. A rise in the cytosolic [Ca^{++}] results in the activation of Ca^{++}-calmodulin–dependent myosin light-chain kinase, which phosphorylates a regulatory light chain on myosin. The phosphorylated myosin then binds actin and undergoes a ratchet action, pulling the thin filaments toward the center of the myosin filament (see text for details of the cross-bridge cycle). A decrease in the cytosolic [Ca^{++}] reduces myosin light-chain phosphorylation and thus promotes relaxation of smooth muscle.

myosin phosphorylation involves cGMP-dependent activation of a myosin phosphatase. In particular, the ability of endothelial cells to relax underlying vascular smooth muscle cells through the release of nitric oxide may entail a nitric oxide–dependent increase of cGMP in the smooth muscle cell, resulting in dephosphorylation of myosin. The inhibitory activity of cGMP has also been used pharmacologically to increase coronary blood flow and to treat erectile dysfunction.

During an asthma attack, constriction of bronchiolar smooth muscle restricts airflow and thus oxygenation of blood. Such attacks can be life-threatening unless they are properly treated. One form of therapy is the administration of an agonist of β_2-adrenergic receptors, which relaxes the smooth muscle and thus restores airflow. Note that bronchiolar smooth muscle contains predominantly β_2-adrenergic receptors, whereas cardiac muscle contains predominantly β_1-adrenergic receptors. Therefore, administration of a β_2-adrenergic receptor agonist can relax smooth muscle without the potentially dangerous side effect of stimulating the heart, which would increase energy consumption at a time when oxygenation of the blood is compromised. The mechanism by which β_2-adrenergic receptors relax smooth muscle cells involves an increase in cAMP level, which inhibits myosin light-chain phosphorylation because of cAMP-dependent phosphorylation of myosin light-chain kinase.

Vasoconstriction of the coronary arteries also represents a life-threatening condition and often precipitates a heart attack. The vasodilator nitroglycerin is administered during the attack to reverse this vasoconstriction and does so by increasing cGMP levels in the smooth muscle. The cGMP can then activate myosin phosphatase, decreasing the level of myosin light-chain phosphorylation and hence relaxing the vascular smooth muscle. As there is normally a basal level of cGMP synthesis and degradation in a given tissue, attention has also been directed to increasing cGMP levels by inhibiting its degradation in a tissue-specific manner. Pharmaceutical companies have identified tissue-specific inhibitors of phosphodiesterases that degrade cGMP, resulting in localized increases in cGMP that can increase blood flow to a specific organ. An example of such a phosphodiesterase inhibitor is sildenafil, which is used to treat erectile dysfunction.

Slight Changes in Membrane Potential Can Dramatically Influence Smooth Muscle Tone

Ca^{++} influx into vascular smooth cells through voltage-gated Ca^{++} channels contributes to vascular tone. Therefore, one means of decreasing vascular tone, and hence decreasing blood pressure, involves the use of Ca^{++} channel blockers. However, studies raise the possibility of a second approach aimed at hyperpolarizing the vascular smooth muscle membrane, thereby closing the voltage-gated Ca^{++} channels and hence relaxing the smooth muscle. In particular, it has been shown that small spontaneous release of Ca^{++} from the SR, called **sparks,** just under the sarcolemma can hyperpolarize the smooth muscle by activating a Ca^{++}-activated K^+ channel. Moreover, the frequency of these Ca^{++} sparks, and hence the degree of hyperpolarization and relaxation, can be increased by activators of cAMP-dependent protein kinase, providing a second mechanism by which cAMP may relax smooth muscle.

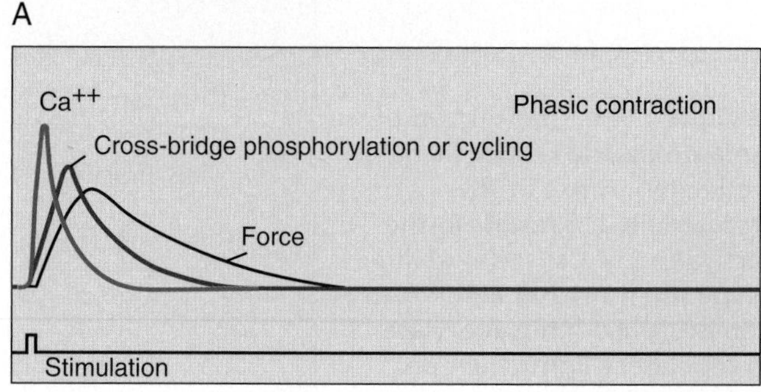

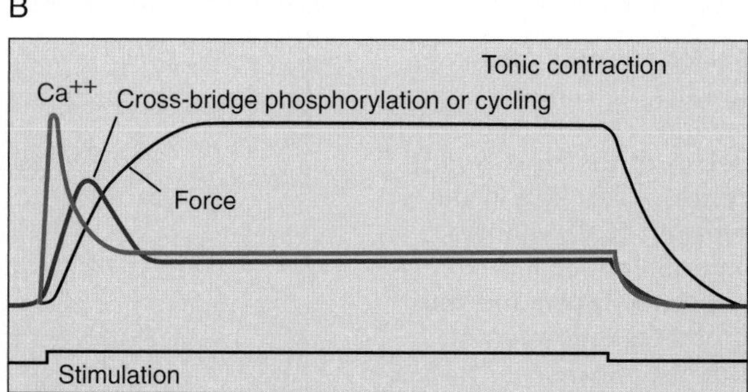

FIGURE 14–5. A, Phasic smooth muscles exhibit a short-lived contraction. Examples of phasic smooth muscle are found in the gastrointestinal tract and the urinary bladder. B, Tonic smooth muscles exhibit a prolonged contraction. Examples include vascular smooth muscle, sphincters, and bronchioles of the lung. The prolonged contraction occurs at low energy cost because of transition to a latch state. Note that phasic contractions are associated with a brief elevation of the cytosolic [Ca^{++}], whereas tonic contractions are characterized by an initial peak of the cytosolic [Ca^{++}] followed by a slight decline during the period of maintained tension. Removal of the stimulus results in a further decline of the cytosolic [Ca^{++}] and relaxation of the smooth muscle.

The Latch State Allows Smooth Muscle to Maintain Tone for Long Periods with Little Energy Use

Phasic smooth muscles exhibit a short-lived contraction, analogous to the twitch in skeletal muscle, whereas tonic smooth muscle is able to maintain tension for prolonged periods **(Figure 14–5).** Importantly, the maintenance of tension by tonic smooth muscle can occur with little ATP use. The mechanism underlying this decrease in ATP use during maintenance of tension involves a transition to the **latch state,** where the myosin stays attached to the actin instead of quickly dissociating and reinitiating the cross-bridge cycle. Recall that one ATP molecule is hydrolyzed during each cross-bridge cycle. Smooth muscle has devised a way to prolong state 3 (the rigor state) in the presence of normal concentrations of ATP. The importance of the latch state is clear, as evidenced by the ability of vascular smooth muscle to exert force for extended periods to sustain blood pressure, without expending a lot of energy or risking fatigue. As shown in **Figure 14–6,** the mechanism by which the latch state occurs is thought to involve dephosphorylation of myosin while it is still attached to the actin (i.e., in state 3). The dephosphorylated myosin is then predicted to detach from actin much slower than phosphorylated myosin, explaining the slow cross-bridge cycling and hence low ATP use. Dephosphorylated "latch" cross-bridges eventually release from actin and must therefore be rephosphorylated by Ca^{++}-calmodulin–dependent myosin light-chain kinase to bind actin and re-enter state 1, before returning to the latch state.

ATP consumption is reduced during the latch state, such that smooth muscle uses 300-fold less ATP than would be required by skeletal muscle to generate the same force. In addition to the use of ATP for myosin cross-bridge cycling, smooth muscle, like striated muscle, requires ATP for ion transport to maintain the resting membrane potential, to sequester Ca^{++} in the SR, and to extrude Ca^{++} from the cell. All of these metabolic needs are readily met by oxidative phosphorylation. Fatigue of smooth muscle does not occur unless the cell is deprived of oxygen.

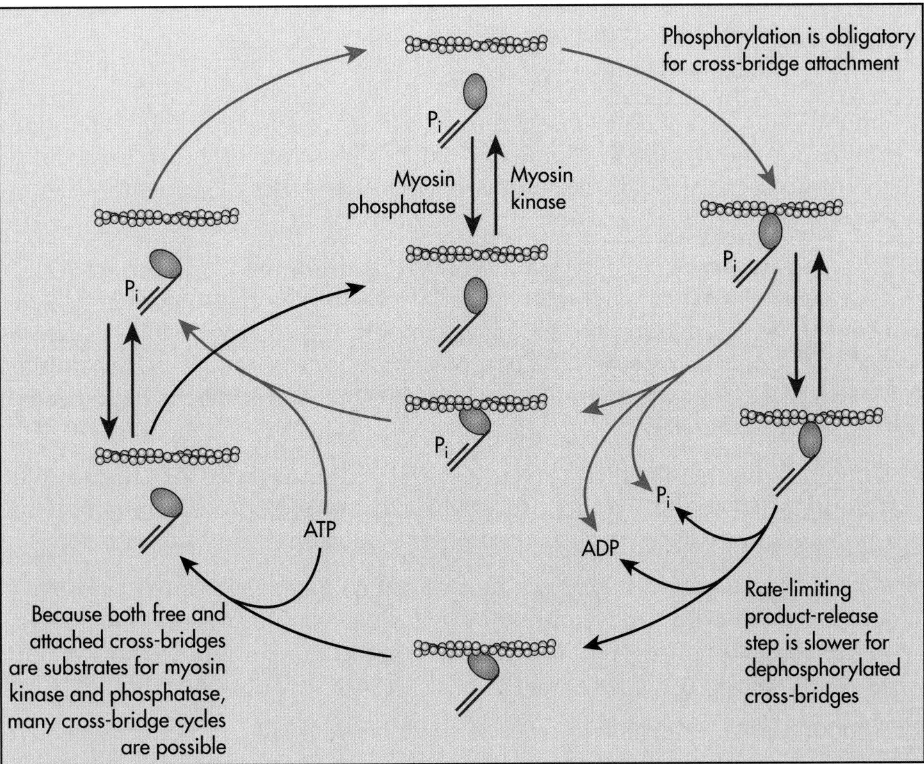

FIGURE 14–6. Tonic smooth muscle can maintain tension at low energy cost because of a transition to a latch state, which is thought to involve dephosphorylation of myosin while it is still attached to actin. Dephosphorylation slows the detachment of myosin from actin, thereby reducing cross-bridge cycling velocity and hence ATP use (see text for details).

The Number and Size of Smooth Muscle Cells Can Increase Under Certain Conditions

During development and growth, the number of smooth muscle cells increases. Smooth muscle tissue mass also increases if an organ is subjected to a sustained increase in mechanical work. This increase in mass is called compensatory hypertrophy. A striking example occurs in the arterial media in hypertension. The increased mechanical load on the muscle cells appears to be the common factor that induces this hypertrophy.

Overstretching of smooth muscle can reduce its ability to contract. For example, when the urethra in a man is compressed because of enlargement of the prostate, urination becomes difficult and the bladder becomes overextended, resulting in urinary bladder hypertrophy. The ability of the smooth muscle to contract is diminished in these distended bladders and is associated with alteration in Ca^{++} mobilization and cross-bridge cycling. Normal contractile function is often restored after alleviation of the compression and obstruction.

Smooth Muscle Cells also Have Synthetic and Secretory Functions

The growth and development of tissues that contain smooth muscles are associated with increases in the connective tissue matrix. Smooth muscle cells can synthesize and secrete the materials that make up this matrix. These components include collagen, elastin, and proteoglycans.

Summary

- Smooth muscle is an involuntary muscle that lacks striations. There are two basic types of smooth muscle, single-unit and multi-unit. Single-unit smooth muscle acts like an electrical syncytium, whereas in multi-unit smooth muscle, cells contract independently. These classifications represent ends of a spectrum, with many smooth muscles exhibiting some degree of coupling.
- Smooth muscles lack sarcomeres, T tubules, and troponin. Smooth muscle, however, contains the functional equivalent of a sarcomere; actin filaments extend from dense bodies, and myosin filaments overlap thin filaments from opposing dense bodies. Smooth muscles also contain caveolae, which are the functional equivalent of T tubules. Contraction of smooth muscle is consistent with the sliding filament theory, but since it lacks troponin, smooth muscle contraction is thick filament regulated, requiring Ca^{++}-dependent myosin phosphorylation.
- Smooth muscle contraction can be initiated with or without a change in membrane potential. The ability of a hormone to contract smooth muscle without changing membrane potential is called pharmacomechanical coupling and typically involves hormonal stimulation of InsP3 production.
- Relaxation of smooth muscle can be induced by a decrease in the cytosolic [Ca^{++}], an increase in cAMP, or an increase in cGMP and is attributable to a decrease in myosin phosphorylation. This decrease in myosin phosphorylation may result from a reduction in the rate of phosphorylation (e.g., at low cytosolic [Ca^{++}] or increased cAMP) or from a stimulation of myosin dephosphorylation (e.g., after elevation of cGMP).
- Smooth muscle exhibits two types of contraction, phasic and tonic. Phasic contraction is characterized by a rapid cycling of the myosin cross-bridges during tension development and shortening. Tonic contraction is characterized by maintenance of tension and is often associated with a transition to the latch state, where the smooth muscle maintains tension at low energy cost because of a decrease in the rate of cross-bridge cycling.

Bibliography

Berridge MJ: Inositol trisphosphate and calcium signalling, *Nature* 361:315, 1993.

Bonnevier J et al: Modulation of Ca^{2+} sensitivity by cyclic nucleotides in smooth muscle from protein kinase G–deficient mice, *J Biol Chem* 279:5146, 2004.

Christ GJ et al: Gap junctions in vascular tissues. Evaluating the role of intercellular communication in the modulation of vasomotor tone, *Circ Res* 79:631, 1996.

Horowitz A et al: Mechanisms of smooth muscle contraction, *Physiol Rev* 76:967, 1996.

Jaggar JH et al: Calcium sparks in smooth muscle, *Am J Physiol Cell Physiol* 278:C235, 2000.

Lotvall J: The long and short of beta$_2$-agonists, *Pulm Pharmacol Ther* 15:497, 2002.

Malmqvist U et al: Slow cycling of unphosphorylated myosin is inhibited by calponin, thus keeping smooth muscle relaxed, *Proc Natl Acad Sci USA* 94:7655, 1997.

Mecham RP et al: Connective tissue production by vascular smooth muscle in development and disease, *Chest* 99(suppl): 43S, 1991.

Murphy RA: What is special about smooth muscle? The significance of covalent crossbridge regulation, *FASEB J* 8:311, 1994.

Owens GK: Regulation of differentiation of vascular smooth muscle cells, *Physiol Rev* 75:487, 1995.

Reed CE: Inhaled corticosteroids: why do physicians and patients fail to comply with guidelines for managing asthma? *Mayo Clin Proc* 79:453, 2004.

Somlyo AP, Somlyo AV: Ca^{2+} sensitivity of smooth muscle and nonmuscle myosin II: modulated by G proteins, kinases, and myosin phosphatase, *Physiol Rev* 83:1325, 2003.

Wellman GC, Nelson MT: Signaling between SR and plasmalemma in smooth muscle: sparks and the activation of Ca^{2+}-sensitive ion channels, *Cell Calcium* 34:211, 2003.

Wellman GC et al: Role of phospholamban in the modulation of arterial Ca^{2+} sparks and Ca^{2+}-activated K^+ channels by cAMP, *Am J Physiol Cell Physiol* 281:C1029, 2001.

Case Studies

Case 14–1

While playing a game of soccer, a 14-year-old girl experiences difficulty in breathing. She exhibits intense anxiety, cyanosis, sweating, and wheezing and has a heart rate of 120 beats/min. A paramedic at the game administers O_2 and then transports her to the hospital. The emergency department physician administers a β_2-adrenergic agonist via an inhaler to relax her bronchiolar smooth muscle. Her breathing improves, but she reports severe fatigue.

1. **The difficulty in breathing before treatment is attributable to which of the following?**
   A. Fatigue of the skeletal muscles involved in breathing
   B. Narrowing of the airways caused by edema
   C. Narrowing of the airways caused by smooth muscle contraction
   D. Decreased levels of ATP in the airway smooth muscle

2. **The β_2-adrenergic agonist was probably able to reverse the difficulty in breathing by which of the following?**
   A. cAMP-dependent phosphorylation of cardiac phospholamban
   B. cGMP-dependent stimulation of airway smooth muscle myosin phosphatase
   C. cAMP-dependent inhibition of airway smooth muscle myosin light-chain kinase
   D. cGMP-dependent stimulation of cardiac sarcolemmal Ca^{++} pump
   E. Phosphorylation of troponin I in cardiac and airway smooth muscle

Case 14–2

A 45-year-old woman told her physician of recurring episodes of cold-induced paleness in her hands, followed by cyanosis, throbbing pain, and then redness. The diagnosis is primary Raynaud's disease.

1. **The cold-induced paleness was caused by which of the following?**
   A. Reduced oxygenation of the blood
   B. Increased oxygen use
   C. Transient vasoconstriction
   D. Transient thrombosis
   E. Increased oxygen dissociation from hemoglobin

2. **The redness of the hands was caused by which of the following?**
   A. An increase in blood flow
   B. Further vasoconstriction
   C. Binding of CO_2 to hemoglobin
   D. A decrease in venous return
   E. Edema

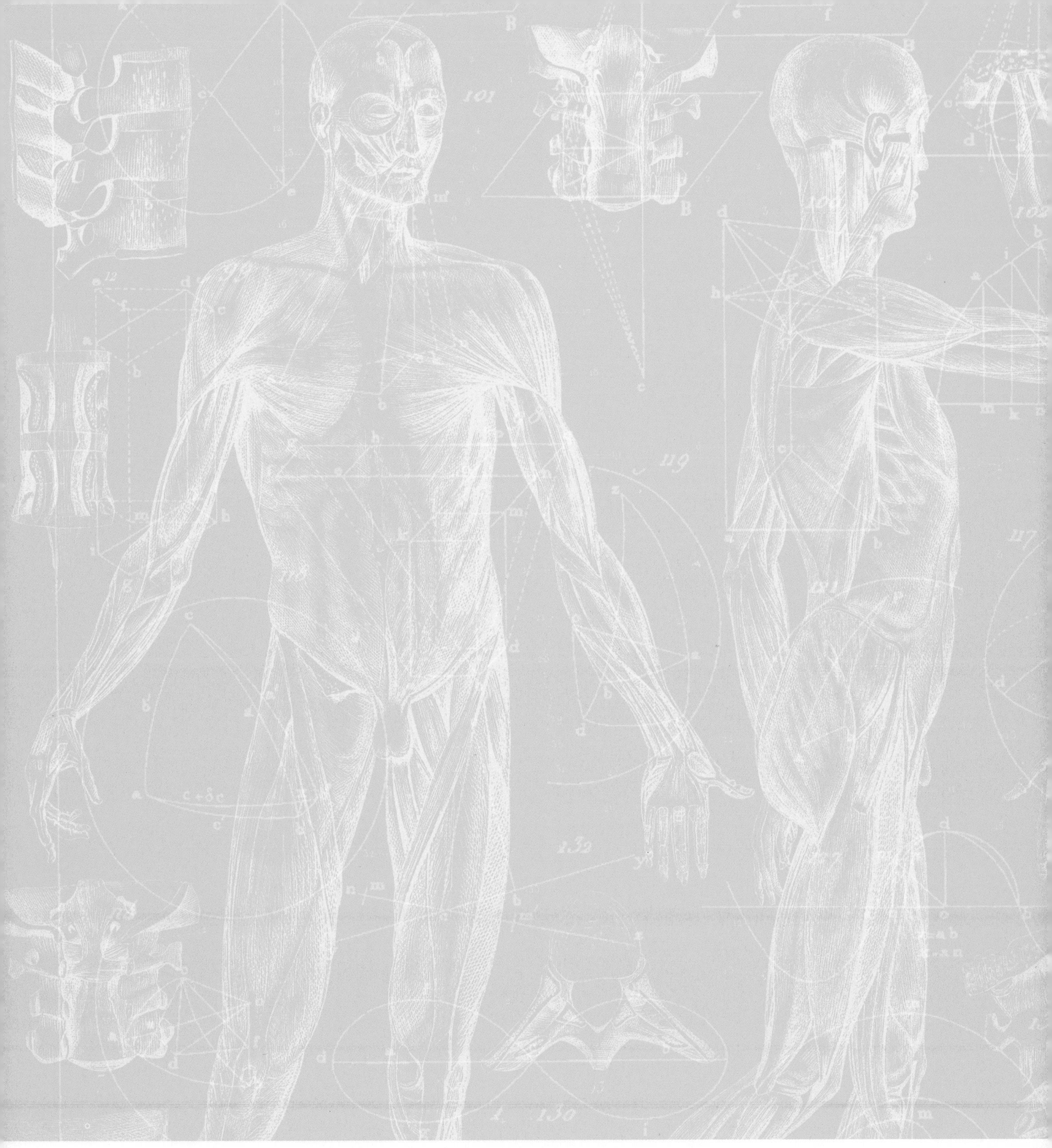

Part Four: Cardiovascular System

Matthew N. Levy and Achilles Pappano

Chapter 15: Overview of the Circulation, Blood, and Hemostasis

Objectives

- Describe the compositions and functions of the blood vessels.
- Define the relationship of the vascular cross-sectional area to the velocity of blood flow in the various vascular segments.
- Explain the pressure changes and pathways of blood flow throughout the vasculature.
- Describe the constituents of blood.
- Explain the functions of the cellular elements of blood.
- Describe the importance of blood group matching before blood transfusions.
- Explain the factors involved in hemostasis, blood coagulation, and clot lysis.

The Heart and Blood Vessels Form the Circulatory System

The circulatory, endocrine, and nervous systems constitute the principal integrating systems of the body. The nervous system facilitates communications, and the endocrine glands regulate certain body functions. The circulatory system (Figure 15–1) is made up essentially of a pump (the **heart**) and a complex series of distributing and collecting tubes (the **blood vessels**). The heart and blood vessels transport essential substances to the various tissues throughout the body and remove the byproducts of metabolism. The circulatory system also participates in certain homeostatic mechanisms, such as the regulation of body temperature, the maintenance of body fluids, and the supply of oxygen and nutrients under various physiological conditions.

The pumping action of the heart and the extensive system of thin blood vessels (the capillaries) permit the rapid exchange of vital substances between the vascular channels and the tissues. In this chapter, the function and regulation of these structures are discussed. The heart and blood vessels can regulate the responses of the tissues to any changes in physiological and pathological conditions by altering the flow of blood to the various tissues. This chapter provides a general, functional overview of the circulatory system; the functions of the various components of the circulatory system are discussed later.

The Heart Is Composed of Two Pumps

The mechanical contractions of the heart constitute two pumps in series (Figure 15–1). One pump, the **right ventricle,** propels blood through the blood vessels in the lungs (the **pulmonary circulation**) and thereby accomplishes the local exchanges of oxygen and carbon dioxide. The second pump, the

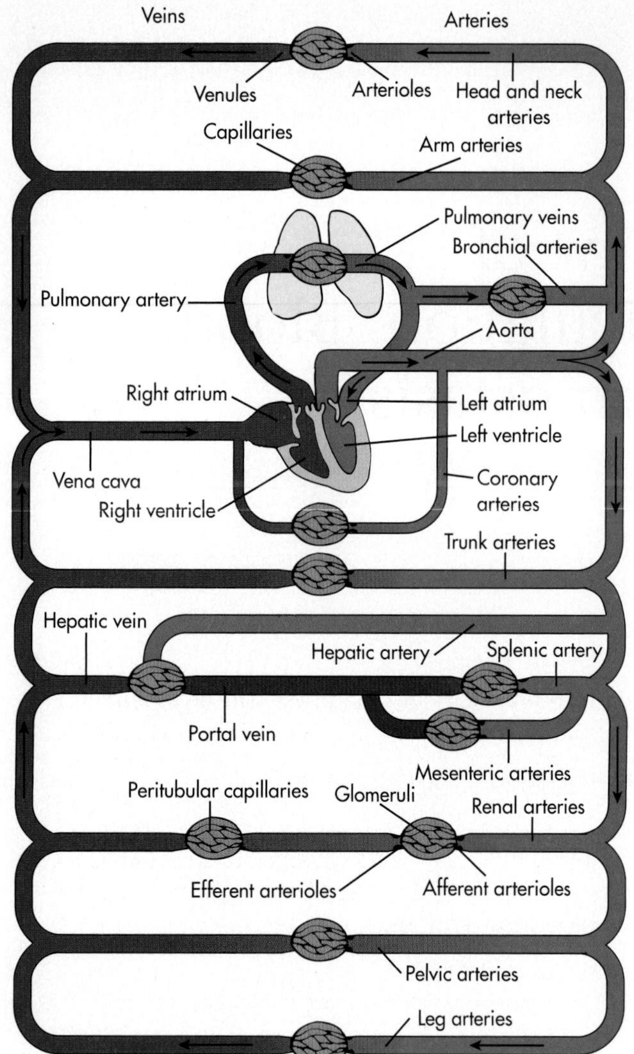

FIGURE 15–1. Parallel and series arrangement of the vessels making up the circulatory system. The capillary beds are represented by thin lines connecting the arteries *(red)* with the veins *(blue)*. The black, crescent-shaped thickenings proximal to the capillary beds represent the arterioles (resistance vessels). (Redrawn from Green HD. In Glasser O, ed: *Medical physics, vol 1,* Chicago, 1944, Mosby.)

left ventricle, propels blood through the blood vessels (the **systemic circulation**) in the other tissues of the body. The flow of blood generated by the heart is unidirectional as a consequence of the **flap valves** in the heart. Although the blood flow generated by each ventricle is intermittent, the blood flows continuously through the blood vessels in the peripheral tissues. This flow is continuous because the large stroke volume ejected by each cardiac contraction distends the aorta and its branches after each ventricular contraction **(systole).** The elastic recoil of the distended arterial walls propels the blood forward during ventricular relaxation **(diastole)** (see also Figure 18–8 in Chapter 18).

Blood Vessels Connect the Heart with Organs

Blood moves rapidly through the aorta and its arterial branches. These branches narrow and their walls become thinner as they approach the periphery. The vessels also change structurally. The large-diameter aorta is predominantly an elastic structure, but the small peripheral arterioles are much less distensible **(Figure 15–2)**.

In the large arteries, frictional resistance **(viscosity)** to blood flow is not pronounced, and pressures are only slightly less than in the aorta **(Figure 15–3)**. However, IN THE SMALL ARTERIES AND ARTERIOLES, RESISTANCE TO BLOOD FLOW IS LARGE, AND THE PRESSURE DROP ACROSS THESE VESSELS IS ALSO LARGE. This resistance to blood flow reaches a maximal level in the small arterioles, which are sometimes referred to as the stopcocks of the vascular system. Hence, the pressure drop is greatest across the terminal segment of the small arteries.

In addition to the reduction in pressure along the arterioles, there is a change from a pulsatile to a steady blood flow **(Figure 15–4)**. THE PULSATILE ARTERIAL BLOOD FLOW, CAUSED BY THE INTERMITTENT EJECTION OF BLOOD FROM THE HEART, IS DAMPED AT THE CAPILLARY LEVEL BY A COMBINATION OF TWO FACTORS: **DISTENSIBILITY** OF THE LARGE ARTERIES AND **FRICTIONAL RESISTANCE** IN THE SMALL ARTERIES AND ARTERIOLES.

In a patient with hyperthyroidism **(Graves' disease),** the basal metabolism (i.e., the total rate of calorie use) is elevated, and the systemic arterioles are usually dilated substantially. The consequent reduction in arteriolar resistance diminishes the damping effect on the pulsatile arterial pressure. This vasodilatation is often manifested as pulsatile flow in the capillaries, which is often observed in the fingernail bed of patients with this ailment.

Many capillaries arise from each arteriole. The total cross-sectional area of the capillary bed is very large, despite the fact that the cross-sectional area of each capillary is much less than that of each arteriole. Consequently, blood flow velocity is very slow in the capillaries. This diminished flow velocity is analogous to the sluggish rate of flow in the wide regions of a tube (see Figure 20–1 in Chapter 20). Conditions in the capillaries are ideal for the exchange of diffusible substances between blood and tissues because capillaries are short tubes with very thin walls and because flow velocity is so slow.

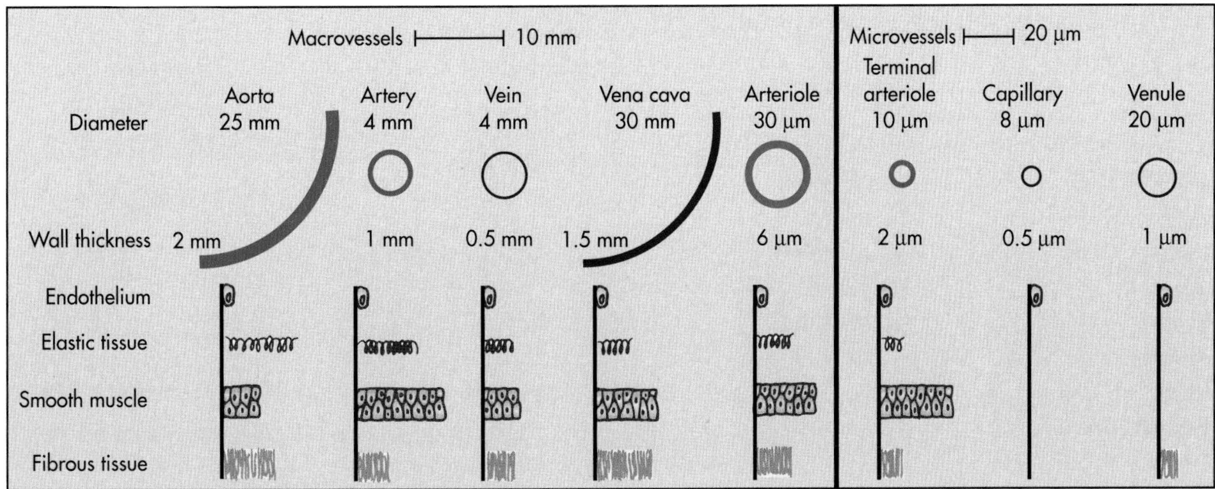

FIGURE 15–2. Internal diameter, wall thickness, and relative amounts of the principal components of the vessel walls of the various blood vessels that make up the circulatory system. Cross sections of the vessels are not drawn to scale because of the huge range from the aorta and venae cavae to the capillaries. (Redrawn from Burton AC: *Physiol Rev* 34:619, 1954.)

On its return to the heart from the capillaries, blood passes through venules and then through veins of increasing size. Pressure within these vessels decreases progressively until the blood reaches the right atrium (Figure 15–3). Near the heart, the number of veins decreases, the wall thickness and composition of the veins change, the total cross-sectional area of the venous channels diminishes, and the velocity of blood flow increases (Figure 15–4). Note that the velocity of blood flow and the cross-sectional area at each level of the vasculature are essentially mirror images (Figure 15–4).

Data from a 20-kg dog **(Table 15–1)** indicate that the number of vessels between the aorta and the capillaries increases about 3 billion–fold and the total cross-sectional area increases about 500-fold. The fractional volume of blood in the systemic vascular system is greatest (67%) in the veins and venules. Only 5% of the total blood volume exists in the capillaries, and 11% of the total blood volume is located in the aorta, arteries, and arterioles. In contrast, the blood volume in the pulmonary vascular bed is about equally divided among the arterial, capillary, and venous blood vessels. The cross-sectional areas of the venae cavae

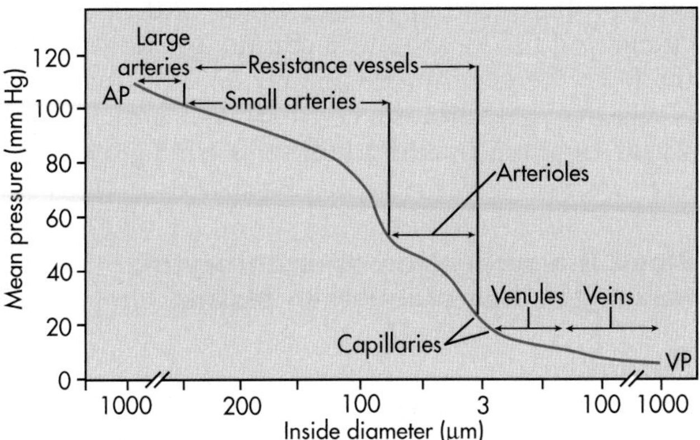

FIGURE 15–3. Pressure drop across the vascular system in the hamster cheek pouch. AP, mean arterial pressure; VP, venous pressure. (Redrawn from Davis MJ et al: *Am J Physiol* 250:H291, 1986.)

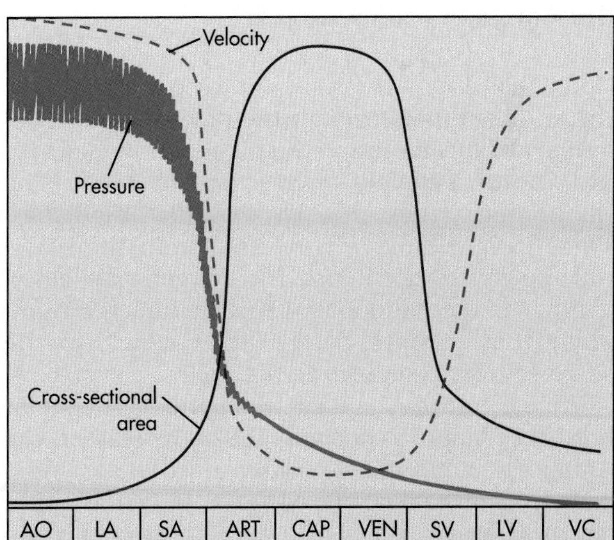

FIGURE 15–4. Phasic pressure, velocity of flow, and cross-sectional area of the systemic circulation. The important features are the inverse relationship among velocity and the cross-sectional area, the major pressure drop across the small arteries and arterioles, and the maximal cross-sectional area and minimal flow rate in the capillaries. AO, aorta; LA, large arteries; SA, small arteries; ART, arterioles; CAP, capillaries; VEN, venules; SV, small veins; LV, large veins; VC, venae cavae.

TABLE 15–1. VASCULAR DIMENSIONS IN A 20-KG DOG

Vessels	No.	Total Cross-sectional Area (cm^2)	Total Blood Volume (%)
Systemic			
Aorta	1	2.8	
Arteries	40-110,000	40	11
Arterioles	2.8×10^6	55	
Capillaries	2.7×10^9	1357	5
Venules	1×10^7	785	
Veins	660,000-110	631	67
Venae cavae	2	3.1	
Pulmonary			
Arteries and arterioles	$1\text{-}1.5 \times 10^6$	137	3
Capillaries	2.7×10^9	1357	4
Venules and veins	1×10^6	210	5
Heart			
Atria	2		
Ventricles	2		5

exceed the cross-sectional area of the aorta. Therefore, the velocity of flow is slower in the venae cavae than in the aorta (Figure 15–4).

How Does Blood Move Through the Cardiovascular Circuit?

Blood that enters the right ventricle via the right atrium is pumped through the pulmonary arterial system at a mean pressure that is about one seventh that in the systemic arteries (Figure 15–1). The blood then passes through the lung capillaries, where carbon dioxide is released from the blood and oxygen is taken up. The oxygen-rich blood returns via the pulmonary veins to the left atrium, where it is pumped by the left ventricle to the periphery, thus completing the cycle.

In the normal, intact circulation, the total volume of blood is constant, and an increase in the volume of blood in one region must be accompanied by an equivalent decrease in some other region. However, the distribution of the circulating blood to the various regions of the body is determined by the output of the left ventricle and by the contractile state of the arterioles in these regions. THE CIRCULATORY SYSTEM IS COMPOSED OF CONDUITS THAT ARE ARRANGED IN SERIES AND IN PARALLEL (Figure 15–1). This arrangement, which is discussed earlier, has important implications for the blood flow, the resistance to flow, and the pressure in the various blood vessels.

Blood and Hemostasis

The main function of the circulating blood is to carry oxygen and nutrients to the various tissues in the body and to remove carbon dioxide and waste products from those tissues. Furthermore, blood transports other substances, such as hormones, white blood cells, and platelets, from their sites of production to their sites of action. Blood also aids in the distribution of fluids, solutes, and heat. Hence, blood contributes to **homeostasis,** which is the maintenance of a constant internal environment.

Blood consists of red blood cells, white blood cells, and platelets. These components are suspended in a complex solution **(plasma)** of various salts, proteins, carbohydrates, lipids, and gases. The circulating blood volume accounts for about 7% of the body weight. Approximately 55% of the blood is plasma; the protein content is 7 g/dL (about 4 g/dL of albumin and 3 g/dL of plasma globulins).

Blood is a suspension of erythrocytes, leukocytes, and platelets in plasma

Erythrocytes

The erythrocytes (red blood cells) are flexible, biconcave disks that transport oxygen to the body tissues (**Figure 15–5**). Mammalian erythrocytes are unusual in that they lack a nucleus. The average erythrocyte is 7 μm in diameter. Erythrocytes arise from **pluripotential stem cells** in the bone

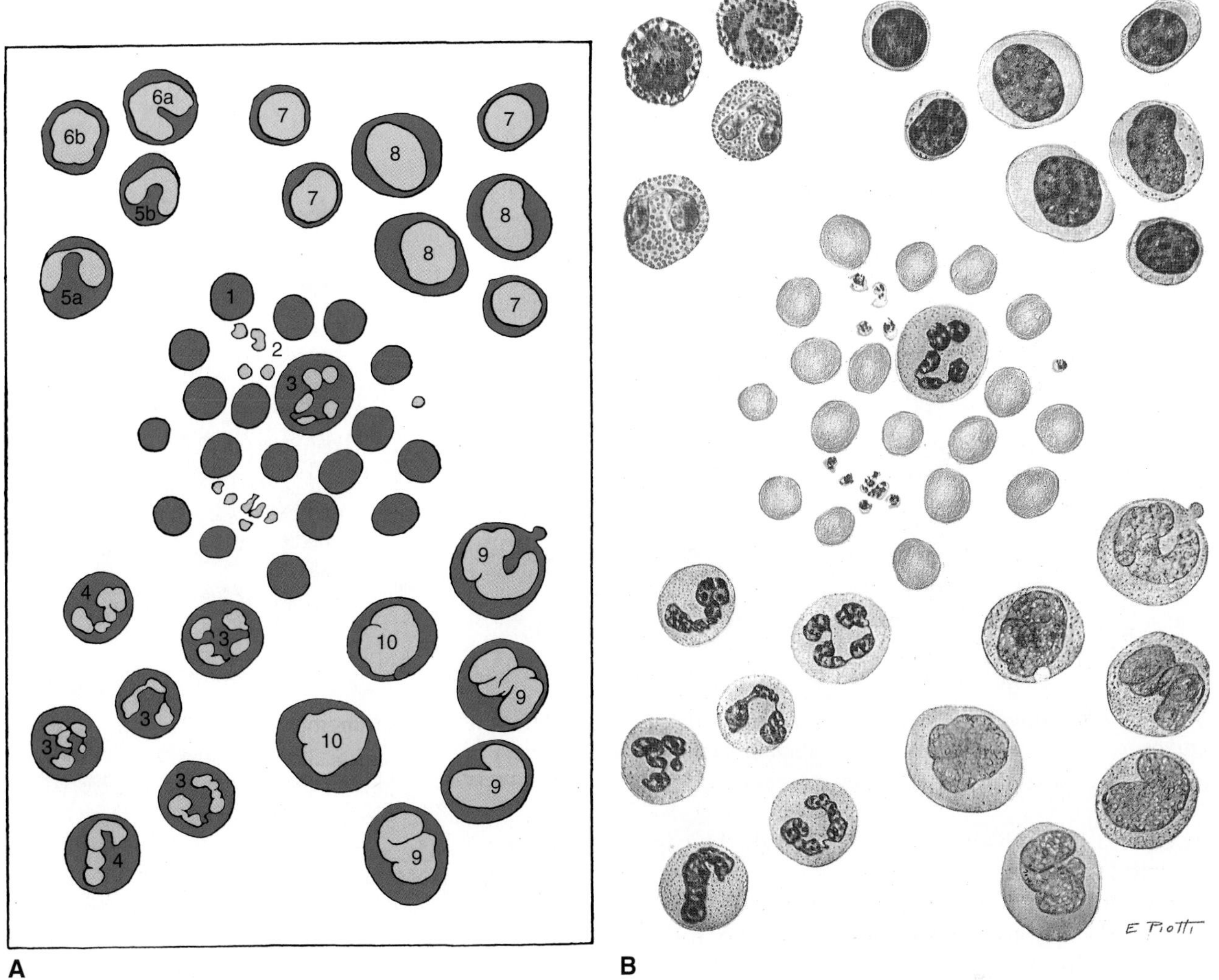

FIGURE 15–5. The morphology of blood cells. 1, normal red cells; 2, platelets; 3, neutrophils; 4, neutrophil, band form; 5a, eosinophil, two lobes; 5b, eosinophil, band form; 6a, basophil, band form; 6b, metamyelocyte, basophilic; 7, lymphocyte, small; 8, lymphocyte, large; 9, monocyte, mature; 10, monocytes, young. (From Daland GA: *A color atlas of morphologic hematology,* Cambridge, Mass, 1951, Harvard University Press.)

marrow. All of the cells in the circulating blood are derived from these stem cells. Most of these immature cells develop into various forms of developed cells, such as **erythrocytes, monocytes, megakaryocytes,** and **lymphocytes.** During maturation, the erythrocytes lose their nuclei before these cells enter the circulation, and their average life span is 120 days. Approximately 5 million erythrocytes are present per microliter of blood. However, a small fraction of the pluripotential stem cells remain in their undifferentiated state.

The main protein in the erythrocytes is **hemoglobin** (about 15 g/dL of blood). Hemoglobin consists of **heme,** which is an iron-containing tetrapyrrole (see Chapter 30). Heme is linked to **globin,** a protein composed of four polypeptide chains (two α chains and two β chains in the normal adult). The iron moiety of hemoglobin binds loosely and reversibly to oxygen to form oxyhemoglobin. The affinity of hemoglobin for oxygen is affected by pH, temperature, and 2,3-diphosphoglycerate concentration. These factors facilitate oxygen uptake in the lungs and its release in the tissues.

Changes in the polypeptide subunits of globin affect the affinity of hemoglobin for oxygen. For example, fetal hemoglobin has two γ chains instead of two β chains. This substitution increases its affinity for oxygen. Changes in the polypeptide subunits of globin may induce certain serious diseases, such as **sickle cell anemia** and **erythroblastosis fetalis** (Figure 15–6). Sickle cell anemia is a disorder associated with the presence of **hemoglobin S,** which is an abnormal form of hemoglobin in the erythrocytes. Many of the erythrocytes in the bloodstream of patients with sickle cell anemia have a sickle-like shape (Figure 15–6). Consequently, many

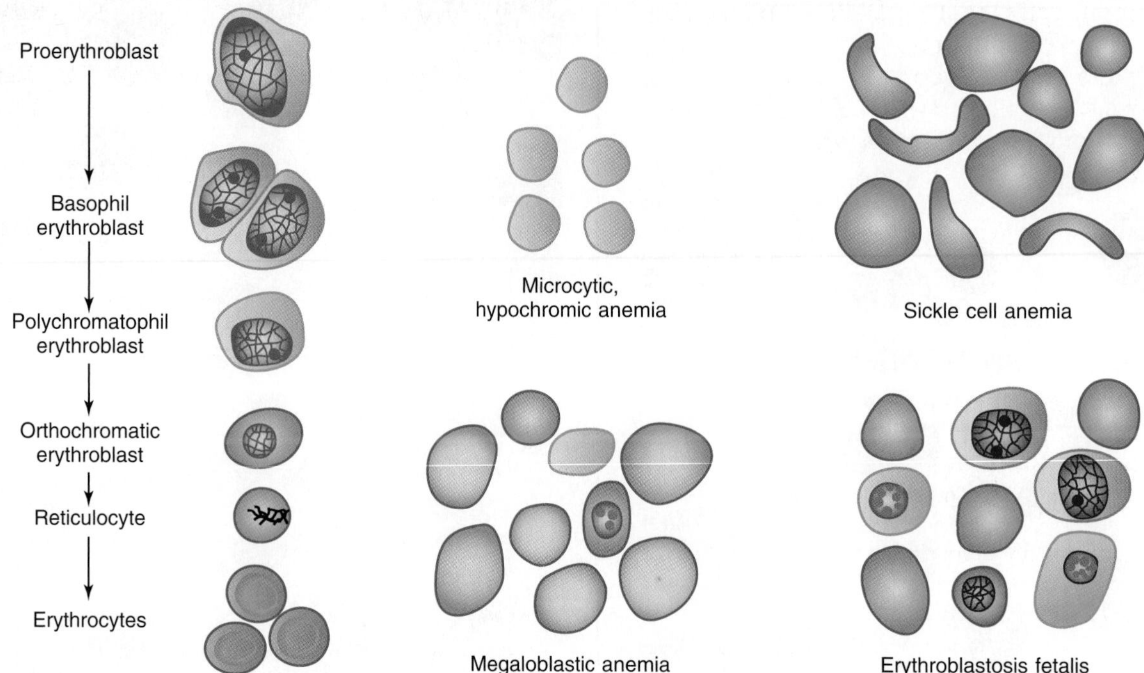

FIGURE 15–6. Genesis of red blood cells and red blood cells in different types of anemias. (From Guyton AC, Hall JE: *Textbook of medical physiology,* ed 10, Philadelphia, 2000, WB Saunders.)

of the abnormal cells cannot pass through the capillaries and therefore cannot deliver adequate oxygen and nutrients to the local tissues. **Thalassemia** is also a genetic disorder of the globin genes; α and β forms exist. In either case, the disorder leads ultimately to a **microcytic** (small-cell), **hypochromic** (inadequate quantity of hemoglobin) anemia (see the upper, central panel of Figure 15–6).

The number of circulating red cells normally remains fairly constant. The production of erythrocytes **(erythropoiesis)** is regulated by the glycoprotein **erythropoietin,** which is secreted mainly by the kidneys. Erythropoietin enhances erythrocyte production by accelerating the differentiation of stem cells in the bone marrow. This substance is often used clinically to increase red blood cell production in anemic patients.

Anemia and chronic hypoxia are prevalent in people who live at high altitudes. Such conditions tend to stimulate erythrocyte production and thereby induce **polycythemia,** which is an abnormally high quantity of circulating red blood cells. When the subjects return to lower altitudes, the elevated red blood cell concentration inhibits erythropoiesis. The red blood cell count is also greatly increased in **polycythemia vera,** a disease of unknown cause. The elevated erythrocyte concentration in this disease increases blood viscosity and thereby impairs the flow to vital tissues.

Leukocytes

There are normally 4000 to 10,000 leukocytes (white blood cells) per microliter of blood. Leukocytes include granulocytes (65%), lymphocytes (30%), and monocytes (5%). Of the granulocytes, about 95% are neutrophils, 4% are eosinophils, and 1% are basophils. White blood cells originate from the primitive stem cells in the bone marrow. After birth, granulocytes and monocytes in humans continue to originate in the bone marrow, whereas lymphocytes originate in the lymph nodes, spleen, and thymus.

Granulocytes and monocytes are motile, nucleated cells that contain **lysosomes,** which in turn contain enzymes capable of digesting foreign material such as microorganisms, damaged cells, and cellular debris. Thus, leukocytes constitute a major defense mechanism against infections. Microorganisms or the products of cell destruction release **chemotactic substances** that attract granulocytes and monocytes. When migrating leukocytes reach the foreign agents, they engulf them **(phagocytosis)** and then destroy them by the action of enzymes that form **oxygen-derived free radicals** and **hydrogen peroxide** (Figure 15–5).

Lymphocytes. Lymphocytes vary in size and have large nuclei. Most lymphocytes lack cytoplasmic granules (Figure 15–5). The two main types of lymphocytes are **B lymphocytes,** which are responsible for **humoral immunity,** and **T lymphocytes,** which are responsible for cell-mediated immunity. When lymphocytes are stimulated by an **antigen** (a foreign protein on the surface of a microorganism or allergen), the B lymphocytes are transformed into **plasma cells,** which synthesize and release antibodies **(gamma globulins).** Antibodies are carried by the bloodstream to a site of infection, where they "tag" foreign invaders for destruction by other components of the immune system.

The principal T lymphocytes are cytotoxic, and they also provide long-term protection against certain viruses, bacteria, and cancer cells. These T lymphocytes may also reject various surgically transplanted organs. Specific T lymphocytes, called **helper T cells,** activate B cells, whereas **suppressor T cells** inhibit B-cell activity. Other types of B and T lymphocytes, called **memory cells,** serve to "remember" specific antigens. These cells can quickly generate an immune response when they are exposed to the specific antigen. Protection against several infectious diseases has been achieved by injection of an appropriate antigen. Also, protective **vaccines** have been developed by the injection of killed or attenuated organisms into suitable hosts, such as horses and sheep. Such vaccines stimulate the production of specific antibodies against a particular microorganism.

Platelets

Platelets are small (3-μm) nuclear cell fragments of **megakaryocytes,** which reside in the bone marrow. When the megakaryocytes mature, they fragment into platelets, which enter the circulation. The platelets are important in hemostasis, as discussed later.

Blood is divided into groups by antigens located on erythrocytes

FOUR PRINCIPAL BLOOD GROUPS, DESIGNATED O, A, B, AND AB, PREVAIL IN HUMAN SUBJECTS. EACH GROUP IS IDENTIFIED BY THE TYPE OF ANTIGEN THAT IS PRESENT ON THE ERYTHROCYTE. People with type A blood have A antigens; those with type B blood have B antigens; those with type AB have both A and B antigens; and those with type O have neither antigen. The plasma of group O blood contains antibodies to A, B, and AB.

Group A plasma contains antibodies to B antigens, and group B plasma contains antibodies to A antigens. Group AB plasma has no antibodies to O, A, or B antigens. In blood transfusions, cross-matching is necessary to prevent agglutination of donor red cells by antibodies in the plasma of the recipient. Because plasma of groups A, B, and AB has no antibodies to group O erythrocytes, people with group O blood are called **universal donors.** Conversely, persons with AB blood are called **universal recipients** because their plasma has no antibodies to the antigens of the other three groups. In addition to the ABO blood grouping, there are **Rh (Rhesus factor)–positive** and **Rh-negative groups.**

An Rh-negative person can develop antibodies to Rh-positive red blood cells if that person is exposed to Rh-positive blood. During pregnancy, for example, a mother who is Rh negative can make antibodies for Rh-positive cells if the fetus is Rh positive (inherited from the father). Rh-positive red cells from the fetus can enter the maternal bloodstream at the time of placental separation and induce Rh-positive antibodies in the mother's plasma. The Rh-positive antibodies from the mother can also reach the fetus via the placenta and can agglutinate and hemolyze fetal red blood cells. This condition is known as **erythroblastosis fetalis,** a hemolytic disease of the newborn (Figure 15–6).

Hemostasis is achieved by vasoconstriction, platelet aggregation, and coagulation of the blood

Hemostasis is defined as the arrest of bleeding. When blood vessels are damaged, bleeding may occur. The following three processes may act to stem the flow of blood: vasoconstriction, platelet aggregation, and blood coagulation.

Vasoconstriction

Physical injury to a blood vessel elicits a contractile response **(vasoconstriction)** of the vascular smooth muscle and thus a narrowing of the vessel. Vasoconstriction in severed arterioles can close the vascular lumen completely and stop the flow of blood. The contraction of the vascular smooth muscle is caused principally by the direct mechanical stimulation of the perivascular nerves.

Platelet aggregation

Damage to the endothelium of a blood vessel causes platelets to adhere to the site of injury. The adherent platelets release **adenosine diphosphate** and **thromboxane A_2,** which cause additional platelets to adhere. The aggregation of platelets may continue in this manner until some of the small blood vessels become blocked by the mass of aggregated platelets. Platelets are prevented from aggregating along the length of a normal vessel by the antiaggregation action of **prostacyclin.** This substance is released from the normal endothelial cells in the adjacent, uninjured part of the vessel. Platelets also release **serotonin (5-hydroxytryptamine),** which enhances vasoconstriction, and **thromboplastin,** which hastens blood coagulation.

Bleeding is an important clinical problem, and trauma is the most common cause of bleeding. Gastrointestinal bleeding can also occur, and it can cause severe anemia or cardiovascular shock. Occult blood in the stool can be the first sign of **peptic ulcer** or of **intestinal bleeding.** When the platelet count is low, as in **thrombocytopenic purpura,** tiny hemorrhages **(petechiae)** or larger hemorrhages **(ecchymoses)** may appear in the skin and mucous membranes. Bleeding occurs into the tissues (especially the joints) in **hemophilia,** a hereditary disease. This disease occurs only in males, but the genetic abnormality is carried by females.

Blood coagulation

Clotting of blood is a complex process consisting of the sequential activation of various factors in the blood. The cascade of reactions in which one activated factor activates another is depicted in **Figure 15–7.** Several of the factors are synthesized in the liver, as is vitamin K, which is essential for the synthesis of these liver-derived clotting factors.

THE KEY STEP IN BLOOD CLOTTING IS THE CONVERSION OF FIBRINOGEN TO FIBRIN BY THROMBIN. The clot formed by this reaction consists of a dense network of fibrin strands in which blood cells and plasma are trapped **(Figure 15–8)**. The two blood coagulation pathways, the **extrinsic pathway** and the **intrinsic pathway,** converge on the activation of factor X, which catalyzes the cleavage of prothrombin to thrombin (Figure 15–7). Tissue damage and the release of tissue thromboplastin initiate blood clotting via the extrinsic pathway. Blood clotting via the intrinsic pathway is initiated by exposure of the blood to a negatively charged surface. This can occur within blood vessels when the endothelium is damaged and blood comes in contact with collagen. It can also occur outside the body when blood comes in contact with negatively charged surfaces such as glass. If blood is carefully

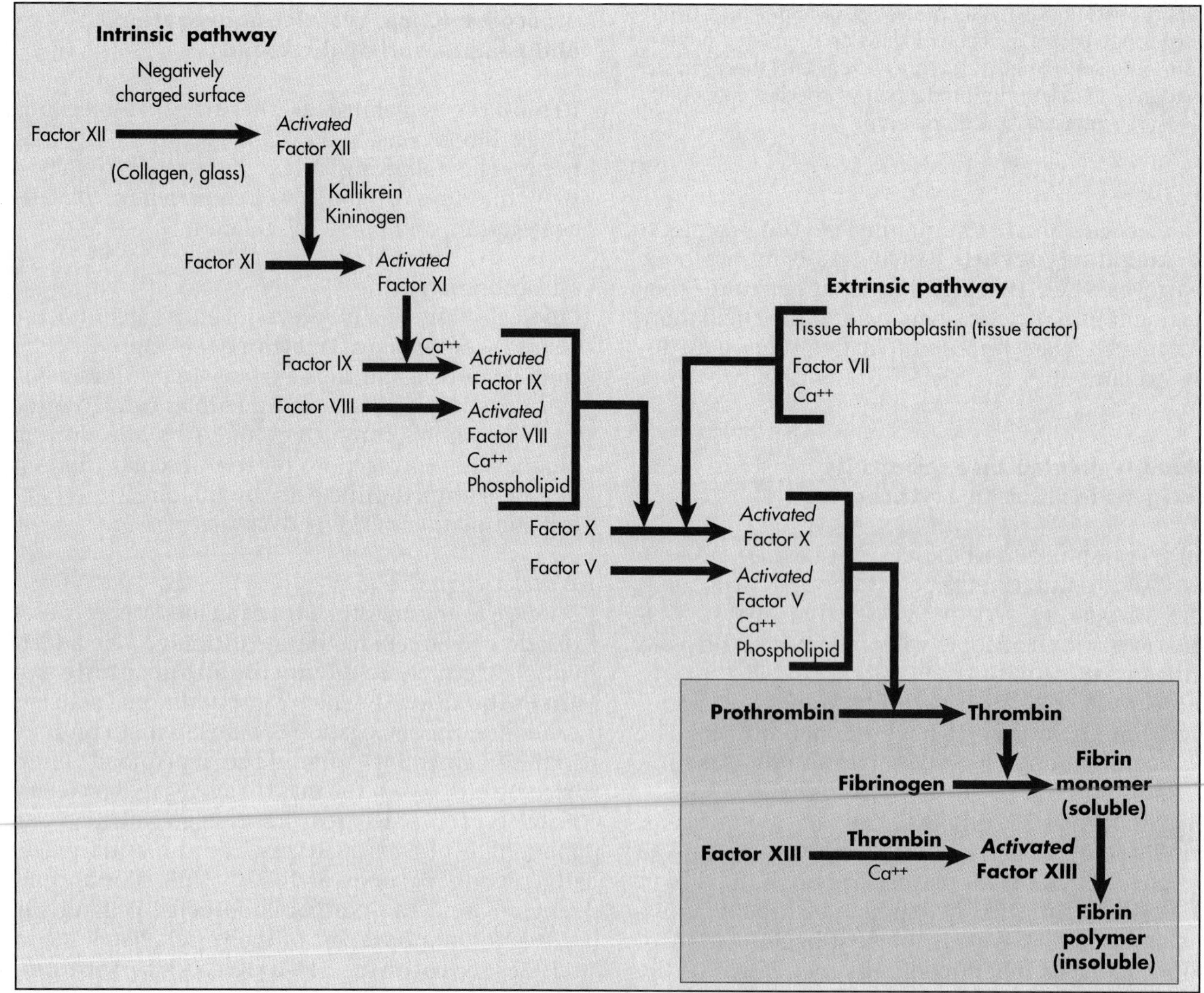

FIGURE 15–7. Intrinsic and extrinsic pathways in the formation of a fibrin clot.

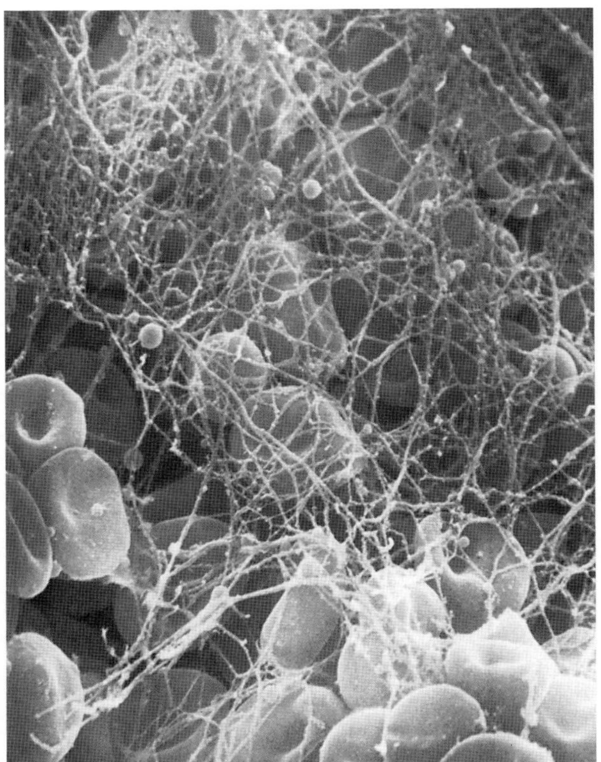

FIGURE 15–8. Scanning electron micrograph of a human blood clot showing red blood cells immobilized within a network of fibrin threads. The small spheres are platelets. (Magnification ×9000.) (From Shelly WB: *JAMA* 249:3089, 1983.)

drawn into a syringe coated with silicone, clotting is greatly delayed.

After a clot is formed, the actin and myosin of the platelets trapped in the fibrin mesh interact in a manner similar to that in muscle. The resultant contraction pulls the fibrin strands toward the platelets and thereby extrudes the **serum** (plasma without fibrinogen) and shrinks the clot. The process is called **clot retraction.** The function of clot retraction is not clear, but it may serve to approximate the edges of severed blood vessels.

Several cofactors are required for blood coagulation (Figure 15–7); the most important is Ca^{++}. If Ca^{++} in the blood is removed or bound, coagulation does not occur.

Blood clots can be lysed, and blood coagulation can be prevented

Clot lysis

Normal blood contains **plasminogen,** an inactive precursor of the proteolytic enzyme **plasmin.** Activators of the conversion of plasminogen to plasmin are found in tissues, plasma, and urine **(urokinase).**

Exogenous plasminogen activators such as **streptokinase** and **tissue plasminogen activator** are used clinically to dissolve intravascular clots. This treatment is used especially to dissolve clots in the coronary arteries of patients with acute **myocardial infarction** (damage to the heart muscle that is most frequently caused by a clot in a major coronary artery).

Anticoagulants

Blood coagulation can be prevented in vitro by the addition of citrate or oxalate, which removes Ca^{++} from the solution. For rapid in vivo anticoagulation, **heparin,** a sulfated polysaccharide produced by mast cells, is injected intravenously.

Heparin is used in extracorporeal circuits during open-heart surgery and in the prevention of intravascular clot extension. For prolonged anticoagulation, **dicumarol** is used. This drug inhibits the synthesis of vitamin K–dependent factors and is used for treatment of conditions such as **thrombophlebitis** (inflammation of a vein associated with an intravascular blood clot).

Summary

- The circulatory system consists of a pump (the heart), a series of distributing and collecting tubes (blood vessels), and an extensive system of thin vessels that permit rapid exchange of substances between the tissues and blood.
- Blood pressure decreases progressively from the aorta to the venae cavae. The greatest resistance to blood flow, and hence the greatest pressure drop, in the arterial system occurs at the level of the small arteries and the arterioles.
- Pulsatile pressure is progressively damped by the elasticity of the arteriolar walls and the frictional resistance to blood flow in the small arteries and arterioles. Hence, capillary blood flow is essentially nonpulsatile.
- The velocity of blood flow is inversely related to the total cross-sectional area of the vasculature at any downstream point along the vascular system.

- Most of the blood in the vascular bed is in the venous side of the circulation.
- Blood consists of red cells (erythrocytes), white cells (leukocytes and lymphocytes), and platelets, all suspended in a solution containing salts, proteins, carbohydrates, and lipids.
- There are four major blood groups: O, A, B, and AB. Type O blood can be given to people with any of the blood groups because the plasma of all of the blood groups lacks antibodies to type O red cells. Hence, people with type O blood are referred to as universal donors. By the same token, people with AB blood are referred to as universal recipients because their plasma lacks antibodies to red cells of all of the blood groups. In addition to O, A, B, and AB blood groups, there are Rh-positive and Rh-negative blood groups.
- A cascade of reactions that constitute an intrinsic pathway and an extrinsic pathway is involved in blood coagulation. The final steps in which the two pathways join are the conversion of prothrombin to thrombin and the conversion of fibrinogen to fibrin, a reaction catalyzed by thrombin.
- Blood clots may be liquefied by plasmin, a proteolytic enzyme whose formation from plasminogen is catalyzed by tissue activators (e.g., urokinase) or exogenous activators (e.g., streptokinase, tissue plasminogen activator).

Bibliography

Christensen KL, Mulvany MJ: Location of resistance arteries, *J Vasc Res* 38:1, 2001.

Le DT et al: Hemostatic factors in rabbit limb lymph: relationship to mechanisms regulating extravascular coagulation, *Am J Physiol* 274:H769, 1998.

Lozano M, Cid J: The clinical implications of platelet transfusions associated with ABO or Rh(D) incompatibility, *Transfus Med Rev* 17:57, 2003.

Mannucci PM: Hemostatic drugs, *N Engl J Med* 339:245, 1998.

Pugsley MK, Tabrizchi R: The vascular system. An overview of structure and function, *J Pharmacol Toxicol Methods* 44:333, 2000.

Reid ME, Lomas-Francis C: Molecular approaches to blood group identification, *Curr Opin Hematol* 9:152, 2002.

Urbaniak SJ, Greiss MA: RhD haemolytic disease of the fetus and the newborn, *Blood Rev* 14:44, 2000.

Yamomoto F: Molecular genetics of ABO, *Vox Sang* 78(suppl 2):91, 2000.

Case Studies

Case 15–1

After a knife wound to the groin, a man develops a large arteriovenous shunt between the iliac artery and vein.

1. **Which of the following changes will occur in his systemic circulation?**
   A. Blood flow in the capillaries of the fingernail bed will be pulsatile.
   B. The circulation time (antecubital vein to tongue) is decreased.
   C. The arterial pulse pressure (systolic pressure minus diastolic pressure) is decreased.
   D. The greatest velocity of blood flow prevails in the vena cava.
   E. Pressure in the right atrium is greater than in the inferior vena cava.

2. **As a consequence of the arteriovenous shunt between iliac artery and vein:**
   A. Perfusion of the coronary artery bed will diminish.
   B. Blood flow to the cerebral arteries decreases.
   C. Blood is shunted from a muscular artery to a muscular vein.
   D. Perfusion of the involved leg capillaries increases.
   E. Intravascular pressure in the iliac vein decreases.

Case 15–2

A 30-year-old man has a long history of epigastric pain that is relieved by eating food, drinking milk, or taking antacid tablets. He went to see his physician because of 3 weeks of progressive fatigue and shortness of breath on exertion. Physical examination revealed only severe pallor and a rapid heart rate. A stool sample was black and guaiac positive (indicative of blood in stool).

1. **A peripheral blood examination showed which of the following?**
   A. Red cells of uniform size
   B. A hematocrit of 45%
   C. A red cell count of 5 million cells/mm^3
   D. Blood hemoglobin of 6 g/dL
   E. A normal hemoglobin/red cell ratio

2. **The blood vessel from which bleeding occurs is found where?**
   A. In the splanchnic circulation to the large intestine
   B. In the renal arteries to glomeruli
   C. In the pelvic arteries to the urinary bladder
   D. In the splanchnic vessels to the gastric artery
   E. In the iliac artery to the leg

Chapter 16: Electrical Activity of the Heart

Objectives

- ❖ Explain the types of cardiac action potentials.
- ❖ Define the ionic basis of cardiac action potentials.
- ❖ Explain the temporal changes in cardiac excitability.

Two centuries ago, Galvani and Volta demonstrated that electrical phenomena are involved in the spontaneous contractions of the heart. In 1855, Kölliker and Müller reported that when they placed the nerve of an innervated skeletal muscle in contact with the surface of a beating frog's heart, the skeletal muscle twitched with each cardiac contraction. These investigators concluded that the spontaneous excitation of the heart had generated sufficient electrical activity to excite the motor nerve fibers and thereby stimulate the skeletal muscle. The electrical events that normally take place in the heart initiate cardiac contraction. Disorders in electrical activity can induce serious and sometimes lethal disturbances in the cardiac rhythm.

Cardiac Transmembrane Potentials Are Prolonged

Microelectrodes have been inserted into the interior and exterior of individual cardiac cells immersed in an electrolyte solution to investigate the electrical behavior of those cells. The microelectrode is attached to a galvanometer, which measures the strength of the electrical current that flows from one electrode to the other. The potential changes recorded from typical fast-response and slow-response ventricular muscle fibers are illustrated in **Figure 16–1**.

When two electrodes are placed in an electrolyte solution near a strip of quiescent cardiac muscle cells, the potential difference (point *a*) measured between the two electrodes is zero (Figure 16–1, *left panel*). When one of the electrodes is then inserted into the interior of the cardiac muscle fiber, the galvanometer immediately records a decreased transmembrane potential (to point *b*) of about −90 mV (Figure 16–1, *left panel*). This electronegativity of the interior of the resting cardiac cell with respect to the cell exterior is also characteristic of skeletal muscle cells, smooth muscle cells, nerve cells, and most other cells within the body (see also Chapter 2).

At point *c* in Figure 16–1, the ventricular cell is excited electrically, and the cell membrane rapidly depolarizes. Near the end of the depolarization **(phase 0),** the potential difference is actually reversed, such that the potential of the interior of the cell exceeds that of the exterior by about 20 mV. The upstroke is followed immediately by a brief period of partial, **early repolarization (phase 1)** and then by a **plateau (phase 2),** which persists for about 200 msec. The membrane then repolarizes **(phase 3)** until the resting state of polarization **(phase 4)** is again attained (at point *e*). **Final repolarization (phase 3)** develops more slowly than does depolarization **(phase 0).**

The temporal relationships between the electrical events in the cardiac muscle and in the mechanical contraction of the muscle are shown in **Figure 16–2**. This rapid depolarization (phase 0 of the

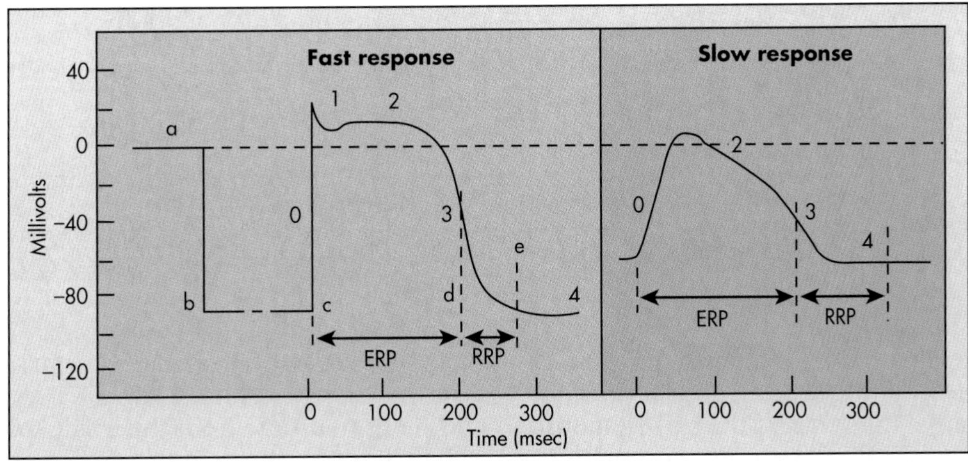

FIGURE 16–1. Changes in transmembrane potential recorded from a fast-response *(left)* and a slow-response *(right)* cardiac fiber in isolated cardiac tissue immersed in an electrolyte solution. The numbers refer to the various phases of the action potentials. ERP, effective refractory period; RRP, relative refractory period.

action potential) occurs well before the contractile force attains its peak, and repolarization is completed well before the cell reaches its full resting value. The relaxation of the cardiac muscle takes place mainly during phase 4 of the action potential.

There Are Two Principal Types of Cardiac Action Potentials

The two main types of cardiac action potentials are shown in Figure 16–1. One action potential type, the **fast response,** occurs in normal atrial and ventricular myocytes and in the specialized conducting fibers **(Purkinje fibers)** of the heart. A fast-response action potential is shown in the left panel of Figure 16–1. The other type of action potential, the **slow response,** occurs in the **sinoatrial (SA) and atrioventricular (AV) nodes.** The SA node is the natural pacemaker region of the heart, and the AV node is the specialized tissue that conducts the cardiac impulse from atria to ventricles. The slow-response action potential is shown in the right panel of Figure 16–1.

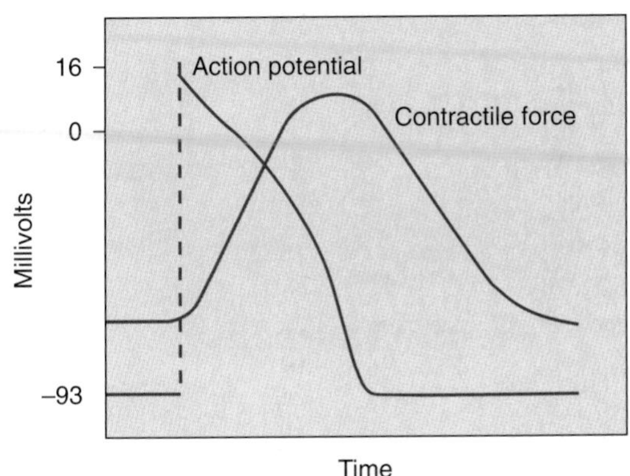

FIGURE 16–2. Relationships between the developed force and the changes in transmembrane potential in a thin strip of ventricular muscle. (Redrawn from Kavaler F, Fisher VJ, Stuckey JH: *Bull N Y Acad Med* 41:592, 1965.)

Fast responses may change to slow responses under certain pathological conditions. For example, in coronary artery disease, a region of cardiac muscle may be deprived of its normal blood supply. As a result, the $[K^+]$ rises in the interstitial fluid that surrounds the affected muscle cells because K^+ is lost from the inadequately perfused, **ischemic** cells. The action potentials in some of these cells may then be converted from fast-response to slow-response action potentials. An experimental conversion from a fast to a slow response is illustrated in **Figure 16–3.**

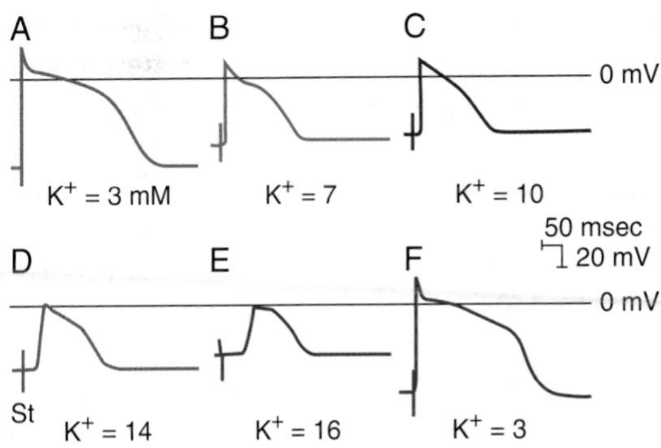

FIGURE 16–3. Effect of changes in external $[K^+]$ on the transmembrane action potentials recorded from a Purkinje fiber. The stimulus artifact (St) appears as a biphasic spike to the left of the upstroke of the action potential. The horizontal lines near the peaks of the action potentials denote 0 mV. (From Myerburg RJ, Lazzara R. In Fisch E, ed: *Complex electrocardiography,* Philadelphia, 1973, FA Davis.)

TABLE 16–1. ION CONCENTRATIONS AND EQUILIBRIUM POTENTIALS IN CARDIAC MUSCLE CELLS

Ion	Extracellular Concentration (mM)	Intracellular Concentration (mM)	Equilibrium Potential (mV)
Na^+	145	10	70
K^+	4	135	–94
Ca^{++}	2	10^{-4}	132

Data from Ten Eick RE et al: *Prog Cardiovasc Dis* 24:157, 1981.

As shown in Figure 16–1, the resting membrane potential (phase 4) of the fast response is considerably more negative than that of the slow response. Furthermore, the slope of the upstroke (phase 0), the amplitude of the action potential, and the extent of the overshoot of the fast response are greater in the fast-response fibers than in the slow-response fibers. The amplitude of the action potential and the steepness of the upstroke are important determinants of how rapidly the action potentials are propagated. In slow-response cardiac tissues, the action potentials are propagated more slowly than in fast-response cardiac tissues. Furthermore, impulse conduction is more likely to be blocked in slow-response cardiac tissue than in fast-response tissue. Slow conduction and a tendency toward conduction block increase the likelihood of certain rhythm disturbances.

The Resting Potential Is Determined by Ionic Diffusion

THE VARIOUS PHASES OF THE CARDIAC ACTION POTENTIAL ARE ASSOCIATED WITH CHANGES IN THE CELL MEMBRANE PERMEABILITY, MAINLY TO Na^+, K^+, AND Ca^{++} IONS. Such changes in cell membrane permeability alter the movement of these ions across the membrane. The permeability of the membrane to a given ion, its transmembrane concentration difference, and the transmembrane electrical potential difference define the net quantity of the ions that will diffuse across the membrane. Permeability changes are accomplished by the opening and closing of specific ion channels.

As with all other cells in the body (see also Chapter 2), the concentration of potassium ions inside a cardiac muscle cell, $[K^+]_i$, is far greater than the potassium concentration outside the cell, $[K^+]_o$ **(Figure 16–4)**. The reverse concentration gradient exists for Na^+ and Ca^{++} ions. Estimates of the extracellular and intracellular concentrations of Na^+, K^+, and Ca^{++} and the equilibrium potentials (this term is defined later in this chapter) for these ions are compiled in **Table 16–1**.

THE RESTING CELL MEMBRANE IS RELATIVELY PERMEABLE TO K^+, BUT MUCH LESS SO TO Na^+ AND Ca^{++}. Hence, K^+ tends to diffuse from the inside to the outside of the cell in the direction of the K^+ concentration gradient, as shown on the right side of the cell in Figure 16–4.

Any flux of K^+ that occurs during phase 4 takes place mainly through specific **K^+ channels.** Several types of K^+ channels exist in cardiac cell membranes. Some of these channels are regulated (i.e., they open and close) according to the transmembrane potential, whereas other channels are regulated by a chemical signal (e.g., the extracellular acetylcholine concentration). One of the specific K^+ channels through which K^+ passes during phase 4 is a voltage-regulated channel that conducts the **inwardly rectifying K^+ current.** This current is symbolized as i_{K1} and is discussed in more detail later **(Figure 16–5)**.

The i_{K1} current is established because many of the anions, such as the proteins inside the cell, are not free to diffuse out with the K^+ (Figure 16–4). Therefore, the K^+ diffuses out of the cell and leaves the impermeant A^- behind. The deficiency of cations then causes the interior of the cell to become electronegative (see also Chapter 2). As a result, the positively charged K^+ ions are attracted to the interior of the cell by the negative potential that exists

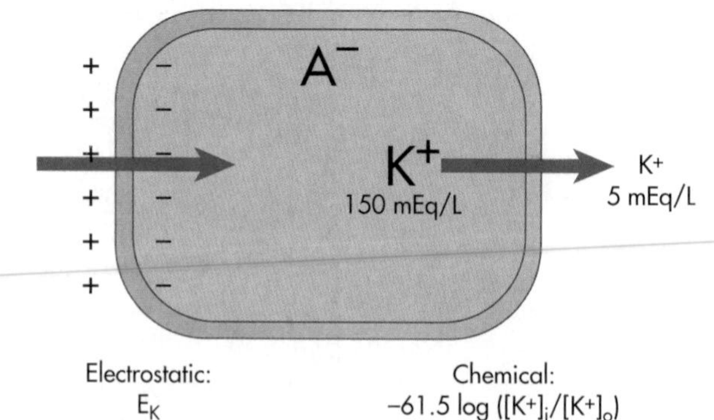

FIGURE 16–4. Balance of chemical and electrostatic forces that act across a resting cardiac cell membrane. The balance is based on a 30:1 ratio of $[K^+]_i$ to $[K^+]_o$ and the presence of a nondiffusible anion (A^-) inside, but not outside, the cell.

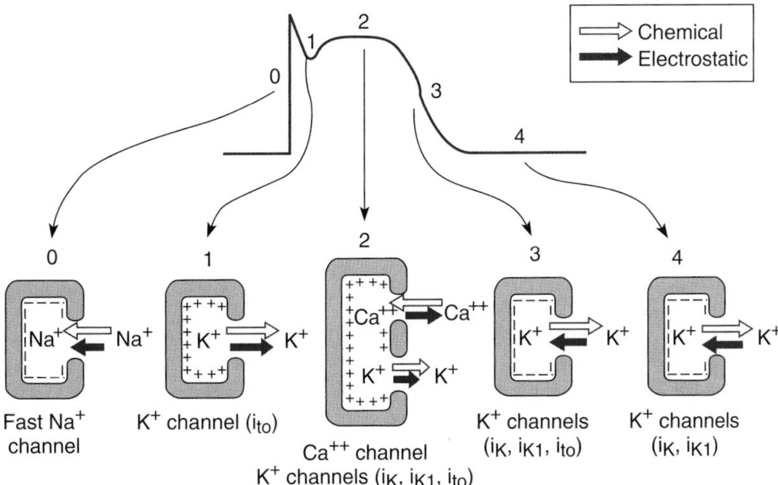

FIGURE 16–5. The principal ionic currents and channels that generate the various phases of the action potential in a cardiac cell. Phase 0: The chemical and electrostatic forces both favor the entry of Na^+ into the cell through fast Na^+ channels to generate the upstroke. Phase 1: The chemical and electrostatic forces both favor the efflux of K^+ through i_{to} channels to generate early, partial repolarization. Phase 2: During the plateau, the net influx of Ca^{++} through Ca^{++} channels is balanced by the efflux of K^+ through i_K, i_{K1}, and i_{to} channels. Phase 3: The chemical forces that favor the efflux of K^+ through i_K, i_{K1}, and i_{to} channels predominate over the electrostatic forces that favor the influx of K^+ through these same channels. Phase 4: The chemical forces that favor the efflux of K^+ through i_K and i_{K1} channels slightly exceed the electrostatic forces that favor the influx of K^+ through these same channels.

there, as shown on the left side of the cell in Figure 16–4.

Therefore, two opposing forces regulate the movement of K^+ across the cell membrane. A chemical force, based on the concentration gradient, results in net outward diffusion of K^+. The counterforce is based on electrostatic differences between the interior and exterior of the cell. If the system comes into equilibrium, the chemical and the electrostatic forces would be equal. As explained in Chapter 2, this equilibrium is expressed by the **Nernst equation** for K^+:

$$E_K = -61.5 \log ([K^+]_i/[K^+]_o)$$

The right-hand term represents the chemical potential difference, whereas the left-hand term, E_K, represents the electrostatic potential difference that would exist across the cell membrane if K^+ were the only diffusible ion. E_K is called the **potassium equilibrium potential.**

When the measured concentrations of $[K^+]_i$ and $[K^+]_o$ for mammalian myocardial cells are substituted into the Nernst equation, the calculated value of E_K equals about −95 mV (Table 16–1). This value is slightly more negative than the resting potential that prevails in the myocardial cells. Therefore, the potential that tends to drive K^+ out of the resting cell is small. The actual resting potential is slightly less negative than the predicted potential because the cell membrane is slightly permeable to other ions, notably to Na^+.

The balance of the forces that act on Na^+ opposes the force that acts on K^+ in resting cardiac cells. The intracellular Na^+ concentration, $[Na^+]_i$, is much less than the extracellular Na^+ concentration, $[Na^+]_o$. The sodium equilibrium potential, E_{Na}, expressed by the Nernst equation, is about 70 mV (Table 16–1). At equilibrium, therefore, the cell interior is about 70 mV more positive than the cell exterior. This potential difference is necessary to counterbalance the chemical potential for Na^+. However, the actual membrane potential of resting myocytes is about −90 mV. Hence, both chemical and electrostatic forces act to favor movement of extracellular Na^+ into the cell. However, the influx of Na^+ through the membrane is not great because the resting cell membrane is not very permeable to Na^+. Nevertheless, this small inward current of Na^+ can cause the potential (V_m) within the resting cell to be slightly greater than the value (E_K) predicted by the Nernst equation for K^+ **(Figure 16–6)**.

The dependence of V_m on the conductances and on the intracellular and extracellular concentrations of K^+, Na^+, and other ions is described by the **chord conductance equation,** as explained in Chapter 2. This equation reveals that the relative membrane conductances to Na^+ and K^+ determine the resting potential of the cell. In the resting cardiac cell, the conductance to K^+ (g_K) is about 100 times greater than the conductance to Na^+ (g_{Na}). Therefore, the chord conductance equation is equivalent to the Nernst equation for K^+. Because g_{Na} is so small in the resting cell, changes in the

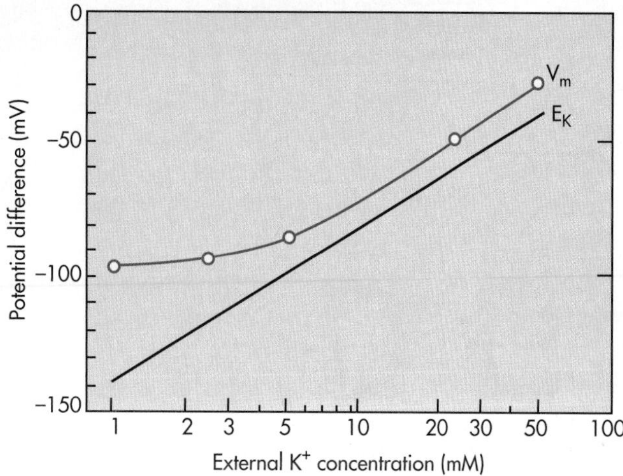

FIGURE 16–6. The V_m of a cardiac muscle fiber varies inversely with the $[K^+]$ of the external medium. The oblique blue line represents the E_K predicted by the Nernst equation.

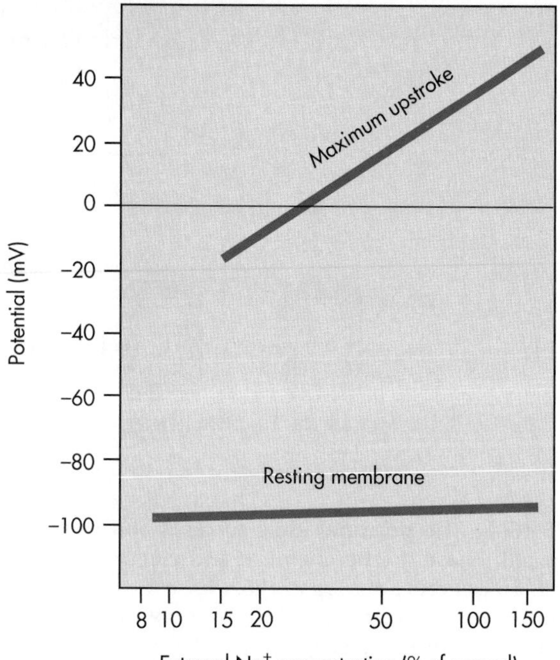

FIGURE 16–7. The $[Na^+]$ in the external medium is the main determinant of the peak value of the upstroke of the action potential *(upper line)* in cardiac muscle, but it has little influence on the resting membrane potential *(lower line)*.

external $[Na^+]$ do not significantly affect V_m **(Figure 16–7)**.

When the $[K^+]_i/[K^+]_o$ ratio is decreased experimentally in a suspension of myocytes by raising $[K^+]_o$, the measured value of V_m approximates the value of E_K that is predicted by the Nernst equation (Figure 16–6). When the extracellular $[K^+]$ exceeds about 5 mM, the measured values correspond closely with the predicted values. The measured levels are only slightly less than those predicted by the Nernst equation because g_K is so much greater than g_{Na}. However, for values of $[K^+]_o$ below about 5 mM, g_K decreases as $[K^+]_o$ is diminished. As g_K decreases, the effect of g_{Na} on the transmembrane potential increases, as predicted by the chord conductance equation. This change in g_K accounts for the greater deviation of the measured V_m from the value predicted by the Nernst equation for K^+ when the levels of $[K^+]_o$ are low.

The Fast Response Depends on Na^+

Phase 0 is genesis of the upstroke

Any stimulus that abruptly changes the resting membrane potential to a critical value (called the **threshold**) results in an action potential. The characteristics of fast-response action potentials are shown in Figure 16–1. The rapid depolarization (phase 0) is related almost exclusively to the influx of Na^+ into the myocyte due to a sudden increase in g_{Na}. The **amplitude** of the action potential (i.e., the potential change during phase 0) varies linearly with the logarithm of $[Na^+]_o$, as shown in Figure 16–7. When $[Na^+]_o$ is increased from about 20% of its normal value (about +40 mV) to about 150% of its normal value, the transmembrane potential at the peak of the action potential increases from about −20 mV to about +40 mV.

The physical and chemical forces responsible for the transmembrane movements of Na^+ are diagrammed in **Figure 16–8.** When the resting membrane potential, V_m, is suddenly changed from −90 mV (Figure 16–8, *A*) to the threshold level of about −65 mV (Figure 16–8, *B*), the properties of the cell membrane change dramatically. Na^+ enters the myocyte through specific **fast Na^+ channels** that exist in the membrane (see also Chapter 3). These channels can be blocked by the puffer fish toxin, **tetrodotoxin.** Also, many of the drugs used to treat certain cardiac rhythm disturbances **(cardiac arrhythmias)** act by blocking these fast Na^+ channels.

THE MANNER IN WHICH Na^+ MOVES THROUGH THESE FAST CHANNELS SUGGESTS THAT THE FLUX IS CONTROLLED BY TWO TYPES OF **GATES** IN EACH CHANNEL. One of these, the ***m* gate,** tends to open the channel as V_m becomes less negative. Hence, this is called an **activation gate.** The other gate, the ***h* gate,** tends to close the channel as V_m becomes less negative.

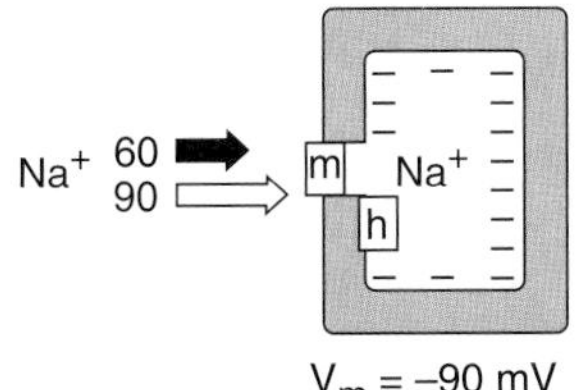

During phase 4, the chemical (60 mV) and electrostatic (90 mV) forces favor influx of Na^+ from the extracellular space. Influx is negligible, however, because the activation *(m)* gates are closed.

A

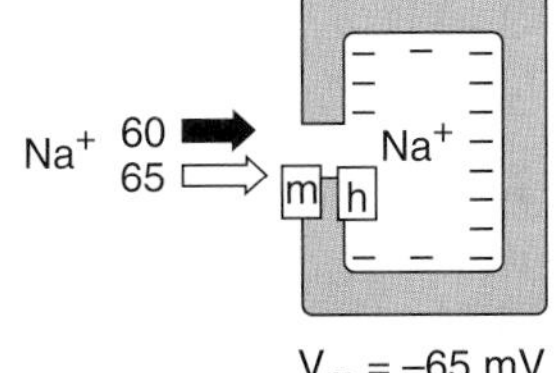

If V_m is brought to about –65 mV, the *m* gates begin to swing open, and Na^+ begins to enter the cell. This reduces the negative charge inside the cell and thereby opens still more Na^+ channels, which accelerates the influx of Na^+. The change in V_m also initiates the closure of inactivation *(h)* gates, which operate more slowly than the *m* gates.

B

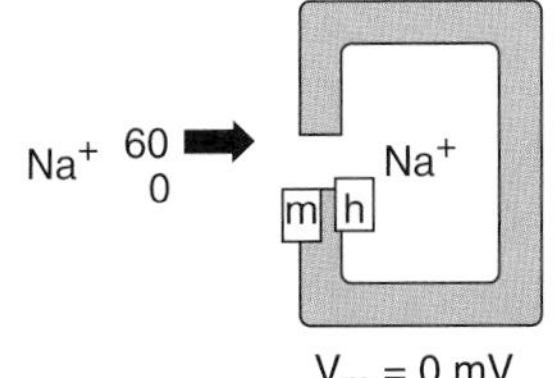

The rapid influx of Na^+ sharply decreases the negativity of V_m. As V_m approaches 0, the electrostatic force attracting Na^+ into the cell is neutralized. Na^+ continues to enter the cell, however, because of the substantial concentration gradient, and V_m begins to become positive.

C

Na+ 60
20
m h
Na+
V_m = +20 mV

When V_m is positive by about 20 mV, Na^+ continues to enter the cell because the diffusional forces (60 mV) exceed the opposing electrostatic forces (20 mV). The influx of Na^+ is slow, however, because the net driving force is small, and many of the inactivation gates have already closed.

D

Na+ 60
30
m
h
Na+
V_m = +30 mV

When V_m reaches about 30 mV, the *h* gates have now all closed, and Na^+ influx ceases. The *h* gates remain closed until the first half of repolarization, and thus the cell is absolutely refractory during this entire period. During the second half of repolarization, the *m* and *h* gates approach the state represented by panel *A*, and thus the cell is relatively refractory.

E

FIGURE 16–8. The gating of an Na^+ channel in a cardiac cell membrane during phase 4 (A) and during various stages of the action potential upstroke (B to E). The positions of the *m* and *h* gates in the fast Na^+ channels are shown at the various levels of V_m. The electrostatic forces are represented by the white arrows and the chemical (diffusional) forces by the black arrows.

Hence, this is called an **inactivation gate.** The *m* and *h* designations were originally employed by Hodgkin and Huxley in their mathematical model of impulse conduction in nerve fibers.

As stated, the V_m of a resting cell is about –90 mV. The *m* gates are closed and the *h* gates are wide open, as shown in Figure 16–8, *A*. Because the $[Na^+]$ outside the cell exceeds the $[Na^+]$ inside the cell, the interior of the cell is electrically negative with respect to the exterior. Hence, both chemical and electrostatic forces act to draw Na^+ into the cell.

The electrostatic force in Figure 16–8, *A*, is a potential difference of 90 mV, and it is represented by the white arrow. The chemical forces evoked by the differences in Na^+ concentrations inside and outside these cells are represented by the black arrows in Figure 16–8. For an $[Na^+]$ difference of about 130 mM, a potential difference of 60 mV (with the potential inside more positive than the potential outside) is necessary to counterbalance the chemical, or diffusional, force, according to the Nernst equation for Na^+ (see also Chapter 2). Therefore, the net chemical force (black arrows) that favors the inward movement of Na^+ in Figure 16–8 is equivalent to a potential difference of 60 mV. In the resting cell (Figure 16–8, *A*), the total electrochemical force that favors the inward movement of Na^+ is 60 + 90, or 150 mV. The *m* gates are closed, however, and therefore the conductance of the resting cell membrane to Na^+ is very low. Hence, when the cell is in the resting state, virtually no Na^+ moves into the cell.

Any stimulus that decreases V_m tends to open the *m* gates and thereby activates the fast Na^+ channels. The precise potential required to open the *m* gates, and thus to activate the Na^+ channels, varies somewhat from one channel to another in the cell membrane. As V_m becomes progressively less negative, more *m* gates swing open, and the influx of Na^+ accelerates (Figure 16–8, *B*). The entry of Na^+ into the interior of the cell neutralizes some of the negative charges within the cell and thereby renders V_m still less negative. The consequent change in V_m opens more *m* gates and augments the inward Na^+ current. This process is considered to be **regenerative.** As V_m approaches about –65 mV, the remaining *m* gates rapidly swing open in the fast Na^+ channels until virtually all the *m* gates are open (Figure 16–8, *C*).

The rapid opening of the *m* gates in the fast Na^+ channels is responsible for the large, abrupt increase in Na^+ conductance (g_{Na}) that occurs in phase 0 (the upstroke) of the action potential (**Figure 16–9**, *A*). The rapid influx of Na^+ accounts for the steepness of the action potential upstroke. The maximal rate of change of V_m varies from 100 to 200 V/sec in myocardial cells and from 500 to 1000 V/sec in Purkinje fibers. The Na^+ that enters the cell during one action potential alters V_m by more than 100 mV. The actual quantity of Na^+ that enters the cell is so small and occurs in only a portion of the cell's volume such that the resulting change in the intracellular $[Na^+]$ cannot be measured precisely. Hence, the chemical force as well as the electrostatic force changes throughout the action potential. In Figure 16–8, note that the lengths of the black arrows remain constant (denoting a chemical force of 60 mV), whereas the white arrows change in magnitude and direction.

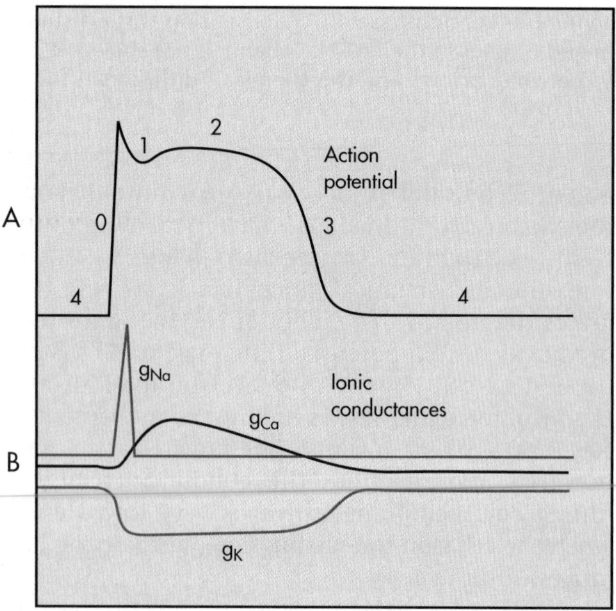

FIGURE 16–9. Changes in g_{Na}, g_{Ca}, and g_K during phases 0 to 4 of the action potential (A) of a fast-response cardiac cell. The conductance diagrams (B) are qualitative, not quantitative.

As Na^+ rushes into the cardiac cell during phase 0, the negative charges inside the cell are neutralized, and V_m becomes progressively less negative. When V_m falls to zero (Figure 16–8, *C*) an electrostatic force no longer exists to pull Na^+ into the cell. As long as the fast Na^+ channels remain open, however, Na^+ continues to enter the cell because of the large concentration gradient. This inward Na^+ current causes the cell interior to become positively charged (Figure 16–8, *D*). This reversal of the membrane polarity is the so-called **overshoot** of the cardiac action potential. Such a reversal of the electrostatic gradient would tend to repel the entry of additional Na^+ (Figure 16–8, *D*). However, as long as the inwardly directed chemical forces exceed the outwardly directed electrostatic forces, the net flux of Na^+ is directed inward, even though the rate at which Na^+ enters the cell diminishes.

The inward Na^+ current finally stops when the *h* (inactivation) gates close (Figure 16–8, *E*). Like the activity of the *m* gates, the activity of the *h* gates is governed by the value of V_m. However, the *m* gates open rapidly (in about 0.1 msec), whereas the closure of the *h* gates requires several milliseconds. Phase 0 finally ends when all of the *h* gates have closed, thereby inactivating the fast Na^+ channels. The closure of the *h* gates so soon after the opening of the *m* gates accounts for the quick return of g_{Na} from its maximum to its resting value (Figure 16–9, *B*).

The *h* gates then remain closed until the cell has partially repolarized during phase 3 (at about time *d* in Figure 16–1). From time *c* to time *d,* the cell is in its **effective refractory period,** and it will not respond to further excitation. This mechanism prevents a sustained, tetanic contraction of cardiac muscle. Tetanic contraction of the ventricular myocytes would retard ventricular relaxation, and therefore it would interfere with the normal intermittent pumping action of the heart.

About midway through phase 3 (time *d* in Figure 16–1), the *m* and *h* gates in some of the fast Na^+ channels have resumed the states shown in Figure 16–8, *A*. Such channels are said to have **recovered from inactivation.** The cell begins to respond to further excitation, but weakly at first (**Figure 16–10**). Throughout the remainder of phase 3, the cell completes its recovery from inactivation. By time *e* in Figure 16–1, the *h* gates have reopened and the *m* gates have reclosed in all the fast Na^+ channels; that is, they have resumed the status depicted in Figure 16–8, *A*.

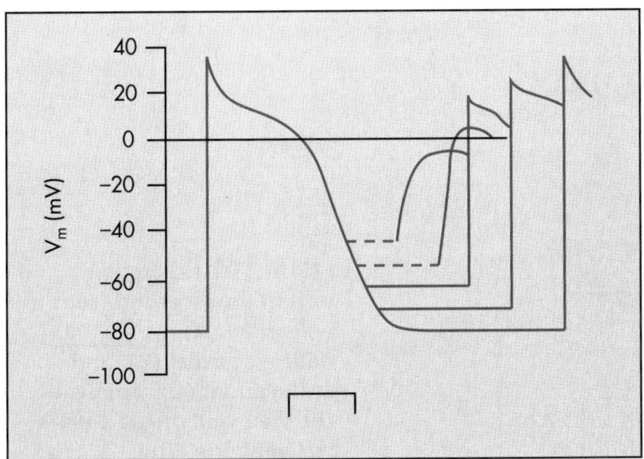

FIGURE 16–10. Changes in action potential amplitude and slope of the upstroke as premature action potentials are initiated at different stages of the relative refractory period of the preceding excitation in a fast-response fiber (bar = 100 msec). (Redrawn from Rosen MR, Wit AL, Hoffman BF: *Am Heart J* 88:380, 1974.)

Phase 1 is genesis of early repolarization

In many cardiac cells that have a prominent plateau, phase 1 constitutes an early, brief period of **limited repolarization.** In Figure 16–1 (left panel), this brief repolarization is represented by a notch that lies between the end of the upstroke and the beginning of the plateau. Repolarization is brief and caused by the activation of a **transient outward current (i_{to}),** which is carried mainly by K^+. Activation of the K^+ channels during phase 1 elicits a brief efflux of K^+ from the cell, for two reasons: the interior of the cell is positively charged, and the internal [K^+] greatly exceeds the external [K^+] (Figure 16–5). As a result of this transient efflux of positively charged ions, the cell is briefly and partially repolarized (phase 1).

The phase 1 notch is prominent in ventricular Purkinje fibers (**Figure 16–11**). The phase 1 notch is also prominent in action potentials recorded from the epicardial and midmyocardial regions of the ventricular myocardium, but not in action potentials recorded from the endocardial regions of the ventricular myocardium (**Figure 16–12**). The cycle length of depolarization also affects phase 1. When the basic cycle length at which the epicardial and midmyocardial fibers are depolarized is increased from 300 to 8000 msec, the phase 1 notch becomes more pronounced, and the action potential duration is increased substantially. The same increase in basic cycle length in endocardial fibers has no effect on phase 1, and its effect on the action potential duration is small (Figure 16–12, *C*). In the presence of 4-aminopyridine, which blocks the K^+ channels that carry i_{to}, the phase 1 notch becomes much less prominent in the action potentials recorded from the epicardial and midmyocardial regions of the ventricles than in the action potentials recorded from the endocardial regions.

Phase 2 is genesis of the plateau

DURING THE PLATEAU OF THE ACTION POTENTIAL, Ca^{++} ENTERS THE MYOCARDIAL CELLS THROUGH **Ca^{++} CHANNELS,** WHICH ACTIVATE AND INACTIVATE MUCH MORE SLOWLY THAN DO THE FAST Na^+ CHANNELS. During the flat portion of phase 2 (Figure 16–5), this influx of positive charge carried by Ca^{++} is counterbalanced by the efflux of positive charge carried by K^+. The K^+ exits through channels that conduct mainly the i_{to}, i_K, and i_{K1} currents. The i_{to} current is responsible for phase 1, as described previously, but it is not completely inactivated until after phase 2 has expired. The i_K and i_{K1} currents are described later in this chapter.

Ca^{++} conductance during the plateau

The Ca^{++} channels are voltage regulated, and they are activated as V_m becomes progressively less negative during the upstroke of the action potential. Various types of Ca^{++} channels have been identified in cardiac tissues (see Chapter 3). However, this discussion concentrates on the predominant channel, the so-called L-type Ca^{++} channel. Some of the important characteristics of this channel are illustrated in **Figure 16–13**, which also shows the Ca^{++} currents that are generated by voltage-clamping an isolated atrial myocyte. Note that when V_m is suddenly increased to +30 mV from a holding potential of 30 mV, an inward Ca^{++} current is activated. After the inward current reaches its minimum value, it gradually returns to zero (i.e., the channel inactivates slowly). Thus, because the current that

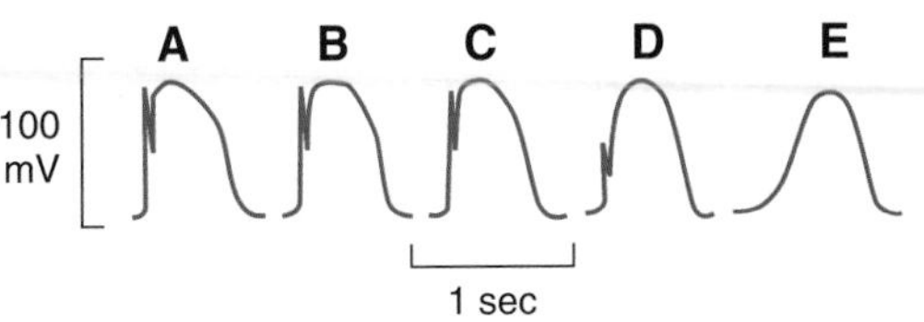

FIGURE 16–11. Effect of tetrodotoxin on the action potentials recorded in a calf Purkinje fiber perfused with a solution containing epinephrine and K^+ (10.8 mM). The concentration of tetrodotoxin was 0 M in A, 3×10^{-8} M in B and later in C, 3×10^{-7} M in D, and 3×10^{-6} M in E. (Redrawn from Carmeliet E, Vereecke J: *Pflugers Arch* 313:300, 1969.)

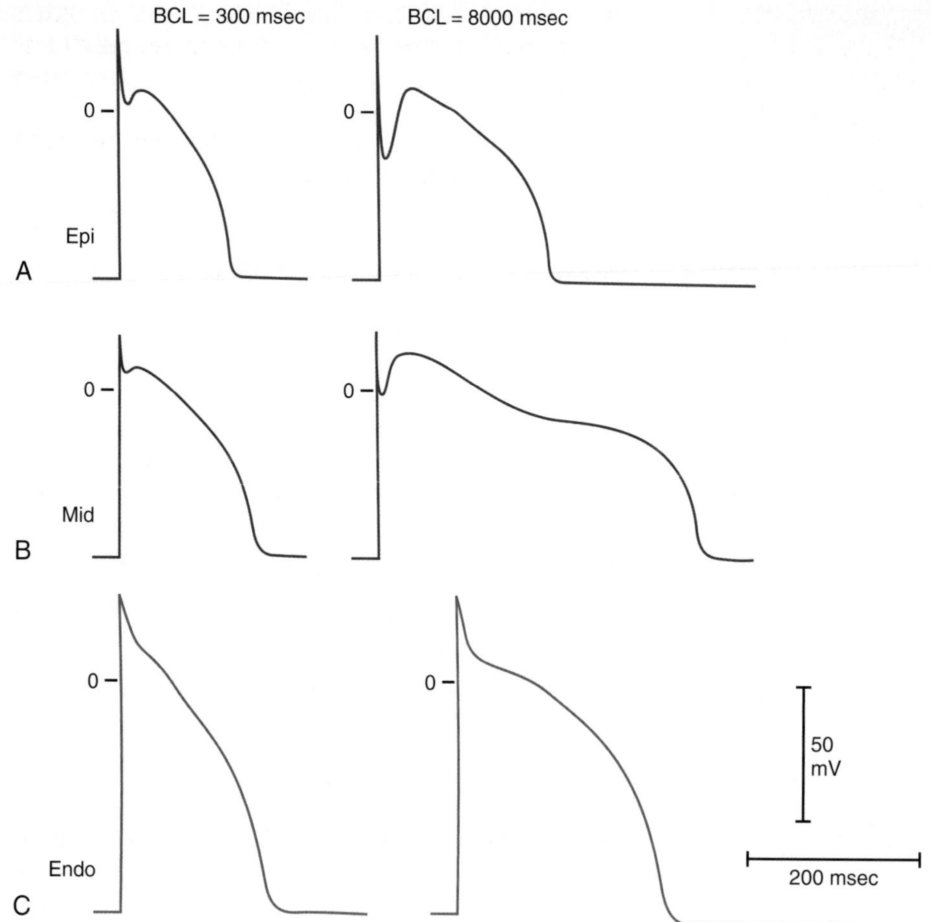

FIGURE 16–12. Action potentials recorded from the epicardial (A), midmyocardial (B), and endocardial (C) regions of the free wall of the canine left ventricle. The preparations were driven at basic cycle lengths (BCL) of 300 and 8000 msec. (From Liu D-W, Gintant GA, Antzelevitch C: *Circ Res* 72:671, 1993, with permission of the American Heart Association.)

passes through these channels is prolonged, the channels are designated **L-type.**

Opening of the Ca^{++} channels is reflected by an increase in Ca^{++} conductance (g_{Ca}) immediately after the upstroke of the action potential (Figure 16–9). At the beginning of the action potential, the intracellular [Ca^{++}] is much less than the extracellular [Ca^{++}] (Table 16–1). Consequently, the increase in g_{Ca} promotes an influx of Ca^{++} into the cell throughout the action potential plateau. Various factors, such as neurotransmitters and drugs, may substantially influence g_{Ca}. The adrenergic neurotransmitter **norepinephrine,** the β-adrenergic receptor agonist **isoproterenol,** and various other **catecholamines** may enhance Ca^{++} conductance, whereas the parasympathetic neurotransmitter **acetylcholine** may decrease Ca^{++} conductance. The enhancement of Ca^{++} conductance by catecholamines is probably the principal mechanism by which the catecholamines enhance cardiac muscle contractility.

To enhance Ca^{++} conductance, catecholamines first interact with **β-adrenergic receptors** in the cardiac cell membrane. This interaction stimulates the membrane-bound enzyme **adenylyl cyclase,** which raises the intracellular concentration of **cyclic adenosine monophosphate (cAMP)** (see also Chapter 5). The rise in the level of cAMP enhances the activation of the L-type Ca^{++} channels in the cell membrane (Figure 16–13) and thus augments the influx of Ca^{++} into the cells from the interstitial fluid. Conversely, acetylcholine interacts

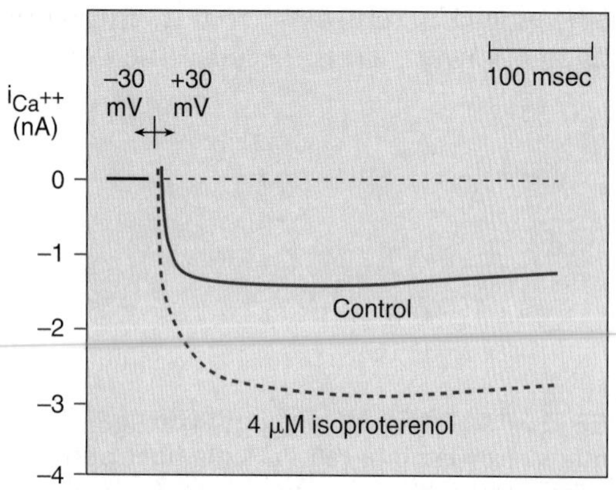

FIGURE 16–13. Effect of isoproterenol on the Ca^{++} current conducted by L-type Ca^{++} channels in voltage-clamped, canine atrial myocytes when the potential was changed from −30 to +30 mV. (Redrawn from Bean BP: *J Gen Physiol* 86:1, 1985.)

with **muscarinic receptors** in the cell membrane and inhibits adenylyl cyclase. In this way, acetylcholine antagonizes the activation of the Ca^{++} channels and thereby diminishes g_{Ca}.

The **Ca^{++} channel antagonists,** such as **verapamil** and **diltiazem,** are substances that block Ca^{++} channels. These drugs decrease g_{Ca} and thereby impede the influx of Ca^{++} into myocardial cells. The Ca^{++} channel antagonists decrease the duration of the action potential plateau and diminish the strength of the cardiac contraction **(Figure 16–14)**. An important consequence of blocking Ca^{++} channels is their use to treat supraventricular arrhythmias. In this condition, many impulses pass from atria to ventricles via the AV node, which has slow-response action potentials dependent on L-type Ca^{++} channels. Verapamil and diltiazem reduce the number of atrial impulses that pass to the ventricles by their blockade of Ca^{++} channels. This reduces the frequency of ventricular contractions, allows more adequate diastolic filling, and improves cardiac output. The Ca^{++} channel antagonists depress the contraction of the vascular smooth muscle and thereby induce generalized vasodilation. This diminished vascular resistance reduces the counterforce **(afterload)** that opposes the propulsion of blood from the ventricles into the arterial system (see Chapters 20 and 21). Hence, vasodilator drugs, such as the Ca^{++} channel antagonists, are often referred to as **afterload-reducing drugs** and are used to **treat hypertension.**

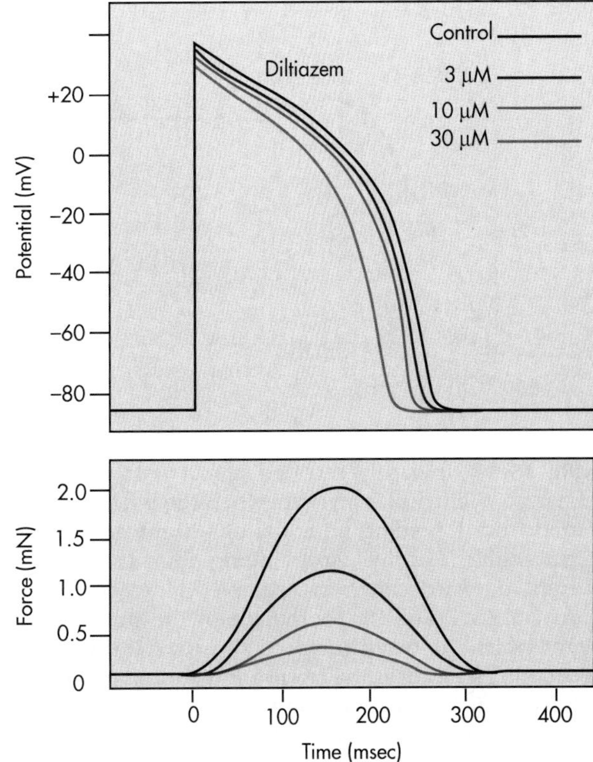

FIGURE 16–14. Effects of diltiazem, a Ca^{++} channel antagonist, on the action potentials (in millivolts) and isometric contractile forces (in millinewtons) recorded from an isolated papillary muscle of a guinea pig. The tracings were recorded under control conditions *(black line)* and in the presence of diltiazem in concentrations of 3 μM/L *(blue line),* 10 μM/L *(red line),* and 30 μM/L *(green line).* (Redrawn from Hirth C, Borchard U, Hafner D: *J Mol Cell Cardiol* 15:799, 1983.)

K^+ conductance during the plateau

During the plateau (phase 2) of the action potential, the concentration gradient of K^+ across the cell membrane is virtually the same as it is during phase 4, but V_m is positive. Therefore, both the chemical and the electrostatic forces favor the efflux of K^+ from the cell (Figure 16–5). If the value of g_K were the same during the plateau as it is during phase 4, the efflux of K^+ during phase 2 would greatly exceed the influx of Ca^{++}, and a plateau could not be achieved (Figure 16–5). However, as V_m approaches and then attains positive values near the peak of the action potential upstroke, g_K suddenly decreases (Figure 16–9). THE DIMINISHED K^+ CURRENT ASSOCIATED WITH THE REDUCTION IN g_K PREVENTS AN EXCESSIVE LOSS OF K^+ FROM THE CELL DURING THE PLATEAU.

This reduction in g_K at both positive and negative values of V_m is called **inward rectification.** This g_K response is a characteristic of several K^+ currents, including the i_{K1} current. The current-voltage relationship of the K^+ channels that conduct i_{K1} has been determined by voltage-clamping the cardiac cells **(Figure 16–15)**. Note that for the cell depicted in Figure 16–15, the current-voltage curve intersects the voltage axis at a V_m of about −80 mV. The absence of ionic current flow at the point of intersection indicates that the electrostatic forces equal the chemical (diffusional) forces at this potential (Figure 16–4). In this ventricular cell preparation, therefore, the Nernst equilibrium potential (E_K) for K^+ is −80 mV. This value reflects the ratio of intracellular $[K^+]$ to extracellular $[K^+]$ in this experimental preparation.

When the membrane potential is clamped at levels negative to −80 mV in this same isolated cardiac cell (Figure 16–15), the electrostatic forces exceed the chemical forces, and an inward K^+ current is induced (as denoted by the negative values of K^+ current over this range of voltages). Note also that if V_m becomes more negative than −80 mV, the slope of the K^+ curve is steep, even at the point on the curve at which $V_m = E_K$. Thus, when V_m equals E_K or is negative to E_K, a small change in V_m induces a substantial change in the K^+ current; that is, g_K is large. During phase 4, the V_m of a myocardial cell is slightly less negative than the E_K (Figure 16–6). The substantial g_K that prevails

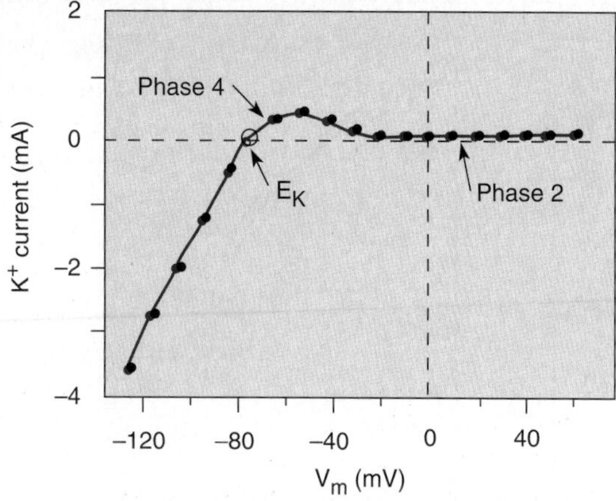

FIGURE 16–15. Inwardly rectified K^+ currents recorded from a rabbit ventricular myocyte when the potential was changed from a holding potential of –80 mV to various test potentials. Positive values along the vertical axis represent outward currents; negative values represent inward currents. The V_m coordinate of the point *(open circle)* at which the curve intersects the *x* axis is the reversal potential; it denotes the Nernst equilibrium potential, at which point the chemical and electrostatic forces are equal. (Redrawn from Giles WR, Imaizumi Y: *J Physiol [Lond]* 405:123, 1988.)

during phase 4 of the cardiac action potential is accounted for mainly by the i_{K1} channels.

When the transmembrane potential is clamped at levels less negative than –80 mV (Figure 16–15), the chemical forces exceed the electrostatic forces. Therefore, the net K^+ currents are directed outward (as denoted by the corresponding positive values of the K^+ current). Note that for V_m values less negative than –80 mV, the curve in Figure 16–15 is relatively flat, and for V_m values less negative than about –30 mV, the K^+ current is virtually zero. Thus, at the V_m values that prevail during the action potential plateau, the efflux of K^+ through the i_{K1} channels is negligible. Conversely, the inwardly directed K^+ current is substantial for those values of V_m that prevail during phase 4. Thus, the i_{K1} current is **inwardly rectified.**

The characteristics of another K^+ channel, the **delayed rectifier (i_K)** channel, also contribute to the low g_K that prevails during the plateau. These K^+ channels are closed during phase 4, but they are activated by the potentials that prevail toward the end of phase 0. However, activation proceeds slowly during the plateau. Hence, activation of these channels tends to increase g_K gradually during phase 2. Thus, these channels play only a minor role during phase 2, but they do contribute to the process of final repolarization (phase 3), as described next.

Phase 3 is genesis of final repolarization

The process of final repolarization (phase 3) starts at the end of phase 2, when the efflux of K^+ from the cardiac cell begins to exceed the influx of Ca^{++}. At least three outward K^+ currents (i_{to}, i_K, and i_{K1}) contribute to the final repolarization (phase 3) of the cardiac cell (Figure 16–5).

The transient outward current (i_{to}) and the delayed rectifier current (i_K) help initiate repolarization. These currents are therefore important determinants of the duration of the plateau. For example, the plateau duration is substantially less in atrial than in ventricular myocytes **(Figure 16–16)**.

Electrophysiological experiments have shown that the intensity of the outward K^+ current during the plateau is greater in atrial than in ventricular myocytes. When the outward K^+ current exceeds

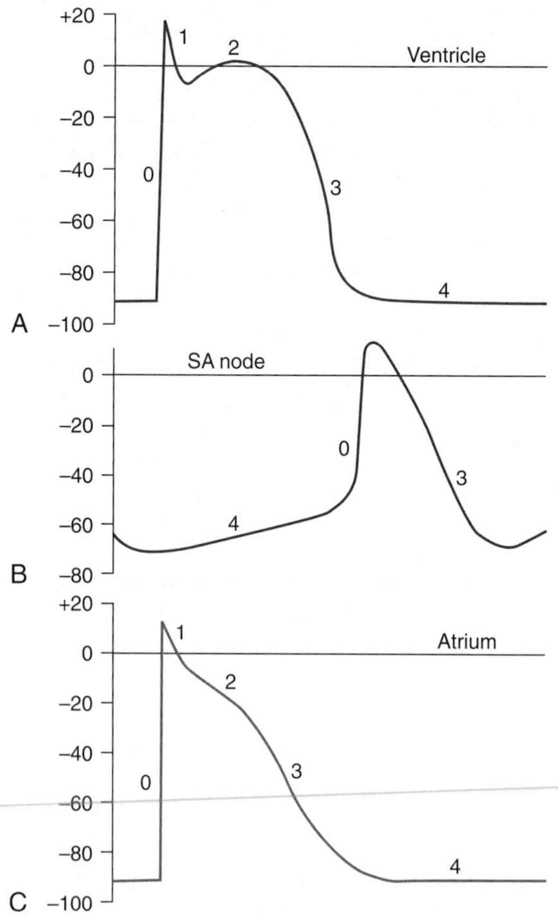

FIGURE 16–16. Typical action potentials (in millivolts) recorded from cells in the ventricle (A), SA node (B), and atrium (C). Sweep velocity in B is half that in A or C. (From Hoffman BF, Cranefield PF: *Electrophysiology of the heart,* New York, 1960, McGraw-Hill.)

the inward Ca^{++} current, repolarization begins. Hence, the greater the K^+ current during phase 2, the earlier repolarization begins. The greater density of the K^+ current in atrial than in ventricular myocytes accounts for the shorter action potentials in atrial than in ventricular myocytes. When the outward K^+ current begins to exceed the inward Ca^{++} current, repolarization begins. Hence, the greater the K^+ current during phase 2, the earlier repolarization begins.

The action potential duration in ventricular myocytes varies considerably with the locations of these myocytes in the ventricular walls (Figure 16–12). The delayed rectifier (i_K) current appears to account for these differences. In endocardial myocytes, where the action potential duration is least, the intensity of i_K is greatest. The converse applies to the midmyocardial myocytes. The intensity of i_K and the action potential duration are intermediate for the epicardial myocytes.

The inwardly rectified K^+ current, i_{K1}, does not participate in the initiation of repolarization because the conductance of these channels is not substantial at the range of V_m values that prevail during the plateau. However, the i_{K1} channels do contribute substantially to the rate of repolarization once phase 3 has begun. As the net efflux of cations causes V_m to become increasingly negative during phase 3, the conductance of the channels that carry the i_{K1} current increases progressively. In Figure 16–15, the hump in the flat portion of the current-voltage curve reflects the increase in i_{K1} conductance as V_m changes from about –20 mV to about –60 mV. Thus, as V_m passes through this range of values positive to the Nernst equilibrium potential (small open circle in Figure 16–15), the outward K^+ current increases and thereby accelerates repolarization.

The Slow Response Is Found in all Cardiac Cells

Fast-response action potentials (Figure 16–1, *left panel*) consist of four principal components: an upstroke (phase 0); an early, partial repolarization (phase 1); a plateau (phase 2); and a final repolarization (phase 3). However, in the slow response (Figure 16–1, *right panel*), the upstroke is much more gradual, the early repolarization (phase 1) is absent, the plateau is less prolonged and less flat, and the transition from the plateau to the final repolarization is less distinct.

Blocking fast Na^+ channels with tetrodotoxin in a fast-response fiber can generate slow responses under appropriate conditions. The Purkinje fiber action potentials shown in Figure 16–11 clearly exhibit the two response types. In the control tracing (*A*), the typical fast-response action potential displays a prominent notch, which separates the upstroke from the plateau. In action potentials *B* to *E,* progressively larger quantities of tetrodotoxin are added to the bathing solution to produce a graded blockade of the fast Na^+ channels. Figure 16–11 shows that the upstroke and notch become progressively less prominent in action potentials *B* to *D*. In action potential *E,* the notch has disappeared and the upstroke is gradual; the action potential resembles a typical slow response.

Certain cells in the heart, notably those in the SA and AV nodes, are normally slow-response fibers. In such fibers, depolarization is achieved mainly by the influx of Ca^{++} through the Ca^{++} channels. Repolarization is accomplished in these fibers by the inactivation of the Ca^{++} channels and by the increased K^+ conductance through the i_{K1} and i_K channels.

The Fast Response Underlies Rapid Conduction of the Cardiac Impulse

In fast-response fibers, the Na^+ channels are activated rapidly when the transmembrane potential of one region of the fiber suddenly changes from a resting value of about –90 mV to the threshold value of about –70 mV. The inward Na^+ current then rapidly depolarizes the cell at that site. This portion of the fiber becomes part of the depolarized zone, and the border is displaced accordingly. The same process then begins at the new border. This process is repeated again and again, and the border moves continuously down the fiber as a wave of depolarization (see Figure 3–9).

The conduction velocity along the fiber varies directly with the amplitude of the action potential and with the rate of change of potential (dV_m/dt) during phase 0. The amplitude of the action potential equals the difference in potential between the fully depolarized and the fully polarized regions of the cell interior. The magnitude of the local currents is proportional to this potential difference. These local currents shift the potential of the resting zone toward the threshold value. Hence, they act as the local stimuli that depolarize the adjacent, resting portion of the fiber to its threshold potential. THE GREATER THE AMPLITUDE OF THE ACTION POTENTIAL, THE MORE EFFECTIVE ARE THE LOCAL STIMULI IN DEPOLARIZING ADJACENT PARTS OF THE MEMBRANE AND THE MORE

RAPIDLY IS THE WAVE OF DEPOLARIZATION PROPAGATED DOWN THE FIBER.

The rate of change of potential (dV_m/dt) during phase 0 is also an important determinant of the conduction velocity. If the active portion of the fiber depolarizes gradually, the local currents between the resting region and the neighboring depolarizing region are small. The resting region adjacent to the active zone is depolarized gradually, and hence more time is required for each new section of the fiber to reach threshold.

The level of the resting membrane potential is also an important determinant of conduction velocity. This factor influences the amplitude of the action potential and the slope of the upstroke. The transmembrane potential just before depolarization may vary for the following reasons: the external $[K^+]$ has changed (Figure 16–3); in intrinsically automatic cardiac fibers, V_m becomes progressively less negative during phase 4 (Figure 16–16, *B*); and if the cell is excited prematurely, the cell membrane is not repolarized fully from the preceding excitation (Figure 16–10).

The V_m level affects conduction velocity because the inactivation or *h* gates (Figure 16–8) in the fast Na^+ channels are voltage dependent. The less negative the V_m, the greater is the number of *h* gates that tend to close. During the normal process of excitation, depolarization proceeds so rapidly during phase 0 that the slow *h* gates do not close until the end of phase 0. However, if partial depolarization proceeds gradually, the gates have ample time to close and thereby some of the Na^+ channels are inactivated. When the cell is partially depolarized, many of the Na^+ channels are already inactivated. Hence, only a fraction of the Na^+ channels is available to conduct the inward Na^+ current during phase 0.

Figure 16–6 illustrates how the resting V_m in a cardiac muscle fiber is affected by the value of E_K. When $[K^+]_o$ is greater than about 5 mM, the measured value of V_m corresponds with the value predicted by the Nernst equation because g_K is much greater than g_{Na}. However, for values of $[K^+]_o$ less than 5 mM, g_K decreases as $[K^+]_o$ diminishes.

When $[K^+]_o$ is increased gradually from 3 mM to 16 mM (Figure 16–3), the resting V_m becomes progressively less negative. This rise in $[K^+]_o$ decreases the amplitudes and durations of the action potentials, and the steepness of the upstrokes diminishes. Consequently, the conduction velocity diminishes progressively. At $[K^+]_o$ levels of 14 and 16 mM (segments *D* and *E*), the resting V_m attains levels that are sufficient to inactivate all the fast Na^+ channels. The action potentials in panels *D* and *E* are characteristic slow responses.

Most of the experimentally induced changes in transmembrane potential shown in Figure 16–3 also take place in patients with **coronary artery disease.** When blood flow to a myocardial region diminishes, the supplies of oxygen and metabolic substrates delivered to the ischemic tissues are insufficient. The ATP-sensitive K^+ channels are kept in a closed state by the nucleotide, whose synthesis requires a continuous supply of oxygen. When blood flow is inadequate, ATP concentration falls and the activity of the ATP-dependent K^+ channel is increased. Also, the ischemic myocytes accumulate excess Na^+ while they lose K^+ to the surrounding interstitial space. Consequently, the $[K^+]$ in the extracellular fluid surrounding the ischemic myocytes is elevated. The myocytes are affected by the elevated $[K^+]$ and permeability in much the same way as is the myocyte that is depicted in Figure 16–3. Such changes may disturb cardiac rhythm and conduction critically.

The Ca^{++} Current Determines Conduction of the Slow Response

Local circuits (see Figure 3–9) are partially responsible for propagation of the slow response. However, the characteristics of the conduction process differ quantitatively from those of the fast response. The threshold potential is about −40 mV for the slow response, and this response is much slower than it is for the fast response. The conduction velocities of the slow responses in the SA and AV nodes are about 0.02 to 0.1 m/sec. The fast-response conduction velocities are about 0.3 to 1 m/sec for myocardial cells, and the velocities are about 1 to 4 m/sec for the specialized conducting (Purkinje) fibers in the ventricles. Slow responses are more likely to be blocked than are fast responses. Also, fast-response fibers can respond at repetition rates that are much greater than the repetition rates of slow-response fibers.

Cardiac Excitability Is Determined by the Availability of Na^+ and Ca^{++} Currents

Artificial pacemakers and other electrical devices for correction of serious cardiac rhythm disturbances have been developed. Therefore, detailed knowledge of cardiac excitability has become essential. The excitability characteristics of cardiac cells differ considerably, depending on whether the prevailing action potentials are generated by fast- or slow-response fibers.

Na^+ current activates and inactivates: the refractory period

Once a fast response has been initiated, the depolarized cell is no longer excitable until the cell is partially repolarized (Figure 16–1, *left panel*). THE INTERVAL FROM THE BEGINNING OF ONE ACTION POTENTIAL UNTIL THE TIME THAT THE FIBER CAN CONDUCT ANOTHER ACTION POTENTIAL IS CALLED THE **EFFECTIVE REFRACTORY PERIOD.** In a **fast-response fiber,** this period extends from the beginning of phase 0 to a point in phase 3 at which repolarization has reached about –50 mV (time *c* to time *d* in Figure 16–1, *left panel*). At about this value of V_m, the electrochemical *m* and *h* gates for many of the fast Na^+ channels have been reset.

However, the cardiac fiber is not fully excitable until it has been completely repolarized (time *e* in Figure 16–1). Before repolarization is complete (period *d* to *e* in Figure 16–1), an action potential may be evoked only when the stimulus is sufficiently strong to evoke a response during phase 4. Period *d* to *e* is called the **relative refractory period.**

When a fast response is evoked during the relative refractory period of a previous excitation, its characteristics vary with the membrane potential that exists at the time of stimulation (Figure 16–10). The later in the relative refractory period that the fiber is stimulated, the greater is the increase in the amplitude of the response and in the slope of the upstroke. Presumably, the number of fast Na^+ channels that have recovered from inactivation increases as repolarization proceeds during phase 3. As a consequence of the greater amplitude and upstroke slope of the evoked response, the increase in propagation velocity varies directly with the time in the relative refractory period at which the fiber is stimulated. Once the fiber is fully repolarized, the response is constant, no matter what time in phase 4 the stimulus is applied.

In a patient who has occasional **premature depolarizations** (Figure 16–10), the timing of these early beats may determine their clinical consequence. If they occur late in the refractory period of the preceding depolarization or after full repolarization, the premature depolarization is probably inconsequential. However, if the premature depolarizations originate early in the relative refractory period of the ventricles, conduction of the premature impulse from the site of origin will be slow, and hence reentry is likely to occur. If that reentry is irregular (i.e., if ventricular fibrillation ensues), the consequence may be grave (see Figure 17–24 in Chapter 17).

Ca^{++} current generates the slow response

IN SLOW-RESPONSE FIBERS, THE RELATIVE REFRACTORY PERIOD FREQUENTLY EXTENDS WELL BEYOND PHASE 3 (Figure 16–1, *right panel*). Even after the cell has completely repolarized, it may be difficult to evoke a propagated response for some time. This characteristic of slow-response fibers is called **post-repolarization refractoriness.**

Action potentials evoked early in the relative refractory period are small, and the upstrokes are not very steep **(Figure 16–17)**. The amplitudes and upstroke slopes progressively improve as action potentials are elicited later in the relative refractory period. The recovery of full excitability is much slower than in the fast response. Impulses that arrive early in the relative refractory period are conducted much more slowly than are those that arrive late in that period. The lengthy refractory periods also lead to conduction blocks. Even when slow responses recur at a slow repetition rate, the fiber may be able to conduct only a fraction of those impulses; for example, only alternate impulses may be propagated.

Stimulus cycle length determines action potential duration

Changes in cycle length alter the duration of action potentials in cardiac cells **(Figure 16–18)** and thus change their refractory periods. Consequently, changes in cycle length are often important factors in the initiation or termination of certain arrhythmias (irregular heart rhythms). The changes in action potential duration produced by stepwise reductions in cycle length from 2000 to 200 msec in a Purkinje fiber are shown in Figure 16–18. Note that as the cycle length diminishes, the action potential duration decreases. The direct correlation between action potential duration and cycle length is mediated by g_K changes that involve at least two types of

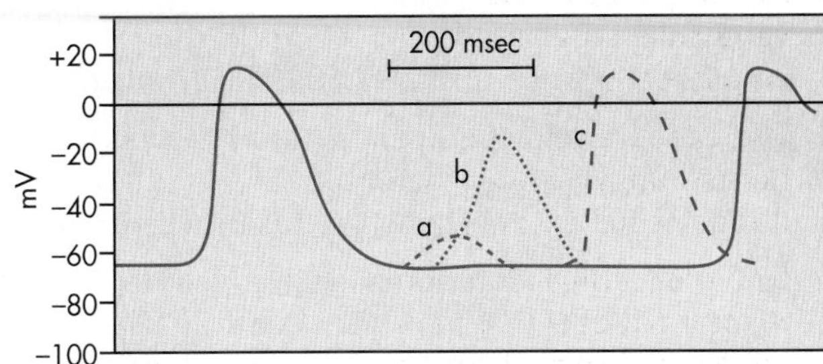

FIGURE 16–17. Effects of excitation at various times after the initiation of an action potential in a slow-response cardiac fiber. (Modified from Singer DH et al: *Progr Cardiovasc Dis* 24:97, 1981.)

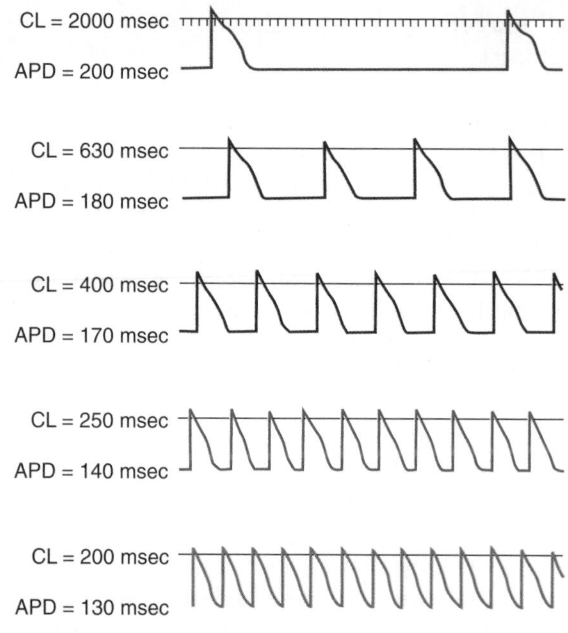

FIGURE 16–18. Effect of changes in cycle length (CL) on the action potential duration (APD) of canine Purkinje fibers. (Modified from Singer D, Ten Eick RE: *Am J Cardiol* 28:381, 1971.)

K^+ channels—namely, those channels that conduct the delayed rectifier K^+ current, i_K, and those that conduct the transient outward K^+ current, i_{to}.

The i_K current is activated at values of V_m near zero, but the current activates slowly and remains activated for hundreds of milliseconds. The i_K current also inactivates slowly. Consequently, as the basic cycle length diminishes, each action potential appears earlier in the inactivation period of the i_K current of the preceding action potential. Therefore, the shorter the basic cycle length, the greater is the outward K^+ current during phase 2, and hence the shorter the duration of the action potential.

The current also influences the relationship between cycle length and action potential duration. The i_{to} current is also activated at near-zero potentials, and its magnitude varies inversely with the cardiac cycle length. Therefore, as cycle length decreases, the resulting increase in the outward K^+ current shortens the plateau. The relative contributions of i_K and of i_{to} to the relationship between action potential duration and cardiac cycle length vary from species to species.

Summary

- ❖ The transmembrane action potentials that can be recorded from cardiac myocytes contain the following five phases:

  Phase 0: The action potential upstroke is produced when a suprathreshold stimulus rapidly depolarizes the membrane by activating the fast Na^+ channels.

  Phase 1: The notch is an early partial repolarization achieved by the efflux of K^+ through transmembrane channels that conduct the transient outward current, i_{to}.

  Phase 2: The plateau represents a balance between the influx of Ca^{++} through transmembrane Ca^{++} channels and the efflux of K^+ through several types of K^+ channels.

  Phase 3: Final repolarization is initiated when the efflux of K^+ exceeds the influx of Ca^{++}. The resultant partial repolarization rapidly increases the K^+ conductance and rapidly restores full repolarization.

  Phase 4: The resting potential of the fully repolarized cell is determined mainly by conductance of the cell membrane to K^+ through i_{K1} channels.

- ❖ Fast-response action potentials are recorded from atrial and ventricular myocardial fibers and from ventricular specialized conducting (Purkinje) fibers. The action potential is characterized by a large amplitude, a steep upstroke, and a relatively long plateau.
- ❖ The effective refractory period of fast-response fibers begins at the upstroke of the action potential and persists until midway through phase 3. The fiber is relatively refractory during the remainder of phase 3, and it regains full excitability when it is fully repolarized (phase 4).
- ❖ Slow-response action potentials are recorded from normal SA and AV nodal cells and from abnormal myocardial cells that have been partially depolarized. The action potential is characterized by a less negative resting potential, a smaller amplitude, a less steep upstroke, and a shorter plateau than in the fast-response action potential. The upstroke is produced by the activation of Ca^{++} channels.
- ❖ Slow-response fibers become absolutely refractory at the beginning of the upstroke, and partial excitability may not be regained until very late in phase 3 or until after the fiber is fully repolarized.

Bibliography

Bers DM, Perez-Reyes E: Ca channels in cardiac myocytes: structure and function in Ca influx and intracellular Ca release, *Cardiovasc Res* 42:339, 1999.

Carmeliet E: Cardiac ionic currents and acute ischemia: from channels to arrhythmias, *Physiol Rev* 79:917, 1999.

Grant AO: Molecular biology of sodium channels and their role in cardiac arrhythmias, *Am J Med* 110:296, 2001.

Hille B: *Ion channels of excitable membranes,* ed 3, Sunderland, Mass, 2001, Sinauer Associates.

Irisawa H, Brown HF, Giles W: Cardiac pacemaking in the sinoatrial node, *Physiol Rev* 73:197, 1993.

Kléber AG, Rudy Y: Basic mechanisms of cardiac impulse propagation and associated arrhythmias, *Physiol Rev* 84:431, 2004.

Nichols CG et al: Inward rectification and implications for cardiac excitability, *Circ Res* 78:1, 1996.

Oudit GY et al: The molecular physiology of the cardiac transient outward potassium current (I_{to}) in normal and diseased myocardium, *J Mol Cell Cardiol* 33:851, 2001.

Sicouri S, Antzelevitch C: Electrophysiologic characteristics of M cells in the canine left ventricular free wall, *J Cardiovasc Electrophysiol* 6:591, 1995.

Tseng GN: I_{Kr}: the hERG channel, *J Mol Cell Cardiol* 33:835, 2001.

Zipes DP, Jalife J: *Cardiac electrophysiology: from cell to bedside,* ed 2, Philadelphia, 1995, WB Saunders.

Case Study

Case 16–1

A 63-year-old man suddenly felt a crushing pain beneath his sternum. He became weak, began to sweat profusely, and noticed that his heart was beating rapidly. He called his physician, who made the diagnosis of myocardial infarction. The tests made at the hospital confirmed the physician's suspicion that the patient had suffered a "heart attack"—that is, a major coronary artery to the left ventricle had suddenly become occluded. An electrocardiogram indicated that the SA node was the source of the rapid heart rate. Two hours after admission to the hospital, the patient suddenly became much weaker. His arterial pulse rate was only about 40 beats/min. An electrocardiogram at this time revealed that the atrial rate was about 90 beats/min and that conduction through the AV junction was completely blocked, undoubtedly because the infarct affected the AV conduction system. Electrodes of an artificial pacemaker were inserted into the patient's right ventricle, and the ventricular contractions were paced at a frequency of 75 beats/min. The patient felt stronger and more comfortable almost immediately.

1. Soon after coronary artery occlusion, the interstitial fluid $[K^+]$ rose substantially in the flow-deprived region. What does the high $[K^+]_o$ in this region mean?

A. It increases the propagation velocity of the myocardial action potentials.
B. It decreases the post-repolarization refractoriness of the myocardial cells.
C. It changes the resting (phase 4) transmembrane potential to a less negative value.
D. It diminishes the automaticity of the myocardial cells.
E. It decreases the likelihood of reentrant arrhythmias.

2. The mechanism by which the SA node generated impulses at a rapid rate during the early stages of the coronary artery occlusion involves which of the following?

A. An increased slope of the action potential upstroke (phase 0) of the automatic cells
B. An increased slope of the slow diastolic depolarization of the automatic cells
C. An increased firing threshold of the automatic cells
D. An increased negativity (hyperpolarization) of the initial portion of the slow diastolic depolarization
E. An increased action potential amplitude of the automatic cells

3. What is the mechanism most likely responsible for the patient's arterial pulse rate of about 40 beats/min after impulse conduction through the AV junction was blocked?

A. Excitation of the ventricles via an AV bypass tract
B. Conversion of ventricular myocardial fibers to automatic cells
C. Firing of ventricular ectopic cells that have the same electrophysiological characteristics as SA node cells
D. Firing of automatic cells (Purkinje fibers) in the specialized conduction system of the ventricles
E. Excitation of ventricular cells by the rhythmic activity in the autonomic neurons that innervate the heart

4. When the heart was being paced, the cardiologist discontinued ventricular pacing periodically to test the patient's cardiac status. The cardiologist found that the ventricles did not begin beating spontaneously until about 5 to 10 seconds after cessation of pacing because the preceding period of pacing led to which of the following?

A. Overdrive suppression of the automatic cells in the ventricles
B. The release of norepinephrine from the cardiac sympathetic nerves
C. The release of neuropeptide Y from the cardiac sympathetic nerves
D. Fatigue of the ventricular myocytes
E. The release of acetylcholine from the cardiac parasympathetic nerves

Chapter 17: Natural Excitation of the Heart

Objectives

- ❖ Discuss the basis of automaticity.
- ❖ Describe the spread of excitation of the heart.
- ❖ Explain the basis of reentry.
- ❖ Describe the components of the electrocardiogram.

The nervous system controls various aspects of cardiac function, such as the heart rate and the strength of cardiac contraction. However, cardiac function does not require an intact innervation. Indeed, a cardiac transplant patient, whose heart has been completely denervated, can still adapt well to stress. The ability of the transplanted heart to function and to adapt to changing conditions depends on certain intrinsic properties of cardiac tissue, especially its automaticity.

THE PROPERTIES OF **AUTOMATICITY** (THE ABILITY TO INITIATE ITS OWN BEAT) AND **RHYTHMICITY** (THE REGULARITY OF SUCH ACTIVITY) ALLOW THE PERFUSED HEART TO BEAT, EVEN WHEN IT IS COMPLETELY REMOVED FROM THE BODY. If the coronary vasculature of an excised heart is artificially perfused with blood or with an oxygenated electrolyte solution, the rhythmic cardiac contractions may persist for many hours. Certain cells in the atria and ventricles can initiate beats; such cells reside mainly in the nodal tissues or in the specialized conducting fibers of the heart.

In the normal mammalian heart, the region that generates impulses at the greatest frequency is the **sinoatrial (SA) node,** which is the main **pacemaker** of the heart. Detailed mapping of the electrical potentials on the surface of the right atrium reveals two or three sites of automaticity. These sites are located near the SA node itself, and they serve along with the SA node as an **atrial pacemaker complex.** At certain times, these loci might initiate impulses simultaneously. At other times, the site of earliest excitation might shift from locus to locus, depending on certain conditions, such as the level of autonomic neural activity.

Regions of the heart other than the SA node may initiate beats under special circumstances. Such regions are called **ectopic foci** or **ectopic pacemakers.** Ectopic foci may become pacemakers when their own rhythmicity is enhanced, the rhythmicity of the higher order pacemakers is depressed, or all conduction pathways between the ectopic focus and the regions with greatest rhythmicity become blocked. Ectopic pacemakers may act as a safety mechanism when normal pacemaking centers fail. However, if an ectopic center fires while the normal pacemaking center still functions, the ectopic activity may induce either sporadic rhythm disturbances, such as **premature depolarizations** (Figure 17–1), or continuous rhythm disturbances, such as **paroxysmal tachycardias** (Figure 17–2).

When the SA node or other components of the atrial pacemaker complex are destroyed, certain pacemaker cells in the atrioventricular (AV) junction usually become the pacemakers for the entire heart. Automatic cells in the atria usually become dominant after a time that varies from minutes to days. Purkinje fibers in the specialized conduction system of the ventricles also display automaticity. Characteristically, these fibers generate impulses at

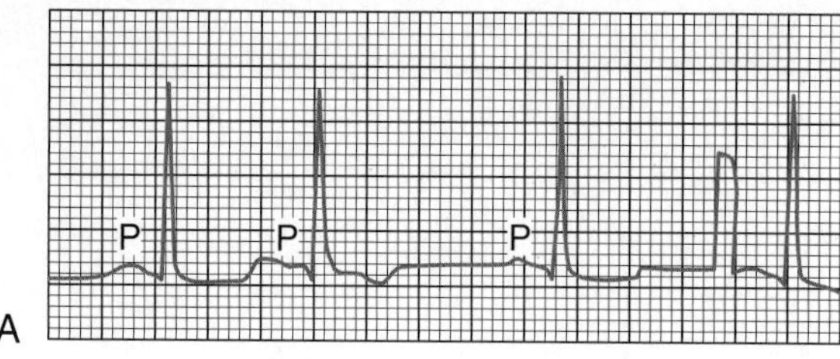

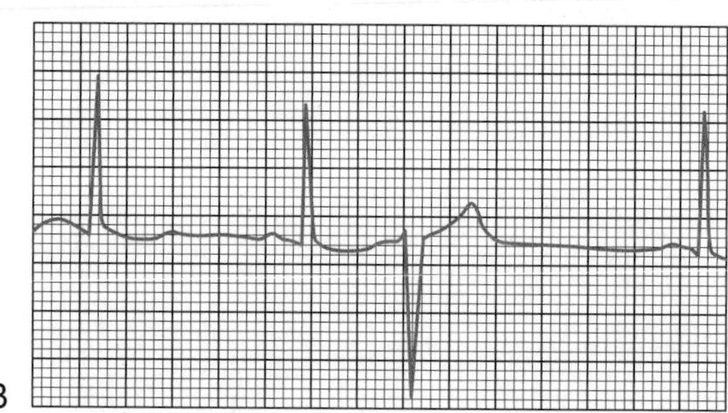

FIGURE 17–1. A premature atrial depolarization (A) and a premature ventricular depolarization (B). The premature atrial depolarization (the second beat in the top tracing) is characterized by an inverted P wave and normal QRS and T waves. The interval after the premature depolarization is not much longer than the usual interval between beats. The brief rectangular deflection just before the last depolarization is a standardization signal. The premature ventricular depolarization is characterized by bizarre QRS and T waves and is followed by a compensatory pause.

a very slow rate. When the AV junction cannot conduct impulses from the atria to the ventricles **(Figure 17–3)**, these **idioventricular pacemakers** in the Purkinje fiber network initiate ventricular contractions, but at a frequency of only 30 to 40 beats/min.

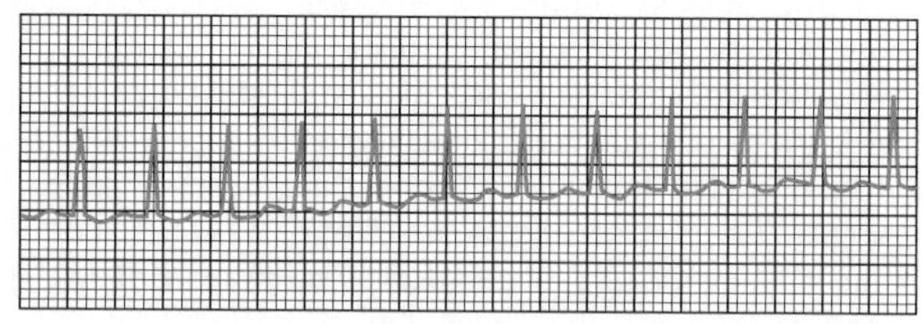

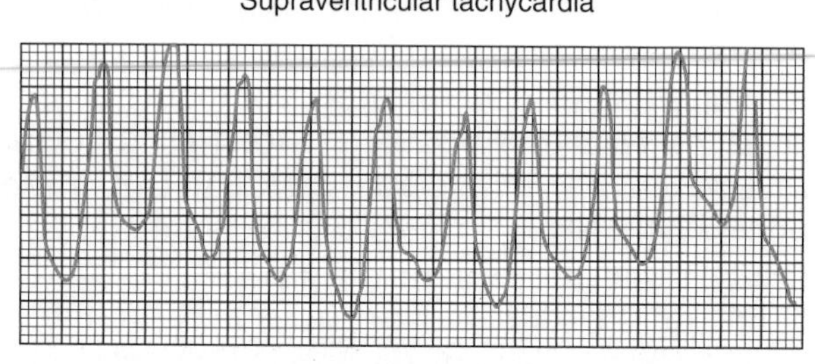

FIGURE 17–2. A and B, Paroxysmal tachycardias.

The Sinoatrial Node Is the Natural Pacemaker of the Heart

In adult humans, the SA node is about 8 mm long and 2 mm thick, and it lies posteriorly in the groove at the junction between the superior vena cava and the right atrium **(Figure 17–4)**. The sinus node artery runs lengthwise through the center of the node. The SA node contains two principal types of cells:

- small, round cells having few organelles and myofibrils; and
- slender, elongated cells, which are intermediate in appearance between the round and slender atrial myocardial cells.

The round cells are probably the pacemaker cells. The slender, elongated cells probably conduct the impulses to the center of the node and to the nodal margins.

A typical transmembrane action potential recorded from a cell in the SA node is depicted in Figure 16–16, *B* (see Chapter 16). Compared with the transmembrane potential recorded from a ventricular myocardial cell (see Figure 16–16, *A*), the resting potential of the SA node cell is usually less negative, the upstroke of the action potential (phase 0) is less steep, the plateau is not sustained, and the repolarization (phase 3) is more gradual. All these attributes are characteristic of the slow response. As in cells that exhibit the slow response, tetrodotoxin has no influence on the SA nodal action potential. Thus, the upstroke of the action potential is not produced by an inward current of Na^+ through fast channels.

The transmembrane potential during phase 4 is much less negative in SA and AV nodal automatic cells than in atrial or ventricular myocytes because nodal cells lack the i_{K1} (inward rectifying) type of K^+ channel. Therefore, the ratio of g_K to g_{Na} during phase 4 is much less in the nodal cells than in the myocytes. During phase 4, therefore, V_m deviates much more from the K^+ equilibrium potential (E_K) in nodal cells than it does in myocytes.

The principal feature that distinguishes a pacemaker fiber from other cardiac fibers resides in phase 4. IN NONAUTOMATIC CELLS, THE POTENTIAL REMAINS CONSTANT DURING PHASE 4, WHEREAS A PACEMAKER FIBER IS CHARACTERIZED BY A SLOW DIASTOLIC DEPOLARIZATION THROUGHOUT PHASE 4. Depolarization proceeds at a steady rate until the threshold is attained, and an action potential is then triggered.

The discharge frequency of pacemaker cells may be determined by changes in the rate of depolarization during phase 4, the maximal negativity during phase 4, or the threshold potential **(Figure**

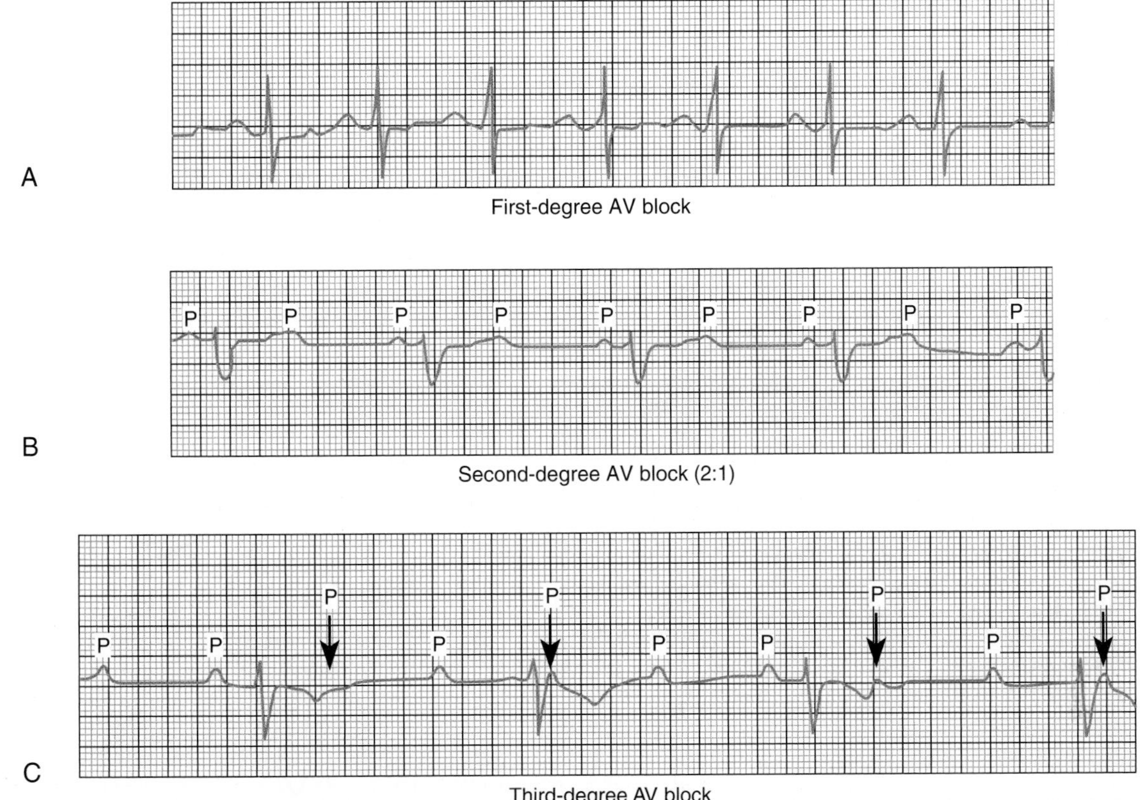

FIGURE 17–3. AV blocks. A, First-degree block; PR interval is 0.28 second. B, Second-degree block (2:1). C, Third-degree block; note the dissociation between the P waves and the QRS complexes.

17–5). When the rate of slow diastolic depolarization is increased (from *b* to *a* in Figure 17–5, *A*), the threshold potential is attained, and the heart rate increases. A rise in the threshold potential (from TP-1 to TP-2 in Figure 17–5, *B*) delays the onset of phase 0 (from time *b* to time *c*), and the heart rate is reduced accordingly. Similarly, when the maximal negative potential is increased (from *a* to *d* in Figure 17–5, *B*), more time is required to reach threshold TP-2 when the slope of phase 4 remains unchanged, and the heart rate therefore diminishes.

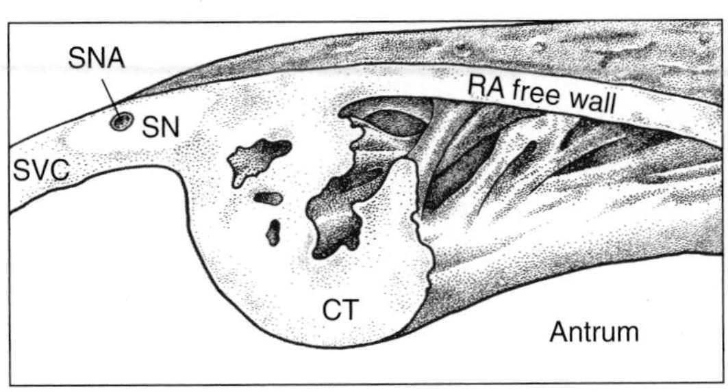

FIGURE 17–4. Location of the sinoatrial node (SN) near the junction between the superior vena cava (SVC) and the right atrium (RA). SNA, sinoatrial artery; CT, crista terminalis. (Redrawn from James TN: *Am J Cardiol* 40:965, 1977.)

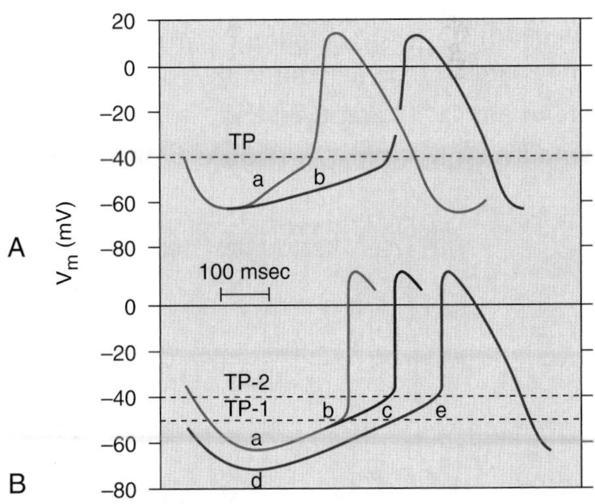

FIGURE 17–5. Mechanisms involved in the changes in frequency of pacemaker firing. In A, a reduction in the slope (from *a* to *b*) of slow diastolic depolarization diminishes the firing frequency. In B, an increase in the threshold potential (from TP-1 to TP-2) or an increase in the magnitude of the resting potential (from *a* to *d*) also diminishes the firing frequency. (Redrawn from Hoffman BF, Cranefield PF: *Electrophysiology of the heart,* New York, 1960, McGraw-Hill.)

Ordinarily, pacemaker firing frequency is controlled by the activity of both divisions of the autonomic nervous system. Increased sympathetic nervous activity, through the release of norepinephrine, raises the heart rate principally by increasing the slope of the slow diastolic depolarization. This mechanism of increasing heart rate occurs during physical exertion, anxiety, or certain illnesses, such as **febrile infectious diseases.**

Increased vagal activity, through the release of acetylcholine, diminishes the heart rate by hyperpolarizing the pacemaker cell membrane and reducing the slope of the slow diastolic depolarization **(Figure 17–6)**. These mechanisms of decreasing heart rate occur when vagal activity is predominant. An extreme example is **vasovagal syncope,** which is a brief period of lightheadedness or loss of consciousness caused by an intense burst of vagal activity. This type of syncope is a reflex response to pain or to certain psychological stimuli.

Changes in autonomic neural activity usually do not change heart rate by altering the threshold level of V_m that initiates the firing of a nodal pacemaker cell. However, certain antiarrhythmic drugs, such as **quinidine** and **procainamide,** do raise the threshold potential of the automatic cells to less negative values.

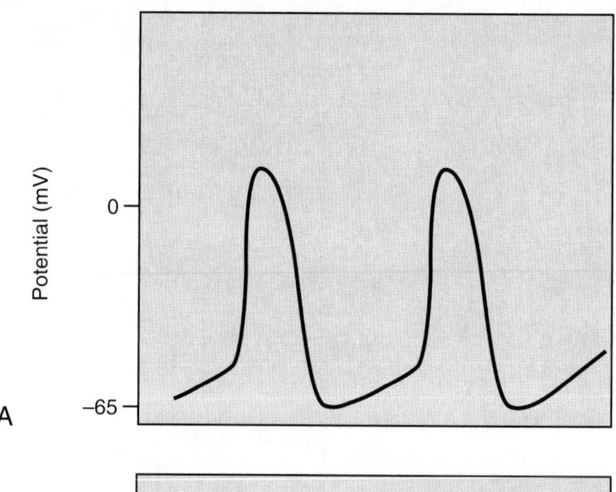

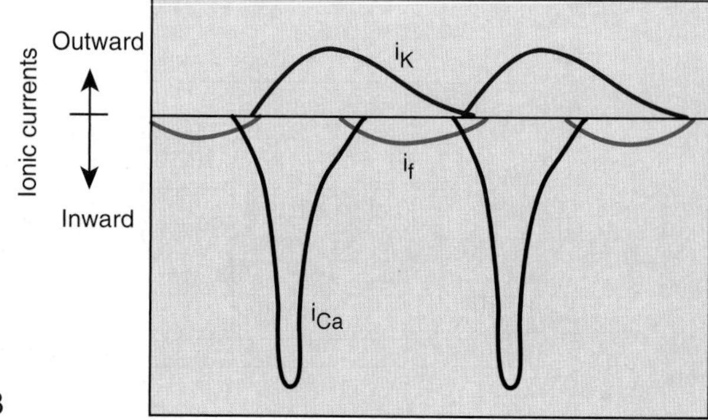

FIGURE 17–7. The transmembrane potential changes (A) that occur in SA node cells are produced by three principal currents (B): (1) an inward Ca^{++} current, i_{Ca}; (2) a hyperpolarization-induced inward current, i_f; and (3) an outward K^+ current, i_K.

Fluxes of K^+, Ca^{++}, and Na^+ underlie automaticity

Several ionic currents contribute to the slow diastolic depolarization that occurs characteristically in the automatic cells of the heart. In SA node pacemaker cells, the slow diastolic depolarization is mediated by at least three ionic currents:

- an inward current, i_f, induced by hyperpolarization;
- an inward Ca^{++} current, i_{Ca}; and
- an outward K^+ current, i_K **(Figure 17–7)**.

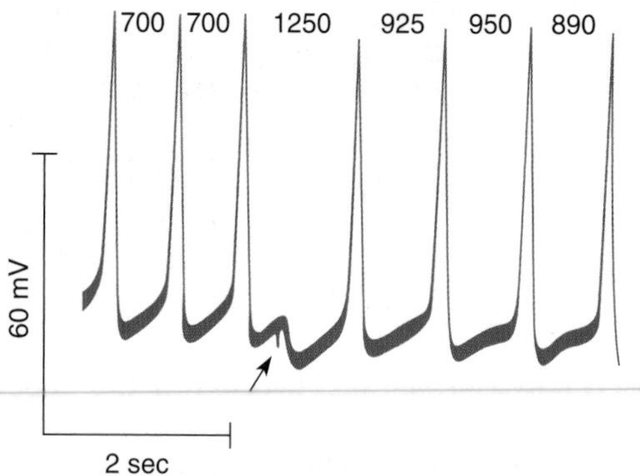

FIGURE 17–6. Effect of a brief vagal stimulus *(arrow)* on the transmembrane potential recorded from an SA node pacemaker cell in an isolated cat atrium preparation. The cardiac cycle lengths, in milliseconds, are denoted by the numbers at the top of the figure. (Modified from Jalife J, Moe GK: *Circ Res* 45:595, 1979, with permission of the American Heart Association.)

The inward current, i_f, is activated near the end of repolarization. The subscript *f* in the preceding sentence alludes to a "funny" current carried mainly by Na^+ through specific channels that differ from the fast Na^+ channels. This current was dubbed "funny" because its discoverers did not expect to find an inward Na^+ current in the pacemaker cells after repolarization had been completed. This i_f current is activated as the membrane potential becomes negative to about −50 mV. The more negative the membrane potential, the greater is the activation of the i_f current.

The second current responsible for diastolic depolarization is the Ca^{++} current, i_{Ca}. This current is activated toward the end of phase 4, as the transmembrane potential reaches a value of about −55 mV (Figure 17–7, *A*). Once the Ca^{++} channels are activated, the Ca^{++} influx increases into the cells. This influx accelerates the rate of diastolic depolarization, which then leads to the upstroke of the action potential. A decrease in the external [Ca^{++}] **(Figure 17–8)** or the addition of Ca^{++} channel antagonists **(Figure 17–9)** diminishes the amplitude of

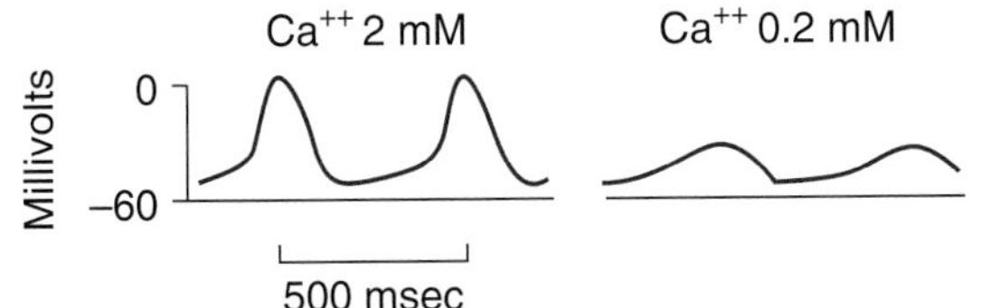

FIGURE 17–8. Transmembrane action potentials recorded from an SA node pacemaker cell in an isolated rabbit atrium preparation. The concentration of Ca^{++} in the bath was reduced from 2 mM to 0.2 mM. (Modified from Kohlhardt M, Figulla HR, Tripathi O: *Basic Res Cardiol* 71:17, 1976.)

the action potential and the slope of the slow diastolic depolarization in SA node cells.

The progressive diastolic depolarization, which is mediated by the two inward currents i_f and i_{Ca}, is opposed by an outward current, the delayed rectifier K^+ current, i_K. This efflux of K^+ tends to repolarize the cell after the upstroke of the action potential has been completed. K^+ continues to leave the cell well beyond the time of maximal repolarization, but its efflux diminishes throughout phase 4 (Figure 17–7, *B*). As the current diminishes, its opposition to the depolarizing effects of the two inward currents (i_{Ca} and i_f) also gradually decreases.

The ionic basis for automaticity in the AV node pacemaker cells resembles that in the SA node cells. Similar mechanisms also account for automaticity in ventricular Purkinje fibers, except that the Ca^{++} current is not involved. The slow diastolic depolarization is mediated principally by the imbalance between the effects of the hyperpolarization-induced inward current, i_f, and the gradually diminishing outward K^+ current, i_K.

The autonomic neurotransmitters affect automaticity by altering membrane ionic currents. The adrenergic transmitters increase all three currents involved in SA nodal automaticity. To increase the slope of diastolic depolarization, the augmentations of i_f and i_{Ca} by the adrenergic transmitters must exceed the enhancement of i_K.

The hyperpolarization induced by the acetylcholine released at the vagus endings in the heart is achieved by an increase in g_K (Figure 17–6). This change in conductance is mediated through activation of specific **acetylcholine-regulated K^+ channels**. Acetylcholine also diminishes the i_f and i_{Ca} currents. The autonomic neural effects on cardiac cells are described in greater detail in Chapter 19.

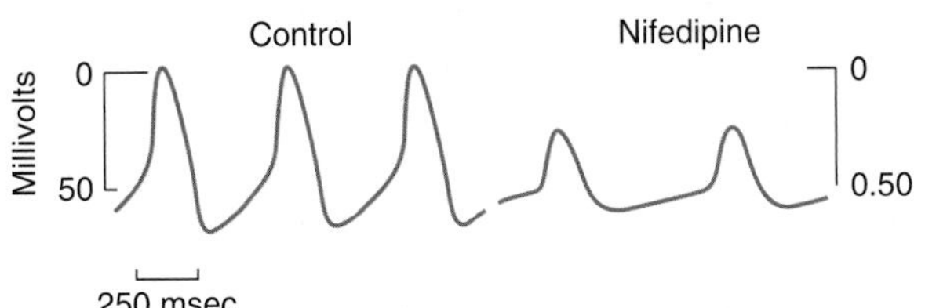

FIGURE 17–9. Effects of nifedipine (5.6×10^{-7} M), a Ca^{++} channel antagonist, on the transmembrane potentials recorded from an AV node cell in a rabbit. (From Ning W, Wit AL: *Am Heart J* 106:345, 1983.)

Overdrive suppresses automaticity

The automaticity of pacemaker cells diminishes after a period of excitation at a high frequency. This phenomenon is known as **overdrive suppression.** The firing of the SA node tends to suppress the automaticity in the other loci because the intrinsic rhythmicity of the SA node is greater than that of the other latent pacemaking sites in the heart.

If an ectopic atrial focus suddenly begins to fire at a high rate (e.g., 150 impulses/min) in an individual whose normal heart rate is 70 beats/min, the ectopic site would become the pacemaker for the entire heart. If that ectopic focus suddenly stopped firing, the SA node might remain quiescent briefly because of overdrive suppression. The interval from the end of the overdrive period until the SA node resumes firing is called the **sinus node recovery time.** In patients with **sick sinus syndrome,** the sinus node recovery time is prolonged and the patient would lose consciousness if the resulting period of **asystole** (absence of a heartbeat) persists for longer than a few seconds.

Overdrive suppression results from the activity of the membrane pump, Na^+,K^+-ATPase, which extrudes three Na^+ from the cell in exchange for two K^+. Normally, a certain amount of Na^+ enters the cardiac cell during each depolarization. The more frequently the cell is depolarized, therefore, the more Na^+ enters the cell per minute. At high excitation frequencies, the activity of the Na^+,K^+-ATPase increases and extrudes a larger amount of Na^+ from the cell interior. The activity of the Na^+,K^+-ATPase hyperpolarizes the cell because the amount of Na^+ extruded by the pump exceeds the amount of K^+ that enters the cell. Therefore, the slow diastolic depolarization requires more time to reach the firing threshold, as shown in Figure 17–5, *B*. Furthermore, when the overdrive suddenly ceases, the activity of the Na^+,K^+-ATPase does not slow instantaneously, but it remains overactive temporarily. This excessive extrusion of Na^+ opposes the gradual depolarization of the pacemaker cell during phase 4 and thereby transiently suppresses the cell's intrinsic automaticity.

Atrial Muscle Conducts the Cardiac Impulse from the Sinoatrial Node to the Atrioventricular Node

From the SA node, the cardiac impulse spreads radially throughout the right atrium (**Figure 17–10**) along ordinary atrial myocardial fibers, at a conduction velocity of approximately 1 m/sec. A special pathway, the anterior interatrial myocardial band (or **Bachmann's bundle**), conducts the impulse from the SA node directly to the left atrium. The wave of excitation that proceeds inferiorly through the right atrium ultimately reaches the AV node, which is normally the sole route of entry of the cardiac impulse to the ventricles.

The configuration of the atrial transmembrane potential is depicted in Figure 16–16, *C* (see Chapter 16). Compared with the potential recorded from a typical ventricular fiber (see Figure 16–16, *A*), the atrial plateau (phase 2) is briefer and less developed, and repolarization (phase 3) is slower. The action potential duration in atrial myocytes is shorter than that in ventricular myocytes because the efflux of K^+ during the plateau is greater in atrial myocytes than in ventricular myocytes.

Atrioventricular Node Connects the Atria to the Ventricular Conducting System

The atrial excitation wave reaches the ventricles via the AV node. In adult humans, this node is approximately 22 mm long, 10 mm wide, and 3 mm thick. The node is situated posteriorly on the right side of the interatrial septum, near the ostium of the coronary sinus. The AV node contains the same two cell types as does the SA node, but the round cells in the AV node are less abundant, and the elongated cells predominate.

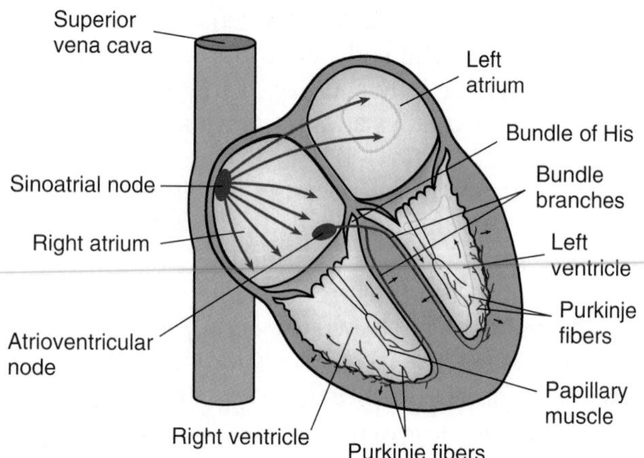

FIGURE 17–10. The cardiac conduction system. (Modified from Berne RM, Levy MN, Koeppen BM, Stanton BA: *Physiology,* ed 5, Philadelphia, 2004, Elsevier.)

The AV node is composed of three functional regions:

- the AN region, which is the transitional zone between the atrium and the remainder of the node;
- the N region, which is the midportion of the AV node; and
- the NH region, in which the nodal fibers gradually merge with the bundle of His (Figure 17–10).

This bundle of fibers is the upper portion of the specialized conducting system for the ventricles. Normally, the AV node and bundle of His are the only pathways along which the cardiac impulse travels from atria to ventricles.

Some people have accessory AV pathways, which often serve as a **reentry loop (Figure 17–11)**. Such pathways can lead to serious cardiac rhythm disturbances, such as the **Wolff-Parkinson-White syndrome.** This congenital syndrome is the most common disorder in which a bypass tract of myocardial fibers serves as an accessory pathway from the atria to the ventricles. Ordinarily, the syndrome causes no functional abnormality. The disturbance is easily detected in the electrocardiogram because a portion of the ventricle is excited via a bypass tract before the remainder of the ventricle is excited via the AV node and His-Purkinje system. This preexcitation can be recognized by the bizarre configuration of the ventricular **QRS** complex in the electrocardiogram. On occasion, however, a reentry loop develops, in which the atrial impulse travels to the ventricles via the AV node or the bypass tract. The impulse may then return to the atria through the other of the two pathways. Continuous circling around the loop leads to a rapid rhythm **(supraventricular tachycardia).** This rhythm may be incapacitating because time for ventricular filling may not be sufficient. The AV node can be blocked transiently by injecting adenosine intravenously or by increasing vagal activity reflexly by pressing on the carotid sinuses in the neck. A normal sinus rhythm is usually restored. Radiofrequency catheter ablation is often used to eliminate the bypass tract and this arrhythmia.

Several features of AV conduction are significant physiologically and clinically. The principal delay in the passage of the impulse from the atria to the ventricles occurs in the AN and N regions of the AV node; the N region is the midregion of the AV node. The conduction velocity is actually slower in the N region than in the AN region. However, the path length is substantially greater in the AN than in the N region. The conduction times through the AN and N zones account for the delay from the beginning of the **P wave** to the beginning of the **QRS complex** in an electrocardiogram (**Figure 17–12**).

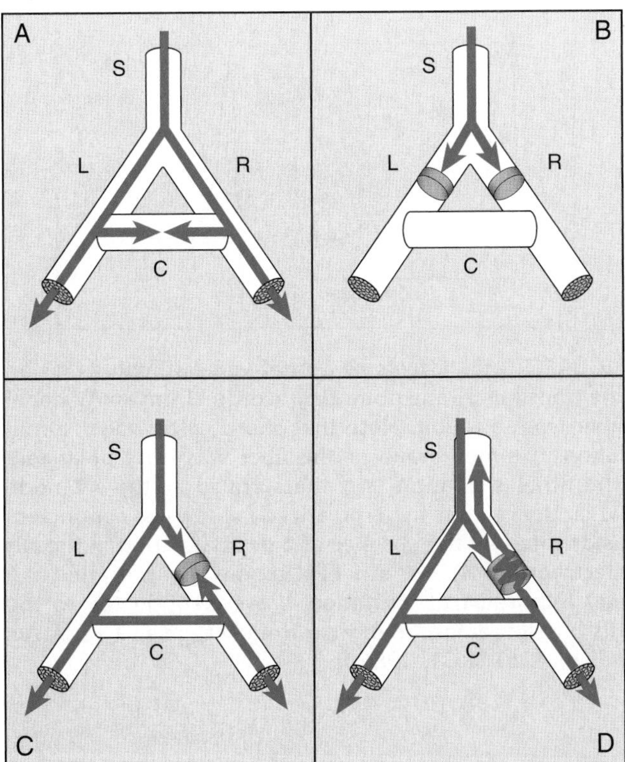

FIGURE 17–11. The role of unidirectional block in reentry. In A, an excitation wave traveling down a single bundle (S) of fibers continues down the left (L) and right (R) branches. The depolarization wave enters the connecting branch (C) from both ends and is extinguished at the zone of collision. In B, the wave is blocked in the L and R branches. In C, antegrade and retrograde (bidirectional) block exists in branch R. In D, unidirectional block exists in branch R. The antegrade impulse that travels downward from S to R is blocked because the region of unidirectional block has not regained its excitability. The retrograde impulse in R arrives at this region later after excitability has recovered and is conducted through and reenters bundle S.

FUNCTIONALLY, THE DELAY BETWEEN THE ATRIAL AND VENTRICULAR EXCITATIONS PERMITS OPTIMAL VENTRICULAR FILLING DURING AN ATRIAL CONTRACTION.

In the N region, slow-response action potentials prevail. The resting potential is about −60 mV, the upstroke velocity is slow (about 5 V/sec), and the conduction velocity is about 0.05 m/sec. **Tetrodotoxin,** which blocks the fast Na^+ channels, has virtually no effect on the action potentials or on the slow-response fibers in this region. Conversely, Ca^{++} channel antagonists depress AV conduction and decrease the amplitude and duration of the action potentials **(Figure 17–13)**. The shapes of the action potentials in the AN region are intermediate between those in the N region and in the atria. Similarly, the action potentials in the NH

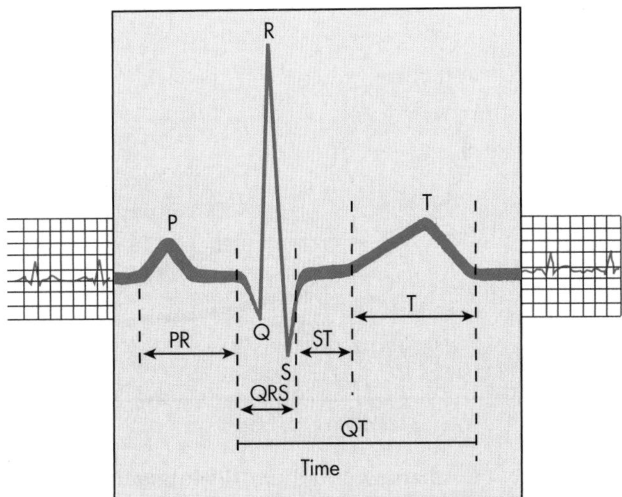

FIGURE 17–12. Important deflections and intervals of a typical electrocardiogram.

region are transitional between those in the N region and the bundle of His.

Like other slow-response action potentials, the relative refractory periods of cells in the N region extend well beyond the period of complete repolarization; that is, these cells display **post-repolarization refractoriness** (see Figure 16–17). As the time between successive atrial depolarizations is decreased, conduction through the AV junction slows **(Figure 17–14)**. An abnormal prolongation of the AV conduction time is called **first-degree AV block** (Figure 17–3, *A*). Most of the prolongation of AV conduction induced by a decrease in atrial cycle length takes place in the N region of the AV node.

Impulses tend to be blocked in the AV node, even when the applied stimulation frequencies are easily conducted in other regions of the heart. If the atria are depolarized at a high repetition rate, only a fraction of the atrial impulses will be conducted through the AV junction to the ventricles. The conduction pattern in which only some of the atrial

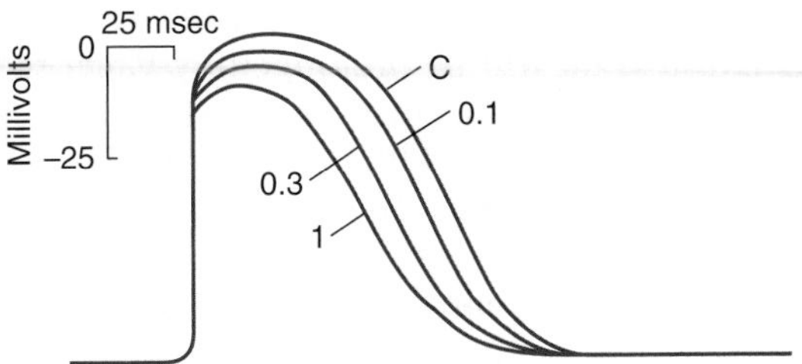

FIGURE 17–13. Transmembrane potentials recorded from a rabbit AV node cell under control conditions (C) and in the presence of the calcium channel antagonist diltiazem in concentrations of 0.1, 0.3, and 1 μmol/L. (Redrawn from Hirth C, Borchard U, Hafner D: *J Mol Cell Cardiol* 15:799, 1983.)

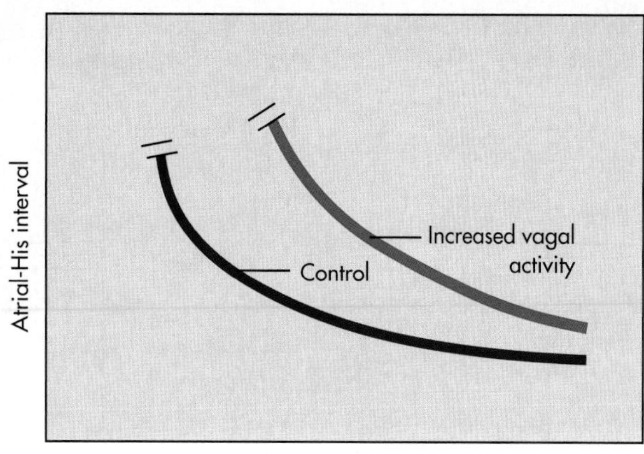

FIGURE 17–14. Changes in atrium-His intervals induced by pacing the atria at various cycle lengths in a group of human subjects under control conditions and during a reflexly induced increase in vagal activity produced by the intravenous infusion of phenylephrine. (Redrawn from Page RL et al: *Circ Res*, 68:1614, 1991, with permission of the American Heart Association.)

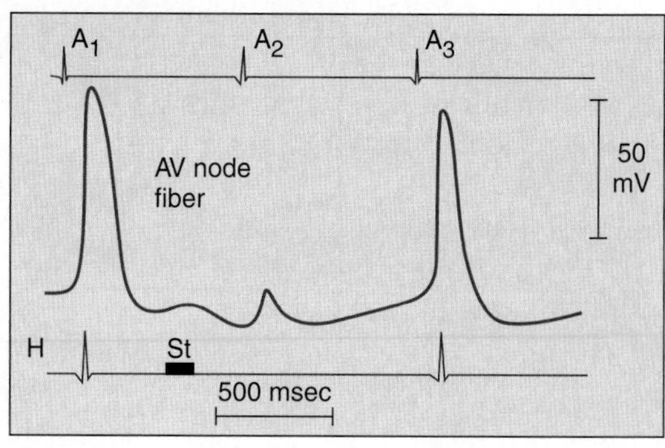

FIGURE 17–15. Effects of a brief vagal stimulus (St) on the transmembrane potential recorded from an AV nodal fiber from a rabbit. Note that shortly after vagal stimulation, the membrane of the fiber was hyperpolarized. The atrial excitation (A_2) that arrived at the AV node when the cell was hyperpolarized failed to be conducted, as denoted by the absence of a depolarization in the His electrogram (H). The atrial excitations that preceded (A_1) and followed (A_3) excitation A_2 were conducted to the His bundle region. (Redrawn from Mazgalev T et al: *Am J Physiol* 251:H631, 1986.)

impulses are conducted to the ventricles is called **second-degree AV block** (Figure 17–3, *B*). This type of block may protect the ventricles from excessive contraction frequencies, wherein the filling time between contractions might be inadequate.

Retrograde conduction can occur through the AV node. However, the propagation time is significantly prolonged and the impulse is blocked at low repetition rates when the impulse is conducted in the retrograde rather than in the antegrade direction. Finally, the AV node is a common site for **reentry;** the underlying mechanisms are explained in Figure 17–11.

The autonomic nervous system regulates AV conduction

Weak vagal activity may simply prolong the AV conduction time. Thus, for any given atrial cycle length, the atrium to His or the atrium to ventricle conduction time will be prolonged by vagal stimulation (Figure 17–14). Stronger vagal activity may cause many or most of the atrial impulses to be blocked in the AV node. The conduction pattern in which all of the atrial impulses are blocked is called **third-degree,** or **complete, AV block** (Figure 17–3, *C*). The vagally induced delay or absence of conduction through the AV junction occurs mainly in the N region of the node.

Acetylcholine, released by vagus nerve fibers, hyperpolarizes the conducting fibers in the AV node region (**Figure 17–15**). The greater the hyperpolarization at the time of arrival of the atrial impulse, the more impaired is the AV conduction. In the experiment shown in Figure 17–15, vagus nerve fibers are stimulated intensely (at St) shortly before the second atrial depolarization (A_2). That atrial impulse arrives at the AV node when its cell membrane is maximally hyperpolarized in response to the vagal stimulus. The absence of a corresponding depolarization of the bundle of His shows that the vagal stimulus prevents the conduction of the second atrial impulse through the AV node. Only a small, nonpropagated response to the second atrial impulse is evident in the recording from the conducting fiber.

The cardiac sympathetic nerves, on the other hand, facilitate AV conduction. They decrease the AV conduction time and enhance the rhythmicity of the latent pacemakers in the AV junction. The norepinephrine released at the sympathetic nerve terminals increases the amplitude and slope of the upstroke of the AV nodal action potentials, principally in the AN and N regions of the node.

Ventricular Conduction Is Rapid

The bundle of His passes subendocardially down the right side of the interventricular septum for about 1 cm, and then it divides into the right and left **bundle branches** (Figure 17–10). The right bundle branch, which is a direct continuation of the bundle of His, proceeds down the right side of the interventricular septum. The left bundle branch, which is considerably thicker than the right, arises almost perpendicularly from the bundle of His and perforates the interventricular septum. On the subendocardial surface of the left side of the interventricular septum, the left bundle branch splits into a thin anterior division and a thick posterior division.

Impulse conduction in the right or left bundle branch, or in either division of the left bundle branch, may be impaired. Conduction blocks may develop in one or more of these conduction pathways as a consequence of **coronary artery disease** or of degenerative processes that are associated with aging. Such conduction blocks may elicit characteristic electrocardiographic patterns. Block of either bundle branch is known as right or left **bundle branch block.** Block of either subdivision of the left bundle branch is called left anterior or left posterior **hemiblock.**

The right bundle branch and the two divisions of the left bundle branch ultimately subdivide into a complex network of conducting fibers, called **Purkinje fibers,** that spread out over the subendocardial surfaces of both ventricles. In certain mammalian species, such as cattle, the Purkinje fiber network is arranged in discrete, encapsulated bundles **(Figure 17–16).**

Purkinje fibers have abundant, linearly arranged sarcomeres, as do myocytes. However, the T-tubular system is absent in the Purkinje fibers of many species, but the T-tubular system is well developed in the myocytes. Purkinje fibers are the broadest cells in the heart; they are 70 to 80 μm in diameter, compared with diameters of 10 to 15 μm for ventricular myocytes. Partly because of the large diameters of the Purkinje fibers, the conduction velocities (1 to 4 m/sec) in those fibers exceed those of any other fiber types within the heart. The increased conduction velocity permits a rapid activation of the entire endocardial surface of the ventricles.

The action potentials recorded from epicardial and endocardial fibers resemble one another. Phase 1 is more prominent in epicardial fibers but less prominent in endocardial fibers **(Figure 17–17).** In general, phase 1 is prominent in Purkinje fiber action potentials (see Figure 16–11 in Chapter 16), and the duration of the plateau (phase 2) is intermediate between that of epicardial and midmyocardial myocytes.

Because Purkinje fibers have long refractory periods, many premature excitations of the atria are conducted through the AV junction, but they are blocked subsequently by the Purkinje fibers. Blockade of these atrial excitations prevents premature contraction of the ventricles. This protection against the effects of premature atrial depolarizations is especially pronounced when the heart rate is slow. The action potential duration and hence the effective refractory period of the Purkinje fibers vary inversely with the heart rate (see Figure 16–18). At slow heart rates, the effective refractory period of the Purkinje fibers is especially prolonged. As the heart rate increases, however, the refractory period diminishes. Similar directional changes in the refractory period occur also in ventricular myocytes in response to changes in basic cycle

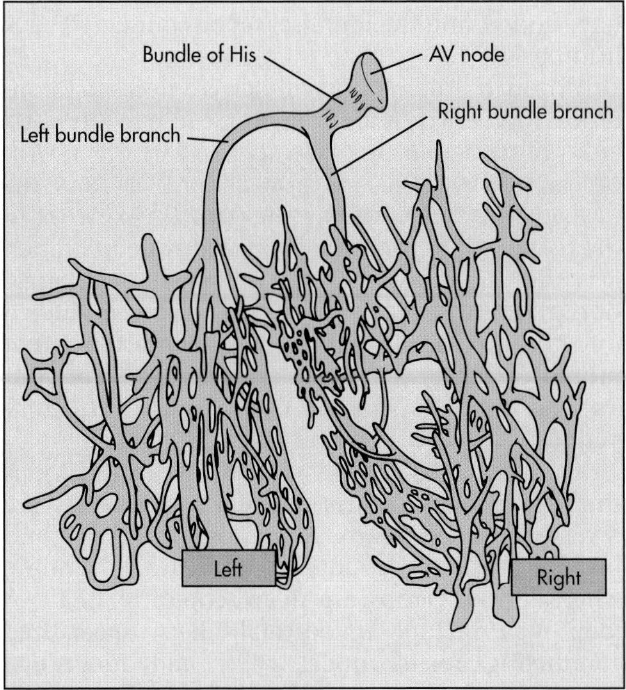

FIGURE 17–16. Atrioventricular and ventricular conduction system of the calf heart.

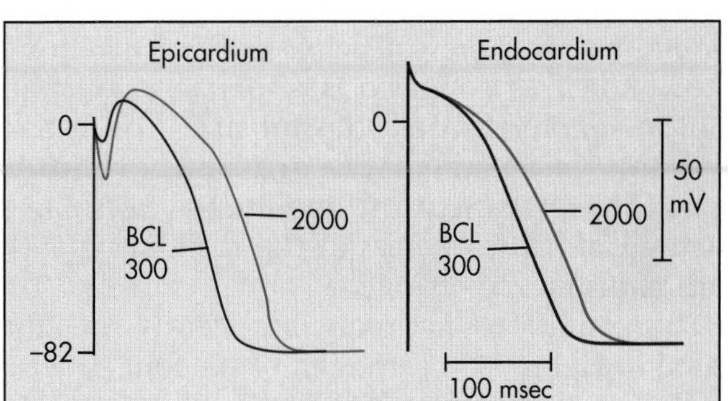

FIGURE 17–17. Action potentials recorded from myocardial cells in the epicardial and endocardial regions of the left ventricles. The preparations were driven at basic cycle lengths (BCL) of 300 and 2000 msec. (Redrawn from Litovsky SH, Antzelevitch C: *J Am Coll Cardiol* 14:1053, 1989.)

length (Figure 17–17). However, in the AV node, the effective refractory period does not change appreciably over the normal range of heart rates, and it actually increases when the heart rate is rapid. THEREFORE, WHEN THE ATRIUM IS EXCITED AT HIGH REPETITION RATES, IT IS THE AV NODE THAT PROTECTS THE VENTRICLES FROM THESE EXCESSIVELY HIGH FREQUENCIES.

The first regions of the ventricles to be excited by impulses arriving from the AV node are the interventricular septum (except the basal portion) and the papillary muscles. The wave of activation spreads into the substance of the septum from both its left and right endocardial surfaces. Early contraction of the septum tends to make it more rigid and allows it to serve as an anchor point for the contraction of the remaining ventricular myocardium. Also, early contraction of the papillary muscles prevents eversion of the AV valves during ventricular systole.

The endocardial surfaces of both ventricles are activated rapidly, but the wave of excitation spreads from endocardium to epicardium at a slower velocity (about 0.3 to 0.4 m/sec). Because the right ventricular wall is appreciably thinner than the left, the epicardial surface of the right ventricle is activated earlier than that of the left ventricle. Also, apical and central epicardial regions of both ventricles are activated earlier than are their respective basal regions. The last portions of the ventricles to be excited are the posterior basal epicardial regions and a small zone in the basal portion of the interventricular septum.

Reentry Is the Cause of Many Rhythm Disturbances

Under certain conditions, a cardiac impulse may reexcite some myocardial regions through which the impulse had previously passed. This phenomenon, known as **reentry,** is responsible for many clinical **arrhythmias** (disturbances of cardiac rhythm). The reentry may be **ordered** or **random.** In the ordered variety, the impulse traverses a fixed anatomical path, whereas in the random type, the path continues to change.

The conditions necessary for reentry are illustrated in Figure 17–11. In each of the four panels, a single bundle (S) of cardiac fibers splits into a left (L) and right (R) branch. A connecting bundle (C) runs between the two branches. The impulse moving down bundle S is normally conducted along the L and R branches (panel *A*). As the impulse reaches connecting link C, the impulse enters from both sides and becomes extinguished at the point of collision. The impulse from the left side cannot proceed farther because the tissue beyond is absolutely refractory; it had just been depolarized from the other direction. The impulse also cannot pass through bundle C from the right, for the same reason.

Panel *B* of Figure 17–11 shows that the impulse cannot complete the circuit if antegrade block exists in the L and R branches of the fiber bundle. Furthermore, if bidirectional block exists at any point in the loop (e.g., branch R in panel *C*), the impulse also cannot reenter.

A necessary condition for reentry is that at some point in the loop, the impulse can pass in one direction but not in the other. This phenomenon is called **unidirectional block.** As shown in Figure 17–11, panel *D*, the impulse may travel down branch L normally and then become blocked in the antegrade direction in branch R. The impulse that was conducted down branch L, and through the connecting branch C, may be able to penetrate the depressed region in branch R from the retrograde direction, even though the antegrade impulse had been blocked previously at this same site.

Why is the antegrade impulse blocked, but not the retrograde impulse? The antegrade impulse arrives at the depressed region in branch R earlier than does the retrograde impulse because the retrograde impulse traverses a longer path. Therefore, the antegrade impulse may be blocked simply because it arrives at the depressed region during its effective refractory period. If the retrograde impulse is delayed sufficiently, the refractory period may have ended, and the impulse can be conducted back into bundle S.

Although unidirectional block is a necessary condition for reentry, it alone cannot cause reentry. FOR REENTRY TO OCCUR, THE EFFECTIVE REFRACTORY PERIOD OF THE REENTERED REGION MUST BE SHORTER THAN THE PROPAGATION TIME AROUND THE LOOP. In panel *D*, if the tissue just beyond the depressed zone in branch R is still refractory from the antegrade depolarization, the retrograde impulse will not be conducted into branch S. Therefore, the conditions that promote reentry are those that prolong the conduction time or shorten the effective refractory period.

The functional components of the reentry loops that are responsible for specific arrhythmias are diverse in intact hearts. Some loops are large and involve entire specialized conduction bundles, whereas other loops are microscopically small. A loop may include myocardial fibers, specialized conducting fibers, nodal cells, and junctional tissues in almost any conceivable arrangement. Also, cardiac cells in the loop may be normal or deranged.

Triggered Activity Can Generate Arrhythmias

TRIGGERED ACTIVITY IS SO NAMED BECAUSE IT IS ALWAYS COUPLED TO A PRECEDING ACTION POTENTIAL. Because reentrant activity is also coupled to a preceding action potential, the arrhythmias induced by triggered activity are usually difficult to distinguish from those induced by **reentry.** Triggered activity is caused by **afterdepolarizations.** Two types of afterdepolarizations are recognized: **early afterdepolarizations (EADs)** and **delayed afterdepolarizations (DADs).** EADs appear at the end of the plateau (phase 2) or about midway through repolarization (phase 3), whereas DADs occur near the very end of repolarization or just after full repolarization (phase 4).

Early afterdepolarizations occur during the plateau

EADs tend to appear near the end of the action potential plateau or during repolarization, but before the cells have fully repolarized. EADs are more likely to occur when the prevailing heart rate is slow; a rapid heart rate suppresses EADs. In the experiment shown in **Figure 17–18**, EADs were induced by the addition of cesium in an isolated Purkinje fiber preparation. Afterdepolarizations were not evident when the preparation was driven at a cycle length of 2 seconds. When the cycle length was increased to 4 seconds, however, EADs appeared. Most of the EADs were subthreshold (first two arrows), but one of the EADs reached threshold and triggered an action potential. When the cycle length was increased to 6 seconds, each driven action potential generated an EAD that triggered a second action potential. Furthermore, when the cycle length was increased to 10 seconds, each driven action potential triggered a salvo of about five additional action potentials.

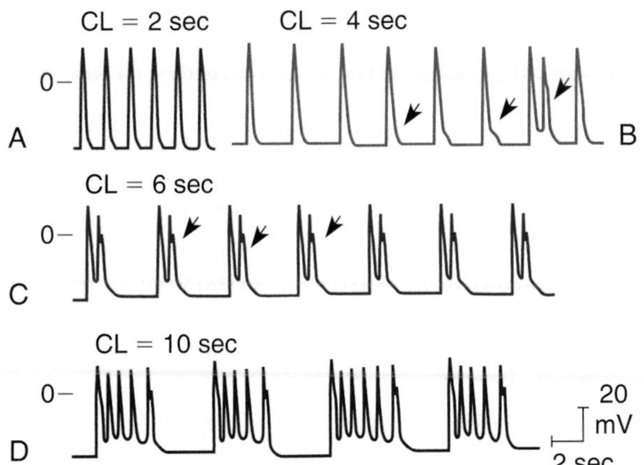

FIGURE 17–18. Effect of pacing at different cycle lengths (CL) on cesium-induced early afterdepolarizations (EADs) in a canine Purkinje fiber. A, EADs not evident. B, EADs first appear *(arrows)*. Third EAD reaches threshold and triggers an action potential *(third arrow)*. C, EADs that appear after each driven depolarization trigger an action potential. D, Triggered action potentials occur in salvos. (Modified from Damiano BP, Rosen M: *Circulation* 69:1013, 1984, with permission of the American Heart Association.)

EADs are more likely to occur in cardiac cells with prolonged action potentials than in cells with short action potentials. For example, EADs can be induced more readily in myocytes from the midmyocardial region of the ventricular walls than in myocytes from the endocardial or epicardial regions. These responses are induced by the disparities in the action potential durations of these cells (see Figure 16–12). Furthermore, EADs may be produced experimentally by interventions that prolong the action potential. As shown in Figure 17–18, EADs are more prevalent when the basic cycle length is increased. Such increases in basic cycle length prolong the action potential, and this prolongation contributes to the generation of the EADs. Certain antiarrhythmic drugs, such as **quinidine,** also prolong the action potential. Consequently, these drugs increase the likelihood that EADs will occur. Hence, antiarrhythmic drugs are frequently proarrhythmic.

The direct correlation between a cell's action potential duration and its susceptibility to EADs is probably related to the time required for the Ca^{++} channels in the cell membranes to recover from inactivation. When action potentials are sufficiently prolonged, some Ca^{++} channels that were activated at the beginning of the plateau have sufficient time to recover from inactivation. Hence, they may be reactivated before the cell repolarizes fully. This secondary activation could then trigger an EAD.

Delayed afterdepolarizations occur toward the end of repolarization

DADs are more likely to occur than are EADs when the heart rate is high. The most important characteristics of DADs are shown in **Figure 17–19.** In the experiment depicted, transmembrane potentials are recorded from Purkinje fibers that are exposed to a high concentration of **acetylstrophanthidin,** a digitalis-like substance. In the absence of any driving stimuli, these fibers are quiescent.

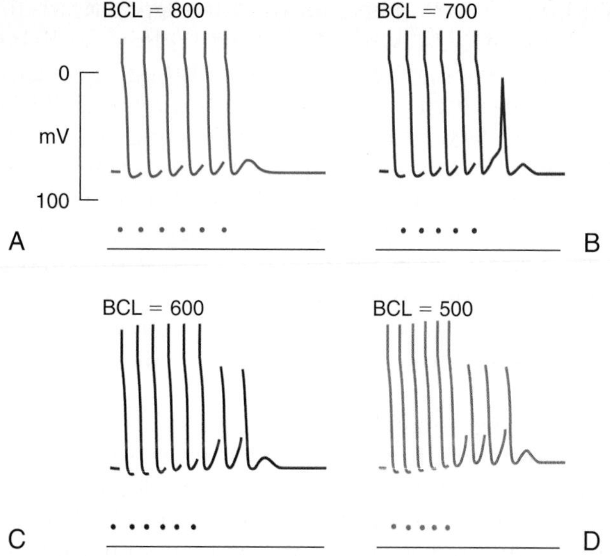

FIGURE 17–19. Transmembrane action potentials recorded from isolated canine Purkinje fibers. Acetylstrophanthidin, a digitalis-like agent, was added to the bath, and sequences of six driven beats (denoted by the dots) were produced at basic cycle lengths (BCL) of 800, 700, 600, and 500 msec. Note that delayed afterpotentials occurred after the driven beats and that these afterpotentials reached threshold after the last driven beat in panels B to D. (From Ferrier GR, Saunders JH, Mendez C: *Circ Res* 32:600, 1973, with permission of the American Heart Association.)

In each panel of Figure 17–19, a sequence of six driven depolarizations is induced at a specific basic cycle length. When the cycle length is 800 msec (*A*), the last driven depolarization is followed by a brief, partial depolarization (DAD) that does not reach threshold. Once that afterdepolarization subsides, the transmembrane potential remains constant until another driving stimulus is given. The upstroke of a DAD can be detected after each of the first five driven depolarizations.

When the basic cycle length is reduced to 700 msec (*B*), the DAD that followed the last driven beat does reach threshold, and a nondriven depolarization (or extrasystole) ensues. This extrasystole is itself followed by an afterpotential that is subthreshold. Reducing the basic cycle length to 600 msec (*C*) also evokes an extrasystole after the last driven depolarization. The afterpotential that follows the extrasystole does reach threshold, however, and a second extrasystole occurs. When the six driven depolarizations are separated by intervals of 500 msec (*D*), a sequence of three extrasystoles follows. Slightly shorter basic cycle lengths, or slightly greater concentrations of acetylstrophanthidin, evoke a long sequence of nondriven beats; such a sequence resembles a paroxysmal tachycardia (Figure 17–2).

DADs are associated with elevated intracellular Ca^{++} concentrations. The amplitudes of the DADs are increased by interventions that raise intracellular Ca^{++} concentrations. Such interventions include increasing the extracellular [Ca^{++}] and administering toxic amounts of digitalis glycosides. The elevated levels of intracellular Ca^{++} provoke the oscillatory release of Ca^{++} from the sarcoplasmic reticulum. Hence, in myocardial cells, DADs are accompanied by small, rhythmic changes in developed force. The high intracellular Ca^{++} concentrations also activate certain membrane channels that permit the passage of Na^+ and K^+. The net flux of these cations constitutes a **transient inward current,** i_{ti}, that is at least partly responsible for the afterdepolarization of the cell membrane. The elevated intracellular [Ca^{++}] may also activate Na^+-Ca^{++} exchange (see Chapter 1). This electrogenic antiporter, which transfers three Na^+ ions into the cell for each Ca^{++} ion it ejects, also creates a net inward cation current that contributes to the DAD.

Electrocardiography Is an Important Clinical Tool

The electrocardiogram enables the physician to infer the course of the cardiac impulse by recording the variations in electrical potential at various loci on the surface of the body. By analyzing the details of these fluctuations of electrical potential, the physician gains valuable insight into the anatomical orientation of the heart, the relative sizes of its chambers, the various disturbances of rhythm and conduction, the extent and location of ischemic damage to the myocardium and its progress, the effects of altered electrolyte concentrations, and the influence of certain drugs (notably digitalis, antiarrhythmic agents, and Ca^{++} channel antagonists). Because electrocardiography is an extensive and complex discipline, only elementary principles are considered in this section.

What is scalar electrocardiography?

In electrocardiography, a **lead** is the electrical connection from the patient's skin to the recording device (an electrocardiograph). The leads are connected to a galvanometer (a device that measures the strength of an electrical current) within the electrocardiograph. The systems of leads used to record routine electrocardiograms are oriented in certain planes of the body. The diverse electromotive forces that exist in the heart at any moment can be represented by a three-dimensional **vector** (a quantity with magnitude and direction). A system of recording leads oriented in a given plane detects the projection of the three-dimensional vector on that plane. The potential difference between two recording electrodes represents the projection of the vector on the line between the two leads. Components of vectors projected on such lines are not vectors but **scalar quantities** (quantities that have magnitude but not direction). Hence, a recording of the temporal potential differences between two points on the skin is called a **scalar electrocardiogram.**

This electrocardiogram records the temporal changes of the electrical potential between some point on the surface of the skin and an indifferent electrode or between pairs of points on the skin surface. The cardiac impulse progresses through the heart in a complex, three-dimensional pattern. Hence, the precise configuration of the electrocardiogram varies among persons, and in any given person, the pattern varies with the location of the leads. The graphic display of the electrical impulse recorded by an electrocardiogram is called a **tracing.**

In general, a tracing consists of P, QRS, and T waves (Figure 17–12). The PR interval (or more precisely, the PQ interval) is a measure of the time from the onset of atrial activation to the onset of ventricular activation; the PR interval normally varies from 0.12 to 0.20 second. A considerable fraction of this time involves passage of the impulse through the AV conduction system. Pathological prolongations of the PR interval are associated with disturbances of AV conduction. Such disturbances may be produced by inflammatory, circulatory, pharmacological, or nervous mechanisms.

The configuration and amplitude of the QRS complex vary considerably among individuals. The duration of the QRS interval usually varies between 0.06 and 0.10 second. An abnormally prolonged QRS complex may indicate a block in the normal conduction pathways through the ventricles; such a block would involve the left or right bundle branch. During the ST interval, the entire ventricular myocardium is depolarized. Therefore, the ST segment normally lies on the **isoelectric line.** Any appreciable deviation of the ST segment from the isoelectric line may indicate ischemic damage of the myocardium. The QT interval is sometimes referred to as the period of "electrical systole" of the ventricles. This interval is closely correlated with the mean action potential duration of the ventricular myocytes. The duration of the QT interval is about 0.4 second, and it varies inversely with the heart rate (see Figure 16–18).

In most leads, the T wave is deflected in the same direction from the isoelectric line as is the major component of the QRS complex. However, biphasic or oppositely directed T waves are perfectly normal in certain leads. When the T wave and QRS complex deviate in the same direction from the isoelectric line, this indicates that the repolarization process proceeds in a direction counter to the depolarization process. T waves that are abnormal either in direction or in amplitude may indicate myocardial damage, electrolyte disturbances, or cardiac hypertrophy.

Limb leads are standardized

The original electrocardiographic lead system was devised by Willem Einthoven. In his lead system, the vector sum of all cardiac electrical activity at any moment is called the **resultant cardiac vector.** This directional electrical force is considered to lie in the center of an equilateral triangle whose apices are located in the left and right shoulders and in the pubic region **(Figure 17–20)**. This triangle, called **Einthoven's triangle,** is oriented in the frontal plane of the body. Hence, only the projection of the resultant cardiac vector on the frontal plane is detected by this system of leads. For convenience, the electrodes are connected to the right and left forearms, rather than to the corresponding shoulders, because the arms represent simple extensions of the leads from the shoulders.

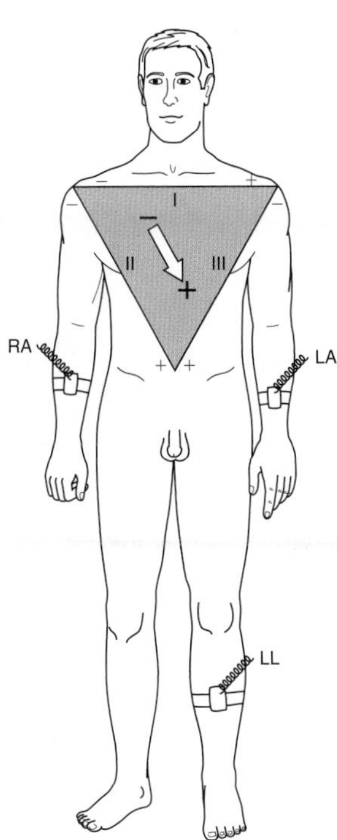

FIGURE 17–20. Einthoven's triangle, illustrating the galvanometer connections for standard limb leads I, II, and III. (Modified from Berne RM, Levy MN, Koeppen BM, Stanton BA: *Physiology*, ed 5, Philadelphia, 2004, Elsevier.)

Similarly, a leg represents an extension of the lead system from the pubis, and thus the third electrode is usually connected to an ankle.

Certain conventions dictate the manner in which these standard limb leads are connected to the galvanometer. Lead I records the potential difference between the left arm (LA) and the right arm (RA). The galvanometer connections are such that when the potential at LA (V_{LA}) exceeds the potential at RA (V_{RA}), the galvanometer stylus is deflected upward from the isoelectric line. In Figure 17–20, this arrangement of the galvanometer connections for lead I is designated by a plus sign at LA and by a minus sign at RA. Lead II records the potential difference between RA and LL (left leg), and the stylus is deflected upward when V_{LL} exceeds V_{RA}. Finally, lead III registers the potential difference between LA and LL, and the stylus is deflected upward when V_{LL} exceeds V_{LA}. These galvanometer connections were chosen arbitrarily so that the QRS complexes are upright in all three standard limb leads in most normal individuals.

Let the frontal projection of the resultant cardiac vector be represented by an arrow (tail negative, head positive), as in **Figure 17–21**. The potential difference, $V_{LA} - V_{RA}$, recorded in lead I is represented by the component of the vector projected along the horizontal line between LA and RA, also shown in Figure 17–20. If the vector makes an angle, θ, of 60 degrees with the horizontal line (as in Figure 17–21, *A*), the magnitude of the potential recorded by lead I equals the vector magnitude times the cosine of 60 degrees. The deflection recorded in lead I is upward because the positive arrowhead lies closer to LA than to RA. The deflection in lead II is also upright because the arrowhead lies closer to LL than to RA. The magnitude of the lead II deflection is greater than that in lead I because in this example, the direction of the vector parallels that of lead II. Therefore, the magnitude of the projection on lead II exceeds that on lead I. Similarly, in lead III, the deflection is upright and its magnitude equals that in lead I.

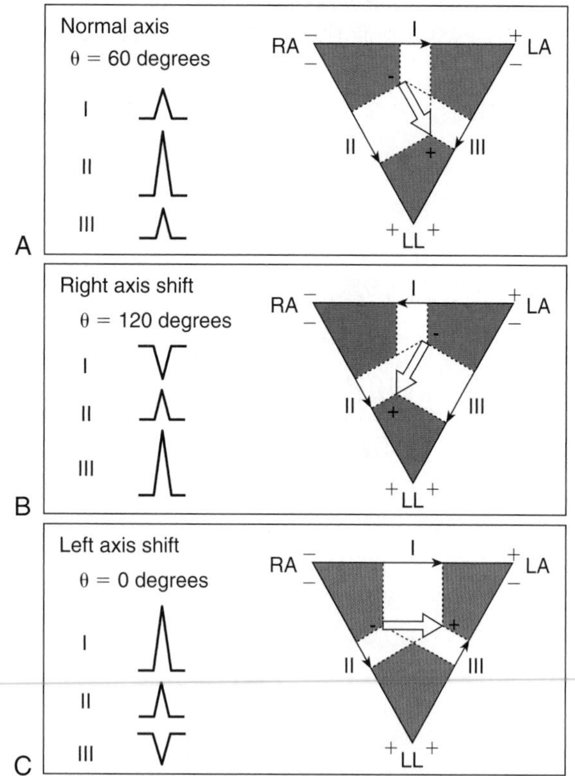

FIGURE 17–21. Magnitude and direction of the QRS complexes in limb leads I, II, and III when the mean electrical axis (Q) is 60 degrees (A), 120 degrees (B), and 0 degrees (C). (Modified from Berne RM, Levy MN, Koeppen BM, Stanton BA: *Physiology,* ed 5, Philadelphia, 2004, Elsevier.)

If the vector in Figure 17–21, *A,* is the result of electrical events that occur during the peak of the QRS complex, the orientation of this vector is said to represent the **mean electrical axis** of the heart in the frontal plane. The positive direction of this axis is taken in the clockwise direction from the horizontal plane (contrary to the usual mathematical convention). In normal individuals, the average mean electrical axis is approximately 60 degrees (as in Figure 17–21, *A*). Therefore, the QRS complexes are usually upright in all three leads, and the largest complex is in lead II.

> Changes in the mean electrical axis may occur if the anatomical position of the heart is altered or in certain cardiovascular disturbances that alter the relative mass of the right and left ventricles. For example, the axis tends to shift toward the left (more horizontal) in short, stocky individuals and toward the right (more vertical) in tall, thin persons. Also, in left or right **ventricular hypertrophy** (an increased myocardial mass of either ventricle), the axis shifts toward the hypertrophied side.

If the mean electrical axis shifts substantially to the right (as in Figure 17–21, *B*, where θ = 120 degrees), the projections of the QRS complexes on the standard leads change considerably. In this case, the largest upright deflection is in lead III. Furthermore, the deflection in lead I is inverted because the arrowhead is closer to RA than to LA. When the axis shifts to the left (Figure 17–21, *C*, where θ = 0 degrees), the largest upright deflection is in lead I, and the QRS complex in lead III is inverted.

In addition to limb leads I, II, and III, other limb leads that are oriented in the frontal plane are routinely recorded in patients. The axes of such **unipolar limb leads** form angles of +90, –30, and –150 degrees with the horizontal axis. Furthermore, the

precordial leads are also recorded to determine the projections of the cardiac vector on the sagittal and transverse planes of the body. These precordial leads are recorded from six selected points on the anterior and lateral surfaces of the chest in the vicinity of the heart. The unipolar and precordial lead systems are described in most textbooks on electrocardiography.

Arrhythmias Arise from Disturbances of Impulse Initiation or Propagation

Cardiac arrhythmias reflect disturbances of either **impulse initiation** or **impulse propagation.** Disturbances of impulse initiation include those that arise from the SA node and those that originate from various ectopic foci. The principal disturbances of impulse propagation are conduction blocks and reentrant rhythms.

Altered sinoatrial rhythms can produce arrhythmias

Mechanisms that vary the firing frequency of cardiac pacemaker cells are illustrated in Figure 17–5. Changes in the SA nodal firing rate are usually produced by the cardiac autonomic nerves. Examples of electrocardiograms of **sinus tachycardia** and **sinus bradycardia** are shown in **Figure 17–22**. The P, QRS, and T deflections are all normal, but the cardiac cycle duration (the P-P interval) is altered. Characteristically, in response to the development of sinus bradycardia or tachycardia, cardiac frequency changes gradually. Several beats are required to attain its new steady-state value. Electrocardiographic evidence of respiratory cardiac arrhythmia is common, and it is manifested as a rhythmic variation in the P-P interval at the respiratory frequency.

There are various forms of atrioventricular conduction block

Various physiological, pharmacological, and pathological processes can impede impulse transmission through the AV conduction tissue. The site of block can be localized precisely by recording the **His bundle electrogram** (Figure 17–23). To obtain such tracings, an electrode catheter is introduced into a peripheral vein and threaded centrally until the electrode lies in the region of the AV junction. When the electrode is properly positioned, a distinct deflection (H in Figure 17–23) is registered as the cardiac impulse passes through the bundle of His. The time intervals required for propagation from the atrium to the bundle of His (A-H interval) and from the bundle of His to the ventricles (H-V interval) may be measured accurately. Abnormal prolongation of the A-H interval or H-V interval indicates block above or below the bundle of His, respectively.

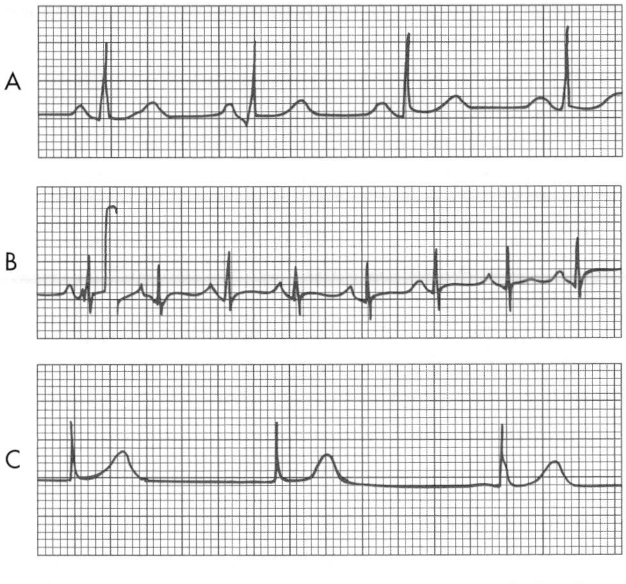

FIGURE 17–22. Electrocardiograms recorded from humans with various SA rhythms. A, Normal sinus rhythm. B, Sinus tachycardia. C, Sinus bradycardia.

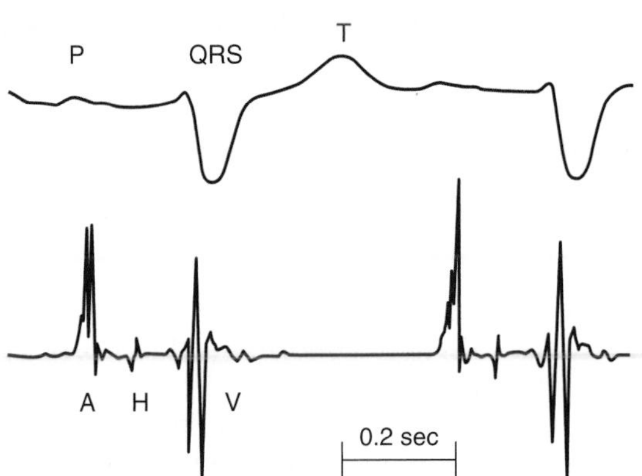

FIGURE 17–23. His bundle electrogram (*lower tracing,* retouched) and lead II of the scalar electrocardiogram *(upper tracing).* The deflection, H, which represents the impulse conduction over the bundle of His, is clearly visible between the atrial (A) and the ventricular (V) deflections. The conduction time from the atria to the bundle of His is denoted by the A-H interval; that from the bundle of His to the ventricles, by the H-V interval. (Courtesy of Dr. J. Edelstein.)

Three degrees of AV block can be distinguished, as shown in Figure 17–3. **First-degree AV block** is characterized by a prolonged PR interval. In Figure 17–3, *A*, the PR interval is 0.28 second; an interval greater than 0.20 second is abnormal. In most cases of first-degree block, the A-H interval is prolonged and the H-V interval is normal. Hence, the delay in a first-degree AV block is located above the His bundle (i.e., in the AV node).

In **second-degree AV block,** all QRS complexes are preceded by P waves, but not all P waves are followed by QRS complexes. The ratio of P waves to QRS complexes is usually the ratio of two small integers (such as 2:1, 3:1, or 3:2). Figure 17–3, *B,* illustrates a typical 2:1 block. The site of block may be above or below the His bundle. A block below the bundle is usually more serious than one above the bundle because the block below the bundle is more likely to evolve into a third-degree block. An artificial pacemaker is frequently implanted when the block is below the bundle.

Third-degree AV block is often referred to as **complete heart block** because the impulse is unable to traverse the AV conduction pathway from atria to ventricles. The most common sites of complete block are distal to the bundle of His. In complete heart block, the atrial and ventricular rhythms are entirely independent, as shown in Figure 17–3, *C*. Because of the slow ventricular rhythm (32 beats/min in this example), the distribution of blood flow to the body is often inadequate, especially during muscle activity. Third-degree block is often associated with **syncope** (lightheadedness), which is caused principally by insufficient cerebral blood flow. Third-degree block is one of the most common conditions that require artificial pacemakers.

Premature depolarizations can generate arrhythmias

Premature depolarizations occur occasionally in most normal individuals, but they arise more commonly under certain abnormal conditions. Such depolarizations may originate in the atria, AV junction, or ventricles. One type of premature depolarization follows a normally conducted depolarization after a constant time interval, called the **coupling interval.** If the normal depolarization is suppressed in some way (e.g., by vagal stimulation), the premature depolarization is also abolished. Such premature depolarizations are called **coupled extrasystoles,** or simply **extrasystoles,** and they probably reflect a reentry phenomenon (Figure 17–11). A second type of premature depolarization occurs as the result of enhanced automaticity in some ectopic focus. This ectopic center may fire regularly, and a zone of tissue that conducts unidirectionally may protect this center from being depolarized by the normal cardiac impulse. If this premature depolarization occurs at a regular interval or at an integer multiple of that interval, the disturbance is called **parasystole.**

A **premature atrial depolarization** is shown in Figure 17–1, *A*. In the tracing, the normal interval between beats is 0.89 second (heart rate, 68 beats/min). The premature atrial depolarization (second P wave in the figure) follows the preceding P wave by only 0.56 second. The configuration of the premature P wave differs from the configuration of the other, normal P waves. The P wave configuration changes because the course of atrial excitation, which originates at some ectopic focus in the atrium, differs from the normal spread of excitation, which originates at the SA node. The configuration of the QRS complex of the premature depolarization is usually normal because the ventricular excitation spreads over the usual pathways.

A **premature ventricular depolarization** appears in Figure 17–1, *B*. Because the premature excitation originates at some ectopic focus in the ventricles, the impulse propagation is abnormal. Hence, the configurations of the QRS and T waves are entirely different from the normal deflections. The premature QRS complex follows the preceding normal QRS complex by only 0.47 second. The interval after the premature excitation is 1.28 seconds, which is considerably longer than the normal interval between beats (0.89 second). The interval (1.75 seconds) from the QRS complex just before the premature excitation to the QRS complex just after it is virtually equal to the duration of two normal cardiac cycles (0.89 + 0.89 = 1.78 seconds).

The prolonged interval that usually follows a premature ventricular depolarization is called a **compensatory pause.** This pause occurs because the ectopic ventricular impulse does not disturb the natural rhythm of the SA node. Either the ectopic ventricular impulse is not conducted retrogradely through the AV conduction system or the SA node had already fired at its natural interval before the ectopic impulse could have reached it and thus depolarized it prematurely. Furthermore, the SA node impulse generated just before or just after the ventricular extrasystole does not usually affect the ventricle. Hence, the AV junction and perhaps also the ventricles may still be refractory from the premature excitation. In Figure 17–1, *B*, the P wave associated with the extrasystole occurs synchronously with the T wave of the premature ventricular depolarization, and therefore it cannot easily be identified in the tracing.

Ectopic foci initiate tachycardias

In contrast to the gradual rate changes that characterize sinus tachycardia, the rapid firing rate that originates from an ectopic focus typically begins and ends abruptly. Hence, such ectopic tachycardias are usually called **paroxysmal tachycardias.** Episodes of paroxysmal tachycardia may persist for only a few beats or for long periods, and such episodes often recur. Paroxysmal tachycardias may result from the rapid firing of an ectopic pacemaker, a triggered activity secondary to afterpotentials, or an impulse that circles a reentry loop repetitively.

Paroxysmal tachycardias that originate in the atria or in the AV junctional tissues (Figure 17–2, *A*) are usually indistinguishable, and therefore both are included in the term **paroxysmal supraventricular tachycardia.** In this tachycardia, the impulse often circles a reentry loop that includes atrial and AV junctional tissue. The QRS complexes are often normal because ventricular activation proceeds over the usual pathways.

As its name implies, **paroxysmal ventricular tachycardia** originates from an ectopic focus in the ventricles. The electrocardiogram is characterized by repeated, bizarre QRS complexes that reflect the abnormal intraventricular impulse conduction (Figure 17–2, *B*). Paroxysmal ventricular tachycardia is much more ominous than supraventricular tachycardia because it is frequently a precursor of **ventricular fibrillation**, a lethal arrhythmia described in the next section.

Fibrillation occurs in atria and ventricles

Under certain conditions, cardiac muscle undergoes an irregular type of contraction that is entirely ineffectual in propelling blood. Such an arrhythmia is termed **fibrillation,** and the disturbance may involve either the atria or the ventricles. Fibrillation probably represents a reentry phenomenon in which the reentry loop fragments into multiple, irregular circuits.

The electrocardiographic changes in **atrial fibrillation** are shown in **Figure 17–24**, *A*. This arrhythmia occurs in various types of chronic heart disease. The atria do not contract and relax sequentially during each cardiac cycle, and thus they do not contribute to ventricular filling. Instead, the atria undergo a continuous, uncoordinated, rippling motion. P waves do not appear in the electrocardiogram; they are replaced by continuous irregular fluctuations of potential called **f waves.** The AV node is activated at intervals that may vary considerably from cycle to cycle. Hence, no constant interval occurs between successive QRS complexes or between successive ventricular contractions. Because the strength of ventricular contraction depends on the interval between beats, the volume and rhythm of the pulse are irregular. In many patients, the atrial reentry loop and the pattern of AV conduction are more regular than they are in atrial fibrillation. The rhythm is then referred to as **atrial flutter.**

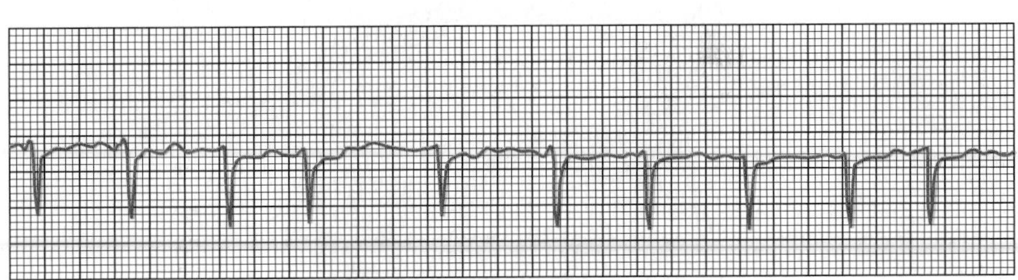

Atrial fibrillation

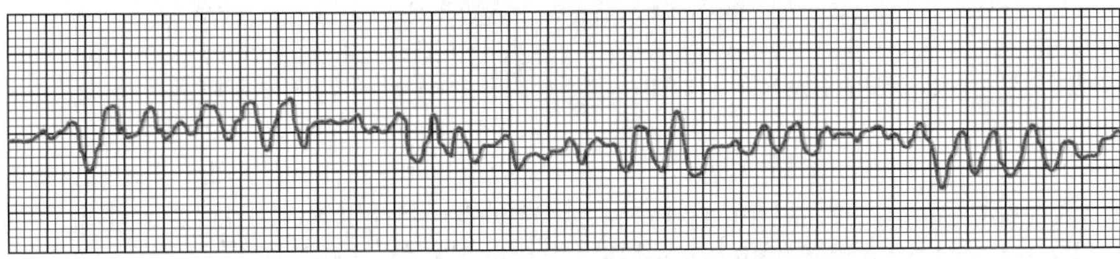

Ventricular fibrillation

FIGURE 17–24. Atrial and ventricular fibrillation. (Modified from Berne RM, Levy MN, Koeppen BM, Stanton BA: *Physiology,* ed 5, Philadelphia, 2004, Elsevier.)

Atrial fibrillation and **atrial flutter** are usually not life-threatening; people with these disturbances can usually perform normally. However, because the atria do not contract and relax fully, blood clots tend to form in the atria. Such clots can then travel to the pulmonary or systemic vascular beds. Patients with atrial flutter or fibrillation are usually treated with anticoagulants to prevent the trapping of clots in these vascular beds.

Ventricular fibrillation, on the other hand, leads to loss of consciousness within a few seconds. The irregular, continuous, uncoordinated twitchings of the ventricular muscle fibers pump no blood. Death ensues unless immediate effective resuscitation is achieved or the rhythm spontaneously reverts to normal, which rarely occurs. Ventricular fibrillation may supervene when the entire ventricle, or some portion of it, is deprived of its normal blood supply. It may also occur as a result of electrocution or in response to certain drugs and anesthetics. In the electrocardiogram (Figure 17–24, *B*), irregular fluctuations of potential are manifested.

Ventricular fibrillation is often initiated when a premature impulse arrives during the **vulnerable period,** which coincides with the downslope of the T wave of the electrocardiogram. During this period, the excitability of the cardiac cells varies spatially. Some fibers are still in their effective refractory periods; others have almost fully recovered their excitability; and still others are able to conduct impulses, but only at slow conduction velocities. Consequently, the action potentials are propagated over the chambers in many irregular wavelets that travel along circuitous paths and at various conduction velocities. As a region of cardiac cells becomes excitable again, it is ultimately reentered by one of the wave fronts that travel around the chamber. Hence, the process is self-sustaining.

Atrial fibrillation may be changed to a normal sinus rhythm by drugs that prolong the refractory period. As the cardiac impulse completes the reentry loop, it may then encounter the myocardial fibers that are no longer excitable. However, dramatic therapy is required in ventricular fibrillation. Conversion to a normal sinus rhythm is accomplished by means of a strong electrical current that places the entire myocardium briefly in a refractory state. Techniques have been developed to administer the current safely through the intact chest wall. In successful cases, the SA node again takes over the normal pacemaker function for the entire heart. When atrial defibrillation does not respond adequately to drugs, electrical defibrillation may also be used to correct this condition.

More recently, **implantable cardioverter defibrillator** devices have been developed to prevent death in patients who have suddenly developed either ventricular fibrillation or paroxysmal ventricular tachycardia **(Figure 17–25)**.

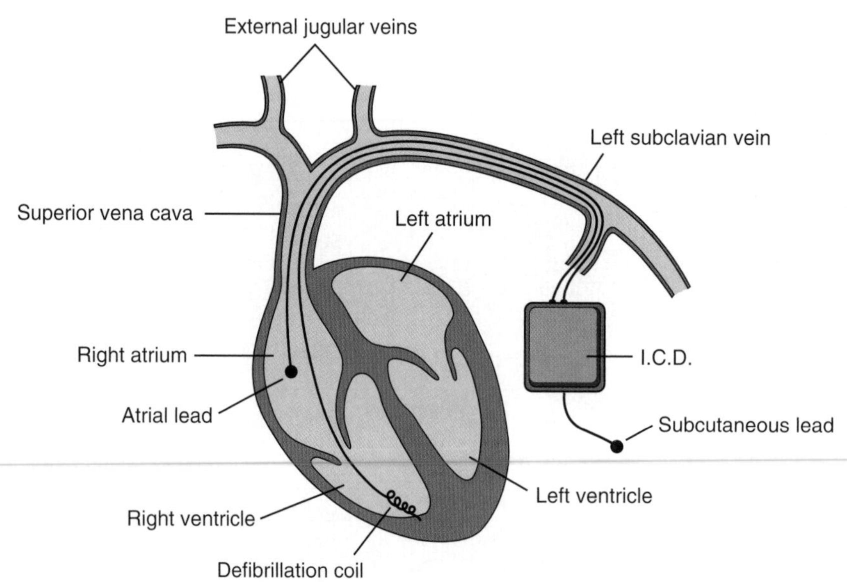

FIGURE 17–25. The main components of an implantable cardioverter defibrillator (I.C.D.). (Modified from Berne RM, Levy MN, Koeppen BM, Stanton BA: *Physiology,* ed 5, Philadelphia, 2004, Elsevier.)

Summary

- Automaticity is characteristic of certain cells in the SA and AV nodes and in the ventricular specialized conducting system. Slow depolarization of the membrane during phase 4 is the hallmark of automaticity.
- The SA node normally initiates the impulse that induces cardiac contraction. This impulse is propagated from the SA node to the atrial tissues and ultimately reaches the AV node. After a delay in the AV node, the cardiac impulse is propagated throughout the ventricles.
- Ectopic foci in the atrium, AV node, or His-Purkinje system may initiate propagated cardiac impulses if the normal pacemaker cells in the SA node are suppressed or if the rhythmicity of the ectopic automatic cells is abnormally enhanced.
- Under certain abnormal conditions, afterdepolarizations may appear early in phase 3 of a normally initiated beat, or the afterdepolarizations may be delayed until near the end of phase 3 or the beginning of phase 4. Such afterdepolarizations may themselves trigger propagated impulses. Early afterdepolarizations are more likely to occur when the basic cycle length of the initiating beats is long and when the cardiac action potentials are abnormally prolonged. Delayed afterdepolarizations are more likely to occur when the basic cycle length of the initiating beats is short and when the cardiac cells are overloaded with Ca^{++}.
- Simple conduction block is the retardation or failure of impulse propagation in a cardiac fiber.
- A cardiac impulse may traverse a loop of cardiac fibers and reenter previously excited tissue when the impulse is conducted slowly around the loop and when the impulse is blocked unidirectionally in some section of the loop.
- The electrocardiogram, which is recorded from the surface of the body, traces the conduction of the cardiac impulse throughout the heart.
- The electrocardiogram may be used to detect and analyze certain cardiac arrhythmias, such as altered SA rhythms, AV conduction blocks, premature depolarizations, ectopic tachycardias, and atrial and ventricular fibrillation.

Bibliography

Anderson RH, Ho SY: The architecture of the sinus node, the atrioventricular conduction axis, and the internodal atrial myocardium, *J Cardiovasc Electrophysiol* 9:1233, 1998.

Antzelevitch C: Basic mechanisms of reentrant arrhythmias, *Curr Opin Cardiol* 16:1, 2001.

Carmeliet E: Cardiac ionic currents and acute ischemia: from channels to arrhythmias, *Physiol Rev* 79:917, 1999.

Hille B: *Ion channels of excitable membranes,* ed 3, Sunderland, Mass, 2001, Sinauer Associates.

Levy MN, Schwartz PJ: *Vagal control of the heart: experimental basis and clinical implications,* Armonk, NY, 1994, Futura Publishing.

Mangrum JM, DiMarco JP: The evaluation and management of bradycardia, *N Engl J Med* 342:703, 2000.

Nattel S: Atrial electrophysiology and mechanisms of atrial fibrillation, *J Cardiovasc Pharmacol Ther* 8(suppl 1):S5, 2003.

Rohr S: Role of gap junctions in the propagation of the cardiac action potential, *Cardiovasc Res* 62:309, 2004.

Shimizu A, Centurion OA: Electrophysiological properties of the human atrium in atrial fibrillation, *Cardiovasc Res* 54:302, 2002.

Shorofsky SR, Balke CW: Calcium currents and arrhythmias: insights from molecular biology, *Am J Med* 110:127, 2001.

Wu J, Zipes DP: Mechanisms underlying atrioventricular nodal conduction and the reentrant circuit of atrioventricular nodal reentrant tachycardia using optical mapping, *J Cardiovasc Electrophysiol* 13:831, 2002.

Case Study

Case 17–1

An 18-year-old high-school student has seen a cardiologist regularly since it was discovered that she had symptoms of the long QT (LQT) syndrome 3 years ago. At that time, she experienced several episodes of lightheadedness during a soccer game. Her family physician found that analysis of systems was normal except for some electrocardiographic abnormalities. She was referred to the cardiologist, whose examination included an electrocardiogram. The cardiologist reported a normal sinus rhythm with a heart rate of 71 beats/min in this patient. Other electrocardiographic data were a PR interval of 0.14 second, QRS duration of 0.10 second, and QT interval of 475 msec. The QT interval, even corrected for heart rate, is abnormally long. Analysis of DNA revealed that she had a mutation in a gene linked to a cardiac K^+ channel. The mutation (loss of function) results in less outward repolarizing current and therefore a longer ventricular action potential. The phenotype of her syndrome is designated LQT1. The cardiologist had the patient walk around the office for light exercise. Immediately after exercising, her heart rate was increased and her QT interval had decreased, as expected. The cardiologist advised her not to participate in competitive athletics and prescribed a β-adrenergic antagonist (atenolol) to be taken daily. She has followed this regimen and remains symptom free since her condition was first diagnosed.

1. **What does the PR interval of 0.14 second indicate?**
   A. Impulse initiation in the SA node is unusually rapid.
   B. Conduction of the impulse through the bundle branches is slower than normal.
   C. Conduction time of the impulse from atria through the AV node and ventricular conducting system to ventricles is normal.
   D. Atrial action potentials are initiated within normal limits.
   E. The contractile state of the left ventricle is weaker than normal.

2. **What does the QT interval measure?**
   A. Interval between successive SA node impulses
   B. Conduction velocity of atrial muscle
   C. Time for impulse conduction through the AV node
   D. Velocity of conduction in the ventricular conducting system
   E. Duration of the ventricular action potential

3. **When the patient exercised, heart rate increased. This can be measured in which of the following?**
   A. Reduced R-R interval
   B. Lengthened PR interval
   C. Increased duration of the QRS complex
   D. Decreased amplitude of P waves
   E. Increased R wave amplitude

4. **The long QT syndrome is associated with early afterdepolarizations and can eventually produce torsades de pointes (a form of ventricular fibrillation). What happened to the patient's QT interval during exercise?**
   A. Increased because of greater closing of repolarizing K^+ channels
   B. Decreased because of greater opening of depolarizing Na^+ channels
   C. Increased because of greater inactivation of Na^+ channels
   D. Decreased because of greater activation of repolarizing K^+ channels
   E. Increased because of greater tendency for reentry

Chapter 18: Cardiac Pump

Objectives

- ❖ Describe how the microscopic and gross anatomy of the heart enable it to pump blood through the systemic and pulmonary circulations.
- ❖ Explain how electrical excitation of the heart is coupled to its contractions.
- ❖ List the factors that determine cardiac contractile force.
- ❖ Discuss the pressure changes in the heart chambers and great vessels during a complete cardiac cycle.

The heart exhibits a wide range of activity and functional capacity and performs a tremendous amount of work over the lifetime of an individual. The heart can function independently, but its performance is influenced by numerous humoral and neural factors. This chapter describes some of the basic intrinsic mechanisms that affect cardiac activity.

The Structure of the Heart Is Designed for Optimal Function

Several important morphological and functional differences exist between myocardial and skeletal muscle cells. However, the contractile elements within the two types of cells are similar. Each skeletal or cardiac muscle cell is made up of sarcomeres that contain thick filaments composed of myosin and thin filaments composed of actin. As in skeletal muscle, shortening of the cardiac sarcomere occurs by the sliding filament mechanism. Actin filaments slide along adjacent myosin filaments via cycling of the intervening cross-bridges, and thereby the Z lines are brought closer together.

A striking difference is that cardiac muscle appears to be a **syncytium** (a single multinucleated cell formed from many fused cells) with branching and interconnecting fibers, whereas skeletal muscle cells do not interconnect. However, the myocardium is not a true anatomical syncytium. The myocardial fibers are separated laterally from adjacent fibers by their respective **sarcolemmas.** Also, the end of each fiber is separated from its neighbor by dense structures, **intercalated disks,** that are continuous with the sarcolemma (**Figure 18–1**). Nevertheless, cardiac muscle functions as a syncytium because a wave of depolarization, followed by contractions of the atria and ventricles **(an all-or-none response),** occurs when a suprathreshold stimulus is applied (see also Chapter 17).

As the wave of excitation approaches the end of a cardiac cell, the spread of excitation to the next cell depends on the electrical conductance of the boundary between the two cells. **Gap junctions (nexuses),** with high conductances, are present in the intercalated disks between adjacent cells (**Figure 18–1**). These gap junctions, which facilitate the conduction of the cardiac impulse from one cell to the next, are made up of **connexons,** which are hexagonal structures that connect the cytosol of adjacent cells. Each connexon consists of six polypeptides, which surround a core channel that serves as a low-resistance pathway for cell-to-cell conductance. Impulse conduction in cardiac tissue progresses more rapidly in a direction parallel to (isotropic) rather than perpendicular to (anisotropic) the long axes of the constituent fibers.

Another difference between cardiac and fast skeletal muscle fibers is in the number of mitochondria **(sarcosomes)** in the two tissues. Fast skeletal muscle has relatively few mitochondria,

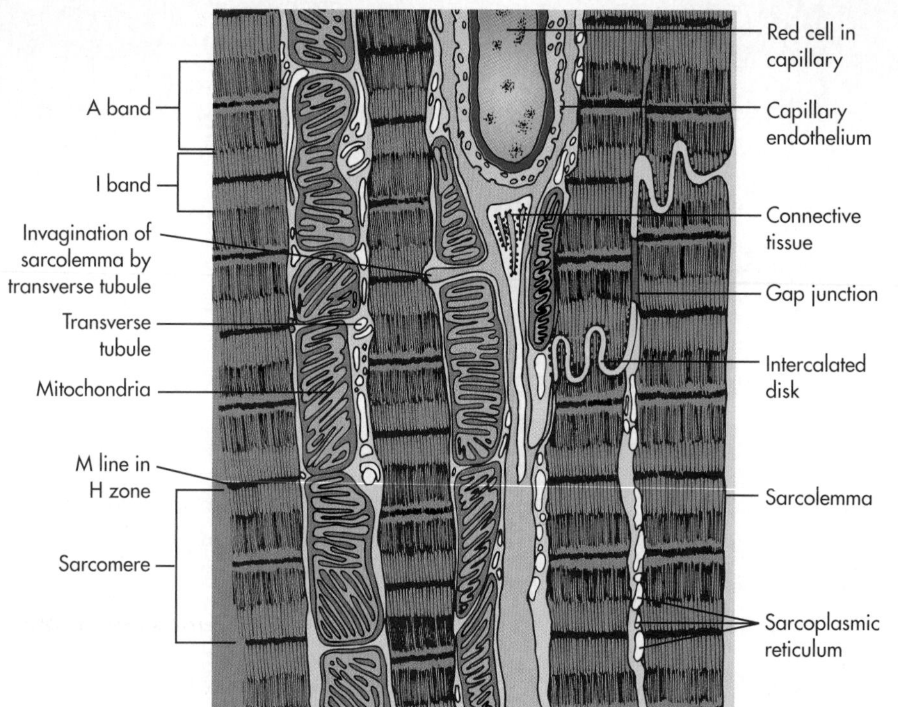

FIGURE 18–1. Diagram of an electron micrograph of cardiac muscle. Note the large number of mitochondria and the intercalated disks with nexuses (gap junctions), transverse tubules, and longitudinal tubules.

and it is called on for relatively short periods of repetitive or sustained contraction. It also can metabolize anaerobically and build up a substantial O_2 debt. In contrast, cardiac muscle is richly endowed with mitochondria (Figure 18–1). Also, it must contract repetitively for a lifetime, and it resists development of a significant O_2 debt. Rapid oxidation of substrates, accompanied by ATP synthesis, can keep pace with the myocardial energy requirements. This can be achieved because of the large number of mitochondria, which contain the respiratory enzymes necessary for oxidative phosphorylation (see also Chapter 13).

To provide adequate O_2 and substrate for its metabolic machinery, the myocardium is also endowed with a rich capillary supply, about one capillary per fiber. Thus, diffusion distances are short, and O_2, CO_2, substrates, and waste material can move rapidly between the myocardial cells and capillaries. With respect to such exchanges, electron micrographs of the myocardium show deep invaginations of the sarcolemma into the fiber at the Z lines (Figure 18–1). These sarcolemmal invaginations constitute the **transverse-tubular (T-tubular) system.** The T-tubule lumina are continuous with the bulk of interstitial fluid, and they play a key role in excitation-contraction coupling.

The sarcoplasmic reticulum network consists of small-diameter sarcotubules that surround the myofibrils. The sarcoplasmic reticulum releases and takes up Ca^{++} and hence is important in myocardial contraction and relaxation.

The force-length relationship of myocardial fibers determines myocardial contractions

Skeletal and cardiac muscle show similar force-length relationships. The developed force is maximal when cardiac muscle begins contracting at resting sarcomere lengths of 2.0 to 2.4 μm. At such lengths, overlap of the thick and thin filaments is optimal, and the number of cross-bridge attachments is maximal. The developed force of cardiac muscle is less than maximal when the sarcomeres are stretched beyond the optimum length because the overlap of the filaments is less. Hence, cross-bridge cycling is less. At resting sarcomere lengths shorter than optimal, the thin filaments that extend from adjacent Z lines overlap one another in the central region of the sarcomere. This arrangement of the thin filaments diminishes contractile force.

The force-length relationship for the intact heart is shown graphically in **Figure 18–2**. Developed force (i.e., the force attained during contraction) may be expressed as ventricular systolic pressure, and myocardial resting fiber length may be expressed as end-diastolic ventricular volume. The

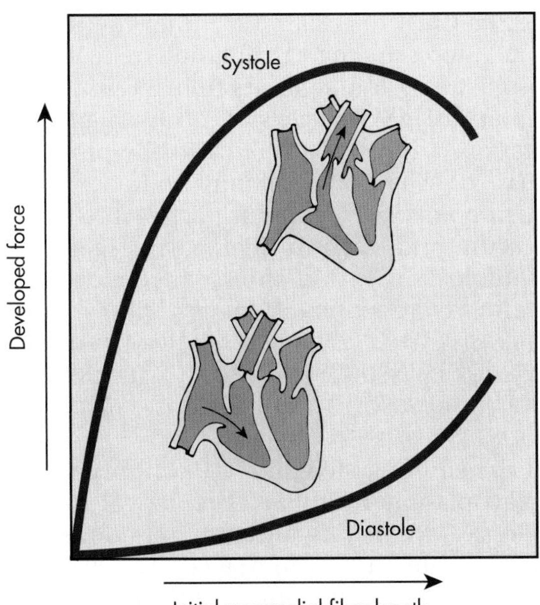

FIGURE 18–2. Relationship of the myocardial resting fiber length (sarcomere length), or end-diastolic volume, to the developed force, or peak systolic ventricular pressure, during ventricular contraction in the intact dog heart. (Redrawn from Patterson SW et al: *J Physiol* 48:465, 1914.)

lower curve in Figure 18–2 depicts the ventricular pressure produced by increments in ventricular volume during diastole (at rest). The upper curve is the peak pressure developed by the ventricle during systole at each filling volume. THE GRAPH ILLUSTRATES THE RELATIONSHIP OF FORCE (OR PRESSURE) DEVELOPMENT BY THE VENTRICLE AS A FUNCTION OF INITIAL FIBER LENGTH (OR INITIAL VOLUME). This is known as the **Frank-Starling relationship,** named after the scientists who first described it.

Stretch of the myocardium by greater ventricular filling enhances the affinity of **troponin C** for Ca^{++} and also may increase Ca^{++} uptake and release from the sarcoplasmic reticulum **(Figure 18–3)**. These two effects increase developed force and thereby contribute to the increase in force when the cardiac muscle fiber length increases.

The pressure-volume curve in diastole is flat at low volumes. Thus, large increases in volume can be accommodated with only small increases in pressure; that is, the ventricle is compliant. Nevertheless, the systolic pressure is considerable at the lower filling pressures. The ventricle becomes much less compliant with greater filling, however, as evidenced by the sharp rise of the diastolic curve at

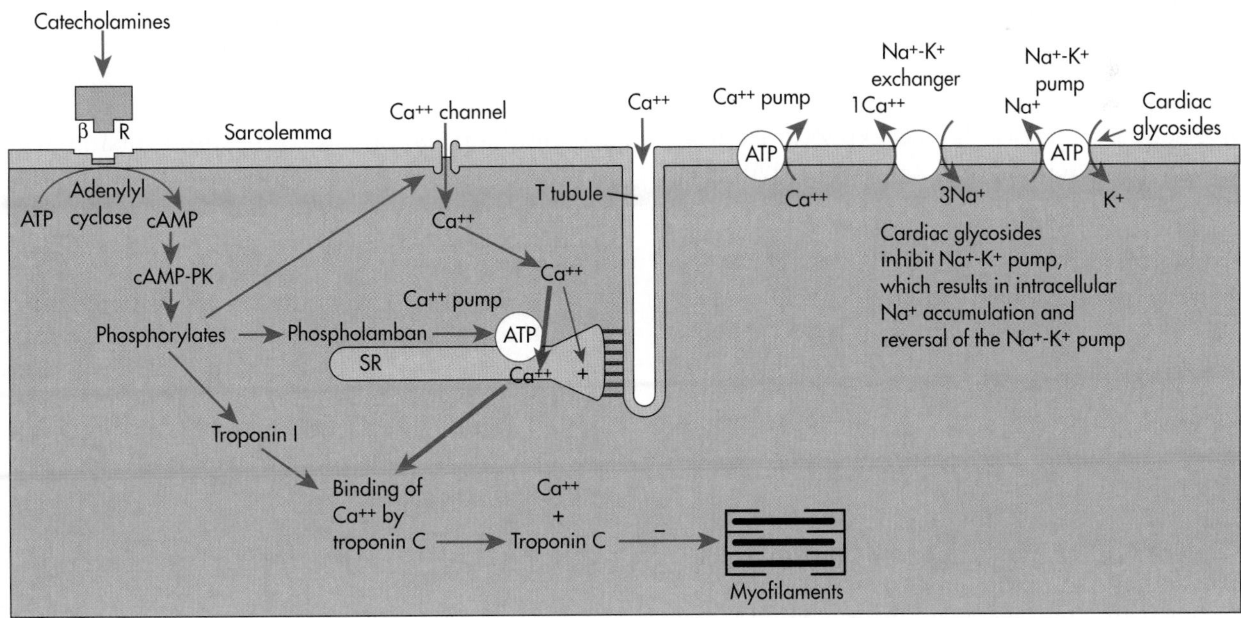

FIGURE 18–3. Movements of Ca^{++} in excitation-contraction coupling in cardiac muscle. The influx of Ca^{++} from the interstitial fluid during excitation triggers the release of Ca^{++} from the sarcoplasmic reticulum (SR). The free cytosolic Ca^{++} activates contraction of the myofilaments (systole). Relaxation (diastole) occurs as a result of the uptake of Ca^{++} by the sarcoplasmic reticulum and the extrusion of intracellular Ca^{++} by Na^{+}-Ca^{++} exchange and, to a limited degree, by the Ca^{++} pump. Negative signs indicate inhibition; positive signs indicate activation. βR, β-adrenergic receptor; cAMP, cyclic adenosine monophosphate; cAMP-PK, cAMP-dependent protein kinase.

large intraventricular volumes. The normal heart operates only on the ascending portion of the Frank-Starling curve depicted in Figure 18–2 (upper curve).

If the heart becomes greatly distended with blood during diastole, as may occur in cardiac failure, it functions less efficiently. **More energy is required** (greater wall tension) for the distended heart to eject a given volume of blood per beat than is required for the normal undilated heart. The less efficient pumping of the distended heart is an example of Laplace's law (see Chapter 19), which states that the tension in the wall of a blood vessel or cardiac chamber equals the transmural pressure (distending pressure) times the radius of the chamber.

Excitation-contraction coupling is mediated by Ca^{++}

The heart requires optimum concentrations of Na^+, K^+, and Ca^{++} to function normally. In the absence of Na^+, the heart is not excitable. It does not beat because the action potential of myocardial fibers depends on the extracellular $[Na^+]$. In contrast, the resting membrane potential is independent of the Na^+ gradient across the membrane (see Figure 16–7). Under normal conditions, the extracellular $[K^+]$ is about 4 mM. A substantial increase in extracellular K^+ produces depolarization, loss of excitability of the myocardial cells, and cardiac arrest. Ca^{++} is also essential for cardiac contraction. Removal of Ca^{++} from the extracellular fluid decreases contractile force and eventually causes arrest in diastole. Conversely, an increase in the extracellular $[Ca^{++}]$ enhances contractile force, but very high $[Ca^{++}]$ induces cardiac arrest in systole (rigor). THE LEVEL OF THE FREE INTRACELLULAR $[Ca^{++}]$ IS MAINLY RESPONSIBLE FOR THE CONTRACTILE STATE OF THE MYOCARDIUM.

A wave of excitation initially spreads rapidly along the sarcolemma from cell to cell via the gap junctions, and graded depolarization spreads into the interior of the cells via the T tubules. During the plateau (phase 2) of the action potential, the Ca^{++} permeability of the sarcolemma increases (see Chapter 16). Ca^{++} flows down its electrochemical gradient and enters the cell through voltage-dependent Ca^{++} channels in the sarcolemma and in the invaginations of the sarcolemma, the T tubules (Figure 18–3). Channel opening can be enhanced by phosphorylation of the channel proteins by a cAMP-dependent protein kinase. The primary source of extracellular Ca^{++} is the interstitial fluid (2 mM Ca^{++}).

The amount of Ca^{++} that enters the cell from the extracellular space is not sufficient to induce contraction of the myofibrils, but it serves as a trigger **(trigger Ca^{++})** to release Ca^{++} from the intracellular Ca^{++} stores in the sarcoplasmic reticulum. The cytosolic free $[Ca^{++}]$ increases from a resting level of less than 0.1 μM to levels of 1.0 to 10 μM during excitation, and the Ca^{++} binds to the protein **troponin C.** The Ca^{++}-troponin complex interacts with tropomyosin to unblock active sites between the actin and myosin filaments (Figure 18–3). This unblocking action allows cross-bridge cycling and thus contraction of the myofibrils (systole). MECHANISMS THAT RAISE THE CYTOSOLIC $[Ca^{++}]$ INCREASE THE DEVELOPED FORCE, AND MECHANISMS THAT LOWER THE CYTOSOLIC $[Ca^{++}]$ DECREASE THE DEVELOPED FORCE.

At the end of systole, the Ca^{++} influx ceases, and the sarcoplasmic reticulum is no longer stimulated to release Ca^{++}. In fact, the sarcoplasmic reticulum avidly takes up Ca^{++} via an ATP-energized Ca^{++} pump that is inhibited by **phospholamban** in the absence of cAMP. Phosphorylation of troponin I inhibits the Ca^{++} binding of troponin C. This action permits tropomyosin to again block the sites for interaction between the actin and myosin filaments, and relaxation (diastole) occurs (Figure 18–3).

The release of norepinephrine at the terminals of cardiac sympathetic nerves, which occurs during emotional stress, accelerates the rates of contraction and relaxation of the heart as well as the force of cardiac contraction. The norepinephrine activates adenylyl cyclase, and the resulting increase in cAMP activates cAMP-dependent protein kinase. The kinase phosphorylates the Ca^{++} channels to enhance the rate and magnitude of Ca^{++} uptake. It also phosphorylates phospholamban, which enhances Ca^{++} uptake by the sarcoplasmic reticulum. Thus, the phosphorylations by the cAMP-dependent kinase increase the speeds of contraction and relaxation.

The Ca^{++} that enters the cell to initiate contraction must be removed during diastole. The removal is accomplished primarily by an electrogenic exchange of three Na^+ for one Ca^{++} (Figure 18–3). Ca^{++} is also removed from the cell by an electrogenic pump that uses energy to transport Ca^{++} across the sarcolemma (Figure 18–3).

Digitalis, a drug used in the treatment of heart failure, also increases contractile force by elevating the level of intracellular Ca^{++}. Digitalis inhibits Na^+,K^+-ATPase; hence, less Na^+ is pumped out of the myocytes. This results in a decreased Na^+ gradient across the cell membrane, and thus less Na^+ can enter the cell. Therefore, less Ca^{++} can leave the cell by Na^+-Ca^{++} exchange (Figure 18–3).

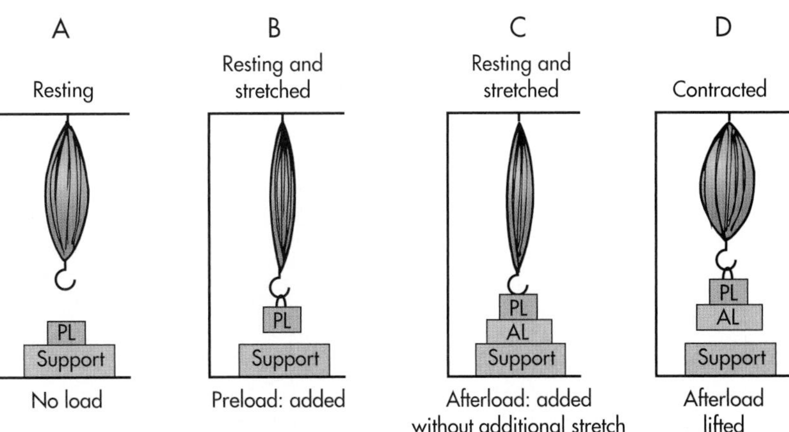

FIGURE 18–4. Preload and afterload in a papillary muscle. A, Resting stage in the intact heart just before opening of the AV valves. B, Preload in the intact heart at the end of ventricular filling. C, Supported preload plus afterload in the intact heart just before opening of the aortic valve. D, Lifting preload plus afterload in the intact heart: ventricular ejection with decreased ventricular volume. AL, afterload; PL, preload; PL and AL, total load.

Preload and afterload are determinants of cardiac performance

Figure 18–4 shows the sequence of events that occur during the contraction of a preloaded and afterloaded papillary muscle. In Figure 18–4, *A,* the muscle is relaxed and bears no weight. For the intact left ventricle, this situation is analogous to the point in the cardiac cycle at which the ventricle has relaxed after ejection has terminated, the aortic valve has closed, and the mitral valve is about to open (at the end of isovolumic relaxation in Figure 18–8). In Figure 18–4, *B,* the resting muscle is stretched by a preload. In the intact heart, this action represents the end of filling of the left ventricle during ventricular diastole; that is, it represents the **end-diastolic volume.** In Figure 18–4, *C,* the resting muscle is still stretched by the preload, but a supported afterload has been added without allowing the muscle to be stretched further. In the intact heart, the analogous condition is the point in the cardiac cycle at which ventricular contraction has just started and the mitral valve has just closed. The aortic valve has not yet opened because the ventricle has not developed enough intraventricular pressure to force it open (isovolumic contraction phase; see Figure 18–8). In Figure 18–4, *D,* the muscle has contracted and lifted the afterload. In the intact heart, this condition represents left ventricular ejection into the aorta. During ejection, the afterload is represented by aortic and intraventricular pressures, which are virtually equal to each other during the periods of rapid and reduced ejection (see Figure 18–8).

The preload can be increased by greater filling of the left ventricle during diastole (Figure 18–2). At lower end-diastolic volumes, increments in filling pressure during diastole elicit a greater systolic pressure during the subsequent contraction. Systolic pressure increases until a maximum systolic pressure is reached at the optimum preload (Figure 18–2). If diastolic filling continues beyond this point, developed pressure does not increase further. At very high filling pressures, peak pressure development in systole is reduced.

When the preload is constant, a higher systolic pressure can be reached during ventricular contractions by raising the afterload (e.g., increasing aortic pressure by restricting the runoff of blood to the peripheral vessels). Increments in afterload produce progressively higher peak systolic pressures **(Figure 18–5).** If the afterload continues to increase, it becomes so great that the ventricle can no longer generate enough force to open the aortic valve (Figure 18–5). At this point, ventricular systole is totally isometric; blood is not ejected, and thus the volume of the ventricle does not change during systole. The maximum pressure developed by the left ventricle under these conditions is the maximum isometric force that the ventricle can generate at a given preload.

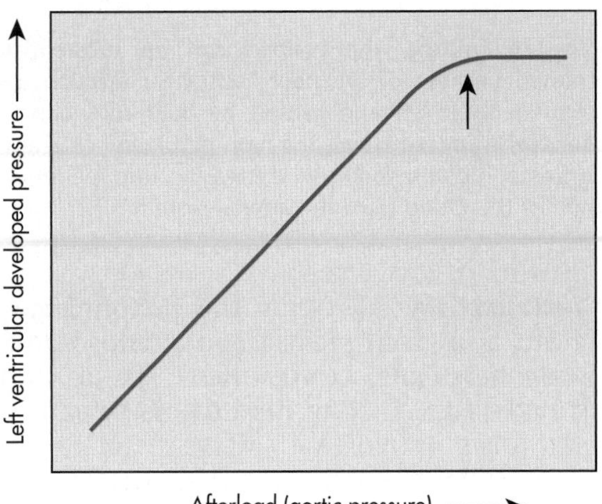

FIGURE 18–5. Effect of increasing afterload on developed pressure at constant preload. At the arrow, the maximum developed pressure is reached. Further increments in afterload prevent opening of the aortic valve.

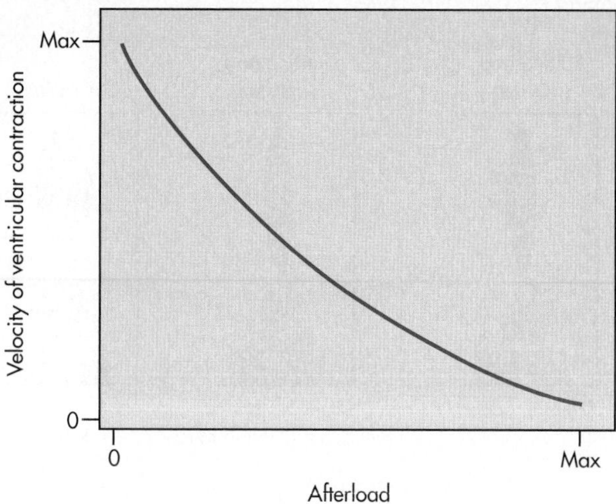

FIGURE 18–6. Effect of increasing afterload on the velocity of contraction at constant preload. Max, maximum.

Force and velocity are functions of the intracellular concentration of free Ca^{++}. When velocity is constant, force equals the afterload during muscle contraction. FORCE AND VELOCITY ARE INVERSELY RELATED. WITH NO LOAD, THE VELOCITY OF THE MUSCLE CONTRACTION IS MAXIMUM, WHEREAS WITH A MAXIMUM LOAD (WHEN CONTRACTION CAN NO LONGER SHORTEN THE MUSCLE), VELOCITY IS ZERO **(Figure 18–6)**.

Preloads and afterloads depend on certain characteristics of the vascular system and on the behavior of the heart. With respect to the vasculature, the degree of venomotor tone and peripheral resistance influence preload and afterload. With respect to the heart, a change in the rate or stroke volume can also alter preload and afterload. Hence, cardiac and vascular factors interact to affect preload and afterload (see Chapter 24).

In **heart failure,** the preload can be substantially increased because of the poor ventricular ejection and increased blood volume caused by fluid retention. In **essential hypertension,** the high peripheral resistance augments the afterload by decreasing the peripheral runoff of the blood from the arterial system.

Contractility represents the performance of the heart at a given preload and afterload and at constant heart rate. CONTRACTILITY MAY BE DETERMINED EXPERIMENTALLY AS THE CHANGE IN PEAK ISOMETRIC FORCE (ISOVOLUMIC PRESSURE) AT A GIVEN INITIAL FIBER LENGTH (END-DIASTOLIC VOLUME). Contractility can be augmented by certain drugs, such as norepinephrine and digitalis, and by an increase in contraction frequency **(tachycardia).** The increase in contractility **(positive inotropic effect)** produced by any of these interventions is

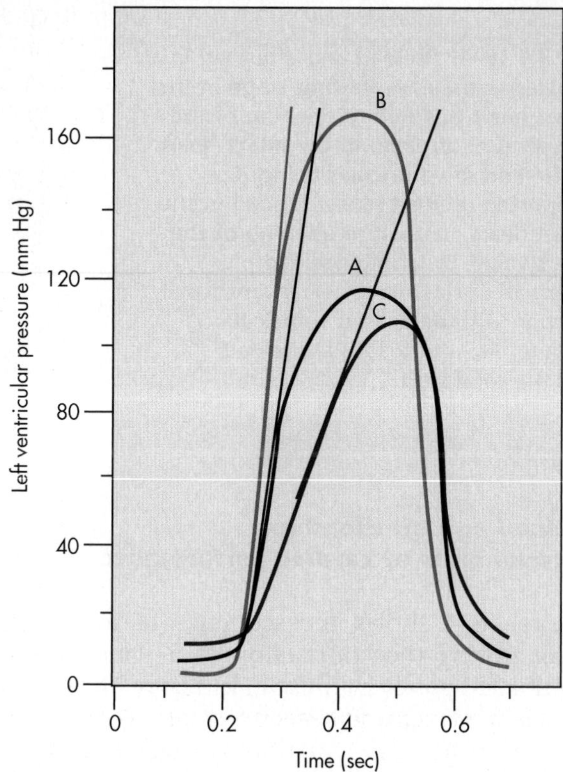

FIGURE 18–7. Left ventricular pressure curves with tangents drawn to the steepest portions of the ascending limbs to indicate the maximum dP/dt value. Curve A, control. Curve B, hyperdynamic heart, such as that which occurs after the administration of norepinephrine. Curve C, hypodynamic heart, such as that which occurs during cardiac failure. See text for details.

reflected by increments in developed force and velocity of contraction.

In rare instances, patients with asthma have accidentally received excessive doses of epinephrine subcutaneously. The patients develop marked tachycardia and increases in myocardial contractility, cardiac output, and total peripheral resistance. The result is dangerously high blood pressure. Treatment consists of a tourniquet on the injected limb with intermittent brief releases of the tourniquet and the use of adrenergic blocking medications.

A reasonable index of myocardial contractility can be obtained from the contour of ventricular pressure curves **(Figure 18–7)**. A hypodynamic heart is characterized by an elevated end-diastolic pressure, a slowly rising ventricular pressure, and a somewhat reduced ejection phase (curve C in Figure 18–7). A hyperdynamic heart (such as a heart stimulated by norepinephrine) shows a reduced end-diastolic pressure, a rapidly rising ventricular pressure, and a brief ejection phase (curve B in

Figure 18–7). The slope of the ascending limb of the ventricular pressure curve indicates the maximum rate of force development by the ventricle. The maximum rate of change in pressure, the **maximum dP/dt,** is illustrated by the tangents to the steepest portion of the ascending limbs of the ventricular pressure curves. The slope is maximal during the isovolumic phase of systole **(Figure 18–8)**. At any given degree of ventricular filling, the slope provides an index of the initial contraction velocity and hence of contractility.

The contractile state of the myocardium can also be derived from the maximum velocity of blood flow in the ascending aorta during the cardiac cycle—that is, the initial slope of the aortic flow curve (Figure 18–8). The **ejection fraction,** which is the ratio of the volume of blood ejected from the left ventricle per beat **(stroke volume)** to the volume of blood in the left ventricle at the end of diastole (end-diastolic volume), is widely used clinically as an index of contractility. Other measurements that reflect the magnitude or velocity of the ventricular contraction have been used to assess the contractile state of the cardiac muscle. No index is entirely satisfactory.

The Cardiac Chambers Consist of Two Atria, Two Ventricles, and Four Valves

The atria are thin-walled, low-pressure chambers. They function as large reservoirs and conduits of blood for their respective ventricles. The ventricles are formed by a substantial layer of muscle fibers that originate from the fibrous skeleton at the base of the heart, mainly around the aortic orifice. These fibers sweep toward the apex at the epicardial surface. They also pass toward the endocardium as they gradually undergo a 180-degree change in direction. These fibers lie parallel to the epicardial fibers and form the endocardium and papillary muscles. At the apex of the heart, the fibers twist and turn inward to form papillary muscles. At the base of the heart and around the valve orifices, the myocardial fibers form a thick, powerful layer of muscles that decrease the ventricular circumference to aid in the ejection of blood and narrow the atrioventricular (AV) valve orifices as an aid to valve closure. Ventricular ejection is implemented not only by a reduction in circumference but also by a decrease in the longitudinal axis; the decrease is accomplished by a descent of the base of the heart. The early contraction of the ventricular apex, coupled with approximation of the ventricular walls, propels the blood toward the outflow tracts.

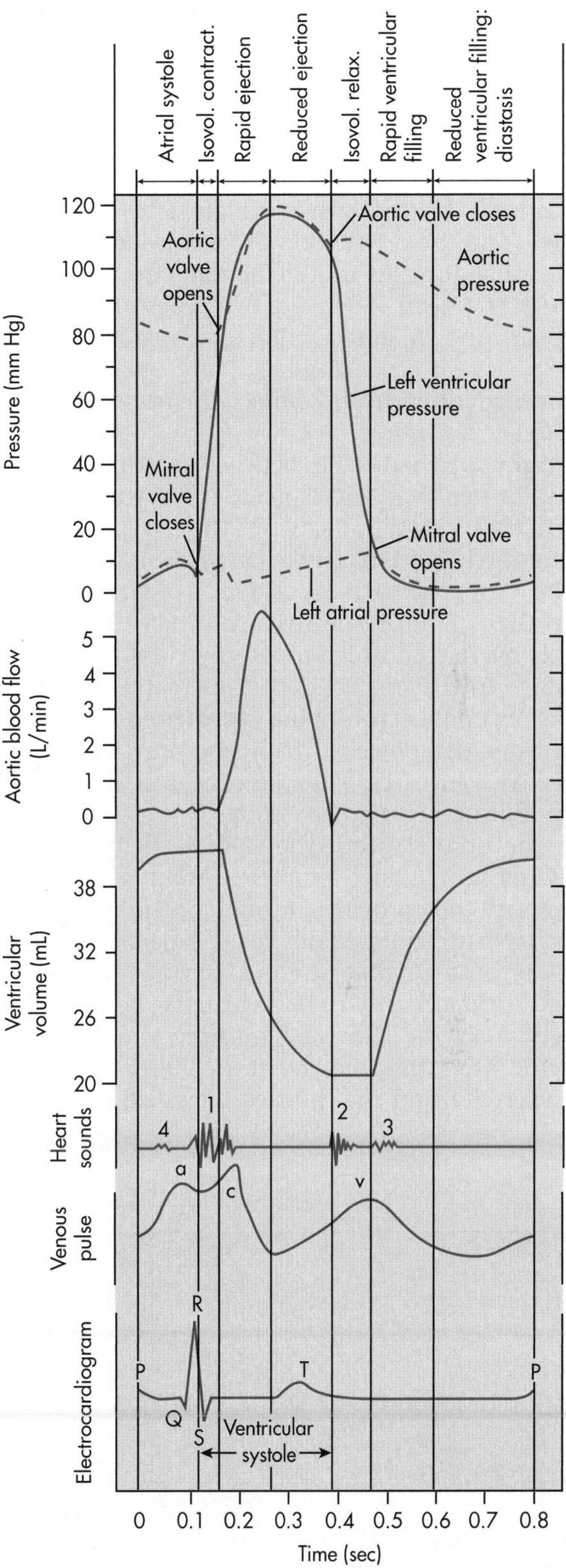

FIGURE 18–8. Left atrial, aortic, and left ventricular pressure pulses correlated in time with aortic flow, ventricular volume, heart sounds, venous pulse, and the electrocardiogram for a complete cardiac cycle in the dog. See text for details.

Cardiac valves are interposed between atria and ventricles

The cardiac valves consist of thin flaps of tough, flexible, endothelium-covered fibrous tissue, firmly attached at the base to the fibrous valve rings. Movements of the valve leaflets are essentially passive, and the orientation of the cardiac valves is responsible for the unidirectional flow of blood through the heart. There are two types of valves in the heart: the AV and semilunar valves.

Atrioventricular valves connect the upper and lower chambers

The **tricuspid valve** lies between the right atrium and right ventricle and is made up of three cusps; the **mitral valve** lies between the left atrium and left ventricle and has two cusps. The total area of the cusps of each AV valve is approximately twice that of the respective AV orifice. Thus, the leaflets overlap considerably in the closed position. Attached to the free edges of these valves are fine, strong filaments **(chordae tendineae),** which arise from the powerful papillary muscles of the respective ventricles. They prevent eversion of the valves during ventricular systole.

In the normal heart, the valve leaflets are relatively close to one another during ventricular filling, and they provide a funnel for the transfer of blood from atrium to ventricle. This partial approximation of the valve surfaces during diastole is caused primarily by eddy currents behind the leaflets. Also, the chordae tendineae and papillary muscles are stretched by the filling ventricle and exert tension on the free edges of the valve leaflets.

Movements of the mitral valve leaflets throughout the cardiac cycle are shown in **Figure 18–9.** In **echocardiography,** short pulses of high-frequency sound waves (ultrasound) are sent through the chest tissues and heart, and the echoes reflected from the various cardiac structures are recorded. The timing and the pattern of the reflected waves provide important clinical information, such as the diameter of the heart, the ventricular wall thickness, and the magnitude and direction of the movements of various components of the heart, including the valves.

In Figure 18–9, the echocardiographic transducer is positioned to depict movement of the anterior leaflet of the mitral valve. The posterior leaflet moves in a pattern that is a mirror image of the anterior leaflet. In the projection shown in Figure 18–9, the excursions of the leaflet appear to be much smaller. At point D, the mitral valve opens, and during rapid filling (point D to point E), the anterior leaflet moves toward the ventricular septum. During the reduced filling phase (point E to point F), the valve leaflets float toward each other, but the valve does not close. The ventricular filling contributed by atrial contraction (point F to point A) forces the leaflets apart, and a second approximation of the leaflets follows (point A to point C). At point C, the valve is closed by ventricular contraction. The valve leaflets, which bulge toward the atrium, stay pressed together during ventricular systole (point C to point D).

Semilunar valves connect the ventricles with arteries

The valves between the right ventricle and pulmonary artery and between the left ventricle and

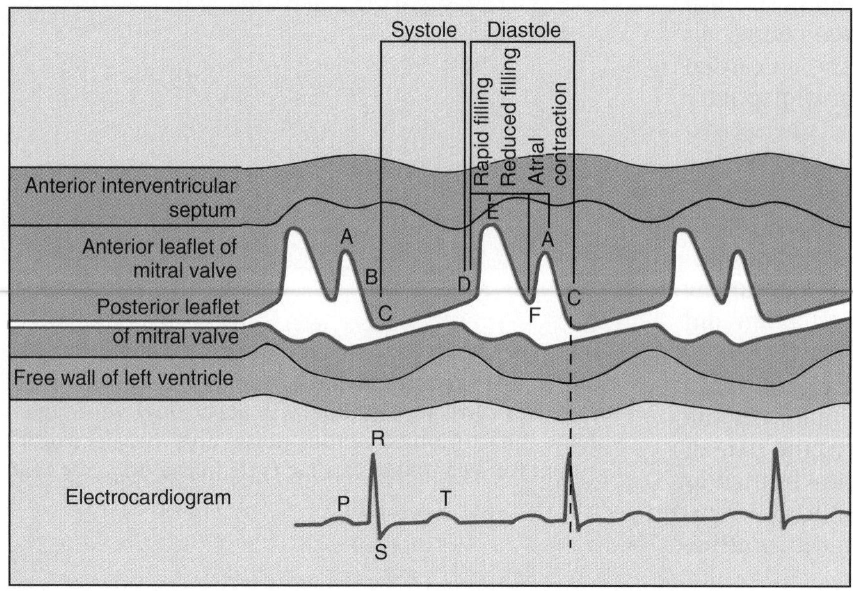

FIGURE 18–9. *Top,* Drawing made from an echocardiogram showing movements of the mitral valve leaflets (particularly the anterior leaflet), changes in the diameter of the left ventricular cavity, and thickness of the left ventricular walls during the cardiac cycles in a healthy person. The mitral valve closes at C and opens at D. C to D, ventricular systole; D to C, ventricular diastole; D to E, rapid filling; E to F, reduced filling (diastasis); F to A, atrial contraction. *Bottom,* Simultaneously recorded electrocardiogram.

aorta consist of three cuplike cusps attached to the valve rings. At the end of the reduced ejection phase of ventricular systole, blood flow reverses briefly toward the ventricles (shown as a negative flow in the phasic aortic flow curve in Figure 18–8). This flow reversal snaps the cusps together and prevents regurgitation of blood into the ventricles. During ventricular systole, the cusps do not lie back against the walls of the pulmonary artery and aorta; instead, they float in the bloodstream approximately midway between the vessel walls and their closed position. Behind the semilunar valves are small outpocketings **(sinuses of Valsalva)** of the pulmonary artery and aorta. Eddy currents develop in these sinuses and keep the valve cusps away from the vessel walls. The orifices of the right and left coronary arteries are located behind the right and left cusps, respectively, of the aortic valve. Were it not for the presence of the sinuses of Valsalva and the eddy currents developed therein, the coronary ostia could be blocked by the valve cusps.

The pericardium is a sac that invests the heart

The pericardium consists of a visceral layer that is adherent to the epicardium and a parietal layer separated from the visceral layer by a thin layer of fluid. The fluid layer provides lubrication for the continuous movement of the enclosed heart. The pericardium is not very distensible and thus strongly resists a large, rapid increase in cardiac size. Therefore, the pericardium helps prevent sudden overdistention of the heart chambers.

In contrast to an acute change in intracardiac pressure, a progressive and sustained enlargement of the heart (as can occur in **cardiac hypertrophy**) or a slow progressive increase in pericardial fluid (as can occur with **pericardial effusion**) gradually stretches the intact pericardium.

The major heart sounds are produced by cardiac valve closure

Four sounds are usually produced by the heart, but only two are ordinarily audible through a stethoscope. With electronic amplification, even the less intense heart sounds can be detected and recorded graphically as a **phonocardiogram.**

The **first heart sound,** initiated at the onset of ventricular systole (Figure 18–8), consists of a series of vibrations of mixed, unrelated low-frequency noises. The first sound is the loudest and longest of the heart sounds, and it has a crescendo-decrescendo quality. The first heart sound is caused primarily by the oscillation of blood in the ventricular chambers and by the vibration of the chamber walls. The vibrations are caused in part by the abrupt rise in ventricular pressure, with acceleration of blood back toward the atria. However, the sound is produced mainly by sudden tension changes and by recoil of the AV valves and of the adjacent structures when the blood is decelerated by closure of the AV valves.

The **second heart sound,** which occurs with closure of the semilunar valves (Figure 18–8), is composed of higher frequency vibrations (higher pitch), is of shorter duration and lower intensity, and has a greater snapping quality than the first heart sound. Abrupt closure of the semilunar valves causes this sound. This closure initiates oscillations of the columns of blood and of the tensed vessel walls by the stretch and recoil of the closed valves.

The **third heart sound** is usually not audible, but it is sometimes heard in children with thin chest walls or in patients with left ventricular failure. This sound consists of a few low-intensity, low-frequency vibrations that are heard best in the region of the cardiac apex. The sound occurs in early diastole, and it is probably the result of vibrations of the ventricular walls caused by the abrupt cessation of ventricular distention and deceleration of blood entering the ventricles.

A **fourth,** or atrial, **sound,** consisting of a few low-frequency oscillations, is occasionally heard in healthy individuals. It is caused by the oscillation of blood in the cardiac chambers during the atrial contraction (Figure 18–8).

Asynchronous AV valve closures can produce **split sounds** over the apex of the heart and over the base of the semilunar valves. Deformities of the valves can produce cardiac **murmurs.** Stenosis or incompetence of the valves may be congenital or produced by disease (e.g., **rheumatic fever**). The timing and character of the murmur provide clues to the type of valve damage.

The Cardiac Cycle Is the Sequential Contraction and Relaxation of Atria and Ventricles

Ventricular systole is initiated by ventricular excitation

The onset of ventricular contraction coincides with the peak of the R wave of the electrocardiogram and with the initial vibration of the first heart sound. The onset of contraction is indicated on the ventricular pressure curve as the earliest rise in ventricular pressure after atrial contraction (Figure 18–8). The interval between the start of ventricular systole and the opening of the semilunar valves (when ventricular pressure rises abruptly) is called **isovolumic contraction** because ventricular volume is constant during this brief period.

Opening of the semilunar valves marks the onset of the **ejection phase,** which may be subdivided into an earlier, shorter phase **(rapid ejection)** and a later, longer phase **(reduced ejection).** The rapid ejection phase is characterized by a sharp rise in ventricular and aortic pressures that terminates at the peak ventricular and aortic pressures, an abrupt decrease in ventricular volume, and a large aortic blood flow (Figure 18–8). During the reduced ejection period, runoff of blood from the aorta to the periphery exceeds ventricular output, and hence aortic and ventricular pressures decline. Throughout ventricular systole, the blood returning to the atria progressively increases the atrial pressure.

During rapid ventricular ejection, left ventricular pressure slightly exceeds aortic pressure, and flow accelerates, whereas during reduced ventricular ejection, the reverse holds true. This reversal of the ventricular-aortic pressure gradient occurs in the presence of the continuous flow of blood from the left ventricle to the aorta. This reversal of the pressure gradient is caused by the momentum of the forward blood flow. The momentum results from the storage of potential energy in the stretched arterial walls, which decelerates the flow of blood into the aorta.

The effect of ventricular systole on left ventricular diameter is shown in Figure 18–9. During ventricular systole (Figure 18–9, point C to point D), the interventricular septum and the free wall of the left ventricle become thicker and move closer to each other.

At the end of ejection, a volume of blood approximately equal to that ejected during systole remains in the ventricular cavities. This **residual volume** is fairly constant in normal hearts. However, it is smaller when heart rate increases or when outflow resistance is reduced, and it is larger when the opposite conditions prevail.

An increase in myocardial contractility may decrease residual volume, especially in the depressed heart. In severely hypodynamic and dilated hearts, as in **heart failure,** the residual volume can become much greater than the stroke volume.

Ventricular filling occurs during diastole

Closure of the aortic valves produces the **incisura** (a notch) on the descending limb of the aortic pressure curve; the incisura marks the end of ventricular systole. The period between closure of the semilunar valves and opening of the AV valves is called **isovolumic relaxation.** It is characterized by a precipitous fall in ventricular pressure without a change in ventricular volume (Figure 18–8).

Most ventricular filling occurs immediately after the AV valves open. The blood that had returned to the atria during the previous ventricular systole is abruptly released into the relaxing ventricles. This period of ventricular filling is called the **rapid filling phase** (Figure 18–8). The atrial and ventricular pressures decrease despite the increase in ventricular volume because the relaxing ventricles exert less and less force on the blood in their cavities.

The rapid filling phase is followed by a phase of slow filling called **diastasis.** During this phase, blood returning from the periphery flows into the right ventricle, and blood from the pulmonary circulation flows into the left ventricle. This slow ventricular filling is indicated by gradual increases in atrial, ventricular, and venous pressures and in ventricular volume (Figure 18–8).

The onset of atrial systole occurs soon after the beginning of the P wave of the electrocardiogram. The transfer of blood from atria to the ventricles, accomplished by the peristalsis-like wave of atrial contraction, completes the period of ventricular filling (Figure 18–8). Throughout ventricular diastole, atrial pressure barely exceeds ventricular pressure. This small pressure gradient indicates that the resistance of the pathway through the open AV valves during ventricular filling is normally very low.

Because there are no valves at the junctions of the venae cavae and right atrium or at the junctions of the pulmonary veins and left atrium, atrial contraction can force blood in both directions. Little blood is pumped back into the venous tributaries during the brief atrial contraction, mainly because of the inertia of the inflowing blood.

Atrial contraction is not essential for ventricular filling. Adequate filling is often observed in patients with **atrial fibrillation** or with **complete heart block,** despite the absence of atrial contraction. However, asynchronous atrial contraction, as occurs in atrial fibrillation, can exacerbate heart failure symptoms because it reduces ventricular filling and thereby cardiac output.

The contribution of atrial contraction to ventricular filling is governed substantially by the heart rate and the structure of the AV valves. At slow heart rates, filling virtually ceases toward the end of diastasis, and atrial contraction contributes little to ventricular filling. When the heart rate is rapid, diastasis is abbreviated, and the atrial contribution can become substantial, especially if the atrium contracts immediately after the rapid filling phase, when the AV pressure gradient is maximal.

When the heart rate becomes so rapid that the period of ventricular relaxation is markedly abbreviated, ventricular filling is seriously impaired, despite the contribution of atrial contraction. In certain diseases (e.g., **mitral stenosis**), the AV valves may be severely narrowed, and atrial contraction becomes more important to ventricular filling than it is in the normal heart.

A Graph of the Cardiac Pressure-Volume Relationship Reveals the Sequence of Dynamic Changes During a Single Cardiac Cycle

The changes in left ventricular pressure and volume throughout the cardiac cycle are summarized in **Figure 18–10.** Time is not considered in this pressure-volume loop. Diastolic filling starts at point A and terminates at point C, when the mitral valve closes. The initial decrease in left ventricular pressure (point A to point B), despite the rapid inflow of blood from the atrium, results from progressive ventricular relaxation and increased distensibility. During the remainder of diastole (point B to point C), the increase in ventricular pressure reflects ventricular filling and the passive elastic characteristics of the ventricle. After the initial phase of ventricular diastole, only a small increase in pressure occurs with the increase in ventricular volume (point B to point C). Atrial systole (the small upward deflection just to the left of point C) contributes to ventricular volume and pressure. With isovolumic contraction (point C to point D), pressure rises steeply and ventricular volume remains constant. At point D, the aortic valve opens. During the rapid ejection phase (point D to point E), the large reduction in volume is associated with a progressive increase in ventricular pressure. This pressure increment is less than the increase that occurs during isovolumic contraction. This phase is followed by reduced ejection (point E to point F) and by a small decrease in ventricular pressure. The aortic valve closes at point F; this is followed by isovolumic relaxation (point F to point A), which is characterized by a sharp drop in pressure and no change in volume. The mitral valve opens at point A to complete one cardiac cycle.

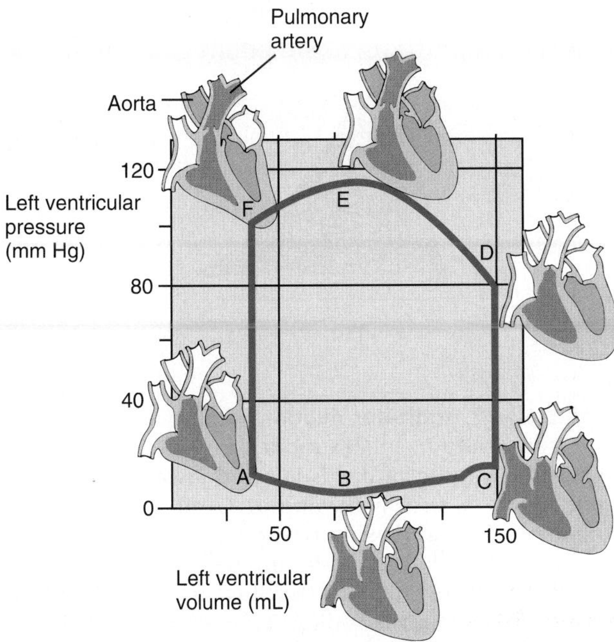

FIGURE 18–10. Pressure-volume loop of the left ventricle for a single cardiac cycle (A to F). See text for details.

The Fick principle is used to measure cardiac output

Adolph Fick contrived the first method for measuring cardiac output in intact animals and humans. The basis for this method, called the **Fick principle,** is simply an application of the law of conservation of mass. The principle is derived from the fact that the quantity of O_2 delivered to the pulmonary capillaries via the pulmonary artery plus the quantity of O_2 that enters the pulmonary capillaries from the alveoli must equal the quantity of O_2 carried away by the pulmonary veins.

The rate of O_2 delivery to the lungs, q_1, equals the O_2 concentration in the pulmonary arterial blood, $[O_2]_{pa}$, multiplied by the pulmonary arterial blood flow, Q, which equals the cardiac output, as follows:

$$q_1 = Q[O_2]_{pa} \qquad \textbf{18-1}$$

At equilibrium, q_2, the net rate of O_2 uptake by the pulmonary capillaries from the alveoli equals the O_2 consumption of the body. The rate at which O_2 is carried away by the pulmonary veins, q_3, equals the O_2 concentration in pulmonary venous blood, $[O_2]_{pv}$, multiplied by the total pulmonary venous flow, which is virtually equal to the pulmonary arterial blood flow, Q, as follows:

$$q_3 = Q[O_2]_{pv} \qquad \textbf{18-2}$$

From the conservation of mass, the following occurs:

$$q_1 + q_2 = q_3 \qquad \textbf{18-3}$$

Therefore, from Equations 18–1 to 18–3, the following occurs:

$$Q[O_2]_{pa} + q_2 = Q[O_2]_{pv} \qquad \textbf{18-4}$$

Solving for cardiac output, one finds the following:

$$Q = q_2/([O_2]_{pv} - [O_2]_{pa}) \qquad \textbf{18-5}$$

Equation 18–5 is the statement of the Fick principle.

In the clinical determination of cardiac output, O_2 consumption is computed from measurements of the volume and O_2 content of expired air over a given interval. Because the O_2 concentration of peripheral arterial blood, $[O_2]_{pa}$, is essentially identical to that in the pulmonary veins, $[O_2]_{pv}$, the O_2 concentration is determined on a sample of peripheral arterial blood that is withdrawn by needle puncture. Pulmonary arterial blood represents mixed systemic venous blood. Samples for O_2 analysis are obtained from the pulmonary artery or right ventricle through a cardiac catheter.

An example of the calculation of cardiac output in a normal, resting adult is illustrated in **Figure 18–11**. When the O_2 consumption is 250 mL/min, the arterial (and pulmonary venous) O_2 content is 0.20 mL of O_2 per milliliter of blood, and the mixed venous (and pulmonary arterial) O_2 content is 0.15 mL of O_2 per milliliter of blood, the cardiac output would be 250/(0.20 – 0.15) = 5000 mL/min.

The Fick principle is also used for estimating the O_2 consumption of organs in situ, when blood flow and the O_2 contents of the arterial and venous blood can be determined. Algebraic rearrangement of Equation 18–5 reveals that O_2 consumption equals the blood flow multiplied by the arteriovenous O_2 concentration difference. For example, if the blood flow through one kidney is 700 mL/min, arterial O_2 content is 0.20 mL of O_2 per milliliter of blood, and renal venous O_2 content is 0.18 mL of O_2 per milliliter of blood, then the rate of O_2 consumption by that kidney must be 700(0.20 – 0.18) = 14 mL/min.

The indicator dilution technique can be used to estimate cardiac output

The **indicator dilution technique** has been widely used to estimate cardiac output in human subjects (**Figure 18–12**). A measured quantity of

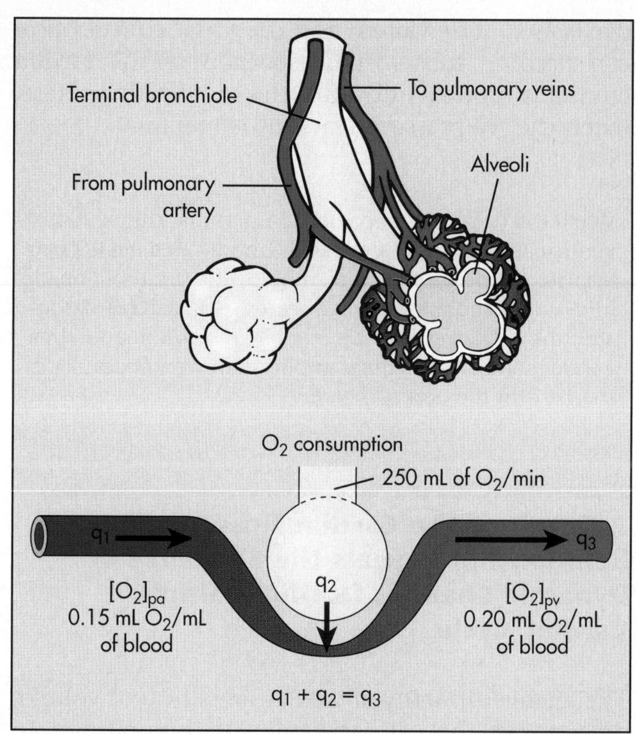

FIGURE 18–11. Diagram illustrating the Fick principle for measuring cardiac output. The change in color from pulmonary artery to pulmonary vein represents the change in color of the blood as venous blood becomes fully oxygenated.

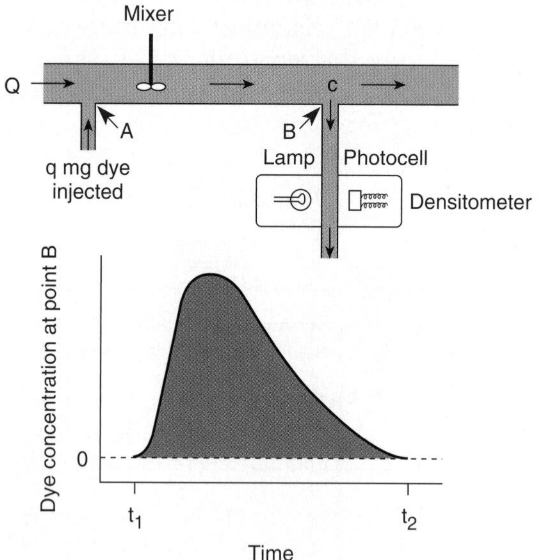

FIGURE 18–12. Indicator dilution technique for measuring cardiac output. In this model, in which there is no recirculation, q mg of dye is injected instantaneously at point A into a stream flowing at Q mL/min. A mixed sample of the fluid flowing past point B is withdrawn at a constant rate through a densitometer; c is concentration of dye in the fluid. The resultant dye concentration curve at point B has the configuration shown in the lower section of the figure. (Modified from Berne RM, Levy MN, Koeppen BM, Stanton BA: *Physiology,* ed 5, Philadelphia, 2004, Elsevier.)

some indicator (a dye or isotope that remains within the circulation) is injected rapidly into a large central vein or into the right side of the heart through a catheter. Arterial blood is continuously drawn through a detector (densitometer or isotope rate counter), and a curve of indicator concentration is recorded as a function of time. The greater the blood flow (cardiac output), the greater the dilution of the injected dye. The most common indicator is a bolus of cold saline injected into the pulmonary artery through a cardiac catheter. The cardiac output can be calculated from the change in the temperature of the blood flowing past the temperature detector at the tip of the catheter. Currently, the most popular indicator dilution technique is **thermodilution.** The principle of the thermodilution technique is the same as that of the indicator dilution technique, except that the change in **temperature,** rather than the change in **color density,** is measured.

Summary

- An increase in myocardial fiber length, such as that occurring with an augmented ventricular filling during diastole (preload), produces a more forceful ventricular contraction. This relationship between fiber length and strength of contraction is known as the Frank-Starling relationship or Starling's law.
- Although the myocardium is made up of individual cells with discrete membrane boundaries, the cardiac myocytes that constitute the ventricles contract almost in unison, as do those of the atria. The myocardium functions as a syncytium with an all-or-none response to excitation. Cell-to-cell conduction occurs through gap junctions that connect the cytosol of adjacent cells.
- During the upstroke of the action potential, voltage-gated Ca^{++} channels open to admit extracellular Ca^{++} into the cell. The influx of Ca^{++} triggers the release of Ca^{++} from the sarcoplasmic reticulum. The elevated intracellular Ca^{++} produces contraction of the myofilaments.
- Relaxation of the myocardial fibers is accomplished by restoration of the resting cytosolic Ca^{++} level by pumping Ca^{++} back into the sarcoplasmic reticulum and exchanging it for extracellular Na^{+} across the sarcolemma.
- The velocity and force of contraction are functions of the intracellular concentration of free Ca^{++}. Force and velocity are inversely related, so with no load, force is negligible and velocity is maximal. In an isometric contraction, in which no external shortening occurs, force is maximal and velocity is zero.
- In the ventricles, the preload is the stretch of the fibers caused by blood during ventricular filling, and the afterload is the aortic pressure against which the left ventricle ejects blood.
- Contractility is an expression of cardiac performance at a given preload and afterload and heart rate. Contractility is increased mainly by interventions that increase intracellular Ca^{++} levels and decreased by interventions that decrease intracellular Ca^{++} levels.
- Simultaneous recording of the left atrial pressure, left ventricular pressure, aortic pressure, ventricular volume, heart sounds, and electrocardiogram graphically portrays the sequential and related electrical and cardiodynamic events throughout a cardiac cycle.
- Cardiac output can be determined, according to the Fick principle, by dividing the O_2 consumption of the body by the difference between the O_2 content of arterial and mixed venous blood. It can also be measured by dye dilution or thermodilution techniques.

Bibliography

Bers DM: *Excitation-contraction coupling and cardiac contractile force*, ed 2, Boston, 2001, Kluwer Academic Publishers.

Brady AJ: Mechanical properties of isolated cardiac myocytes, *Physiol Rev* 71:413, 1991.

Brette F, Orchard C: T-tubule function in mammalian cardiac myocytes, *Circ Res* 92:1182, 2003.

Franzini-Armstrong C, Protasi F, Ramesh V: Comparative ultrastructure of Ca^{2+} release units in skeletal and cardiac muscle, *Ann N Y Acad Sci* 853:20, 1998.

Guatimosim S et al: Local Ca^{2+} signaling and EC coupling in heart: Ca^{2+} sparks and the regulation of the $[Ca^{2+}]_i$ transient, *J Mol Cell Cardiol* 34:941, 2002.

Kamp TJ, Hell JW: Regulation of cardiac L-type calcium channels by protein kinase A and protein kinase C, *Circ Res* 87:1095, 2000.

Muller FU et al: Junctional sarcoplasmic reticulum transmembrane proteins in the heart, *Basic Res Cardiol* 97(suppl 1):I52, 2002.

Rapundalo ST: Cardiac protein phosphorylation: functional and pathophysiological correlates, *Cardiovasc Res* 38:559, 1998.

Scoote M, Poole-Wilson PA, Williams AJ: The therapeutic potential of new insights into myocardial excitation-contraction coupling, *Heart* 89:371, 2003.

Todaka K et al: Effect of ventricular stretch on contractile strength, calcium transient, and cAMP in intact canine hearts, *Am J Physiol* 274:H990, 1998.

Case Study

Case 18–1

A 60-year-old woman entered the hospital complaining of shortness of breath, fatigue, and swelling of her ankles and lower legs. She had these symptoms for about 3 years but refused medical treatment until they became severe. As a child, she had rheumatic fever and developed a murmur, which was diagnosed as mitral stenosis. Physical examination revealed a dyspneic, slightly cyanotic woman with ankle and pretibial edema, distended neck veins, enlarged tender liver, ascites, and rales at the lung bases. The electrocardiogram showed atrial fibrillation and right axis deviation. A chest x-ray film showed an enlarged heart and shadows at the lung bases that were compatible with pulmonary edema. A cardiac work-up revealed a low cardiac output. After a week of treatment for congestive heart failure, her symptoms abated, and she was sent home with a prescription for medication.

1. What did auscultation of the heart reveal?

A. Harsh systolic murmur heard best at the cardiac apex
B. Harsh systolic murmur heard best in the second interspace to the left of the sternum
C. Soft, high-pitched diastolic murmur heard best in the second interspace to the left of the sternum
D. Rumbling, low-pitched diastolic murmur heard best at the cardiac apex
E. High-pitched systolic murmur heard best in the second interspace to the right of the sternum

2. Which of the following is observed in atrial fibrillation?

A. A regular heartbeat
B. A heart rate measured by auscultation over the precordium lower than that measured by palpation of the radial artery
C. A very rapid irregular pulse
D. A constant strength of the heartbeats as palpated at the wrist
E. Regular P waves in the electrocardiogram

3. Which of the following therapeutic measures would help this patient?

A. Insertion of a pacemaker to correct the arrhythmia
B. Phlebotomy (blood removal via a peripheral vein)
C. Saline infusion to increase preload and hence cardiac output
D. Intravenous administration of norepinephrine to restore normal cardiac rhythm
E. Administration of a Ca^{++} uptake blocker such as diltiazem

4. Which of the following findings would be true for this patient?

A. Increased serum albumin level
B. Increased pulmonary wedge pressure (obtained by threading a catheter through a peripheral vein as far as it will go into a branch of the pulmonary artery)
C. Increased Na^+ excretion
D. Reduced peripheral resistance
E. Increased pulse pressure

5. **Which of the following drugs would *not* be prescribed for this patient?**
   A. Dicumarol
   B. Digoxin
   C. Procainamide
   D. Hydrochlorothiazide
   E. Nitroglycerin

6. **The patient's whole-body O_2 consumption was 300 mL/min, and the pulmonary artery and the brachial artery blood O_2 contents were, respectively, 8 mL/dL and 18 mL/dL. What was the patient's cardiac output?**
   A. 2.0 L/min
   B. 4.8 L/min
   C. 3.0 L/min
   D. 1.3 L/min
   E. 1.2 L/min

Chapter 19: Regulation of the Heartbeat

Objectives

- Describe the neural control of heart rate.
- Explain the role of preload in the regulation of myocardial contraction.
- Describe the neural regulation of myocardial contraction.
- Discuss the effects of hormones on myocardial contraction.
- Explain the effects of blood gases on myocardial contraction.

The quantity of blood pumped by the heart each minute **(cardiac output)** equals the volume of blood pumped each beat **(stroke volume)** multiplied by the number of heartbeats per minute **(heart rate).** Thus, the cardiac output may be varied by changing the heart rate or the stroke volume. The control of cardiac activity may therefore be subdivided into the regulation of pacemaker activity and the regulation of contractile strength. The control of pacemaker activity is mediated mainly by the autonomic nervous system. The cardiac nerves also regulate contractile strength, but a number of mechanical and other humoral factors are also important.

Autonomic Nerves Control Heart Rate

In normal adults, the average heart rate at rest is about 70 beats/min, but the rate is significantly greater in children. During sleep, the heart rate diminishes by 10 to 20 beats/min, but during exercise or emotional excitement, the rate may rise to well above 100 beats/min. In various types of heart failure and in febrile diseases, the heart rate may also be high. In well-trained athletes at rest, the heart rate is often very slow, about 45 beats/min.

The sinoatrial (SA) node is usually under the tonic influence of both divisions of the autonomic nervous system. STIMULATION OF THE SYMPATHETIC SYSTEM INCREASES HEART RATE, WHEREAS STIMULATION OF THE PARASYMPATHETIC SYSTEM DECREASES IT. Changes in heart rate usually involve a reciprocal action of the two divisions of the autonomic nervous system. Thus, an increased heart rate is usually achieved by a waning of parasympathetic activity and a concomitant increase in sympathetic activity; deceleration is usually accomplished by the opposite changes in neural activity. The sympathetic and parasympathetic innervation on the right side of the heart in humans is shown in **Figure 19–1**.

Parasympathetic activity usually predominates in healthy, resting individuals. Abolition of the parasympathetic influence by the drug **atropine** (a **muscarinic receptor antagonist**) usually increases the heart rate substantially **(Figure 19–2)**. Conversely, abolition of sympathetic regulation by the drug **propranolol** (a **β-adrenergic receptor antagonist**) usually slows the heart only slightly (Figure 19–2). Thus, IN HEALTHY, RESTING PEOPLE, THE INHIBITORY PARASYMPATHETIC EFFECTS ON HEART RATE USUALLY PREDOMINATE OVER THE FACILITATORY SYMPATHETIC EFFECTS. When the effects of both divisions of the autonomic nervous system are blocked by the combination of these two drugs in adults, the heart rate averages about 100 beats/min. The rate that prevails after complete autonomic blockade is called the **intrinsic heart rate.**

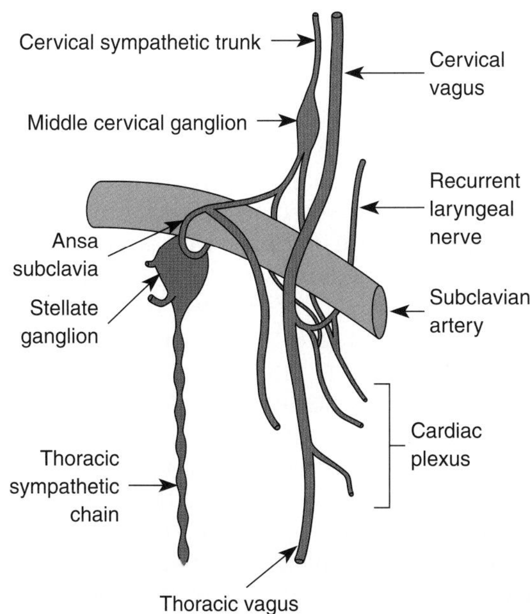

FIGURE 19–1. Sympathetic and parasympathetic (vagal) innervation of the heart on the right side of the body in humans.

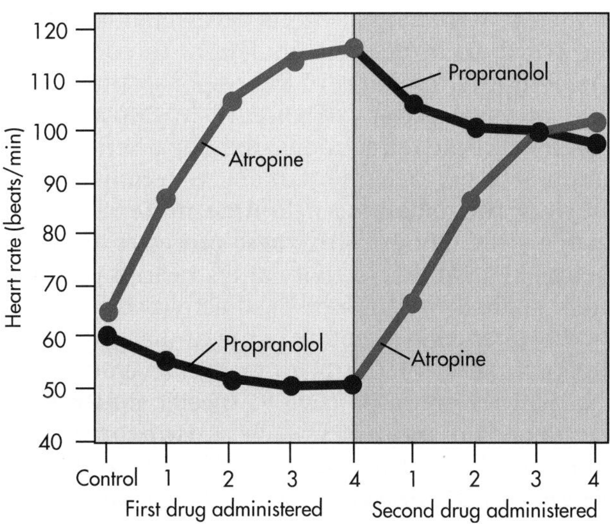

FIGURE 19–2. The mean effects of four equal doses of atropine and of propranolol, given sequentially, on the heart rate of 10 healthy young men. In half of the trials, atropine was given first (*top curve*); in the other half, propranolol was given first (*bottom curve*). (Redrawn from Katona PG et al: *J Appl Physiol* 52:1652, 1982.)

Neural Regulation Involves the Autonomic Nervous System

Sympathetic neural effects are facilitatory

The cardiac sympathetic fibers originate in the upper five or six thoracic and lower one or two cervical segments of the spinal cord (see also Chapter 10). Preganglionic fibers emerge from the spinal column through the white communicating branches and enter the paravertebral chains of ganglia. Most of the preganglionic fibers ascend the paravertebral chains and synapse with postganglionic neurons, mainly in the stellate and middle cervical ganglia. Postganglionic sympathetic fibers then join with parasympathetic fibers to form the **cardiac plexus.** This plexus is a complex network of nerve trunks that contain sympathetic and parasympathetic efferent nerves to the heart as well as afferent nerves from sensory receptors in the heart and great vessels.

Sympathetic fibers from the right and left sides of the body are distributed asymmetrically to heart tissues. In the dog, for example, right cardiac sympathetic nerve stimulation increases the heart rate more than does equivalent stimulation of sympathetic fibers on the left side; the asymmetry is reversed for the control of ventricular contractile force.

The facilitatory effects of sympathetic stimulation on heart rate develop much more slowly than do the inhibitory effects of vagal stimulation (**Figure 19–3**). The onset of the cardiac response to sympathetic stimulation is gradual for two reasons. First, the sympathetic neurotransmitter norepinephrine is released relatively slowly from the cardiac sympathetic nerve terminals. Second, norepinephrine achieves its cardiac effects via a slow second-messenger system, principally the adenylyl cyclase system (see Chapter 5). Further-

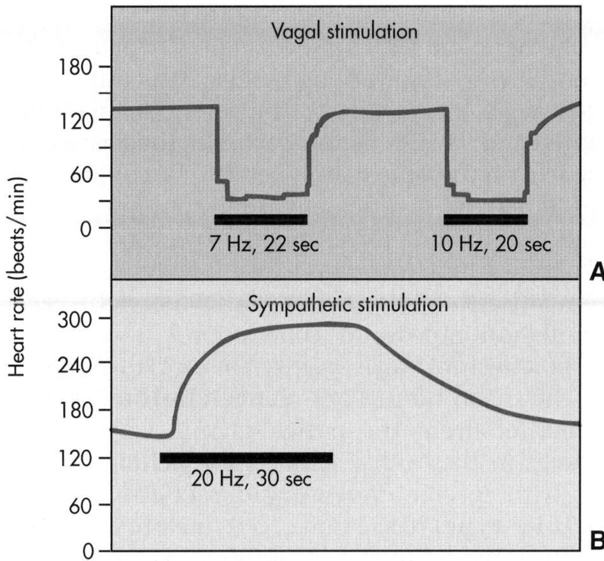

FIGURE 19–3. Changes in heart rate evoked by stimulation (*horizontal bars*) of the vagus (A) and sympathetic (B) nerves in an anesthetized dog. (Modified from Warner HR, Cox A: *J Appl Physiol* 17:349, 1962.)

more, the sympathetic effects decay gradually after the cessation of neural stimulation, in contrast to the abrupt termination of the response after cessation of vagal activity (Figure 19–3). Most of the norepinephrine released during sympathetic stimulation is taken back up by the nerve terminals, and much of the remaining neurotransmitter is carried away by the bloodstream; these processes are slow. Hence, sympathetic activity alters heart rate much more gradually than does vagal activity.

The adrenergic receptors in the cardiac tissues are predominantly of the β-adrenergic receptor type; that is, they are responsive to specific **β-adrenergic receptor agonists,** such as **isoproterenol,** and are inhibited by other specific **β-adrenergic receptor antagonists,** such as **propranolol.**

Parasympathetic neural effects are inhibitory

Preganglionic parasympathetic fibers to the heart originate in the medulla oblongata, in neurons that lie in the **dorsal motor nucleus of the vagus** or in the **nucleus ambiguus** (see also Chapter 10). The precise location of these neurons varies from species to species. Centrifugal fibers from these nuclei pass inferiorly through the neck via the vagus nerves (the tenth cranial nerves), which lie close to the common carotid arteries. The nerve fibers then travel through the mediastinum and synapse with postganglionic cells that are located on the epicardial surface of the heart or within the walls of the heart itself. Many of the parasympathetic cardiac ganglion cells are located in epicardial fat pads near the SA and atrioventricular (AV) nodes.

The right and left vagi are usually distributed differentially to the various cardiac structures. The right vagus nerve affects the SA node predominantly, and its stimulation decreases the firing rate. The left vagus nerve mainly retards AV conduction, and its activity may actually interrupt impulse conduction from atria to ventricles. However, the bilateral innervation overlaps considerably; left vagal stimulation inhibits the SA node, and right vagal stimulation impedes AV conduction.

The effects of vagal activity are mediated mainly by the neurotransmitter **acetylcholine,** which is released from the postganglionic vagus nerve endings in the cardiac tissues. Acetylcholine interacts with specific **cholinergic receptors (muscarinic type)** on cardiac cell membranes. The action of the released acetylcholine can be blocked by the muscarinic receptor antagonist **atropine.** The cardiac tissues are rich in the enzyme **acetylcholinesterase,** which rapidly hydrolyzes the neurally released acetylcholine. Hence, after vagal activity ceases, the effects decay quickly (Figure 19–3, *A*). Furthermore, the effects of vagal activity on heart rate have a short latency (less than 100 msec). The response to the vagal activity attains a steady state quickly, and the released acetylcholine activates special **acetylcholine-regulated K^+ channels** in the cardiac cells. Opening of these channels is prompt because this action does not require an intermediate second-messenger system, such as the adenylyl cyclase system. THE COMBINATION OF THE BRIEF LATENCY AND THE RAPID DECAY OF THE RESPONSE PROVIDES THE POTENTIAL FOR THE VAGUS NERVES TO EXERT A BEAT-BY-BEAT CONTROL OF HEART RATE AND AV CONDUCTION.

Parasympathetic effects preponderate over sympathetic effects at the SA node. In an experiment on an anesthetized dog, the frequencies of neural stimulation were adjusted so that the steady-state increase in the heart rate evoked by cardiac sympathetic stimulation alone equaled the steady-state decrease in heart rate induced by vagal stimulation alone (**Figure 19–4**). In this experiment, the heart rate increased by about 80 beats/min during sympathetic stimulation at a frequency of 4 Hz (S = 4), and the heart rate decreased by about 80 beats/min during vagal stimulation at 8 Hz (V = 8). However, during **concurrent** sympathetic and vagal stimulation at these same frequencies (S = 4; V = 8), heart rate decreased by about 80 beats/min. Thus, the effects of combined vagal and sympathetic stimulation did not differ perceptibly from the effects of vagal stimulation alone; that is, the sympathetic effects were scarcely detectable during combined sympathetic and vagal stimulation. The mechanisms responsible for this overwhelming vagal predominance are discussed later (see "Parasympathetic nerves influence atrial and ventricular contractions").

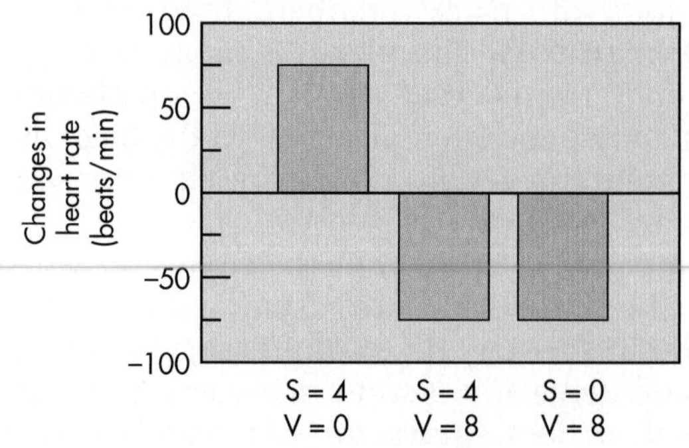

FIGURE 19–4. The changes in heart rate evoked by cardiac sympathetic (S) and vagal (V) stimulation in an anesthetized dog. The numerical values of S and V represent the stimulation frequencies (in hertz). (Modified from Levy MN, Zieske H: *J Appl Physiol* 27:465, 1969.)

Cerebral centers regulate autonomic control

Several cerebral centers help regulate cardiac rate, rhythm, and contractile strength (see also Chapter 10). Excitation of specific nuclei in the **thalamus** or **hypothalamus** alters the heart rate. Hypothalamic centers are also involved in the circulatory responses to fluctuations in environmental temperature. Experimentally induced temperature changes in the anterior hypothalamus markedly affect heart rate and peripheral resistance (see also Chapter 10). Stimuli applied to the H_2 fields of Forel in the **diencephalon** elicit cardiovascular responses that resemble those observed during muscular exercise. In the **cerebral cortex,** the centers that influence cardiac function are located mostly in the frontal and temporal lobes, the motor cortex, the premotor cortex, the orbital cortex, the insula, and the cingulate gyrus.

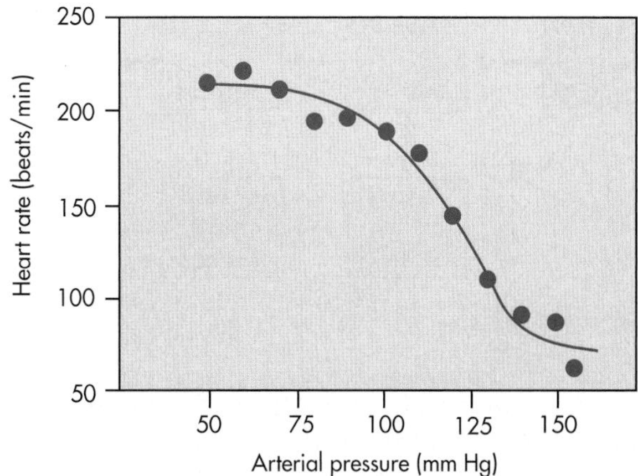

FIGURE 19–5. Heart rate as a function of mean arterial pressure in a group of five conscious, chronically instrumented monkeys. Arterial pressure was increased by phenylephrine infusions and decreased by nitroprusside infusions. (Modified from Cornish KG et al: *Am J Physiol* 257:R595, 1989.)

Autonomic Reflexes Regulate Cardiac Function

Baroreceptor reflexes integrate cardiac function with arterial blood pressure

Acute changes in blood pressure alter heart rate reflexly. Such changes in heart rate are mediated mainly by the pressure receptors **(baroreceptors),** which are located in the carotid sinuses and aortic arch (see also Chapter 23). An example of the heart rate changes elicited by vasodilator and vasoconstrictor drugs in a group of conscious, chronically instrumented monkeys is shown in **Figure 19–5.** As the arterial blood pressure was elevated from about 50 to about 150 mm Hg in these experiments, the heart rate decreased progressively. Changes in blood pressure above and below this range had little additional effect on heart rate.

Moderate deviations in blood pressure from the normal level are usually accomplished by reciprocal changes in sympathetic and parasympathetic activity. For example, a moderate reduction in blood pressure will evoke a rise in heart rate, and this change in rate is mediated usually by a concomitant increase in sympathetic activity and a decrease in vagal activity. Sudden, large changes in blood pressure, however, are usually accompanied by activity in only one autonomic division. When the arterial blood pressure is markedly reduced, the sympathetic nerves become very active, and the vagus nerves are virtually quiescent. However, when the arterial pressure is markedly elevated, the sympathetic nerves become quiescent, and the vagus nerves are hyperactive.

Atrial sensory receptors regulate cardiac and renal function

In 1915, the British physiologist Francis Bainbridge reported that infusions of blood or saline solution increased the heart rate, regardless of whether the infusions did or did not raise the arterial blood pressure. Cardiac acceleration was observed whenever central venous pressure rose sufficiently to distend the right side of the heart. The effect was abolished by cutting both vagi. Bainbridge postulated that increased cardiac filling raised the heart rate reflexly and that the afferent impulses were conducted by the vagi.

Many investigators have confirmed that the heart may accelerate in response to the intravenous administration of fluid. However, the magnitude and direction of the response depend on a number of factors, especially the prevailing heart rate. When the heart rate is relatively slow, intravenous infusions usually accelerate the heart. When the heart rate is more rapid, however, infusions will usually slow the heart. Acute increases in blood volume not only evoke the Bainbridge reflex but also activate other reflexes (notably the baroreceptor reflex) that tend to change heart rate in the opposite direction **(Figure 19–6).** The actual change in heart rate induced by an intravenous infusion is therefore the result of these antagonistic reflex effects.

Sensory receptors in both atria influence heart rate. The receptors are located principally in the

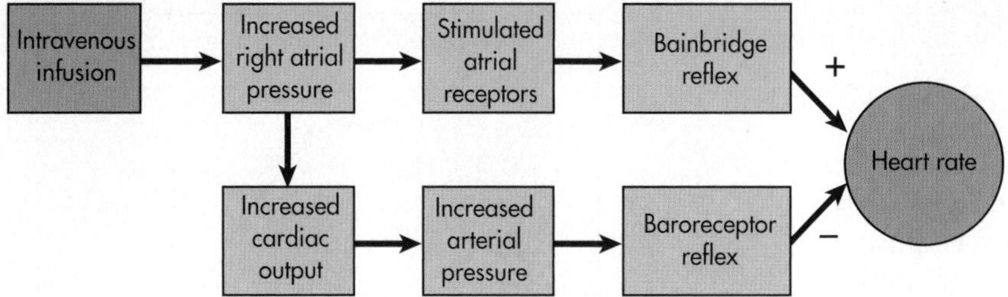

FIGURE 19–6. Intravenous infusions of blood or electrolyte solutions tend to increase heart rate via the Bainbridge reflex and to decrease heart rate via the baroreceptor reflex. The actual change in heart rate induced by such infusions is the result of these two opposing reflex actions.

venoatrial junctions. Distention of these receptors sends impulses centrally in the vagi. The efferent impulses are carried by sympathetic and parasympathetic fibers to the SA node. Stimulation of the atrial receptors also increases urine flow. A reduction in renal sympathetic nerve activity might be partially responsible for this diuresis. However, the principal mechanisms appear to be a neurally mediated reduction in the secretion of **vasopressin (antidiuretic hormone)** by the posterior pituitary gland (see Chapter 45) and the release of another peptide, **atrial natriuretic peptide,** from the atrial tissues in response to atrial contraction and stretch (see Chapter 38).

Respiration reflexly modulates sinus node activity

Cardiac cycle length often fluctuates rhythmically at the frequency of respiration. Such fluctuations are detectable in most resting adults, and they are more pronounced in children. The cycle length typically decreases during inspiration and increases during expiration **(Figure 19–7)**. Recordings of action potentials from the autonomic nerves to the heart in experimental animals reveal that the neural activity increases in the sympathetic nerve fibers during inspiration but that it increases in the vagal fibers during expiration. Acetylcholine released at the vagal endings quickly alters the firing of the pacemaker cells in the SA node, and the acetylcholine is removed rapidly from the nodal tissue. Therefore, periodic bursts of vagal activity can cause the heart rate to vary rhythmically.

Conversely, norepinephrine released at the sympathetic endings affects the pacemaker cells much more gradually than does acetylcholine, and norepinephrine is removed from the cardiac tissues more slowly than is acetylcholine. Thus, the effects of rhythmic variations in sympathetic activity on heart rate are damped. Hence, THE RHYTHMIC CHANGES IN HEART RATE ASSOCIATED WITH RESPIRATION ARE ASCRIBABLE ALMOST ENTIRELY TO THE OSCILLATIONS IN VAGAL ACTIVITY. Respiratory sinus arrhythmia is exaggerated when vagal tone is enhanced.

Reflex and central factors both contribute to the genesis of the respiratory cardiac arrhythmia. During inspiration, the lung volume increases and the intrathoracic pressure decreases (see Chapter 28). Lung distention stimulates pulmonary stretch receptors and tends to increase heart rate reflexly. The reduction in intrathoracic pressure during inspiration increases venous return to the right side of the heart (see Figure 24–12). The resulting distention of the right atrium elicits the Bainbridge reflex (Figure 19–6). After the time delay required for the increased systemic venous return to reach the left side of the heart, left ventricular stroke volume increases and thereby raises systemic arterial blood pressure. These alterations in blood flow reduce heart rate reflexly through baroreceptor stimulation (Figure 19–6).

The respiratory center in the medulla oblongata directly influences the nearby cardiac autonomic centers. This influence has been established in anesthetized animals placed on a heart-lung machine. In such preparations, the chest is open, the lungs are collapsed, and the arterial blood pressure and central venous pressure do not fluctuate rhythmically. Nevertheless, respiratory movements of the

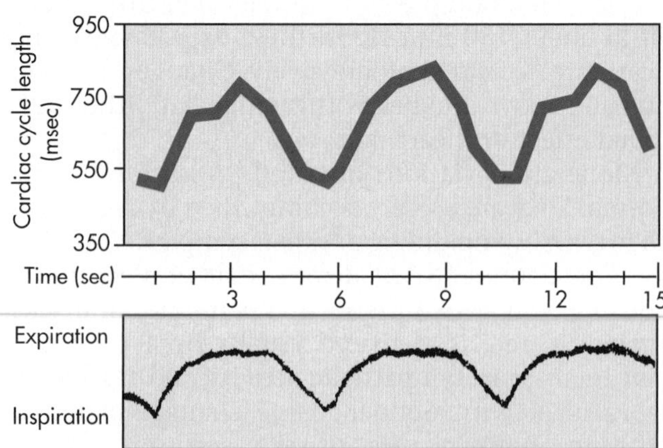

FIGURE 19–7. Respiratory sinus arrhythmia in a resting, unanesthetized dog. Note that the cardiac cycle length increases during expiration and decreases during inspiration. (Modified from Warner MR et al: *Am J Physiol* 251:H1134, 1986.)

rib cage and diaphragm demonstrate that the medullary respiratory center is still active. Cyclic heart rate changes accompany the respiratory movements. These rhythmic changes in heart rate are almost certainly induced by a direct interaction between the respiratory and cardiac centers in the medulla.

Arterial chemoreceptor reflexes affect cardiac function

The cardiac response to peripheral chemoreceptor stimulation (see Chapter 23) merits special consideration because it illustrates the complexity that may be introduced when one stimulus excites two organ systems simultaneously. In intact animals, stimulation of the carotid body chemoreceptors consistently increases ventilatory rate and depth (see Chapter 31) but usually has little effect on heart rate. The small, directional changes in heart rate are related to the enhancement of pulmonary ventilation. When chemoreceptor stimulation augments respiration only slightly, heart rate usually decreases; when the increment in pulmonary ventilation is more pronounced, heart rate usually increases.

The cardiac response to peripheral chemoreceptor stimulation is influenced by primary and secondary reflex mechanisms **(Figure 19–8)**. THE PRIMARY REFLEX EFFECT OF CAROTID CHEMORECEPTOR EXCITATION IS TO STIMULATE THE MEDULLARY VAGAL CENTERS AND THEREBY TO INHIBIT THE AUTOMATICITY OF THE SA NODE. This primary effect becomes evident when the usual respiratory response is absent. THE SECONDARY REFLEX EFFECTS OF RESPIRATORY EXCITATION TEND TO INHIBIT THE MEDULLARY VAGAL CENTERS AND THEREBY TO INCREASE HEART RATE. Therefore, the respiratory effects of chemoreceptor stimulation tend to mask the primary inhibitory effects that chemoreceptor stimulation exerts on the SA node (Figure 19–8).

A dramatic example of the primary inhibitory influence of chemoreceptor stimulation on heart rate in a human subject is displayed in **Figure 19–9**. This electrocardiogram was recorded from a quadriplegic patient who was unable to breathe naturally. The patient required tracheal intubation and artificial respiration. When the tracheal cannula was disconnected briefly to permit removal of excess tracheal secretions, a marked bradycardia developed within seconds. The bradycardia reflects the primary inhibitory effects of the chemoreceptor stimulation on heart rate. These inhibitory effects were evoked by the hypoxia (diminished arterial O_2 tension) and hypercapnia (increased arterial CO_2 tension) that resulted from the patient's inability to breathe (Figure 19–8). The primary inhibitory effects were not opposed by the blood gas changes and the pulmonary stretch effects that ordinarily prevail in patients who can breathe normally. The bradycardia could be abolished temporarily in this patient by injecting the muscarinic receptor antagonist **atropine.** Furthermore, the onset of the bradycardia could be delayed substantially by mechanically hyperventilating the patient before disconnecting him from the tracheal cannula.

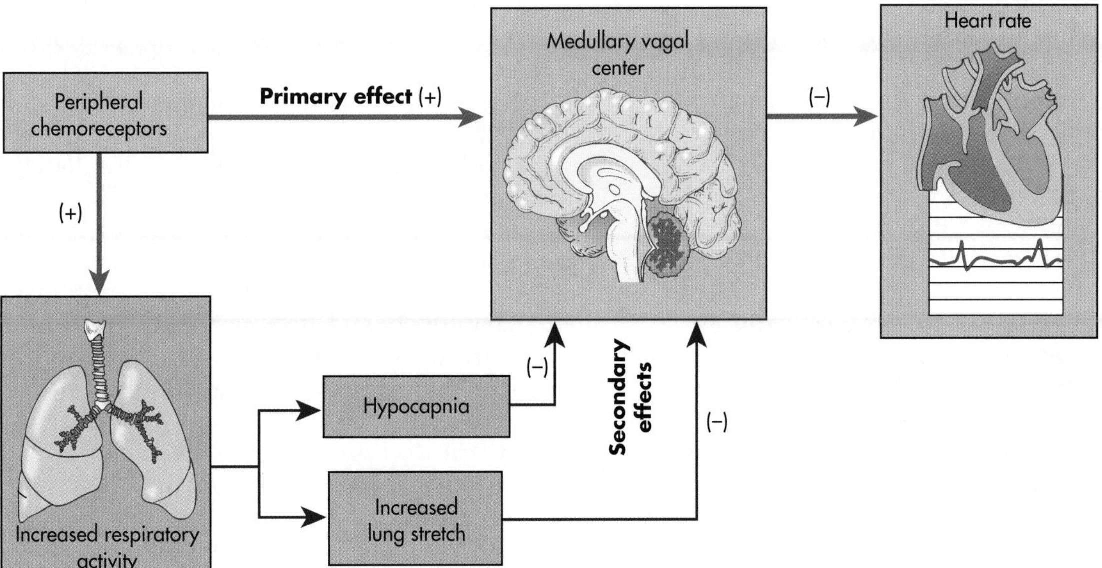

FIGURE 19–8. The primary effect of arterial chemoreceptor stimulation on heart rate is to excite the cardiac vagal center in the medulla and thus to decrease heart rate. Chemoreceptor stimulation also excites the respiratory center in the medulla. The consequent hypocapnia and increases in lung inflation tend to inhibit the medullary vagal center. Thus, the overall heart rate response is the result of these opposing influences.

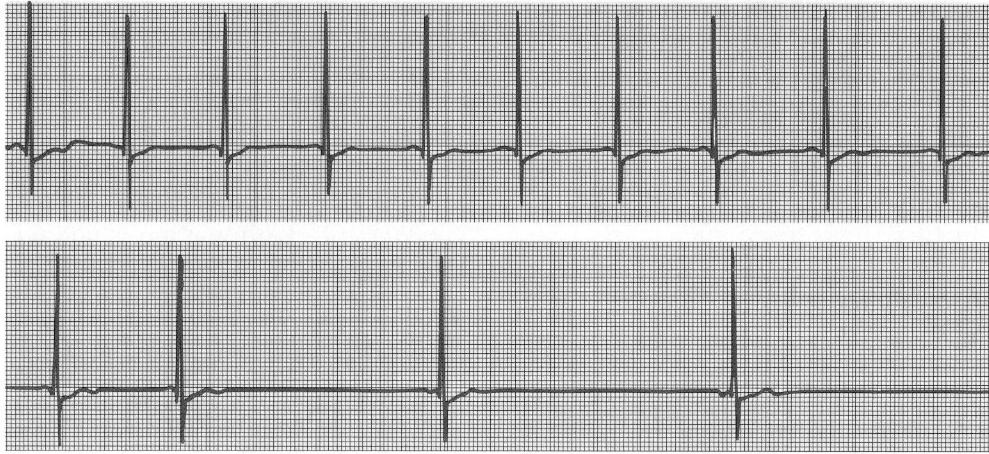

FIGURE 19–9. Electrocardiogram of a 30-year-old man who could not breathe spontaneously and required tracheal intubation and artificial respiration because of injury to his cervical spine. The two strips are continuous. When his tracheal catheter was temporarily disconnected from the respirator (at the beginning of the top strip), his heart rate quickly decreased from 65 beats/min to about 20 beats/min. (Modified from Berke JL, Levy MN: *Eur Surg Res* 9:75, 1977.)

Ventricular sensory receptors reflexly affect cardiac function

Sensory receptors located in the ventricular endocardium initiate reflex effects similar to those elicited by the arterial baroreceptors. Excitation of these endocardial receptors diminishes heart rate and peripheral vascular resistance. The receptor discharge pattern parallels the changes in ventricular pressure. Impulses originating in these receptors are transmitted to the medulla oblongata via the vagus nerves.

Other sensory receptors have been identified in the epicardial regions of the ventricles. These receptors discharge in patterns unrelated to the changes in ventricular pressure. Various mechanical and chemical stimuli excite these ventricular receptors, but their physiological functions are not clear.

Regulation of Myocardial Performance

Intrinsic and extrinsic factors regulate cardiac performance

Just as the heart can initiate its own beat in the absence of any nervous or hormonal control, so also can the myocardium adapt to changing hemodynamic conditions by mechanisms intrinsic to cardiac muscle itself. Experiments on animals with denervated hearts as well as observations in human subjects with cardiac transplants reveal that this organ adjusts remarkably well to various types of stress, even in the absence of any cardiac innervation. For example, racing greyhounds with denervated hearts performed almost as well as those with an intact innervation. The maximal running speed in the denervated animals was only 5% less than it was before cardiac denervation. In these dogs, the fourfold increase in cardiac output when the animals ran was achieved principally by an increase in stroke volume. In normal dogs, the increase in cardiac output during exercise is accompanied by a proportionate increase in heart rate; stroke volume does not change much (see also Chapter 26). The cardiac adaptation in the denervated animals was not achieved entirely by intrinsic mechanisms because circulating catecholamines contributed significantly. When the β-adrenergic receptors were blocked by propranolol in greyhounds with denervated hearts, their racing performance was severely impaired.

The principal intrinsic cardiac adaptation involves changes in the resting length of the myocardial fibers. This adaptation is designated **Starling's law of the heart** or the **Frank-Starling mechanism.** The mechanical and structural bases for this mechanism are explained in Chapters 13 and 18. However, intrinsic mechanisms that do not depend on changes in resting length also help regulate myocardial performance.

Myocardial fiber length determines cardiac contraction (Frank-Starling mechanism)

In 1895, the German physiologist **Otto Frank** described the response of the isolated heart of the frog to alterations in the stretching force **(preload)** on the myocardial fibers just before contraction. He observed that as the preload was increased, the heart responded with a more forceful contraction. About

20 years later, the English physiologist **Ernest Starling** described the intrinsic response of the canine heart to changes in right atrial and aortic pressure in the isolated heart-lung preparation.

In this preparation, the right ventricular filling pressure is varied by altering the height of a reservoir connected to the right atrium. The filling pressure just before ventricular contraction constitutes the preload for the myocardial fibers in the ventricular wall. The right ventricle then pumps this blood through the pulmonary vessels to the left atrium. The lungs are artificially ventilated. Blood is pumped by the left ventricle into the aortic arch and then through some external tubing back to the right atrial reservoir. A resistance device in the external tubing allows the investigator to control the aortic pressure. This pressure constitutes the **afterload** for left ventricular ejection (see also Chapter 18).

One of Starling's recordings of the changes in ventricular volume evoked by a sudden increase in right atrial pressure is shown in **Figure 19–10.** Aortic pressure in this experiment was permitted to increase only slightly when the right atrial pressure (preload) was increased. In the top tracing, an increase in ventricular volume is registered as a downward deflection. Hence, the upper border of the tracing represents the systolic ventricular volume, the lower border indicates the diastolic ventricular volume, and the width of the tracing reflects the **stroke volume** (i.e., the volume of blood ejected by a ventricle during each heartbeat).

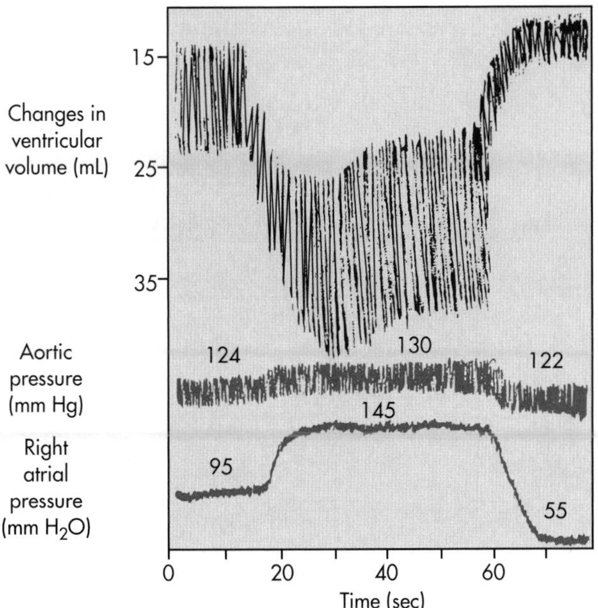

FIGURE 19–10. Changes in ventricular volume in a canine heart-lung preparation when the right atrial pressure was suddenly increased from 95 to 145 mm H_2O and subsequently lowered to 55 mm H_2O. Note that an increase in ventricular volume is registered as a downward shift in the volume tracing. (Redrawn from Patterson SW, Piper H, Starling EH: *J Physiol [Lond]* 48:465, 1914.)

For several beats after the rise in preload, the ventricular volume progressively increased. This indicates that a disparity must have existed between ventricular inflow during diastole and ventricular outflow during systole. During a given systole, the volume of blood expelled by the ventricles was not as great as the volume that had entered the ventricles during the preceding diastole. This progressive accumulation of blood dilated the ventricles and lengthened the individual myocardial fibers in the walls of the ventricles.

The increased diastolic volume and fiber length somehow facilitate ventricular contraction and enable the ventricles to pump a greater stroke volume. Diastolic volume and fiber length continue to increase on successive heartbeats in response to a sustained increase in preload. At equilibrium, the cardiac output exactly matches the augmented filling volume. The mechanism by which increased fiber length enhances the stroke volume depends in part on a change in the number of interacting cross-bridges between the thick and thin filaments. However, a more important factor is that changes in myocardial fiber length substantially change the sensitivity of the contractile proteins to Ca^{++}. An optimum fiber length exists, however, beyond which contraction is actually impaired (see Chapters 13 and 18). Therefore, excessively high preloads may depress rather than enhance the pumping capacity of the ventricles by overstretching the myocardial fibers.

Pronounced changes in preload occur most commonly as a consequence of changes in blood volume. For example, the acute loss of blood **(hemorrhage)** is accompanied by reductions in pressure in the great central veins. Hence, the cardiac filling pressure (preload) is also diminished. Even though blood loss usually leads to a concomitant reduction in arterial blood pressure (afterload), the influence of the preload on cardiac output usually predominates over the influence of the afterload. Furthermore, cardiac output usually decreases in response to hemorrhage (see also Chapters 24 and 26). Large blood transfusions, on the other hand, will increase the cardiac filling pressure, and therefore the transfusions act to increase cardiac output.

Changes in diastolic fiber length also permit the isolated heart to compensate for an increase in afterload. In Starling's experiments on the heart-lung preparation, the arterial pressure (the **afterload**) was abruptly raised, whereas the ventricular filling pressure (the **preload**) was held constant. Initially, the increased afterload diminished the ventricular stroke volume. Because venous return to the right atrium was held constant in these experiments, the volume of blood in the ventricles progressively increased for the next several heartbeats. Consequently, the lengths of the ventricular myocardial fibers increased. This change in end-diastolic fiber length finally enabled the ventricles to pump a stroke volume that was equal to the control stroke volume, despite the greater ventricular afterload.

When cardiac compensation involves ventricular dilatation, the force required by each myocardial fiber to generate a given intraventricular systolic pressure must be appreciably greater than that developed by the fibers in a ventricle of normal size. The relationship between the ventricular volume, the intraventricular pressure, and the force that prevails in the ventricular myocardial fibers resembles the relationship (see **Laplace's law**, Chapter 22) for cylindrical tubes in that for a constant internal pressure, the intramural force (wall tension) varies directly with the radius of the tube (see Figure 22–3). Consequently, to attain a given intraventricular pressure, the myocardial fibers in a dilated heart must develop considerably more force than do the fibers in a normal-sized heart. Therefore, these fibers require considerably more oxygen to perform a given amount of external work than do those fibers in a normal-sized heart (see also Chapter 25).

The most common clinical condition that is characterized by a chronic increase in afterload is **essential hypertension,** which is a sustained increase in arterial blood pressure of unknown cause. The principal hemodynamic change causing the elevated blood pressure is a generalized arteriolar vasoconstriction. The heart adapts initially to this increased afterload by an increase in diastolic ventricular volume, as explained before. Ultimately, however, the mass of ventricular muscle cells also increases; that is, the heart **hypertrophies.** This constitutes an additional mechanism by which the heart adapts to a sustained increase in afterload.

The Frank-Starling mechanism is ideally suited for matching the cardiac output to the venous return. This mechanism also ensures that the amount of blood pumped by one ventricle over a substantial series of heartbeats equals the amount of blood pumped by the other ventricle over that same series of beats. Any sudden, excessive output by one ventricle soon results in a greater venous return to the other ventricle. The consequent increase in diastolic fiber length in this other ventricle serves as the stimulus to increase the output of the second ventricle to a value that approaches the output of its mate. For this reason, IT IS THE FRANK-STARLING MECHANISM THAT MAINTAINS A PRECISE BALANCE OVER TIME BETWEEN THE OUTPUTS OF THE RIGHT AND LEFT VENTRICLES. Even a small but maintained imbalance in the outputs of the two ventricles would be catastrophic because the two ventricles are arranged in series in a closed circuit. The blood volume in the systemic or pulmonic vascular beds would progressively increase, and the blood volume in the remaining vascular beds would progressively diminish.

Heart frequency regulates myocardial contraction

The effects of contraction frequency on the force developed in an isometrically contracting cat papillary muscle are shown in **Figure 19–11**, *A*. Initially, the strip of cardiac muscle was stimulated to contract only once every 20 seconds. When the pacing cycle length was decreased to once every 0.63 second, the developed force increased progressively over the next several beats. This progressive increase in developed force induced by a change in contraction frequency is known as the **staircase** (or **treppe**) **phenomenon.** At the new steady state, the developed force was more than five times greater than it was at the longer pacing cycle length. A return to the shorter cycle length had the opposite influence on developed force.

The effect of a wide range of pacing cycle length on the steady-state level of developed force is shown in Figure 19–11, *B*. As the cycle length was

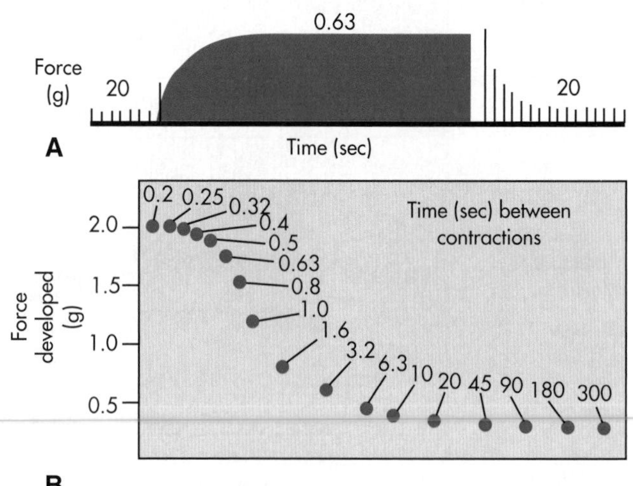

FIGURE 19–11. A, Changes in force development in an isolated papillary muscle from a cat as the interval between contractions was changed from 20 seconds to 0.63 second and then back to 20 seconds. B, The steady-state forces developed at the indicated intervals (in seconds). (Redrawn from Koch-Weser J, Blinks JR: *Pharmacol Rev* 15:601, 1963.)

diminished from 300 seconds to about 10 seconds, developed force increased only slightly. However, as the cycle length was reduced further, to a value of about 0.5 second, the developed force increased sharply. Further reduction of the cycle length to 0.2 second had little additional effect on developed force.

The progressive rise in developed force as the interval between contractions is suddenly decreased (e.g., from 20 seconds to 0.63 second in Figure 19–11, *A*) is mediated by a gradual rise in the intracellular Ca^{++} content. Ca^{++} enters the cell during each action potential plateau (see Chapter 16). Hence, when the time between contractions is reduced (i.e., when the contraction frequency is increased), the Ca^{++} influx per minute increases. As contraction frequency increases, the action potential plateau shortens, and therefore less Ca^{++} enters the myocardial cell per contraction. However, the fractional increment in the number of beats per minute exceeds the fractional decrement in the Ca^{++} influx per beat. Therefore, the intracellular Ca^{++} content rises when the contraction frequency is raised and the contractile force is augmented, as shown in Figure 19–11.

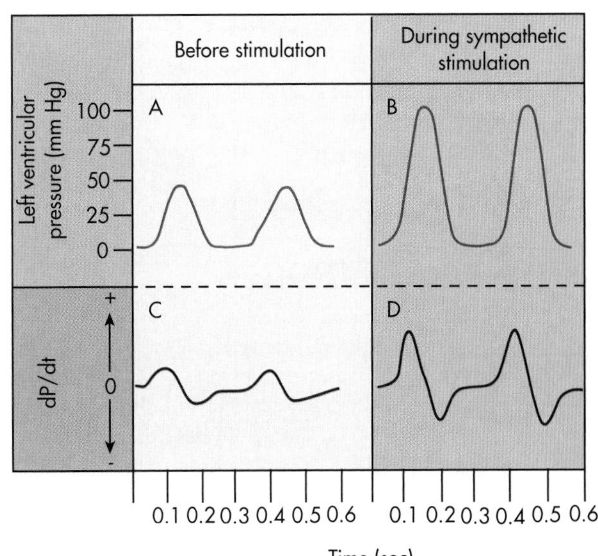

FIGURE 19–12. In an isovolumic canine left ventricle preparation, stimulation of the cardiac sympathetic nerves increases the peak left ventricular pressure and increases the maximum rates of intraventricular pressure rise and fall (dP/dt). (Unpublished tracing from experiments of Levy MN et al: *Circ Res* 19:5, 1966.)

Neurohumoral factors regulate contractility

Although the heart possesses effective intrinsic mechanisms of adaptation, various extrinsic mechanisms are also important in regulating myocardial contractility. Under various natural conditions, the extrinsic mechanisms dominate the intrinsic mechanisms. The extrinsic regulatory factors may be subdivided into nervous and humoral components.

Autonomic nerves regulate cardiac contraction

Sympathetic nerves affect contraction and relaxation

Sympathetic neural activity enhances atrial and ventricular contractility. The density of the sympathetic innervation of the atria and of the SA and AV nodes is about three times that of the ventricles. Alterations in ventricular contraction evoked by electrical stimulation of the cardiac sympathetic nerves in an anesthetized dog are shown in **Figure 19–12.** In this experiment, the heart and lungs were functionally isolated from the rest of the body, and the heart rate was maintained constant by electrical pacing of the right atrium. All venous return to the heart was interrupted. The coronary arteries were then perfused with oxygenated blood at a constant arterial pressure by a heart-lung perfusion apparatus similar to that used clinically for open heart operations. This perfusion apparatus was also used to maintain an adequate perfusion of the entire systemic circulation.

To determine the effects of sympathetic neural activity on cardiac performance, a balloon was inserted into the left ventricle, and enough saline was instilled into the balloon to fill the entire cardiac chamber. Because the saline is virtually incompressible, the ventricular contractions were isovolumic. When the cardiac sympathetic nerves were stimulated in this preparation, the peak ventricular pressure (Figure 19–12, *B*) and the maximum rate of pressure rise (dP/dt) during systole (Figure 19–12, *D*) were markedly increased. Also, the rate of ventricular relaxation (indicated by the minimum value of dP/dt) was increased (Figure 19–12, *D*).

Sympathetic stimulation not only enhances the mechanical contraction of the heart but also facilitates ventricular filling. For example, in an experiment (**Figure 19–13**) on an intact, anesthetized dog (not placed on heart-lung bypass), the animal's heart was paced at a constant rate. Stimulation of the cardiac sympathetic nerves increased the aortic blood pressure substantially (Figure 19–13, *B*), and it increased the stroke volume (not shown). Concurrently, the sympathetic stimulation shortened ventricular systole (Figure 19–13, *D*) and diminished the left ventricular pressure during diastole (Figure 19–13, *D*). Both of these responses

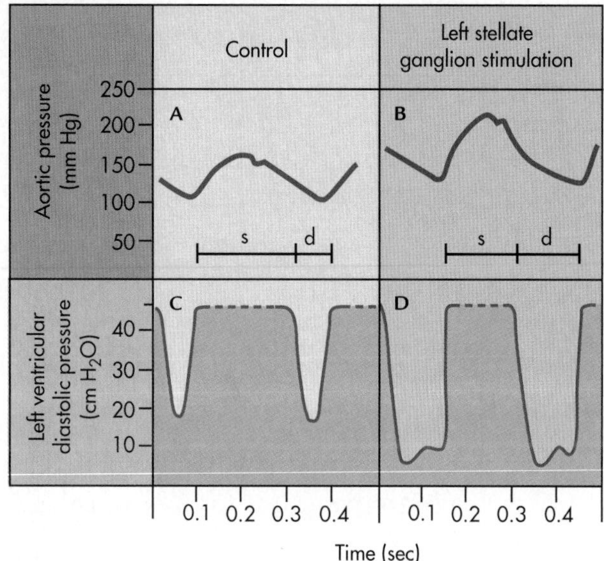

FIGURE 19–13. Stimulation of the cardiac sympathetic nerves (left stellate ganglion) of an anesthetized dog increases aortic pressure (B) but decreases the left ventricular diastolic pressure. Note also the abridgment of systole (s), which allows more time in diastole (d) for ventricular filling (D); the heart was paced at a constant rate. In the ventricular pressure tracings (C and D), the pen excursion cannot exceed 45 mm Hg (*dashed horizontal lines*); actual peak ventricular pressures during systole can be estimated from the aortic pressure tracings. (Redrawn from Mitchell JH, Linden RJ, Sarnoff SJ: *Circ Res* 8:1100, 1960.)

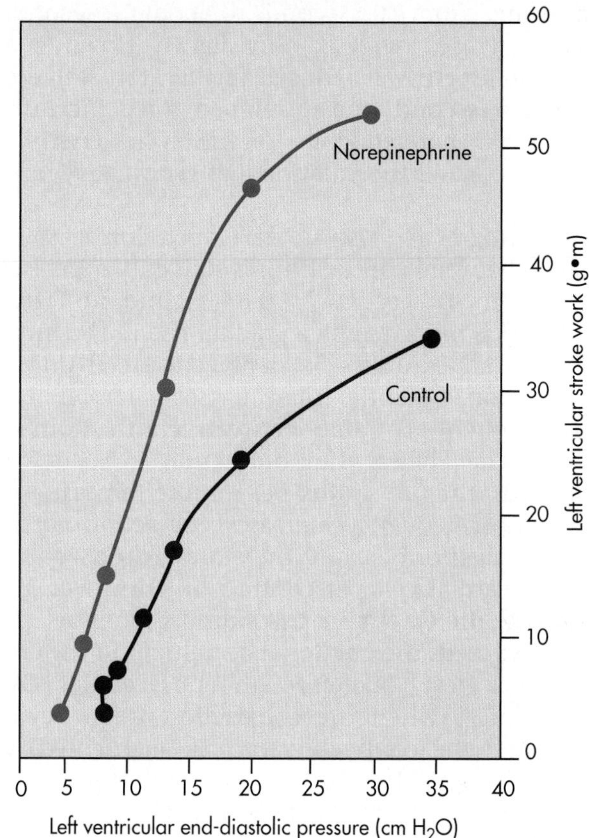

FIGURE 19–14. During a constant infusion of norepinephrine in an anesthetized dog, the left ventricle accomplishes more stroke work than it does under control conditions. This effect of norepinephrine is reflected by a shift to the left of the ventricular function curve. (Redrawn from Sarnoff SJ et al: *Circ Res* 8:1108, 1960.)

facilitated ventricular filling. The reason for the sympathetically induced reduction in the ventricular diastolic pressure (i.e., the preload) is explained in Chapter 24.

The overall effect of increased cardiac sympathoadrenal activity on ventricular performance in intact animals can best be appreciated in terms of families of **ventricular function curves** (see also Chapter 24). Such curves depict the changes in left ventricular performance as a function of the end-diastolic pressure (preload) in the ventricle. In the experiment shown in **Figure 19–14, stroke work** (which is the product of stroke volume and mean aortic pressure) was used as the index of performance. When sympathoadrenal activity was increased by the infusion of norepinephrine, the ventricle was able to accomplish more stroke work at any given level of ventricular end-diastolic pressure; that is, the ventricular function curves are shifted to the left (Figure 19–14).

SYMPATHOADRENAL ACTIVITY ENHANCES MYOCARDIAL PERFORMANCE MAINLY BY FACILITATING THE INFLUX OF Ca^{++} INTO THE MYOCYTES. The adrenergic agonists norepinephrine and epinephrine interact with β-adrenergic receptors in the cardiac cell membranes. This interaction activates **adenylyl cyclase,** which raises the intracellular levels of **cAMP** (see also Chapters 5, 18, and 48).

Changes in myocardial contractility induced by norepinephrine infusions have been tested in resting, unanesthetized dogs. The maximum rate of rise of left ventricular pressure (dP/dt), an index of myocardial contractility, varies directly with the norepinephrine concentration in the blood **(Figure 19–15)**. The increase in dP/dt was proportional to the concentration of norepinephrine in the blood. In these same animals, moderate exercise increased the maximum dP/dt by almost 100%, but it raised the circulating catecholamines by only 0.5 ng/mL. By itself, such a rise in norepinephrine concentration would have had only a negligible effect on left ventricular dP/dt. Therefore, the pronounced change in dP/dt observed during exercise must have been mediated mainly by the norepinephrine released from the cardiac sympathetic fibers rather than by the catecholamines released from the adrenal medulla.

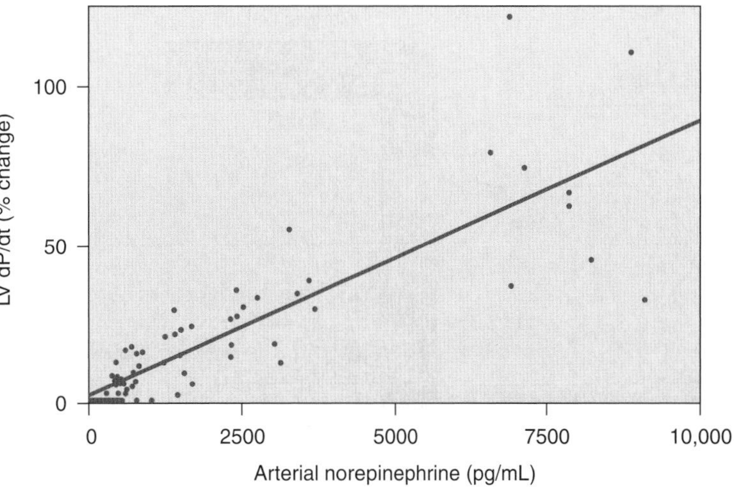

FIGURE 19–15. Effect of norepinephrine infusions on ventricular contractility in a group of resting, unanesthetized dogs. The plasma concentrations of norepinephrine (pg/mL) plotted along the abscissa are the increments above the control values. The maximal rate of rise of left ventricular pressure (LV dP/dt), an index of contractility, is plotted along the ordinate as percentage change from the control value. (Redrawn from Young MA, Hintze TH, Vatner SF: *Am J Physiol* 178:H82, 1985.)

Parasympathetic nerves influence atrial and ventricular contractions

The vagus nerves strongly inhibit the SA node, atrial myocardium, and AV conduction tissue. These parasympathetic nerves also depress the ventricular myocardium, but the effects are less pronounced. In the total heart bypass preparation (such as that used to derive Figure 19–12), vagal stimulation decreases the peak left ventricular pressure and the maximum rates (dP/dt) of pressure development and of pressure decline. The effects are opposite to those elicited by sympathetic stimulation (see Figures 19–3 and 19–12).

The effects of increased vagal activity on the ventricular myocardium are achieved largely by antagonizing the facilitatory effects of any concurrent sympathetic activity. This antagonism takes place at two levels. At the level of the autonomic nerve endings in the heart, the acetylcholine released from vagal endings inhibits the release of norepinephrine from nearby sympathetic endings. At the level of the cardiac cell membranes, the rise in intracellular cAMP that would ordinarily be produced in response to a given quantity of neurally released norepinephrine is attenuated by the acetylcholine released from nearby vagal endings.

These antagonistic interactions between the sympathetic and vagal effects on the ventricular myocardium also take place in other cardiac structures, such as the SA node. For example, in the experiment shown in Figure 19–4, sympathetic stimulation alone at a frequency of 4 Hz increased heart rate substantially. However, during combined sympathetic and vagal stimulation, the vagal influence was so predominant that the heart rate response to combined stimulation did not differ perceptibly from the effects of vagal stimulation alone. The intraneuronal and intracellular mechanisms responsible for the interactions between the sympathetic and parasympathetic systems in the neural control of cardiac function are shown in **Figure 19–16**.

Chemical components of the blood modulate cardiac contractions

Hormones have marked effects on cardiac contractility

Various hormones influence cardiac function. The principal hormone secreted by the adrenal medulla is **epinephrine,** although a small quantity of norepinephrine is also released (see Chapter 48). The rate of catecholamine secretion by the adrenal medulla is regulated by essentially the same mechanisms that control the activity of the sympathetic nervous system. The effects of those catecholamines on the heart are qualitatively similar to the effects of those released from the sympathetic nerve endings. However, the concentrations of circulating catecholamines rarely rise sufficiently high to affect cardiac function appreciably.

Numerous studies on intact animals and humans have demonstrated that **thyroid hormones** enhance myocardial contractility (see Chapter 46). The rates of calcium uptake and of ATP hydrolysis by the sarcoplasmic reticulum are increased in experimental hyperthyroidism, and the opposite effects occur in hypothyroidism. Thyroid hormones increase protein synthesis in the heart, which leads to cardiac hypertrophy. These hormones also affect the composition of myosin isoenzymes in cardiac muscle. They increase principally those isoenzymes with the greatest ATPase activity and thereby enhance myocardial contractility substantially.

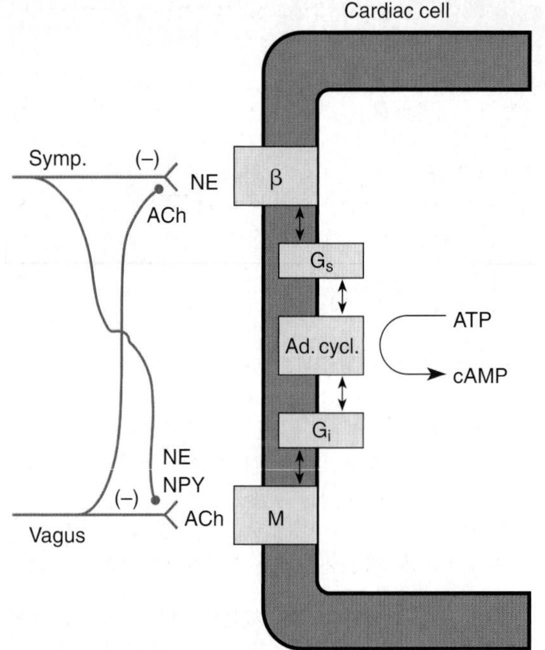

FIGURE 19–16. The interneuronal and intracellular mechanisms responsible for the interactions between the sympathetic and parasympathetic systems in the neural control of cardiac function. NE, norepinephrine; ACh, acetylcholine; NPY, neuropeptide Y; β, β-adrenergic receptor; M, muscarinic receptor; G_s and G_i, stimulatory and inhibitory G proteins; Ad. cycl., adenylyl cyclase; ATP, adenosine triphosphate; cAMP, cyclic adenosine monophosphate. (From Levy MN. In Kulbertus HE, Franck G, eds: *Neurocardiology,* Mt. Kisco, NY, 1988, Futura.)

Cardiac activity is sluggish in patients with inadequate thyroid function **(hypothyroidism);** that is, the heart rate is slow and cardiac output is diminished. The converse is true in patients with overactive thyroid glands **(hyperthyroidism).** Characteristically, such patients exhibit tachycardia, high cardiac output, palpitations, and arrhythmias.

Insulin enhances myocardial contractility in several mammalian species. The effect of insulin is evident even when hypoglycemia is prevented by glucose infusions and when the β-adrenergic receptors are blocked. In fact, the insulin-induced enhancement of contractility is potentiated by β-adrenergic receptor blockade. The improved contractility cannot be explained satisfactorily by the concomitant increase of glucose transport into the myocardial cells.

Glucagon has potent positive inotropic and chronotropic effects on the heart. The endogenous hormone is probably not involved in the normal regulation of the cardiovascular system, but it has been used pharmacologically to treat various cardiac conditions. The effects of glucagon on the heart closely resemble those of the catecholamines because they arise from activation of the adenylyl cyclase–cAMP system.

Blood gases affect the heart directly and indirectly

Changes in oxygen tension ($Pa{O_2}$) of the blood perfusing the brain and the peripheral chemoreceptors affect the heart through nervous mechanisms, as described earlier in this chapter. These indirect effects of hypoxia are usually prepotent. Moderate degrees of hypoxia characteristically increase heart rate, cardiac output, and myocardial contractility by increasing sympathetic nervous activity. These changes are largely abolished by β-adrenergic receptor blockade. The $Pa{O_2}$ of the blood perfusing the myocardium also influences myocardial performance directly. The effect of hypoxia is biphasic; moderate degrees are stimulatory and more severe degrees are depressant.

Changes in CO_2 tension ($Pa{CO_2}$) in the blood also affect the myocardium directly and indirectly. The indirect, neurally mediated effects produced by increased $Pa{CO_2}$ are similar to those evoked by a decrease in $Pa{O_2}$. The direct effects on myocardial performance elicited by changes in $Pa{CO_2}$ in the coronary arterial blood are illustrated in **Figure**

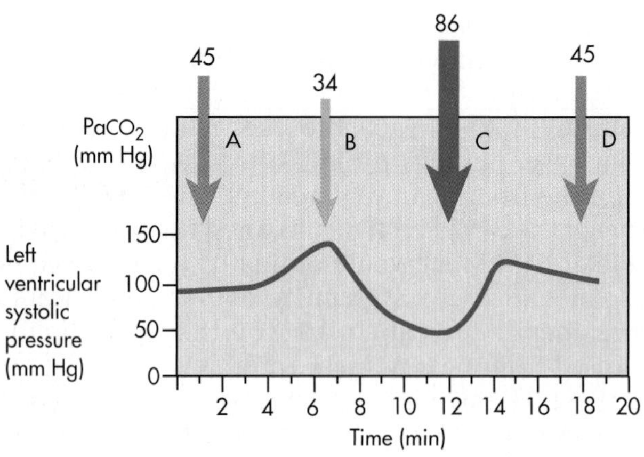

FIGURE 19–17. A decrease in the arterial blood tension of CO_2 ($Pa{CO_2}$) from 45 to 34 mm Hg increases left ventricular systolic pressure (*arrow B*) in an isovolumic canine left ventricle preparation. A subsequent rise in $Pa{CO_2}$ to 86 mm Hg has the reverse effect. When the $Pa{CO_2}$ is returned to the control level (45 mm Hg), left ventricular systolic pressure returns to its original value. (Derived from experiments by Ng ML et al: *Am J Physiol* 213:115, 1967.)

19–17. In this experiment on an isolated left ventricle preparation, the control Pa_{CO_2} was 45 mm Hg (arrow A). Decreasing the Pa_{CO_2} to 34 mm Hg (arrow B) was stimulatory, whereas increasing Pa_{CO_2} to 86 mm Hg (arrow C) was depressant. In intact animals, systemic increases in Pa_{CO_2} activate the sympathoadrenal system, and this change compensates for the direct depressant effect of the increased Pa_{CO_2} on the heart.

Neither the Pa_{CO_2} nor the blood pH is a primary determinant of myocardial behavior; the induced change in intracellular pH is the critical factor. The reduced intracellular pH diminishes the influx of Ca^{++} into the cell via the Ca^{++} channels and the Na^{+}-Ca^{++} antiporter, decreases the amount of Ca^{++} released from the sarcoplasmic reticulum in response to excitation of the myocytes, and affects myofilament sensitivity to Ca^{++} directly. When they are exposed to a given concentration of Ca^{++}, the myofibrils develop less force as the prevailing intracellular pH decreases.

Figure 19–18 shows the changes in contractile performance and in intracellular pH when perfusion is halted in an isolated, perfused rabbit heart. When flow ceased, the left ventricular pressure diminished rapidly until the contraction virtually halted within about 4 minutes. These changes were accompanied by a progressive reduction in intracellular pH, from a control value of 7.0 to a value of about 6.3 after 4 minutes of ischemia.

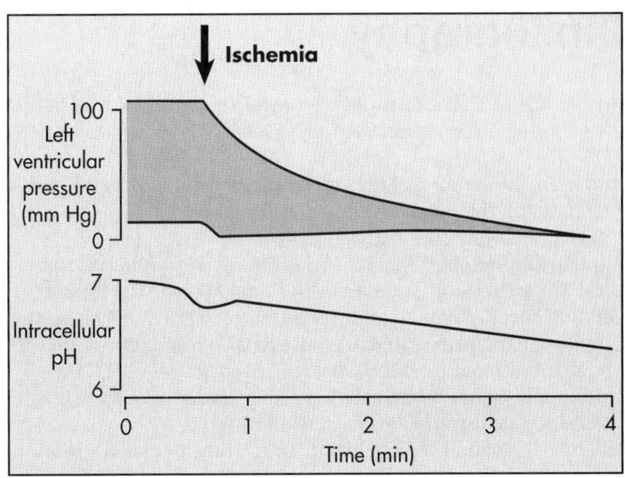

FIGURE 19–18. Effect of ischemia on left ventricular pressure and intracellular pH in an isolated perfused rabbit heart. (Modified from Mohabir R et al: *Circ Res* 69:1525, 1991.)

In patients with coronary artery disease, a narrowed region of a major coronary artery may suddenly become occluded by a blood clot; this is the most common cause of a "heart attack." The consequent inadequacy of blood flow **(myocardial ischemia)** to the myocardium leads to progressive impairment of the contractility of the deprived myocardial cells. This impairment of contractility is mediated by a combination of extracellular and intracellular changes in the blood gases and in the pH of the ischemic region of the heart. These changes include reductions in P_{O_2} and pH and increases in P_{CO_2}.

Summary

- Cardiac function is regulated by various intrinsic and extrinsic mechanisms.
- Heart rate is regulated mainly by the autonomic nervous system. Sympathetic activity increases heart rate, and parasympathetic (vagal) activity decreases heart rate.
- The baroreceptor, chemoreceptor, pulmonary inflation, atrial receptor (Bainbridge), and ventricular receptor reflexes all serve to regulate heart rate.
- The principal intrinsic mechanisms that regulate myocardial contraction are the Frank-Starling and rate-related mechanisms.
- The autonomic nervous system regulates myocardial performance mainly by varying the Ca^{++} conductance of the cell membrane via the adenylyl cyclase system.
- Various hormones, including epinephrine, adrenocortical steroids, thyroid hormones, insulin, and glucagon, regulate myocardial performance.
- Changes in the blood concentrations of O_2, CO_2, and H^{+} alter cardiac function directly and reflexly.

Bibliography

Ally A: Ventrolateral medullary control of cardiovascular activity during muscle contraction, *Neurosci Biobehav Rev* 23:65, 1998.

Andresen MC et al: Cellular mechanisms of baroreceptor integration at the nucleus tractus solitarius, *Ann N Y Acad Sci* 940:132, 2001.

Billman GE: Aerobic exercise conditioning: a nonpharmacological antiarrhythmic intervention, *J Appl Physiol* 92:446, 2002.

DiBona GF: Peripheral and central interactions between the renin-angiotensin system and the renal sympathetic nerves in control of renal function, *Ann N Y Acad Sci* 940:395, 2001.

Grimm DR: Neurally mediated syncope: a review of cardiac and arterial receptors, *J Clin Neurophysiol* 14:170, 1997.

Iellamo F: Neural mechanisms of cardiovascular regulation during exercise, *Auton Neurosci* 90:66, 2001.

Lanfranchi PA, Somers VK: Arterial baroreflex function and cardiovascular variability: interactions and implications, *Am J Physiol Regul Integr Comp Physiol* 283:R815, 2002.

Paton JF, Kasparov S, Paterson DJ: Nitric oxide and autonomic control of heart rate: a question of specificity, *Trends Neurosci* 25:626, 2002.

Segar JL: Ontogeny of the arterial and cardiopulmonary baroreflex during fetal and postnatal life, *Am J Physiol* 273:R457, 1997.

Sved AF, Ito S, Madden CJ: Baroreflex dependent and independent roles of the caudal ventrolateral medulla in cardiovascular regulation, *Brain Res Bull* 51:129, 2000.

Zimmerman MC, Davisson RL: Redox signaling in central neural regulation of cardiovascular function, *Prog Biophys Mol Biol* 84:125, 2004.

Case Study

Case 19–1

A 48-year-old woman was susceptible to occasional, usually brief episodes of lightheadedness. She noticed that her heart rate was very rapid during these episodes and that the lightheadedness disappeared when the heart rate returned to normal. Her physician noted no significant abnormalities during the physical examination of the patient. The physician obtained a 24-hour recording of the patient's electrocardiogram. On review of this recording, the physician detected a 7-minute period during which the patient's heart rate increased abruptly from a resting value of about 75 beats/min to a steady level of about 145 beats/min. At the end of the 7-minute period of tachycardia, the heart rate decreased abruptly and attained the resting value again of about 75 beats/min within 1 minute. The patient's problem was diagnosed as paroxysmal supraventricular tachycardia, which is a sudden, pronounced increase in heart rate; this problem is mediated usually by a reentry circuit in the AV junction. During a subsequent visit to her physician, the patient's paroxysmal tachycardia appeared spontaneously. The physician was able to terminate the tachycardia promptly by carotid sinus massage (i.e., massaging the patient's neck just below the angles of the jaw, in the region of the bifurcations of the common carotid arteries). The physician noted that the patient's arterial blood pressure was 95/75 mm Hg during the tachycardia and that it returned to a value of 130/85 mm Hg (the patient's usual resting blood pressure) soon after the termination of the tachycardia.

1. A reduction in the patient's mean arterial pressure during the paroxysmal tachycardia would have what reflex effect?

A. Decrease in myocardial contractility
B. Increase in cardiac cycle duration
C. Decrease in AV conduction velocity
D. Increase in norepinephrine release from the cardiac sympathetic nerves
E. Decrease in Ca^{++} conductance of myocytes during the action potential plateau

2. A sudden, substantial increase in efferent vagal activity (induced by carotid sinus massage, for example) would do which of the following?

A. Strengthen the contraction of atrial myocytes
B. Strengthen the stimulatory action of any concurrent sympathetic activity
C. Increase the speed of impulse conduction in the ventricular Purkinje fibers
D. Decrease the heart rate within one or two cardiac cycles
E. Shorten the AV conduction time

3. When the patient was in a normal sinus rhythm, what would administration of a drug that antagonizes the muscarinic cholinergic receptors do?

A. Abolish or dampen any rhythmic changes in heart rate that occur at the subject's respiratory frequency
B. Weaken the contractions of the atrial myocytes

C. Delay AV conduction
D. Decrease the action potential duration in atrial myocytes
E. Hyperpolarize the atrial myocytes during the resting phase (phase 4) of the action potential

4. **If the patient had a prominent respiratory sinus arrhythmia when she was not afflicted by the paroxysmal tachycardia, which of the following functional changes would take place?**
   A. Efferent vagal activity would decrease during inspiration.
   B. Efferent cardiac sympathetic activity would decrease during inspiration.
   C. The slope of the slow diastolic depolarization of the sinoatrial cells would decrease during inspiration.
   D. The respiratory sinus arrhythmia would become more pronounced in response to hemorrhage.
   E. Propranolol would abolish the respiratory sinus arrhythmia.

5. **When neural activity in the vagus nerves suddenly ceases, why does the heart rate response to that vagal activity rapidly disappear?**
   A. The cardiac cells gradually become more responsive to acetylcholine.
   B. The vagus nerve endings rapidly take up the released acetylcholine.
   C. The cardiac myocytes rapidly take up the released acetylcholine.
   D. The acetylcholine in the nerve endings is rapidly depleted.
   E. The abundant acetylcholinesterase rapidly degrades the released acetylcholine.

Chapter 20: Hemodynamics

Objectives

- ❖ Define the relationship between the velocity of blood flow and cross-sectional area of the vascular bed.
- ❖ Describe the factors that govern the relationship between blood flow and pressure gradient.
- ❖ Distinguish between resistances in series and resistances in parallel.
- ❖ Compare laminar and turbulent flow.
- ❖ Describe the influence of the particulates in blood on blood flow.

The electrical and mechanical characteristics of the heart have been described in the preceding chapters. The generation of the signal that initiates the cardiac contraction has been described, the processes involved in excitation-contraction coupling have been explained, and the factors that regulate the cardiac contraction have been identified. In this chapter, we begin to describe the physical factors that regulate blood flow through the various vascular beds. In subsequent chapters, we will describe how the behavior of the blood vessels is regulated.

Physical Factors Govern Blood Flow

The fluid mechanics of the circulatory system are complicated and therefore difficult to analyze precisely. The heart is an intermittent pump, and its behavior is regulated by many physical and chemical factors. The blood vessels are branched, distensible conduits of continuously varying dimensions. The blood is a suspension mainly of erythrocytes but also of leukocytes, platelets, and lipid globules. All of these structures are dispersed in the plasma, which is a colloidal solution of proteins. Despite this complexity, however, an understanding of the relevant, elementary principles of fluid mechanics provides considerable insight into the physical behavior of the vascular system. Certain basic principles are expounded in this chapter to illuminate the interrelationships among vascular geometry, blood velocity, blood flow, and blood pressure.

Bloodstream Velocity Depends on Cross-sectional Area

The relationship between the velocity of the bloodstream and the dimensions of the vascular bed is illustrated by the wide and narrow pair of conduits, aligned in series, in **Figure 20–1**. In this diagram, **velocity (v)** refers to the rate of displacement of a particle of the incompressible fluid per unit of time. Consider that the conduit is rigid and that it has a wide section (area $A_1 = 5\ cm^2$) and a narrow section (area $A_2 = 1\ cm^2$). Also, let the incompressible fluid enter the wide end of the tube at a flow, Q_1, of $5\ cm^3/sec$. The **flow (Q)** refers to the volume of fluid that passes a given cross section of the conduit per unit time. Then, the velocity, v_1, of a fluid particle as it passes through the broad cross section, A_1, would be

$$v_1 = Q_1/A_1 = 1\ cm/sec \qquad \textbf{20-1}$$

Thus, a particle of fluid advances a distance (ΔL_1) of 1 cm each second (Figure 20–1). When the fluid enters the narrow section of the tube, the volume (Q_2) of fluid that passes cross section A_2 each second

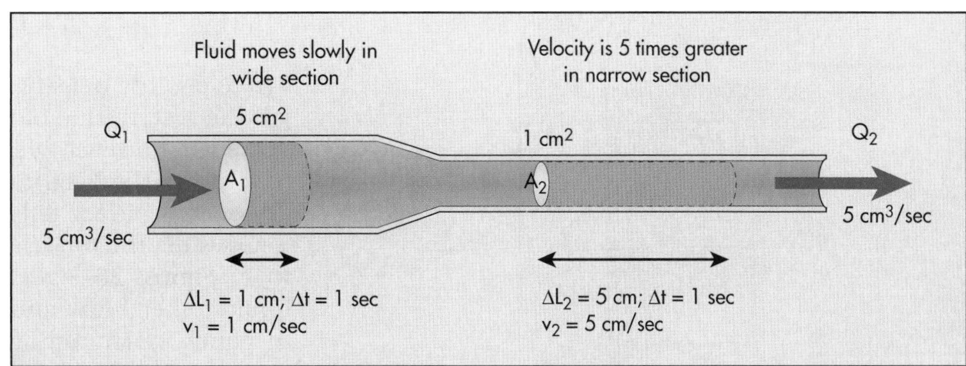

FIGURE 20–1. In a conduit that contains a wide segment and a narrow segment, the fluid velocities in the two segments are inversely proportional to the cross-sectional areas of the segments.

must equal the volume (Q_1) that had passed cross section A_1 each second; that is, $Q_2 = Q_1$. The velocity, v_2, in the narrow section would be

$$v_2 = Q_2/A_2 = 5 \text{ cm/sec} \qquad \text{20-2}$$

Thus, each particle of fluid must move past section A_2 five times faster than it did past section A_1. By the law of conservation of mass,

$$Q_1 = Q_2 \qquad \text{20-3}$$

From Equations 20-1 to 20-3, therefore,

$$v_1/v_2 = A_2/A_1 \qquad \text{20-4}$$

Hence, when the caliber of a tube varies with the axial location along the tube, the fluid velocities at these axial sites are inversely proportional to the corresponding cross-sectional areas. This relationship also holds for more complex hydraulic systems, such as the circulatory system, which is composed of numerous conduits of different calibers and in which the tubes are aligned both in series and in parallel.

As shown in Figure 15–4, the velocity of the blood decreases progressively as the blood flows rapidly through the large arteries and then through the smaller arteries, arterioles, capillaries, and venules. The velocity of the blood in each of these components of the vascular system varies inversely with the **total** cross-sectional area of the various components of the cardiovascular system. The total cross-sectional areas of the small veins, large veins, and venae cavae flow increase in proportion to the total cross-sectional areas for these various components of the cardiovascular system. As the blood then passes through the venules and continues centrally through the intermediate veins toward the venae cavae, the velocity increases progressively again. The velocities in the various serial sections of the circulatory system are inversely proportional to the total cross-sectional areas of the respective sections. The total cross-sectional area of all the parallel systemic capillaries greatly exceeds the total cross-sectional area of any of the other serial sections of the systemic vascular bed. Hence, the velocity of the bloodstream in the capillaries is much less than that in any other vascular segment. THE VERY SLOW MOVEMENT OF THE BLOOD THROUGH THE CAPILLARIES ALLOWS AMPLE TIME FOR EXCHANGE OF MATERIALS BETWEEN THE TISSUES AND THE BLOOD.

The Relationship Between Pressure and Flow Depends on Characteristics of the Blood and Conduits

The most useful equation that defines the relationships among the various physical factors that govern pressure and flow in hydraulic systems (including the circulatory system) was derived by the French physician Poiseuille more than a century ago. This equation, known as **Poiseuille's law,** applies to the flow of fluids through cylindrical tubes, but it applies precisely only under restricted conditions. The equation applies specifically to the steady, laminar flow of newtonian fluids. The term **steady flow** signifies the absence of variations of flow in time. **Laminar flow** is the type of motion in which the fluid moves as a series of infinitesimally thin layers, with each layer moving at a velocity different from that of its neighboring layers (**Figure 20–2**, *A*). A **newtonian fluid** has certain critical physical properties that are described later. A newtonian fluid is essentially a homogeneous fluid, such as an electrolyte solution.

Flow is proportional to pressure difference

Pressure is a salient determinant of flow. The pressure P (in dynes/cm^2) at a distance h cm below the surface of a liquid is

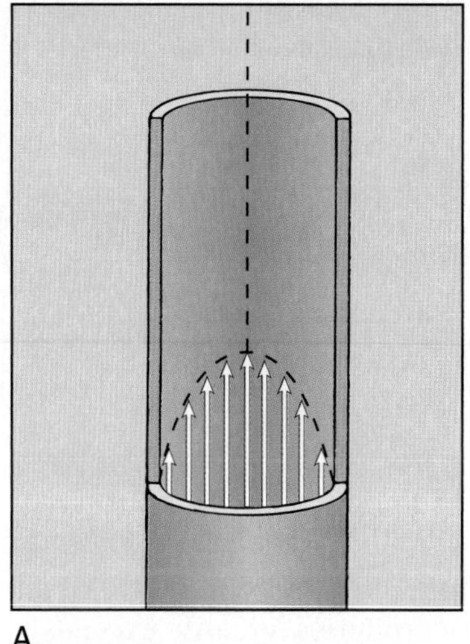

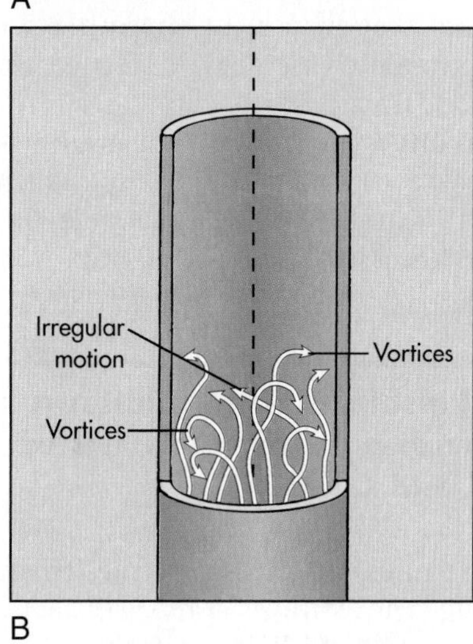

FIGURE 20–2. A, In laminar flow, all elements of the fluid move in streamlines that are parallel to the axis of the tube; no fluid moves in a radial or circumferential direction. B, In turbulent flow, various elements of the fluid move irregularly in axial, radial, and circumferential directions.

$$P = h\rho g \qquad 20\text{-}5$$

where ρ is the density of the liquid (in g/cm^3) and g is the acceleration of gravity (in cm/sec^2). For convenience, however, pressure is frequently expressed in terms of the height, h, of a column of the liquid above an arbitrary reference level.

Consider the tube that connects reservoirs R_1 and R_2 in **Figure 20–3**. Let reservoir R_1 be filled with liquid to height h_1, and let reservoir R_2 be empty, as in panel *A*. The outflow pressure, P_o, is therefore equal to the atmospheric pressure, which is designated the zero, or reference, level. The inflow pressure, P_i, is then equal to the same reference level plus the height, h_1, of the column of liquid in reservoir R_1. Under these conditions, let the flow, Q, through the tube be 5 mL/sec.

If reservoir R_1 is now filled to twice the height, h_2 (as in panel *B*), and reservoir R_2 is again empty, the flow will be twice as great (i.e., 10 mL/sec) as it is in panel *A*. Thus, with reservoir R_2 empty, the flow through the tube will be directly proportional to the inflow pressure, P_i.

If reservoir R_2 is now allowed to fill to height h_1 and the fluid level in R_1 is maintained at h_2 (as in panel *C*), the flow will again become 5 mL/sec. If the fluid level in R_2 attains the same height as in R_1, flow will cease; that is, Q = 0 mL/sec (panel *D*). THUS, FLOW IS DIRECTLY PROPORTIONAL TO THE DIFFERENCE BETWEEN THE INFLOW AND OUTFLOW PRESSURES:

$$Q \propto P_i - P_o \qquad 20\text{-}6$$

The blood flow through specific vascular beds is affected by the difference between the inflow (arterial) and outflow (venous) pressures that prevail for that vascular bed. Such pressure differences may be

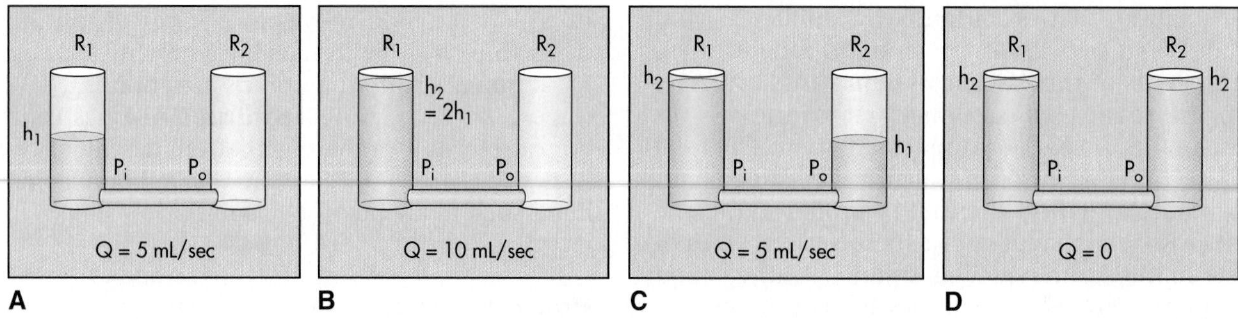

FIGURE 20–3. The flow, Q, of fluid through a tube connecting two reservoirs, R_1 and R_2, is proportional to the difference between the pressure at the inflow end (P_i) and the pressure at the outflow end (P_o) of the tube. A, When R_2 is empty, fluid flows from R_1 to R_2 at a rate proportional to the pressure in R_1. B, When the fluid level in R_1 is increased twofold, the flow increases proportionately. C, Flow from R_1 to R_2 is proportional to the difference between the pressures in R_1 and R_2. D, When pressure in R_2 rises to equal the pressure in R_1, flow ceases.

affected substantially by gravitational forces and by the competence of the venous valves, as explained in Chapter 24.

The blood flow through the legs and feet may be entirely different during standing and during recumbency. In standing subjects, the arterial blood pressure in the legs will be considerably higher than the arterial blood pressure in the thorax; this difference will, of course, depend on the subject's height. In people with normal venous valves, the venous blood pressure in the legs and feet may be only slightly above the atmospheric pressure (see also Chapters 24 and 25). However, in patients with **varicose veins** (abnormally dilated veins) in the legs, the venous valves are incompetent. Therefore, the blood pressure in the varicose veins in the legs of standing subjects may be elevated by the same amount as is the arterial blood pressure in the legs. Thus, the arteriovenous pressure difference and the blood flow in the legs will be substantially greater in standing people with normal venous valves than in those with varicose veins.

Blood flow depends on tube dimensions

For any given pressure difference between the two ends of a tube, the flow will depend on the dimensions of the tube. Consider the tube connected to the reservoir in **Figure 20–4**, *A*. If the tube's length is L_1 and its radius is r_1, the flow Q_1 is observed to be 10 mL/sec.

The tube connected to the reservoir in panel *B* of Figures 20–3 and 20–4 has the same radius as that in panel *A*, but it is twice as long. Under these conditions, the flow Q_2 is found to be 5 mL/sec, or only half as great as flow Q_1. Conversely, for a tube half as long as L_1, the flow would be twice as great as Q_1. In other words, flow is inversely proportional to the length of the tube:

$$Q \propto 1/L \qquad 20\text{-}7$$

The length L_3 of the tube connected to the reservoir in Figure 20–4, *C*, is the same as L_1, but the radius r_3 is twice as great as r_1. Under these conditions, the flow Q_3 increases to a value of 160 mL/sec, which is 16 times greater than Q_1. The precise measurements of Poiseuille revealed that flow varies directly as the fourth power of the radius (just as in the preceding example):

$$Q \propto r^4 \qquad 20\text{-}8$$

Blood flow depends on viscosity

Finally, for a given pressure difference across a cylindrical tube of given dimensions, the flow will be affected by the nature of the fluid itself. This flow-determining property of fluids is termed **viscosity, η.** Consider that the fluid level in the reservoir in panel *D* of Figure 20–4 equals that in panel *A* and that the tubes connected to the bottoms of both reservoirs are identical. However, if the viscosity η_4 of the fluid in the reservoir in panel *D* is twice the viscosity η_1 of the fluid in the reservoir of panel *A*, then flow Q_4 through the tube in panel *D* will be only half the flow Q_1 through the tube in panel *A*. Thus,

$$Q \propto 1/\eta \qquad 20\text{-}9$$

For most homogeneous liquids, such as water itself or true solutions in water, this inverse proportionality prevails during laminar flow. Such fluids are said to be **newtonian.** For heterogeneous liquids, notably suspensions such as blood, the inverse proportionality is not so precise. Such fluids are said to be **non-newtonian.**

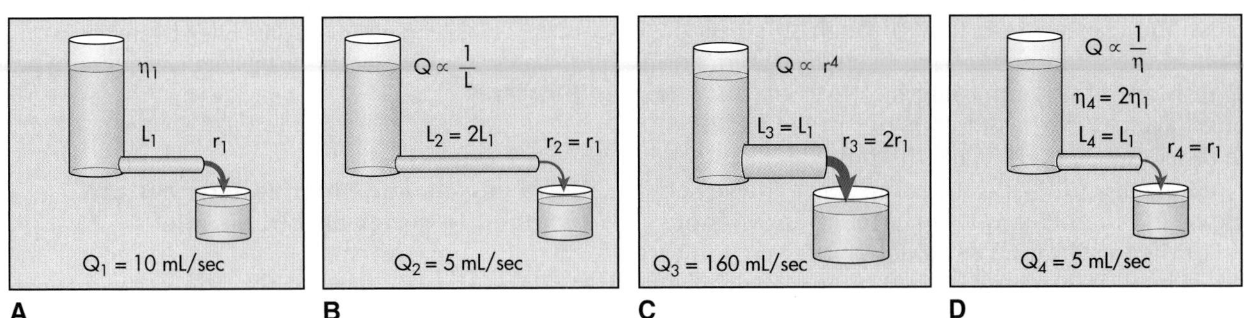

FIGURE 20–4. The flow, Q, of fluid through a tube is inversely proportional to the length, L, and the viscosity, η, and directly proportional to the fourth power of the radius, r. A, Reference condition: for a given pressure, length, radius, and viscosity, let the flow Q_1 equal 10 mL/sec. B, If the tube length doubles, flow decreases by 50%. C, If the tube radius doubles, flow increases 16-fold. D, If viscosity doubles, flow decreases by 50%.

Poiseuille's law relates pressure, tube dimension, and viscosity to blood flow

Poiseuille's law takes into account the various factors that influence the flow of a fluid through a tube; the law applies under restricted conditions. Poiseuille's law states that for the steady, laminar flow of a newtonian fluid through a cylindrical tube, the flow, Q, varies directly as the difference between the inflow and outflow pressures, $P_i - P_o$, and the fourth power of the radius, r, of the tube. The flow also varies inversely as the length, L, of the tube and as the viscosity, η, of the fluid. The full statement of Poiseuille's law is

$$Q = \pi(P_i - P_o)r^4/8\eta L \quad \text{20-10}$$

where π/8 is the constant of proportionality.

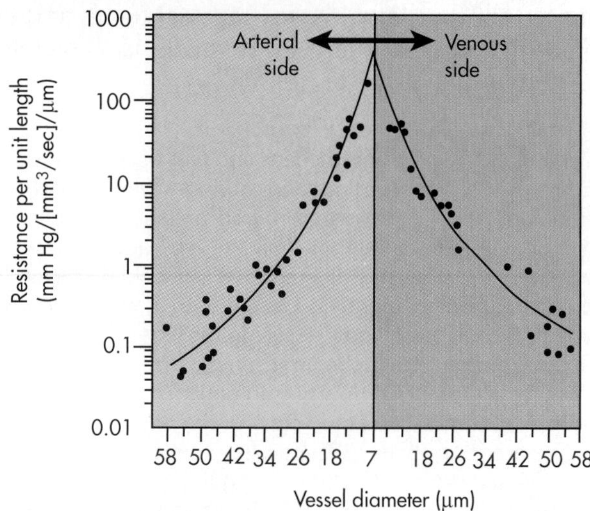

FIGURE 20–5. The resistance per unit length (R/L) of individual small blood vessels in the cat mesentery. The capillaries (diameter, 7 μm) are denoted by the vertical line between the red and blue panels. The solid circles represent the actual data. The two curves through the data represent the regression equations for the arteriole and venule data. Note that for both types of vessels, the calculated resistance per unit length is inversely proportional to the fourth power of the vessel diameter. (Redrawn from Lipowsky HH, Kovalcheck S, Zweifach BW: *Circ Res* 43:738, 1978.)

Resistance to Flow Depends on Flow and Pressure Difference

In electrical theory, resistance, R, is defined as the ratio of voltage drop, E, to electrical current flow, I. By analogy, the hydraulic resistance, R, may be defined as the ratio of pressure drop, $P_i - P_o$, to fluid flow, Q. For the steady, laminar flow of a newtonian fluid through a cylindrical tube, the physical components of hydraulic resistance may be identified by rearranging Poiseuille's law to yield the hydraulic resistance equation:

$$R = (P_i - P_o)/Q = 8\eta L/\pi r^4 \quad \text{20-11}$$

Thus, when Poiseuille's law applies, the resistance to flow depends only on the dimensions (L and r) of the tube and on the viscosity (η) of the fluid.

THE PRINCIPAL DETERMINANT OF THE RESISTANCE TO BLOOD FLOW THROUGH ANY INDIVIDUAL VESSEL WITHIN THE CIRCULATORY SYSTEM IS ITS CALIBER because resistance varies inversely as the fourth power of the radius. The resistance to flow through small blood vessels in the cat mesentery has been measured, and the resistance per unit length of vessel (R/L) is plotted against the vessel diameter in **Figure 20–5.** The resistance is highest in the individual capillaries (diameter, 7 μm), and it diminishes as the vessels increase in diameter on the arterial and venous sides of the capillaries. The values of R/L were found to be virtually proportional to the fourth power of the diameter for the larger vessels on both sides of the capillaries.

The small arteries and arterioles possess a thick coat of circularly arranged smooth muscle fibers, by means of which the lumen radius may be varied. Changes in vascular resistance are induced mainly by nervous and humoral factors that alter the contractile state of the arteriolar smooth muscle cells. The control of vascular resistance is described in Chapter 23.

In severe **arteriosclerosis,** a lipid deposit in the intima of a major artery forms a plaque that may protrude into the lumen and severely narrow it. In this event, the major resistance to flow in the vascular bed supplied by that diseased artery may reside in that large artery itself, rather than in the small arteries and arterioles of that vascular bed. Such occlusive lesions in important large arteries, such as the coronary arteries, are often treated by balloon dilatation **(angioplasty)** or by coronary artery **bypass surgery.**

Blood vessels and their resistances are arranged in series and in parallel

In the cardiovascular system, the various types of vessels listed along the horizontal axis in Figure 15–4 lie in **series** with one another. In vessels aligned in series, a red blood cell travels sequentially from one vessel in the series to the next vessel and then on to the next one, as illustrated in **Figure**

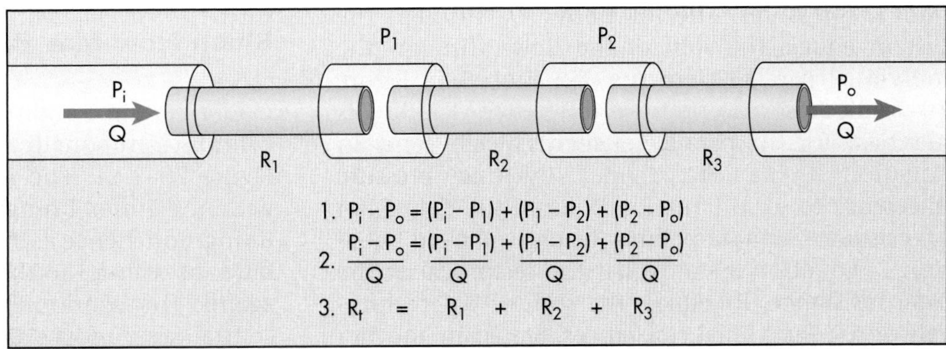

FIGURE 20–6. For resistances R_1, R_2, and R_3 arranged in series, the total resistance, R_t, equals the sum of the individual resistances.

20–6. Furthermore, the individual members within each category of vessels are ordinarily arranged in **parallel** with one another. In a parallel arrangement, a red blood cell that arrives at the junction of a number of parallel vessels would have the immediate option of traveling through just one of these parallel channels, as illustrated in **Figure 20–7**. The capillaries throughout the lungs are in parallel with one another, and similarly the capillaries throughout the systemic circulation are also largely in parallel with one another. Notable exceptions are the capillaries in the renal vasculature (wherein the peritubular capillaries are in series with the glomerular capillaries) and in the splanchnic vasculature (wherein the hepatic capillaries are in series with the intestinal capillaries). Formulas for the total hydraulic resistance of conduits arranged in series and in parallel can be derived in the same manner as for electrical resistances.

Three hydraulic resistances, R_1, R_2, and R_3, are aligned in series in Figure 20–6. The pressure drop across the entire system (i.e., the difference between inflow pressure, P_i, and outflow pressure, P_o) consists of the sum of the pressure drops across each of the individual resistances (Equation 1 in Figure 20–6). Under steady-state conditions, the flow, Q, through any given cross section must equal the flow through any other cross section. By dividing each component in Equation 1 by Q (Equation 2), it becomes evident from the definition of resistance—that is, $R = (P_i - P_o)/Q$—that the total resistance, R_t, of the entire system of resistances in series equals the sum of the individual resistances:

$$R_t = R_1 + R_2 + R_3 \qquad \textbf{20-12}$$

For resistances in parallel (Figure 20–7), all tubes have the same inflow pressures and the same

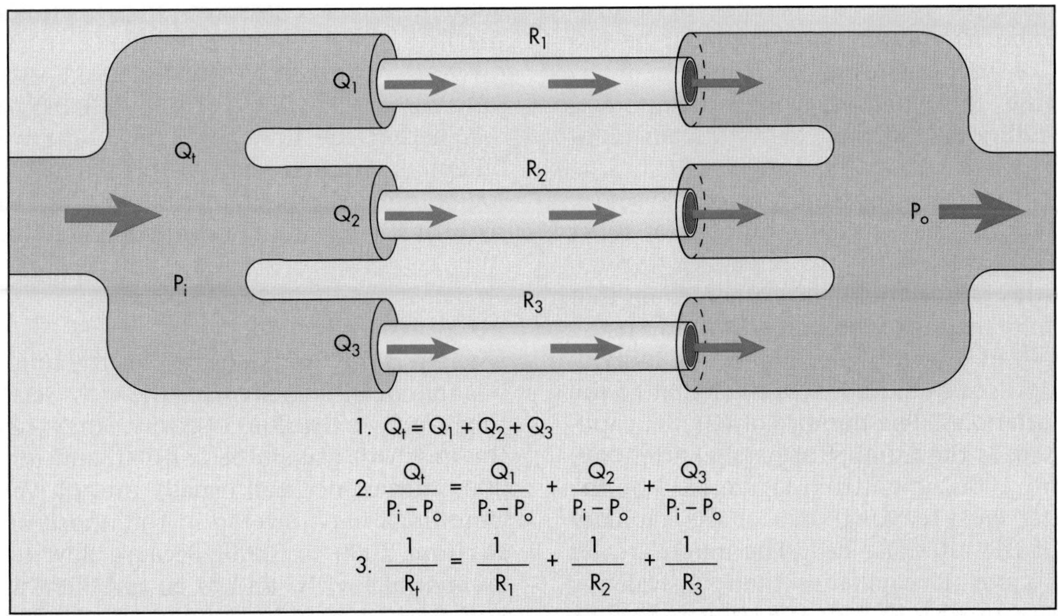

FIGURE 20–7. For resistances R_1, R_2, and R_3 arranged in parallel, the reciprocal of the total resistance, R_t, equals the sum of the reciprocals of the individual resistances.

outflow pressures. The total flow, Q_t, through the system equals the sum of the flows through the individual parallel elements (Equation 1 in Figure 20–7). Because the pressure difference ($P_i - P_o$) is identical for all parallel elements, each term in Equation 1 may be divided by that pressure difference to yield Equation 2. From the definition of resistance, Equation 3 may be derived from Equation 2. Equation 3 states that the reciprocal of the total resistance, R_t, equals the sum of the reciprocals of the individual resistances. Stated in another way, if we define hydraulic **conductance** as the reciprocal of resistance, it becomes evident that FOR TUBES IN PARALLEL, THE TOTAL CONDUCTANCE IS THE SUM OF THE INDIVIDUAL CONDUCTANCES.

A few examples will illustrate some of the fundamental properties of parallel hydraulic systems. For example, if the resistances of the three parallel elements in Figure 20-7 were all equal, then

$$R_1 = R_2 = R_3 \qquad \textbf{20-13}$$

Therefore, from Equation 3 in Figure 20–7

$$1/R_t = 3/R_1 \qquad \textbf{20-14}$$

and hence

$$R_t = R_1/3 \qquad \textbf{20-15}$$

Thus, the total resistance is less than any of the individual resistances. Furthermore, for any parallel arrangement, the total resistance must be less than that of any of the individual parallel tubes. For example, consider a system in which a high-resistance tube is added in parallel to a low-resistance tube. The total resistance must be less than that of the low-resistance component by itself because the high-resistance component affords an additional pathway, or conductance, for fluid flow.

Similarly, the total resistance across a set of parallel tubes diminishes as the number of tubes increases. This explains why the resistance through the total array of arterioles is greater than that through the total array of capillaries in the systemic circulation, even though the caliber of the individual capillaries is substantially less than that of the individual arterioles. The number of parallel capillaries far exceeds the number of parallel arterioles. This disparity is documented in Figure 15–4 by the much greater cross-sectional area of the capillary bed than of the arteriolar bed. The much greater number of systemic capillaries than of systemic arterioles accounts for the lower resistance to flow through the total array of capillaries than through the total array of arterioles.

Blood Flow May Be Laminar or Turbulent

Under certain conditions, the flow of a fluid in a cylindrical tube will be **laminar,** as illustrated in Figure 20–2, *A*. The thin layer of fluid in contact with the inner lining of the tube adheres to the lining and hence is motionless. The thin layer of fluid just central to this external lamina must shear against this motionless layer. Therefore, this more central layer moves slowly, but with a finite velocity. Similarly, the next more central layer travels still faster such that the longitudinal velocity profile is a parabola. The velocity of the fluid adjacent to the wall is zero, whereas the velocity at the center of the stream is maximum. The maximum velocity of the central component is twice the mean velocity of flow across the entire cross section of the tube. In laminar flow, fluid elements remain in one lamina, or streamline, as the fluid progresses longitudinally along the tube. Flow occurs only in an axial direction—that is, parallel to the axis of the tube. Particles of fluid do not move in either a radial or a circumferential direction.

Irregular motions of the fluid elements may develop as fluid flows through a tube; this irregular flow is called **turbulent flow** (Figure 20–2, *B*). Under such conditions, fluid elements do not remain confined to definite laminae. Rapid radial and circumferential mixing occurs, and vortices may develop. More pressure is required to force a given flow of fluid through the same tube when the flow is turbulent than when it is laminar. In turbulent flow, the pressure drop is approximately proportional to the square of the flow, whereas in laminar flow, the pressure drop is proportional to the first power of the flow. HENCE, TO PRODUCE A GIVEN FLOW, A PUMP, SUCH AS THE HEART, MUST DO CONSIDERABLY MORE WORK IF TURBULENCE DEVELOPS.

Whether the flow through a tube will be turbulent or laminar may be predicted by computing a dimensionless number, called **Reynolds' number, N_R,** which is defined as follows:

$$N_R = \rho D\bar{v}/\eta \qquad \textbf{20-16}$$

where ρ is the fluid density, D is the tube diameter, $\bar{v}$ is the mean velocity over the cross section of the tube, and η is the fluid viscosity. For N_R below 2000, the flow will usually be laminar, and for N_R above 3000, turbulence will usually prevail. Various flow conditions may develop in the transition range of N_R from 2000 to 3000. Because flow tends to be laminar at low N_R and to be turbulent at high N_R, Equation 20-16 indicates that large diameters, high velocities, and low viscosities predispose to the development of turbulence.

In addition to these factors, abrupt variations in tube dimensions or irregularities in the tube walls may produce turbulence. Turbulence is usually accompanied by vibrations of the fluid and surrounding structures. Some of these vibrations within the cardiovascular system are in the auditory frequency range and may be detected as **murmurs.**

The factors that predispose to turbulence may account for some of the **cardiac murmurs** that are heard clinically. In certain cardiac disorders, the valves are **stenotic** (narrowed). As the blood passes through such narrowed valves, the flow becomes turbulent, and a cardiac murmur can be detected with a stethoscope. In severe anemia, **functional cardiac murmurs** (murmurs that are not caused by structural abnormalities) are often detectable. Such murmurs are caused by the high-flow velocities that usually prevail in severely anemic patients and by the reduced viscosity of the blood (because of the low red blood cell content).

Blood Is a Non-newtonian Fluid

The viscosity of a newtonian fluid, such as water, may be determined by measuring the flow that prevails at a given pressure difference through a cylindrical tube of known length and radius. As long as the flow is laminar, the viscosity may be computed by substituting these values into Poiseuille's equation. If the flow is laminar, the calculated viscosity of a given newtonian fluid at a specified temperature will be constant, regardless of the tube dimensions and flows. However, for a non-newtonian fluid, the viscosity calculated from Poiseuille's equation may vary considerably when different tube dimensions and flows are used. Therefore, in considering the rheological (flow-related) properties of a suspension, such as blood, the term *viscosity* does not have a unique meaning. The term **apparent viscosity** is frequently applied to the value of viscosity obtained for non-newtonian fluids, such as blood, under the particular conditions of measurement.

Rheologically, blood is a suspension, principally of erythrocytes, in a relatively homogeneous liquid, the blood plasma. For this reason, the apparent viscosity of blood varies as a function of the **hematocrit ratio** (the ratio of erythrocyte volume to whole blood volume). In **Figure 20–8**, the upper curve represents the ratio of the apparent viscosity of whole blood to that of blood plasma over a range of hematocrit ratios from 0% to 80%. The data were derived from measurements of flow through a glass tube 1 mm in internal diameter. The viscosity of plasma is 1.2 to 1.3 times that of water.

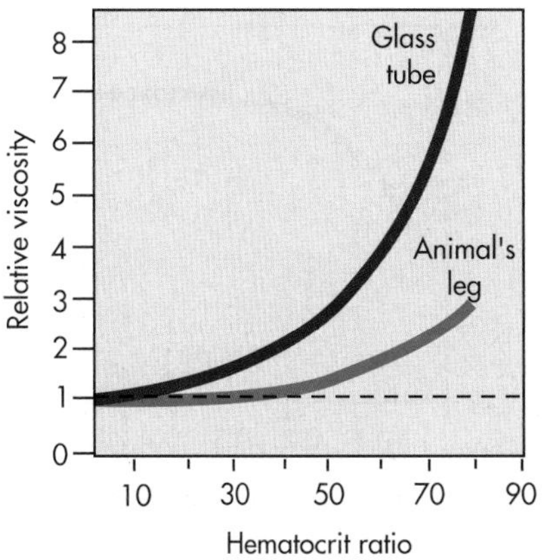

FIGURE 20–8. The viscosity of whole blood, relative to that of plasma, increases progressively as the hematocrit ratio rises. For any given hematocrit ratio, the apparent viscosity of blood is less when it is measured in a biological viscometer (such as the tissues of an anesthetized dog) than in a glass capillary tube with a lumen diameter of 1 mm. (Redrawn from Levy MN, Share L: *Circ Res* 1:247, 1953.)

When the apparent viscosity of blood with a normal hematocrit ratio of 45% is measured with a glass tube viscometer (Figure 20–8, upper curve), the apparent viscosity of the blood is about 2.5 times that of plasma. In severe anemia, blood viscosity is low. As the hematocrit ratios are increased, the slope of the curve increases progressively; it is especially steep at the high range of hematocrit ratios. If the hematocrit ratio rises to about 70%, which it may in patients with **polycythemia vera,** the apparent viscosity may increase by considerably more than twofold (Figure 20–8). The vascular resistance to blood flow increases proportionately. The effect of such a change in hematocrit ratio on peripheral vascular resistance may be substantial. Severe **essential hypertension** is the most common cause of a chronically elevated arterial blood pressure. In patients with this disorder, the total peripheral resistance (ratio of the systemic arteriovenous pressure difference to the cardiac output) rarely increases more than twofold.

For any given hematocrit ratio, the apparent viscosity of blood depends on the dimensions of the tube used to estimate the viscosity. **Figure 20–9** demonstrates that the apparent viscosity of blood is not affected appreciably by changes in tube diameter when the diameters exceed 0.3 mm. However, the apparent viscosity does diminish progressively as the tube diameter is decreased to values below this level. The major resistance to blood flow in vascular beds normally resides in the very small arteries and arterioles, which have diameters substantially less than 0.3 mm. Thus, these small vessels would be the principal determinants of the

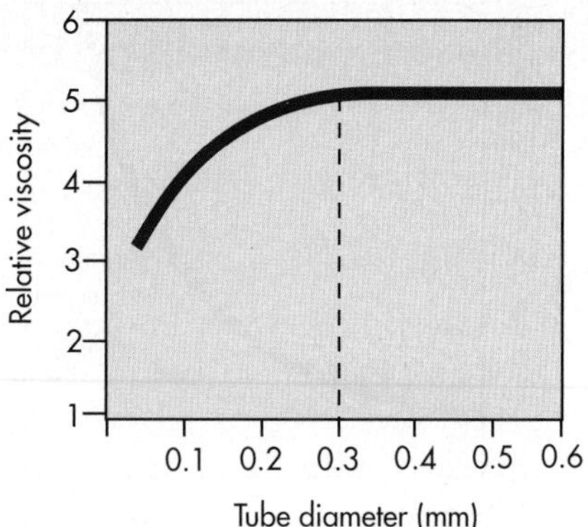

FIGURE 20–9. The viscosity of blood, relative to that of water, increases as a function of tube diameter, up to a diameter of about 0.3 mm. (Redrawn from Fahraeus R, Lindqvist T: *Am J Physiol* 96:562, 1931.)

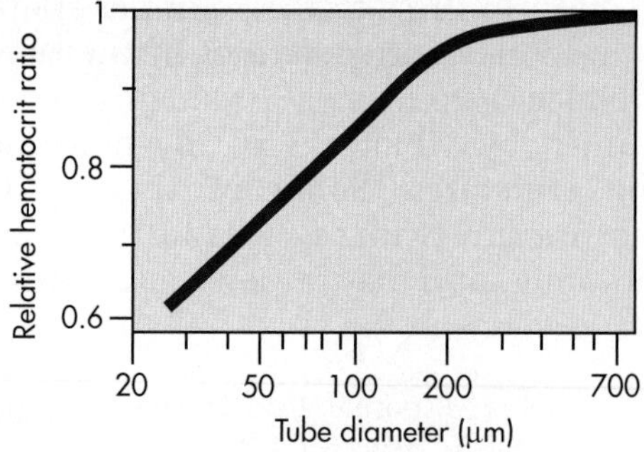

FIGURE 20–10. The relative hematocrit ratio of blood flowing from a feed reservoir through capillary tubes of various calibers as a function of the tube diameter. The relative hematocrit ratio is the ratio of the hematocrit of the blood in the outlet tube to that of the blood in the feed reservoir. (Redrawn from Barbee JH, Cokelet GR: *Microvasc Res* 3:6, 1971.)

apparent viscosity of the blood flowing through living tissues.

The tendency for such small tubes to diminish the apparent viscosity of the blood, as shown in Figure 20–9, explains why the apparent viscosity is less when a biological tissue is used as a viscometer (lower curve, Figure 20–8) than when a glass tube with a lumen diameter of 1 mm is used as a viscometer (upper curve, Figure 20–8). The influence of tube diameter on apparent viscosity is explained in part by the difference in the actual composition of the blood as it flows from large tubes into small tubes. The composition changes because in the small tubes, the red blood cells tend to accumulate in the faster axial stream. When the plasma is mainly consigned to the slower marginal layers of the bloodstream, the differences in velocity with radial location in the tube are shown in Figure 20–2, *A*. Because the red blood cells traverse the tube more quickly than does the plasma, the hematocrit ratio of the blood in the capillary tube is actually less than the hematocrit ratio of the blood in the reservoir to which the tube is connected **(Figure 20–10)**.

The apparent viscosity of blood diminishes as the shear rate is increased **(Figure 20–11)**, a phenomenon called **shear thinning.** The **shear rate** is the rate at which one layer of fluid moves with respect to the adjacent layers; the shear rate varies directly with the flow. The greater tendency of the erythrocytes to accumulate in the axial laminae at higher flow rates is partly responsible for the nonnewtonian behavior of blood. However, a more important factor is that at very slow rates of shear, the suspended cells tend to aggregate, and this tendency increases the viscosity. This tendency to aggregate diminishes as the flow is increased.

The deformability of the erythrocytes is also a factor in shear thinning, especially when the hematocrit ratio is high. The mean diameter of human red blood cells is about 7 μm. However, these cells are able to pass through openings with a diameter of only 3 μm. As blood that is densely packed with erythrocytes is caused to flow at progressively greater rates, the erythrocytes become more deformable. The greater deformability diminishes the apparent viscosity of the blood.

The flexibility of human erythrocytes is enhanced when the concentration of fibrinogen in the plasma is elevated. Conversely, the erythrocytes are misshapen and inflexible in patients with **sickle cell anemia.** This disorder often causes serious disturbances of regional blood flow. (See also Chapter 15.)

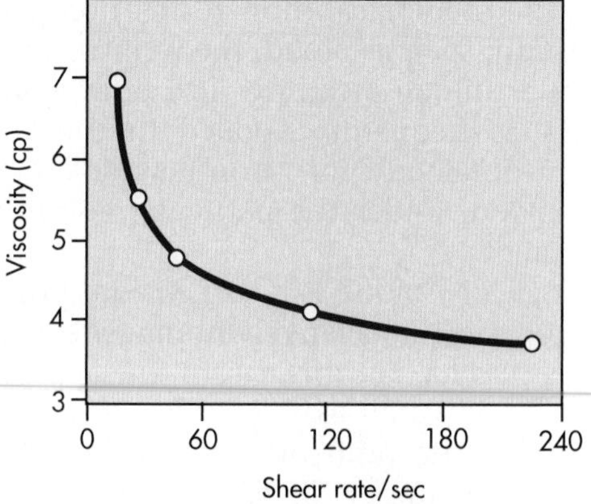

FIGURE 20–11. The viscosity (in centipoise) of blood as a function of the shear rate, which is the ratio of the velocity of one layer of fluid to that of the adjacent layers. The shear rate is directionally related to the flow. (Redrawn from Amin TM, Sirs JA: *Q J Exp Physiol* 70:37, 1985.)

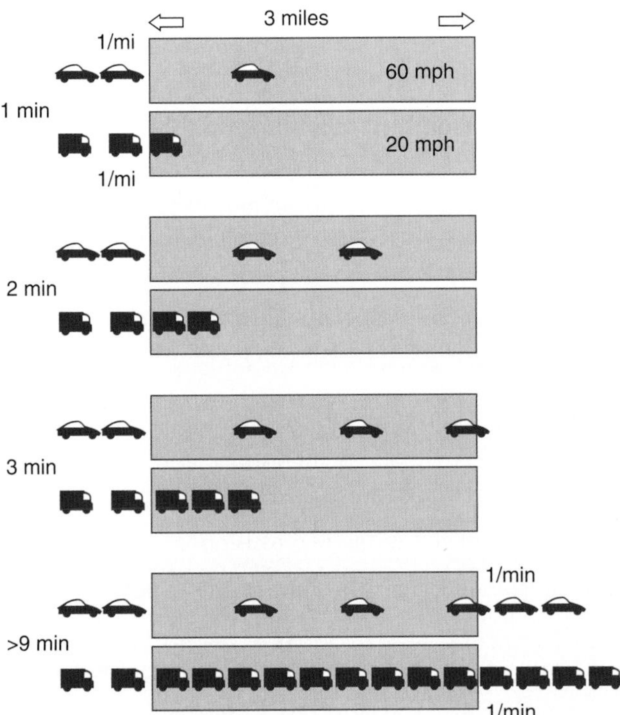

FIGURE 20–12. When the car velocity is three times as great as the truck velocity, the ratio of cars to trucks on the bridge will be 1:3 after 9 minutes, even though one of each type of vehicle enters and leaves the bridge each minute.

The disparity in the relative velocities of the red blood cells and plasma in the small blood vessels can be appreciated in the following analogy. Consider the flow of automobile traffic across a bridge that is 3 miles long **(Figure 20–12)**. Let the cars move in one lane at a speed of 60 mph and the trucks in another lane at 20 mph, as shown in Figure 20–12. If one car and one truck start out across the bridge each minute, then except for the initial few minutes of traffic flow across the bridge, one car and one truck will arrive at the other end each minute. Yet, if one counts the actual number of cars and trucks on the bridge at any moment, three times as many slowly moving trucks as rapidly traveling cars will be on the bridge.

Because the axial portions of the bloodstream contain a greater proportion of red cells, and this axial portion will move with a greater velocity, the red cells tend to traverse the tube in less time than does the plasma. Therefore, the red cells correspond to the rapidly moving cars in the analogy, and the plasma corresponds to the slowly moving trucks. Measurement of transit times of the different blood constituents through the vascular beds of various organs has shown that red cells do travel faster than the plasma through these vascular beds. Furthermore, the hematocrit ratios of the blood contained in the small blood vessels of various tissues are lower than those in blood samples withdrawn from large arteries or veins in the same animal **(Figure 20–13)**.

The physical forces responsible for the drift of the erythrocytes toward the axial stream and away from the vessel walls when blood is flowing at normal rates are not fully understood. One factor is the great flexibility of the red blood cells. At low flow rates, comparable to those in the microcirculation, rigid particles do not migrate toward the axis of the tube, whereas flexible particles do migrate. The concentration of flexible particles near the tube axis is enhanced by increasing the shear rate.

The tendency for the erythrocytes to aggregate at low flows depends on the concentration of the larger protein molecules, especially fibrinogen, in the plasma. For this reason, the changes in blood viscosity with flow rate are much more pronounced when the concentration of fibrinogen is high. Also, when flow rates are low, leukocytes tend to adhere to the endothelial cells of the microvessels and thereby to increase the apparent viscosity of the blood.

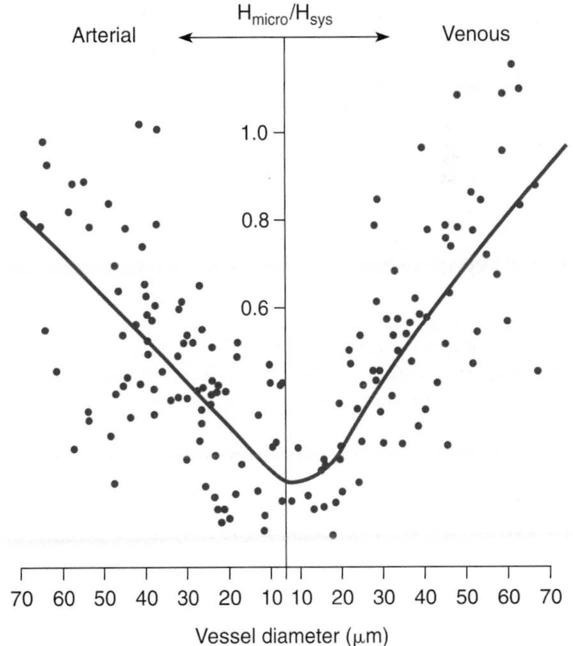

FIGURE 20–13. The hematocrit ratio (H_{micro}) of the blood in various-sized arterial and venous microvessels in the cat mesentery relative to the hematocrit ratio (H_{sys}) in the large systemic vessels. The hematocrit ratio is least in the capillaries and tiny venules. (Modified from Lipowsky HH, Usami S, Chien S: *Microvasc Res* 19:297, 1980.)

Summary

- The vascular system is composed of two major subdivisions, the systemic and pulmonary circulations, which are in series with one another.
- Each subdivision is composed of a number of types of vessels (e.g., arteries, arterioles, and capillaries) that are aligned in series with one another. In general, most vessels of a given type (e.g., capillaries) are arranged in parallel with each other.
- The mean velocity of the bloodstream in a given type of vessel is directly proportional to the total blood flow through all the vessels of that type, and it is inversely proportional to the cross-sectional area of all the parallel vessels of that type.
- When blood flow is steady and laminar in vessels larger than arterioles, the flow is proportional to the difference between the inflow and outflow pressures and to the fourth power of the radius, and it is inversely proportional to the length of the vessel and to the viscosity of the fluid (Poiseuille's law).
- For resistances aligned in series, the total resistance equals the sum of the individual resistances.
- For resistances aligned in parallel, the reciprocal of the total resistance equals the sum of the reciprocals of the individual resistances.
- Flow tends to become turbulent when flow velocity is high, when fluid viscosity is low, when tube diameter is large, or when the lumen of the vessel is irregular.
- Blood flow is non-newtonian in very small vessels; that is, Poiseuille's law is not applicable.
- The apparent viscosity of the blood diminishes as shear rate (flow) increases and as the tube dimensions decrease.

Bibliography

Ajmani RS, Rifkind JM: Hemorheological changes during human aging, *Gerontology* 44:111, 1998.

Alonso C et al: Transient rheological behavior of blood in low-shear tube flow: velocity profiles and effective viscosity, *Am J Physiol* 268:H25, 1995.

Baskurt OK, Meiselman HJ: Blood rheology and hemodynamics, *Semin Thromb Hemost* 29:435, 2003.

Brun JF: Hormones, metabolism and body composition as major determinants of blood rheology: potential pathophysiological meaning, *Clin Hemorheol Microcirc* 26:63, 2002.

Hoeks AP et al: Noninvasive determination of shear-rate distribution across the arterial wall, *Hypertension* 26:26, 1995.

Iordache BE, Remuzzi A: Numerical analysis of blood flow in reconstructed glomerular capillary segments, *Microvasc Res* 49:1, 1995.

Kwaan HC, Wang J: Hyperviscosity in polycythemia vera and other red cell abnormalities, *Semin Thromb Hemost* 29:451, 2003.

London M: The role of blood rheology in regulating blood pressure, *Clin Hemorheol Microcirc* 17:93, 1997.

Pries AR, Secomb TW, Gaetgens P: Design principles of vascular beds, *Circ Res* 77:1017, 1995.

Reinhart WH: Molecular biology and self-regulatory mechanisms of blood viscosity: a review, *Biorheology* 38:203, 2001.

Case Study

Case 20–1

A 70-year-old man reported to his physician that he experienced severe pain in his right leg whenever he walked briskly and that the pain disappeared soon after he discontinued walking. The physician referred him to a vascular surgeon, who carried out several hemodynamic tests on the patient. Angiography showed that the patient had a large arteriosclerotic plaque about 3 cm distal to the origin of the right femoral artery; the left femoral artery appeared to be normal. The mean arterial pressure in the resting patient's left femoral artery was 100 mm Hg, and the blood flow in this artery was 500 mL/min. The mean arterial pressure in the resting patient's right femoral artery proximal to the plaque was 100 mm Hg, and just distal to the plaque, it was 80 mm Hg. The blood flow in this artery was 300 mL/min. The mean venous pressure was 10 mm Hg in the left and right femoral veins.

1. **What is the resistance to blood flow in the vascular bed perfused by the right femoral artery?**
   A. 0.03 mm Hg/mL/min
   B. 0.30 mm Hg/mL/min
   C. 3.00 mm Hg/mL/min
   D. 3.33 mm Hg/mL/min
   E. 33.3 mm Hg/mL/min

2. **What is the resistance to blood flow (R_t) in the combined vascular beds perfused by both femoral arteries?**
   A. 0.48 mm Hg/mL/min
   B. 0.84 mm Hg/mL/min
   C. 1.10 mm Hg/mL/min
   D. 0.11 mm Hg/mL/min
   E. 11.1 mm Hg/mL/min

3. **What is the resistance to flow imposed by the arteriosclerotic plaque in the right femoral artery?**
   A. 0.066 mm Hg/mL/min
   B. 0.660 mm Hg/mL/min
   C. 0.15 mm Hg/mL/min
   D. 1.50 mm Hg/mL/min
   E. 15.0 mm Hg/mL/min

Chapter 21: Arterial System

Objectives

- ❖ Explain how the pulsatile blood flow in the large arteries is converted into a steady flow in the capillaries.
- ❖ Explain the factors that determine the mean, systolic, and diastolic arterial pressures and the arterial pulse pressure.
- ❖ Describe the common procedure for measuring the arterial blood pressure in humans.

Preceding chapters describe how the heart operates to provide the pumping action required to distribute blood to the peripheral tissues. Chapter 20 presents elementary physical principles that provide some quantitative insight into the relationships between pressure, flow, and vascular dimensions. This chapter describes the operation of the large distributing arteries, which serve as conduits between the heart and the microcirculation, where the exchange of nutrients and waste products takes place.

Arteries Serve as Hydraulic Filters

The principal function of the systemic and pulmonary arterial systems is to distribute blood to the capillary beds throughout the body. The arterioles, which are the terminal components of the arterial system, regulate the distribution of blood to the capillary beds. The aorta and pulmonary artery and their major branches constitute a system of conduits between the heart and the arterioles. These conduits have a substantial volume, and in normal individuals, they are very compliant.

Because the normal arteries are so compliant and the arterioles present such a high resistance to blood flow, the arterial system constitutes a **hydraulic filter,** so called because THE ARTERIAL SYSTEM CONVERTS THE INTERMITTENT FLOW GENERATED BY THE HEART TO A VIRTUALLY STEADY FLOW THROUGH THE CAPILLARIES **(Figure 21–1)**. The entire ventricular stroke volume is discharged into the arterial system during ventricular systole, which occupies approximately one third of the cardiac cycle duration. In fact, most of the stroke volume is pumped during the rapid ejection phase of ventricular systole (see Figure 18–8), which constitutes about half of total systole. Part of the energy released by the cardiac contraction is kinetic energy that is dissipated as forward capillary flow during ventricular systole. The remainder is stored as potential energy because much of the stroke volume is retained by the distensible arteries during systole (Figure 21–1, *A*). During diastole, the elastic recoil of the arterial walls converts this potential energy into capillary blood flow, and this flow continues through the capillaries at a fairly steady rate throughout diastole (Figure 21–1, *B*).

In a patient with severe **arteriosclerosis** (the arterial walls are rigid), capillary flow is more pulsatile than normal. Ventricular ejection leads to an appreciable increase in capillary flow during ventricular systole, and flow virtually ceases during diastole. Similarly, the hydraulic filter is less effective in people with abnormally large stroke volumes than in normal people. For example, in patients with **chronic aortic valve regurgitation** (a leaky aortic valve), the volume of blood ejected during systole is usually greater than the normal stroke volume because much of the ejected volume leaks back into the left ventricle through the incompetent valve during diastole. Such a supernormal stroke volume induces a pulsatile flow in all the systemic capillaries. In such patients, a **capillary pulse** can be perceived in the patient's nail beds during physical examination. Application of a slight force at the distal tip of a fingernail blanches the adjacent region of the nail. In patients with aortic regurgitation, the margin between the pink and blanched regions of the nail bed is perceptibly pulsatile with each heartbeat.

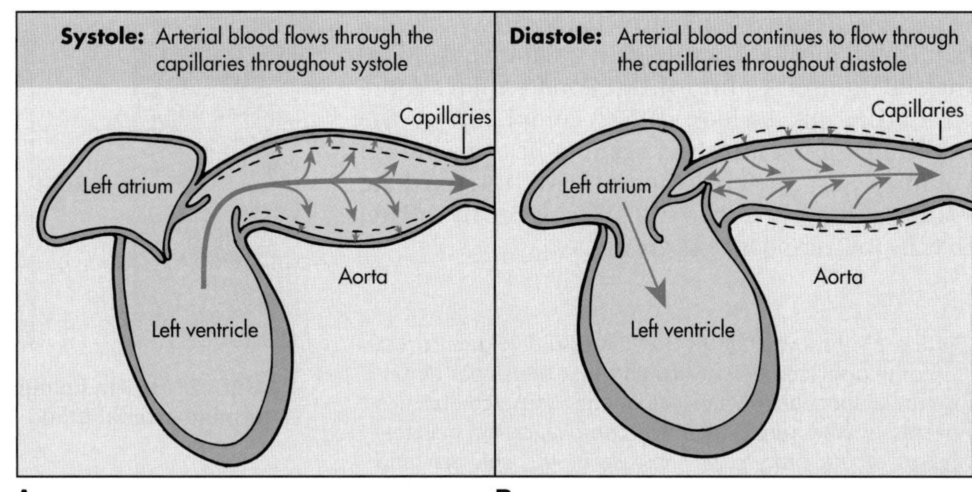

FIGURE 21–1. A, When the arteries are normally compliant, a substantial fraction of the stroke volume is stored in the arteries during ventricular systole; the arterial walls are stretched. B, During ventricular diastole, the previously stretched arteries recoil. The volume of blood displaced by the recoil ensures continuous capillary flow throughout diastole.

Arteries Are Compliant Tubes

The elastic properties of the arterial wall may be appreciated by first considering the static pressure-volume relationship for the aorta. For one study **(Figure 21–2)**, aortae were obtained at autopsy from people of different ages. All aortic branches were tied, and successive volumes of liquid were injected into this closed elastic system, just as a liquid might be introduced into a balloon. After each increment of volume was injected, the internal pressure in the aorta was measured **(Table 21–1)**.

FIGURE 21–2. Pressure-volume relationships for aortae obtained at autopsy from humans in different age groups (denoted by the numbers at the right end of each curve). (Data from Hallock P, Benson IC: *J Clin Invest* 16:595, 1937.)

In Figure 21–2, the pressure-volume curve for the youngest group (20 to 24 years) is sigmoidal. The curve is approximately linear over most of its extent, but the slope ($\Delta V_a/\Delta P_a$) decreases at the upper and lower ends. At any given point, the slope represents the **arterial compliance (C_a):**

$$C_a = \Delta V_a/\Delta P_a \qquad \textbf{21-1}$$

Figure 21–2 reveals that in normal young people, C_a is least at very high and very low pressures and is greatest over the normal range of pressure

TABLE 21–1. GLOSSARY OF SYMBOLS

Symbol	Meaning
Capacitance (C)	
C_a	Arterial compliance
C_v	Venous compliance
Flow (Q)	
Q_h	Cardiac output
Q_r	Peripheral runoff
Pressure (P)	
$\bar{P}_a$	Mean arterial pressure
P_a	Arterial pressure
P_d	Diastolic arterial pressure
P_{ra}	Right atrial pressure
P_s	Systolic arterial pressure
P_v	Venous pressure
Resistance (R)	
R_t	Total systemic resistance
Volume (V)	
V_a	Arterial volume
V_h	Volume pumped by the heart
V_r	Runoff volume
V_v	Venous volume

variations. These compliance changes resemble the familiar changes encountered in inflating a balloon. Introduction of air into the balloon requires more effort (i.e., the balloon is less compliant) at the beginning of inflation and again at near-maximum volume, just before rupture. At intermediate volumes, however, the balloon is easier to inflate; that is, its compliance is greater.

Figure 21–2 shows that the aortic pressure-volume curves become displaced downward and that the slopes diminish as a function of advancing age; thus, compliance decreases with age. Diminished compliance is a manifestation of the progressive increase in the collagen and decrease in the elastin contents of arterial walls. The heart cannot eject a given stroke volume as rapidly into a rigid arterial system as it can into a more compliant system.

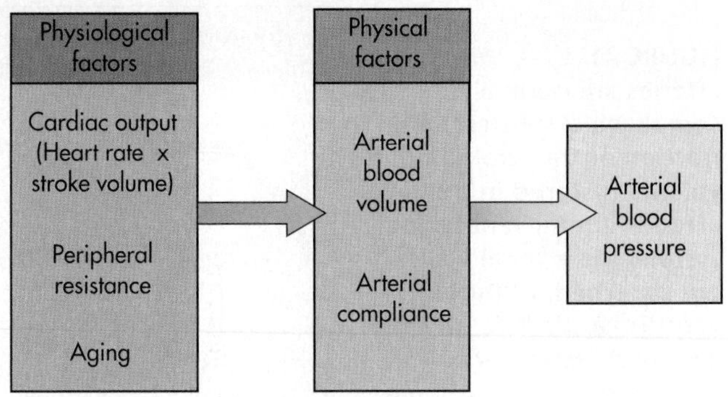

FIGURE 21–3. Physiological and physical factors that determine arterial blood pressure.

Arterial Blood Pressure Is Determined by Several Factors

The arterial blood pressure is routinely measured when a physician examines a patient, and this measurement provides valuable information about the patient's cardiovascular status. The factors that determine the arterial blood pressure cannot be evaluated precisely. Therefore, this chapter takes a simplified approach in an attempt to understand the principal determinants of arterial blood pressure.

The determinants of arterial blood pressure are arbitrarily subdivided into physical and physiological components (**Figure 21–3**). For simplicity, the arterial system is assumed to be a static, elastic system, much like a tubular balloon. The only two **physical factors** considered are the **blood volume** within the arterial system and the elastic characteristics **(compliance)** of the system, just as the pressure in a balloon depends on the volume of fluid (air or liquid) in the balloon and the compliance of the balloon. The **physiological factors** to be considered are **cardiac output** (the product of **heart rate** and **stroke volume**), **peripheral resistance,** and **aging.** Such physiological factors operate through one or both of the physical factors.

The mean arterial pressure is determined by cardiac output and peripheral resistance

THE MEAN ARTERIAL PRESSURE (**$\bar{P}_a$**) IS THE BLOOD PRESSURE IN THE ARTERIES AVERAGED OVER TIME. It may be precisely determined by inserting a needle directly into a peripheral artery and recording the arterial blood pressure with a transducer. The $\bar{P}_a$ can be determined from the arterial blood pressure tracing by dividing the area under the tracing by the elapsed time interval, as shown in **Figure 21–4**. In the absence of a precise intraarterial pressure tracing, however, the $\bar{P}_a$ can usually be estimated satisfactorily from the measured values of the **systolic pressure (P_s)** and the **diastolic pressure (P_d)** obtained indirectly by use of a sphygmomanometer (described later). The value of the $\bar{P}_a$ can be estimated by the following formula:

$$\bar{P}_a \approx P_d + (P_s - P_d)/3 \qquad \textbf{21-2}$$

The physical factors (Figure 21–3) that determine the level of the arterial pressure (P_a) can be estimated from a rearrangement of Equation 21–1:

$$\Delta P_a = \Delta V_a / C_a \qquad \textbf{21-3}$$

Thus, ANY CHANGE IN P_a VARIES DIRECTLY WITH A CHANGE IN ARTERIAL BLOOD VOLUME (V_a) AND INVERSELY WITH A CHANGE IN C_a.

Many physiological factors regulate the P_a. These factors operate through the physical factors—namely, V_a and C_a (Equation 21-3).

Any temporal change in the volume (dV_a/dt) of blood in the arteries depends on the balance between the rate at which the heart pumps blood into the arteries **(cardiac output [Q_h])** and the rate at which the blood flows out of the arteries **(peripheral runoff [Q_r])** through the arterioles and capillaries and into the veins, as follows:

$$dV_a/dt = Q_h - Q_r \qquad \textbf{21-4}$$

This equation, an expression of the **law of conservation of mass,** states that ANY CHANGE IN V_a SIMPLY REFLECTS THE DIFFERENCE IN THE RATES AT WHICH BLOOD ENTERS AND LEAVES THE ARTERIAL SYSTEM. If arterial inflow (Q_h) exceeds the runoff (Q_r), then the

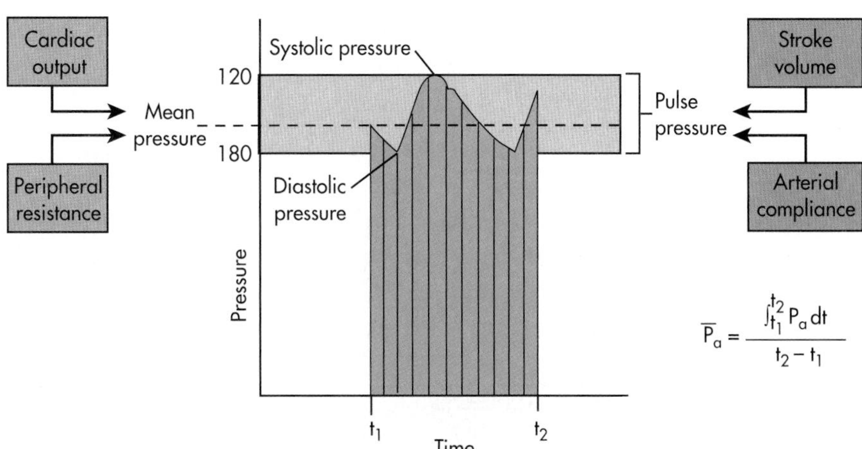

FIGURE 21–4. Arterial systolic pressure, diastolic pressure, pulse pressure, and mean pressure and the factors that determine them.

arterial volume (V_a) increases, the arterial walls distend, and pressure rises. The converse happens when Q_r exceeds Q_h. Finally, if Q_h equals Q_r, $\bar{P}_a$ remains constant.

Cardiac output is the blood flow into the arterial system

How an alteration in Q_h changes $\bar{P}_a$ can be appreciated by considering some simple examples. Under control conditions, let Q_h be 5 L/min and $\bar{P}_a$ be 100 mm Hg (**Figure 21–5,** *A*). Under steady-state conditions, $Q_h = Q_r$. The **total peripheral resistance (R_t)** is the resistance to blood flow in the systemic vascular bed:

$$R_t = (\bar{P}_a - \bar{P}_{ra})/Q_r \qquad \textbf{21-5}$$

where $\bar{P}_{ra}$ is the mean right atrial pressure. Because $\bar{P}_{ra}$ is usually close to zero, the following occurs:

$$R_t \approx \bar{P}_a/Q_r \qquad \textbf{21-6}$$

Therefore, in the example shown in Figure 21–5, *A*, R_t is 100/5 mm Hg, or 20 mm Hg/L/min.

Now suppose Q_h suddenly increases to 10 L/min (Figure 21–5, *B*) so that Q_h exceeds Q_r. In the first one or two heartbeats, however, the increment in blood volume in the arteries is negligible, and $\bar{P}_a$ is unchanged. Because Q_r from the arteries depends on $\bar{P}_a$ and R_t, Q_r also does not change appreciably at first. Therefore, Q_h, now 10 L/min, exceeds Q_r, still only 5 L/min, and V_a progressively increases.

The increase in V_a raises the arterial blood pressure. In this example of a sudden increase in Q_h, blood continues to accumulate in the arteries until the pressure rises high enough to force through the peripheral resistance a runoff, Q_r, that equals the elevated Q_h (Figure 21–5, *C*). If Equation 21-6 is solved for Q_r:

$$Q_r = \bar{P}_a/R_t \qquad \textbf{21-7}$$

This equation makes it evident that Q_r does not attain a value of 10 L/min until the $\bar{P}_a$ reaches 200 mm Hg, provided R_t remains constant at 20 mm Hg/L/min. Thus, $\bar{P}_a$ DEPENDS ONLY ON Q_h AND PERIPHERAL RESISTANCE. C_a does not affect the steady-state level that $\bar{P}_a$ attains in response to a change in Q_h or peripheral resistance; the compliance affects only the rate at which the new steady-state value of $\bar{P}_a$ is attained.

Peripheral resistance regulates the flow out of the arterial system

Similar reasoning may now be applied to explain the changes in $\bar{P}_a$ that accompany alterations in R_t. Suppose the control conditions are identical to the control conditions of the preceding example (Figure 21–5, *A*). If R_t suddenly increases to 40 mm Hg/L/min from the control value of 20 mm Hg/L/min (Figure 21–5, *D*), the $\bar{P}_a$ is virtually unchanged over the duration of the first one or two heartbeats because sufficient time has not passed to allow V_a to change substantially. Although $\bar{P}_a$ is still virtually equal to 100 mm Hg, the Q_r suddenly decreases to 2.5 L/min when R_t is increased to 40 mm Hg/L/min. If the Q_h remains constant at 5 L/min, Q_h will exceed Q_r, and thus V_a will increase. Consequently, $\bar{P}_a$ rises and continues to rise until it reaches 200 mm Hg (Figure 21–5, *E*). At this pressure level (Q_r = 200/40 mm Hg = 5 L/min), which equals the Q_h, $\bar{P}_a$ then remains at the new steady-state level of 200 mm Hg as long as Q_h and R_t do not change.

These findings therefore confirm that $\bar{P}_a$ depends only on Q_h and R_t (Figure 21–5). It is immaterial whether the change in Q_h is accomplished by an alteration in heart rate, stroke volume, or both. Because Q_h equals heart rate multiplied by stroke volume, any change in heart rate that is balanced by an inverse change in stroke volume does not alter Q_h, and therefore $\bar{P}_a$ is not affected.

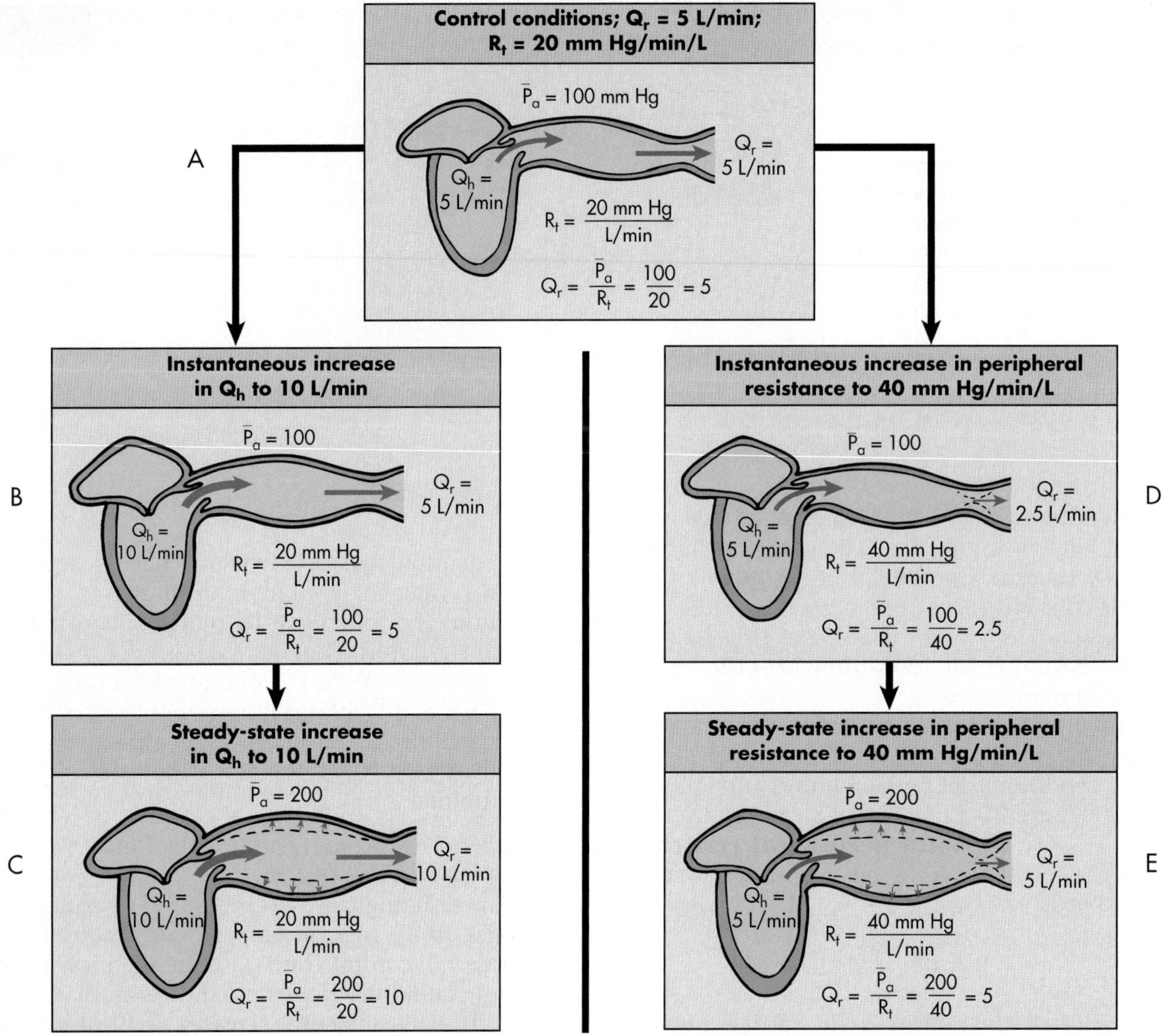

FIGURE 21–5. Relationship of $\bar{P}_a$ to Q_h, Q_r, and R_t under controlled conditions (A), in response to an increase in Q_h (B and C), and in response to an increase in R_t (D and E).

Arterial pulse pressure is the amplitude of the arterial pressure fluctuation

The arterial pulse pressure for a given heartbeat equals the difference between $\mathbf{P_s}$ and $\mathbf{P_d}$ for that heartbeat; P_s and P_d are the maximum and minimum values, respectively, of the P_a during that heartbeat (Figure 21–4). **ARTERIAL PULSE PRESSURE** IS DETERMINED BY STROKE VOLUME AND C_a (Figure 21–4).

Stroke volume determines the arterial volume fluctuation

The effect of a change in stroke volume on pulse pressure may be analyzed more clearly under conditions in which C_a remains constant. C_a is constant over any linear region of a pressure-volume curve (Figure 21–2). If the V_a is plotted along the vertical axis and P_a is plotted along the horizontal axis, the slope of the pressure-volume curve (dV_a/dP_a) is by definition the C_a.

The effect of a change in stroke volume on arterial pulse pressure can be appreciated by considering a healthy person who initially has a heart rate of 100 beats/min, a stroke volume of 50 mL, and an R_t of 20 mm Hg/L/min. Because Q_h equals heart rate multiplied by stroke volume, this person's Q_h is 5 L/min. As shown in Figure 21–5, *A,* this person would have a $\bar{P}_a$ of 100 mm Hg. The P_s of course exceeds 100 mm Hg, and the P_d is less than 100 mm Hg. Suppose P_s and P_d for this person are 120 mm Hg and

90 mm Hg, respectively; the values for $\bar{P}_a$, P_s, and P_d satisfy Equation 21–2. The average normal P_d is about 80 mm Hg; the value of 90 mm Hg is used here only to simplify certain computations.

Several hemodynamic events take place just before and during the rapid ejection phase of systole of a normal heartbeat (see Chapter 18). Throughout the ventricular diastole of the preceding heartbeat and during the brief period of isovolumic contraction, the heart has pumped no blood into the arteries, but blood has flowed out of the arteries and through the resistance vessels continuously. Hence, V_a has been declining, and consequently $\bar{P}_a$ has been falling continuously throughout these nonejection phases of the cardiac cycle. In a person whose P_d is 90 mm Hg, this minimum pressure will have been attained at the end of the isovolumic contraction phase of systole (see Figure 18–8).

Under steady-state conditions, the volume of blood that flows out of the arteries and through the peripheral resistance vessels during each cardiac cycle equals the stroke volume. In healthy people, most of the stroke volume is ejected during the rapid ejection phase of ventricular systole (see Figure 18–8). If a person has a stroke volume of 50 mL and 80% of that volume is expelled during rapid ejection (i.e., $Q_h = 0.80 \times 50 = 40$ mL, as illustrated in **Figure 21–6**, *A*), the fractional volume flowing out of the arteries during rapid ejection is approximately equal to the fraction of the cardiac cycle duration occupied by the rapid ejection phase. Assume that during the rapid ejection phase, 16% of the stroke volume exits the arteries through the peripheral resistance; that is, the Q_r during rapid ejection is 0.16×50 mL, or 8 mL (Figure 21–6, *A*).

Hence, the **volume increment** (ΔV_a) that prevails in the arteries during the rapid ejection phase of the cardiac cycle equals the quantity of blood (Q_h = 40 mL) pumped into the aorta during this phase of the cardiac cycle minus the quantity of blood (Q_r = 8 mL) that has exited through the peripheral resistance vessels during this same period; that is, the ΔV_a equals 32 mL (Figure 21–6, *A*). In this hypothetical subject, the ΔV_a causes P_a to rise from the diastolic level of 90 mm Hg to the systolic level of 120 mm Hg (Figure 21–6). In other words, the ΔV_a of 32 mL produces a pressure increment (ΔP_a) of 30 mm Hg; this pressure increment is by definition the **pulse pressure** (Figure 21–4).

Thus, the magnitude of the pulse pressure (ΔP_a) is determined simply by the values of ΔV_a and C_a. The relationship is evident from a rearrangement of Equation 21-1:

$$\Delta P_a = \Delta V_a / C_a \qquad \textbf{21-8}$$

The pulse pressure equals the V_a increment during the rapid ejection phase of ventricular systole divided by C_a. In the previous example, C_a was equal to $\Delta V_a/\Delta P_a$ = 32/30 mm Hg, or 1.07 mL/mm Hg (Figure 21–6, *A*).

Suppose that the cardiovascular status changes such that the heart rate decreases to 50 beats/min, the stroke volume increases to 100 mL (Figure 21–6, *B*), but the peripheral resistance (20 mm Hg/L/min) and C_a (1.07 mL/mm Hg) remain unchanged. Because Q_h (heart rate × stroke volume) still equals 5 L/min and the peripheral resistance is also unchanged, the $\bar{P}_a$ remains at 100 mm Hg (Equation 21–6).

To determine the new pulse pressure, assume that the fraction of the stroke volume (100 mL) expelled during rapid ejection is still 80%; that is, $Q_h = 0.80 \times 100$ mL, or 80 mL (Figure 21–6, *B*). Suppose again that 16% of the stroke volume exits the arterial system through the peripheral resistance during rapid ejection. Hence, Q_r during rapid ejection is 0.16×100 mL, or 16 mL. Thus, the ΔV_a during rapid ejection is 80 – 16 mL, or 64 mL.

A ΔV_a of 64 mL in an arterial system with a compliance of 1.07 mL/mm Hg produces a pressure increment (i.e., a pulse pressure) of 60 mm Hg (Figure 21–6, *B*), which is twice the pulse pressure that prevailed under control conditions (Figure 21–6, *A*). If the relationships among the mean pressure, P_s, and P_d satisfy Equation 21–2, this person's P_s and P_d would equal 140 mm Hg and 80 mm Hg, respectively. Hence, if Q_h, peripheral resistance, and C_a remain constant, an increase in stroke volume would raise P_s and lower P_d but would not affect the mean pressure ($\bar{P}_a$) (Figure 21–6, *D*).

Arterial pulse pressure provides valuable clues about a patient's stroke volume, provided the C_a is essentially normal. Patients who have severe **congestive heart failure** or who have had a severe **hemorrhage** are likely to have very small arterial pulse pressures because their stroke volumes are abnormally small. Conversely, individuals with large stroke volumes are likely to have above-average arterial pulse pressures. For example, well-trained athletes at rest tend to have low heart rates. Thus, the prolonged ventricular filling times induce the ventricles to pump more blood per heartbeat. Consequently, the pulse pressures of such athletes tend to be higher than average. Similarly, in patients with **chronic aortic valve regurgitation,** blood leaks back into the left ventricle from the aorta during diastole. This backflow into the ventricle diminishes the aortic P_d and increases the blood volume in the left ventricle during diastole. The augmented ventricular filling volume increases the stroke volume during systole. Characteristically, a patient with aortic valve regurgitation has a low arterial P_d, an elevated arterial P_s, and consequently a greatly increased arterial pulse pressure.

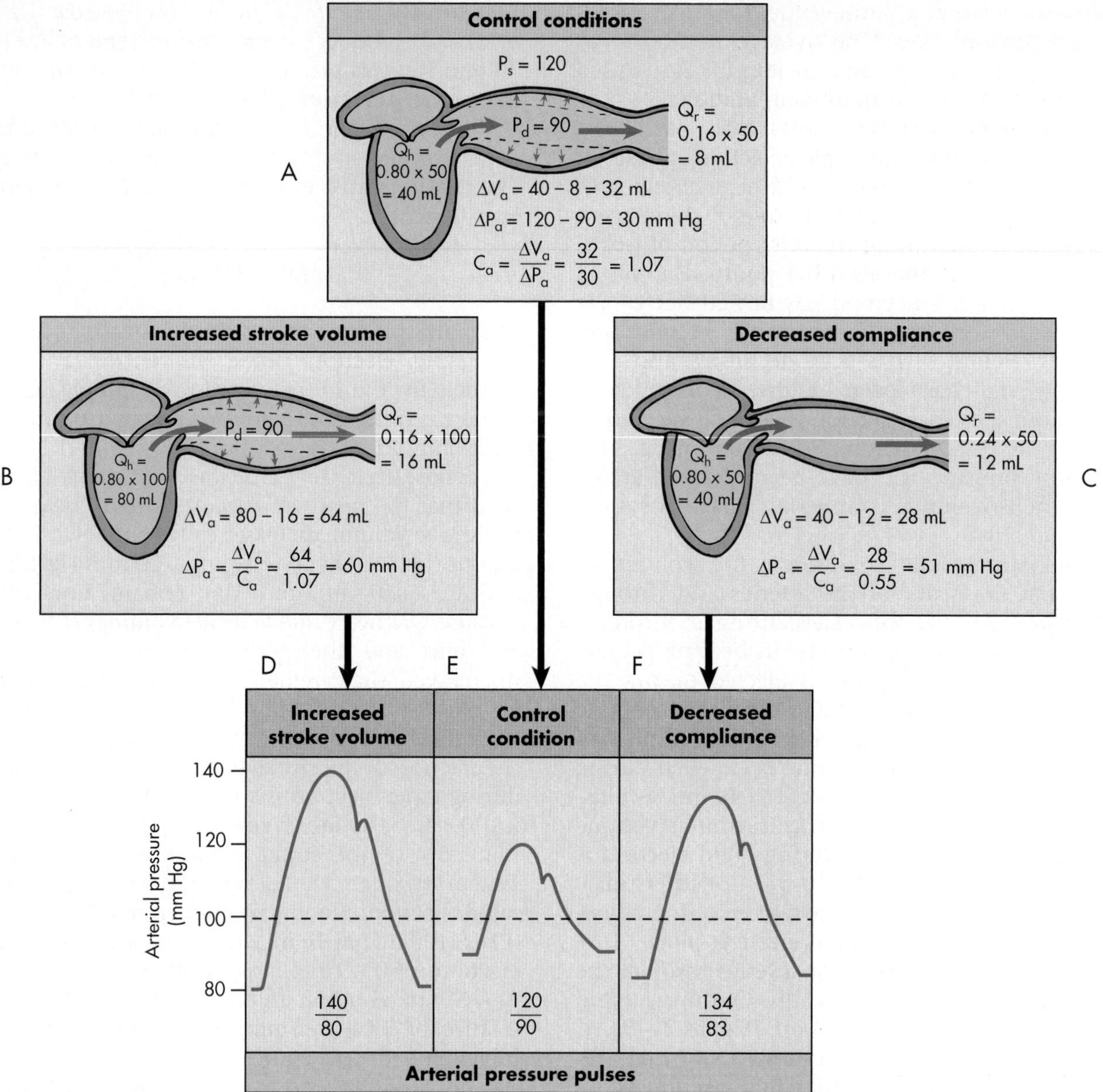

FIGURE 21–6. Effects of an increase in stroke volume and a decrease in C_a on the arterial pulse pressure. The heart pumps a volume (Q_h) of 40 mL of blood into the arterial system with each heartbeat during rapid ejection (A). Concomitantly, a volume (Q_r) of 8 mL runs out of the arteries through the peripheral resistance. The heart now pumps 80 mL with each beat into the arteries during rapid ejection, and 16 mL runs out of the arteries during the same period (B). The heart still pumps 80% of the stroke volume (50 mL) during the rapid ejection phase despite a decreased C_a (0.55 mL/mm Hg) (C). Under conditions that do not alter the $\bar{P}_a$, an increase in stroke volume (D) or a decrease in C_a (F) causes the arterial pulse pressure to exceed the control value (E) of the arterial pulse pressure.

Arterial compliance affects arterial pressure fluctuation

A change in C_a affects the pulse pressure (Figure 21–6, *C*). Assume that heart rate, stroke volume, and peripheral resistance are the same as in the control condition (Figure 21–6, *A*). However, the arteries are about half as compliant as before (i.e., C_a = 0.55 mL/mm Hg). Because the Q_h and peripheral resistance are the same as in the two preceding examples (Figure 21–6, *A* and *B*), the $\bar{P}_a$ still is 100 mm Hg (Figure 21–6, *F*).

Even though the C_a is much less than the control value, the heart can still pump 80% of the stroke volume during rapid ejection (i.e., Q_h = 40 mL). Because the less compliant arteries accommodate a smaller increment in volume during rapid ejection, the fraction (24%) of the stroke volume that will run out of the arteries during the rapid ejection period (Q_r = 12 mL) will exceed the fraction (16%) that runs out of the arteries in the same period under control conditions (Q_r = 8 mL). In arteries whose compliance is only 0.55 mL/mm Hg, the V_a increment (V_a = 40 − 12 = 28 mL) produces a pressure increment (pulse pressure) of 51 mm Hg (Figure 21–6, *C*). If the relationships among P_s, P_d, and mean pressure satisfy Equation 21–2, P_s and P_d will be approximately 134 mm Hg and 83 mm Hg, respectively (Figure 21–6, *F*). Thus, when C_a is diminished, P_s will exceed the control P_s, P_d will be lower than the control P_d, and pulse pressure will be substantially greater than the control pulse pressure (Figure 21–6, *E*).

The C_a of old people in general (Figure 21–2) and of young people with substantial **arteriosclerosis** (hardening of the arteries) is low, and this condition is reflected by the pulse pressures in such individuals. The P_s tends to be abnormally high (so-called **systolic hypertension**), but the P_d tends to be less than average (80 mm Hg) for normal young people.

The characteristic changes in arterial blood pressure in patients with **essential hypertension** (the most common form of chronic hypertension in humans) are a moderate increase in P_d and a substantially greater increase in P_s. Thus, the $\bar{P}_a$ and the arterial pulse pressure are augmented. The $\bar{P}_a$ is elevated because the R_t is increased; the reasons for this increase remain to be established. The principal reason for the increase in arterial pulse pressure is that the arteries become less compliant when they are stretched by the elevated arterial blood pressure. The reduced compliance is reflected by the decrease in the slope of the pressure-volume curve when P_a is elevated (Figure 21–2).

Indirect Methods Are Often Used to Measure Blood Pressure

Needles or catheters may be introduced into peripheral arteries of patients in the cardiac catheterization laboratories or intensive care units of hospitals. Arterial blood pressure can then be measured directly by electronic pressure transducers. Ordinarily, however, blood pressure is estimated indirectly by use of a **sphygmomanometer.** This instrument consists of a sturdy cuff and an inflatable bag. The cuff is wrapped around the arm above the elbow, and the inflatable bag, which lies between the cuff and the skin, is positioned over the brachial artery. When the patient's blood pressure is measured, a rubber squeeze bulb is used to raise the pressure in the bag to a value that exceeds the patient's arterial P_s. The elevated pressure in the cuff occludes the brachial artery. Air is then slowly released from the bag by use of a needle valve in the inflation bulb.

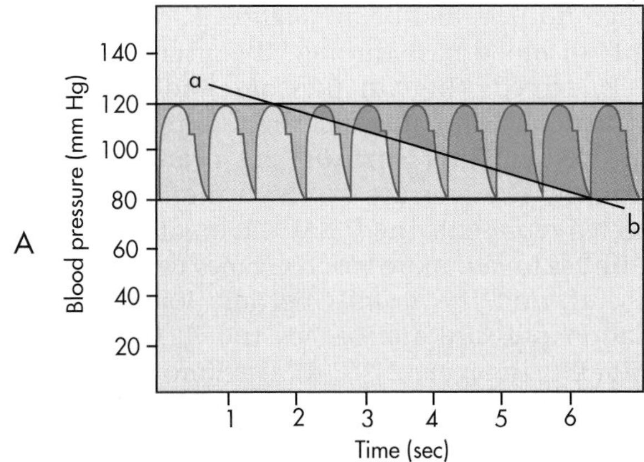

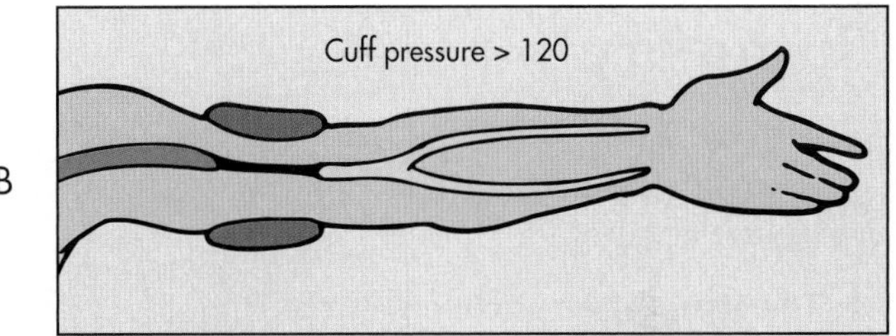

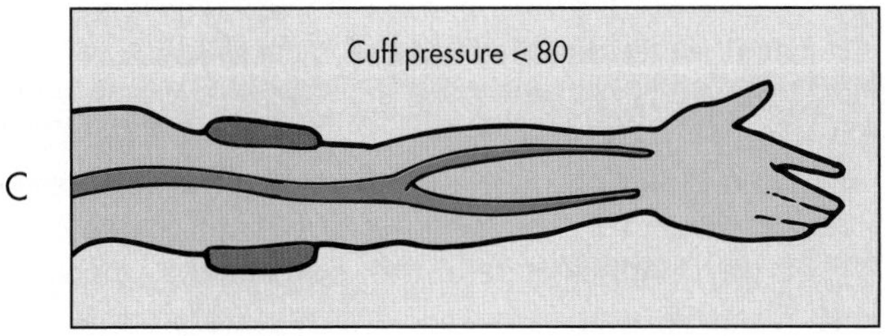

FIGURE 21–7. Measurement of arterial blood pressure with a sphygmomanometer. A, If the patient's arterial blood pressure is 120/80 mm Hg, the pressure *(oblique line)* in a cuff around the patient's arm is allowed to fall from above 120 mm Hg (point a) to below 80 mm Hg (point b) in about 6 seconds. B, When the cuff pressure exceeds 120 mm Hg, no blood passes through the arterial segment under the cuff, and no sounds can be detected with a stethoscope bell placed on the arm distal to the cuff. C, When the cuff pressure falls below 80 mm Hg, arterial flow through the region surrounded by the cuff is continuous, and no sounds are audible. When the cuff pressure is between 120 and 80 mm Hg, spurts of blood traverse the artery segment under the cuff during each heartbeat, and Korotkoff sounds are heard through the stethoscope.

The health care worker listens with a stethoscope applied to the skin in the antecubital space over the brachial artery. While the pressure in the bag exceeds the P_s, the brachial artery is occluded and no sounds are heard (**Figure 21–7,** *B*). When the inflation pressure falls just below the arterial P_s

(upper horizontal line in Figure 21–7, *A*), small spurts of blood pass through the artery each time the P_a exceeds the cuff pressure, and they create turbulence. Consequently, slight tapping sounds (called **Korotkoff sounds**) are heard with each heartbeat. The pressure at which the first sound is detected represents the $\mathbf{P_s}$. As the inflation pressure continues to fall, more blood escapes per beat under the cuff, and the sounds become louder. As the inflation pressure approaches the P_d (lower horizontal line in Figure 21–7, *A*), the Korotkoff sounds become muffled. As the inflation pressure falls just below the minimum pressure in the artery, the sounds disappear; this indicates the $\mathbf{P_d}$ (Figure 21–7, *C*).

Korotkoff sounds are generated by the impact of the spurt of blood that passes under the cuff and meets the static column of blood beyond the cuff. The impact creates turbulence and generates audible vibrations. Once the inflation pressure is less than the P_d, flow is continuous in the brachial artery, and sounds are no longer heard.

Summary

- The arteries not only conduct blood from the heart to the capillaries but also store some of the ejected blood during each cardiac systole. Consequently, flow can continue through the capillaries throughout cardiac diastole.
- The aging process diminishes the compliance of the arteries.
- The less compliant the arteries, the more work the heart must do to pump a given Q_h.
- The $\bar{P}_a$ varies directly with the Q_h and R_t.
- The arterial pulse pressure varies directly with the stroke volume but inversely with C_a.
- When blood pressure is measured with a sphygmomanometer, the P_s is signaled by a tapping sound that originates in the artery distal to the cuff as the cuff pressure falls below the peak P_a, and the P_d is manifested by the disappearance of the sound as the cuff pressure falls below the minimum P_a.

Bibliography

Armentano RL et al: Arterial wall mechanics in conscious dogs, *Circ Res* 76:468, 1995.

Burattini R, Campbell KB: Effective distributed compliance of the canine descending aorta estimated by modified T-tube model, *Am J Physiol* 264:H1997, 1993.

Folkow B, Svanborg A: Physiology of cardiovascular aging, *Physiol Rev* 73:725, 1993.

Frasch HF, Kresh JY, Noordergraaf A: Two-port analysis of microcirculation: an extension of windkessel, *Am J Physiol* 270:H376, 1996.

Fung YC: *Biodynamics: circulation,* Heidelberg, Germany, 1984, Springer-Verlag.

Kelly RP, Tunin R, Kass DA: Effects of reduced aortic compliance on cardiac efficiency and contractile function of in situ canine left ventricle, *Circ Res* 71:490, 1992.

Laskey WK et al: Estimation of total systemic arterial compliance in humans, *J Appl Physiol* 69:112, 1990.

Lee RT, Kamm RD: Vascular mechanics for the cardiologist, *J Am Coll Cardiol* 23:1289, 1994.

Mulvany MJ, Aalkjaer C: Structure and function of small arteries, *Physiol Rev* 70:921, 1990.

O'Rourke M, Kelly R, Avolio A: *Arterial pulse,* Baltimore, 1992, Williams & Wilkins.

Piene H: Pulmonary arterial impedance and right ventricular function, *Physiol Rev* 66:606, 1986.

Stergiopolis N, Meister J-J, Westerhof N: Determinants of stroke volume and systolic and diastolic aortic pressure, *Am J Physiol* 270:H2050, 1996.

Van Gorp AD et al: Technique to assess aortic distensibility and compliance in anesthetized and awake rats, *Am J Physiol* 270:H780, 1996.

Case Study

Case 21–1

A 33-year-old man complained about chest pain on exertion. He was referred to a cardiologist, who performed a number of studies, including right- and left-sided cardiac catheterization for hemodynamic information and coronary angiography to image the status of the coronary arteries. Among the data obtained during these studies were the findings that the patient's pulmonary artery and aortic pressures were as follows:

Pressure	Pulmonary Artery (mm Hg)	Aorta (mm Hg)
Systolic	30	120
Diastolic	15	80
Pulse	15	40
Mean	20	93

The hemodynamic and angiographic studies disclosed no serious abnormalities. The patient's physicians recommended certain changes in lifestyle and diet, and the patient continued to do well for about 20 years, when systemic arterial blood pressure was found to be 190/100 mm Hg and $\overline{P}_a$ was estimated to be 130 mm Hg. These and other findings led his physicians to the diagnosis of essential hypertension.

1. **Why was the patient's aortic $\overline{P}_a$ (93 mm Hg) much higher than his pulmonary $\overline{P}_a$ (20 mm Hg) at the time of the initial examination?**
   A. His systemic vascular resistance is much greater than his pulmonary vascular resistance.
   B. His aortic compliance is much greater than his pulmonary compliance.
   C. His left ventricular stroke volume is much greater than his right ventricular stroke volume.
   D. The total cross-sectional area of his pulmonary capillary bed is much greater than the total cross-sectional area of his systemic capillary bed.
   E. The duration of the rapid ejection phase of the left ventricle exceeds the duration of the rapid ejection phase of the right ventricle.

2. **When the patient became hypertensive, his arterial pulse pressure (90 mm Hg) increased to a value higher than his pulse pressure (40 mm Hg) before the hypertension. Why?**
   A. His systemic vascular resistance is less than it was before he became hypertensive.
   B. The duration of the reduced ejection phase of the left ventricle decreases as the arterial blood pressure rises.
   C. His C_a was diminished in part because of the hypertension and in part because of the effects of aging.
   D. The total cross-sectional area of the systemic capillary bed increases substantially in hypertensive subjects.
   E. His aortic compliance became greater than his pulmonary C_a.

Chapter 22: Microcirculation and Lymphatics

Objectives

- ❖ Describe the regulation of regional blood flow by the arterioles.
- ❖ Enumerate the physical and chemical factors affecting the microvessels.
- ❖ Explain the roles of diffusion, filtration, and pinocytosis in transcapillary exchange.
- ❖ Describe the balance between hydrostatic and osmotic forces under normal and abnormal conditions.
- ❖ Describe the lymphatic circulation.

The entire circulatory system is designed to supply the body tissues with blood in amounts commensurate with their requirements for O_2 and nutrients and to remove CO_2 and other waste products for excretion by the lungs and kidneys. The exchange of gases, water, and solutes between the vascular and interstitial fluid compartments occurs mainly across the capillaries, which consist of a single layer of endothelial cells. The arterioles, capillaries, and venules constitute the microcirculation, and blood flow through the microcirculation is regulated by the arterioles, also known as the **resistance vessels** (see Chapter 20). The large arteries serve solely as blood conduits, whereas the veins serve as storage or **capacitance vessels** as well as blood conduits.

Functional Anatomy of Circulation Includes Arterioles and Capillaries

Arterioles are the stopcocks of circulation

The arterioles, which range in diameter from about 5 to 100 µm, have a thick smooth muscle layer, a thin adventitial layer, and an endothelial lining (see Figure 15–2). The arterioles give rise directly to the **capillaries** (diameter, 5 to 10 µm) or in some tissues to **metarterioles** (diameter, 10 to 20 µm), which then give rise to capillaries **(Figure 22–1)**. The metarterioles can serve either as thoroughfares to the venules, bypassing the capillaries, or as conduits for supplying the capillary bed. There are often cross-connections from arteriole to arteriole and from venule to venule as well as in the capillary network. Arterioles that give rise directly to capillaries regulate flow through their cognate capillaries by constriction or dilation. The capillaries form an interconnecting network of tubes of different lengths; the average length is 0.5 to 1 mm.

The diameter of the resistance vessels is determined by the balance between the contractile force of the vascular smooth muscle and the distending force produced by the intraluminal pressure. The greater the contractile activity of the vascular smooth muscle of an arteriole, the smaller its diameter. At times, the small arterioles may be completely occluded, partly because of infolding of the endothelium **(Figure 22–2)**. When the intravascular pressure diminishes, vessel diameter decreases, as does tension in the vessel wall (Laplace's law;

Figure 22–3). When perfusion pressure is progressively reduced, a point is reached at which a segment of the vessel is occluded and blood flow ceases even though a positive pressure gradient from the afferent to the efferent end of the vessel may still exist. The transmural pressure at which flow ceases is called the **critical closing pressure.**

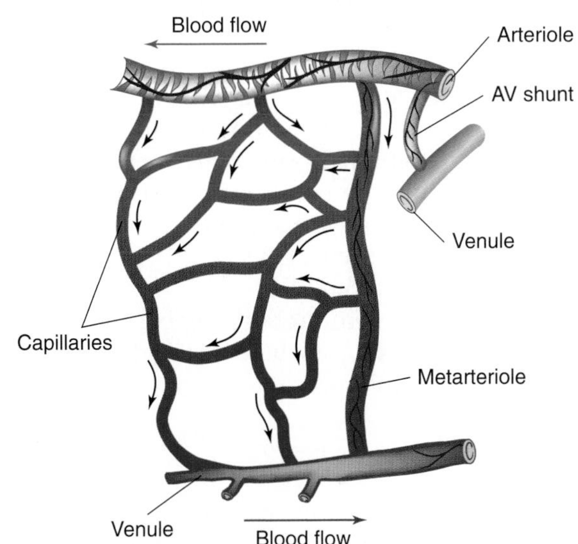

FIGURE 22–1. Microcirculation. The circular structures on the arteriole and venule represent smooth muscle fibers, and the branching solid lines represent sympathetic nerve fibers. The arrows indicate the direction of blood flow. AV, arteriovenous.

Capillaries permit the exchange of solutes, water, and gases

Capillary distribution varies from tissue to tissue. Metabolically active tissues such as cardiac and skeletal muscle and glands have numerous capillaries, whereas less active tissues such as subcutaneous tissue and cartilage have few capillaries. Also, not all capillaries have the same diameter. Because some capillaries have diameters smaller than those of erythrocytes, the red cells must become temporarily deformed to pass through them. Normal red cells are flexible and readily change their shape to conform to that of the small capillaries (see Chapter 20).

Blood flow in the capillaries is not uniform and depends chiefly on the contractile state of the arterioles. The average velocity of capillary blood flow is 1 mm/sec; however, it can quickly vary from zero to several millimeters per second in the same vessel. Capillary blood flow may vary randomly, or it may oscillate rhythmically at different frequencies as determined by contraction and relaxation **(vasomotion)** of the precapillary vessels. This vasomotion is partly an intrinsic contractile behavior of the vascular smooth muscle. Furthermore, changes in **transmural pressure** (intravascular pressure minus extravascular pressure) affect the contractile state of the precapillary vessels. An increase in the transmural pressure, whether it is produced by an

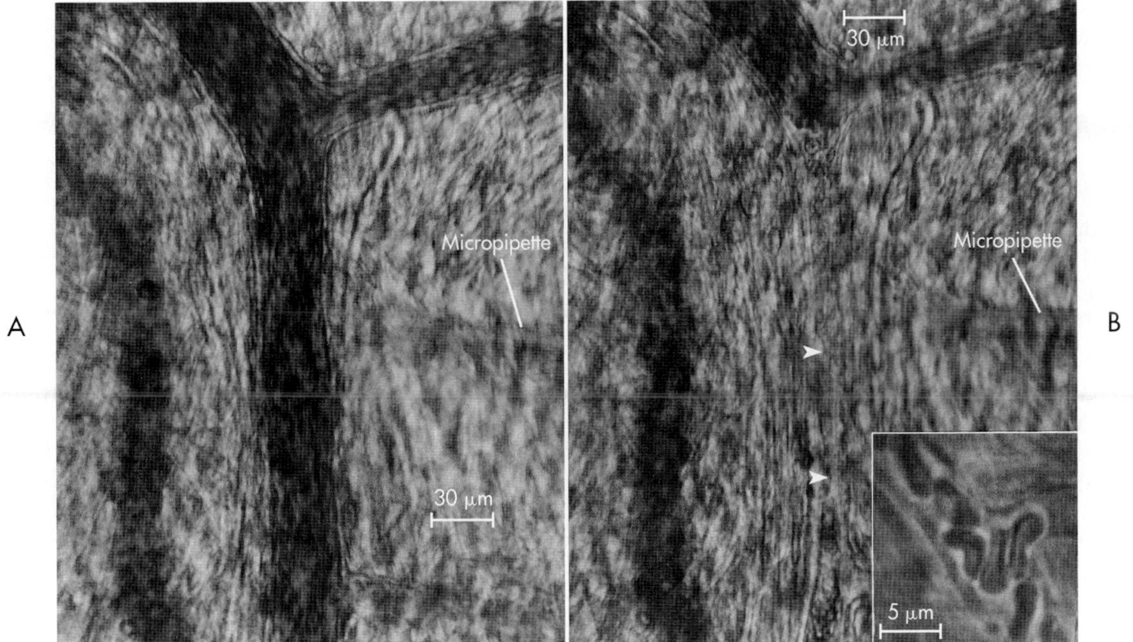

FIGURE 22–2. Arterioles of a hamster cheek pouch. A, Before the microinjection of norepinephrine. B, After the injection. Note the complete closure of the arteriole between the arrows and the narrowing of a branch arteriole at the upper right. *Inset,* Capillary with red cells during a period of complete closure of the feeding arteriole. (Courtesy of David N. Damon.)

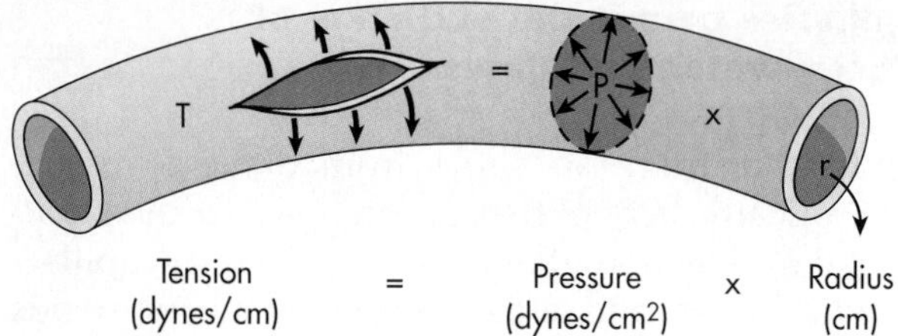

FIGURE 22–3. Diagram of a small blood vessel illustrating Laplace's law (T = Pr), in which force tends to pull apart a theoretical longitudinal slit in the vessel. P, intraluminal pressure; r, radius of the vessel; T, wall tension as the force per unit length tangential to the vessel wall.

increase in venous pressure or by the dilation of arterioles, elicits contraction of the terminal arterioles at the points of origin of the capillaries. Conversely, a decrease in the transmural pressure elicits precapillary vessel relaxation. In addition, humoral and neural factors affect vasomotion.

Although reduced transmural pressure relaxes the terminal arterioles, blood flow through the capillaries cannot increase if the reduced intravascular pressure is caused by severe constriction of the parent arterioles or metarterioles. Large arterioles and metarterioles also exhibit vasomotion. However, contraction of these vessels usually does not occlude the lumen and arrest blood flow, whereas contraction of the terminal arterioles may arrest blood flow. Blood flow through the capillaries has been termed **nutritional flow** because it provides for the exchange of gases and solutes between blood and tissue, whereas blood flow that bypasses the capillaries in traveling from the arterial to the venous side of the circulation has been termed **nonnutritional,** or **shunt, flow** (Figure 22–1). In some areas of the body (e.g., fingertips), true arteriovenous shunts exist (see Chapter 25). In many tissues such as muscle, however, evidence of anatomical shunts is lacking.

The true capillaries lack smooth muscle and are therefore incapable of active constriction. Nevertheless, the endothelial cells that form the capillary wall contain actin and myosin and can alter their shape in response to certain chemical stimuli. However, such changes in endothelial cell shape do not regulate blood flow through the capillaries. CHANGES IN CAPILLARY DIAMETER ARE PASSIVE AND ARE CAUSED BY ALTERATIONS IN PRECAPILLARY AND POSTCAPILLARY RESISTANCE.

For many years, it was believed that endothelial cells were inert and merely served as barriers to blood cells and large molecules such as plasma proteins. However, it is now known that the endothelium can synthesize substances that affect the contractile state of the arterioles (**Figure 22–4**). One such vasodilator is **endothelium-derived relaxing factor (EDRF),** identified as the gas **nitric oxide (NO).** The discoverers of NO as a signal molecule were awarded the 1998 Nobel Prize for Medicine and Physiology. NO, formed and released in response to stimulation of the endothelium by various agents (e.g., acetylcholine, ATP, serotonin, bradykinin, histamine, substance P), can also interfere with platelet aggregation. **Prostacyclin,** another vasodilator that is synthesized by endothelial cells, also inhibits platelet adherence to the endothelium and platelet aggregation. Thereby, it aids in the prevention of intravascular thrombosis (see Chapter 15). A vasoconstrictor substance, **endothelin,** has also been isolated from endothelial cells.

The thin-walled capillaries can withstand high internal pressures without bursting because of their narrow lumens. This can be explained in terms of Laplace's law, as follows:

$$T = Pr \qquad \textbf{22-1}$$

where T is tension in the vessel wall (dynes/cm), P is transmural pressure (dynes/cm^2), and r is radius

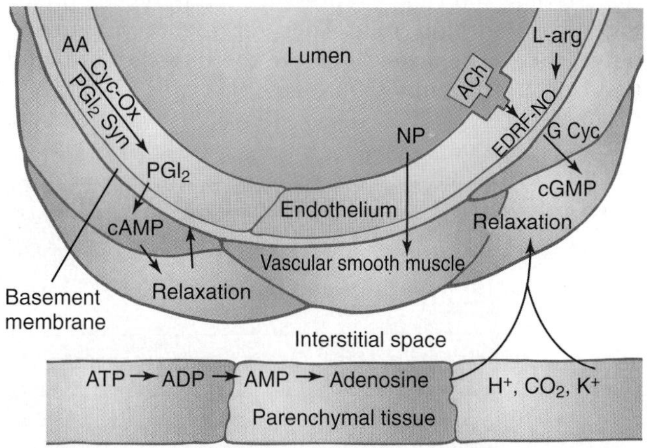

FIGURE 22–4. Arteriole illustrating endothelium- and nonendothelium-mediated vasodilation. Prostacyclin (PGI_2) is formed from arachidonic acid (AA) by the action of cyclooxygenase (Cyc-Ox) and prostacyclin synthetase (PGI_2 Syn) in the endothelium and elicits relaxation of the adjacent vascular smooth muscle via increases in cAMP. Stimulation of the endothelial cells with acetylcholine (ACh) or other agents (see text) results in the formation and release of an EDRF (NO). The EDRF stimulates guanylyl cyclase (G Cyc) to increase cGMP in the vascular smooth muscle to produce relaxation. The vasodilator agent nitroprusside (NP) acts directly on the vascular smooth muscle. Substances such as adenosine, H^+, CO_2, and K^+ can arise in the parenchymal tissue and elicit vasodilation by direct action on the vascular smooth muscle. L-arg, L-arginine.

of the vessel (cm). Wall tension (T) is the force per unit length tangential to the vessel wall. This force opposes the distending force (Pr) that tends to pull apart a theoretical longitudinal slit in the vessel (Figure 22–3). Transmural pressure is essentially equal to intraluminal pressure because extravascular pressure is usually negligible.

At normal aortic (100 mm Hg) and capillary (25 mm Hg) pressures, the wall tension of the aorta is about 12,000 times greater than that of the capillary (100 mm Hg × radius of 1.5 cm for the aorta versus 25 mm Hg × radius of 5×10^{-4} cm for the capillary). In a person standing quietly, capillary pressure in the feet may reach 100 mm Hg (see Chapter 24). Under such conditions, capillary wall tension increases to a value that is only 0.003 that of the wall tension in the aorta at the same internal pressure.

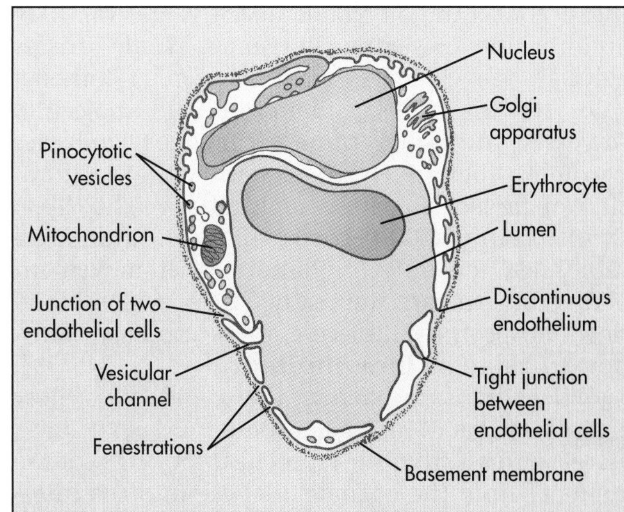

FIGURE 22–5. Sketch of an electron micrograph showing a composite capillary in cross section.

According to Laplace's equation, wall tension increases as vessels dilate, even when internal pressure remains constant. Such is the case in **aneurysm** (local widening) **of the aorta,** in which wall tension may become high enough to rupture the vessel.

Capillary permeability varies among body tissues

The permeability of the capillary endothelial membrane is not the same in all body tissues. For example, liver capillaries are very permeable, and albumin escapes at a much greater rate than from the less permeable muscle capillaries. Also, permeability is not uniform along the whole capillary; the venous ends are more permeable than the arterial ends, and permeability is greatest in the venules. The greater permeability at the venous end of the capillaries and in the venules is caused by the greater number of **pores (clefts).** In most tissues, the clefts are sparse and occupy only about 0.02% of the capillary surface area **(Figure 22–5)**. In the brain, clefts are absent in the capillaries, and a **blood-brain barrier** to many small molecules exists.

In addition to clefts, some of the more porous capillaries (e.g., in the kidney and intestine) contain fenestrations 20 to 100 nm wide, whereas other capillaries (e.g., in the liver) have a discontinuous endothelium. The fenestrations appear to be sealed by a thin diaphragm, but they are permeable to large molecules. In contrast, only small molecules can pass through the intercellular clefts of the endothelium.

Transcapillary Exchange Encompasses a Few Processes

Solvents and solutes move across the capillary endothelial wall via three processes: diffusion, filtration, and pinocytosis.

Diffusion is the most important means for solute transfer across the capillary endothelium

Normally only about 0.06 mL of water per minute moves back and forth across the capillary wall per 100 g of tissue as a result of filtration and absorption. In contrast, 300 mL of water per minute per 100 g of tissue moves by diffusion, a 5000-fold difference (see Chapter 1). Only about 2% of the plasma passing through the capillaries is filtered. In contrast, the rate that water diffuses back and forth across the endothelium is 40 times greater than the rate at which it is delivered to the capillaries via blood flow. The transcapillary exchange of solutes is also governed by diffusion. Thus, DIFFUSION IS THE KEY FACTOR IN THE EXCHANGE OF GASES, SUBSTRATES, AND WASTE PRODUCTS BETWEEN THE CAPILLARIES AND THE TISSUE CELLS. However, the **net transfer** of fluid across the capillary endothelium is primarily attributable to filtration and absorption.

Diffusion of lipid-insoluble substances is affected by size

The capillary pores do not restrict diffusion for small molecules such as water, NaCl, urea, and glucose. Diffusion proceeds so rapidly that the mean concentration gradient across the capillary endothelium is extremely small. Water passes through the capillary pores between endothelial cells. As the size of lipid-insoluble molecules increases, diffusion through muscle capillaries becomes progressively more restricted. The diffusion of molecules with a molecular weight (MW) greater than 60,000 becomes minimal. With small molecules, the only limitation to net movement across the capillary wall is the rate at which blood flow transports the molecules to the capillary; transport is said to be **flow limited.**

When transport across the capillary is flow limited, a small-molecule solute (e.g., an inert tracer) diffuses from the blood near the origin of the capillary from the cognate arteriole into the interstitial fluid and parenchymal cells **(Figure 22–6)**. A somewhat larger molecule moves farther along the capillary before its concentration in the blood becomes insignificant, and a still larger molecule cannot pass at all through the capillary pores (Figure 22–6, *A*). An increase in blood flow velocity extends the detectable concentration of small molecules farther down the capillary and increases the capillary diffusion capacity.

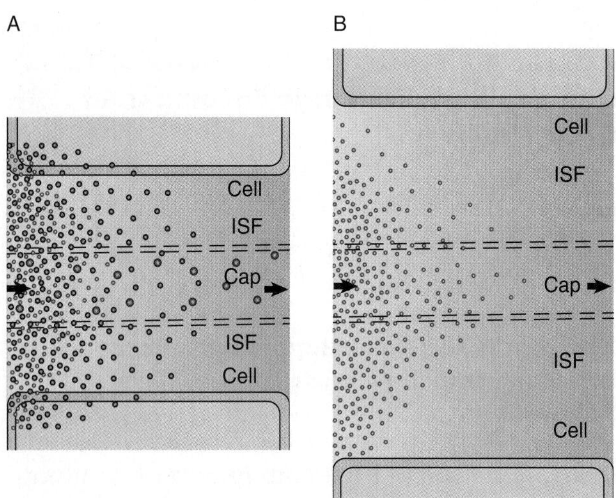

FIGURE 22–6. Flow- and diffusion-limited transport from capillaries (Cap) to tissue. A, Flow-limited transport. The smallest water-soluble inert tracer particles *(red dots)* reach negligible concentrations after passing only a short distance down the capillary. Larger particles with similar properties *(blue dots)* travel farther along the capillary before reaching insignificant intracapillary concentrations. Both substances cross the interstitial fluid (ISF) and reach the parenchymal tissue. Because of their size, more of the smaller particles are taken up by the tissue cells. The largest particles *(purple dots)* cannot penetrate the capillary pores and thus do not escape from the capillary lumen except by pinocytotic vesicle transport. An increase in the volume of blood flow or an increase in capillary density increases tissue supply for the diffusible solutes. Note that capillary permeability is greater at the venous end of the capillary (also in the venule, not shown) because of the larger number of pores in this region. B, Diffusion-limited transport. When the distance between the capillaries and the parenchymal tissue is large as a result of edema or low capillary density, diffusion becomes a limiting factor in the transport of solutes from capillary to tissue, even at high rates of capillary blood flow.

With large molecules, diffusion across the capillaries is the factor that limits exchange **(diffusion limited).** In other words, capillary permeability to a large-molecule solute limits the transport of the solute across the capillary wall (Figure 22–6, *A*).

Under normal conditions, the diffusion of small lipid-insoluble molecules is so rapid that the exchange of such molecules between blood and tissue is never a problem. Such an exchange can become limited when the distances between capillaries and tissue cells are great—for example, when capillary density is very low or tissue edema is extensive (Figure 22–6, *B*).

Lipid-soluble molecules move easily between blood and tissue

In contrast to the movement of lipid-insoluble molecules, the movement of lipid-soluble molecules across the capillary wall is not limited to capillary pores because such molecules can pass directly through the lipid membranes of the entire capillary endothelium. Consequently, lipid-soluble molecules move rapidly between blood and tissue. Lipid solubility (oil-to-water partition coefficient) is a good index of the ease of transfer of lipid molecules through the capillary endothelium.

Both O_2 and CO_2 are lipid soluble and readily pass through the endothelial cells. Calculations based on the diffusion coefficient for O_2, capillary density and diffusion distances, blood flow, and tissue O_2 consumption indicate that the O_2 supply of normal tissue at rest and during activity is not limited by diffusion or by the number of open capillaries.

Measurements of the O_2 tension and O_2 saturation of hemoglobin in the microvessels indicate that in many tissues, the blood O_2 content at the entrance of the capillaries has already decreased to about 80% of that in the aorta. This reduction is a result of the diffusion of O_2 from the arterioles. Furthermore, CO_2 loading and the resulting intravascular shifts in the oxyhemoglobin dissociation curve (see Chapter 30) occur in the precapillary vessels. These findings indicate that O_2 and CO_2 pass directly between adjacent arterioles, venules, and possibly arteries and veins (countercurrent exchange; see Chapter 38). This exchange of gas represents a diffusional shunt of gas around the capillaries; at low blood flow rates, it may limit the supply of O_2 to the tissue.

Capillary filtration is regulated by the hydrostatic and osmotic forces across the endothelium

The direction and the magnitude of the movement of water across the capillary wall are determined by the algebraic sum of the hydrostatic and osmotic pressures that exist across the membrane. An increase in the intracapillary hydrostatic pressure favors the movement of fluid from the vessel to the interstitial space. Conversely, an increase in the concentration of osmotically active particles within the vessels favors the movement of fluid into the vessels from the interstitial space.

Hydrostatic force is dependent on pressure and resistance

The hydrostatic pressure (blood pressure) within the capillaries is not constant; it depends on the arterial pressure, the venous pressure, and the precapillary (arterioles) and postcapillary (venules and small veins) resistances. A rise in the arterial or venous pressure increases capillary hydrostatic pressure (P_c), whereas a reduction in either has the opposite effect. An increase in arteriolar resistance reduces capillary pressure, whereas an increase in venous resistance raises capillary pressure.

CAPILLARY HYDROSTATIC PRESSURE IS THE PRINCIPAL FORCE IN CAPILLARY FILTRATION, and the pressure varies from tissue to tissue and even within the same tissue. Average values, which were obtained from many direct measurements in human skin, are about 32 mm Hg at the arterial end of the capillaries and about 15 mm Hg at the venous end of the capillaries at the level of the heart (**Figure 22–7**). When an individual stands, the hydrostatic pressures in the capillaries of the lower extremities are higher and those of capillaries in the head are lower than when the individual is recumbent.

Tissue pressure, or more specifically **interstitial fluid pressure** (P_i), outside the capillaries, opposes capillary filtration. Hydrostatic pressure minus interstitial fluid pressure ($P_c - P_i$) constitutes the driving force for filtration. In the absence of edema, the P_i is essentially zero.

Osmotic forces restrain fluid loss

THE KEY FACTOR THAT RESTRAINS FLUID LOSS FROM THE CAPILLARIES IS THE OSMOTIC PRESSURE OF THE PLASMA PROTEINS, USUALLY TERMED THE **COLLOID OSMOTIC PRESSURE** OR **ONCOTIC PRESSURE** (**π_p**) (see Chapter 1). The total osmotic pressure of plasma is about 6000 mm Hg, whereas the oncotic pressure is only

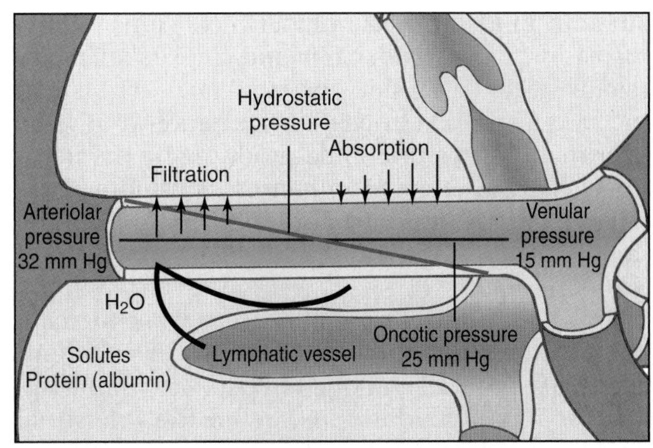

FIGURE 22–7. Factors responsible for filtration and absorption across the capillary wall and for the formation of lymph.

about 25 mm Hg. However, this small oncotic pressure is important in fluid exchange across the capillary wall because the plasma proteins are essentially confined to the intravascular space. The electrolytes that are mainly responsible for the total osmotic pressure of plasma are virtually equal in concentration on both sides of the capillary endothelium. The relative permeability of solute to that of water influences the actual magnitude of the osmotic pressure.

The **reflection coefficient** is the relative impediment to the passage of a substance through the capillary membrane. The reflection coefficient of water is 0 and that of albumin (to which the endothelium is almost impermeable) is 1. Filterable solutes have reflection coefficients between 0 and 1 (see Chapter 1).

Of the plasma proteins, albumin preponderates in determining oncotic pressure. The average albumin molecule (MW, 69,000) is approximately half the size of the average globulin molecule (MW, 150,000), and it is present in a greater concentration than the globulins (4.0 versus 3.0 g/dL of plasma). Albumin also exerts a greater osmotic force than can be accounted for solely on the basis of the number of molecules dissolved in the plasma. Therefore, albumin cannot be completely replaced by inert substances of the same molecular size (e.g., dextran). This additional osmotic force becomes disproportionately greater at high concentrations of albumin (as in plasma), and it is weak to absent in dilute solutions of albumin (as in interstitial fluid).

One reason for the behavior of albumin is its negative charge at a normal blood pH. The negatively charged albumin attracts and retains cations (principally Na^+) in the vascular compartment (the Gibbs-Donnan effect; see Chapter 2). Furthermore, albumin binds a small number of Cl^- ions, which increases its negative charge and thus its ability to retain more Na^+ inside the capillaries. The small increase in the electrolyte concentration of plasma over that of interstitial fluid produced by the negatively charged albumin enhances its osmotic force relative to that of an ideal solution containing the same concentration of a solute with an MW of 37,000.

Small amounts of albumin escape from the capillaries and enter the interstitial fluid. This albumin exerts a very small osmotic force (0.1 to 5 mm Hg) because its concentration is low in the interstitial fluid, and at low concentrations, the osmotic force of albumin becomes simply a function of the number of albumin molecules per unit volume of interstitial fluid; the additional osmotic force caused by albumin's negative charge is absent.

Starling's hypothesis describes the balance of hydrostatic and osmotic forces

The relationship between hydrostatic pressure and oncotic pressure and the role of these pressures in regulating fluid passage across the capillary endothelium were expounded by Ernest Starling in 1896. Starling's hypothesis is expressed by the following equation:

$$Q_f = k[(P_c + \pi_i) - (P_i + \pi_p)] \qquad 22\text{-}2$$

where

Q_f = fluid movement across the capillary wall

k = filtration constant for the capillary membrane

P_c = capillary hydrostatic pressure (mm Hg)

π_i = interstitial fluid oncotic pressure (mm Hg)

P_i = interstitial fluid hydrostatic pressure (mm Hg)

π_p = plasma oncotic pressure (mm Hg)

Net filtration occurs when the algebraic sum of the hydrostatic and osmotic pressures across the capillaries is positive, and net absorption occurs when the sum is negative.

Classically, filtration was thought to occur at the arterial end of the capillary and absorption at its venous end because of the gradient of hydrostatic pressure along the capillary. This is true for the idealized capillary, as depicted in Figure 22–7. However, in some vascular beds (e.g., the renal glomerulus), hydrostatic pressure in the capillary is high enough to result in filtration along the entire length of the capillary. In other vascular beds (e.g., in the intestinal mucosa), the hydrostatic and oncotic forces are such that absorption occurs along the whole capillary.

In the normal steady state, arterial pressure, venous pressure, postcapillary resistance, interstitial fluid hydrostatic and oncotic pressures, and plasma oncotic pressure remain relatively constant, and changes in precapillary resistance determine the movement of fluid across the capillary wall. Because water moves so quickly across the capillary endothelium, the hydrostatic and osmotic forces are nearly in steady state along the entire capillary. Thus, filtration and absorption normally occur with very small imbalances of pressure across the capillary wall. Only about 2% of the plasma flowing through the vascular system is filtered, and of this, about 85% is absorbed in the capillaries and venules. The remainder returns to the vascular system in the lymph, along with the albumin that escapes from the capillaries.

In the lungs, the mean capillary hydrostatic pressure is only about 8 mm Hg. Because the plasma oncotic pressure is 25 mm Hg and interstitial fluid oncotic pressure is approximately 15 mm Hg, the net force slightly favors reabsorption. Pulmonary lymph is formed, however, and it consists of fluid that is osmotically drawn out of the capillaries by the small amount of plasma protein that escapes through the capillary endothelium.

> In pathological conditions such as **left ventricular failure** or **mitral valve stenosis,** the pulmonary capillary hydrostatic pressure may exceed plasma oncotic pressure. Accordingly, **pulmonary edema,** a condition that can seriously interfere with gas exchange in the lungs, may occur.

The capillary filtration coefficient is a convenient way to estimate the rate of fluid movement across the capillary endothelium

The rate of fluid movement (Q_f) across the capillary membrane depends not only on the algebraic sum of the hydrostatic and osmotic pressures (ΔP) across the endothelium but also on the area (A_m) of the capillary wall available for filtration, the distance (Δx) across the capillary wall (i.e., the thickness), the viscosity (η) of the filtrate, and the filtration constant (k) of the membrane, as follows:

$$Q_f = kA_m\Delta P/\eta\Delta x \qquad 22\text{-}3$$

Because the thickness and area of the capillary wall and the viscosity of the filtrate are relatively constant for a given preparation, they can be incorporated with the filtration constant in a total filtration constant (k_t), which is expressed per unit weight of tissue. Hence, the equation can be simplified to the following:

$$Q_f = k_t \Delta P \qquad 22\text{-}4$$

where k_t is the total capillary filtration coefficient and the units for Q_f are milliliters per minute per 100 g of tissue.

In any given tissue, the filtration coefficient per unit area of capillary surface—and thus capillary permeability—is changed neither by physiological conditions such as arteriolar dilation and capillary distention nor by adverse conditions such as hypoxia, hypercapnia, and acidosis.

Capillary injury (e.g., toxins, severe burns) increases capillary permeability greatly (as indicated by an increased filtration coefficient), and significant amounts of fluid and protein leak out of the capillaries into the interstitial space. One of the important therapeutic measures used in the treatment of extensive **burns** is the replacement of lost fluid and plasma proteins.

Physiological states can disturb hydrostatic-osmotic balance

Modest changes in arterial pressure may have little effect on filtration because the change may be countered by adjustments of the precapillary resistance vessels (autoregulation; see Chapter 23).

In a condition such as **hemorrhage,** in which arterial and venous pressures are severely reduced, the capillary hydrostatic pressure falls. Furthermore, the low arterial blood pressure in hemorrhage decreases blood flow (and thus O_2 supply) to the tissues; therefore, vasodilator metabolites accumulate and relax the arterioles. The reduced transmural pressure also induces precapillary vessel relaxation. Consequently, absorption predominates over filtration and thereby constitutes one of the body's compensatory mechanisms for restoring blood volume (see also Chapter 26).

An increase in venous pressure, as occurs in the feet when a person changes from the lying to the standing position, elevates capillary pressure and enhances filtration (see Chapter 24). However, the increase in transmural pressure causes precapillary vessel closure (myogenic mechanism; see Chapter 23); therefore, the capillary filtration coefficient decreases. This reduction in the capillary surface available for filtration protects against the extravasation of large amounts of fluid into the interstitial space.

The elevation of venous pressure (e.g., in **pregnancy** or **congestive heart failure,** combined with standing) enhances filtration beyond the capacity of the lymphatic system in the legs to remove the capillary filtrate from the interstitial space. **Edema** of the ankles and lower legs results.

The protein concentration in plasma may also change in pathological states. Thus, it may alter the osmotic force and movement of fluid across the capillary membrane.

The plasma protein concentration is increased in **dehydration** (e.g., from water deprivation, prolonged sweating, severe vomiting, or diarrhea), and water moves by osmotic forces from the tissues to the vascular compartment. In contrast, the plasma protein concentration is reduced in **nephrosis** (a renal disease in which protein is lost in the urine), and edema may occur. When capillaries are injured, as in burns, protein along with fluid escapes from the plasma into the interstitial space and increases the oncotic pressure of the interstitial fluid. This greater osmotic force outside the capillaries causes additional fluid loss from the vascular system and may lead to severe intravascular **hypovolemia.**

Pinocytosis enables large molecules to cross the capillary endothelium

Some transfer of substances across the capillary wall can occur in tiny vesicles; this process is called **pinocytosis** (see Chapter 1). Pinocytotic vesicles, formed by pinching off a section of the surface membrane, can take up substances on one side of the capillary endothelial cell, move by thermal kinetic energy across the cell, and deposit their contents at the other side of the endothelial cell. The amount of material that can be transported in this way is much less than that moved by diffusion. However, pinocytosis may move large (30 nm) lipid-insoluble molecules between the blood and interstitial fluid. The number of pinocytotic vesicles in the endothelium varies with the tissue (muscle > lung > brain) and increases from the arterial to the venous end of the capillary.

The Lymphatics Return Fluid, and Solutes May Escape from the Capillaries to the Circulating Blood

The terminal lymphatic vessels consist of a widely distributed closed-end network of highly permeable lymph capillaries that resemble blood capillaries in appearance. However, they generally lack tight junctions between endothelial cells, and they possess fine filaments that anchor them to the surrounding connective tissue. During skeletal muscle contraction, these fine strands may distort the lymphatic vessel and open spaces between the endothelial cells. This distortion permits protein, large particles, and cells in the interstitial fluid to enter the lymphatic capillaries.

The blood capillary filtrate and the protein and cells that have passed from the intravascular compartment to the interstitial fluid compartment are returned to the circulation by virtue of tissue pressure. This process is facilitated by intermittent skeletal muscle contractions, contractions of the lymphatic vessels, and an extensive system of one-way valves. The lymph flows through thin-walled vessels of progressively larger diameter and finally enters the right and left subclavian veins at their junctions with the respective internal jugular veins. Only cartilage, bone, epithelium, and tissues of the central nervous system are devoid of lymphatic vessels.

The volume of fluid that flows through the lymphatic system in 24 hours is about equal to an animal's total plasma volume. The protein returned by the lymphatics to the blood in a day is about one fourth to one half of the circulating plasma proteins. Lymphatic return is the only means whereby protein (mainly albumin) leaving the vascular compartment can be returned to the blood because back-diffusion into the capillaries is negligible against the large albumin concentration gradient. If the protein was not removed from the interstitial spaces by the lymph vessels, it would accumulate in the interstitial fluid and act as an oncotic force to draw fluid from the blood capillaries to the interstitial spaces and produce edema.

In addition to returning fluid and protein to the vascular bed, the lymphatic system filters the lymph at the lymph nodes and removes foreign particles such as bacteria. Thus, the lymphatic system is an important component of the body's defense against bacterial invasion.

The largest lymphatic vessel, the thoracic duct, drains the lower extremities, returns protein lost through the permeable liver capillaries, and carries substances (principally fat in the form of chylomicrons) that are absorbed from the gastrointestinal tract to the circulating blood.

Lymph flow varies considerably; it is almost nil in resting skeletal muscle but increases during exercise in proportion to the degree of muscle activity. Lymph flow is increased by any mechanism that enhances the rate of blood capillary filtration; such mechanisms include increased capillary pressure, increased capillary permeability, and decreased plasma oncotic pressure.

If the volume of interstitial fluid exceeds the drainage capacity of the lymphatics or if the lymphatic vessels become blocked, such as in **elephantiasis** (caused by **filariasis,** a worm infestation), interstitial fluid accumulates (edema), chiefly in the more compliant tissue (e.g., subcutaneous tissue).

Summary

- Blood flow through the capillaries is regulated chiefly by contraction and relaxation of the arterioles (resistance vessels).
- The capillaries, which consist of a single layer of endothelial cells, can withstand high transmural pressure by virtue of their small diameter. According to Laplace's law, wall tension equals the transmural pressure multiplied by the radius of the capillary ($T = Pr$).
- The endothelium is the source of EDRF (shown to be NO) and of prostacyclin, which relax vascular smooth muscles and oppose platelet aggregation.
- The movement of water and small solutes between the vascular and interstitial fluid compartments occurs through capillary pores mainly by diffusion but also by filtration and absorption.
- Because the rate of diffusion is about 40 times greater than the blood flow in the tissue, the exchange of small lipid-insoluble molecules is flow limited. The larger the molecules, the slower the diffusion, until the lipid-insoluble molecules become diffusion limited. Molecules larger than about 60,000 MW are essentially confined to the vascular compartment.
- Lipid-soluble substances such as CO_2 and O_2 pass directly through the lipid membranes of the capillary endothelial cells, and the ease of transfer is directly proportional to the degree of lipid solubility of the substance.

- Capillary filtration and absorption are described by Starling's equation: $Q_f = k[(P_c + \pi_i) - (P_i + \pi_p)]$. Net filtration occurs when the algebraic sum of $(P_c + \pi_i)$ and $(P_i + \pi_p)$ is positive, and net absorption occurs when it is negative.
- By a process called pinocytosis, large molecules can move across the capillary wall in vesicles formed from the lipid membrane of the capillaries.
- Fluid and protein that have escaped from the blood capillaries enter the lymphatic capillaries and are transported via the lymphatic system back to the blood vascular compartment.

Bibliography

Aukland K: Why don't our feet swell in upright position? *News Physiol Sci* 9:214, 1994.

Aukland K, Reed RK: Interstitial-lymphatic mechanisms in the control of extracellular fluid volume, *Physiol Rev* 73:1, 1993.

Bert JL, Pearce RH: The interstitium and microvascular exchange. In Renkin EM, Michel CC, eds: *Handbook of physiology, section 2, The cardiovascular system, vol 4, parts 1 and 2, Microcirculation,* Bethesda, Md, 1984, American Physiological Society.

Crone C, Levitt DG: Capillary permeability to small solutes. In Renkin EM, Michel CC, eds: *Handbook of physiology, section 2, The cardiovascular system, vol 4, parts 1 and 2, Microcirculation,* Bethesda, Md, 1984, American Physiological Society.

Curry FRE: Regulation of water and solute exchange in microvessel endothelium: studies in single perfused capillaries, *Microcirculation* 1:11, 1994.

Furchgott RF: Endothelium-derived relaxing factor: discovery, early studies, and identification as nitric oxide, *Biosci Rep* 19:235, 1999.

Ignarro LJ et al: Nitric oxide as a signaling molecule in the vascular system: an overview, *J Cardiovasc Pharmacol* 34:879, 1999.

Luscher TF, Vanhoutte PM: *The endothelium: modulator of cardiovascular function,* Boca Raton, Fla, 1990, CRC Press.

Michel CC: Fluid movements through capillary walls In Renkin EM, Michel CC, eds: *Handbook of physiology, section 2, The cardiovascular system, vol 4, parts 1 and 2, Microcirculation,* Bethesda, Md, 1984, American Physiological Society.

Pries AR et al: Resistance to blood flow in microvessels in vivo, *Circ Res* 75:904, 1994.

Renkin EM: Control of microcirculation and blood-tissue exchange. In Renkin EM, Michel CC, eds: *Handbook of physiology, section 2, The cardiovascular system, vol 4, parts 1 and 2, Microcirculation,* Bethesda, Md, 1984, American Physiological Society.

Rippe B, Haraldsson B: Transport of macromolecules across microvascular walls: the two-pore theory, *Physiol Rev* 74:163, 1994.

Rosell S: Neuronal control of microvessels, *Annu Rev Physiol* 42:359, 1980.

Welsh DG, Segal SS: Endothelial and smooth muscle cell conduction in arterioles controlling blood flow, *Am J Physiol* 274:H178, 1998.

Xia J, Duling BR: Patterns of excitation-contraction coupling in arterioles: dependence on time and concentration, *Am J Physiol* 274:H323, 1998.

Case Studies

Case 22–1

A 45-year-old man with a long history of alcoholism (average 1 L/day of whiskey) was admitted to the hospital as an emergency because he vomited blood and fainted. In the past few months, he noted progressive anorexia, fatigue, jaundice, generalized itching, and abdominal swelling. Physical examination revealed a semicomatose man with pallor, jaundice, and ascites. The blood pressure was 90/40 mm Hg, the heart rate was 100 beats/min, and the hematocrit was 35%. Results of liver function tests indicated severe liver damage. The diagnosis was advanced cirrhosis of the liver. Immediate treatment was transfusion with 3 units of blood. The following pressures were noted before the transfusion:

Mesenteric capillary hydrostatic pressure (estimated)	44 mm Hg
Plasma oncotic pressure	23 mm Hg
Pressure in peritoneal cavity	8 mm Hg
Peritoneal fluid oncotic pressure	2 mm Hg

1. **Which transcapillary pressure was responsible for the ascites?**
   A. 11 mm Hg
   B. 21 mm Hg
   C. 8 mm Hg
   D. 15 mm Hg
   E. 13 mm Hg

2. **After lost blood was replaced by transfusion, how was this condition treated?**
   A. Dialysis
   B. High-fat diet
   C. Portacaval shunt
   D. Cholecystectomy
   E. Erythromycin

3. **Which substance is mainly responsible for the oncotic pressure of the patient's plasma?**
   A. Na^+
   B. Albumin
   C. Cl^-
   D. Globulin
   E. K^+

Case 22–2

A 25-year-old man suffered third-degree burns over the upper three fourths of his body in a fire in his home. Several hours elapsed before he reached the hospital. On admission, he was in a shock-like state. His heart rate was 110 beats/min, his blood pressure was 90/70 mm Hg, and his hematocrit was 55%. Blood analysis revealed a Na^+ level of 145 mEq/L, a K^+ level of 4 mEq/L, a Cl^- level of 105 mEq/L, and an albumin level of 3.5 g/dL.

1. **The *most* effective treatment is an intravenous infusion of which fluid?**
   A. Saline
   B. Whole blood
   C. 5% glucose
   D. Dextran
   E. Plasma

2. **After several months of treatment with extensive artificial skin grafts, the patient was able to walk and resume an almost normal life. However, after prolonged standing, he noted slight ankle swelling but no ecchymoses in his feet. Why did the capillaries in his feet not rupture when he stood?**
   A. Arterioles reflexly constrict and prevent exposure of the capillaries to high pressure.
   B. The tissue pressure rises and opposes an increase in the capillary pressure.
   C. The total capillary cross-sectional area is large enough to distribute the pressure and thereby compensate for the high intracapillary pressure.
   D. The capillary diameter is so small that the capillary wall tension is low.
   E. Capillaries constrict by a myogenic mechanism.

Chapter 23: Peripheral Circulation and Its Control

Objectives

- ❖ Indicate the intrinsic and extrinsic (neural and humoral) factors that regulate peripheral blood flow.
- ❖ Explain the autoregulation of blood flow and the myogenic mechanism for local adjustments of blood flow.
- ❖ Explain the metabolic regulation of blood flow.
- ❖ Explain the role of the sympathetic nerves in blood flow regulation.
- ❖ Describe vascular reflexes in the control of blood flow.
- ❖ Describe the role of humoral agents in the regulation of blood flow.

The function of the heart and large blood vessels is to pump and carry blood to the tissues of the body. The distribution of blood to the regions of the body where it is needed and away from where it is not needed rests with the small arteries and arterioles. THE REGULATION OF PERIPHERAL BLOOD FLOW IS ESSENTIALLY UNDER DUAL CONTROL: CENTRALLY BY THE NERVOUS SYSTEM AND LOCALLY IN THE TISSUES BY THE CONDITIONS IN THE IMMEDIATE VICINITY OF THE BLOOD VESSELS. In some areas of the body, such as the skin and the splanchnic regions, neural regulation of blood flow predominates; in others, such as the heart and the brain, local factors are dominant.

The small arteries and arterioles that regulate blood flow throughout the body are called the **resistance vessels.** These vessels offer the greatest resistance to the flow of blood pumped to the tissues by the heart and thereby are important in the maintenance of arterial blood pressure. Smooth muscle fibers are the main component of the walls of the resistance vessels (see Figure 15–2). Therefore, the vessel lumen can be varied from complete obliteration (by strong contraction of the smooth muscle with infolding of the endothelial lining) to maximal dilation (by full relaxation of the smooth muscle). At any given time, some resistance vessels are closed by partial contraction **(tone)** of the arteriolar smooth muscle. If all the resistance vessels in the body dilated simultaneously, the blood pressure would fall precipitously.

Contraction and Relaxation of Arteriolar Vascular Smooth Muscle Regulate Peripheral Blood Flow

Vascular smooth muscle controls total peripheral resistance and arterial and venous tone. The smooth muscle cells are small, mononucleate, and spindle shaped. They are generally arranged in several helical or circular layers around the larger vessels and in a thick circular layer around the arterioles (see Chapter 14). Passive stretching of the microvessels caused by an increase in intravascular pressure decreases vascular resistance, whereas a decrease in intravascular pressure increases vascular resistance via the recoil of the stretched vascular muscle.

Peripheral Blood Flow Is Controlled by Intrinsic Factors

Autoregulation and the myogenic mechanism tend to keep blood flow constant in the face of changes in perfusion pressure

Blood flow is adjusted to the existing metabolic activity in certain tissues. Furthermore, at constant levels of tissue metabolism, imposed changes in the perfusion pressure are met with vascular resistance changes that maintain a constant blood flow. This mechanism, which is illustrated in **Figure 23–1**, is commonly referred to as the **autoregulation of blood flow.** In the skeletal muscle preparation from which these data were gathered, the muscle was completely isolated from the rest of the animal and was in a resting state. The pressure was abruptly increased or decreased from a control pressure of 100 mm Hg. The blood flows observed immediately after the change in perfusion pressure are represented by the blue curve. Maintenance of the pressure at each new level was followed within 60 seconds by a return of flow to or toward the control level; the red curve represents those steady-state flows. Over the pressure range of 20 to 120 mm Hg, the steady-state flow is relatively constant. Calculation of resistance (pressure/flow) across the vascular bed during steady-state conditions indicates that when the perfusion pressure was elevated, the resistance vessels constricted, whereas when it was reduced, they dilated.

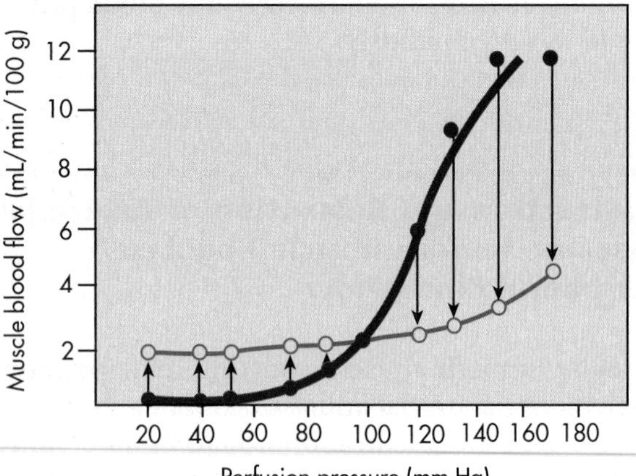

FIGURE 23–1. Pressure-flow relationship in the skeletal muscle vascular bed of the dog. The closed circles *(blue line)* represent the flows obtained immediately after abrupt changes in perfusion pressure from the control level (point where lines cross). The open circles *(red line)* represent the steady-state flows obtained at the new perfusion pressure. (Data from Jones RD, Berne RM: *Circ Res* 14:126, 1964.)

A **myogenic mechanism** appears to be responsible for this constancy of blood flow in the presence of an altered perfusion pressure. ACCORDING TO THE MYOGENIC MECHANISM, THE VASCULAR SMOOTH MUSCLE CONTRACTS IN RESPONSE TO STRETCH AND RELAXES WITH A REDUCTION IN STRETCH. An abrupt increase in perfusion pressure initially distends the blood vessels. This passive vascular distention is followed by contraction of the smooth muscles of the resistance vessels and a return of blood flow to the previous control level.

The operation of a myogenic mechanism would be expected to be minimal because blood pressure is reflexly maintained at a fairly constant level under normal conditions. However, when a person changes from a lying to a standing position, a large increase in transmural pressure occurs in the vessels of the lower extremities. The precapillary vessels constrict in response to this imposed stretch. The constriction diminishes capillary filtration until the increase in plasma oncotic pressure and the increase in interstitial fluid pressure balance the elevated capillary hydrostatic pressure associated with the vertical position (see Chapters 22 and 24).

If arteriolar resistance did not increase with standing, the hydrostatic pressure in the lower parts of the legs would reach such high levels that large volumes of fluid would pass from the capillaries into the interstitial fluid compartment and produce **edema.** In a patient with elevated venous pressure, as in **heart failure,** the added hydrostatic pressure in the standing position produces edema of the feet, ankles, and lower legs.

The endothelium actively regulates blood flow

The endothelial lining of blood vessels produces vasoactive factors (NO, endothelin) that regulate vascular caliber. Production and release of these factors are regulated by chemical (acetylcholine, bradykinin) and physical factors. An example of physical control by the endothelium is shown in **Figure 23–2** taken from an experiment with an isolated arteriole perfused at constant transmural pressure. In isolated coronary arterioles perfused at constant transmural pressure, rapid blood flow elicits vasodilation (Figure 23–2, *A*). The vasodilation is caused by **endothelium-derived relaxing factor (NO),** which is released by the endothelial cells in response to the shear stress that the rapid flow exerts on the vascular endothelium. The vessel does not dilate in response to increased flow after the endothelium has been removed

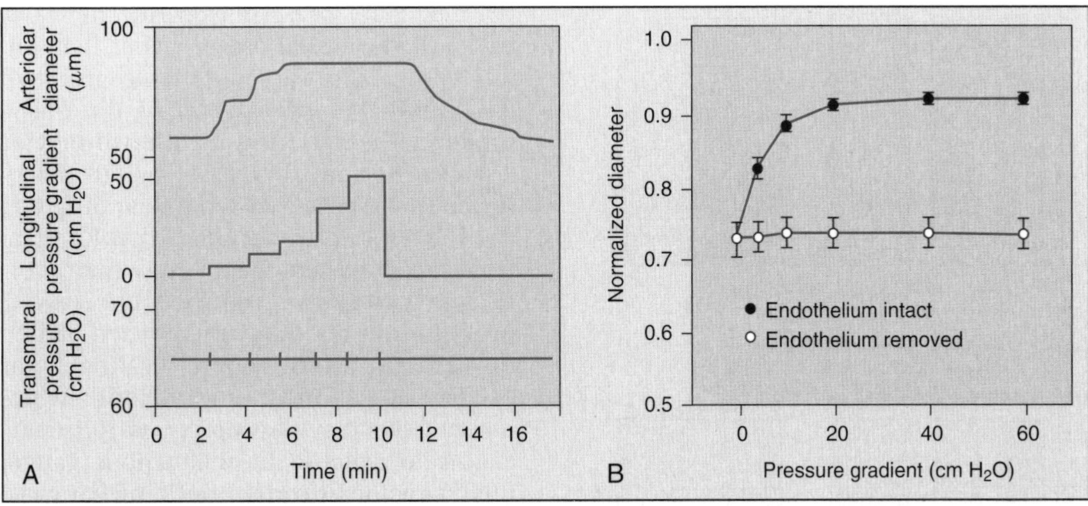

FIGURE 23–2. A, Flow-induced vasodilation in an isolated cardiac arteriole perfused at constant transmural pressure. The flow rate was increased by raising a reservoir connected to the proximal end of the cannulated arteriole. The transmural pressure *(bottom line)* was held constant by lowering a reservoir connected to the distal end of the arteriole by the same amount as the proximal reservoir was raised. The longitudinal pressure gradient *(center line)* was elevated in steps by raising the proximal reservoir and lowering the distal reservoir. The flow rate (not shown) was increased proportionately to the increase in the longitudinal pressure gradient (driving pressure). The arteriolar diameter *(top line)* increased with the rise in driving pressure. B, Flow-induced vasodilation is abolished when the endothelium is removed from the arteriole. (Data from Kuo L, Davis MJ, Chilian WM: *Am J Physiol* 259:H1063, 1990.)

(Figure 23–2, *B*). Presumably, the release of NO caused by increased shear stress is absent in the endothelium-denuded vessel.

Tissue metabolic activity is the main factor in the local regulation of blood flow

According to the metabolic hypothesis, BLOOD FLOW IS GOVERNED BY THE METABOLIC ACTIVITY OF THE TISSUE. ANY INTERVENTION THAT IMPEDES O_2 SUPPLY TO THE TISSUE RELEASES VASODILATOR METABOLITES FROM THE TISSUE. When the metabolic rate of the tissue increases or the O_2 delivery to the tissue decreases, more vasodilator substance is formed, and blood flow increases. If perfusion pressure is constant, a decrease in metabolic activity will decrease the concentration of the vasodilator in the tissue and thereby increase precapillary resistance. Similarly, if metabolic activity is constant, an increase in perfusion pressure and consequently in blood flow will decrease the tissue concentration of the vasodilator agent (metabolite washout) and increase precapillary resistance. An attractive feature of the metabolic hypothesis is that in most tissues, blood flow closely parallels metabolic activity. Thus, even when blood pressure is kept fairly constant, tissue metabolic activity and blood flow may vary together under physiological conditions.

Many substances, including lactic acid, CO_2, H^+, Na^+, inorganic phosphate ions, interstitial fluid osmolarity, adenosine, and NO, have been proposed as mediators of metabolic vasodilation. However, none of these agents alone fulfills all of the criteria for a physiological vasodilator in skeletal muscle.

Metabolic control of vascular resistance by the release of a vasodilator is predicated on the existence of **basal tone**—that is, the partial contraction (tonic activity) of vascular smooth muscle. In contrast to basal tone in skeletal striated muscle, basal tone in vascular smooth muscle is independent of the nervous system, and the factor responsible is not known. It could be related to the muscles, a vasoconstrictor substance in the blood, or both.

If arterial inflow to a vascular bed is stopped for a few seconds to several minutes, blood flow immediately after the release of the occlusion exceeds the flow before the occlusion, and it returns only gradually to the control level. This increase in blood flow **(reactive hyperemia)** is illustrated in **Figure 23–3**, in which blood flow to the leg was stopped by clamping the femoral artery for 15, 30, and 60 seconds. Release of the 60-second occlusion resulted in a peak blood flow that was 70% greater than the control flow, and the flow returned to the control level within about 110 seconds.

When this same experiment is done in humans by inflation of a blood pressure cuff on the upper arm, dilation of the resistance vessels of the hand

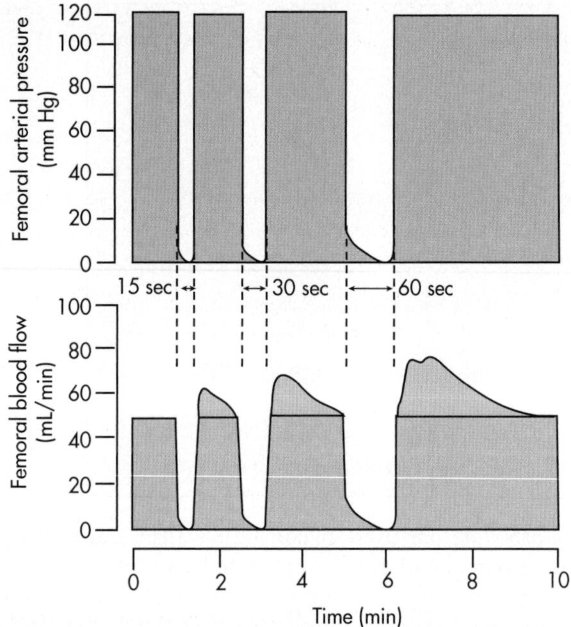

FIGURE 23–3. Reactive hyperemia in the hind limb of a dog after 15-, 30-, and 60-second occlusions of the femoral artery. (From Berne RM: Unpublished observations.)

and forearm is evident as a bright red skin color and a fullness of the veins, which occur immediately after the cuff is released. Within limits, the peak flow and particularly the duration of the reactive hyperemia are proportional to the duration of the occlusion (Figure 23–3). If the arm is exercised during the occlusion period, reactive hyperemia is increased. These observations and the close relationship that exists between metabolic activity and blood flow in the unoccluded limb are consonant with the concept of metabolic regulation of tissue blood flow.

Extrinsic Control of Peripheral Blood Flow Is Mediated Mainly by the Sympathetic Nervous System

Impulses in regions of the medulla descend in the sympathetic nerves to increase vascular resistance

Several regions in the medulla oblongata influence cardiovascular activity (see Chapter 19). Stimulation of the dorsal lateral medulla causes vasoconstriction, cardiac acceleration, and enhanced myocardial contractility. Caudal and ventromedial to the pressor region in the medulla is a zone that decreases blood pressure on stimulation. This **depressor area** exerts its effect by the direct inhibition of spinal neurons and by the inhibition of the medullary **pressor region.** These areas constitute a physiological center rather than an anatomical center because no discrete group of cells is discernible, yet stimulation of the pressor region produces the responses mentioned previously.

From the vasoconstrictor regions, fibers descend in the spinal cord and synapse at different levels of the thoracolumbar region (T1 to L2 or L3). Fibers from the intermediolateral gray matter of the cord emerge with the ventral roots but leave the motor fibers to join the paravertebral sympathetic chains through the white communicating branches (see Chapter 10). These preganglionic white (myelinated) fibers may pass up or down the sympathetic chains to synapse in the various ganglia within the chains or in certain outlying ganglia. Postganglionic gray branches (unmyelinated) then join the corresponding segmental spinal nerves and accompany them to the periphery to innervate the arteries and veins. Postganglionic sympathetic fibers from the various ganglia join the large arteries and accompany them as an investing network of fibers to the resistance (arterioles) and capacitance (veins) vessels.

The vasoconstrictor regions are tonically active. Reflexes or humoral stimuli that enhance this activity increase the frequency of impulses reaching the terminal branches of the vessels. A neurohumor (norepinephrine) is released from the postganglionic nerve endings and constricts (α-adrenergic effect) the resistance vessels. Inhibition of the vasoconstrictor area diminishes the frequency of impulses in the efferent fibers, and this effect results in vasodilation. In this manner, NEURAL REGULATION OF THE PERIPHERAL CIRCULATION IS ACCOMPLISHED MAINLY BY ALTERING THE NUMBER OF IMPULSES PASSING DOWN THE VASOCONSTRICTOR FIBERS OF THE SYMPATHETIC NERVES TO THE BLOOD VESSELS. The tonic activity of the vasomotor regions may vary rhythmically, which is manifested as oscillations of arterial pressure. Some oscillations occur at the frequency of respiration **(Traube-Hering waves)** because sympathetic impulses to the resistance vessels increase during inspiration. Other oscillations **(Mayer waves)** occur at a lower frequency than that of respiration.

An increase in sympathetic nerve activity constricts resistance and capacitance vessels

The vasoconstrictor fibers of the sympathetic nervous system supply the arteries, arterioles, and veins, but the neural influence on the large vessels is far less important functionally than it is on the microcirculation. Capacitance vessels (veins) are more responsive than resistance vessels to sympathetic nerve stimulation; they are maximally constricted at a lower frequency of stimulation than resistance vessels are. However, capacitance vessels respond less to vasodilator metabolites. Norepinephrine is the neurotransmitter released at the sympathetic nerve terminals at the blood vessels. Many other factors, such as circulating hormones and particularly locally released substances, modify the liberation of norepinephrine from the nerve terminals.

At basal vascular tone, approximately one third of the blood volume in a tissue can be mobilized from the capacitance vessels on stimulation of the sympathetic nerves at physiological frequencies. Only small increases in tissue blood volume are obtained with maximum doses of the potent vasodilator acetylcholine because basal tone is very low in capacitance vessels. Hence, at basal tone, the tissue blood volume is close to maximum. In exercise, activation of the sympathetic nerve fibers constricts veins and augments central venous pressure and hence the cardiac filling pressure.

In **arterial hypotension,** such as that induced by hemorrhage, the capacitance vessels constrict and thereby aid in overcoming the associated decrease in central venous pressure. In addition, the resistance vessels constrict in **hemorrhagic shock** and thereby assist in the restoration of arterial pressure (see Chapter 26). Furthermore, extravascular fluid is mobilized by a greater reabsorption of fluid from the tissues into the capillaries in response to the lowered capillary hydrostatic pressure caused by the lower arterial pressure.

Parasympathetic neural influence is apparent only in blood vessels in the cranial and sacral regions

The efferent fibers of the cranial division of the parasympathetic nervous system supply the blood vessels of the head and viscera; fibers of the sacral division supply the blood vessels of the genitalia, bladder, and large bowel. Skeletal muscle and skin do not receive parasympathetic innervation. The effect of these cholinergic fibers on total vascular resistance is small because only a small proportion of the resistance vessels of the body receives parasympathetic fibers.

Epinephrine and norepinephrine are the chief humoral factors that affect vascular resistance

Epinephrine and norepinephrine exert a profound effect on the peripheral blood vessels. In skeletal muscle, epinephrine in low concentrations dilates resistance vessels (β-adrenergic effect) and in high concentrations constricts them (α-adrenergic effect). However, in skin, only vasoconstriction occurs with epinephrine. In contrast, norepinephrine elicits vasoconstriction in all vascular beds. When stimulated, the adrenal gland releases mainly epinephrine but also some norepinephrine into the systemic circulation (see Chapter 48). Under physiological conditions, however, the effect of catecholamine release from the adrenal medulla is much less important than the effect of norepinephrine release from the sympathetic nerves.

Vascular reflexes are responsible for rapid adjustments of blood pressure

Areas of the medulla oblongata that mediate sympathetic and vagal effects are under the influence of neural impulses (arising in the baroreceptors, chemoreceptors, hypothalamus, cerebral cortex, and skin) and of local CO_2 and O_2 concentrations.

Baroreceptors

The **baroreceptors** (or **pressoreceptors**) are stretch receptors located in the **carotid sinuses** (slightly widened areas of the internal carotid arteries at their points of origin from the common carotid arteries; **Figure 23–4**) and in the **aortic arch.** Impulses arising in the carotid sinus travel up afferent fibers in the **carotid sinus nerve,** which is a branch of the glossopharyngeal nerve. Impulses arising in the baroreceptors of the aortic arch reach the medulla via afferent fibers in the vagus nerves. These fibers from both sets of baroreceptors travel to the **nucleus of the tractus solitarius (NTS)** in the medulla. The NTS is the site of central projection of the chemoreceptors and baroreceptors. Its stimulation inhibits sympathetic nerve impulses to the peripheral blood vessels and produces vasodilation **(depressor effect),** whereas experimental destruction of the NTS produces vasoconstriction **(pressor effect).**

THE BARORECEPTOR NERVE TERMINALS IN THE WALLS OF THE CAROTID SINUS AND AORTIC ARCH RESPOND TO THE VASCULAR STRETCH AND DEFORMATION INDUCED BY ARTERIAL PRESSURE. The frequency of firing is enhanced by an increase in blood pressure and diminished by a reduction in blood pressure. An increase in the impulse frequency inhibits the medullary vasoconstrictor regions and results in peripheral vasodilation and a lowering of blood pressure. Contributing to a lowering of the blood pressure is bradycardia caused by stimulation of the vagal nuclei in the medulla. The carotid sinus baroreceptors are more sensitive to pressure change

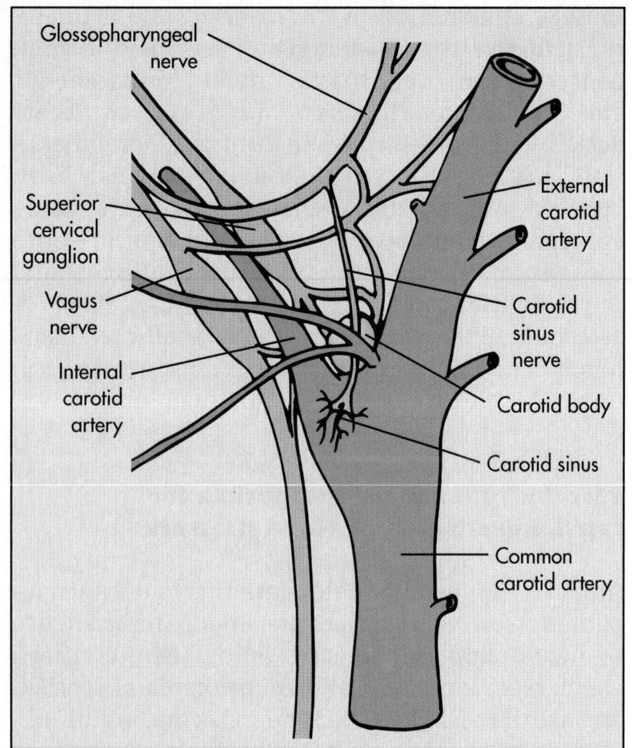

FIGURE 23–4. Carotid sinus and carotid body and their innervation in the dog. (Modified from Adams WE: *The comparative morphology of the carotid body and carotid sinus,* Springfield, Ill, 1958, Charles C Thomas.)

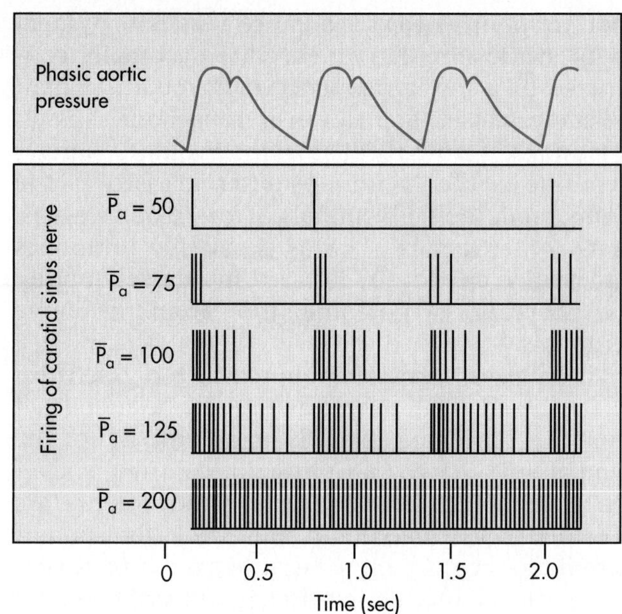

FIGURE 23–5. Relationship of phasic aortic blood pressure to the firing of a single afferent nerve fiber from the carotid sinus at different levels of mean arterial pressure ($\bar{P}_a$).

than the aortic baroreceptors are. However, when the blood pressure changes are pulsatile, the two sets of baroreceptors respond similarly.

The carotid sinus with the sinus nerve intact can be isolated from the rest of the circulation and artificially perfused. Under these conditions, changes in the pressure within the carotid sinus elicit reciprocal changes in the blood pressure of the experimental animal. The receptors in the walls of the carotid sinus adapt, and therefore they are more responsive to constantly changing pressures than to sustained constant pressures; this is illustrated in **Figure 23–5**. At normal levels of blood pressure, a barrage of impulses from a single fiber of the carotid sinus nerve is initiated in early systole by the pressure rise; only a few spikes are observed during late systole and early diastole (Figure 23–5). At lower pressures, these phasic changes are even more evident, but the overall frequency of discharge is reduced. The blood pressure threshold for eliciting sinus nerve impulses is about 50 mm Hg, and a maximum level of sustained firing is reached at approximately 200 mm Hg.

The baroreceptor response is greater to a large than to a small pulse pressure because baroreceptors adapt. This is illustrated in **Figure 23–6**, which shows the effects of damping pulsations in the carotid sinus on the frequency of firing in a sinus nerve fiber and on the systemic arterial pressure. When the pulse pressure in the carotid sinuses is reduced but mean pressure remains constant, the frequency of the neural impulses recorded from a sinus nerve fiber decreases, and the systemic arterial pressure increases. Restoration of the pulse

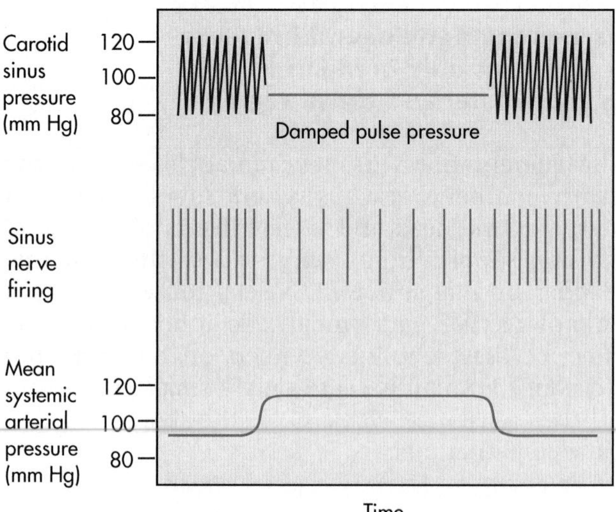

FIGURE 23–6. Effect of reducing pulse pressure in the vascularly isolated perfused carotid sinuses *(top)* on impulses recorded from a fiber of a sinus nerve *(middle)* and on the mean systemic arterial pressure *(bottom)*. The mean pressure in the carotid sinuses *(red line, top)* is constant when pulse pressure is damped.

pressure in the carotid sinus returns the frequency of sinus nerve discharge and systemic arterial pressure to control levels (Figure 23–6).

The resistance increases that occur in the peripheral vascular beds in response to reduced pressure in the carotid sinus vary from one vascular bed to another and thereby redistribute blood flow. For example, the resistance changes elicited in the dog by altering the carotid sinus pressure are greatest in the femoral vessels, less in the renal vessels, and least in the mesenteric and celiac vessels.

The sensitivity of the carotid sinus reflex can be altered. For example, in **hypertension,** when the carotid sinus becomes stiffer and less deformable as a result of the high intraarterial pressure, baroreceptor sensitivity decreases. A reduction in baroreceptor sensitivity is also observed in **chronic heart failure.** In some individuals, the carotid sinus is overly sensitive to pressure; tight collars or other forms of external pressure over the region of the carotid sinus may elicit **hypotension** and **fainting.**

THE BARORECEPTORS PLAY A KEY ROLE IN SHORT-TERM ADJUSTMENTS OF BLOOD PRESSURE WHEN THE CHANGES IN BLOOD VOLUME, CARDIAC OUTPUT, AND PERIPHERAL RESISTANCE ARE RELATIVELY ABRUPT (AS IN EXERCISE). HOWEVER, LONG-TERM CONTROL OF BLOOD PRESSURE (i.e., OVER DAYS OR WEEKS) IS DETERMINED MAINLY BY THE INDIVIDUAL'S FLUID BALANCE—NAMELY, THE BALANCE BETWEEN FLUID INTAKE AND OUTPUT. When peripheral resistance is constant, an increased blood volume raises blood pressure by augmenting cardiac output (see Chapter 24). BY FAR, THE MOST IMPORTANT ORGAN IN CONTROL OF BODY FLUID VOLUME AND THUS BLOOD PRESSURE IS THE KIDNEY. With overhydration, the excess fluid is excreted, whereas with dehydration, urine output is reduced.

Cardiopulmonary baroreceptors

In addition to the carotid sinus and aortic baroreceptors, cardiopulmonary receptors also exist; both types of receptors are necessary for the full expression of blood pressure regulation. Cardiopulmonary receptors initiate reflexes via vagal and sympathetic afferent and efferent nerves. These reflexes are tonically active, and they can alter peripheral resistance in response to changes in intracardiac, venous, and pulmonary vascular pressures.

Peripheral chemoreceptors are stimulated by decreases in arterial blood O_2 tension and increases in arterial blood CO_2 tension

The **peripheral chemoreceptors** consist of the carotid body (at the bifurcation of the carotid artery) and several small, highly vascular bodies in the regions of the aortic arch. THE CHEMORECEPTORS ARE SENSITIVE TO CHANGES IN ARTERIAL BLOOD O_2 TENSION ($Pa{O_2}$), CO_2 TENSION ($Pa{CO_2}$), AND pH. Although they are concerned mainly with the regulation of respiration (see Chapter 31), the peripheral chemoreceptors reflexly influence the circulatory system to a minor degree.

A reduction in $Pa{O_2}$ stimulates the chemoreceptors. The resulting increase in the frequency of impulses in the afferent nerve fibers from the carotid and aortic bodies stimulates the vasoconstrictor regions; this action increases tone in the resistance and capacitance vessels. The **reflex** vascular effect induced by an increased $Pa{CO_2}$ and by a reduced pH is much less than the **direct** effect of **hypercapnia** (an elevated $Pa{CO_2}$) and of H^+ on the vasomotor regions in the medulla. When hypoxia and hypercapnia coexist **(asphyxia),** stimulation of the chemoreceptors is greater than the sum of the two blood gas stimuli acting independently. Simultaneous stimulation of the chemoreceptors and reduction of arterial pressure (reduced stimulation of the baroreceptors) enhance the vasoconstrictor response of the peripheral vessels. However, when both the baroreceptors and chemoreceptors are stimulated together (e.g., high carotid sinus pressure and low $Pa{O_2}$), the cardiovascular effects of the baroreceptors predominate.

Chemoreceptors with sympathetic afferent fibers exist in the heart. These cardiac chemoreceptors are activated by myocardial ischemia, and they transmit the precordial pain **(angina pectoris)** associated with an inadequate blood supply to the myocardium.

Hypothalamus

Optimal function of the cardiovascular reflexes requires the integrity of pontine and hypothalamic structures. Furthermore, these structures are responsible for behavioral and emotional control of the cardiovascular system. Stimulation of the anterior hypothalamus decreases blood pressure and heart rate, whereas stimulation of the posterolateral region increases blood pressure and heart rate. The hypothalamus also contains a temperature-regulating center that affects the skin vessels. Cooling of the skin or of the blood perfusing the hypothalamus results in constriction of the skin vessels and heat conservation; warm stimuli have the opposite effects.

Cerebrum

The cerebral cortex can also affect the blood flow distribution in the body. Stimulation of the motor and premotor areas can affect blood pressure; a pressor response is usually obtained. However, vasodilation and hypotensive responses may be evoked (e.g., blushing, fainting) in response to an emotional stimulus.

Skin and viscera

Painful stimuli can elicit either an increase or a decrease in blood pressure, depending on the magnitude and location of the stimulus. Distention of the viscera often decreases blood pressure, whereas painful stimuli on the body surface usually raise blood pressure.

Pulmonary reflexes

Inflation of the lungs reflexly dilates systemic resistance vessels and decreases arterial blood pressure. Conversely, collapse of the lungs causes the constriction of systemic vessels. Afferent fibers that mediate this reflex are carried in the vagus nerves. Stimulation of the pulmonary stretch receptors inhibits the vasomotor areas. The magnitude of the depressor response to lung inflation is directly related to the degree of inflation and to the existing level of vasoconstrictor tone; the greater the vascular tone, the greater the hypotension produced by lung inflation.

Chemosensitive regions of the medulla

Increases in Pa_{CO_2} stimulate the medullary vasoconstrictor regions and thereby increase peripheral resistance. Reduction in Pa_{CO_2} below normal levels (as with hyperventilation) decreases the tonic activity in these areas and thus decreases peripheral resistance. The chemosensitive regions are also affected by changes in pH. A lowering of blood pH stimulates and a rise in blood pH inhibits these areas.

Changes in Pa_{O_2} usually have little direct effect on the vasomotor region in the medulla. The reflex effect of hypoxia is mediated mainly by the carotid and aortic chemoreceptors. A moderate reduction of Pa_{O_2} stimulates the vasomotor region, but severe reduction depresses vasomotor activity, just as a very low Pa_{O_2} depresses other areas of the brain.

Cerebral ischemia, such as that which can occur with an expanding **intracranial tumor,** results in severe peripheral vasoconstriction. The stimulation is probably caused by a local accumulation of CO_2 and a reduction of O_2 in certain regions of the brain. With prolonged severe ischemia, extreme depression of cerebral function eventually supervenes, and the blood pressure falls.

Regulation of Peripheral Blood Flow Is Achieved by Balance Between Intrinsic and Extrinsic Factors

Dual control of the peripheral vessels by intrinsic and extrinsic mechanisms constitutes a complex system of vascular regulation. This system enables the body to direct blood flow to areas where the need is greater and to divert it away from areas where the need is less. In some tissues, the relative potency of extrinsic and intrinsic mechanisms is constant. However, in other tissues, the ratio is changeable, depending on that tissue's state of activity. In the brain and heart, which are vital structures with limited tolerance for a reduced blood supply, intrinsic flow-regulating mechanisms are dominant.

Massive discharge of the medullary vasoconstrictor region (which might occur in response to a severe, acute hemorrhage) has negligible effects on the cerebral and cardiac resistance vessels, but it greatly constricts the skin, renal, and splanchnic blood vessels.

In the skin, extrinsic vascular control is dominant. Not only do the cutaneous vessels participate strongly in a general vasoconstrictor discharge, but they also respond selectively through the hypothalamic pathways that subserve body temperature regulation. However, intrinsic control can be demonstrated by local changes of skin temperature that can modify or override the central influence on the resistance and capacitance vessels.

In skeletal muscle, the changing balance between extrinsic and intrinsic mechanisms can be clearly seen. In resting skeletal muscle, neural control (vasoconstrictor tone) is dominant. This can be demonstrated by the large increment in blood flow that occurs immediately after the sympathetic nerves to the muscle are cut. Just before and at the start of running, blood flow increases in the leg muscles. After the onset of exercise, the intrinsic flow-regulating mechanism assumes control. Because of the local increase in metabolites, vasodilation occurs in the active muscles. Vasoconstriction occurs in the inactive muscles and other tissues as a manifestation of the general sympathetic discharge associated with exercise. However, the constrictor impulses that reach the resistance vessels of the active muscles are overridden by the local metabolic effect, which dilates the vessels. Operation of this dual-control mechanism thus provides more blood where it is required and shunts it away from the inactive areas.

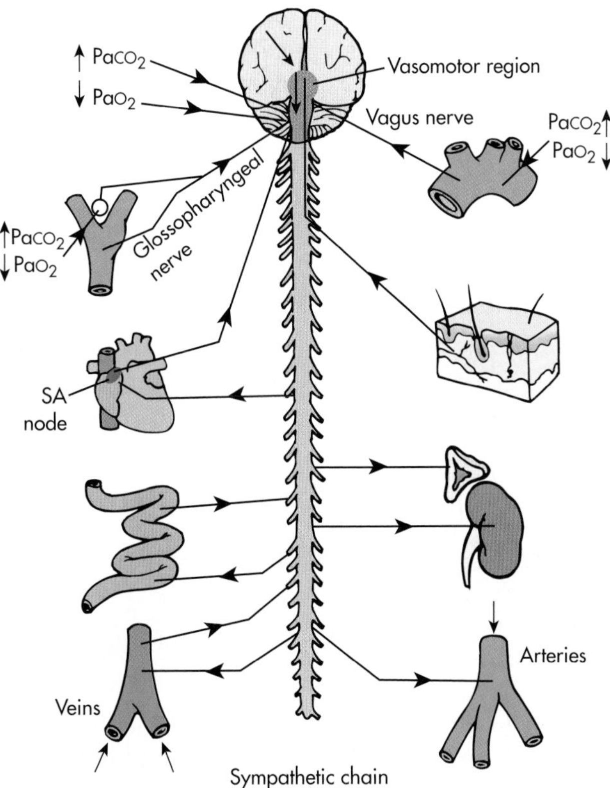

FIGURE 23–7. Neural input and output of the vasomotor region. SA node, sinoatrial node.

Similar effects may be achieved by a general increase in Pa_{CO_2}. Normally, the hyperventilation associated with exercise keeps the Pa_{CO_2} at normal levels. However, if the Pa_{CO_2} increases during exercise, generalized vasoconstriction occurs because of the stimulation of the medullary vasoconstrictor region by CO_2. In the active muscles, where the CO_2 concentration is highest, the smooth muscle of the arterioles relaxes in response to the high Pa_{CO_2} concentration locally. Factors that affect and that are affected by the medullary vasomotor region are summarized in **Figure 23–7**.

Summary

- The arterioles, often referred to as the *resistance vessels,* are important in the regulation of blood flow through their cognate capillaries. Smooth muscle, which constitutes a major fraction of the wall of the arterioles, contracts and relaxes in response to neural and humoral stimuli.
- Most tissues show autoregulation of blood flow, a phenomenon characterized by a relatively constant blood flow in the face of a substantial change in perfusion pressure. A logical explanation of autoregulation is the myogenic mechanism, by which an increase in transmural pressure elicits a direct contractile response of the vascular smooth muscle, whereas a decrease in transmural pressure directly elicits relaxation.
- The striking parallelism between tissue blood flow and tissue O_2 consumption indicates that blood flow is regulated largely by a metabolic mechanism. A decrease in the O_2 supply/demand ratio of a tissue releases one or more vasodilator metabolites that dilate arterioles and thereby enhance the O_2 supply.
- Neural regulation of blood flow is accomplished mainly by the sympathetic nervous system. Sympathetic nerves to blood vessels are tonically active; inhibition of the vasoconstrictor center in the medulla reduces peripheral vascular resistance. Stimulation of the sympathetic nerves constricts resistance and capacitance vessels.

- In the organs and tissues supplied by the cranial and sacral divisions of the parasympathetic nervous system, blood vessels are under parasympathetic (as well as sympathetic) control. Parasympathetic activity usually induces vasodilation, but the effect is ordinarily weak.
- The baroreceptors (or pressoreceptors) in the internal carotid arteries and aorta are tonically active and regulate blood pressure on a moment-to-moment basis. Stretch of these receptors caused by an increase in arterial pressure reflexly inhibits the vasoconstrictor center in the medulla and induces vasodilation, whereas a decrease in arterial pressure disinhibits the vasoconstrictor center and induces vasoconstriction.
- The carotid baroreceptors predominate over those in the aorta, and both respond more vigorously to pulsatile pressure (stretch) than to steady (nonpulsatile) pressures.
- Baroreceptors are also present in the cardiac chambers and large pulmonary vessels (cardiopulmonary baroreceptors); they have less influence on blood pressure than arterial baroreceptors do, but they participate in blood volume regulation.
- Peripheral chemoreceptors in the carotid bodies and aortic arch and central chemoreceptors in the medulla oblongata are stimulated by a decrease in Pa_{O_2} and by an increase in Pa_{CO_2}. Stimulation of these chemoreceptors generally increases the rate and depth of respiration but also produces peripheral vasoconstriction.
- Peripheral vascular resistance and hence blood pressure can be affected by stimuli arising in the skin, viscera, lungs, and brain.
- The combined effect of neural and local metabolic factors is to distribute blood to active tissues and to divert it from inactive tissues. In vital structures such as the heart and brain and in contracting skeletal muscle, metabolic factors predominate over neural factors.

Bibliography

Berg BR, Cohen KD, Sarelius IH: Direct coupling between blood flow and metabolism at the capillary level in striated muscle, *Am J Physiol* 272:H2693, 1997.

Cowley AW Jr: Long-term control of blood pressure, *Physiol Rev* 72:231, 1992.

Doyle MP, Duling BR: Acetylcholine induces conducted vasodilation by nitric oxide–dependent and –independent mechanisms, *Am J Physiol* 272:H1364, 1997.

Hainsworth R: Reflexes from the heart, *Physiol Rev* 71:617, 1991.

Hickner RC et al: Role of nitric oxide in skeletal muscle blood flow at rest and during dynamic exercise in humans, *Am J Physiol* 273:H405, 1997.

Kuo L, Davis JJ, Chilian WM: Endothelium-dependent flow-induced dilation of isolated coronary arterioles, *Am J Physiol* 259:H1063, 1990.

Marshall JM: Peripheral chemoreceptors and cardiovascular regulation, *Physiol Rev* 74:543, 1994.

Persson PB: Modulation of cardiovascular control mechanisms and their interaction, *Physiol Rev* 76:193, 1996.

Persson PB, Kirchheim HR, eds: *Baroreceptor reflexes,* Berlin, 1991, Springer-Verlag.

Porter VA et al: Frequency modulation of Ca^{2+} sparks is involved in regulation of arterial diameter by cyclic nucleotides, *Am J Physiol* 274:C1346, 1998.

Shepard JT: Cardiac mechanoreceptors. In Fozzard HA et al, eds: *The heart and cardiovascular system: scientific foundations,* ed 2, Philadelphia, 1991, Raven Press.

Shoemaker JK et al: Contributions of acetylcholine and nitric oxide to forearm blood flow at exercise onset and recovery, *Am J Physiol* 273:H2388, 1997.

Zucker IH, Gilmore JP, eds: *Reflex control of the circulation,* Boca Raton, Fla, 1991, CRC Press.

Case Studies

Case 23–1

A 40-year-old man goes to see his physician because of pain in the calves of both legs when he walks moderate distances; the pain is especially noticeable when he walks uphill or when he climbs stairs. The onset of the pain was insidious and has progressively increased in frequency and severity. He has had no other symptoms. He eats a normal diet, drinks two cocktails before dinner, and has smoked two packs of cigarettes per day for the past 22 years. The findings on physical examination were essentially normal except for the absence of pulses in the dorsalis pedis and posterior tibial arteries in both legs. Arteriography revealed a narrowing of the major arteries of both lower legs. He was diagnosed as having **thromboangiitis obliterans,** a severe progressive obstructive disease of large arteries.

1. **What do the arterioles in the lower legs show at rest in this subject?**
   A. Myogenic constriction
   B. Metabolic dilation
   C. Autoregulation
   D. Myogenic dilation
   E. Metabolic constriction

2. **What will the physician probably recommend?**
   A. Stopping smoking
   B. A vasodilator medication
   C. Bilateral sympathectomy of the lower extremities
   D. Application of heat to the lower legs three or four times a day
   E. A vasoconstrictor medication

Case 23–2

A 72-year-old man was admitted to the hospital for repeated brief episodes of loss of consciousness.

1. **Which of the following diagnoses should *not* be considered?**
   A. Carotid sinus hypersensitivity
   B. Complete heart block
   C. Orthostatic hypotension
   D. Atrial or ventricular tachycardia
   E. Diabetic coma

2. **The electrocardiogram indicated supraventricular (atrial) tachycardia (SVT) as the cause of his syncope, a rare complication of SVT. Which of the following would *not* be prescribed for treatment of this arrhythmia?**
   A. Intravenous adenosine
   B. Valsalva's maneuver
   C. Digitalis
   D. Carotid sinus massage
   E. Electrical ablation of the atrial ectopic focus

Chapter 24: Control of Cardiac Output: Coupling of the Heart and Blood Vessels

Objectives

- ❖ Describe the principal determinants of cardiac output.
- ❖ Describe the principal determinants of cardiac preload and afterload.
- ❖ Explain the mechanical coupling between the heart and blood vessels.
- ❖ Explain the effects of gravity on venous function.

The first few chapters in this part of the book deal with the operation of the heart, the energy source responsible for pumping blood to all the tissues of the body. The next several chapters deal with the operation and control of the various types of blood vessels that serve as the conduits for blood delivery to the tissues. This chapter describes and explains the principal interactions between the cardiac and vascular components of the cardiovascular system. Whereas the heart determines how much blood is pumped through the blood vessels, the blood vessels concurrently influence the quantity of blood that the heart pumps to the tissues.

Critical Cardiac and Vascular Factors Regulate Cardiac Output

FOUR MAJOR FACTORS CONTROL CARDIAC OUTPUT (Q_h): HEART RATE, MYOCARDIAL CONTRACTILITY, PRELOAD, AND AFTERLOAD (**Figure 24–1**). Heart rate and myocardial contractility are strictly **cardiac factors.** They are intrinsic characteristics of the cardiac tissues, although they are modulated by various neural and humoral mechanisms. As explained in Chapter 18, **preload** is the stretching force that acts on cardiac muscle before contraction, whereas **afterload** is the force that opposes cardiac muscle shortening. The preload and afterload depend on the characteristics of both the heart and the vascular system. NOT ONLY ARE PRELOAD AND AFTERLOAD IMPORTANT DETERMINANTS OF Q_h, BUT THESE FEATURES ARE ALSO DETERMINED BY Q_h. Hence, preload and afterload may be designated **coupling factors** (Figure 24–1) because they constitute a functional coupling between the heart and blood vessels.

The heart pumps blood around the vascular system, which is a closed circuit. The rate at which the blood is pumped around the circuit (i.e., Q_h) is an important determinant of preload and afterload. Concomitantly, the physical characteristics of the blood vessels determine preload and afterload. Hence, these coupling factors regulate the quantity of blood that the heart pumps around the circuit per unit time. Understanding the regulation of Q_h thus requires an appreciation of the nature of the coupling between the heart and vascular system.

Graphs that relate Q_h to preload are used to analyze some of the critical interactions between the heart and blood vessels. This graphic analysis involves two independent functional relationships between Q_h and preload. In this analysis, attention is directed to the right ventricular preload, which is the pressure in the right atrium and thoracic venae

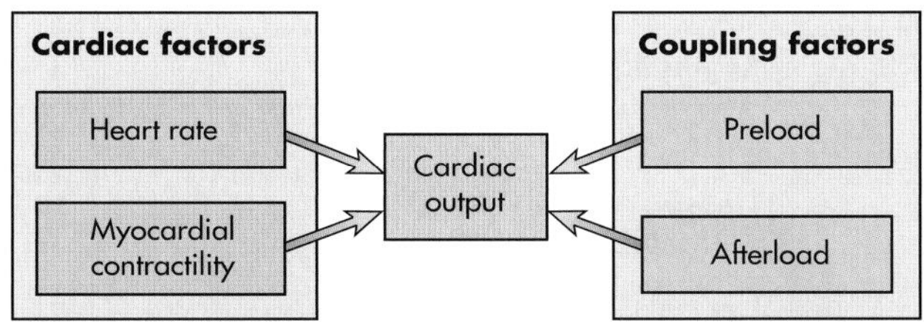

FIGURE 24–1. Determinants of cardiac output (Q_h).

cavae; this pressure is often called the **central venous pressure (P_v).**

The **cardiac function curve** defines the dependence of Q_h on preload—that is, the well-known Frank-Starling relationship (see Chapters 18 and 19). The cardiac function curve is a characteristic of the heart itself; classically, it was studied in hearts completely isolated from the rest of the circulatory system. Over the normal range of Q_h and P_v, this curve indicates that a rise in P_v leads to an increase in Q_h; that is, Q_h ORDINARILY VARIES DIRECTLY WITH P_v.

The other functional relationship between P_v and Q_h is defined by a second curve. THIS CURVE, THE **VASCULAR FUNCTION CURVE,** DEPICTS HOW Q_h AFFECTS P_v. This relationship depends on certain critical characteristics of the vascular system—namely, peripheral resistance, arterial (C_a) and venous (C_v) compliances, and blood volume. The vascular function curve is entirely independent of the characteristics of the heart; it applies even if the heart is replaced by a mechanical pump. The vascular function curve indicates that if the Q_h is increased, the P_v decreases; that is, P_v VARIES INVERSELY WITH Q_h.

Thus, the cardiac function curve indicates that Q_h ordinarily varies directly with P_v, whereas the vascular function curve indicates that P_v varies inversely with Q_h. These assertions seem contradictory, but as the following discussion indicates, this is not the case.

Cardiac Output Affects Central Venous Pressure

The vascular function curve defines the changes in P_v generated by changes in Q_h. Therefore, in this relationship, P_v is the dependent variable (or response) and Q_h is the independent variable (or stimulus).

The simplified schema of the circulation in **Figure 24–2** helps elucidate how the Q_h determines the level of the P_v. The essential components of the cardiovascular system have been lumped into four elements. The right and left sides of the heart and the pulmonary vascular bed are considered simply to be a pump-oxygenator, much as that used during open-heart surgery. In Figure 24–2, the energy source is simply called a pump. The high-resistance microcirculation is designated the peripheral resistance. Finally, the entire compliance of the system is subdivided into the following components: total C_a and total C_v (see Table 21–1). As defined in Chapter 21, compliance is the increment of volume (ΔV) accommodated per unit change of pressure (ΔP), as follows:

$$C \equiv \Delta V/\Delta P \qquad \textbf{24-1}$$

C_v normally is about 20 times greater than C_a. In the following example, the ratio of C_v to C_a is set at 19:1 to simplify certain calculations. Thus, if it were necessary to add *x* mL of blood to the arterial system to increase the arterial pressure (P_a) by 1 mm Hg, then it would be necessary to add 19*x* mL of blood to the venous system to raise P_v by the same amount.

Figure 24–2 illustrates simply why P_v varies inversely with Q_h. In this example, the model is endowed with characteristics that resemble those of a normal, resting adult (Figure 24–2, *A*). Suppose Q_h is 5 L/min, P_a is 102 mm Hg, and P_v is 2 mm Hg. The total peripheral resistance (R_t) is the ratio of pressure difference ($P_a - P_v$) to flow (runoff) through the peripheral resistance (Q_r). At equilibrium, Q_r equals Q_h. Hence, R_t equals 100/5 mm Hg, or 20 mm Hg/L/min. From heartbeat to heartbeat, the volume of blood in the arteries (V_a) and the volume of blood in the veins (V_v) remain constant because the volume of blood transferred from the veins to the arteries each minute by the heart (Q_h) equals the volume of blood that flows each minute from the arteries through the resistance vessels and into the veins (Q_r).

Imposing cardiac arrest in this model (Figure 24–2, *B*) helps explain the inverse relationship between Q_h and P_v in the vascular function curves. At the very moment that the heart stops, V_a and V_v have not had time to change appreciably. The P_a and P_v depend on V_a and V_v, respectively. Therefore, these pressures are identical to the respective pressures in Figure 24–2, *A* (i.e., P_a = 102 mm Hg, P_v = 2 mm Hg). The arteriovenous pressure gradient of 100 mm Hg forces a flow of 5 L/min through the peripheral resistance of 20 mm Hg/L/min. Thus, although Q_h now equals zero, the flow (Q_r) through the microcirculation equals 5 L/min (Figure 24–2, *B*). In other words, AT THE VERY BEGINNING OF CARDIAC ARREST, THE POTENTIAL ENERGY STORED IN THE ARTERIES BY THE PREVIOUS CONTRACTIONS OF THE HEART CAUSES BLOOD TO BE TRANSFERRED FROM ARTERIES TO VEINS CONTINUOUSLY, INITIALLY AT THE NORMAL CONTROL RATE, EVEN THOUGH THE HEART CAN NO

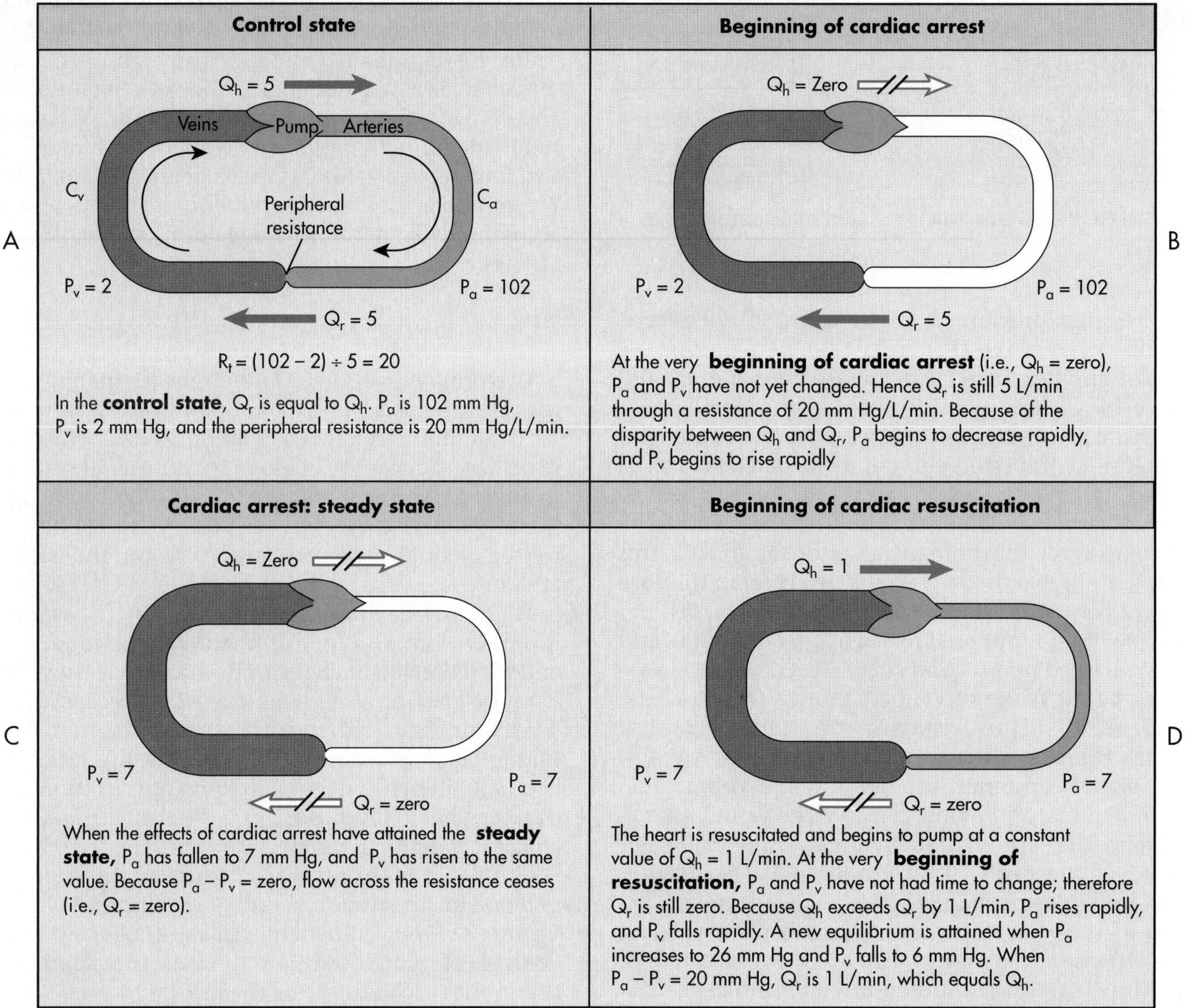

FIGURE 24–2. Simplified model of the cardiovascular system, which consists of a heart that generates a flow (Q_h), an arterial compliance (C_a), a total peripheral resistance (R_t), a flow through that resistance (Q_r), and a venous compliance (C_v).

LONGER TRANSFER BLOOD FROM THE VEINS BACK INTO THE ARTERIES.

After cardiac arrest is imposed, blood continues to flow from the systemic arteries to the systemic veins as long as P_a exceeds P_v (Figure 24–2, *B*). Therefore, V_a progressively decreases, and V_v progressively increases. Because the vessels are elastic structures, P_a progressively falls, and P_v progressively rises. This process continues until P_a and P_v become equal (Figure 24–2, *C*). Once this condition is reached, the flow (Q_r) from arteries to veins through the resistance vessels is zero, as is the Q_h.

At zero flow equilibrium (Figure 24–2, *C*), P_a and P_v depend on the relative compliances of these vessels. Had the C_a and C_v been equal, the decline in P_a would have been equal to the rise in P_v because the decrement in V_a equals the increment in V_v (principle of conservation of mass). P_a and P_v would have both attained the average of P_a plus P_v in Figure 24–2, *A* and *B;* that is, $P_a = P_v$ = (102 mm Hg + 2 mm Hg)/2 = 52 mm Hg.

In actual subjects, however, veins are much more compliant than arteries; the ratio is approximately equal to that assumed for the model (C_v:C_a = 19). Hence, the transfer of blood from arteries to veins at equilibrium would induce a fall in P_a 19 times greater than the concomitant rise in P_v. As Figure 24–2, *C*, shows, P_v increases by 5 mm Hg (to an equilibrium value of 7 mm Hg), whereas P_a falls by 19 × 5 = 95 mm Hg (to an equilibrium value of 7 mm Hg). This equilibrium pressure that exists in the absence of flow is referred to as the **mean**

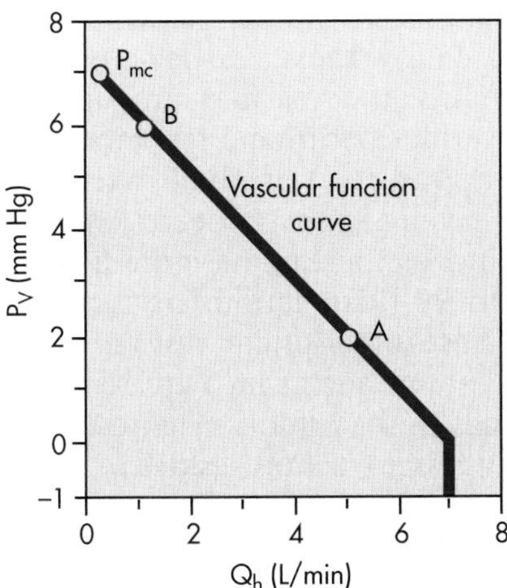

FIGURE 24–3. Changes in P_v produced by changes in Q_h. P_{mc} is the equilibrium pressure throughout the cardiovascular system when Q_h = zero. Points B and A represent P_v when Q_h = 1 and 5 L/min, respectively.

circulatory pressure (static pressure) (P_{mc}). The pressure in the static system reflects the total volume of blood in the system and the overall compliance of the system.

Two important points on the vascular function curve have already been derived, as shown in **Figure 24–3.** One point represents the normal status (depicted in Figure 24–2, *A*). Under control conditions, when Q_h was 5 L/min, P_v was 2 mm Hg. When flow stopped ($Q_h = 0$), P_v became 7 mm Hg at equilibrium; this pressure is the P_{mc}. This point is the *y*-axis intercept in Figure 24–3.

The inverse relationship between P_v and Q_h simply expresses the fact that when Q_h is suddenly decreased, the rate (Q_r) at which blood flows from arteries to the veins through the resistance vessels is temporarily greater than the rate (Q_h) at which the heart pumps it from the veins back into the arteries. During that transient period, a net volume of blood is translocated from the arteries to veins; hence, P_a falls and P_v rises.

In the circulation model shown in Figure 24–2, *D,* when the heart has been resuscitated after a period of cardiac arrest, it immediately begins to generate a Q_h of 1 L/min. Instantaneously, virtually no blood has yet been transferred from the veins to the arteries; therefore, the arteriovenous pressure gradient is zero (Figure 24–2, *D*). Consequently, blood does not flow at first from the arteries through the capillaries and into the veins; that is, $Q_r = 0$. When pumping resumes, blood is being transferred from the veins to the arteries at the rate of 1 L/min; P_v begins to fall, and P_a begins to rise. Because of the difference in compliances, P_a rises 19 times more rapidly than P_v falls.

The resulting arteriovenous pressure gradient causes blood to flow through the resistance vessels. If the pump maintains a constant output of 1 L/min, the P_a will continue to rise and the P_v will continue to fall until the pressure gradient becomes 20 mm Hg. It forces a flow of 1 L/min through a resistance of 20 mm Hg/L/min. This gradient is achieved by a rise of 19 mm Hg (to 26 mm Hg) in P_a and a fall of 1 mm Hg (to 6 mm Hg) in P_v. This equilibrium value of P_v = 6 mm Hg for a Q_h of 1 L/min appears as point B in Figure 24–3. It reflects a net transfer of blood from the venous to the arterial side of the circuit and a consequent reduction of the P_v.

The vascular function curve shows that as Q_h is increased, P_v is diminished (Figure 24–3). The reduction of P_v that can be achieved by an increase in Q_h is limited, however. At some critical maximum value of Q_h, sufficient fluid is translocated from the venous to the arterial side of the circuit to reduce the P_v below the ambient pressure (i.e., the intrathoracic pressure). In a system of very distensible vessels, such as the venous system, the vessels are collapsed by the greater external pressure. This venous collapse constitutes an impediment to venous return to the heart. Hence, it limits the maximum value of Q_h regardless of the strength of the pump. Note that in Figure 24–3, Q_h remains constant as P_v decreases below zero.

Blood volume affects the relationship between cardiac output and central venous pressure

The vascular function curve is affected by changes in total blood volume. As previously stated, P_{mc} depends only on overall vascular compliance and total blood volume. Thus, for a given vascular compliance, P_{mc} increases when the blood volume is expanded **(hypervolemia),** and it decreases when the blood volume is diminished **(hypovolemia).** In the three vascular function curves shown in **Figure 24–4,** for example, blood was either transfused into the static system (Q_h = 0) until P_{mc} reached 9 mm Hg at equilibrium (top curve) or withdrawn from the static system until P_{mc} reached 5 mm Hg at equilibrium (bottom curve). P_{mc} is the *y*-axis intercept in Figure 24–4.

The various vascular function curves in Figure 24–4 are all parallel to one another. To understand why the curves are parallel, consider the example of hypervolemia (top curve), in which P_{mc} had been raised to 9 mm Hg. When the system is static, P_a and P_v would both be 9 mm Hg. If Q_h were then suddenly increased to 1 L/min (as in Figure 24–2, *D*) and if the peripheral resistance were still 20 mm

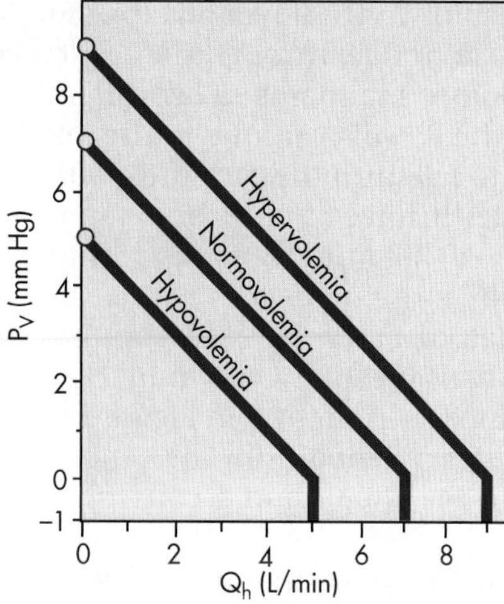

FIGURE 24–4. Effects of increased blood volume (hypervolemia) and decreased blood volume (hypovolemia) on the vascular function curve.

Hg/L/min, an arteriovenous pressure gradient of 20 mm Hg would still be necessary for 1 L/min to flow through the resistance vessels. This does not differ from the example for normovolemia. Assuming the same ratio of C_v to C_a of 19:1, the pressure gradient would be achieved by a decline of 1 mm Hg in P_v and a rise of 19 mm Hg in P_a.

Therefore, a change in Q_h from 0 to 1 L/min would evoke the same reduction in P_v irrespective of the total blood volume as long as the C_v:C_a ratio and the peripheral resistance remain constant. The slope of the vascular function curve is by definition the change in P_v per unit change in Q_h. The vascular function curves that represent different blood volumes are parallel to one another, as shown in Figure 24–4, because the change in P_v induced by a unit change in Q_h is not affected by the blood volume.

Figure 24–4 also shows that the Q_h at which P_v becomes zero varies directly with the blood volume. Therefore, the maximum value that Q_h can attain becomes progressively more limited as the total blood volume is reduced. However, the pressure at which the veins collapse (sharp change in slope of the vascular function curve) is not altered appreciably by changes in blood volume. This pressure depends only on the ambient pressure. When P_v falls below the ambient pressure, the veins collapse, and venous return to the heart is thereby limited.

Peripheral resistance affects the relationship between cardiac output and central venous pressure

The modifications of the vascular function curve that are associated with changes in R_t are shown in **Figure 24–5**. The arterioles contain only about 3% of the total blood volume. Hence, changes in the contractile state of these vessels do not significantly alter P_{mc}. Thus, the vascular function curves that represent various peripheral resistances converge at a common point (P_{mc}) on the P_v axis.

For any given Q_h, the P_v decreases as the peripheral resistance is increased (Figure 24–5). The principal reason for this relationship is that for a given Q_h, an increase in peripheral resistance redistributes the blood volume such that a greater fraction of the blood resides in the arteries (Figure 21–5), and consequently a lesser fraction resides in the veins. This reduction in V_v would be attended by a proportional fall in P_v.

Increases in peripheral resistance are associated with a clockwise rotation of the vascular function curves about a common intercept on the P_v axis because an increase in peripheral resistance tends to decrease P_v without affecting P_{mc} (Figure 24–5). Conversely, arteriolar vasodilation is associated with a counterclockwise rotation. A higher maximum Q_h is attainable when the arterioles are dilated than when they are normal or constricted (Figure 24–5).

The Heart and Blood Vessels Interact with Each Other

The P_v constitutes the filling pressure (essentially, the preload) for the right ventricle. In accordance with the Frank-Starling mechanism (see Chapters 18 and 19), P_v is a cardinal determinant of the Q_h. Ordinarily, Q_h varies directly with P_v; that is, OVER A WIDE RANGE OF VENOUS PRESSURES, A RISE IN P_v INCREASES Q_h. In the discussion to follow, graphs of Q_h as a function of P_v are called **cardiac function curves.** Alterations in myocardial contractility are represented by shifts in these curves.

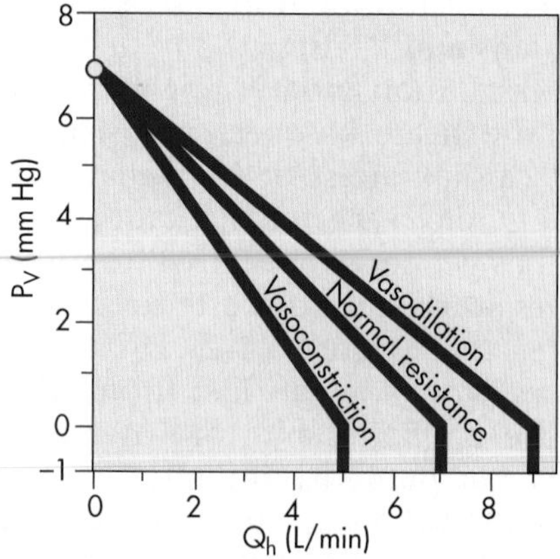

FIGURE 24–5. Effects of arteriolar vasodilation and vasoconstriction on the vascular function curve.

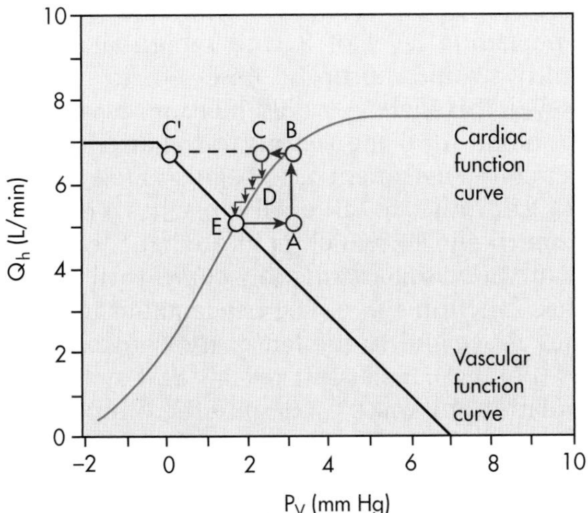

FIGURE 24–6. Typical vascular and cardiac function curves plotted on the same coordinate axes. The coordinates of the equilibrium point, at the intersection of the two curves, represent the stable values of Q_h and P_v at which the system tends to operate. Any perturbation (such as when P_v is suddenly increased to point A) initiates a sequence of changes in Q_h and P_v such that these variables gradually approach their equilibrium values.

Appreciation of the coupling between the heart and blood vessels requires an examination of the interrelationship of the cardiac function and vascular function curves **(Figure 24–6)**. Both curves reflect the relationship between Q_h and P_v. As stated previously, THE CARDIAC FUNCTION CURVE EXPRESSES HOW Q_h VARIES IN RESPONSE TO A CHANGE IN P_v. Hence, Q_h is the **dependent variable** (or response) and P_v is the **independent variable** (or stimulus). By convention, the dependent variable is scaled along the *y* axis and the independent variable is scaled along the *x* axis. Note that in Figure 24–6, the assignment of *x* and *y* axes is conventional for the cardiac function curve.

THE VASCULAR FUNCTION CURVE, CONVERSELY, REFLECTS HOW P_v IS AFFECTED BY A CHANGE IN Q_h. For the vascular function curve, P_v is the dependent variable (or response) and Q_h is the independent variable (or stimulus). By convention, P_v should be scaled along the *y* axis and Q_h along the *x* axis. Note that this convention was observed for the vascular function curves displayed in Figures 24–3 to 24–5.

So that the vascular function curve can be included on the same set of coordinate axes with the cardiac function curve, as in Figure 24–6, the plotting convention for one of these curves must be violated. In this case, the convention for the vascular function curve has been arbitrarily violated. NOTE THAT THE VASCULAR FUNCTION CURVE IN FIGURE 24–6 REFLECTS HOW P_v (SCALED ALONG THE *x* AXIS) VARIES IN RESPONSE TO A CHANGE OF Q_h (SCALED ALONG THE *y* AXIS).

Simultaneous examination of the two curves, one that characterizes cardiac function and the other that characterizes vascular function, provides some insight about the coupling between the heart and vessels. Theoretically, the heart can operate at all combinations of P_v and Q_h that fall on the appropriate cardiac function curve. Similarly, the vascular system can operate at all combinations of P_v and Q_h that fall on the appropriate vascular function curve. AT EQUILIBRIUM, THEREFORE, THE ENTIRE CARDIOVASCULAR SYSTEM (i.e., THE COMBINATION OF HEART AND VESSELS) MUST OPERATE AT THE POINT OF INTERSECTION OF THESE TWO CURVES. Only at this point of intersection does the prevailing P_v evoke the specific Q_h defined by the cardiac function curve. Similarly, only at this point of intersection does the prevailing Q_h evoke the specific P_v defined by the vascular function curve.

The tendency for the cardiovascular system to operate about such an equilibrium may best be illustrated by examining its response to a sudden perturbation. Let us impose a sudden rise in P_v from the equilibrium point to point A in Figure 24–6. Such a change in P_v might be induced during ventricular systole by the rapid injection of a given volume of blood on the venous side of the circuit accompanied by the rapid withdrawal of an equal volume from the arterial side; the total blood volume would remain constant.

As defined by the cardiac function curve in Figure 24–6, this elevated P_v would increase Q_h (from point A to point B) during the very next ventricular systole. The increased Q_h would in turn result in the net transfer of blood from the venous to the arterial side of the circuit, with a consequent reduction in P_v. In one heartbeat, this reduction would be small (from point B to point C) because the heart would transfer only a small fraction of the total V_v over to the arterial side. Because of this reduction in P_v, the Q_h during the very next beat would diminish (from point C to point D) by an amount dictated by the cardiac function curve. Because point D is still above the intersection point, the heart pumps blood from the veins to the arteries at a rate greater than the blood flows across the peripheral resistance from arteries to veins. Because the venoarterial transport exceeds the arteriovenous transport, P_v continues to fall. This process continues in ever-diminishing steps until the point of intersection (point E) is reached. Only one specific combination of Q_h and P_v (denoted by the coordinates of the point of intersection) simultaneously satisfies the conditions defined by the cardiac and vascular function curves.

Changes in myocardial contractility are reflected by shifts in the cardiac function curves

Graphs of cardiac and vascular function curves help explain the effects of alterations in ventricular contractility. **Contractility** refers to an alteration in myocardial performance based on processes (such as a change in responsiveness to intracellular Ca^{++}) that involve the contractile proteins. Semantically, the term specifically excludes any effects imposed by a change in preload or afterload, even if those changes are mediated by an altered responsiveness to Ca^{++}.

In **Figure 24–7**, the lower cardiac function curve represents the control state of contractility, whereas the upper curve reflects an enhanced state of contractility. This pair of hypothetical cardiac function curves is analogous to the experimentally derived pair of ventricular function curves shown in Figure 19–14. The change in contractility reflected by the two hypothetical cardiac function curves might be achieved experimentally by selective stimulation of the sympathetic nerves only to the heart. Such selective stimulation would not directly affect the vasculature, so only one vascular function curve need be included in Figure 24–7.

During the control state, the equilibrium values for Q_h and P_v in Figure 24–7 are designated by point A. At the beginning of cardiac sympathetic nerve stimulation (assuming the effects to be instantaneous and constant), the combination of the prevailing level of P_v and the enhanced contractility would abruptly raise Q_h to point B. However, this high Q_h would increase the net transfer of blood from the venous to the arterial side of the circuit; consequently, P_v begins to fall (to point C). Q_h continues to fall until it reaches a new equilibrium (point D), which is located at the intersection of the vascular function curve with the new cardiac function curve. The new equilibrium (point D) lies above and to the left of the control equilibrium (point A). This shift reveals that sympathetic stimulation increases Q_h despite the diminution of the ventricular filling pressure (i.e., P_v). Such a change accurately describes the true response. In the experiment shown in **Figure 24–8**, stimulation of the left stellate ganglion in an anesthetized dog increased Q_h but decreased the right and left atrial pressures.

Similar changes occur in patients with **congestive heart failure** when they are treated with drugs that improve myocardial contractility, such as dobutamine. Classically, patients with congestive heart failure had a high P_v and an abnormally low Q_h. Drugs that exert a **positive inotropic effect** (i.e., drugs that enhance contractility) raise the Q_h and decrease the P_v. Such observations, when first made, were interpreted to be incompatible with Starling's law. Now it is recognized that this important physiological principle is more faithfully represented by a family of cardiac function curves and that changes in contractility are reflected by shifts from one component curve to another.

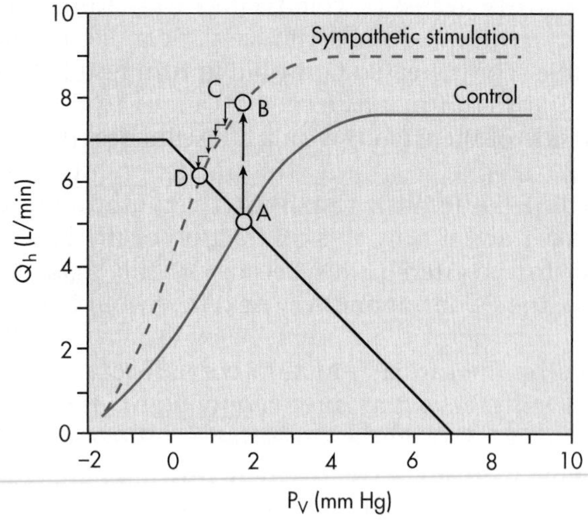

FIGURE 24–7. When myocardial contractility is enhanced (e.g., by cardiac sympathetic nerve stimulation), the equilibrium values of Q_h and P_v shift from the intersection (point A) of the vascular function curve with the control cardiac function curve to the intersection (point D) of the same vascular function curve with the cardiac function curve, which represents the effects of cardiac sympathetic nerve stimulation.

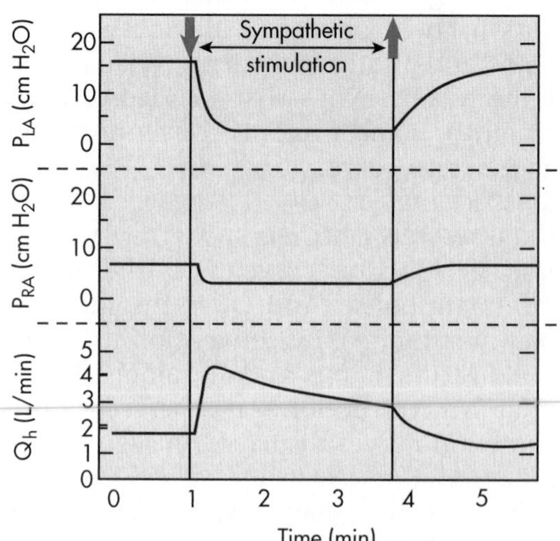

FIGURE 24–8. During electrical stimulation of the cardiac sympathetic nerves in an anesthetized dog, Q_h increased while pressures in the left atrium (P_{LA}) and right atrium (P_{RA}) diminished. (Data from Sarnoff SJ et al: *Circ Res* 8:1108, 1960.)

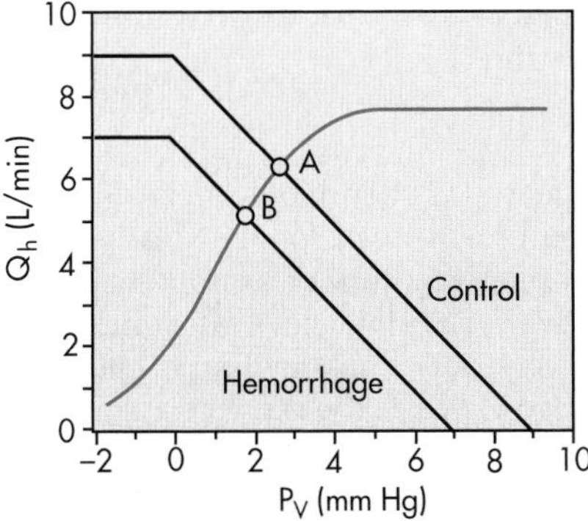

FIGURE 24–9. Hemorrhage is reflected by a shift of the vascular function curve to the left. Therefore, the equilibrium values of Q_h and P_v are both decreased, as denoted by the translocation of the equilibrium from point A to point B.

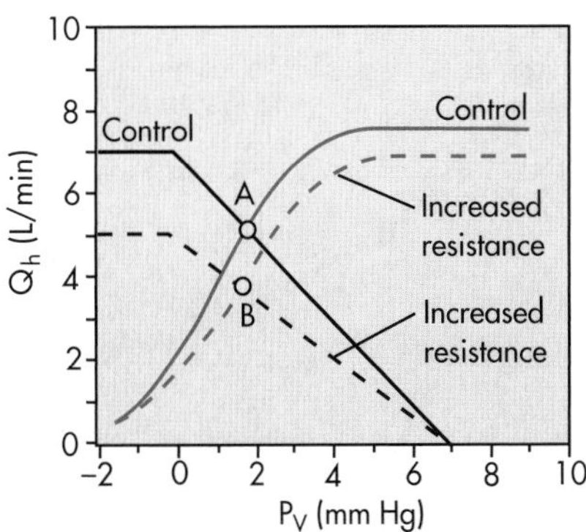

FIGURE 24–10. An increase in peripheral resistance is reflected by downward shifts of the cardiac and vascular function curves. At equilibrium, Q_h is less (point B) when the peripheral resistance is high than when it is normal (point A).

Changes in blood volume mainly affect the vascular function curve

Changes in blood volume do not directly affect the cardiac function curve, but they do influence the vascular function curve in the manner shown in Figure 24–4. For a clear understanding of the circulatory alterations evoked by a given change in blood volume, the appropriate cardiac function curve must be plotted along with the vascular function curves that represent the control and altered vascular states, as shown in **Figure 24–9**.

The parallel shift in the vascular function curve in Figure 24–9 reflects the response to **acute hemorrhage.** Equilibrium (point B), which denotes the values for Q_h and P_v immediately after sudden hemorrhage, lies below and to the left of control equilibrium (point A). Thus, a pure, sudden reduction in blood volume decreases both Q_h and P_v.

Changes in peripheral resistance affect cardiac output relatively more than central venous pressure

Predictions concerning the effects of changes in peripheral resistance on Q_h and P_v are complex because changes in peripheral resistance are associated with shifts in both the cardiac and vascular function curves **(Figure 24–10)**. Recall that in Figure 24–5, vasoconstriction was accompanied by a clockwise rotation of the vascular function curve. The axes are reversed in Figure 24–10, however, and therefore vasoconstriction is associated with a counterclockwise rotation of the vascular function curve depicted. Hence, for any given value of P_v, Q_h is diminished by vasoconstriction. The cardiac function curve is also shifted downward because at any given cardiac filling pressure (P_v), the heart pumps less blood when the peripheral resistance is increased; an increase in peripheral resistance characteristically raises the P_a (the afterload). The new equilibrium (point B) falls below control (point A) because both curves are displaced downward by vasoconstriction.

Changes in Heart Rate Have Variable Effects on Cardiac Output

Q_h IS THE PRODUCT OF STROKE VOLUME AND HEART RATE. Analysis of the effects of changes in heart rate on Q_h is complicated because a change in heart rate alters the other factors (namely, the preload, afterload, and contractility) that determine stroke volume (Figure 24–1). For example, an increase in the heart rate decreases the duration of diastole. Hence, the time available for ventricular filling is abridged, and preload is reduced. If the proposed increase in heart rate did alter Q_h, P_a (afterload) would change. Finally, an increase in heart rate would augment the net influx of Ca^{++} into the cardiac myocytes, and this would enhance myocardial contractility (see Figure 19–11).

Many investigators have varied heart rate by artificial pacing in experiments on animals and in humans. The effects on Q_h qualitatively resemble the experimental results shown in **Figure 24–11**. In that experiment, as the atrial pacing frequency was gradually increased in an anesthetized dog, the stroke volume progressively diminished (Figure 24–11, *A*). Presumably, the reduction in stroke volume was induced by the decreased time for

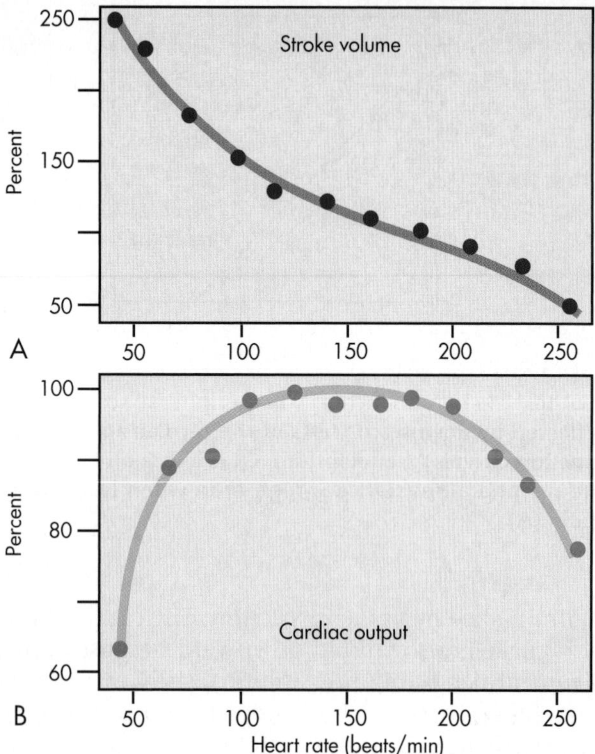

FIGURE 24–11. Changes in stroke volume (A) and in cardiac output (B) induced by changes in the rate of atrial pacing in an anesthetized dog. (Data from Kumada M, Azuma T, Matsuda K: *Jpn J Physiol* 17:538, 1967.)

ventricular filling. However, the change in Q_h evoked by a change in heart rate was influenced markedly by the actual level of the heart rate. In this experiment, for example, as the pacing frequency was raised within the range of 50 to 100 beats/min, an increase in heart rate increased the Q_h. Presumably, at these lower frequencies, the decrement in stroke volume (SV) evoked by a given increase in heart rate (HR) was proportionately less than the increment in heart rate itself. Stated mathematically, the equation $Q_h = SV \times HR$ signifies that if an increment in heart rate exceeds the consequent decrement in stroke volume, then the consequent value of Q_h will exceed the initial value of Q_h.

Over the frequency range from about 100 to 200 beats/min, however, Q_h in these experiments (Figure 24–11, *B*) was not affected appreciably by changes in pacing frequency. Hence, as the pacing frequency was increased, the decrease in stroke volume was proportional to the increase in heart rate. Finally, at excessively high pacing frequencies (>200 beats/min), increments in heart rate diminished Q_h. Therefore, the induced decrement in stroke volume must have exceeded the applied increment in heart rate over this high pacing frequency range. The characteristic inverted U relationship of Q_h to heart rate varies quantitatively among subjects and among physiological states in any given subject.

The characteristic relationship between Q_h and heart rate explains the urgent need for the treatment of patients who have excessively slow or excessively fast heart rates. Profound **bradycardias** (slow rates) may occur as the result of a very slow sinus rhythm in patients with **sick sinus syndrome** or as the result of a slow **idioventricular rhythm** in patients with **complete atrioventricular block.** In either rhythm disturbance, the capacity of the ventricles to fill during a prolonged diastole is limited (often by the noncompliant pericardium). These rhythm disturbances often require the installation of an artificial pacemaker.

Excessively high heart rates in patients with **supraventricular** or **ventricular tachycardias** may also require emergency treatment. The Q_h may be critically low because of the diminished filling time. Reversion of the tachycardia to a more normal rhythm may be accomplished pharmacologically or, in emergencies, by applying a strong electrical current across the thorax or directly to the heart through an implanted device.

Ancillary Factors also Regulate Cardiac Output

In the preceding discussion, the interrelationship between P_v and Q_h has been oversimplified because the effects elicited by changes in just one factor were explained. However, an isolated change in a single variable rarely occurs because many feedback control mechanisms regulate the cardiovascular system. A change in blood volume, for example, reflexly alters cardiac function, peripheral resistance, and venomotor tone. Furthermore, several auxiliary factors also contribute to the regulation of Q_h. Among these, some serve as additional energy sources to help the heart pump blood around the body.

Gravity affects cardiac output

Soldiers standing at attention for long periods, particularly in hot weather, may faint because the Q_h decreases substantially. Under such conditions, gravity impedes venous return from the dependent regions of the body, but it also promotes flow on the arterial side of the same circuit. Therefore, in the dependent regions of the body, the vascular system behaves much like a U-shaped tube, where the effects of gravity in the descending limb (arteries) and ascending limb (veins) of the tube neutralize each other. Such neutralization does not take place in the vessels above the level of the heart because the pressure in the veins at some level above the heart might fall below the ambient pressure, thus collapsing these veins.

The compliance of the blood vessels accounts for the gravitational effects on Q_h. When a person stands, the blood vessels below the level of the heart are distended by the gravitational forces that act on the columns of blood in the vessels. The distention is more prominent on the venous than on the arterial side of the circuit because C_v is much higher than C_a (as explained earlier). Such venous distention is readily observed on the backs of the hands when the arms are allowed to hang below the level of the heart. The hemodynamic effects of distention of the veins **(venous pooling)** below the heart level resemble those caused by the loss of an equivalent volume of blood from the body. When a person shifts from a supine position to a relaxed standing position, 300 to 800 mL of blood may be pooled in the legs. This may reduce Q_h by about 2 L/min.

The compensatory adjustments to the erect position are similar to the adjustments to blood loss. For example, venous pooling and other gravitational effects tend to lower the pressure in the regions of the arterial baroreceptors. The resulting diminution in baroreceptor excitation reflexly speeds the heart, strengthens cardiac contraction, and constricts arterioles and veins (see Chapters 19 and 23). The baroreceptor reflex has a greater effect on the resistance vessels (arterioles) than on the capacitance vessels (veins). On hot days, the compensatory vasomotor reactions are less efficacious, and the absence of muscle activity exaggerates the pooling effects of gravity, as explained later.

Many of the vasodilator drugs used to treat **essential hypertension** and other circulatory disorders also interfere with the reflex adaptation to standing. Similarly, astronauts exposed to weightlessness lose their adaptations after a few days, and they experience difficulties when they first return to a normal gravitational field. When individuals with impaired reflex adaptations stand, their blood pressures may fall dramatically. This response is called **orthostatic hypotension,** which may cause lightheadedness or fainting.

Muscle activity and venous valves constitute an auxiliary blood pump

When a relaxed individual stands, the pressure in the veins below the heart rises. P_v in the legs increases gradually and does not reach equilibrium until almost 1 minute after the subject stands. The slowness of the rise in P_v is attributable to the **venous valves,** which permit flow only toward the heart. When a person stands, the valves prevent blood in the veins from actually falling toward the feet. Hence, the column of venous blood is supported at numerous levels by these valves; temporarily, the venous column consists of many separate segments. However, blood continues to enter the column from many venules and small tributary veins, and pressure continues to rise. As soon as the pressure in one segment exceeds that in the segment just above it, the valve between the two segments is forced open. Ultimately, all the valves in the dependent veins are open, and the column is continuous.

Precise measurement reveals that the final level of P_v in the feet of an individual during quiet standing is only slightly greater than that in a static column of blood extending from the right atrium to the feet. When the person begins to walk or run, the P_v in the legs and feet decreases appreciably. Because of the intermittent venous compression produced by the contracting muscles and because of the presence of the venous valves, blood is forced from the veins toward the heart (see Figure 25–2). Hence, MUSCLE CONTRACTION LOWERS THE P_v IN THE LEGS AND SERVES AS AN AUXILIARY BLOOD PUMP. Furthermore, muscle activity prevents venous pooling and lowers capillary hydrostatic pressure and thereby reduces the tendency for edema fluid to collect in the feet during standing. This mechanism operates effectively in normal people in that not much motion is required for appreciable auxiliary pumping to occur. Thus, if a standing person shifts weight periodically, the pressure in the foot veins is considerably less than the pressure that prevails if he or she remains absolutely still.

This auxiliary pumping mechanism is not very effective in people with **varicose veins** in the legs. The valves in such veins do not operate properly; therefore, when the leg muscles contract, the blood in the leg veins can be forced in the retrograde as well as in the antegrade direction. Thus, when such an individual stands or walks, the P_v in the ankles and feet is excessively high. The consequent high capillary pressure leads to the accumulation of extracellular fluid **(edema)** in the ankles and feet.

Respiration alters venous return

The normal, periodic activity of the respiratory muscles causes rhythmic variations in vena caval flow, and it constitutes an auxiliary pump to promote venous return of blood to the heart. Coughing, straining at stool, and other activities that require the respiratory muscles may affect Q_h substantially.

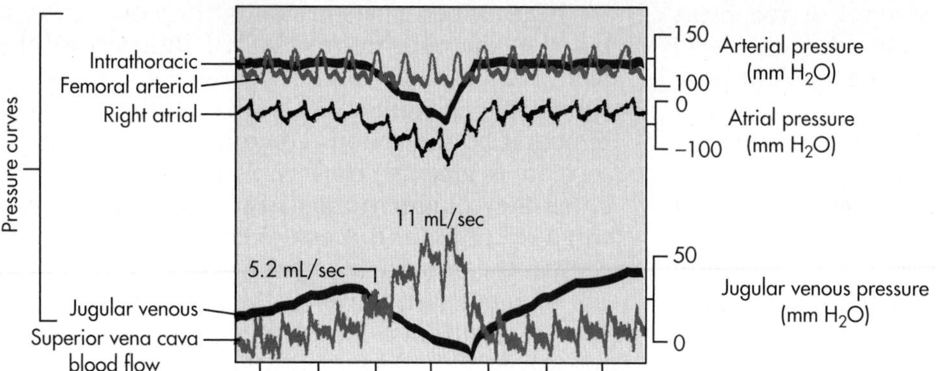

FIGURE 24–12. In an anesthetized dog, intrathoracic, right atrial, and jugular venous pressures decrease and flow in the superior vena cava increases (from 5.2 to 11 mL/sec) during inspiration. (Data from Brecher GA: *Venous return,* New York, 1956, Grune & Stratton.)

The changes in blood flow in the superior vena cava during the respiratory cycle of an anesthetized dog are shown in **Figure 24–12**. During respiration, the changes in intrathoracic pressure are transmitted to the lumens of the thoracic blood vessels. The reduction in P_v during inspiration increases the pressure gradient between the extrathoracic and intrathoracic veins. The consequent acceleration of venous return to the right atrium is displayed in Figure 24–12 as an increase in superior vena caval blood flow from 5.2 mL/sec during expiration to 11 mL/sec during inspiration.

During expiration, flow into the central veins decelerates. However, the mean rate of venous return during normal respiration exceeds the venous flow that occurs in the temporary absence of respiration. Hence, normal inspiration facilitates venous return more than normal expiration impedes it. This facilitation is partly attributable to the valves in the veins of the extremities and neck. These valves prevent any reversal of flow during expiration. Thus, the respiratory muscles and venous valves also constitute an auxiliary pump for venous return.

Summary

- Two important relationships between Q_h and P_v prevail in the cardiovascular system. One applies to the heart and the other to the vascular system.
- With respect to the heart, Q_h varies directly with P_v (preload) over a wide range of P_v. This relationship is represented by the cardiac function curve, and it expresses the Frank-Starling mechanism.
- With respect to the vascular system, P_v varies inversely with Q_h. This relationship is represented by the vascular function curve, and it reflects the fact that an increase in Q_h, for example, augments total blood volume in the arteries and hence decreases blood volume in the veins.
- The principal mechanisms that govern the cardiac function curve are the changes in contractility and afterload.
- The principal factors that govern the vascular function curve are C_a and C_v, peripheral vascular resistance, and total blood volume.
- The equilibrium values of Q_h and P_v that prevail under a given set of physiological conditions are determined by the intersection of the cardiac and vascular function curves.
- At very low and very high heart rates, the heart cannot pump an adequate Q_h.
- Gravity influences Q_h because the veins are very compliant, and substantial quantities of blood tend to pool in the veins of the dependent portions of the body.
- Respiration changes the pressure gradient between the intrathoracic and extrathoracic veins and hence alters venous return.

Bibliography

Aukland K: Why don't our feet swell in the upright position? *News Physiol Sci* 9:214, 1994.

Geddes LA, Wessale JL: Cardiac output, stroke volume, and pacing rate: a review of the literature and a proposed technique for selection of the optimum pacing rate for an exercise responsive pacemaker, *J Cardiovasc Electrophysiol* 2:408, 1991.

Hainsworth R: The importance of vascular capacitance in cardiovascular control, *News Physiol Sci* 5:250, 1990.

Lacolley PJ et al: Microgravity and orthostatic intolerance: carotid hemodynamics and peripheral responses, *Am J Physiol* 264:H588, 1993.

Rothe CF: Mean circulatory filling pressure: its meaning and measurement, *J Appl Physiol* 74:499, 1993.

Rothe CF, Gaddis ML: Autoregulation of cardiac output by passive elastic characteristics of the vascular capacitance system, *Circulation* 81:360, 1990.

Sagawa K et al: *Cardiac contraction and the pressure-volume relationship,* New York, 1988, Oxford University Press.

Seymour RS, Hargens AR, Pedley TJ: The heart works against gravity, *Am J Physiol* 265:R715, 1993.

Sheriff DD et al: Dependence of cardiac filling pressure on cardiac output during rest and dynamic exercise in dogs, *Am J Physiol* 265:H316, 1993.

Smith JJ, ed: *Circulatory response to the upright posture,* Boca Raton, Fla, 1990, CRC Press.

Stick, C, Jaeger H, Witzleb E: Measurements of volume changes and venous pressure in the human lower leg during walking and running, *J Appl Physiol* 72:2063, 1992.

Tyberg JV: Venous modulation of ventricular preload, *Am Heart J* 123:1098, 1992.

Yin FCP, ed: *Ventricular/vascular coupling,* New York, 1987, Springer-Verlag.

Case Study

Case 24–1

A 44-year-old woman had been extremely ill with severe coronary artery disease, and she underwent cardiac transplantation. She recovered well, and 1 month after surgery her cardiovascular function was normal even though her new heart was entirely denervated. About 3 months after surgery, she developed a duodenal ulcer, which suddenly began to bleed. The patient was estimated to have lost about 600 mL of blood in 1 hour. Her physician treated her with diet and antibiotics, and her ulcer was cured in about 2 weeks. The patient appeared to be healthy for about 3 years but then gradually lost some of her strength and energy. Her physician determined that the cardiac transplant was slowly being rejected. Her physician began to treat her with a new drug that substantially and specifically increased myocardial contractility. On occasion, the patient experienced brief periods of tachycardia with a rate of about 250 beats/min; the electrocardiogram indicated that the tachycardia originated in the atrioventricular junction.

1. How would acute blood loss from the duodenal ulcer affect the patient?

A. Decrease P_v and increase Q_h
B. Increase P_v and decrease P_a
C. Decrease P_v and decrease Q_h
D. Increase P_a and decrease Q_h
E. Decrease P_v and increase aortic pulse pressure

2. What would the administration of a drug that acts specifically to improve myocardial contractility do?

A. Decrease P_v and increase Q_h
B. Decrease P_v and decrease P_a
C. Increase P_v and increase aortic pulse pressure
D. Decrease P_v and decrease Q_h
E. Increase P_v and increase C_a

3. Strapping the patient to a tilt table and tilting her to the vertical, head-up position would do what?

A. Increase the pressure in a foot vein and increase P_v
B. Decrease the pressure in a foot vein and decrease Q_h
C. Decrease P_v and increase P_a
D. Decrease the pressure in a foot vein and decrease the arterial pulse pressure
E. Increase the pressure in a foot vein and decrease Q_h

4. When the patient was experiencing tachycardia, what critical hemodynamic changes would be expected?

A. Increase in P_a and increase in P_v
B. Decrease in stroke volume and decrease in Q_h
C. Increase in stroke volume and increase in aortic compliance
D. Increase in P_v and increase in Q_h
E. Decrease in P_v and increase in arterial pulse pressure

Chapter 25: Special Circulations

Objectives

- ❖ Describe the regulation of cutaneous blood flow and the role of the skin in maintaining a constant body temperature.
- ❖ Indicate the relative importance of the local and neural factors in adjustments of skeletal muscle blood flow at rest and during exercise.
- ❖ Explain the physical, neural, and chemical factors that affect coronary blood flow.
- ❖ Describe the regulation of cerebral blood flow.
- ❖ Relate the intestinal and hepatic components of the splanchnic circulation.
- ❖ Explain the changes in the fetal circulation that occur at birth.

Previous chapters on the circulatory system described how the heart and vessels provide the tissues of the body with O_2 and nutrients and remove CO_2 and waste products. The circulations of the various organs of the body differ to some degree with respect to their function and regulation. Thus, it is necessary to include this chapter on special circulations, which discusses the regulatory mechanisms in the cutaneous, skeletal muscle, coronary, cerebral, splanchnic, and fetal circulations. The circulations of the kidneys and lungs are described in the sections on the renal and respiratory systems.

Cutaneous Circulation Is the Flow of Blood to the Skin

The skin has relatively small O_2 and nutrient requirements. The supply of these essential materials is not the chief governing factor in the regulation of cutaneous blood flow, in contrast to the regulation in most other body tissues. THE PRIMARY FUNCTION OF THE CUTANEOUS CIRCULATION IS MAINTENANCE OF A CONSTANT BODY TEMPERATURE. Consequently, blood flow to the skin fluctuates widely, depending on the need for loss or conservation of body heat. The mechanisms responsible for alterations in skin blood flow are activated mainly by changes in ambient and internal body temperatures.

Skin blood flow is regulated mainly by the sympathetic nervous system

The skin has essentially two types of resistance vessels: **arterioles** and **arteriovenous (AV) anastomoses.** The arterioles are similar to those found elsewhere in the body. AV anastomoses shunt blood from the arterioles to the venules and venous plexuses; thus, they bypass the capillary bed (**Figure 25–1**). AV anastomoses are found mainly in the fingertips, palms, toes, soles of the feet, ears, nose, and lips. Unlike arterioles, AV anastomoses are either short and straight vessels or long and coiled vessels, about 20 to 40 μm in lumen diameter. They have thick muscular walls and are richly supplied with nerve fibers. These vessels are almost exclusively under sympathetic neural control, and they dilate maximally when their nerve supply is interrupted. Conversely, reflex stimulation of the sympathetic fibers to these vessels may constrict them to the point that the vascular lumen is completely

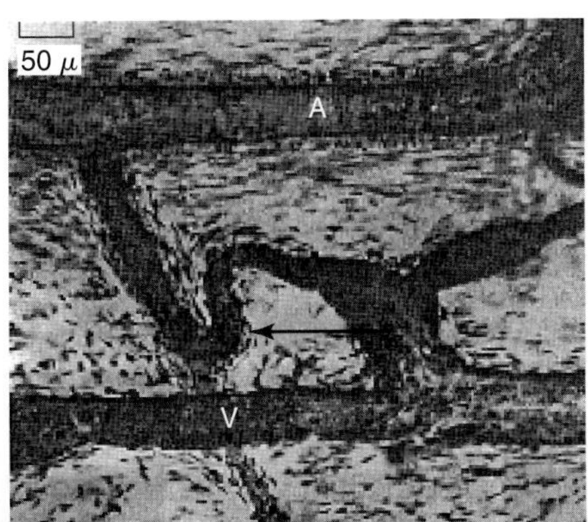

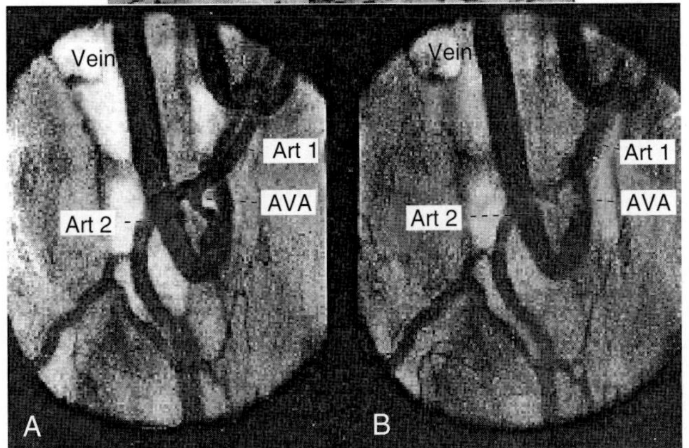

FIGURE 25–1. ***Top,*** **AV anastomosis** ***(arrow)*** **in a human ear injected with Berlin blue. The walls of the AV anastomoses in the fingertips are thicker and more cellular. A, artery; V, vein.** ***Bottom,*** **Two frames from a motion-picture record of the same relatively large AV anastomosis (AVA) in a stable rabbit ear chamber installed 3½ months previously. On the left (A), the AV anastomosis is dilated; on the right (B), it is contracted. On this day, the lumen measured 51 μm dilated and 5 μm contracted at its narrowest point. Arrows indicate the direction of blood flow. Art, artery. (From Berne RM, Levy MN, Koeppen BM, Stanton BA:** ***Physiology,*** **ed 5, Philadelphia, 2004, Elsevier.)**

obliterated (Figure 25–1, *B*). Although AV anastomoses do not exhibit basal tone (tonic activity of the vascular smooth muscle independent of innervation), they are highly sensitive to vasoconstrictor agents such as epinephrine and norepinephrine. Furthermore, AV anastomoses are not under metabolic control, and they fail to show reactive hyperemia or autoregulation of blood flow. Thus, the regulation of blood flow through these anastomotic channels is governed mainly by temperature receptors or by higher centers of the central nervous system.

THE BULK OF THE SKIN RESISTANCE VESSELS EXHIBIT SOME BASAL TONE. IN THE SKIN, VASCULAR RESISTANCE IS UNDER DUAL CONTROL OF THE SYMPATHETIC NERVOUS SYSTEM AND LOCAL REGULATORY FACTORS, much the same as in other vascular beds. IN THE SKIN, HOWEVER, NEURAL CONTROL IS MORE IMPORTANT THAN LOCAL FACTORS. Stimulation of sympathetic nerve fibers to skin blood vessels (i.e., arteries, veins, arterioles) induces vasoconstriction, and severance of the sympathetic nerves induces vasodilation. After chronic denervation of the cutaneous blood vessels, the degree of tone that existed before denervation is gradually regained during several weeks. This is accomplished by an enhanced basal tone that compensates for the degree of tone previously contributed by sympathetic nerve fiber activity. Epinephrine and norepinephrine elicit only vasoconstriction in cutaneous vessels.

Parasympathetic vasodilator nerve fibers do not supply the cutaneous blood vessels. However, stimulation of the sweat glands, which are innervated by cholinergic fibers of the sympathetic nervous system, causes dilation of the skin resistance vessels. Sweat contains an enzyme that acts on a tissue fluid protein to release bradykinin, a polypeptide with vasodilator properties. Bradykinin formed in the tissue can act locally to dilate the arterioles and increase blood flow to the skin.

The skin vessels of certain body regions, particularly the head, neck, shoulders, and upper chest, are under the influence of the higher centers of the central nervous system. For example, blushing (e.g., that caused by embarrassment or anger) is attributable to the inhibition of sympathetic nerve fibers to the face, whereas blanching (e.g., that caused by fear or anxiety) is attributable to the stimulation of the sympathetic nerve fibers to the face.

In contrast to AV anastomoses in the skin, the cutaneous resistance vessels show autoregulation of blood flow and reactive hyperemia. If the arterial inflow to a limb is stopped by brief inflation of a blood pressure cuff, the skin reddens greatly below the point of vascular occlusion when the cuff is deflated. This increased cutaneous blood flow **(reactive hyperemia)** is also manifested by distention of the superficial veins in the erythematous extremity.

Under normal conditions, ambient temperature is the main factor in the regulation of skin blood flow

The primary function of the skin is to preserve the internal milieu and protect it from adverse changes in the environment. Ambient temperature is one of the most important external variables with which the body must contend. Not surprisingly, the skin vasculature is chiefly influenced by environmental temperature. Exposure to cold elicits a generalized cutaneous vasoconstriction that is most pronounced in the hands and feet. This response is chiefly mediated by the nervous system because arrest of the circulation to the hand caused by inflation of a pressure cuff and then immersion of that hand in cold water results in vasoconstriction in the skin of the other extremities that have been exposed only to room temperature. When circulation to the chilled hand is not occluded, the reflex vasoconstriction is caused partly by the cooled blood returning to the general circulation and stimulating the temperature-regulating center in the anterior hypothalamus. Direct application of cold to this region of the brain produces cutaneous vasoconstriction.

The skin vessels of the cooled hand also respond directly to cold. Moderate cooling or exposure of the hand to severe cold (up to 15°C) for brief periods constricts the resistance and capacitance vessels, including AV anastomoses. However, prolonged exposure of the hand to severe cold has a secondary vasodilator effect. Prompt vasoconstriction and severe pain are elicited by immersion of the hand in water near 0°C, but these reactions are soon followed by dilation of the skin vessels, reddening of the immersed part, and alleviation of the pain. With continued immersion of the hand, alternating periods of constriction and dilation occur, but the skin temperature rarely drops as low as it did during the initial vasoconstriction. Prolonged severe cold damages the tissue.

Direct application of heat produces not only local vasodilation of resistance and capacitance vessels and AV anastomoses but also reflex dilation in other parts of the body. The local effect is independent of the vascular nerve supply; the reflex vasodilation is a combination of anterior hypothalamic stimulation by the returning warmed blood and stimulation of receptors in the heated part.

> The rosy faces of people outdoors in the cold are examples of cold vasodilation. However, blood flow through the skin of the face may be very low despite the flushed appearance. The redness of the slowly flowing blood is largely the result of the reduced O_2 uptake by the cold skin and the change in the affinity of hemoglobin for O_2 as reflected by the cold-induced shift to the left of the oxyhemoglobin dissociation curve (see Chapter 30).

The proximity of the major arteries and veins to each other permits considerable heat exchange **(countercurrent)** between the artery and vein. Cold blood that flows in veins from a cooled hand toward the heart takes up heat from adjacent arteries; this warms the venous blood and cools the arterial blood. Heat exchange occurs in the opposite direction when the extremity is exposed to heat. Thus, heat conservation is enhanced during exposure of the extremities to cold, and heat gain is minimized during exposure of the extremities to warmth.

> In patients with **Raynaud's disease,** exposure to cold or emotional stimuli may initiate ischemic attacks in the extremities (especially the fingers). The response is characterized by blanching, followed by cyanosis and then redness. The attacks are often associated with numbness, tingling, pain, and burning sensations.

In light skin, the color is a function of the amount of blood in the skin and subcutaneous tissue and the O_2 content of that blood

The color of the skin is determined in large part by pigment, but in all but very dark skin, the pallor or ruddiness depends on the color and amount of blood in the skin. With little blood in the venous plexus, the skin appears pale; with larger quantities of blood in the venous plexus, the skin has more color. Whether this color is bright red, blue, or some intermediate shade is determined by the degree of oxygenation of blood in the subcutaneous vessels. For example, a combination of vasoconstriction and reduced hemoglobin can make the skin an ashen gray, whereas a combination of venous engorgement and reduced hemoglobin can make it dark purple. Skin color provides little information about the rate of cutaneous blood flow. Rapid blood flow and pale skin may coexist when the AV anastomoses are open, and slow blood flow and red skin may coexist when the extremity is exposed to cold.

Skeletal Muscle Circulations Are Intertwined

Blood flow to skeletal muscle varies directly with the type and contractile activity of the muscle. Blood flow and capillary density are greater in red (slow-twitch, high-oxidative) muscle than in white (fast-twitch, low oxidative) muscle. In resting muscle, the arterioles exhibit asynchronous intermittent contractions and relaxations. Thus, at any given moment, a large percentage of the capillary bed is not perfused. Consequently, the total blood flow through quiescent skeletal muscle is low (1.4 to 4.5 mL/min/100 g). During exercise, the resistance vessels relax, and the muscle blood flow may increase manyfold (≤15 to 20 times the resting level); the magnitude of the increase depends largely on the severity of the exercise.

Control of muscle circulation is achieved by neural and local factors

The relative contribution of neural and local factors is dictated by muscle activity. IN SUBJECTS AT REST, NEURAL AND MYOGENIC REGULATIONS ARE PREDOMINANT; DURING EXERCISE, METABOLIC CONTROL SUPERVENES. As with all tissues, physical factors such as arterial pressure, tissue pressure, and blood viscosity influence blood flow to muscle. However, another physical factor plays a role during exercise: the squeezing effect of the active muscle on the vessels (see also Chapter 24). With intermittent contractions, inflow is restricted and venous outflow is enhanced during each brief contraction. The venous valves prevent the backflow of blood in the veins between contractions, and thus the valves aid in the forward propulsion of blood (**Figure 25–2**). With strong sustained contractions, the vascular bed can be compressed to the point at which blood flow ceases temporarily.

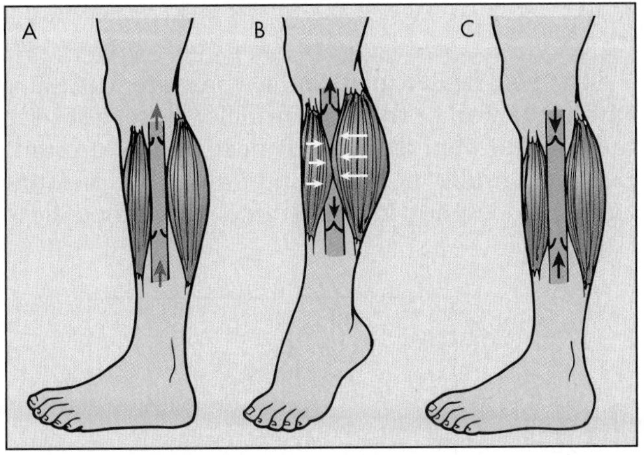

FIGURE 25–2. Action of the muscle pump in venous return from the legs. A, Standing at rest. The venous valves are open, and blood flows upward toward the heart by virtue of the pressure generated by the heart, which is transmitted through the capillaries to the veins from the arterial side of the vascular system (vis à tergo). B, Contraction of the muscle compresses the vein so that the increased pressure in the vein drives blood toward the thorax through the upper valve and closes the lower valve in the uncompressed segment of the vein just below the point of muscle compression. C, Immediately after muscle relaxation, the pressure in the previously compressed venous segment falls, and the reversed pressure gradient causes the upper valve to close. The valve below the previously compressed segment opens because the pressure below it exceeds that above it, and the segment fills with blood from the foot. As blood flow continues from the foot, the pressure in the previously compressed segment rises. When it exceeds the pressure above the upper valve, this valve opens, and continuous flow occurs as in A.

Basal tone and sympathetic nerve activity to muscle vessels regulate blood flow in resting subjects

Although the resistance vessels of muscle have a high basal tone, they also display a tone attributable to continuous low-frequency activity in sympathetic vasoconstrictor nerve fibers. The tonic activity of the sympathetic nerves is greatly influenced by the baroreceptor reflex. An increase in carotid sinus pressure dilates the vascular bed of the muscle, and a decrease elicits vasoconstriction. The reflex participation of resistance vessels in the muscles is important in maintaining a constant arterial blood pressure because muscle is the major body component on the basis of mass and thereby represents the largest vascular bed.

Metabolic activity is the main factor in regulating muscle blood flow during exercise

It has already been stressed that neural regulation of muscle blood flow is superseded by metabolic regulation (see Chapter 23) when the muscle changes from the resting to the contracting state. However, local control also occurs in innervated resting skeletal muscle when the vasomotor nerves are not active. Thus, autoregulation (see Figure 23–1) can be observed in innervated as well as in denervated muscle. In both conditions, autoregulation is characterized by a low venous blood O_2 saturation.

Coronary Circulation Is Dependent on Several Factors and Conditions

Coronary blood flow is under the influence of physical, neural, and metabolic factors

The main force responsible for perfusion of the myocardium is aortic pressure, which is generated by the heart itself. Changes in aortic pressure generally shift coronary blood flow in the same direction. However, alterations of cardiac work, which are produced by increased or decreased aortic pressure, have a considerable effect on coronary resistance. Increased metabolic activity of the heart decreases coronary resistance, whereas a reduction in cardiac metabolism increases coronary resistance. Under normal conditions, blood pressure is kept within relatively narrow limits by the baroreceptor reflex. Therefore, CHANGES IN CORONARY

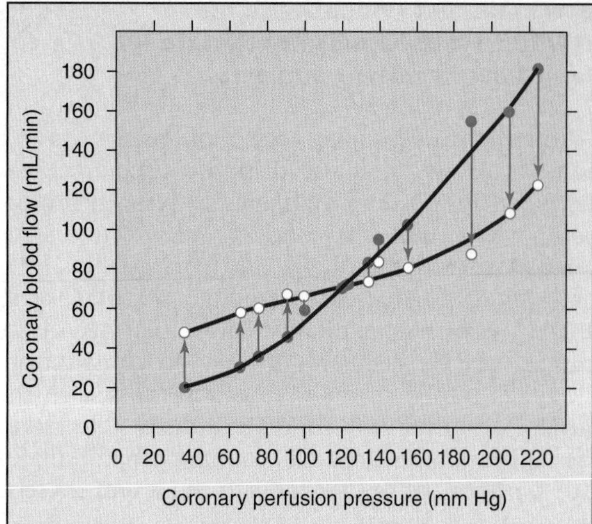

FIGURE 25–3. Pressure-flow relationships in the coronary vascular bed. At constant aortic pressure, cardiac output, and heart rate, coronary artery perfusion pressure was abruptly increased or decreased from the control level indicated by the point where the two lines cross. The closed circles represent the flows that were obtained immediately after the change in perfusion pressure; the open circles represent the steady-state flows at the new pressures. Blood flow tends to return to the control level, a feature most prominent between 60 and 180 mm Hg. (From Berne RM, Levy MN, Koeppen BM, Stanton BA: *Physiology,* ed 5, Philadelphia, 2004, Elsevier.)

BLOOD FLOW ARE CAUSED PRIMARILY BY CALIBER CHANGES OF THE CORONARY RESISTANCE VESSELS IN RESPONSE TO THE METABOLIC DEMANDS OF THE HEART. When the rate of myocardial metabolism is unchanged and coronary perfusion pressure is raised or lowered, coronary blood flow remains relatively constant **(autoregulation of blood flow).** Autoregulation is evident in a cannulated coronary artery perfused at constant aortic pressure and cardiac work. Abrupt changes in perfusion pressure promptly cause marked alterations in coronary blood flow as shown in **Figure 25–3**. When the perfusion pressure is maintained at the new level, blood flow returns toward the initial level. This indicates that autoregulation arises from factors within the system that are able to adjust coronary vascular resistance.

In addition to providing the head of pressure to drive blood through the coronary vessels, the heart also influences its own blood supply by the squeezing effect of the contracting myocardium on the blood vessels that course through it (**extravascular compression** or **extracoronary resistance**). This force is so great during early ventricular systole that blood flow in a large coronary artery supplying the left ventricle is briefly reversed. Left coronary inflow is maximal in early diastole, when the ventricles have relaxed and extravascular compression of the coronary vessels is virtually absent. This flow pattern is seen in the phasic coronary flow curve for the left coronary artery **(Figure 25–4)**. After an initial reversal in early systole, left coronary blood flow parallels the aortic pressure until early diastole, when it rises abruptly. It then declines slowly as aortic pressure falls during the remainder of diastole.

The minimum extravascular resistance and absence of left ventricular work during diastole are used to advantage clinically to improve myocardial perfusion in patients with damaged myocardium and low blood pressure. The method is called **counterpulsation,** and it consists of the insertion of an inflatable balloon into the thoracic aorta through a femoral artery. The balloon is inflated during ventricular diastole and deflated during systole. This procedure enhances coronary blood flow during diastole by raising diastolic pressure when coronary extravascular resistance is lowest. Furthermore, it reduces cardiac energy requirements by lowering aortic pressure (afterload) during ventricular ejection.

Left ventricular myocardial pressure (pressure within the wall of the left ventricle) is greatest near the endocardium and lowest near the epicardium. However, under normal conditions, this pressure gradient does not impair endocardial blood flow

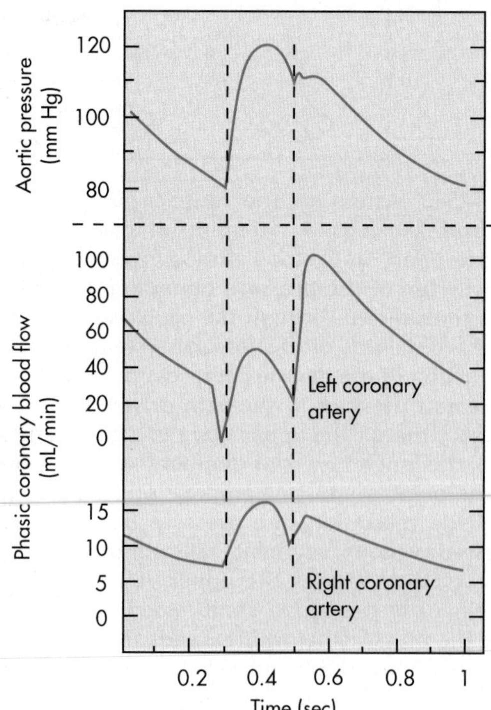

FIGURE 25–4. Comparison of phasic coronary blood flow in the left and right coronary arteries.

because a greater blood flow to the endocardium during diastole compensates for the greater blood flow to the epicardium during systole. In fact, blood flow is slightly higher in the endocardium than in the epicardium under normal conditions. The equality of epicardial and endocardial blood flow must mean that the tone of the endocardial resistance vessels is less than that of the epicardial vessels because extravascular compression is greatest at the endocardial surface of the ventricle.

Under abnormal conditions, when diastolic pressure in the coronary arteries is low, such as in **severe hypotension, partial coronary artery occlusion,** or **severe aortic stenosis,** blood flow is more severely impaired to the endocardial regions than to the epicardial regions of the ventricle. For this reason, myocardial damage after occlusion of the anterior descending branch of the left coronary artery is usually greatest in the inner wall of the left ventricle.

Flow in the right coronary artery shows a similar pattern (Figure 25–4), but because of the lower pressure developed by the thin right ventricle during systole, blood flow does not reverse in early systole. Systolic blood flow in the right coronary artery constitutes a much greater proportion of total coronary inflow than it does in the left coronary artery.

Tachycardia and bradycardia have dual effects on coronary flow. A change in heart rate is accomplished chiefly by shortening or lengthening diastole. During tachycardia, the proportion of time the heart spends in systole (when the vessels are compressed and flow is restricted) increases. However, this mechanical reduction in mean coronary flow is overridden by the coronary dilation associated with the increased metabolic activity of the more rapidly beating heart. During bradycardia, the opposite is true; restriction of coronary inflow is less (diastole is longer), but the metabolic (O_2) requirements of the myocardium are also less.

Neural and neurohumoral factors

THE PRIMARY EFFECT OF STIMULATION OF THE SYMPATHETIC NERVES TO THE CORONARY VESSELS IS VASOCONSTRICTION. HOWEVER, THE OBSERVED EFFECT IS A GREAT INCREASE IN CORONARY BLOOD FLOW. The increase in flow is associated with cardiac acceleration and a more forceful systole. The stronger myocardial contractions and the tachycardia (when a greater fraction of the cardiac cycle consists of systole) tend to restrict coronary flow. However, the increase in myocardial metabolic activity, as evidenced by the changes in rate and in contractility, tends to dilate the coronary resistance vessels. The increase in coronary blood flow elicited by cardiac sympathetic nerve stimulation is the algebraic sum of these factors.

Metabolic factors

One of the most striking characteristics of the coronary circulation is the close parallelism between the level of myocardial metabolic activity and the magnitude of the coronary blood flow. This relationship is also found in the denervated heart. The link between cardiac metabolic rate and coronary blood flow remains unsettled. However, it appears that A DECREASE IN THE RATIO OF O_2 SUPPLY TO O_2 DEMAND (whether it is produced by a reduction in O_2 supply or by an increment in O_2 demand) RELEASES A VASODILATOR SUBSTANCE FROM THE MYOCARDIUM INTO THE INTERSTITIAL FLUID, WHERE THE SUBSTANCE CAN RELAX THE CORONARY RESISTANCE VESSELS.

As diagrammed in **Figure 25–5**, a decrease in arterial blood O_2 content, a decrease in coronary blood flow, or an increase in metabolic rate decreases the O_2 supply/demand ratio. A reduction of oxidative metabolism in vascular smooth muscle reduces ATP, which in turn opens ATP-sensitive K^+ channels and causes hyperpolarization. This potential change reduces Ca^{++} entry and relaxes coronary vascular smooth muscle to increase flow. Also, the release of vasodilators, such as nitric oxide and adenosine, dilates the arterioles and thereby adjusts the O_2 supply to the O_2 demand. A decreased O_2 demand would sustain the ATP level and also reduce the amount of vasodilator substances released and permit greater expression of basal tone.

Numerous other agents, generally referred to as **metabolites,** have been suggested as mediators of the vasodilation evoked by increased cardiac work. Among the substances implicated are CO_2, O_2 (reduced O_2 tension), H^+ (lactic acid), and K^+. Accumulation of vasoactive metabolites may also be

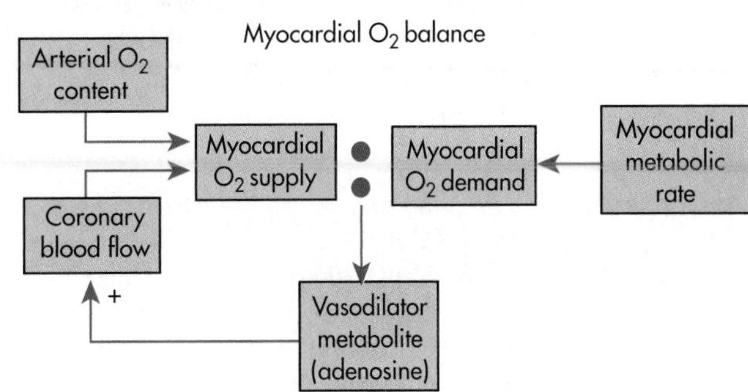

FIGURE 25–5. An imbalance in the O_2 supply/demand ratio alters coronary blood flow by changing the rate of release of a vasodilator metabolite (adenosine) from the cardiomyocytes. A decrease in the ratio elicits an increase in vasodilator release, whereas an increase in the ratio has the opposite effect.

responsible for reactive hyperemia in the heart because the duration of coronary flow after the release of the briefly occluded vessel is, within certain limits, proportional to the duration of the period of occlusion.

Cardiac O_2 consumption is determined by the kind of work done by the heart

The volume of O_2 consumed by the heart is determined by the amount and type of activity the heart performs. Under basal conditions, myocardial O_2 consumption is about 8 to 10 mL/min/100 g of heart. It can increase severalfold with exercise and decrease moderately under conditions such as hypotension and hypothermia. The cardiac venous blood normally has a low O_2 content (about 5 mL/dL), and the myocardium can therefore receive little additional O_2 by further O_2 extraction from the coronary blood.

Left ventricular work per beat **(stroke work)** is approximately equal to the product of the stroke volume and the mean aortic pressure against which blood is ejected by the left ventricle. At resting levels of cardiac output, the kinetic energy component is negligible (see Chapter 20). However, at high cardiac outputs, as in strenuous exercise, the kinetic component can account for up to 50% of total cardiac work. One can simultaneously halve the aortic pressure and double the cardiac output, or vice versa, and still arrive at the same value for cardiac work. However, the O_2 requirements are greater for any given increment of cardiac work when it is achieved by a rise in pressure than when it is achieved by an increase in stroke volume. Pumping an increase in cardiac output at a constant aortic pressure **(volume work)** is accomplished with a small increase in left ventricular O_2 consumption. Conversely, pumping against an increased arterial pressure at a constant cardiac output **(pressure work)** is accompanied by a large increment in myocardial O_2 consumption.

The greater energy demand of pressure work over volume work is clinically important. For example, in **aortic stenosis** (a narrowed aortic valve), left ventricular O_2 consumption is increased because of the high intraventricular pressure developed during systole to overcome the resistance of the stenotic valve, whereas coronary perfusion pressure is normal or reduced because of the pressure drop across the narrowed orifice of the diseased aortic valve. The result is a greater O_2 need by the myocardium in the face of a reduced O_2 supply. This can produce **angina pectoris** (chest pain) and eventually left ventricular failure.

Coronary collateral vessels develop in response to the impairment of coronary blood flow

In the normal human heart, there are virtually no functional intercoronary channels, and an abrupt occlusion of a coronary artery or one of its branches leads to **ischemic necrosis** (tissue death caused by inadequate blood flow) and eventual fibrosis of the areas of myocardium supplied by the occluded vessel.

If a coronary artery narrows slowly during a period of weeks, months, or years, as often occurs in **coronary atherosclerosis,** collateral vessels develop, and they may furnish sufficient blood to the ischemic myocardium to prevent or reduce the extent of myocardial injury if a major coronary artery is occluded abruptly.

Collateral vessels develop between branches of occluded and nonoccluded arteries. They originate from preexisting small vessels that undergo proliferative changes of the endothelium and smooth muscle, possibly in response to wall stress and chemical agents, including vascular endothelial growth factor and fibroblast growth factor released by the ischemic tissue.

When disease causes discrete occlusions or severe narrowing in coronary arteries (lumen diameters as small as 1 mm), the lesions can be bypassed with an artery or vein graft, or the narrow segment can be dilated by insertion of a balloon-tipped catheter into the diseased vessel through a peripheral artery and inflation of the balloon. Distention of the vessel by balloon inflation **(percutaneous transluminal coronary angioplasty)** can produce a lasting dilation of a narrowed coronary artery **(Figure 25–6)**.

Cerebral Circulation Is Regulated by Local and Neural Factors

Blood reaches the brain through the internal carotid and vertebral arteries. The vertebral arteries join to form the basilar artery, which in conjunction with branches of the internal carotid arteries forms the **circle of Willis.** A unique feature of the cerebral circulation is that it all lies within a rigid structure, the cranium. Any increase in arterial inflow, such as that occurring with arteriolar dilation, must be associated with a comparable increase in venous outflow because intracranial contents are incompressible. The volume of blood and extravascular fluid can vary considerably in most tissues. In brain, the volume of blood and extravascular fluid is relatively constant; change in either of these fluid

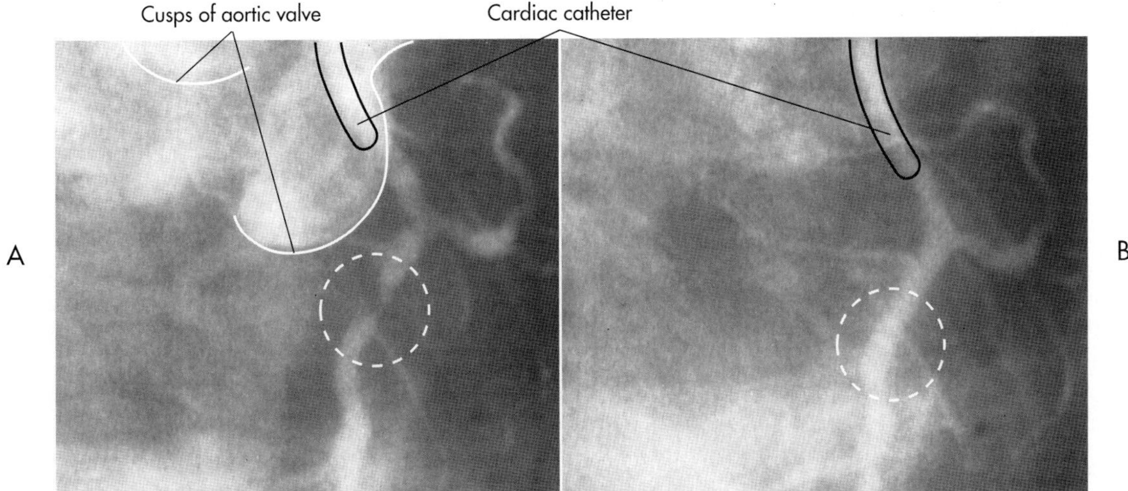

FIGURE 25–6. A, Angiogram (intracoronary radiopaque dye) of a person with marked narrowing of the circumflex branch of the left coronary artery *(circle)*. Reflux of dye into the root of the aorta outlines two of the aortic valve cusps. B, Same segment of the coronary artery after angioplasty. (Courtesy of Dr. Eric R. Powers.)

volumes must be accompanied by a reciprocal change in the other. In contrast to blood flow in most other organs, the total cerebral blood flow is held within a relatively narrow range; in humans, it averages 55 mL/min/100 g of brain.

Local factors predominate over neural factors in the regulation of cerebral blood flow

Of the various body tissues, the brain is the least tolerant of ischemia. Interruption of cerebral blood flow for as little as 5 seconds results in loss of consciousness. Ischemia lasting just a few minutes results in irreversible tissue damage. Fortunately, regulation of the cerebral circulation is mainly under the direction of the brain itself. Local regulatory mechanisms and reflexes that originate in the brain tend to maintain cerebral circulation relatively constant. This constancy prevails even in the presence of adverse extrinsic effects such as sympathetic vasomotor nerve activity, circulating vasoactive agents, and changes in arterial blood pressure. Under certain conditions, the brain also regulates its blood flow by initiating changes in systemic blood pressure.

> The elevation of intracranial pressure, such as that which may occur with a brain tumor, results in an increased systemic blood pressure. This response, called **Cushing's phenomenon,** is apparently caused by ischemic stimulation of vasomotor regions of the medulla. It aids in maintaining cerebral blood flow in the face of elevated intracranial pressure.

Neural factors

The cerebral vessels are innervated by cervical sympathetic nerve fibers that accompany the internal carotid and vertebral arteries into the cranial cavity. Compared with the control of other vascular beds, sympathetic control of the cerebral vessels is weak, and the contractile state of the cerebrovascular smooth muscle depends mainly on local metabolic factors. There are no known sympathetic vasodilator nerves to the cerebral vessels. However, the vessels do receive parasympathetic fibers from the facial nerve, and stimulation of these fibers produces slight vasodilation.

Local factors

IN GENERAL, TOTAL CEREBRAL BLOOD FLOW IS CONSTANT. HOWEVER, REGIONAL CORTICAL BLOOD FLOW IS ASSOCIATED WITH REGIONAL NEURAL ACTIVITY. For example, movement of one hand results in increased blood flow only in the hand area of the contralateral sensorimotor and premotor cortex. Also, talking, reading, and other stimuli to the cerebral center are associated with increased blood flow in the appropriate regions of the cortex (**Figure 25–7**). The mediator of the link between cerebral activity and blood flow has not been established, but nitric oxide and adenosine may be involved.

The cerebral vessels are very sensitive to CO_2 tension. Increases in arterial blood CO_2 tension ($PaCO_2$) elicit marked cerebral vasodilation; inhalation of 7% CO_2 increases cerebral blood flow twofold. By the same token, decreases in $PaCO_2$, which may be elicited by hyperventilation, decrease the cerebral blood flow. CO_2 changes arteriolar resistance by altering the perivascular pH and

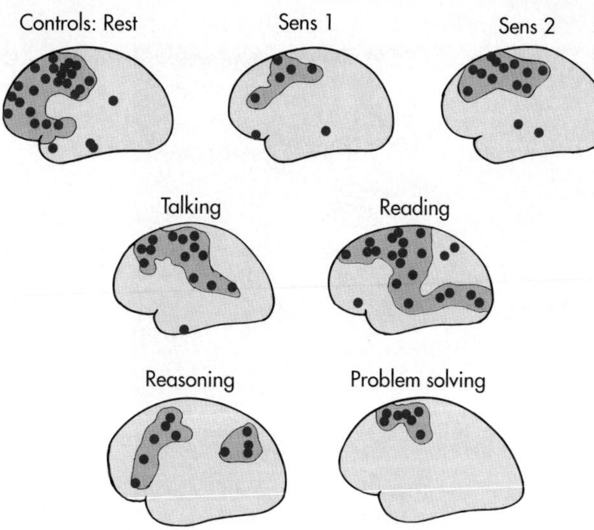

FIGURE 25–7. Effects of different stimuli on the regional blood flow in the contralateral human cerebral cortex. Sens 1, low-intensity electrical stimulation of the hand; Sens 2, high-intensity electrical stimulation of the hand (pain). (Data from Ingvar DG: *Brain Res* 107:181, 1976.)

probably the intracellular pH of the vascular smooth muscle. By independently changing the Pa_{CO_2} and $[HCO_3^-]$, it has been demonstrated that pial vessel diameter (and presumably blood flow) and pH are inversely related, regardless of the level of the Pa_{CO_2}.

The cerebral circulation shows reactive hyperemia and excellent autoregulation between pressures of about 60 and 160 mm Hg. Mean arterial pressures less than 60 mm Hg result in reduced cerebral blood flow and syncope, whereas mean pressures greater than 160 mm Hg may increase the permeability of the blood-brain barrier and cause cerebral edema.

Splanchnic Circulation Includes Intestinal and Hepatic Circulation

The splanchnic circulation consists of the blood supply to the gastrointestinal tract, liver, spleen, and pancreas. The most noteworthy feature of the splanchnic circulation is that two large capillary beds are partly in series with each other. The small splanchnic arterial branches supply the capillary beds in the gastrointestinal tract, spleen, and pancreas. From these capillary beds, the venous blood ultimately flows into the portal vein, which normally provides most of the blood supply to the liver. However, the hepatic artery also supplies blood to the liver.

Intestinal circulation is dependent on regulation and functional hyperemia

Neural regulation

Neural control of the mesenteric circulation is almost exclusively sympathetic. Increased sympathetic activity constricts the mesenteric arterioles and capacitance vessels. These responses are mediated by α receptors, which are prepotent in the mesenteric circulation; however, β receptors are also present. Infusion of a β-receptor agonist, such as isoproterenol, causes vasodilation.

Autoregulation

Autoregulation in the intestinal circulation is less well developed than in certain other vascular beds, such as those in the brain and kidney. The principal mechanism responsible for autoregulation is metabolic, although a myogenic mechanism probably also participates.

Functional hyperemia

Food ingestion increases intestinal blood flow, as does the secretion of the gastrointestinal hormones gastrin and cholecystokinin. The absorption of food also increases intestinal blood flow; the principal mediators of mesenteric hyperemia are glucose and fatty acids.

Hepatic circulation regulates and otherwise controls blood flow

Regulation of flow

Blood flow in the portal venous and hepatic arterial systems varies reciprocally. When blood flow is curtailed in one system, the flow increases in the other. However, the resultant increase in flow in one system usually does not fully compensate for the initiating reduction in flow in the other.

The portal venous system does not autoregulate. As the portal venous pressure and flow are raised, resistance either remains constant or decreases. However, the hepatic arterial system does autoregulate.

The sympathetic nerves constrict the presinusoidal resistance vessels in the portal venous and hepatic arterial systems. However, neural effects on the capacitance vessels are more important. The effects are mediated mainly by α receptors.

Capacitance vessels

The liver contains about 15% of the total blood volume of the body, making it an important blood reservoir in humans. Under appropriate conditions, such as in response to hemorrhage, about half of the hepatic blood volume can be rapidly expelled.

In certain species, notably the dog, the spleen may also serve as an effective blood reservoir. It does not play an important role in humans, however.

Extensive fibrosis of the liver, such as that which occurs in **hepatic cirrhosis,** increases hepatic vascular resistance, which raises portal venous pressure substantially. The consequent increase in the capillary pressure throughout the splanchnic circulation leads to extensive fluid transudation **(ascites)** into the peritoneal cavity.

Fetal Circulation Supplies the Tissues with O_2 and Nutrients from the Placenta and Bypasses the Fetal Lungs

The fetal circulation differs from the circulation of the postnatal infant. The fetal lungs are functionally inactive, and the fetus depends completely on the placenta for O_2 and nutrients. Oxygenated fetal blood from the placenta passes through the umbilical vein to the liver. Approximately half passes through the liver, and the remainder bypasses the liver to the inferior vena cava through the **ductus venosus** (Figure 25–8). In the inferior vena cava, blood from the ductus venosus joins blood returning from the lower trunk and extremities, and this combined stream is in turn joined by blood from the liver through the hepatic veins.

The streams of blood tend to maintain their identity in the inferior vena cava, but they are divided into two streams of unequal size by the edge of the interatrial septum **(crista dividens).** The larger stream, which is mainly blood from the umbilical vein, is shunted to the left atrium through the **foramen ovale,** which lies between the inferior vena cava and the left atrium (Figure 25–8, upper inset). The other stream passes into the right atrium, where it is joined by superior vena caval blood returning from the upper parts of the body and by blood from the myocardium.

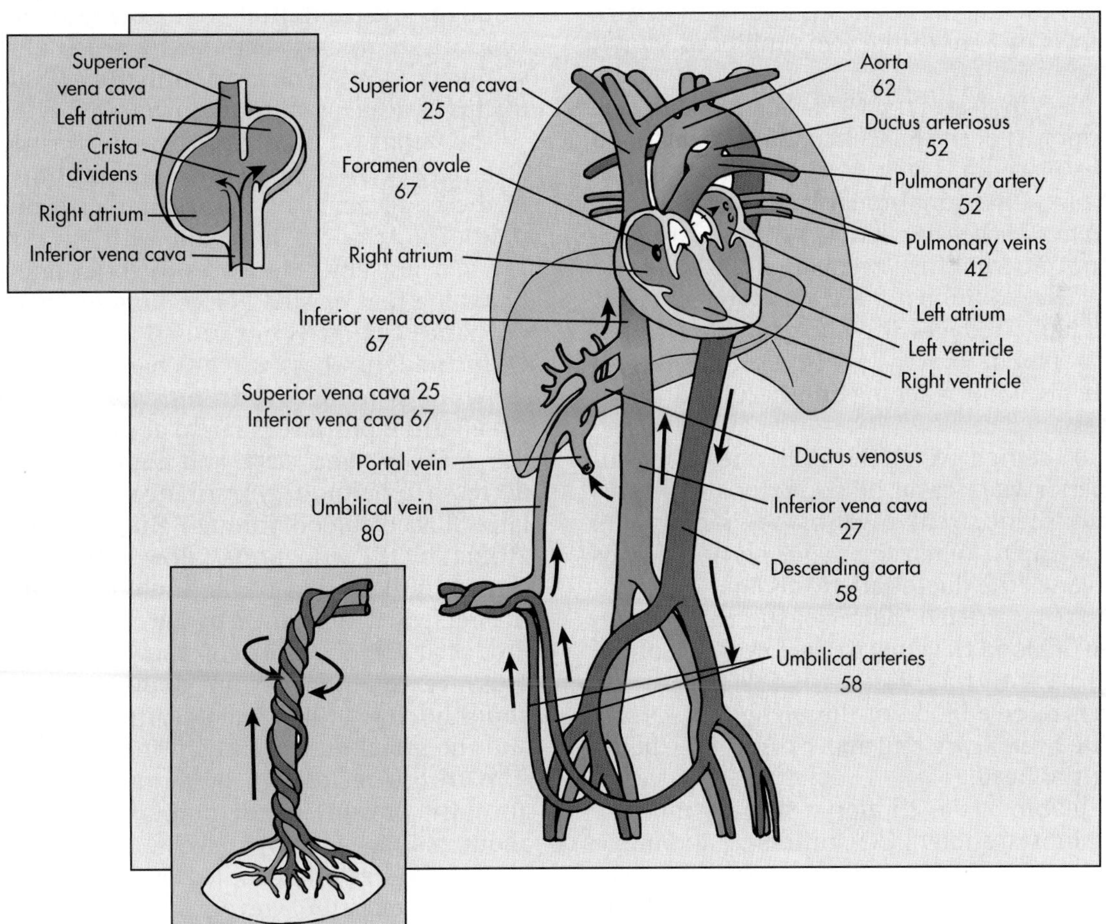

FIGURE 25–8. Fetal circulation. The numbers represent the percentage of O_2 saturation of blood flowing in the indicated blood vessel. *Upper inset,* Direction of flow of a major portion of the inferior vena caval blood through the foramen ovale to the left atrium. *Bottom inset,* Umbilical vessels and placenta. (Data for O_2 saturations from Dawes GS et al: *J Physiol* 126:563, 1954.)

In the adult, the right and left ventricles pump in series; in contrast, the ventricles in the fetus operate essentially in parallel. Because of the large pulmonary resistance, only one tenth of the right ventricular output goes through the lungs. The remainder passes through the **ductus arteriosus** from the pulmonary artery to the aorta at a point distal to the origins of the arteries to the head and upper extremities. Blood flows from the pulmonary artery to the aorta because the pulmonary artery resistance is high and the diameter of the ductus arteriosus is as large as the descending aorta.

The large volume of blood coming through the foramen ovale into the left atrium is joined by blood returning from the lungs, and it is pumped out by the left ventricle into the aorta. Most of the blood in the ascending aorta goes to the head, upper thorax, and arms; the remainder joins blood from the ductus arteriosus and supplies the rest of the body and the placenta. The amount of blood pumped by the left ventricle is about half of that pumped by the right ventricle. The major fraction of the blood that passes down the descending aorta comes from the ductus arteriosus and right ventricle and flows by way of the two umbilical arteries to the placenta.

Figure 25–8 indicates the O_2 saturations of blood at various points of the fetal circulation. Fetal blood leaving the placenta is 80% saturated, but the saturation of blood passing through the foramen ovale is reduced to 67% because it mixes with desaturated blood returning from the lower part of the body and the liver. The addition of the desaturated blood from the lungs reduces the O_2 saturation of left ventricular blood to 62%, which is the level of saturation of blood reaching the head and upper extremities.

Blood in the right ventricle, a mixture of desaturated superior vena caval blood, coronary venous blood, and inferior vena caval blood, is only 52% saturated with O_2. When the major portion of this blood traverses the ductus arteriosus and joins that pumped out by the left ventricle, the resulting O_2 saturation of blood traveling to the lower part of the body and back to the placenta is 58%. Thus, the tissues that receive blood of the highest O_2 saturation are the liver, heart, and upper parts of the body, including the head.

At the placenta, the chorionic villi dip into the maternal sinuses, and O_2, CO_2, nutrients, and metabolic waste products exchange across the membranes. The barrier to exchange is large, and the equilibrium of O_2 tension (P_{O_2}) between the two circulations is not reached at normal rates of blood flow. Therefore, the P_{O_2} of the fetal blood leaving the placenta is low. If fetal hemoglobin did not have a greater affinity for O_2 than that of adult hemoglobin, the fetus would not receive an adequate O_2 supply (see Chapter 30). The fetal oxyhemoglobin dissociation curve is shifted to the left. Therefore, at equal O_2 pressures, fetal blood carries significantly more O_2 than maternal blood does.

In early fetal life, the high cardiac glycogen levels that prevail may protect the heart from acute periods of hypoxia. The glycogen levels gradually decrease to adult levels by term.

At birth, several changes occur in the circulatory system

The umbilical vessels have thick muscular walls that are reactive to trauma, tension, sympathomimetic amines, bradykinin, angiotensin, and changes in P_{O_2}. In animals in which the umbilical cord is not tied, hemorrhage of the newborn is prevented because these large vessels constrict in response to one or more of the stimuli just listed. Closure of the umbilical vessels increases total peripheral resistance and blood pressure. When blood flow through the umbilical vein ceases, the ductus venosus, a thick-walled vessel with a muscular sphincter, closes. The factor initiating closure of the ductus venosus is still unknown.

The asphyxia that starts with constriction or clamping of the umbilical vessels, plus the cooling of the body, activates the respiratory center of the newborn. After the lungs fill with air, pulmonary vascular resistance decreases to about one tenth of the value that existed before lung expansion. This resistance change is not caused by the presence of O_2 in the lungs because the change is just as great if the lungs are filled with nitrogen.

Left atrial pressure is raised above the pressure in the inferior vena cava and right atrium by the decrease in pulmonary resistance with the resulting large flow of blood through the lungs to the left atrium, by the reduction of flow to the right atrium caused by occlusion of the umbilical vein, and by the increased resistance to left ventricular output produced by occlusion of the umbilical arteries. This reversal of the pressure gradient across the atria abruptly closes the valve over the foramen ovale, and the septal leaflets fuse during several days.

With the decrease in pulmonary vascular resistance, the pressure in the pulmonary artery falls to about half its previous level (≈35 mm Hg). This change in pressure, coupled with a slight increase in aortic pressure, reverses the flow of blood through the ductus arteriosus. However, within several minutes, the large ductus arteriosus begins to constrict, producing turbulent flow, which manifests as a murmur in the newborn. Constriction of the ductus arteriosus is progressive and usually complete within 1 to 2 days after birth. Closure of the ductus arteriosus appears to be initiated by the high Po_2 of the arterial blood passing through it; pulmonary ventilation with O_2 closes the ductus, whereas ventilation with air low in O_2 opens this shunt vessel. Whether O_2 acts directly on the ductus or mediates the release of a vasoconstrictor substance is unknown.

At birth, the walls of the two ventricles are about equally thick, or the right ventricle is slightly thicker. Also, in the newborn, the pulmonary arterioles are thick, which is partly responsible for the high pulmonary vascular resistance of the fetus. After birth, the thickness of the walls of the right ventricle diminishes, as does the muscle layer of the pulmonary arterioles; the left ventricular walls become thicker. These changes are progressive for several weeks after birth.

The **ductus arteriosus** occasionally fails to close after birth. This constitutes a common congenital cardiac abnormality that is amenable to surgical correction.

SUMMARY

- Most of the resistance vessels in the skin are under the dual control of the sympathetic nervous system and local vasodilator metabolites, but the AV anastomoses found in the skin of the hands, feet, and face are solely under neural control.
- The main function of skin blood vessels is to aid in the regulation of body temperature either by constricting, which conserves heat, or by dilating, which loses heat.
- Skin blood vessels dilate directly and reflexly in response to heat and constrict directly and reflexly in response to cold.
- Skeletal muscle blood flow is regulated centrally by the sympathetic nerves and locally by the release of vasodilator metabolites.
- Neural regulation of skeletal blood flow in resting subjects is paramount, but metabolic regulation prevails during muscle contractions.
- The physical factors that influence coronary blood flow are the viscosity of the blood, frictional resistance of the vessel walls, aortic pressure, and extravascular compression of the vessels within the walls of the left ventricle.
- Left coronary blood flow is restricted during ventricular systole as a result of extravascular compression, and it is greatest during diastole, when the intramyocardial vessels are not compressed.
- Neural regulation of coronary blood flow is much less important than metabolic regulation. Activation of the cardiac sympathetic nerves directly constricts the coronary resistance vessels. However, the enhanced myocardial metabolism caused by the associated increase in heart rate and contractile force produces vasodilation, which overrides the direct constrictor effect of sympathetic nerve stimulation. Stimulation of the cardiac branches of the vagus nerves slightly dilates the coronary arterioles.
- The metabolic activity of the heart parallels the coronary blood flow. A decrease in O_2 supply or an increase in O_2 demand apparently releases vasodilators that decrease coronary resistance.
- Gradual occlusion of a coronary artery causes collateral vessels to develop from adjacent unoccluded arteries, and they supply blood to the compromised myocardium distal to the point of occlusion.
- Cerebral blood flow is regulated predominantly by metabolic factors, especially CO_2, K^+, and adenosine.
- Increased regional cerebral activity produced by stimuli such as touch, pain, hand motion, talking, reading, reasoning, and problem solving is associated with enhanced blood flow in the activated areas of the cerebral cortex.

- ❖ The microcirculation in the intestinal villi constitutes a countercurrent exchange system for O_2. This places the villi in jeopardy in states of low blood flow.
- ❖ The splanchnic resistance and capacitance vessels are responsive to changes in sympathetic neural activity.
- ❖ The liver receives about 25% of the cardiac output; about three fourths of this comes via the portal vein and about one fourth via the hepatic artery.
- ❖ When blood flow is diminished in either the portal or the hepatic system, flow in the other system usually increases but not proportionately.
- ❖ The liver tends to maintain a constant O_2 consumption, in part because its mechanism for extracting O_2 from the blood is so efficient.
- ❖ The liver normally contains about 15% of the total blood volume. It serves as an important blood reservoir for the body.
- ❖ In the fetus, a large percentage of the right atrial blood passes through the foramen ovale to the left atrium, and a large percentage of the pulmonary artery blood passes through the ductus arteriosus to the aorta.
- ❖ At birth, the umbilical vessels, ductus venosus, and ductus arteriosus close by contraction of their muscle layers.
- ❖ The reduction in the pulmonary vascular resistance caused by lung inflation is the main factor that reverses the pressure gradient between the atria, thereby closing the foramen ovale.

Bibliography

Faber JJ, Thornburg KL: *Placental physiology,* New York, 1983, Raven Press.

Faraci FM, Heistad DD: Regulation of the cerebral circulation: role of endothelium and potassium channels, *Physiol Rev* 78:53, 1998.

Fozzard HA et al, eds: *The heart and cardiovascular system,* ed 2, New York, 1991, Raven Press.

Greenway CV, Lautt WW: Hepatic circulation. In Schultz SG, ed: *Handbook of physiology, section 6, The gastrointestinal system, vol 1, Motility and circulation,* Bethesda, Md, 1989, American Physiological Society.

Guissani DA et al: Dynamics of cardiovascular responses to repeated partial umbilical cord compression in late-gestation sheep fetus, *Am J Physiol* 273(pt 2):H2351, 1997.

Hudetz AG, Shen H, Kampine JP: Nitric oxide from neuronal NOS plays critical role in cerebral capillary flow response to hypoxia, *Am J Physiol* 274:H982, 1998.

Ishibashi Y et al: ATP-sensitive K^+ channels, adenosine, and nitric oxide–mediated mechanisms account for coronary vasodilation during exercise, *Circ Res* 82:346, 1998.

Lautt WW, Legare DJ: Passive autoregulation of portal venous pressure: distensible hepatic resistance, *Am J Physiol* 263:G702, 1992.

Lederer WJ, Nichols CG: Regulation and function of adenosine triphosphate–sensitive potassium channels in the cardio vascular system. In Zipes DP, Jalife J, eds: *Cardiac electrophysiology: from cell to bedside,* ed 2, Philadelphia, 1995, WB Saunders.

Miller FJ, Dellsperger KC, Gutterman DD: Myogenic constriction of human coronary arterioles, *Am J Physiol* 273:H257, 1997.

Mubagwa K, Flameng W: Adenosine, adenosine receptors and myocardial protection: an updated overview, *Cardiovasc Res* 52:25, 2001.

Olsson RA, Bunger R, Spaan JAE: Coronary circulation. In Fozzard HA et al, eds: *The heart and cardiovascular system,* ed 2, New York, 1991, Raven Press.

Park KH et al: Nitric oxide is a mediator of hypoxic coronary vasodilatation, *Circ Res* 71:992, 1992.

Phillis JW, ed: *The regulation of cerebral blood flow,* Boca Raton, Fla, 1993, CRC Press.

Rådegran G, Saltin B: Muscle flow at onset of dynamic exercise in humans, *Am J Physiol* 274:H314, 1998.

Risau W: Mechanisms of angiogenesis, *Nature* 386:671, 1997.

Schaper W et al: Collateral circulation. In Fozzard HA et al, eds: *The heart and cardiovascular system,* ed 2, New York, 1991, Raven Press.

Welsh DG et al: Transient receptor potential channels regulate myogenic tone of resistance arteries, *Circ Res* 90:248, 2002.

Case Studies

Case 25–1

A 70-year-old man with a long history of angina pectoris has been treated successfully with nitroglycerin. He entered the hospital because of short episodes of lightheadedness and occasional loss of consciousness. The findings on physical examination were unremarkable, except for a pulse rate of 35 beats/min. His blood pressure was 130/50 mm Hg. The electrocardiogram showed an atrial rate of 72 beats/min and a ventricular rate of 35 beats/min, with complete disassociation of the P and R waves. The chest x-ray film showed a moderately enlarged heart. The diagnosis was coronary artery disease with complete (third-degree) heart block. A pacemaker was inserted, and the patient was discharged from the hospital.

1. **What did the severe bradycardia produce?**
   A. Myogenic constriction of the coronary vessels
   B. Metabolic dilation of the coronary vessels
   C. Reflex dilation of the coronary vessels
   D. A decrease followed by an increase in coronary resistance
   E. Reversal of the endocardial to epicardial blood flow ratio

2. **Within 2 to 3 months after leaving the hospital, the patient experienced more frequent and more severe bouts of angina pectoris, and he was admitted to the hospital for study. An angiogram showed advanced coronary artery disease with almost complete occlusion of the three main coronary arteries. He was then scheduled for coronary bypass surgery. During the operation, the surgeon electrically stimulated the right and left stellate ganglia. What did this stimulation cause?**
   A. No change in coronary blood flow
   B. An increase in ventricular rate and a decrease in atrial rate
   C. A decrease in ventricular rate and an increase in atrial rate
   D. Sustained coronary dilation in one of the partially occluded vessels
   E. Sustained coronary constriction in one of the partially occluded vessels

3. **Shortly after bypass surgery, the reactivity of his coronary vessels was tested by intracoronary administration (through a catheter) of several vasoactive agents. Which of the following substances elicited an increase in coronary resistance?**
   A. Nitroglycerin
   B. Endothelin
   C. Prostacyclin
   D. Adenosine
   E. Acetylcholine

4. **Despite the coronary bypass surgery, the patient's cardiac function progressively deteriorated. He became severely short of breath (dyspneic) and developed intractable cardiac failure. A suitable donor was found, and he had a heart transplant. After cardiac transplantation, which of the following is true?**
   A. Coronary blood flow increases with vagus nerve stimulation.
   B. Coronary blood flow decreases with sympathetic nerve stimulation.
   C. Heart rate increases with inspiration.
   D. Heart rate decreases with inspiration.
   E. Stroke volume increases with exercise.

Case 25–2

A 53-year-old man has consumed substantial amounts of alcohol during the past 3 decades. For the past 2 or 3 years, he has noticed that his belt size has progressively increased and that his abdomen was distended. His physician was able to evoke a fluid wave across the abdomen when he tapped the patient's abdomen. The physician made the diagnosis of hepatic cirrhosis, which is associated with extensive fibrosis of the liver.

1. **What is the reason for the large accumulation of fluid in the patient's abdomen?**
   A. The hydrostatic pressure in the splanchnic capillaries was abnormally high.
   B. The hydrostatic pressure in the hepatic artery was abnormally high.
   C. The hydrostatic pressure in the hepatic veins exceeded that in the portal vein.
   D. The hydrostatic pressure in the hepatic veins exceeded that in the splenic vein.
   E. The hepatic vascular resistance was subnormal.

Chapter 26: Interplay of Central and Peripheral Factors in Control of the Circulation

Objectives

- ❖ Describe the sequence of cardiovascular events during exercise.
- ❖ Describe how most cardiovascular functions are integrated in exercise.
- ❖ Explain the effects of blood loss on the cardiovascular system.
- ❖ Explain the various compensatory mechanisms that protect against hemorrhagic shock.
- ❖ Explain the various decompensatory mechanisms that intensify the effects of blood loss.

The primary function of the circulatory system is to deliver the nutrients needed for tissue metabolism and growth and to remove metabolic products. How the heart and blood vessels serve this function requires a morphological and functional analysis of the system and a discussion of how the component parts contribute to maintain adequate tissue perfusion under different physiological conditions.

Once the functions of the various components are understood, one must consider their interrelationships in the overall role of the circulatory system. Tissue perfusion depends on arterial pressure and local vascular resistance, and arterial pressure in turn depends on cardiac output and total peripheral resistance (TPR). Arterial pressure is maintained within a relatively narrow range in the healthy individual, a feat accomplished by reciprocal changes in cardiac output and TPR. However, cardiac output and TPR are each influenced by a number of factors, and it is the interplay among these factors that determines the level of these two variables. The autonomic nervous system and the baroreceptors play the key role in regulating blood pressure. However, from the long-range point of view, control of fluid balance by the kidney, adrenal cortex, and central nervous system is crucial in maintaining a constant blood volume.

In a well-regulated system, one may study the extent and sensitivity of the regulatory mechanism by disturbing the system and observing how it restores the preexisting steady state. Disturbances in the form of physical exercise and hemorrhage are used in this chapter to illustrate the effects of the factors that regulate the circulatory system.

Exercise Has Many Benefits for Circulation

Cardiovascular adjustments in exercise require an integration of neural and local chemical factors. The neural factors consist of central command, reflexes originating in the contracting muscle, and the baroreceptor reflex. **Central command** is the cerebrocortical activation of the sympathetic nervous system that produces cardiac acceleration, increased myocardial contractile force, and peripheral vasoconstriction. Reflexes can be activated via stimulation of intramuscular mechanoreceptors (stretch, tension) and chemoreceptors (products of metabolism) in response to muscle contraction. Impulses from these receptors travel centrally via small myelinated (group III) and unmyelinated (group IV) afferent nerve fibers. The central connections of this reflex are unknown, but the efferent limb consists of the sympathetic nerve fibers to the heart and peripheral blood vessels. The baroreceptor reflex is described in Chapters 19 and 23, and the local factors that influence skeletal muscle blood flow (metabolic vasodilators) are described in Chapters 23 and 25.

Exercise activates the autonomic nervous system

The concerted inhibition of parasympathetic control areas and activation of sympathetic control areas in the medulla oblongata increase the heart rate and myocardial contractility. The tachycardia and enhanced contractility increase cardiac output.

Total peripheral resistance is decreased in whole-body exercise

At the same time that the sympathetic nervous system stimulates the heart, it also changes vascular resistance in the periphery. In the skin, kidneys, splanchnic regions, and inactive muscle, sympathetic-mediated vasoconstriction increases vascular resistance, which diverts blood away from these areas. This increased resistance in vascular beds of inactive tissues persists throughout exercise.

As cardiac output and blood flow to active muscles increase with the progressive increase in the intensity of exercise, blood flow to the splanchnic and renal vasculatures decreases. Blood flow to the myocardium increases, whereas that to the brain is unchanged. Skin blood flow initially decreases during exercise and then increases as body temperature rises with the length and intensity of exercise. Skin blood flow finally decreases when the skin vessels constrict as the total body O_2 consumption nears maximum.

THE MAJOR CIRCULATORY ADJUSTMENT TO PROLONGED EXERCISE INVOLVES THE VASCULATURE OF THE ACTIVE MUSCLES. Local formation of vasoactive metabolites markedly dilates the resistance vessels; this dilation progresses as the intensity of exercise is raised. The local accumulation of metabolites relaxes the terminal arterioles. Blood flow through the muscle may increase to 15 to 20 times above the resting level. This metabolic vasodilation of the precapillary vessels in active muscles occurs very soon after the onset of exercise, and the decrease in TPR enables the heart to pump more blood more efficiently at a lesser load (less pressure work; see Chapter 25) than if TPR were unchanged.

Only a small number of the capillaries are perfused in resting muscle, whereas in actively contracting muscle, all or nearly all of the capillaries contain flowing blood **(capillary recruitment).** The surface available for the exchange of gases, water, and solutes increases manyfold. Furthermore, the hydrostatic pressure in the capillaries is increased because of the relaxation of the resistance vessels. Hence, there is a net movement of water and solutes into the muscle tissue. Tissue pressure rises and remains elevated during exercise as fluid continues to move out of the capillaries and is carried away by the lymphatic system. Lymph flow is increased as a result of the rise in capillary hydrostatic pressure and the massaging effect of the contracting muscles on the valve-containing lymphatic vessels (Chapter 22).

The contracting muscle avidly extracts O_2 from the perfusing blood (increased arteriovenous O_2 difference; **Figure 26–1**), and the release of O_2 from the blood is facilitated by the nature of oxyhemoglobin dissociation (see Chapter 30). The reduction in pH caused by the high concentration of CO_2 and the formation of lactic acid and the increase in temperature in the contracting muscle diminish the affinity of hemoglobin for O_2, as reflected by a shift in the oxyhemoglobin dissociation curve to the right. At any given partial pressure of O_2, less O_2 is held by the hemoglobin in the red cells; consequently, O_2 removal from the blood is more effective. O_2 consumption may increase as much as 60-fold with only a 15-fold increase in muscle blood flow. However, the partial pressures of arterial O_2 and arterial CO_2 are normal during exercise. Muscle myoglobin serves as a limited O_2 store in exercise and can release bound O_2 at very low partial pressures. It also facilitates O_2 transport from the capillaries to the mitochondria by serving as an O_2 carrier.

Heart rate, cardiac output, and venous return increase with exercise

The enhanced sympathetic drive and the reduced parasympathetic inhibition of the sinoatrial node continue during exercise; consequently, tachycardia persists. If the workload is moderate and constant, the heart rate reaches a certain level and remains there throughout exercise. However, if the workload increases, the heart rate increases concomitantly until a plateau at about 180 beats/min is reached in severe exercise (Figure 26–1). In contrast to the large increase in heart rate, the increase in stroke volume is only about 10% to 35% (Figure 26–1), the larger

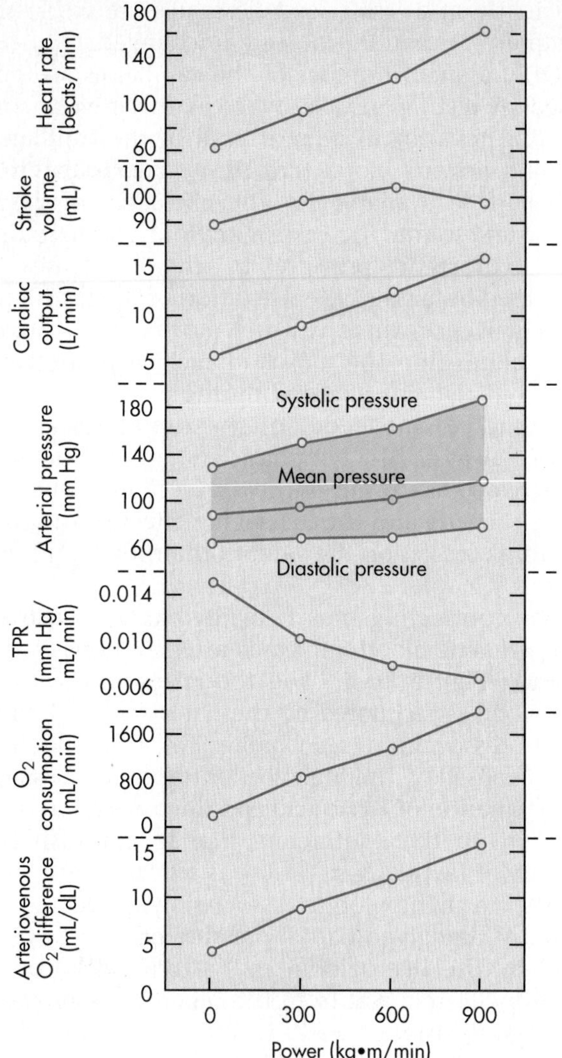

FIGURE 26–1. Effect of different levels of exercise on several cardiovascular variables. (Data from Carlsten A, Grimby G: *The circulatory response to muscular exercise in man,* Springfield, Ill, 1966, Charles C Thomas.)

values occurring in trained individuals. In well-trained distance runners, whose cardiac outputs attain six to seven times the resting level, stroke volume reaches about twice the resting value.

If the baroreceptors are denervated, the cardiac output and heart rate responses to exercise are more sluggish than in animals with normally innervated baroreceptors. However, in the absence of cardiac autonomic innervation, such as that which occurs experimentally after total cardiac denervation, exercise still elicits an increment in cardiac output comparable to that observed in normal animals, but then it is associated with an elevated stroke volume.

In addition to the contribution made by sympathetically mediated constriction of the capacitance vessels in both exercising and nonexercising parts of the body, venous return to the heart is aided by the working skeletal muscles and the muscles of respiration (see also Chapters 24 and 25). The intermittently contracting muscles compress the vessels that course through them. The valves in the compressed veins permit blood flow only toward the right atrium (see Figure 25–2). The flow of venous blood to the heart is also aided by the increase in the pressure gradient developed by the more negative intrathoracic pressure produced by deeper and more frequent respirations.

In a healthy resting person, an increase in heart rate does not usually increase cardiac output appreciably (see Chapter 24). However, in whole-body exercise, the enhanced venous return caused by a decreased TPR (Figure 26–1) in concert with the skeletal muscle pump (see Figure 25–2) is associated mainly with an increase in heart rate. If the heart rate cannot increase normally in response to exercise (e.g., in a patient with complete atrioventricular block), the patient's ability to exercise will be severely limited. HENCE, AN INCREASE IN HEART RATE IS NECESSARY TO ENABLE THE REDUCED TPR AND SKELETAL MUSCLE PUMP TO APPROPRIATELY AUGMENT CARDIAC OUTPUT DURING EXERCISE.

In humans, little evidence exists that blood reservoirs contribute much to the circulating blood volume, with the exception of the skin, lungs, and liver. In fact, blood volume is usually reduced slightly during exercise, as evidenced by a rise in the hematocrit ratio, because of water loss externally through sweating and enhanced ventilation and through fluid movement into the contracting muscle. The fluid loss from the vascular compartment into the interstitium of contracting muscle reaches a plateau as interstitial fluid pressure rises and opposes the increased hydrostatic pressure in the capillaries of the active muscle. The fluid loss is partially offset by the movement of fluid from the splanchnic regions and inactive muscle into the bloodstream. This influx of fluid occurs as a result of a decrease in the hydrostatic pressure in the capillaries of these tissues and an increase in the plasma osmolarity because of movement of osmotically active particles into the blood from the contracting muscle. In addition, reduced urine formation by the kidneys helps conserve body water.

In light to moderate exercise, blood returning to the heart is so rapidly pumped through the lungs and out into the aorta that the central venous pressure (diastolic filling pressure) increases only slightly. In fact, CHEST X-RAY FILMS OF INDIVIDUALS AT REST AND AT EXERCISE REVEAL A DECREASE IN HEART SIZE DURING EXERCISE, which is in harmony with the observations of a constant ventricular diastolic volume. However, in maximal or near-maximal exercise, right atrial pressure and end-diastolic ventricular volume increase. Thus, the Frank-Starling mechanism contributes to the enhanced stroke volume in vigorous exercise.

Arterial pressure increases with exercise

If exercise involves a large proportion of the body musculature, such as in running or swimming, the reduction in total vascular resistance can be considerable (Figure 26–1). Nevertheless, arterial pressure starts to rise with the onset of exercise, and the increase in blood pressure roughly parallels the severity of the exercise performed (Figure 26–1). Therefore, the increase of vascular resistance in the inactive tissues by the sympathetic nervous system (and to some extent by adrenal medullary catecholamine release) is important for maintaining normal or increased blood pressure; sympathectomy or drug-induced block of the adrenergic sympathetic nerve fibers results in a decreased arterial pressure **(hypotension)** during exercise.

Sympathetic-mediated vasoconstriction also occurs in active muscle when additional muscles are activated after about half the total skeletal musculature is contracting. In experiments in which one leg is working at maximal levels and then the other leg starts to work, blood flow decreases in the first working leg. Furthermore, blood levels of norepinephrine rise significantly in exercise, and most of it comes from sympathetic nerves in the active muscles.

As body temperature rises during exercise, the skin vessels dilate in response to the thermal stimulation of the heat-regulating center in the hypothalamus, and TPR decreases further. Blood pressure would decrease were it not for the increased cardiac output and constriction of arterioles in the renal, splanchnic, and other tissues.

In general, the mean arterial pressure rises during exercise as a result of the increased cardiac output. However, the effect of enhanced cardiac output is offset by the overall decrease in TPR, so the increase in mean blood pressure is relatively small (Figure 26–1). Vasoconstriction in inactive vascular beds contributes to the maintenance of a normal arterial blood pressure for adequate perfusion of the active tissues. The actual pressure attained represents a balance between the cardiac output and TPR. Systolic pressure usually increases more than diastolic pressure, which results in an increased pulse pressure (Figure 26–1). The larger pulse pressure is primarily attributable to a greater stroke volume and to a lesser degree to a more rapid ejection of blood by the left ventricle, with less peripheral runoff during the brief ventricular ejection period.

In exercise taken to the point of exhaustion, the compensatory mechanisms begin to fail. The heart rate attains a maximum level of about 180 beats/min, and stroke volume reaches a plateau and often decreases, resulting in a fall in blood pressure. Dehydration occurs. Sympathetic vasoconstrictor activity supersedes the vasodilator influence on the cutaneous vessels, and its effect on the capacitance vessels produces a slight increase in effective blood volume. However, cutaneous vasoconstriction also decreases the rate of heat loss. Body temperature is normally elevated, and the reduction in heat loss through cutaneous vasoconstriction can, under these conditions, lead to very high body temperatures with associated feelings of acute distress (**heat exhaustion** or **heat stroke**). The pH of tissue and blood decreases because of increased lactic acid and CO_2 production. The reduced pH is probably the key determinant of the maximal amount of exercise an individual can tolerate because of muscle pain and the subjective feeling of exhaustion.

A summary of the neural and local effects of exercise on the cardiovascular system is presented in **Figure 26–2**.

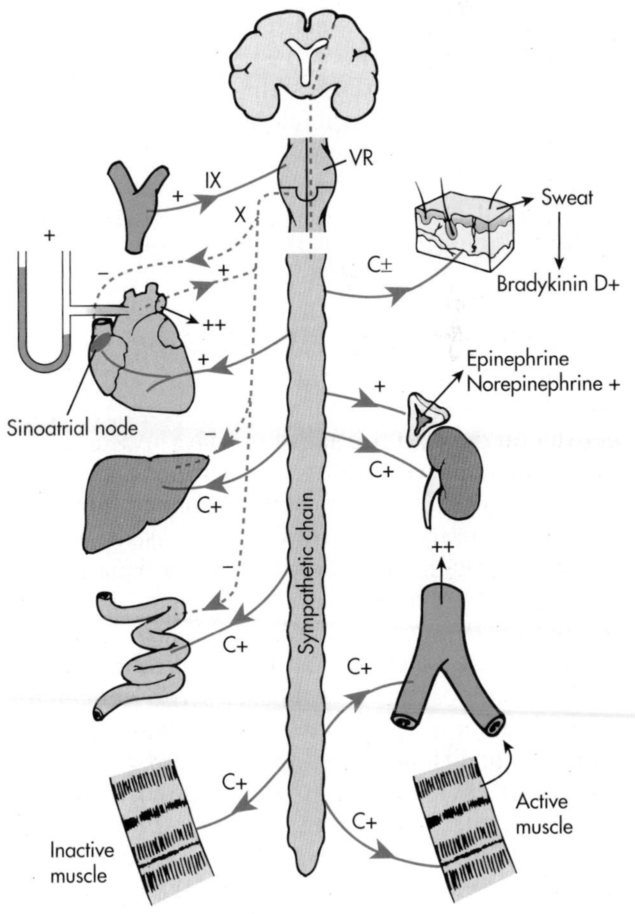

FIGURE 26–2. Cardiovascular adjustments in exercise. C, vasoconstrictor activity; D, vasodilator activity; IX, glossopharyngeal nerve; VR, vasomotor region; X, vagus nerve; +, increased activity; –, decreased activity.

Heart rate and cardiac output abruptly decrease when exercise stops

The TPR remains low for some time after exercise ends, presumably because vasodilator metabolites accumulate in the muscles during the exercise. As a result of the reduced cardiac output and persistence of vasodilation in the muscles, arterial pressure may fall briefly below preexercise levels. Blood pressure is then stabilized at normal levels by the baroreceptor reflexes.

Inadequate O_2 supply limits exercise performance

The two main forces that could limit skeletal muscle performance are the rate of O_2 use by the muscles and the O_2 supply to the muscles. Muscle O_2 use is probably not critical because when maximum O_2 consumption ($V\text{O}_2$max) is reached during exercise of a large percentage of the body muscle mass, the recruitment of additional muscles does not produce a further increase in O_2 consumption. If muscle O_2 use were limiting, the recruitment of more contracting muscle would use additional O_2 to meet the enhanced O_2 requirements and would thereby increase total body O_2 consumption. Therefore, O_2 supply to the active muscles must be inadequate. The limited O_2 supply could be caused by inadequate oxygenation of blood in the lungs or by limitation of the supply of O_2-laden blood to the muscles. Failure of the lungs to fully oxygenate blood can be excluded because even with the most strenuous exercise in subjects at sea level, arterial blood is fully saturated with O_2. Therefore, O_2 delivery (blood flow) to the active muscles appears to be the limiting factor in muscle performance.

This limitation in muscle performance translates into the inability of the heart to increase its output beyond a certain level. Cardiac output equals heart rate multiplied by stroke volume, and heart rate reaches maximum levels before $V\text{O}_2$max is reached. Hence, stroke volume must be the limiting factor. However, blood pressure provides the energy for skeletal muscle perfusion, and blood pressure depends on TPR as well as on cardiac output. During intense exercise at peak $V\text{O}_2$max and peak cardiac output, blood pressure falls as more muscle vascular beds dilate in response to locally released vasodilator metabolites if some centrally mediated vasoconstriction (via the baroreceptor reflex) does not occur in the resistance vessels of the active muscles. Hence, adjustment of resistance in the active muscles appears to be an important factor that limits whole-body exercise (e.g., swimming, running). However, THE MAJOR FACTOR IS THE PUMPING CAPACITY OF THE HEART. When the exercise involves only a small group of muscles (e.g., those of the hand), the cardiovascular system is not taxed, and the limiting factor, although unknown, lies within the muscle.

Physical training and conditioning increase peak O_2 consumption

The response of the cardiovascular system to regular exercise is to increase its capacity to deliver O_2 to the active muscles and improve the ability of the muscle to use O_2. The $V\text{O}_2$max is reproducible in a given individual, and it varies with the level of physical conditioning. Training progressively increases the $V\text{O}_2$max, which reaches a plateau at the highest level of conditioning. Highly "trained" athletes have a lower resting heart rate, greater stroke volume, and lower TPR than they had before training or after deconditioning (becoming sedentary). The low resting heart rate is caused by a higher vagal tone and a lower sympathetic tone. With exercise, the maximum heart rate of the trained individual is the same as that in "untrained" persons, but it occurs at a higher exercise level. The trained person also exhibits a low vascular resistance that is inherent in the muscle. For example, if an individual exercises one leg regularly during an extended period and does not exercise the other leg, the vascular resistance is lower and the $V\text{O}_2$max is higher in the trained leg than in the untrained leg. Also, the well-trained athlete has a lower resting sympathetic outflow to the viscera than a sedentary counterpart does.

Physical conditioning is also associated with greater extraction of O_2 from the blood (greater arteriovenous O_2 difference) by the muscles. With long-term training, capillary density in skeletal muscle increases, as do the concentrations of oxidative enzymes in the mitochondria. Also, the levels of ATPase, myoglobin, and enzymes involved in lipid metabolism appear to increase with physical conditioning.

> Endurance training, such as running or swimming, increases left ventricular volume without increasing left ventricular wall thickness. In contrast, strength exercises, such as weightlifting, increase left ventricular wall thickness **(hypertrophy)** but have little effect on ventricular volume. However, this increase in wall thickness is small relative to that observed in **chronic hypertension,** in which the elevation of afterload persists because of the high TPR.

Hemorrhaging Is a Dangerously Rapid Loss of Blood

In an individual who has lost a large quantity of blood, the arterial systolic, diastolic, and pulse pressures are reduced, and the arterial pulse is rapid and feeble. The skin is pale, moist, and slightly **cyanotic** (blue). The cutaneous veins are collapsed and fill slowly when they are compressed centrally. Respiration is rapid, but the depth of respiration may be shallow or deep.

Arterial blood pressure declines when blood is lost

The changes in mean arterial pressure evoked by acute hemorrhage in animals are illustrated in **Figure 26–3**. If an animal is bled rapidly to bring mean arterial pressure to 50 mm Hg, the arterial pressure tends to rise spontaneously toward control during the subsequent 20 to 30 minutes. In some animals (curve A in Figure 26–3), this trend continues, and normal pressures are regained within a few hours. These animals tend to survive even if their shed blood is not returned to them. In other animals (curve B in Figure 26–3), the pressure begins to decline after the initial rise and continues to fall at an accelerating rate until death ensues. If blood is transfused early in the phase of declining arterial pressure, the animals usually survive. However, at some point later in this phase of declining pressure, the deterioration becomes irreversible.

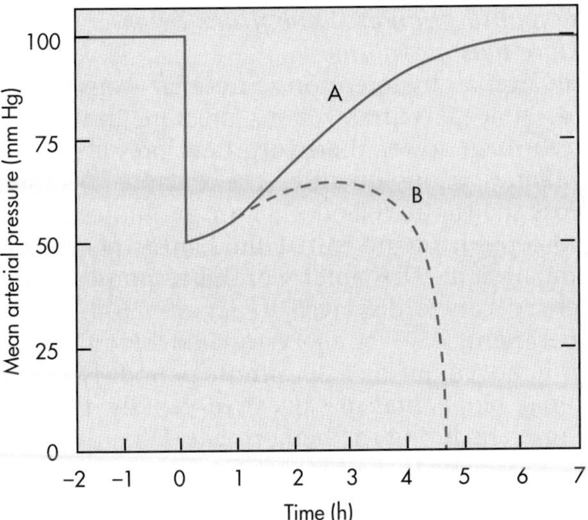

FIGURE 26–3. Changes in mean arterial pressure after rapid hemorrhage. At time zero, the animal is bled rapidly to a mean arterial pressure of 50 mm Hg. The arterial pressure tends to return toward normal at first. In some animals *(curve A),* the pressure continues to improve until the normal pressure is attained even though none of the shed blood has been transfused back into the animal. In other animals *(curve B),* after a temporary period of apparent improvement, the arterial blood pressure begins to decline and falls at a steeper and steeper rate until death ensues.

When the arterial blood pressure fails to return to normal, the state is known as **hemorrhagic shock.** This state usually has a lethal outcome regardless of whether the animal already in shock receives a transfusion of its own shed blood or a transfusion of a larger quantity of matched blood from a donor.

Compensatory mechanisms protect against blood loss

The prominent tendency for arterial blood pressure to rise toward normal levels immediately after acute blood loss (Figure 26–3) indicates that potent compensatory mechanisms must be invoked. Any mechanism that acts to restore normal levels of arterial blood pressure in response to blood loss may be designated a **negative-feedback mechanism.** The term *negative* is applied because the direction of the induced change in pressure is opposite to that of the initiating change. The following negative-feedback mechanisms are evoked by hemorrhage:

- Baroreceptor reflexes
- Chemoreceptor reflexes
- Cerebral ischemia responses
- Reabsorption of tissue fluids into the plasma compartment
- Release of endogenous vasoconstrictor substances
- Renal conservation of salt and water

Baroreceptor reflexes minimize arterial pressure declines

The reductions in the mean arterial and pulse pressures during hemorrhage decrease the excitation of the baroreceptors in the carotid sinuses and aortic arch (see Chapter 23). Several cardiovascular responses are thus evoked reflexly, all of which act to restore the normal arterial blood pressure. Unloading of the arterial baroreceptors decreases vagal tone and augments sympathetic tone, and both of these changes in efferent neural activity increase the heart rate and enhance myocardial contractility (see Chapter 19).

Diminished baroreceptor stimulation evokes generalized arteriolar vasoconstriction as the principal mechanism and that protects the subject from a critical reduction in arterial blood pressure in response to hemorrhage. Although the arteriolar vasoconstriction is widespread throughout the systemic vascular bed, it is not uniform. Hemorrhage-induced vasoconstriction is most severe in the skin, skeletal muscle, and splanchnic vascular beds.

In the early states of mild to moderate hemorrhage, the changes in renal resistance are usually slight. The tendency for increased sympathetic activity to constrict the renal vessels is counteracted by autoregulatory mechanisms (see Chapter 36). In response to more prolonged and more severe hemorrhage, however, renal vasoconstriction becomes intense. Reductions in renal circulation are most severe in the outer layers of the renal cortex; the inner zones of the cortex and outer zones of the medulla are spared.

If renal vasoconstriction persists too long, it is harmful. Frequently, patients who have lost substantial amounts of blood survive the acute hypotensive period, only to die several days later of **kidney failure** resulting from renal ischemia.

Reflexly induced arteriolar vasoconstriction tends to be slight or absent in the cerebral and coronary circulations. In many instances, the cerebral and coronary vascular resistances are diminished. Thus, the reduced cardiac output is redistributed to favor flow through the brain and heart, which are certainly among the most crucial of the body's organs.

The increased sympathetic discharge also evokes a generalized venoconstriction, which has the same hemodynamic consequences as a transfusion of blood (see Chapter 24). Sympathetic activation constricts certain blood reservoirs. This constriction provides an autotransfusion of blood into the circulation. In the dog, considerable quantities of blood are mobilized by contraction of the spleen. In humans, the spleen is not an important blood reservoir. Instead, constriction of the cutaneous and hepatic vasculatures in response to blood loss contributes blood volume to the circulating bloodstream. Therefore, these tissues act as blood reservoirs.

Severe cutaneous vasoconstriction accounts for the characteristic pale, cold skin of patients suffering from blood loss. Warming the skin of such patients improves their appearance considerably, much to the satisfaction of well-meaning individuals who might render first aid. However, it also inactivates an effective, natural compensatory mechanism, to the patient's possible detriment.

Chemoreceptor reflexes help sustain arterial blood pressure

Hemorrhage-induced reductions in arterial pressure below about 60 mm Hg do not evoke any additional baroreceptor-mediated responses because this pressure level constitutes the threshold for baroreceptor stimulation (see Chapter 23). However, low arterial pressure may lead to arterial chemoreceptor stimulation because the resulting inadequate blood flow to the aortic and carotid bodies diminishes the partial pressure of O_2 in the chemoreceptor tissues. Chemoreceptor excitation augments the prevailing vasoconstriction evoked by the baroreceptor reflexes. Also, the respiratory stimulation induced by chemoreceptor excitation assists venous return by the auxiliary pumping mechanism described in Chapter 24.

Cerebral ischemia helps sustain arterial blood pressure

Cerebral ischemia activates the sympathetic nervous system when hemorrhage lowers the arterial blood pressure below about 40 mm Hg. The resulting sympathetic nervous discharge is intense; it is several times greater than the maximal activity that occurs when the baroreceptors cease to be stimulated. Therefore, the vasoconstriction and facilitation of myocardial contractility evoked by cerebral ischemia may be pronounced. When cerebral ischemia is severe, the vagal centers also become activated. The resulting bradycardia may aggravate the hypotension that initiated the cerebral ischemia.

The reabsorption of tissue fluids helps restore plasma volume

The arterial hypotension, arteriolar constriction, and reduced central venous pressure induced by hemorrhage lower the hydrostatic pressure in the capillaries. Consequently, the balance of forces across the capillary endothelium promotes the net reabsorption of interstitial fluid into the vascular compartment. The rapidity of this response in anesthetized cats is displayed in **Figure 26–4**. In this experiment, 45% of the estimated blood volume was removed during a 30-minute period. The mean arterial blood pressure declined rapidly to about 45 mm Hg during the hemorrhage. When bleeding was terminated, the arterial pressure rose rapidly but only temporarily to near the control level. About 2½ hours after cessation of the hemorrhage, the arterial pressure began to fall, and it declined progressively until the animals died. The time course of this response to hemorrhage resembles that of curve B in Figure 26–3.

Associated with these changes in arterial blood pressure, the plasma colloid osmotic pressure declines markedly during bleeding and continues to decrease more gradually for several hours (Figure 26–4). The reduction in the colloid osmotic pressure reflects the dilution of the blood by tissue fluids.

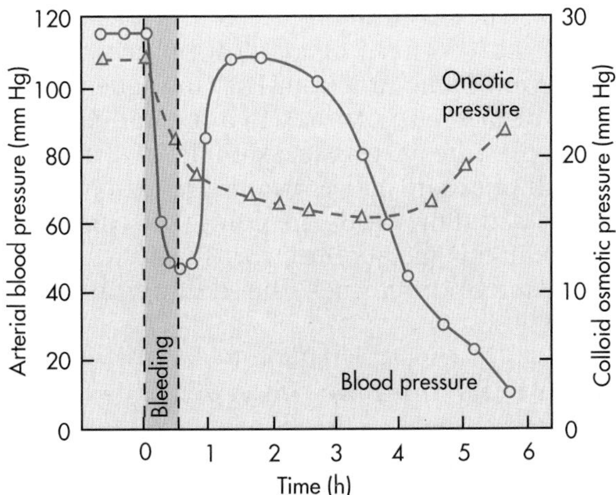

FIGURE 26–4. Changes in arterial blood pressure *(circles)* and plasma colloid osmotic pressure *(triangles)* in response to the withdrawal of 45% of the estimated blood volume during a 30-minute period, beginning at time zero, in a group of anesthetized cats. (Data from Zweifach BW: *Anesthesiology* 41:157, 1974.)

Considerable quantities of fluid may be drawn into the circulation during hemorrhage. Approximately 1 L/hr of fluid might be autoinfused from the interstitial fluid into the circulatory system of an average individual after acute blood loss.

Considerable quantities of fluid also may be slowly shifted from the intracellular to the extracellular spaces. This fluid exchange is probably mediated by the secretion of cortisol from the adrenal cortex in response to hemorrhage.

Endogenous vasoconstrictors help maintain arterial blood pressure

Catecholamines (epinephrine and norepinephrine) are released from the adrenal medulla and postganglionic sympathetic nerve endings in response to acute blood loss (see Chapter 48). The concentrations of epinephrine and norepinephrine increase substantially in the arterial blood within the first minute of hemorrhage and remain elevated (up to 50 times normal) throughout hemorrhage. Retransfusion of the shed blood reduces the blood catecholamine levels to normal.

Vasopressin, a potent vasoconstrictor, is actively secreted by the posterior pituitary gland in response to hemorrhage (see Chapter 45). Removal of about 20% of the blood volume in animals increases vasopressin secretion about 40-fold. The sensory receptors responsible for the augmented release are the sinoaortic baroreceptors and the stretch receptors in the left atrium.

Diminished renal perfusion during hemorrhagic hypotension leads to the secretion of **renin** from the juxtaglomerular apparatus (see Chapters 38 and 47). Consequently, the concentration of renin in the peripheral blood rises as a function of the volume of shed blood. Renin is an enzyme that acts on the plasma protein **angiotensinogen** to form **angiotensin I,** which is converted to angiotensin II, a powerful vasoconstrictor, by the action of angiotensin-converting enzyme.

The kidneys conserve water during hemorrhage

The diminution in arterial blood pressure induced by the loss of blood decreases the glomerular filtration rate and thus curtails water and electrolyte excretion (see Chapter 38). During hemorrhage, fluid and electrolytes are also conserved by the kidneys in response to the release of various hormones, including vasopressin and renin, as noted in the preceding section. The peptide angiotensin II, which is formed by the action of renin and angiotensin-converting enzyme, accelerates the release of aldosterone from the adrenal cortex. Aldosterone in turn stimulates Na^+ reabsorption by the renal tubules, and water accompanies the Na^+ that is actively reabsorbed (see Chapters 37 and 38).

Decompensatory mechanisms intensify the effects of hemorrhage

In contrast to the negative-feedback mechanisms just described, hemorrhage also evokes latent **positive-feedback mechanisms.** Such mechanisms exaggerate the primary changes initiated by the blood loss. Specifically, positive-feedback mechanisms aggravate the hypotension induced by blood loss and tend to initiate vicious cycles that may be fatal. The operation of positive-feedback mechanisms is manifested in the accelerating and eventually lethal decline in blood pressure reflected by curve B of Figure 26–3.

Whether a positive-feedback mechanism leads to a vicious cycle depends on the **gain** of that mechanism; the gain is the ratio of the secondary change evoked by a given feedback mechanism to the primary change itself. A gain greater than 1 induces a vicious cycle; a gain less than 1 does not. For example, consider a positive-feedback mechanism with a gain of 2. If an intervention such as the rapid loss of a specific volume of blood causes the mean arterial blood pressure to decrease quickly by 10 mm Hg, a positive-feedback mechanism (with a gain of 2) subsequently evokes a secondary pressure reduction of 20 mm Hg. This secondary change in turn causes a further decrement of 40 mm Hg; that is, each change induces a subsequent change of twice the magnitude. Hence, mean arterial pressure declines at an ever-increasing rate until death, as depicted by curve B in Figure 26–3.

A positive-feedback mechanism with a gain less than 1 also amplifies the effect of any initiating intervention, but it probably does not generate a vicious cycle. For example, if a primary intervention suddenly decreases the arterial blood pressure by 10 mm Hg, a positive-feedback mechanism with a gain of 0.5 initiates a secondary, additional pressure decline of 5 mm Hg. This, in turn, provokes a decrease of 2.5 mm Hg. The process continues in ever-diminishing steps, and the arterial blood pressure approaches some steady-state value asymptotically. Some of the important positive-feedback mechanisms evoked in response to hemorrhage include cardiac failure, acidosis, inadequate cerebral blood flow, aberration of blood clotting, and depression of the reticuloendothelial system (RES).

Cardiac failure exaggerates the effects of hemorrhage

Whether cardiac failure plays a significant role in the progression of hemorrhagic shock is controversial. All investigators agree that the heart fails terminally, but the importance of cardiac failure during earlier stages of hemorrhagic hypotension remains to be established. Rightward shifts in ventricular function curves (**Figure 26–5**) constitute experimental evidence of a progressive depression of myocardial contractility during a sustained reduction in blood volume.

The hypotension induced by hemorrhage reduces the coronary blood flow, which tends to depress ventricular function. The consequent reduction in cardiac output leads to a further decline in arterial pressure, a classic example of a positive-feedback mechanism. Furthermore, the reduced tissue blood flow leads to a local accumulation of vasodilator metabolites, which decreases TPR and therefore intensifies the decline in arterial pressure.

Acidosis exaggerates the effects of blood loss

Inadequate blood flow during hemorrhage affects the metabolism of all cells in the body. The resulting stagnant anoxia accelerates the tissue production of lactic acid and other acid metabolites. Furthermore, impaired kidney function prevents adequate excretion of the excess H^+, and generalized metabolic acidosis ensues (**Figure 26–6**). Metabolic acidosis depresses the heart and thereby further reduces tissue perfusion and thus aggravates the acidosis. Hypotension is intensified because the acidosis diminishes the reactivity of the heart and arterioles to neurally released and circulating catecholamines.

Central nervous system depression impairs the response to hemorrhage

The arterial hypotension associated with hemorrhagic shock reduces cerebral blood flow. Moderate degrees of cerebral ischemia evoke a pronounced

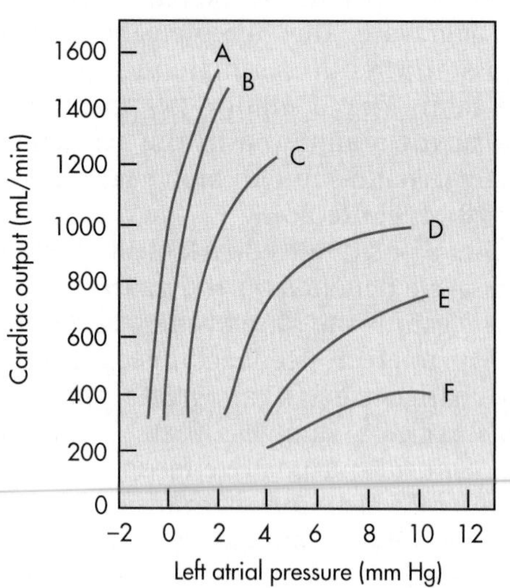

FIGURE 26–5. Left ventricular function curves in an anesthetized dog during hemorrhagic shock. Curve A represents the control curve. Curves B through F represent the curves at 117, 247, 280, 295, and 310 minutes, respectively, after the initial hemorrhage. (Data from Crowell JW, Guyton AC: *Am J Physiol* 203:248, 1962.)

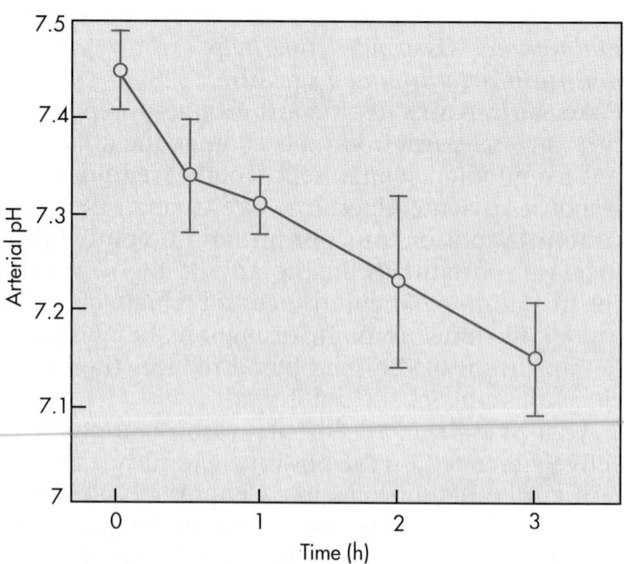

FIGURE 26–6. Reduction in arterial blood pH (mean plus or minus standard deviation) in 11 anesthetized dogs whose blood pressure had been held at 35 mm Hg by arterial bleeding into a reservoir, beginning at time zero. (Data from Markov AK et al: *Circ Shock* 8:9, 1981.)

sympathetic nervous stimulation of the heart, arterioles, and veins. Hence, moderate cerebral ischemia mobilizes various salutary negative-feedback mechanisms, as previously explained. When hypotension is severe, however, the cardiovascular centers in the brainstem are depressed because the reduction in blood flow to the brain is so pronounced. The resulting curtailment of sympathetic neural activity then exaggerates the diminution of cardiac output and TPR. The consequent decline in mean arterial pressure intensifies the inadequate cerebral perfusion.

Various endogenous **opioids,** such as **enkephalins** and **β-endorphin,** may be released into the brain or into the circulation in response to the same stresses that provoke circulatory shock. Enkephalins exist along with catecholamines in secretory granules in the adrenal medulla, and they are released together in response to stress (see Chapter 48). Similar stimuli release β-endorphin from the anterior pituitary gland (see Chapter 45). These opioids depress the brainstem centers that mediate some of the compensatory autonomic adaptations to blood loss and other shock-provoking stresses. Conversely, the opioid antagonist **naloxone** improves cardiovascular function and survival in various forms of shock.

Aberrations of blood clotting intensify the effects of hemorrhage

THE ALTERATIONS OF BLOOD CLOTTING AFTER HEMORRHAGE ARE TYPICALLY BIPHASIC; AN INITIAL PHASE OF HYPERCOAGULABILITY IS FOLLOWED BY A SECONDARY PHASE OF HYPOCOAGULABILITY AND FIBRINOLYSIS (see Chapter 15). In the initial phase, intravascular clots, or **thrombi,** develop within a few minutes of the onset of severe hemorrhage, and coagulation may be extensive throughout the microcirculation.

Thromboxane A_2, which is released from various ischemic tissues, aggregates platelets. The trapped platelets release more thromboxane A_2, which then traps additional platelets. This positive-feedback response intensifies the clotting process. The mortality rate from certain standard shock-provoking procedures has been reduced considerably by the administration of anticoagulants such as **heparin.**

In the later stages of hemorrhagic hypotension, the clotting time is prolonged, and fibrinolysis is prominent. Hemorrhage into the intestinal lumen is common after several hours of hemorrhagic hypotension in various species of animals. Blood loss into the intestinal lumen, of course, aggravates the hemodynamic effects of the original hemorrhage.

Blood loss depresses the reticuloendothelial system

Hemorrhage curtails the phagocytic activity of the RES. Consequently, the antibacterial and antitoxic defense mechanisms of the body are impaired. **Endotoxins** from the normal bacterial flora of the intestine constantly enter the circulation. Ordinarily they are inactivated by the RES, principally in the liver. When the RES is depressed, however, these endotoxins invade the general circulation.

ENDOTOXINS TEND TO LOWER ARTERIAL BLOOD PRESSURE BY AUGMENTING THE SYNTHESIS OF NITRIC OXIDE SYNTHASE, MAINLY IN THE VASCULAR SMOOTH MUSCLE. The nitric oxide generated by the activity of this enzyme is a potent vasodilator that intensifies the hypotension caused by the blood loss.

Positive- and negative-feedback mechanisms interact

Hemorrhage alters a multitude of circulatory and metabolic activities. As previously stated, some of these alterations constitute compensatory or decompensatory feedback systems having either a high gain or a low gain. Furthermore, the gain of any specific system usually varies with the severity of the hemorrhage. For example, when the loss of blood is minimal, the mean arterial pressure is usually within the normal range, and the gain of the baroreceptor reflexes is high. When hemorrhage is more severe, the mean arterial pressure may be below about 60 mm Hg (i.e., below the threshold for the baroreceptors), and therefore further reductions have no additional influence via the baroreceptor reflexes. Hence, below this critical pressure, the baroreceptor reflex gain is near zero.

When blood loss is minor, the gains of the negative-feedback mechanisms are usually high, whereas those of the positive-feedback mechanisms are usually low. The converse is true when hemorrhage is more severe. In a specific, complex pathophysiological state, such as severe blood loss, the generation of a vicious cycle depends on whether the overall gain of the various compensatory and decompensatory systems exceeds 1. The development of a vicious cycle is, of course, more likely when blood losses are severe. Therefore, to avert a vicious cycle in a subject who has suffered a severe hemorrhage, the subject must be treated quickly and intensively, mainly by blood replacement, before the process becomes irreversible.

Summary

- In anticipation of exercise, vagus nerve impulses to the heart are inhibited, and the sympathetic nervous system is activated by central command. The result is an increase in heart rate, myocardial contractile force, and regional vascular resistance.
- With exercise, vascular resistance increases in the skin, kidneys, splanchnic regions, and inactive muscles and decreases in active muscles.
- During exercise, the increase in cardiac output is accomplished mainly by the increase in heart rate. Stroke volume increases only slightly.
- During exercise, TPR decreases, O_2 consumption and blood O_2 extraction increase, and systolic and mean blood pressures increase slightly.
- As body temperature rises during exercise, the skin blood vessels dilate. However, when the heart rate becomes maximal during severe exercise, the skin vessels constrict. This increases the effective blood volume but causes greater increases in body temperature and a feeling of exhaustion.
- The limiting factor in exercise performance is the delivery of blood to the active muscles.
- Acute blood loss induces the following hemodynamic changes: tachycardia, hypotension, generalized arteriolar vasoconstriction, and generalized venoconstriction.
- Acute blood loss invokes various negative-feedback (compensatory) mechanisms such as baroreceptor and chemoreceptor reflexes, responses to moderate cerebral ischemia, reabsorption of tissue fluids, release of endogenous vasoconstrictors, and renal conservation of water and electrolytes.
- Acute blood loss also invokes various positive-feedback (decompensatory) mechanisms such as cardiac failure, acidosis, central nervous system depression, aberrations of blood coagulation, and depression of the RES.
- The outcome of acute blood loss depends on the gains of the various feedback mechanisms and the interactions between the positive- and negative-feedback mechanisms.

Bibliography

Astiz ME, Rackow EC, Weil MH: Pathophysiology and treatment of circulatory shock, *Crit Care Clin* 9:183, 1993.

Buckwalter JB, Clifford PS: Autonomic control of skeletal muscle blood flow at the onset of exercise, *Am J Physiol* 277:H1872, 1999.

Cameron JD, Dart AM: Exercise training increases total systemic arterial compliance in humans, *Am J Physiol* 266:H693, 1994.

Cheng K-P, Igarashi Y, Little WC: Mechanism of augmented rate of left ventricular filling during exercise, *Circ Res* 70:9, 1992.

Collins HL, DiCarlo SE: Daily exercise attenuates the sympathetic component of the atrial baroreflex control of heart rate, *Am J Physiol* 273:H2613, 1997.

Geerdes BP, Frederick KL, Brunner MJ: Carotid baroreflex control during hemorrhage in conscious and anesthetized dogs, *Am J Physiol* 265:R195, 1993.

Herbertson MJ, Werner HA, Walley KR: Nitric oxide synthase inhibition partially prevents decreased LV contractility during endotoxemia, *Am J Physiol* 270:H1979, 1996.

Iellamo F et al: Baroreflex control of sinus node during dynamic exercise in humans: effects of central command and muscle reflexes, *Am J Physiol* 272:H1157, 1997.

Kulics JM, Collins HL, DiCarlo SE: Postexercise hypertension is mediated by reductions in sympathetic nerve activity, *Am J Physiol* 276:H27, 1999.

Rowell LB: *Human cardiovascular control,* New York, 1993, Oxford University Press.

Schadt JC, Ludbrook J: Hemodynamic and neurohumoral responses to acute hypovolemia in conscious mammals, *Am J Physiol* 260:H305, 1991.

Share L: Control of vasopressin release: an old but continuing story, *News Physiol Sci* 11:7, 1996.

Sheriff DD et al: Dependence of cardiac filling pressure on cardiac output during rest and dynamic exercise in dogs, *Am J Physiol* 265:H316, 1993.

Szabo C: Alterations in nitric oxide production in various forms of circulatory shock, *New Horizons* 3:2, 1995.

Tscharkosy ME, Hughson RL: Ischemic muscle chemoreflex response elevates blood flow in nonischemic exercising human forearm muscle, *Am J Physiol* 277:H635, 1999.

Vissing SF, Scherrer U, Victor RG: Stimulation of skin sympathetic nerve discharge by central command: differential control of sympathetic outflow to skin and skeletal muscle during static exercise, *Circ Res* 69:229, 1991.

Yao Y-M et al: Significance of NO in hemorrhage-induced hemodynamic alterations, organ injury, and mortality in rats, *Am J Physiol* 270:H1616, 1996.

Case Studies

Case 26–1

A 23-year-old male track star decided to enter the Boston Marathon. He had run only in short-distance events, up to 10 km, before entry in the marathon. At the 15–mile mark, he was leading the race, but he was soon passed by one of his competitors. This inspired him to make a strong effort to retake the lead, but he was unable to increase his speed. At the 20–mile mark, he began to feel faint; within the next mile, he became sick to his stomach and somewhat disoriented, and he finally staggered and fell to the ground, exhausted.

1. **When the runner was at the 17-mile mark, what limited him from achieving his goal of retaking the lead?**
   A. His leg muscles were unable to use more O_2.
   B. His respiratory system was unable to saturate the arterial blood with O_2.
   C. He had inadequate vasoconstriction in the splanchnic regions and inactive muscles.
   D. His stroke volume became inadequate.
   E. His arteriovenous O_2 difference was decreased.

2. **At the time of his collapse, which of the following did *not* occur?**
   A. His body temperature fell.
   B. His heart rate reached a maximum level.
   C. His skin blood vessels constricted.
   D. His blood pH decreased.
   E. His blood pressure decreased.

Case 26–2

A 47-year-old woman had an acute episode of severe abdominal pain, and she suddenly vomited a large amount of bloody material. Her husband called for an ambulance to take her to the hospital. The emergency department physician learned that the patient had frequent, severe episodes of upper abdominal pain during the past 6 weeks. Physical examination revealed that the patient's skin was very pale and cold, her heart rate was 110 beats/min, and her blood pressure was 85/65 mm Hg. Examination of the patient's blood revealed that the hematocrit ratio (i.e., the ratio of red cell volume to whole blood volume) was 40%. The physician made the tentative diagnosis of a bleeding peptic ulcer.

1. **Why was the patient's skin pale and cold?**
   A. The arterial baroreceptors reflexly induced the parasympathetic nerves to the skin to release acetylcholine.
   B. The arterial chemoreceptors reflexly induced the parasympathetic nerves to the skin to release vasoactive intestinal peptide.
   C. The arterial chemoreceptors reflexly induced the parasympathetic nerves to the skin to release neuropeptide Y.
   D. The arterial baroreceptors reflexly induced the sympathetic nerves to the skin to release nitric oxide.
   E. The arterial baroreceptors reflexly induced the sympathetic nerves to the skin to release norepinephrine.

2. **What does the patient's arterial blood pressure of 85/65 mm Hg indicate?**
   A. The patient's left ventricle was producing an abnormally low cardiac output and low stroke volume.
   B. The patient's left ventricle was pumping more blood than her right ventricle.
   C. The patient's left ventricle was producing an abnormally low cardiac output but a normal stroke volume.
   D. The patient's left ventricle was producing a normal cardiac output and an abnormally low stroke volume.
   E. The patient's left ventricle was pumping less blood than her right ventricle.

3. **If the patient's bleeding had stopped before she arrived at the hospital, which of the following changes would be expected in the blood 1 hour after the patient arrived at the hospital?**
   A. The individual red blood cells would be larger than normal.
   B. The hematocrit ratio would be reduced.
   C. The lymphocyte count would be abnormally high.
   D. The plasma albumin concentration would be increased.
   E. The plasma globulin concentration would be increased.

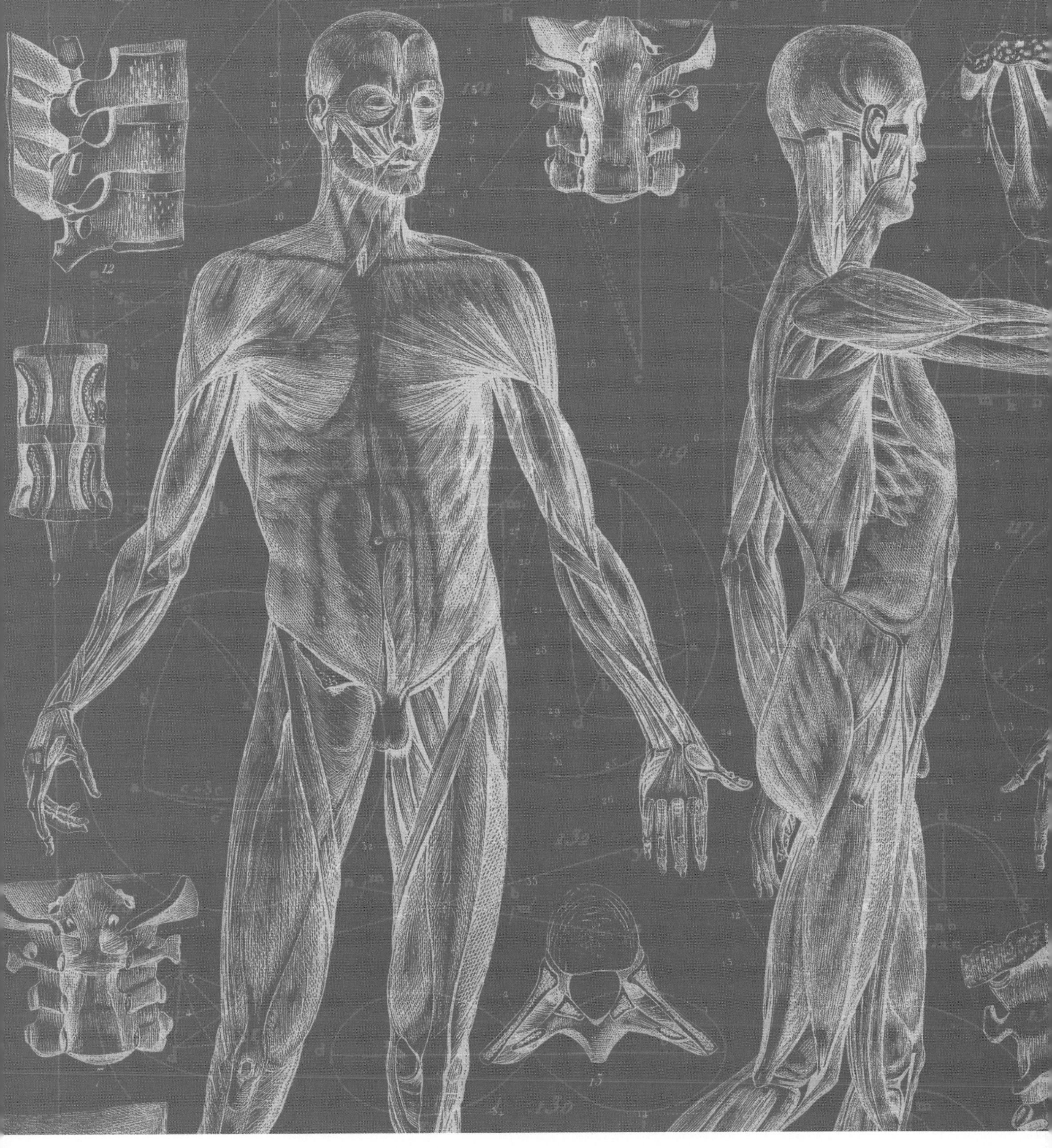

Part Five: Respiratory System

Michelle M. Cloutier and Roger S. Thrall

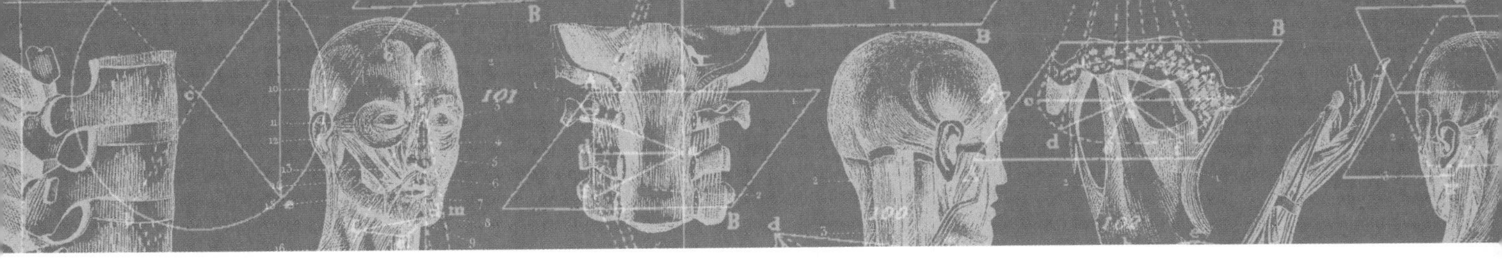

Chapter 27: Overview of the Respiratory System

Objectives

- ❖ Describe the components of respiration, including ventilation and its distribution, perfusion and its distribution, the process of gas exchange, O_2 and CO_2 transport, and control of breathing.
- ❖ Relate the structure of the respiratory system to its unique functions and to disease.

The Major Function of the Lung Is Gas Exchange

The lung has three major functions: gas exchange, host defense, and metabolism. The primary function of the lung is gas exchange, the process by which O_2 is brought into the body and the waste product of breathing, CO_2, is removed.

Breathing is automatic, rhythmic, and under the control of the central nervous system. Gas exchange begins with inspiration, which is initiated by the contraction of the diaphragm, the major muscle of respiration. On contraction, the diaphragm protrudes into the abdominal cavity; this protrusion creates a negative pressure inside the chest. The upper airway (glottis) opens, creating a portal from the outside world to the inside of the lung. Because gases always flow from areas of higher pressure to areas of lower pressure and since the pressure inside the lung and airways during inspiration is less than atmospheric pressure, air moves into the lung in the same way that a vacuum cleaner sucks air into the canister. The volume of air inside the lung increases and gas moves into the alveoli, the gas-exchanging unit of the body, where O_2 is taken up and CO_2 is eliminated. During exhalation, the diaphragm and other muscles of respiration relax, the pressure inside the chest and airways increases and becomes greater than atmospheric pressure, the glottis opens, and gas flows passively out of the lungs.

The lung demonstrates functional unity

Ventilation is the process by which fresh gas moves in and out of the lung. It is responsible for maintaining normal concentrations of O_2 and CO_2 in the alveoli and in the blood. **Tidal volume** is the volume of air inspired (or exhaled) per breath, and **minute ventilation** is the volume of air that enters or leaves the lung per minute. Minute ventilation can be increased either by taking a bigger breath (increasing tidal volume) or by increasing respiratory frequency (the number of breaths each minute). Increases both in tidal volume and in respiratory frequency occur during times of increased metabolic need in the body, such as during fever or exercise.

During inspiration, air moves through the nose or mouth into the trachea, which bifurcates into two main stem bronchi that enter the lung parenchyma (tissue) inside the chest. The right lung, located in the right hemithorax, has three lobes (the right upper lobe, the right middle lobe, and the right lower lobe); the left lung, located in the left hemithorax, has two lobes (the left upper lobe and the left lower lobe). These lobar bronchi then divide (like the branches of a tree) into segmental bronchi **(Figure 27–1)** and further divide into smaller and smaller branches (bronchioles) until the alveolus is reached. The region of the lung supplied by a segmental bronchus is the functional

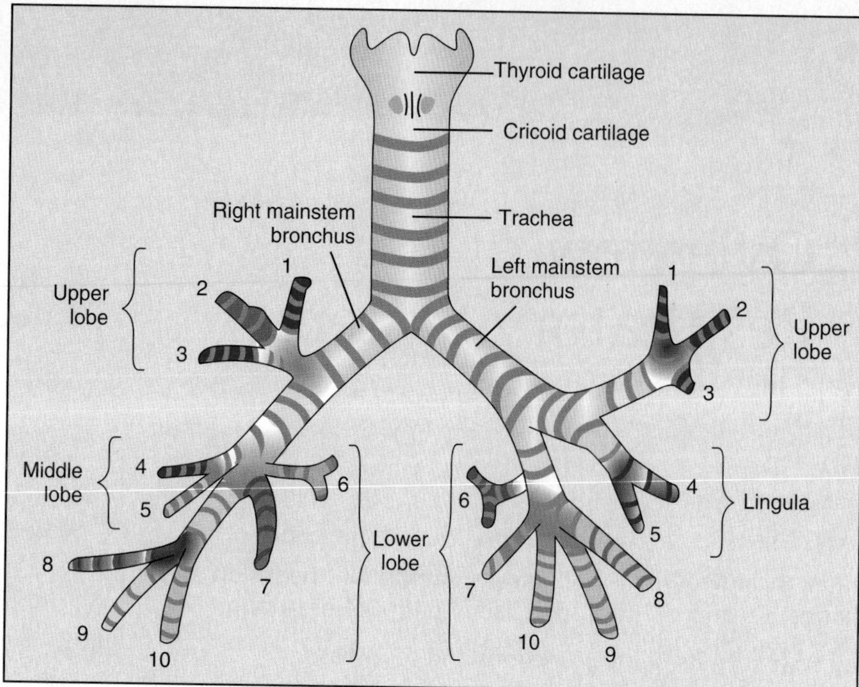

FIGURE 27–1. Anterior view of the bronchopulmonary segments: 1, apical; 2, posterior; 3, anterior; 4, lateral (superior); 5, medial (inferior); 6, superior; 7, medial basal; 8, anterior basal; 9, lateral basal; 10, posterior basal. (From Berne RM, Levy MN, Koeppen BM, Stanton BA: *Physiology,* ed 5, Philadelphia, 2004, Elsevier.)

anatomical unit of the lung. Disease affects different areas of the tracheobronchial tree, and knowledge of their unique anatomy and histology is essential. Bronchi and bronchioles differ not only by size but also by the presence of cartilage, the type of epithelium, and their blood supply. THE LUNG DEMONSTRATES FUNCTIONAL UNITY, THAT IS, THE ANATOMY AND FUNCTION OF EACH ALVEOLAR UNIT ARE IDENTICAL **(Table 27–1).**

Both the right and left lungs are covered by a thin membrane called the **visceral pleura** and are encased by another membrane called the **parietal pleura.** The interface of these two pleurae allows the smooth gliding of the lung as it expands in the chest and produces a potential space. Air can enter between the visceral and parietal pleurae because of trauma, surgery, or rupture of a group of alveoli, creating a **pneumothorax.** Fluid can also enter this space and create a **pleural effusion** or, in the case of severe infection, an **empyema.**

The lung has a dual circulation

The lung has two separate blood supplies. The pulmonary circulation brings deoxygenated blood from the right ventricle to the gas-exchanging units **(alveoli). Perfusion** refers to blood flow in the pulmonary circulation, which equals the heart rate times the right ventricular stroke volume. The bronchial or lesser circulation arises from the aorta and provides nourishment to the lung parenchyma. The dual circulation to the lung is unique, as is the ability of the lung to accommodate large volumes of blood at low pressures.

In normal individuals, ventilation and perfusion are closely matched

Ventilation and perfusion are matched when the pulmonary blood flow is proportionally matched to the pulmonary ventilation. This provides the optimal opportunity and the greatest efficiency for gas exchange to occur. The **ventilation-perfusion ratio** ($\dot{V}/\dot{Q}$) is the ratio of ventilation to blood flow, and it can be defined for a single alveolus or for an entire lung. At the level of a single alveolus, the ratio is defined as the alveolar ventilation divided by the capillary blood flow. At the level of the lung, the ratio is defined as the total alveolar ventilation divided by the cardiac output and is graphically depicted in **Figure 27–2.**

Gas exchange occurs in the alveolar-capillary network

Gas exchange occurs in the alveoli through a dense meshlike network of capillaries and alveoli called the **alveolar-capillary network.** The barrier between the gas in the alveoli and the red blood cell is only 1 to 2 μm in thickness and consists of type I alveolar epithelial cells, capillary endothelial cells, and their respective basement membranes. O_2 and CO_2 passively diffuse across this barrier into plasma

TABLE 27–1. ABBREVIATIONS FOR THE RESPIRATORY SYSTEM

Abbreviation	Meaning
CaO_2	Arterial O_2 content
$C\bar{v}O_2$	Mixed venous O_2 content
DLCO	Diffusion capacity of lung for carbon monoxide
F	Frequency
Fe^{++}	Ferrous iron (reduced state)
Fe^{+++}	Ferric iron
FEV_1	Forced expiratory volume in 1 second
FIO_2	Fraction of inspired O_2
FRC	Functional residual capacity
Hgb	Hemoglobin
$HgbO_2$	Oxyhemoglobin
HCO_3^-	Bicarbonate
H_2CO_3	Carbonic acid
MbO_2	Oxymyoglobin
N_2	Nitrogen
$NaHCO_3$	Sodium bicarbonate
NH_3	Ammonia
NHCOO	Carbamino group
NO	Nitric oxide
PB	Barometric pressure
$PaCO_2$	Arterial blood CO_2 tension
PaO_2	Arterial blood O_2 tension
PAO_2	Alveolar O_2 tension
PCO_2	Partial pressure of CO_2 (in gas or liquid [does not specify arterial or venous])
$\bar{P}la$	Mean left atrial pressure
PO_2	Partial pressure of O_2 (in gas or liquid [does not specify arterial or venous])
$\bar{P}pa$	Mean pulmonary artery pressure
Ppl	Pleural pressure
$PpvO_2$	Pulmonary vein blood O_2 tension
PtO_2	Tissue O_2 tension
PvO_2	Pulmonary artery blood O_2 tension (mixed venous blood O_2 tension)
PVR	Pulmonary vascular resistance
$\dot{Q}$	Perfusion
Raw	Airway resistance
RDS	Respiratory distress syndrome
RQ	Respiratory quotient
RV	Residual volume
SO_2	Relative amount of O_2 to hemoglobin (saturation)
TLC	Total lung capacity
$\dot{V}$	Ventilation
VC	Vital capacity
VDS	Physiological dead space
$\dot{V}O_2$	O_2 consumption
$\dot{V}/\dot{Q}$	Ventilation-perfusion ratio
VT	Tidal volume

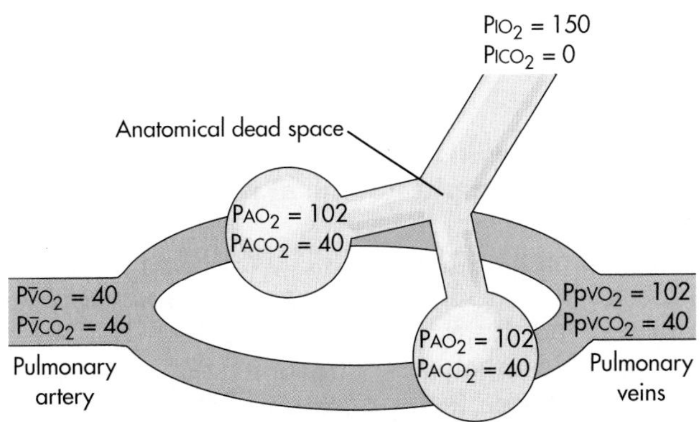

FIGURE 27–2. Model of the normal ventilation-perfusion process. The normal matching of ventilation to perfusion is simplified by showing only two parallel lung units, which are arranged vertically so that the reader will not automatically think of right and left lungs. Each unit receives equal quantities of fresh air ($\dot{V}$) and blood flow ($\dot{Q}$) for its size. The numbers indicate normal human adult resting values in millimeters of mercury (mm Hg) for the gas partial pressures (P) in inspired air (I), alveolar gas (A), and mixed venous ($\bar{v}$) blood arriving at the capillaries from the right ventricle via the pulmonary artery. pv, pulmonary venous.

and red blood cells. Red blood cells pass through the network in less than 1 second, which is sufficient time for CO_2 and O_2 gas exchange.

O_2 and CO_2 transport in blood occurs by specialized mechanisms

The body has developed specialized transport mechanisms to facilitate and optimize both O_2 and CO_2 gas exchange within the alveolar-capillary network and within the tissue capillary bed. The major transport mechanism for O_2 occurs within red blood cells, where oxygen is bound to hemoglobin (Hgb) to form oxyhemoglobin ($HgbO_2$). THE O_2-CARRYING CAPACITY OF BLOOD IS INCREASED 65-FOLD BY BINDING TO HEMOGLOBIN. In contrast to the single $HgbO_2$ molecular structure for O_2 transport, CO_2 is transported in three chemical forms in blood and plasma: HCO_3^- within red blood cells, dissolved CO_2 in plasma, and carbamino protein complexes in plasma and within red blood cells. The majority of CO_2 is transported in the form of HCO_3^- within the red blood cells, where the process is catalyzed by enzymatic activity. The binding and dissociation of O_2 and CO_2 to and from their carrier molecules are facilitated by each other. The dissociation curves of O_2 and CO_2 from their carrier complexes are distinctively different. It is linear for CO_2 and S-shaped for O_2. The differences between these curves have dramatic effects in gas exchange and implications for various diseases and their management (see Chapter 30).

Fluids line the lung epithelium and play important physiological roles

The respiratory system is lined with three different but highly significant fluids: periciliary fluid, mucus, and surfactant. The periciliary fluid and mucus are components of the mucociliary transport system and line the epithelium of the conducting airways from the trachea to the terminal bronchioles. They form a fluid layer that aids in the removal of particulates from the lung. Surfactant lines the epithelium of the alveolus and provides an "anti-stick" function, which decreases surface tension in the alveolus.

The mucociliary transport system captures and removes particles from the conducting airways

The mucociliary transport system provides the major mechanism for the removal of inhaled particles from the lung. It is composed of two fluid layers: the periciliary fluid (sol phase) and mucus (gel phase). The periciliary fluid is nonviscid and is produced by columnar, ciliated epithelial cells. It provides a thin fluid environment for the cilia to beat in and propels the mucus layer up toward the mouth. The mucus layer sits on top of the periciliary fluid and is produced by goblet cells and submucosal tracheobronchial glands (**Figure 27–3**). Mucus is a mixture of macromolecules, primarily glycoproteins, which provide a "sticky" environment for capture of particles from the airways, where they are eventually swallowed.

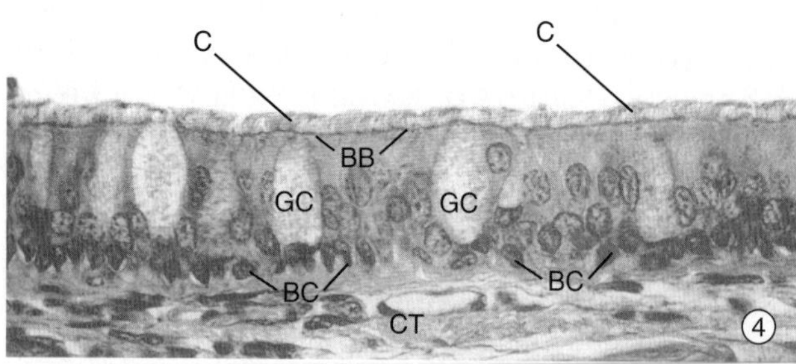

FIGURE 27–3. Scanning electron micrograph of airway: the ciliated, pseudostratified, columnar epithelium of a bronchus. Each cilium is connected to a basal body (BB), which collectively appear at the base of the cilia (C) as a dark band. Goblet cells (GC) and basal cells (BC), the potential precursors of the ciliated cells, are shown. CT, connective tissue. (From Berne RM, Levy MN, Koeppen BM, Stanton BA: *Physiology,* ed 5, Philadelphia, 2004, Elsevier.)

Surfactant diminishes surface tension in the alveolus

The alveoli are lined by a thin fluid film known as **surfactant.** Surfactant is a type of soap or detergent that acts to decrease surface tension. Pulmonary surfactant is a complex mixture of phospholipids, neutral lipids, fatty acids, and proteins. It acts as a barrier at the air-liquid interface in the alveolus.

Surface tension is a measure of the attractive force of surface molecules per unit length of the material to which they are attached. Surface tension forces at the alveolar-capillary (air-liquid) interface are high and influence function. When the volume-pressure curves of a saline-filled and air-filled lung are compared, higher pressure is required to fully inflate the lung with air than with saline because of the different surface tension forces in the air-filled and saline-filled lungs (**Figure 27–4**).

In the absence of surfactant, the surface tension at the air-liquid interface would remain constant,

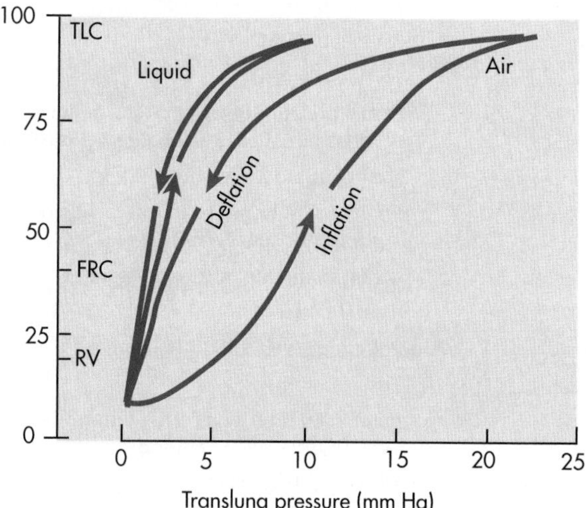

FIGURE 27–4. Pressure-volume loops of a normal human lung for the liquid- and air-filled states. Conventionally, each loop begins and ends at a translung pressure (P_L) equal to zero (minimum lung volume). The blue lines show the liquid-filled lung. The curve is steep, and the inflation and deflation lines are nearly the same. Total lung capacity (TLC), the maximal volume of air in the lung, is achieved at a P_L of 11 mm Hg. The air-filled pressure-volume curve is indicated by the red lines. The inflation limb is displaced far to the right of the curve of the liquid-filled lung, whereas the deflation limb is closer to it. This means that the pressure-volume curve of the lung depends on something that is different between inflation and deflation: alveolar surface tension. FRC, functional residual capacity; RV, residual volume.

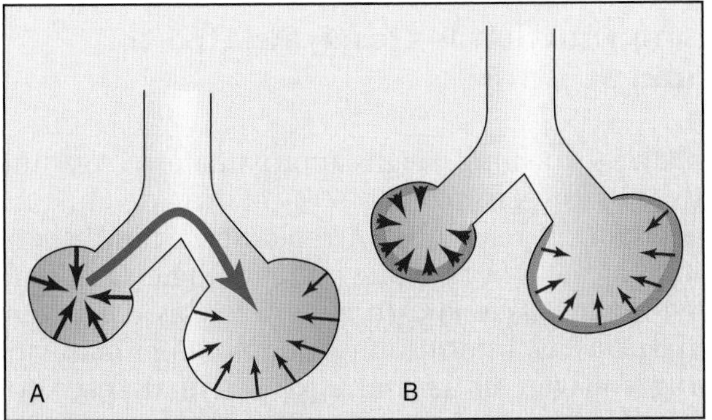

FIGURE 27–5. Surface tension in spheres. Surface forces in a sphere attempt to reduce the area of the surface and generate a pressure within the sphere. By Laplace's law, the pressure generated is inversely proportional to the radius of the sphere. A, Surface forces in a smaller sphere generate a higher pressure (P_S; *heavier arrows*) than those in the larger sphere (P_L; *lighter arrows*). As a result, air moves from the small sphere (higher pressure) to the larger sphere (lower pressure; *red arrow*). This causes the small sphere to collapse and the large sphere to become overdistended. B, Surfactant *(blue layer)* lowers surface tension and lowers it more in the smaller sphere than in the larger sphere. The net result is that P_S is approximately equal to P_L, and the spheres are stabilized. (From Berne RM, Levy MN, Koeppen BM, Stanton BA: *Physiology,* ed 5, Philadelphia, 2004, Elsevier.)

and the pressure needed to maintain the alveolus at that volume would be greater at lower lung volumes **(Figure 27–5)**. Thus, it would require a greater pressure across the wall of the alveolus to produce a given increase in alveolar volume at lower lung volumes than at higher lung volumes. This would create instability of alveolar inflation and alveolar collapse.

SURFACTANT STABILIZES THE INFLATION OF ALVEOLI BECAUSE IT ALLOWS THE SURFACE TENSION TO DECREASE AS THE ALVEOLI BECOME SMALLER (FIGURE 27–5, *B*). As a result, the pressure across the wall required to maintain an alveolus in an inflated state increases as lung volume increases and decreases as lung volume decreases. This is why the inflation limb of the pressure-volume curve in Figure 27–4 is displaced to the right (higher pressure at any volume). In the absence of surfactant, alveoli would collapse **(atelectasis)** as lung volume decreases.

Surfactant is produced by alveolar **type II epithelial cells** and is stored as preformed units in lamellar bodies in the cytoplasm. The major constituent of surfactant is dipalmitoyl phosphatidylcholine, a phospholipid with detergent-like "anti-stick" properties. The second most abundant phospholipid is phosphatidylglycerol, which accounts for 1% to 10% of the surfactant and provides spreading properties to enable the surfactant to cover the large surface area of the alveolus.

In 1959, Avery and Mead discovered that the lungs of premature babies who died of **hyaline membrane disease** were deficient in surfactant. Hyaline membrane disease, or **respiratory distress syndrome,** is characterized by progressive atelectasis and respiratory failure in premature infants. It is the major cause of morbidity and mortality in the neonatal period. The major surfactant deficiency in respiratory distress syndrome is the lack of phosphatidylglycerol with failure of the type II alveolar epithelial cells to secrete adequate quantities of surfactant. As a result, the lungs are more difficult to inflate, but the main problem is that during deflation, the alveoli collapse because the surface tension remains high. The increased work required to inflate the lungs contributes to respiratory fatigue and failure. Surfactant replacement therapy improves ventilation and has decreased the mortality of premature infants. It is now the standard of care.

Breathing Is Regulated in the Central Nervous System

The medulla oblongata, located in the brainstem in the central nervous system, is the main control center for respiration. Within the brainstem, the central pattern generator or respiratory pacemaker integrates peripheral input from the lung and from oxygen receptors in the carotid and aortic bodies with central input from the hypothalamus and amygdala to generate a rhythmic respiratory pattern that responds to the widely varying demands for O_2 uptake and CO_2 removal **(Figure 27–6)**. Neural impulses from the respiratory control center stimulate the diaphragm and intercostal muscles to contract during inspiration, the active phase of breathing.

Mechanoreceptors located within the chest wall and lungs monitor muscle effort and the rate of lung volume change and aid in terminating inspiration. CHEMORECEPTORS LOCATED AT THE BIFURCATION OF THE CAROTID ARTERY IN THE NECK (CAROTID BODY) AND IN THE AORTIC ARCH (AORTIC BODY) SENSE ARTERIAL BLOOD OXYGENATION, AND CHEMORECEPTORS NEAR THE VENTRAL LATERAL SURFACE OF THE BRAINSTEM SENSE CO_2 TENSION WITHIN THE BRAIN TISSUE.

Bronchial tone (constriction and relaxation) and mucus secretion are regulated by the peripheral nervous system

The peripheral nervous system integrates the central nervous system with the environment and

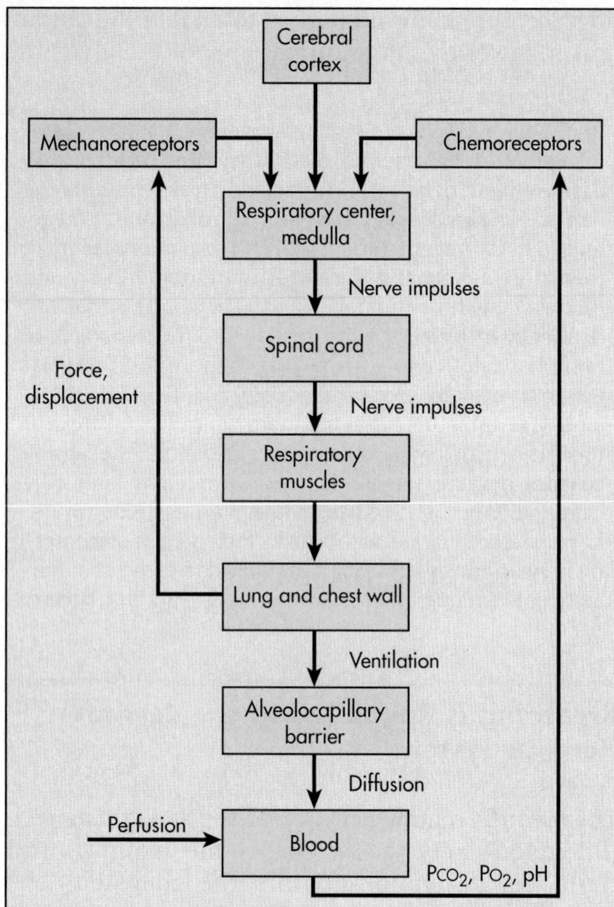

FIGURE 27–6. Diagram showing overall regulation of breathing. The respiratory center neurons, dispersed into several groups in the medulla, show spontaneous cyclic activity but are strongly influenced by stimuli descending from the cerebral cortex (volitional control) and from two sensory loops, mechanoreceptors and chemoreceptors (automatic control). P_{CO_2}, partial pressure of carbon dioxide; P_{O_2}, partial pressure of oxygen.

includes both sensory and motor components. The smooth muscles and glands of the conducting airways are innervated by autonomic neurons, whereas skeletal muscles are innervated by somatic neurons. The autonomic nervous system (parasympathetic—*constriction,* sympathetic—*relaxation,* nonadrenergic noncholinergic inhibitory—*relaxation,* nonadrenergic noncholinergic stimulatory—*constriction*) of the peripheral nervous system innervates the lung and plays a major role in bronchial tone and glandular secretions. Stimulation of the sparse (so sparse it may be nonexistent in humans) sympathetic nerves in the lung results in modest bronchial smooth muscle relaxation. In contrast, stimulation of the parasympathetic pathway leads to airway constriction, blood vessel dilation, and increased glandular secretions (**Figure 27–7**).

Lung Function Is Closely Related to Lung Structure

In adults, the lung weighs approximately 1 kg; lung tissue is responsible for 60% of the weight and blood for the remainder. Alveolar spaces are responsible for most of the lung volume; these spaces are divided by tissue known collectively as the **interstitium.** The interstitium is composed primarily of lung collagen fibers and is a potential space for accumulation of fluid and cells.

The region of the lung supplied by a segmental bronchus is called a **bronchopulmonary segment** (**Figure 27–8**), the functional anatomical unit of the lung. Disease usually involves a segment at a time, resulting in localized changes in breath sounds heard with the stethoscope (i.e., auscultation), and surgical resection follows along segments. Thus, knowledge of lung anatomy is essential since sites of disease are designated by their anatomical locations (e.g., right middle lobe pneumonia). In contrast, the basic physiological unit of the lung is the respiratory or gas-exchanging unit **(alveolar unit),** which consists of the respiratory bronchioles, the alveolar ducts, and the alveoli. Bronchi that contain cartilage and nonrespiratory (i.e., lacking alveoli) bronchioles that lack cartilage serve as conductors of the gas stream. This area of the lung is approximately 150 mL in volume (or ≈30% of a normal breath), does not participate in gas exchange, and forms the **anatomical dead space.** The area from the terminal or nonrespiratory bronchiole to the alveolus is where all gas exchange occurs. This area is only about 5 mm long, but it is the single largest volume of the lung at approximately 2500 mL and is responsible for the surface area of the lung at 70 m^2 when the lung and chest wall are at the resting volume, the **functional residual capacity.**

A chest radiograph is frequently used to diagnose lung disease. A normal chest film shows the larger airways (trachea and bronchi) and blood in the arteries and veins (**Figure 27–9**). A chest radiograph is obtained after maximal inspiration, and as a result, the alveolar walls and capillaries in normal people are too thin to be affected by the penetration of the x-ray beam. Disease resulting in changes in the airways, air spaces, or spaces between alveoli is demonstrated by changes in the penetration of the x-ray beam in specific anatomical areas. Diseased areas such as a pneumonia or atelectasis (absence of air in a lung segment) do not allow the x-ray beam to penetrate and appear as white areas on the film. These white areas are called infiltrates or areas of consolidation. Inflamed and thickened airways also prevent the penetration of the x-ray beam and appear as white streaks on the film. These are known as increased markings.

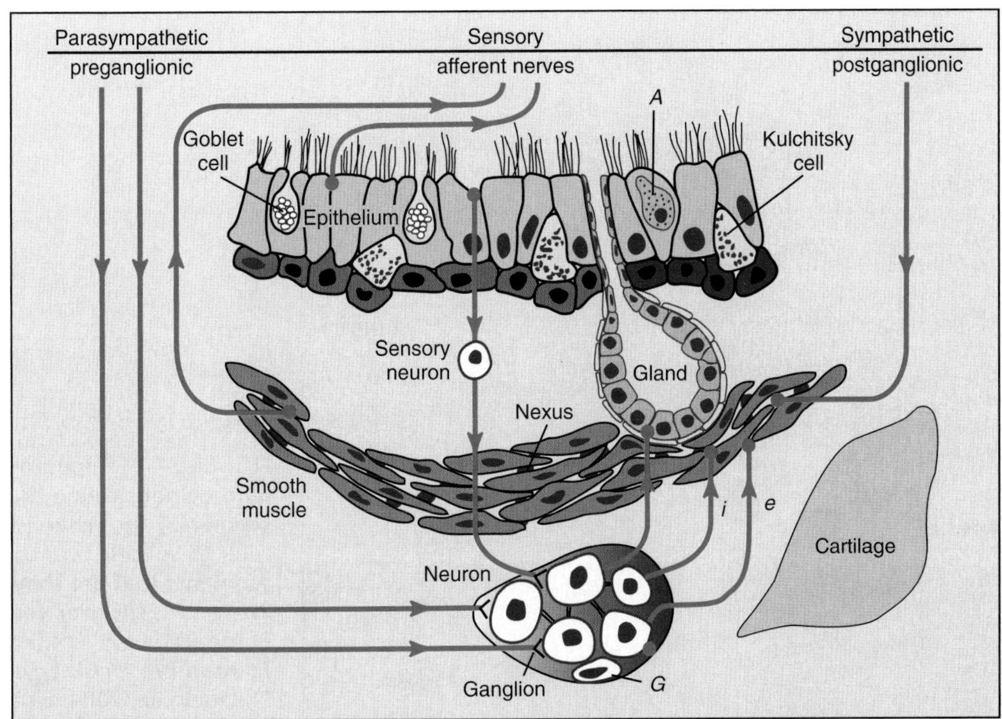

FIGURE 27–7. Schematic summary of the innervation of the airways. In the human lung, parasympathetic, preganglionic fibers descend into the vagus and terminate in the ganglia. The ganglia contain excitatory neurons that are cholinergic and inhibitory neurons that are nonadrenergic. Other neurons with an integrative function are probably also present. Glial cells *(G)* are present in the ganglia. Blood vessels and collagen are excluded from the neuropil. Postganglionic fibers to the smooth muscle are excitatory *(e)* or inhibitory *(i)*. Excitatory fibers may also terminate in the glands. Sensory afferent endings are present in the epithelium and the smooth muscle. The neurons associated with these endings may be in the vagus or the vagal nuclei. Sensory neurons may also be present in the mucosa, and fibers from these neurons may terminate in the ganglia, as in the gastrointestinal tract. Sympathetic postganglionic fibers terminate on airway smooth muscle. In the epithelium, there are cells, such as the Kulchitsky-type cell and the granular cell *(A)*, found only in chickens, whose functions are unknown. Nerves may be related to these cells. The human airway smooth muscle cells are connected by low-resistance junctions, and these connections may permit muscle mass to act as a syncytium. (From Berne RM, Levy MN, Koeppen BM, Stanton BA: *Physiology,* ed 5, Philadelphia, 2004, Elsevier.)

Bronchi are lined with a ciliated, columnar epithelium, which rests on a basement membrane, and are surrounded by smooth muscle. These ciliated cells rhythmically beat in a thin, watery liquid layer produced by the epithelium and transport secreted mucus and inhaled particles toward the trachea, where they are swallowed. Bronchioles are the continuation of the bronchi. They are smaller than 1 mm in diameter, contain no cartilage, and are lined by a simple cuboidal epithelium. Airflow in the bronchi is turbulent and rapid; airflow in the bronchioles is slower and more likely to be laminar. Only turbulent airflow is audible with the stethoscope. Thus, **disease in small airways, where airflow is laminar, is silent.**

The lung is a secondary lymphoid tissue

Although the primary function of the lung is to transport O_2 and CO_2, it also plays a major role in host defense in response to inhaled substances. It is considered a secondary lymphoid organ into which mature lymphocytes migrate and typically contact antigens locally. Although the lung in the upper regions (i.e., carina) has lymph nodes and lymphatic drainage, the primary immune defense resides in what is referred to as the **mucosa-associated lymphoid tissue.** The lung, gastrointestinal system, and urinary system are part of the **mucosal immune system,** which has unique

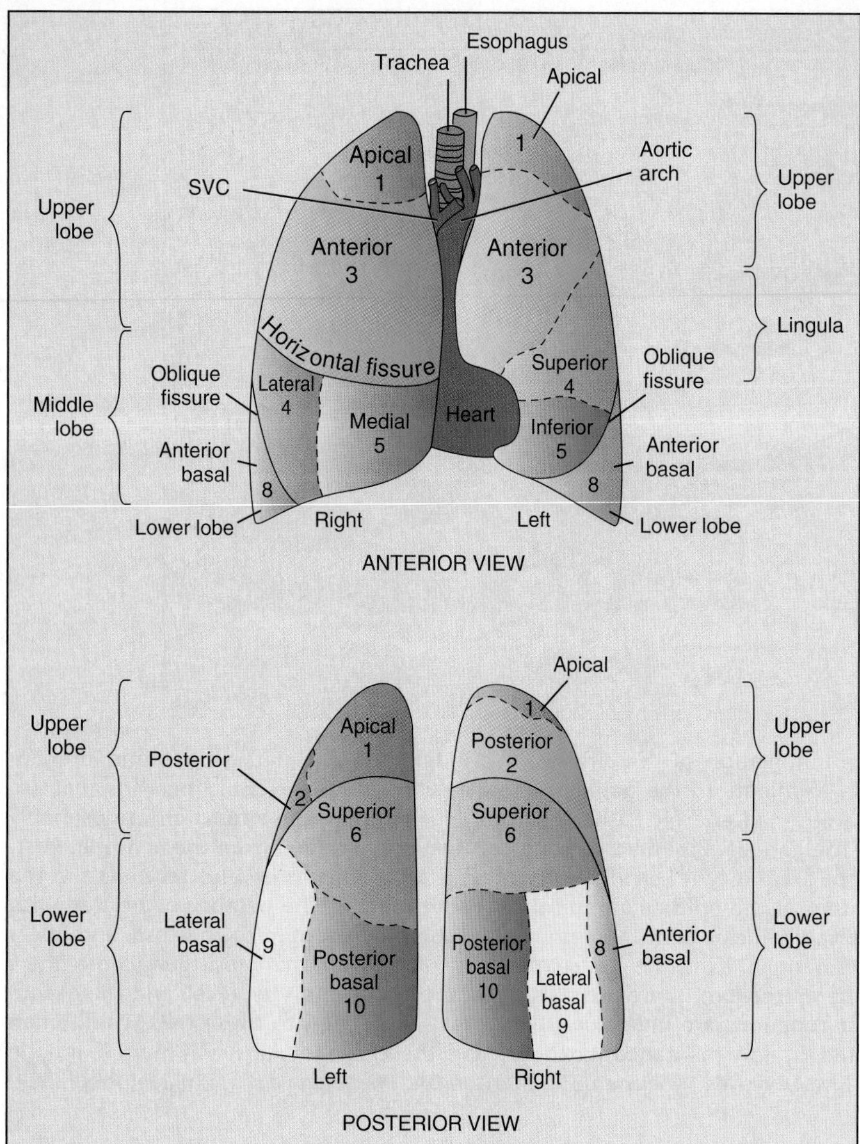

FIGURE 27–8. Topography of the lung demonstrating the lobes, segments, and fissures. Numbers refer to specific bronchopulmonary segments that are shown in Figure 27–1. SVC, superior vena cava. (From Berne RM, Levy MN, Koeppen BM, Stanton BA: *Physiology,* ed 5, Philadelphia, 2004, Elsevier.)

features to protect against the constant insult of environmental antigens and toxins.

The regional lymph nodes of the lung are part of the mediastinal network, which also drains the head, neck, and esophagus. These nodes are common sites to receive cancer cells and thus have important clinical diagnostic value for the spread of cancer (metastasis).

Asthma is a chronic airway disease characterized by inflammation (lymphocytes and eosinophils with a small number of polymorphonuclear cells) of the airways and reversible airway smooth muscle constriction (bronchospasm). Asthma involves both large and small airways. **Bronchiolitis** is a disease of small airways. It usually occurs in young infants and is caused by viruses, particularly **respiratory syncytial virus.** In **emphysema,** a disease primarily of smokers, the alveolar walls, septa, and pulmonary capillary bed are destroyed. This results in large air spaces and a decrease in surface area for gas exchange (demonstrated by a decreased diffusion capacity for carbon monoxide). **Chronic bronchitis,** another disease of smokers, is associated with a marked increase in mucus-secreting cells in the airways and an increase in mucus production.

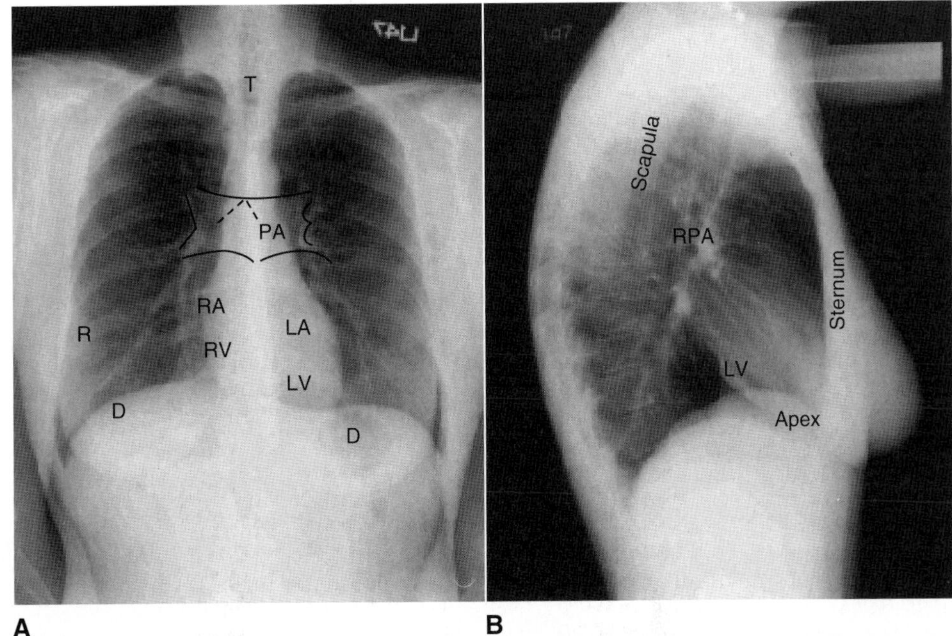

FIGURE 27–9. Normal posteroanterior *(left)* and lateral *(right)* chest radiographs taken at the end of a deep inspiration. The chest wall (ribs [R] and diaphragm [D]) can be seen. The lungs fill all of the thoracic cavity, except for the heart and mediastinum (which contains the trachea [T] dividing into the right and left main stem bronchi [inverted V-shaped dashed line]). Some of the larger distributing pulmonary vessels in the lung can be seen because they contain blood, in contrast to the air-filled lung. Normally, no detail of the alveolar structures can be seen. Outlined are the main pulmonary artery (PA) and the left atrium (LA), into which the pulmonary veins empty. RPA, right pulmonary artery; LV, left ventricle.

Summary

- ❖ The main function of the lung is to bring fresh gas into the lung in close apposition to the blood flowing through the lung so that O_2 can be taken up into the body and the waste product, CO_2, can be removed from the body by passive diffusion efficiently.
- ❖ The lung demonstrates anatomical and physiological unity; that is, each unit is structurally identical and functions just like every other unit.
- ❖ Ventilation is the process by which fresh gas moves in and out of the lung. Tidal volume is the volume of air inspired (or exhaled) per breath, and minute ventilation is the volume of air that enters or leaves the lung per minute. Perfusion is the heart rate multiplied by the right ventricular stroke volume.
- ❖ The lung is unique in its dual circulation and in its ability to accommodate large volumes of blood at low pressure. The pulmonary circulation brings deoxygenated blood from the right ventricle to the gas-exchanging units. The bronchial circulation arises from the aorta and provides nourishment to the lung parenchyma.
- ❖ In healthy individuals, ventilation and perfusion are well matched, resulting in nearly optimal O_2 transport.
- ❖ The hemoglobin in red blood cells is responsible for the enhanced ability of blood to transport O_2.
- ❖ CO_2 is transported out of the cells in the body to the lung mainly as HCO_3^- in plasma.
- ❖ Inspiration is the active phase of breathing; the muscles of the chest wall, mainly the diaphragm, contract and move down into the abdomen, resulting in a negative pressure inside the chest. Gas then flows from higher to lower pressure.

- ❖ As a result of surfactant, the pressure required to keep an alveolus inflated increases as lung volume increases and decreases as lung volume decreases.
- ❖ The respiratory center is located in the medulla in the brainstem. It regulates respiration with input from sensory feedback loops and reflexes in the lung and chest wall and from chemoreceptors that respond to changes in O_2 and CO_2.
- ❖ Conducting airways include the cartilaginous bronchi and the bronchioles to the level of the terminal bronchiole. They do not participate in gas exchange but form the anatomical dead space. The airways, beginning with the respiratory bronchioles that contain alveoli, the alveolar ducts, and the alveoli, are collectively termed the gas-exchanging unit.

Bibliography

Baile EM: The anatomy and physiology of the bronchial circulation, *J Aerosol Med* 9:1, 1996.

Boggs DS, Kinasewitz GT: Review: pathophysiology of the pleural space, *Am J Med Sci* 309:53, 1995.

Creuwels LA, van Golde LM, Haagsman HP: The pulmonary surfactant system: biochemical and clinical aspects, *Lung* 175:1, 1997.

Gandevia SC et al: Human respiratory muscles: sensations, reflexes and fatiguability, *Clin Exp Pharmacol Physiol* 25:757, 1998.

Horsfield K, Cumming G: Morphology of the bronchial tree in man, *J Appl Physiol* 24:373, 1968.

Jeffrey PK: The development of large and small airways, *Am J Respir Crit Care Med* 157(pt 2):S174, 1998.

Massaro D, Massaro GD: Invited review: pulmonary alveoli: formation, the "call for oxygen," and other regulators, *Am J Physiol Lung Cell Mol Physiol* 282:L345, 2002.

Rogers DE: Airway goblet cells: responsive and adaptable frontline defenders, *Eur Respir J* 7:1690, 1994.

Case Studies

Case 27–1

A 20-year-old man presented to the student health clinic with a 24-hour history of high fever, chills, cough, and left-sided chest pain. On listening to his chest with a stethoscope (auscultation), the examiner noted markedly decreased breath sounds with a few abnormal sounds due to opening of airways that closed during the previous exhalation (crackles) posteriorly at the lower edge of the left rib cage.

1. **What will a chest x-ray examination most likely reveal?**
   A. Nothing abnormal
   B. An infiltrate in the right middle lobe
   C. An infiltrate in the basilar segments of the left lower lobe
   D. An infiltrate in the superior segment of the left lower lobe
   E. An infiltrate in the lingula segment of the left upper lobe

Case 27–2

A 50-year-old man who has smoked two packs of cigarettes per day for the past 20 years experiences increased cough productive of copious amounts of yellow-green mucus and increased shortness of breath.

1. **Which of the following statements about $\dot{V}/\dot{Q}$ is most likely to be true in this man?**
   A. Perfusion to the lung will be affected more than ventilation to the alveoli.
   B. Both perfusion and ventilation to the lung are decreased equally.
   C. Ventilation to the alveoli will be affected greater than any changes to perfusion.
   D. There is no effect on ventilation or perfusion.
   E. Perfusion to the lung will be increased while ventilation will be normal.

Case 27–3

A 28-year-old man is infertile because of immotile sperm. This condition affects all ciliated structures within the body.

1. **Which of the following statements about this man are most likely true?**
   A. He is at risk for the development of emphysema with destruction of alveoli and septa and the formation of large air spaces.
   B. He is at risk for abnormalities in immune defense in association with changes in mucociliary transport resulting in mucus retention and secondary infection.
   C. He is at no greater risk for lung disease than are other individuals his age.
   D. He is at risk for localized lung disease because of a localized abnormality in the structure of his lung.

Case 27–4

An infant boy is born after 28 weeks of gestation (normal is 40 weeks) and weighs 2 pounds.

1. **Which of the following statements would not be true about this infant?**
   A. Surfactant replacement therapy should be administered.
   B. This infant will experience significant atelectasis.
   C. Ventilation in this infant will be decreased.
   D. This infant will have a normal level of oxygen and carbon dioxide.

Chapter 28: Mechanical Properties of the Lung and Chest Wall

Objectives

- ❖ Describe lung volumes and the determinants of lung volumes.
- ❖ Define compliance and resistance and their measurement.
- ❖ Characterize the pressure-volume relationships in the lung and chest wall.
- ❖ Describe the determinants of airflow in the airways and the concept of flow limitation.

In this chapter, we discuss lung mechanics, the study of the mechanical properties of the lung and chest wall. In lung mechanics, the chest wall includes all of the structures outside of the lung that move with respiration, including the rib cage and its muscles, the diaphragm, the abdominal cavity, and the anterior abdominal muscles. There are two types of lung mechanics: static mechanics, which describe the mechanical properties of a lung whose volume is not changing with time (lung volumes); and dynamic mechanics, in which lung volume is changing with time (resistance, expiratory flow rates).

Lung Volume Determines Many Properties of the Lung

The interaction between the lung and the chest wall determines lung volumes, and lung volumes play a major role in gas exchange and in the work of breathing. Many lung volumes in medicine are measured with a spirometer. First, the subject breathes normally into the spirometer, and the volume of air that is exhaled with each breath is measured (tidal volume). The subject then takes a maximal inspiration and forcefully exhales fully and completely. The total volume of exhaled air from a maximal inspiration to a maximal exhalation is called the **vital capacity** (VC) **(Figure 28–1).** The volume of air remaining in the lung after a full exhalation is the **residual volume** (RV). Residual volume is the volume of gas trapped in the lung; it cannot be measured with a spirometer, but it can be measured by other techniques, such as helium dilution or plethysmography. The **total lung capacity** (TLC) is the total volume of air contained in the lung and is the sum of the VC and RV. The volume of air remaining in the lung at the end of a normal exhalation is the **functional residual capacity** (FRC). The FRC is the resting volume of the lung.

CHANGES IN LUNG VOLUMES ARE SOME OF THE EARLIEST INDICATORS OF LUNG DISEASE. Of these, one of the most informative is the relationship between RV and TLC, the **RV/TLC ratio.** Normally, RV/TLC is less than 0.25, that is, the volume of air trapped in the lung (RV) is approximately 25% of the total lung volume (TLC). In a group of diseases known as obstructive pulmonary disease, RV/TLC increases because of an increase in the volume of gas trapped in the lung (RV) out of proportion to any increase in the TLC. In restrictive lung disease, the other major group of lung diseases, RV/TLC is also increased but for a different reason. In restrictive lung diseases, the volume of the TLC is *reduced* out of proportion to any decrease in RV.

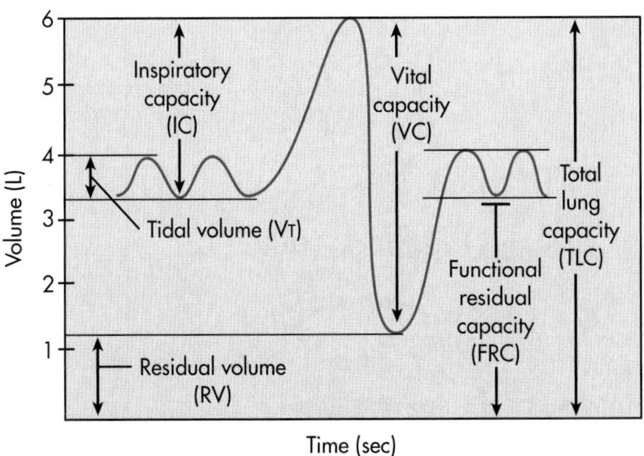

FIGURE 28–1. Real-time tracing of lung volume changes during two normal tidal breaths (VT), after which the subject made a maximal inspiration to total lung capacity (TLC), then an expiration to the residual volume (RV). (The volume exhaled between the total lung capacity and the residual volume is the vital capacity [VC].) The tracing ends with two more tidal breaths. The inspiratory capacity (IC) is the volume between the end expiration of a tidal breath and the total lung capacity. The functional residual capacity (FRC) is the volume of gas that remains in the lung after passive expiration. The left-hand *y* axis shows the average volumes of each of these measurements. Note that normal tidal breathing is near the middle of the total lung capacity.

Lung volumes are determined by the elastic recoil of the lung and by the properties of the chest wall

The lungs are elastic, like a rubber band; that is, they expand when stresses are applied, and they recoil passively (get smaller) when stresses are released. The pressure they create when stresses are applied is called the **elastic recoil pressure.** The lungs are enclosed within the chest wall, which is also capable of expanding and contracting, although to a lesser extent. The chest wall changes volume through chest wall muscle lengthening and shortening. The lungs and chest wall always move together as a unit in healthy individuals.

LUNG VOLUMES ARE DETERMINED THEN BY THE BALANCE BETWEEN THE LUNG'S ELASTIC RECOIL PROPERTIES AND THE PROPERTIES OF THE CHEST WALL. TLC is achieved when the inspiratory forces decrease as the muscles of the chest wall have been stretched to a point where they are insufficient to further expand the lung and chest wall. RV is achieved when the expiratory muscle force is insufficient to further reduce the chest wall volume. FRC is the resting volume of the lung and chest wall. It is also determined by the balance between the elastic recoil of the lung to become smaller and the pressure generated by the chest wall to become larger and is achieved when these two forces are equal and opposite. When the chest wall muscles are weak, the FRC decreases (lung elastic recoil > chest wall muscle force). In the presence of airway obstruction, the FRC increases because more gas is trapped in the lung (elevated RV).

Compliance is a measure of the pressure-volume relationship

Lung compliance (C_L) is a measure of the elastic properties of the lung. It is defined as the change in lung volume produced by a 1-cm change in the pressure across the lung and has the units of mL/cm H_2O. Lung compliance varies with lung volume. As the elastic tissue of the lung is stretched, its capacity for further stretching decreases, just like a rubber band. Therefore, a lung that is expanded or stretched close to TLC has a lower compliance than a lung that is expanded to FRC. In emphysema, elastic tissue is destroyed and the lung is more compliant; as a result, for every 1 cm H_2O increase in pressure, the change in volume is greater than the change in a normal lung (**Figure 28–2**). In contrast, in pulmonary fibrosis, the lung is noncompliant ("stiff"); that is, for every 1 cm H_2O change in pressure, the change in lung volume is less.

Pressure changes in the respiratory system affect lung volumes

Separated by the pleural space, the lung and chest wall move together in healthy individuals. Air flows

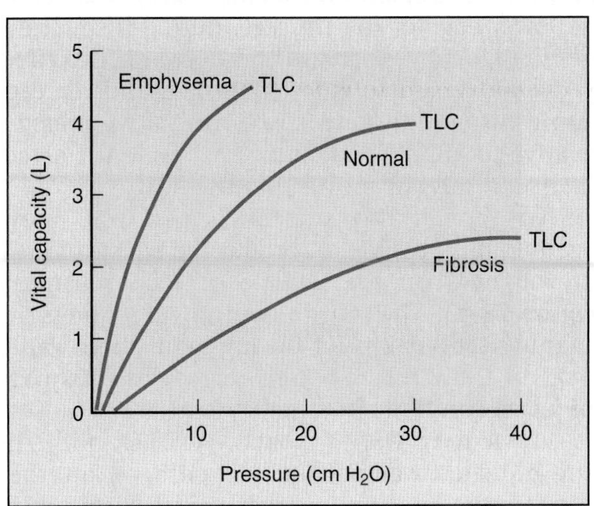

FIGURE 28–2. Fibrosis and emphysema pressure-volume compliance curves. (From Berne RM, Levy MN, Koeppen BM, Stanton BA: *Physiology,* ed 5, Philadelphia, 2004, Elsevier.)

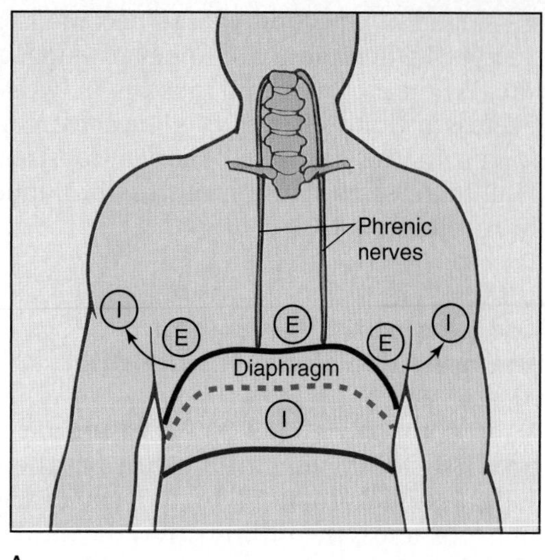

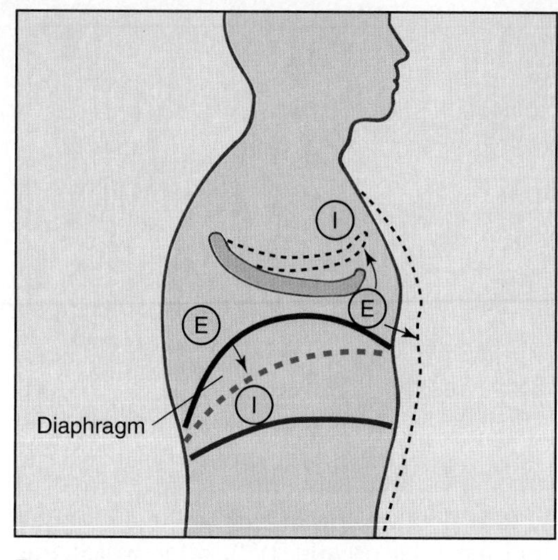

FIGURE 28–3. A, Front view in an upright human showing the descent of the diaphragm and the flaring of the lower ribs caused by the contraction of the diaphragm at its rib attachments during inspiration (I) *(dashed line)*. The phrenic motor nerves to the diaphragm are also shown from their origin in the neck. E, exhalation *(blue line)*. B, Lateral view showing the outward bulge of the abdominal wall as the contracting diaphragm shortens and moves caudally. The limited rotatory motion (pail-handle action) permitted for the rib cage is also shown. In severe emphysema, the diaphragm excursion is limited even in expiration, resulting in a flattened diaphragm *(purple line)*. (B redrawn from Staub NC: *Basic respiratory physiology,* New York, 1991, Churchill Livingstone.)

in and out of the lung when a pressure gradient is created. Gas always flows from higher to lower pressure. That is, when the pressure inside the lung is lower than the pressure in the atmosphere, gas flows into the lung. During quiet breathing, the diaphragm is responsible for 75% of the pressure gradient. During inspiration, this dome-shaped muscle contracts and moves into the abdominal cavity, displacing the abdominal contents caudally (downward) and ventrally (out) **(Figure 28–3).** Since the anterior surface of the diaphragm is attached to the lower edge of the rib cage, during inspiration, the rib cage moves upward and outward. The effect of the movement of the diaphragm and rib cage during inspiration is to create a negative pressure (relative to atmospheric pressure) inside the alveolus. As a result, air moves into the lung.

Even though the lung and chest wall move together, it is possible to sort out the effects of pressure changes on the volume of each separately **(Figure 28–4).** The sum of the individual pressure-volume relationships for the lung and chest wall is equal to the pressure-volume across the **respiratory system.** NOTE THAT AT FRC, THE PRESSURE ACROSS THE RESPIRATORY SYSTEM IS ZERO. At TLC, both the lung and chest wall pressures are positive, and they both require positive distending pressures across their surfaces to maintain their volume. The resting volume of the chest wall alone is the volume at which the pressure across the chest wall is zero, and it is approximately 60% of the TLC. At volumes greater than 60% of the TLC, the chest wall is recoiling inward; at volumes less than 60% of the TLC, the chest wall is recoiling outward.

When the chest wall is opened during thoracic surgery, air enters the pleural space because the pleural pressure is less than the atmospheric or barometric pressure (PB). The condition is called a **pneumothorax** (air in the thoracic cavity outside the lung). A traumatic or spontaneous pneumothorax may be life-threatening because ventilation is inadequate when the pressure in the pleural space is greater than PB, and the increased intrathoracic pressure (known as **tension pneumothorax**) compromises venous return to the heart.

The changes in alveolar and pleural pressure during a tidal volume breath are shown in **Figure 28–5.** In normal individuals, during a tidal volume maneuver, intrapleural (PPL) and alveolar (PA) pressures decrease at the start of inspiration. Gas flows into the lung, and lung volume increases. As the lung inflates, the pressure drops along the airways as gas flows from atmospheric pressure (zero by convention) to the pressure in the alveolus (negative, relative to atmospheric pressure). Airflow stops when the alveolar pressure and the atmospheric pressure (PB) become equal.

On exhalation, the diaphragm moves higher into the chest, intrapleural pressure increases (i.e., becomes less negative), alveolar pressure becomes

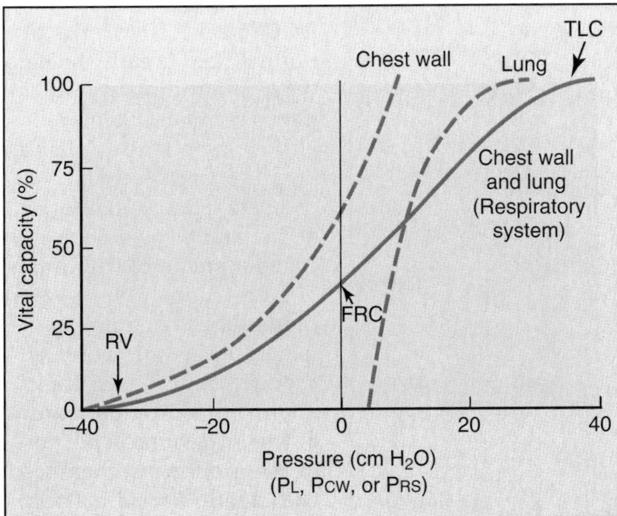

FIGURE 28–4. Distensibilities (compliances) of the lungs and chest wall and their sum, the respiratory system. The curve for the lung is the same as in Figure 28–2. The curves are known as passive, static pressure-volume curves because the pressures are obtained during relaxation at points of no airflow. From below the FRC up to about 75% of the TLC, the compliance of the lung is linear and approximately parallel to the compliance of the chest wall. As TLC approaches, the lungs become less compliant (stiffer) because of stretching of the noncompliant collagen fibers. Also as TLC approaches, the chest wall muscles are maximally stretched and are unable to generate further pressure. Note that over the tidal volume, the respiratory system has a lower compliance (lower slope) than either the lungs or the chest wall. FRC is the point of no pressure in the respiratory system (i.e., the point where the forces of the lung and chest wall are equal and opposite). PL, translung pressure; PCW, trans–chest wall pressure; PRS, trans–respiratory system pressure. (From Berne RM, Levy MN, Koeppen BM, Stanton BA: *Physiology,* ed 5, Philadelphia, 2004, Elsevier.)

positive, the glottis opens, and gas again flows from a higher (alveolus) to a lower (atmospheric) pressure. In the alveolus, the driving force for exhalation is the sum of the elastic recoil pressure of the lung and the intrapleural pressure **(Figure 28–6)**.

In obstructive pulmonary diseases such as chronic bronchitis, there is obstruction to airflow. This obstruction results in air trapping in the lung and lung overinflation (increased RV/TLC). The chest wall becomes barrel shaped and the diaphragm may flatten. This causes the diaphragm to maintain a flattened configuration even during exhalation and results in impaired movement of the diaphragm as the length-force relationship of the muscle fibers is no longer optimal. Impaired movement of the diaphragm is responsible for some of the shortness of breath experienced by patients with obstructive pulmonary diseases.

Turbulent Airflow Creates a Sound Heard with the Stethoscope

Air flows through a tube when there is a pressure difference between the two ends of the tube. Two different types of airflow occur in the airways. At low flow rates, flow is parallel to the walls of the airways and is laminar. Laminar flow occurs in small airways. Turbulent flow is disorganized flow and occurs as the flow rates increase and particularly as the airways divide. Turbulent flow occurs in large airways. Laminar flow is silent, and thus disease involving small airways does not create a sound heard by the stethoscope. The stethoscope detects only turbulent flow.

Asthma is characterized by chronic inflammation of the airways, airflow obstruction that is reversible (although not completely in some patients) either spontaneously or with treatment, and increased airway responsiveness or sensitivity to a variety of stimuli (such as allergens, histamine, exercise, and cold air). These substances cause contraction of the smooth muscle around the airways, swelling of the lining of the airways, and increased secretion of mucus. The overall result of these responses is narrowing of the cross-sectional area of the airways and plugging of the airways with mucus. In asthma, the lung compliance is normal (as opposed to emphysema or pulmonary fibrosis), although the FRC may be increased. The main symptoms that the patient experiences are wheezing, shortness of breath, and cough (which may be productive of thick mucous plugs). If the lung becomes markedly hyperinflated, the diaphragm will become flattened and will work inefficiently. **Bronchodilator drugs** stimulate the sympathetic nerves or inhibit the parasympathetic nerves and dilate the airways.

Airway resistance is determined by the driving pressure and flow

Resistance to airflow occurs in the airways as gas moves from the trachea to the alveolus. The resistance of an airway to airflow (Raw) is defined as the change in pressure from the start to the end of the airway (driving pressure) divided by the flow rate through the airway. For the respiratory system, the difference in pressure is the difference between the barometric pressure (PB) at the open mouth (or zero pressure by convention) and the pressure at the alveolus (PA). During tidal inspiration, the average difference between PB and PA is 0.4 mm Hg, and the average airflow rate during tidal volume inspiration is approximately 0.25 L/sec. Thus, airway resistance (Raw) = 0.4 mm Hg/0.25 L/sec = 1.6 mm Hg/L/sec.

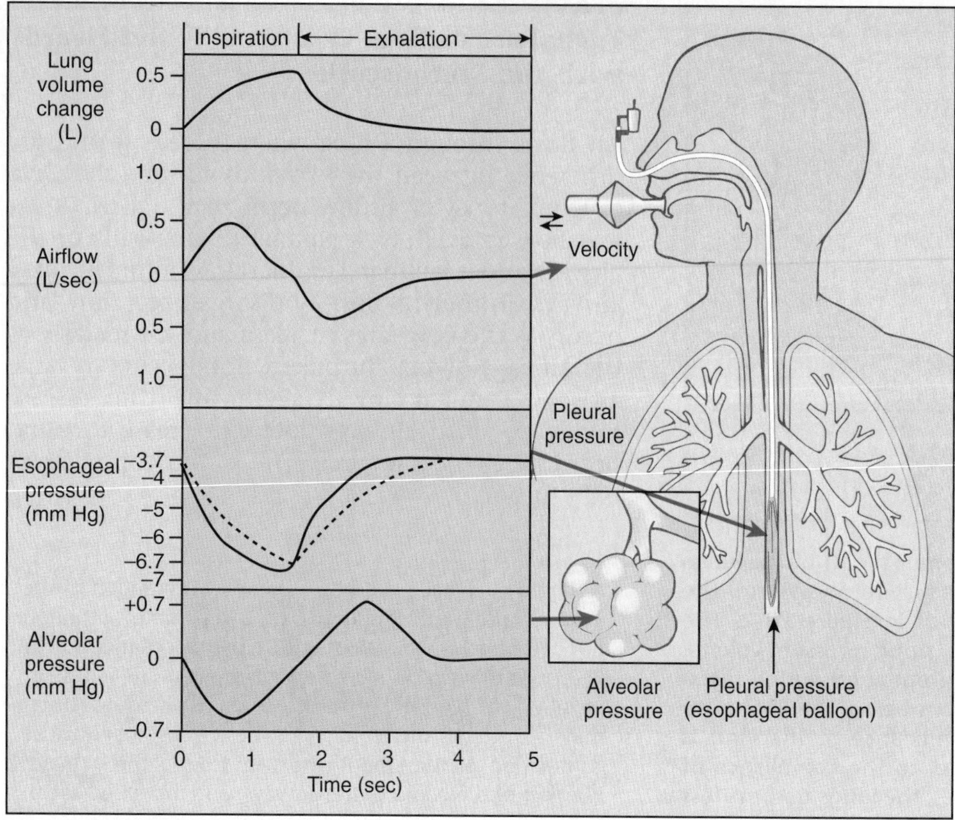

FIGURE 28–5. Dynamics of a normal tidal breath showing the relationships among changes in lung volume, airflow, esophageal (pleural) pressure, and alveolar pressure. Flow is measured at the mouth by a device called a pneumotachograph. The flow signal is integrated (added up over time) to generate the lung volume change. Pleural pressure is approximated by pressure in the intrathoracic portion of the esophagus, measured with a long flaccid balloon. The duration of the breath is 5 seconds (frequency = 12 breaths/min). Inspiration lasts 2 seconds. The curve for pleural pressure includes the pressure required to change volume *(dashed line)* plus the pressure needed to generate airflow; total pressure is the solid line.

Airway resistance differs in the large airways (>2 mm diameter; first eight airway generations), the medium-sized airways (subsegmental bronchi; ≈2 mm), and the small airways (<2 mm; bronchioles). Because of their smaller size and Poiseuille's equation (that resistance varies with the inverse of the fourth power of the radius), one might conclude that the major site of resistance along the bronchial tree is in the smallest airways. The opposite is true. That is, the major site of resistance along the bronchial tree is the large bronchi. THE SMALLEST AIRWAYS CONTRIBUTE VERY LITTLE TO THE OVERALL RESISTANCE OF THE BRONCHIAL TREE **(Figure 28–7).** This is true for two reasons. First, airflow velocity decreases as the effective cross-sectional area increases, and cross-sectional area increases at higher airway generations. Second, the airways exist in parallel rather than in series, and the total resistance is the inverse of the individual resistances.

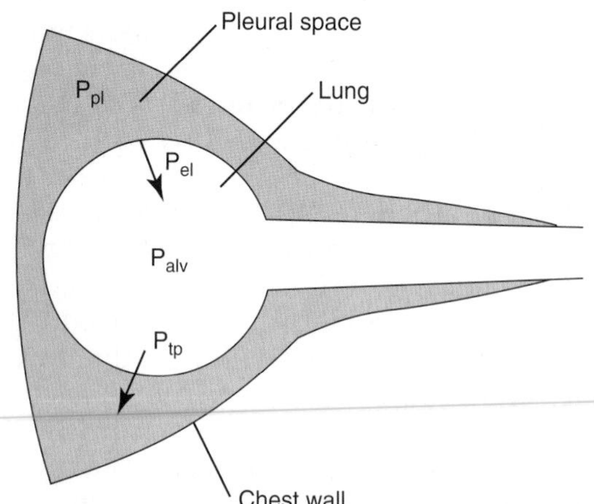

FIGURE 28–6. The relationship between the transpulmonary pressure (P_{tp}) and the pleural (P_{pl}), alveolar (P_{alv}), and elastic recoil (P_{el}) pressures of the lung. The alveolar pressure is the sum of the pleural pressure and the elastic recoil pressure. (From Berne RM, Levy MN, Koeppen BM, Stanton BA: *Physiology,* ed 5, Philadelphia, 2004, Elsevier.)

Lung volume affects airway resistance

Lung volume is the most important factor affecting resistance because the caliber of the airways increases with increasing lung volume **(Figure 28–8).** In the presence of increased airway resistance, breathing at a higher lung volume will reduce airway resistance. Patients with increased airway resistance frequently have high lung volumes. Airway resistance is also affected by the density and viscosity of the inspired gas. For example, during a dive, the increased gas density increases airway resistance. Patients with asthma experiencing a

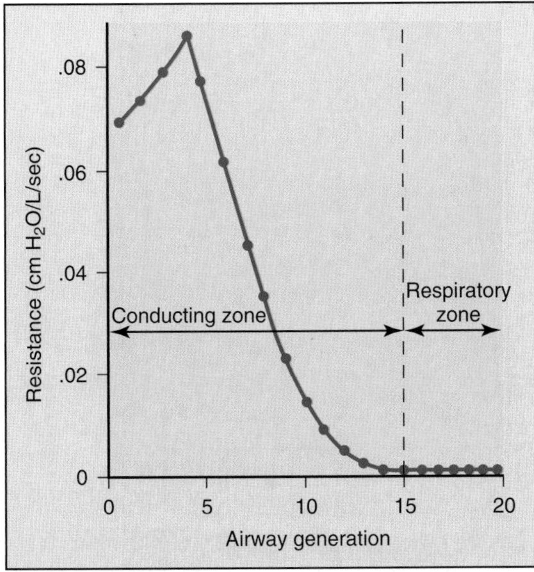

FIGURE 28–7. Airways resistance as a function of the airway generation. In the normal lung, most of the resistance to airflow occurs in the first eight airway generations. (From Berne RM, Levy MN, Koeppen BM, Stanton BA: *Physiology,* ed 5, Philadelphia, 2004, Elsevier.)

severe attack known as **status asthmaticus** are sometimes treated with a gas mixture of helium and oxygen. The decrease in gas density decreases airway resistance and improves oxygenation compared with a gas mixture of oxygen and nitrogen.

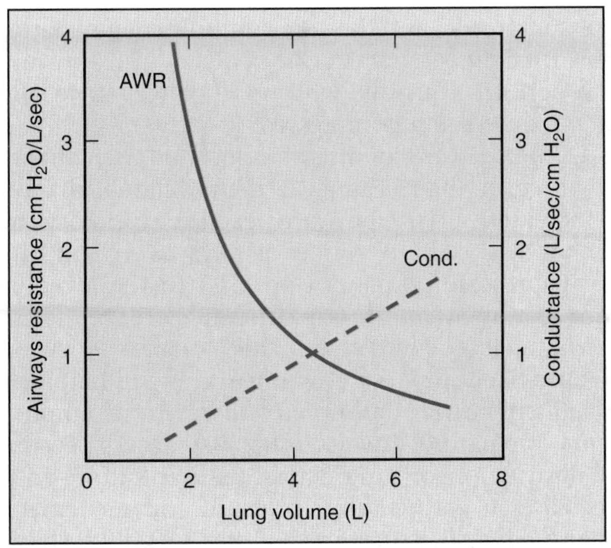

FIGURE 28–8. Airway resistance (AWR) and conductance (Cond.) as a function of lung volume. Conductance is the reciprocal of resistance. (From Berne RM, Levy MN, Koeppen BM, Stanton BA: *Physiology,* ed 5, Philadelphia, 2004, Elsevier.)

Important Clinical Tests of Pulmonary Function Include the Spirogram and the Flow-Volume Curve

The results from taking a maximal inspiration and fully and forcefully exhaling to residual volume can be displayed either as a spirogram or as a flow-volume curve. In the spirogram, volume is displayed as a function of time; in the flow-volume curve, instantaneous flow rate is displayed as a function of volume **(Figure 28–9)**. Both tests can be derived from the same maneuver.

The spirogram provides four major test results: the **forced vital capacity** (FVC); the volume of air exhaled in the first second, known as the **forced expiratory volume in 1 second** (FEV_1); the ratio of the FEV_1 to the FVC **(FEV_1/FVC)**; and the average flow rate over the midportion of the maneuver, the forced expiratory flow (**FEF_{25-75},** also known as the **MMEF,** or midmaximal expiratory flow).

The flow-volume curve or loop records the instantaneous flow rate both during exhalation (expiratory flow-volume loop) and during inspiration (inspiratory flow-volume loop). The flow-volume curve provides four major test results: the FVC; the greatest flow rate achieved during the maneuver, the **peak expiratory flow rate** (PEFR); the instantaneous flow rate at which 50% of the vital capacity has been exhaled **($\dot{V}max_{50}$)**; and the instantaneous flow rate at which 75% of the vital capacity has been exhaled **($\dot{V}max_{75}$)**.

Normal values for each of the pulmonary function tests have been generated. These predicted normal values and their ranges in normal individuals vary with age, gender, ethnicity, and height and to a lesser extent with weight. Abnormalities in values indicate abnormal pulmonary function and can be used to predict abnormalities in gas exchange. Abnormalities in pulmonary function frequently precede changes in other tests, such as chest radiographs. Repeated measurements of pulmonary function determine disease severity and progression and the response to therapy. For example, a 12% or greater increase in FEV_1 after bronchodilator administration is indicative of reversible airway obstruction.

Flow limitation is due to airway compression

PEFR is effort dependent. Greater effort during the expiratory maneuver will result in greater flow. The same, however, is not true for $\dot{V}max_{75}$. A maximum flow rate is achieved with modest effort, and greater effort will not result in greater flow. This

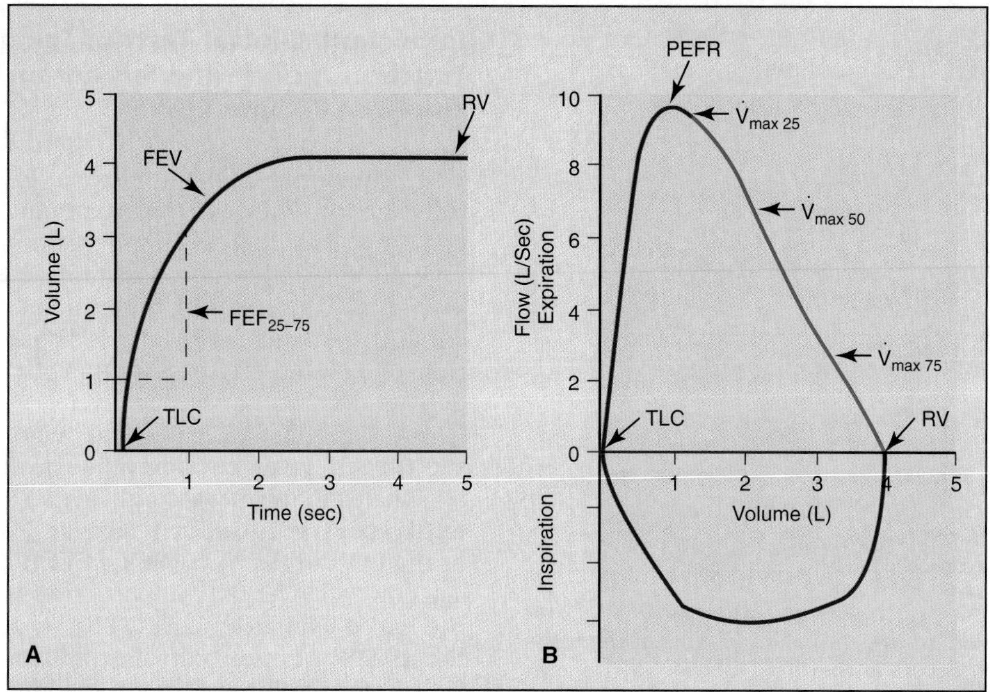

FIGURE 28–9. The clinical spirogram (A) and expiratory flow-volume curve (B). The subject takes a maximal inspiration and then exhales as rapidly, as forcibly, and as maximally as possible. The volume exhaled is plotted as a function of time. In the spirogram that is reported in clinical settings, exhaled volume increases from the bottom of the trace to the top. The most important information from the flow-volume curve is contained in the expiratory portion shown in red. This portion of the curve is effort independent and is a function of dynamic compression. Note the locations of TLC and RV on both tracings. PEFR, peak expiratory flow rate. (From Berne RM, Levy MN, Koeppen BM, Stanton BA: *Physiology,* ed 5, Philadelphia, 2004, Elsevier.)

maximum flow with modest effort is called **flow limitation** (Figure 28–10).

As exhalation begins, the driving pressure for expiratory gas flow is the sum of the elastic recoil pressure of the lung and the pressure inside the pleural space, which is produced by expiratory muscle contraction by the chest wall components. As gas flows out of the lung, this driving pressure decreases for two reasons: the resistance to airflow in the airways, which increases as lung volume decreases; and the decrease in the elastic recoil pressure, which decreases as lung volume decreases. As a result, there is a point inside the chest cavity at which the pressure inside the airways is equal to the pressure outside the airways (the pleural space). This point is called the **equal pressure point,** and in healthy individuals it occurs in the large airways, which are surrounded by cartilage. All airways toward the mouth from the equal pressure point but still inside the chest cavity have a pressure outside (pleural pressure) that is greater than the pressure inside, and they are compressed. No matter how much greater effort one achieves, the flow rate through that airway will not change since the airways are being compressed.

In the presence of disease associated with airway obstruction, the resistance of the individual airways is increased and the pressure head for expiratory gas flow is dissipated in smaller airways; as a result, the equal pressure point moves closer to the alveolus into airways that do not contain cartilage. These airways close completely. This collapse is called **premature airway closure** and is the hallmark of all obstructive pulmonary diseases. In emphysema, premature airway closure also occurs because of destruction of lung elastic tissue resulting in a decrease in elastic recoil pressure and movement of the equal pressure point closer to the alveolus. Premature airway closure also produces the auscultatory sound known as **crackles.** Crackles are produced by the opening of airways that closed on the previous breath.

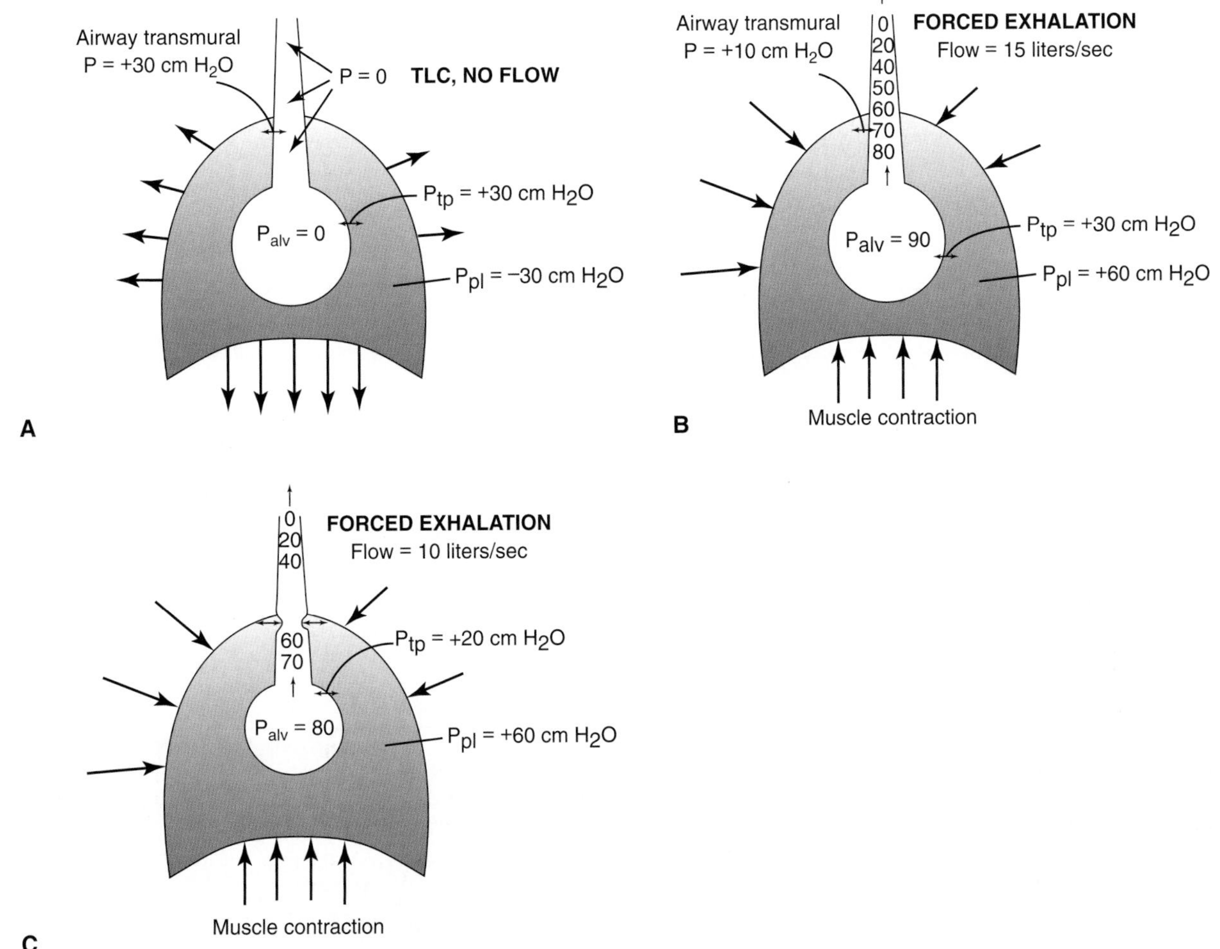

FIGURE 28–10. Flow limitation. A, End inspiration, before the start of exhalation. B, At the start of a forced exhalation. C, Expiratory flow limitation later in forced exhalation. Expiratory flow limitation occurs at locations where airway diameter is narrowed as a result of a negative transmural pressure. (From Berne RM, Levy MN, Koeppen BM, Stanton BA: *Physiology,* ed 5, Philadelphia, 2004, Elsevier.)

The Work of Breathing Occurs Primarily During Inspiration

Breathing requires the use of respiratory muscles, which expend energy. The work or energy cost of breathing is accomplished primarily by the inspiratory muscles and is required to overcome the inherent mechanical properties of the lung (i.e., elastic and flow-resistive forces) to move both the lungs and the chest wall. Under normal circumstances, this work is only 1% to 2% of the total respiratory oxygen consumption, but it increases considerably during activity and with disease. In restrictive lung disease, the increased work is due to a loss of lung compliance; in obstructive diseases, the increased work is due to an increase in airway resistance.

WE BREATHE AT A RESPIRATORY FREQUENCY THAT MINIMIZES OUR WORK **(Figure 28–11).** Patients with pulmonary fibrosis (a restrictive disease associated with increased elastic work) breathe more shallowly and rapidly, and those with obstructive lung disease (e.g., emphysema with normal or low elastic work but high resistance) breathe more slowly and deeply.

TABLE 28–1. PATTERNS OF ABNORMALITIES IN PULMONARY FUNCTION TESTS

Pulmonary Function Measurement	Obstructive Pulmonary Disease	Restrictive Pulmonary Disease
FVC (L)	↓	↓
FEV_1 (L)	↓	↓
FEV_1/FVC	↓	N
FEF_{25-75} (L/sec)	↓	N
PEFR (L/sec)	↓	N
FEF_{50} (L/sec)	↓	N
FEF_{75} (L/sec)	↓	N
Slope of flow-volume curve	↓	N to ↑

Changes in pulmonary function, respiratory patterns, and work of breathing are associated with different types of lung disease

In **emphysema**, a chronic obstructive pulmonary disease (COPD), the alveolar and capillary walls are progressively destroyed. This results in larger than normal changes in lung volume for small changes in transpulmonary pressure because of increased lung compliance. The decrease in elastic recoil also results in movement of the equal pressure point toward the alveolus and premature airway closure. This produces air trapping and increases in RV, FRC, and TLC.

Airway resistance is also increased as the floppy airways close during exhalation. These changes in lung volume increase work of breathing by stretching the respiratory muscles and flattening the diaphragm and decreasing their efficiency. In addition, there is a decrease in the surface area for gas exchange measured as a decrease in the diffusion capacity for carbon monoxide (DLCO).

In **chronic bronchitis,** the other large category of diseases in COPD, mucus and airway inflammation produce an increase in airway resistance and cause the equal pressure point to move toward the alveolus, which leads to increases in RV, FRC, and TLC. Compliance and the surface area for gas exchange (DLCO), however, are normal.

In restrictive lung diseases, such as **pulmonary fibrosis,** lung compliance is decreased, and changes in transpulmonary pressure produce smaller than normal changes in lung volume. Some of the important changes in pulmonary function values in obstructive and restrictive pulmonary diseases are shown in **Table 28–1**.

In **kyphoscoliosis** (a distorted spinal column), the movement of the chest wall is restricted. Hence, lung volumes and chest wall compliance are reduced. In the third trimester of pregnancy, the enlarged uterus increases intraabdominal pressure and restricts the movement of the diaphragm. The FRC, as a result, decreases. This change in lung volume results in decreased lung compliance and increased airway resistance in otherwise healthy women.

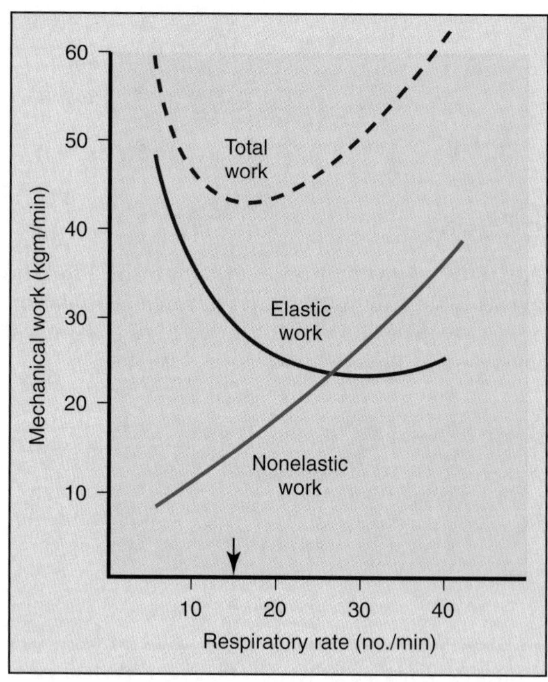

FIGURE 28–11. The effect of respiratory rate on the elastic, nonelastic, and total mechanical work of breathing (the sum of elastic and nonelastic work) at a given level of alveolar ventilation. Subjects tend to adopt the respiratory rate at which the total work of breathing is minimal *(arrow)*. (From Berne RM, Levy MN, Koeppen BM, Stanton BA: *Physiology,* ed 5, Philadelphia, 2004, Elsevier.)

Summary

- Lung volumes are determined by the balance between the lung's elastic recoil properties and the properties of the muscles of the chest wall.
- The vital capacity is the single most important pulmonary function measurement; it is the maximal amount of air that an individual can inhale or exhale.
- The FRC, the volume of air in the lungs at the end of a normal exhalation, is the resting volume of the lung. It is determined by the balance between the lung elastic recoil pressure operating to decrease lung volume and the pressure generated by the chest wall to become larger. At FRC, the forces are equal and opposite and the pressure across the respiratory system is zero.
- Lung compliance is a measure of the elastic properties of the lung. A loss of elastic recoil as seen in patients with emphysema is associated with an increase in lung compliance. In contrast, in diseases associated with pulmonary fibrosis, lung compliance is decreased.
- Gas flows from higher to low pressure. A positive transpulmonary pressure (pressure outside greater than pressure inside the alveolus) is needed to increase lung volume. The pressure across the respiratory system is zero at points of no airflow (end inspiration and end exhalation).
- Resistance is the change in pressure per unit of flow. Airway resistance is determined by airway caliber and length as well as by gas velocity and density. Airway resistance is highly sensitive to changes in airway radius and varies with the inverse of the fourth power of the radius. Resistance is higher in turbulent than in laminar flow.
- The first eight airway generations are the major site of airway resistance. Airway resistance decreases with increases in lung volume and with decreases in gas density.
- The equal pressure point is the point at which the pressures inside and surrounding the airway are the same. As lung volume and elastic recoil pressure decrease, the equal pressure point moves toward the alveolus in normal individuals, resulting in dynamic compression and expiratory flow limitation. In individuals with COPD, at any lung volume, the equal pressure point is closer to the alveolus, resulting in greater expiratory flow limitation and decreased expiratory flow rates.
- Pulmonary function tests (spirometry, flow-volume loop) can detect abnormalities in lung function before individuals become symptomatic. Predicted values for lung volumes and expiratory flow rates vary by age, gender, ethnicity, and height and to a lesser extent by weight.
- Chronic obstructive lung disease (COPD) is characterized by increases in lung volume and airway resistance and decreases in expiratory flow rates. Emphysema, a specific type of COPD, is further characterized by increased lung compliance and decreased surface area for gas exchange (decreased D_{LCO}).
- Restrictive lung diseases are characterized by decreases in lung volume, normal expiratory flow rates and resistance, and a marked decrease in lung compliance.

Bibliography

Altose MD: Pulmonary mechanics. In Fishman AP et al, eds: *Pulmonary diseases and disorders,* ed 3, New York, 1998, McGraw-Hill.

D'Angelo E, Agostoni E: Statics of the chest wall. In Roussos C, ed: *The thorax,* ed 2, New York, 1995, Marcel Dekker.

George RB et al, eds: *Chest medicine: essentials of pulmonary and critical care medicine,* ed 3, Baltimore, 1995, Williams & Wilkins.

Hyatt RE, Scanlon PD, Nakamura M, eds: *Interpretation of pulmonary function tests. A practical guide,* Philadelphia, 1997, Lippincott Williams & Wilkins.

Murray JF: *The normal lung,* ed 2, Philadelphia, 1986, WB Saunders.

Case Studies

Case 28–1

A 75-year-old man complains of shortness of breath with activities of daily living. He has smoked one pack of cigarettes per day for the past 55 years. He has a barrel chest and breath sounds are distant, especially over the apices. His FVC, FEV_1, and FEV_1/FVC are markedly reduced with a significant elevation in the RV/TLC due to a marked increase in RV. His diffusion capacity for carbon monoxide (DLCO) is reduced.

1. **What lung disease does this man most likely have?**
   A. Asthma
   B. Chronic bronchitis
   C. Emphysema
   D. Pulmonary fibrosis
   E. Respiratory distress syndrome

2. **On chest x-ray examination, what would you most likely find?**
   A. A dome-shaped diaphragm with clear lung fields
   B. A dome-shaped diaphragm with increased lung markings
   C. A flattened diaphragm with bullae in the apices and few visible lung markings
   D. A flattened diaphragm with increased lung markings in both lung fields
   E. Increased lung markings localized to the apices of both lungs

Case 28–2

A 60-year-old man is admitted to the intensive care unit for shortness of breath caused by an exacerbation of emphysema. He previously smoked two packs of cigarettes per day for 40 years. His respiratory rate is 40 breaths/min, and he uses accessory muscles to breathe. His physician decides to mechanically ventilate him and temporarily paralyzes him with medication. The ventilator is set for 12 breaths/min with a tidal volume of 1000 mL. The ventilator measures airway pressure at the end of each delivered breath (at a point of no airflow); at this point, the airway pressure is 25 cm H_2O. The ventilator then allows him to passively exhale, and the airway pressure returns to zero (PB).

1. **What is the compliance of his respiratory system?**
   A. 5 mL/cm H_2O
   B. 100 mL/cm H_2O
   C. 20 mL/cm H_2O
   D. 40 mL/cm H_2O
   E. 55 mL/cm H_2O

2. **On further examination, the physician notes that the patient has bilateral wheezes when she listens to his chest. His Raw is measured. The peak airway pressure is 35 cm H_2O, and airflow is 1 L/sec. The physician occludes the airway at the point of peak airway pressure (end inspiration), and it measures 25 cm H_2O. What is the total Raw (including the endotracheal tube)?**
   A. 2 cm H_2O/L/sec
   B. 5 cm H_2O/L/sec
   C. 8 cm H_2O/L/sec
   D. 10 cm H_2O/L/sec
   E. 20 cm H_2O/L/sec

Case 28–3

A 32-year-old woman, a nonsmoker, presents with a 1-week history of an upper respiratory infection and coughing up blood. She has a history of two previous episodes of pneumonia in the right lung. On physical examination, her pulse is 90/min, respirations are 24/min, and blood pressure is 110/72. On lung auscultation, inspiratory and expiratory wheezes are noted over the right upper lobe. On the chest radiograph, a small patchy infiltrate in the right upper lobe with a suggestion of a mass lesion and volume loss is observed. On bronchoscopy, a nodular tumor mass protruding into the lumen of the right upper lobe bronchus is found.

1. **This patient demonstrates which of the following?**
   A. Obstructive pulmonary disease associated with a loss of elastic recoil
   B. Obstructive pulmonary disease associated with an increase in airway resistance
   C. Restrictive pulmonary disease associated with interstitial pneumonitis
   D. Restrictive pulmonary disease associated with muscle weakness
   E. Pulmonary vascular disease associated with pulmonary hypertension

2. **If esophageal pressure changes from –5 cm H_2O to –10 cm H_2O as the patient breathes from FRC to FRC +1 L, what is the compliance of the lung?**
   A. 0.1 L/cm H_2O
   B. 5 cm L/H_2O
   C. 0.2 L/cm H_2O
   D. 10 cm L/H_2O

Case 28–4

A 16-year-old athlete is referred to you for evaluation of chest tightness. The chest tightness primarily occurs with activity but also occasionally at rest. On physical examination, the lungs are clear; a grade 1/6 systolic murmur is noted along the right border of the heart without radiation.

1. **Interpret the following pulmonary function test results (NL = normal for height, gender, and age).**

	Before Bronchodilator Administration	After Bronchodilator Administration
FVC	104% predicted (NL)	108% predicted
FEV_1	88% predicted (NL)	103% predicted
FEV_1/FVC	85% (NL)	95%
FEF_{25-75}	48% predicted (↓)	90% predicted (NL)

   A. Obstructive pulmonary disease with reversibility
   B. Obstructive pulmonary disease without reversibility
   C. Restrictive pulmonary disease with reversibility
   D. Restrictive pulmonary disease without reversibility
   E. Pulmonary vascular disease

Case 28–5

A 17-year-old young woman with asthma presents to your office with an acute asthma exacerbation of moderate severity.

1. **Pulmonary function tests at this time might reveal which of the following?**
   A. Decreased FVC, FEV_1, FEV_1/FVC, and expiratory flow rates with increased RV
   B. Decreased FVC, FEV_1, and expiratory flow rates with normal FEV_1/FVC and normal RV
   C. Normal FVC, FEV_1, and FEV_1/FVC; decreased expiratory flow rates and decreased RV
   D. Normal pulmonary function
   E. Normal FVC, FEV_1, and expiratory flow rates with increased FEV_1/FVC and RV

Case 28–6

A 35-year-old man is seen for a physical examination by his primary care provider. His history is remarkable for a 15-year history of smoking one pack of cigarettes per day. He denies any respiratory symptoms including cough or increased mucus production. He is physically active and denies physical limitation.

1. **Which of the following statements is most likely true?**
   A. A chest radiograph will reveal abnormalities in the lungs.
   B. Pulmonary function tests will reveal early airway obstruction with decreased expiratory flow rates.
   C. The diffusion capacity for carbon monoxide (DLCO) will be abnormal.
   D. A sputum culture will demonstrate evidence of infection.
   E. An exercise stress test will demonstrate coronary artery syndrome.

Chapter 29: Ventilation, Perfusion, and Their Relationship

Objectives

- Explain alveolar ventilation and the gas equations.
- Describe the pulmonary and bronchial circulation in normal individuals and its regulation.
- Explain the importance of ventilation-perfusion relationships in the lung in health and disease.
- Describe the four major mechanisms of hypoxemia and the two major mechanisms of hypercapnia.

The relationship between ventilation and perfusion (as determined by the $\dot{V}/\dot{Q}$ ratio) is the major determinant of normal gas exchange. In this chapter, we examine ventilation and perfusion first individually before discussing the relationship between the two. Finally, we discuss the major mechanisms of hypoxemia and hypercapnia.

Ventilation Is Determined by the Tidal Volume and the Respiratory Frequency

Minute (or total) ventilation is the volume of gas entering or leaving the lung per unit of time (usually a minute). Tidal volume or the volume of gas entering and leaving the lung per breath varies with age, gender, body position, and metabolic activity but is approximately 500 mL in an average-sized adult.

Alveolar ventilation is the part of each breath that participates in gas exchange

Alveolar ventilation is that portion of the minute ventilation that reaches the alveoli and participates in gas exchange. It is composed of the volume of gas that fills the conducting airways (airways that do not participate in gas exchange and known as the **anatomical dead space**) and the volume of gas that participates in gas exchange. Here we describe the composition of the gas mixture as it moves from the ambient environment to the alveolus.

Ambient air is a gas mixture composed of nitrogen (≈79%) and oxygen (≈21%) with minute quantities of carbon dioxide, argon, and other inert gases. Because ambient air is a gas, it obeys the gas laws. All gases can be described either in terms of fractions (e.g., 0.79 N_2) or in terms of partial pressures (e.g., 600 mm Hg). Dalton's gas law states that the sum of the partial pressures (or fractions) of individual gases in air must equal the total pressure (or 1.0). Thus, at sea level, where the total ambient (or barometric) pressure of all the gases is 760 mm Hg, the sum of the partial pressures of all of the gases in the atmosphere must equal 760 mm Hg. For nitrogen, this partial pressure is 600 mm Hg (0.79 × 760 mm Hg). For oxygen, the partial pressure is 160 mm Hg (0.21 × 760 mm Hg); 160 mm Hg is the partial pressure of oxygen at the start of inspiration at the mouth at sea level.

As inspiration begins, the ambient gases are brought into the airways, where they are warmed to body temperature and humidified and become saturated with water. Water vapor pressure at body temperature is 47 mm Hg; this water vapor pressure dilutes the total pressure of the other gases, reducing the partial pressure of oxygen to 150 mm Hg [(760 mm Hg − 47 mm Hg) × 0.21] and the partial pressure of nitrogen to 563 mm Hg [(760 mg Hg − 47 mm Hg) × 0.79]. Note that the total pressure of all the gases is still 760 mm Hg (150 + 563 + 47 mm Hg). Since the conducting airways do not participate in gas exchange, the partial pressures of oxygen, nitrogen, and water vapor remain unchanged in the airways until the gas reaches the alveoli.

O_2 and CO_2 are exchanged in the alveolus

When the inspired gas reaches the alveolus, O_2 is transported across the alveolar membrane and CO_2 moves from the capillary into the alveolus. As a consequence of gas exchange, the fraction of O_2 in the alveolus decreases and the fraction of CO_2 in the alveolus increases. The relationship between O_2 and CO_2 in the alveolus (P_{AO_2} and P_{ACO_2}, respectively) is described by the **alveolar air equation:**

$$P_{AO_2} = (P_B - P_{H_2O}) \times F_{IO_2} - \frac{P_{ACO_2}}{R}$$

where P_B is the barometric pressure; P_{H_2O} is the water vapor pressure; F_{IO_2} is the fraction of oxygen in inspired air (0.21 in room air); and R is the respiratory quotient, which is the relationship between CO_2 production and O_2 consumption (usually 0.8). BECAUSE OF THE DIFFUSIBILITY OF CARBON DIOXIDE, THE ALVEOLAR (A) PARTIAL PRESSURE (P_{ACO_2}) AND THE ARTERIAL (a) PARTIAL PRESSURE (P_{aCO_2}) ARE EQUIVALENT.

The **alveolar air equation** describes the ideal case of what the partial pressure of O_2 *should be* in the alveolus. In a situation of perfect transport and no venous admixture, the alveolar partial pressure (P_{AO_2}) would be the same as the arterial partial pressure (P_{aO_2}). As we will see later, the P_{aO_2} is affected by disease, and the difference between what it should be (P_{AO_2}) and what it actually is in the arterial blood (P_{aO_2}) is indicative of pulmonary disease. In normal individuals, the difference between the ideal alveolar O_2 partial pressure and the partial pressure of O_2 in arterial blood (known as the **Aa gradient**) is less than 15 mm Hg.

The adequacy of alveolar ventilation ($\dot{V}_A$) is measured in terms of P_{aCO_2}, which is tightly regulated by central and peripheral chemoreceptors at 40 mm Hg. **Hyperventilation** (overventilation) is defined as a P_{aCO_2} less than 35 mm Hg and means that alveolar ventilation is excessive for the level of metabolic CO_2 production. **Hypoventilation** (underventilation) is a P_{aCO_2} greater than 45 mm Hg and means that $\dot{V}_A$ is too low for the level of metabolic CO_2 production. Respiratory failure due either to chronic lung disease or to muscle weakness or central nervous system depression is the most common cause of hypoventilation.

Ventilation increases from the apex of the lung to the base during tidal volume breathing

Ventilation is not uniformly distributed in the lung in large part because of the effects of gravity; alveoli in the top of the lung are more expanded than alveoli at the bottom of the lung in the upright position. The pleural pressure is less (more negative) at the apex of the lung than at the base because the weight of the lung tends to pull it downward away from the chest wall. With inspiration, the pleural pressure decreases further. This further decrease in pleural pressure is associated with an increase in the pressure across the lung ($P_L = P_A - Ppl$), and the alveolar volume increases in this area (**Figure 29–1**).

As inspiration begins, the alveoli in the lung are at different lung volumes and are therefore at different locations along the pressure-volume curve of the lung. The smaller alveoli at the base are located along the steep portion of the pressure-volume curve and as a result have a greater compliance and receive more of the tidal volume. In contrast, the expanded alveoli at the apex are closer to the top of the pressure-volume curve. They have a lower compliance, and thus they receive proportionately less of the tidal volume. Thus, in upright individuals, the base of the lung receives more of the tidal volume than the apex.

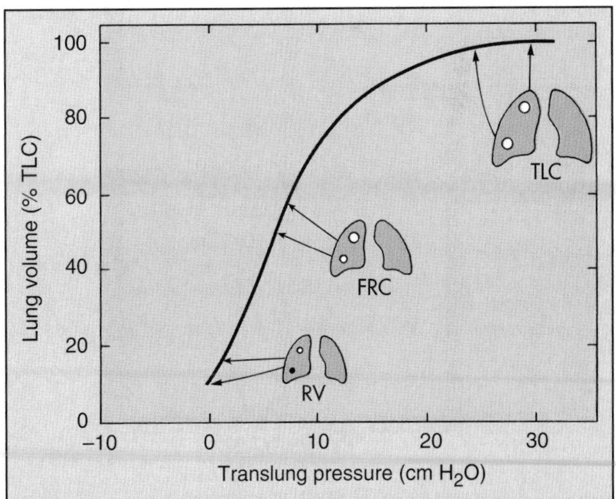

FIGURE 29–1. Regional distribution of lung volume. Because of suspension of the lung from top (i.e., apex in the upright position or anterior in the supine position) to bottom (i.e., base in the upright position or posterior in the supine position), pleural pressure (Ppl) and translung pressure (P_L) of units at the top (apex or anterior) will be greater than those at the bottom (base or posterior). The effect is greatest at residual volume (RV), is less at functional residual capacity (FRC), and disappears at total lung capacity (TLC). (From Berne RM, Levy MN, Koeppen BM, Stanton BA: *Physiology*, ed 5, Philadelphia, 2004, Elsevier.)

Perfusion Is the Process by Which Deoxygenated Blood Passes Through the Lung and Becomes Reoxygenated

The pulmonary circulation begins with the right atrium, where deoxygenated blood enters the right ventricle and is then pumped under low pressure (mean pressure range, 9 to 24 mm Hg) through the pulmonic valve into the main pulmonary artery **(Figure 29–2).** THE ARTERIES OF THE PULMONARY CIRCULATION ARE THE ONLY ARTERIES IN THE BODY THAT CARRY DEOXYGENATED BLOOD. The pulmonary artery quickly divides into a right and left main artery before entering the parenchyma (tissue) of the right and left lung, respectively. The deoxygenated blood in the pulmonary arteries passes through a progressively smaller series of branching vessels that follow the airway branching pattern and end in a complex meshlike network of capillaries where red blood cells flow single file through the alveolus.

A major design feature of the lung is the short distance between alveolar gas and the hemoglobin in red blood cells—a distance of only 1 μm **(Figure 29–3).** This barrier is composed of the type I alveolar epithelial cell, the capillary endothelial cell, and their respective basement membranes. In addition, the flow through the pulmonary circulation is such that the red blood cell remains in the capillary a sufficient time to ensure optimal equilibration between alveolar gas and blood. As a result, the diffusive exchange of O_2 and CO_2 is not rate limiting under most conditions.

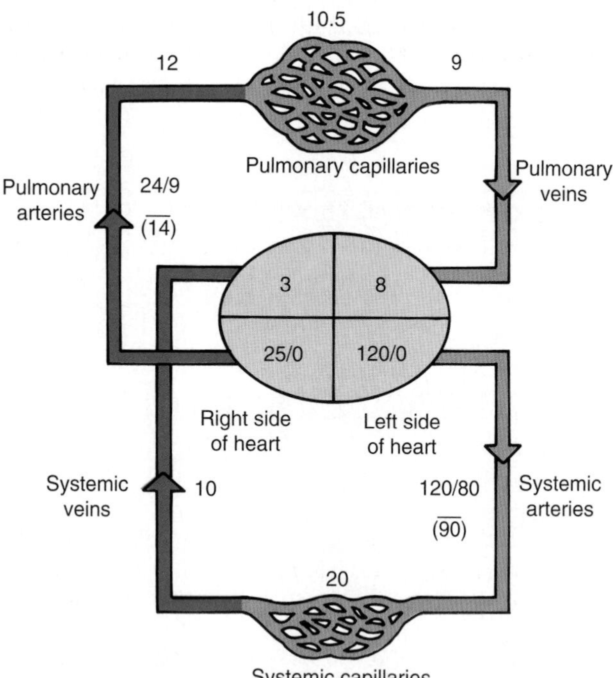

FIGURE 29–2. Schematic representation of the pressures within the systemic and pulmonary circulations in a normal human adult in the resting, supine position. The driving pressure in the systemic circuit ($P_{ao} - P_{ra}$) = 90 − 3 = 87 mm Hg, whereas the driving pressure in the pulmonary circuit ($P_{pa} - P_{la}$) = 14 − 8 = 6 mm Hg. Because the cardiac output must be the same in both circuits, the resistance to flow through the lungs is less than 10% that of the rest of the body. (From Berne RM, Levy MN, Koeppen BM, Stanton BA: *Physiology,* ed 5, Philadelphia, 2004, Elsevier.)

The lung is leaky

In addition to gas exchange, the pulmonary capillaries and alveoli (known as the **alveolar-capillary network**) also function in fluid regulation in the lung. At the pulmonary capillary level, the balance between hydrostatic pressure and oncotic pressure **(Starling forces)** results in a small net movement of fluid out of the capillaries and into the interstitial space. This fluid is then removed from the lung interstitium by the lymphatic system and enters the circulation via the vena cava. An average of 30 mL of fluid per hour is returned to the circulation by this route.

The accumulation of excess fluid in the interstitium of the lung is called **pulmonary edema** and is potentially life-threatening because it interferes with gas exchange and results in ventilation-perfusion mismatching. Excess pulmonary fluid can be caused by congestive heart failure with increased left atrial pressure or by injury to the type I epithelial cells that can occur in some types of interstitial lung diseases.

The pulmonary circulation accommodates the entire cardiac output, but the work associated with this pumping is less than 10% of that required for the systemic circulation. The difference is attributed to the parallel array of pulmonary resistance arteries that are normally dilated and maintain a low **pulmonary vascular resistance** (PVR). Pulmonary blood flow is regulated by potent local mechanisms, of which alveolar PO_2 is the most important.

Imagine a person aspirating (inhaling) a piece of steak (sometimes called a café coronary because the person appears to have had a heart attack) into the right main stem bronchus. All ventilation to the right lung has been cut off. If the right lung continued to receive blood flow, half of the cardiac output going to the lungs would not receive oxygen. The alveolar PO_2 in the right lung decreases, PVR throughout the right lung increases, and as a result, pulmonary blood flow to the right lung decreases. This is one of the major homeostatic (self-regulating) mechanisms in the body, regulating blood flow to areas that are not being ventilated.

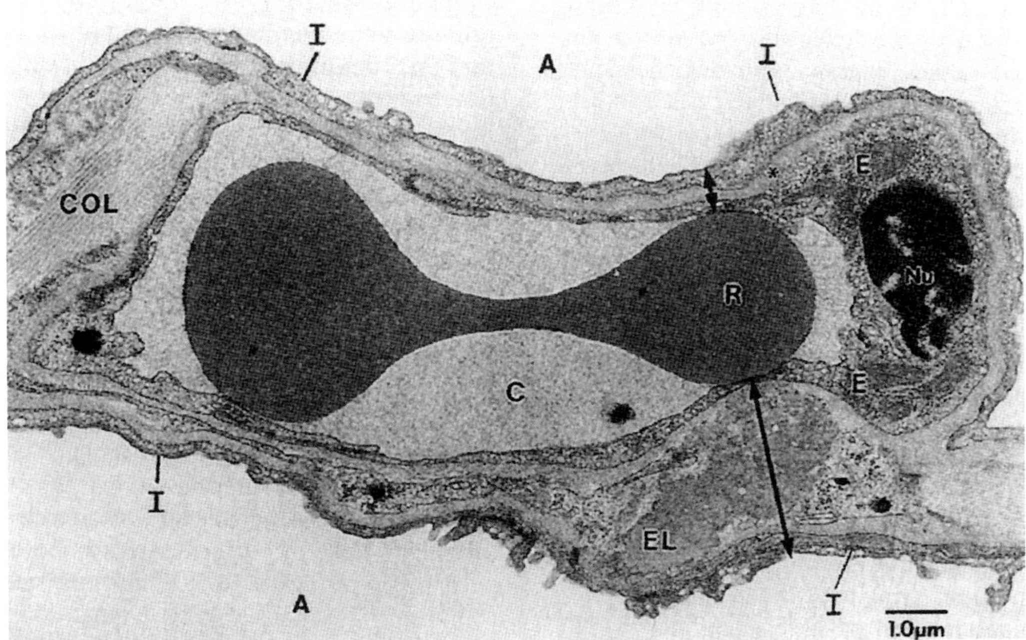

FIGURE 29–3. Cross section of an alveolar wall showing the path for O_2 and CO_2 diffusion. The thin side of the alveolar wall barrier *(short double arrow)* consists of type I epithelium (I), interstitium formed by the fused basal laminae of the epithelial and endothelial cells, capillary endothelium (E), plasma in the alveolar capillary (C), and finally the cytoplasm of the red blood cell (R). The thick side of the gas exchange barrier *(long double arrow)* has an accumulation of elastin (EL), collagen (COL), and matrix that jointly separates the alveolar epithelium from the alveolar capillary endothelium. As long as the red blood cells are flowing, O_2 and CO_2 diffusion probably occurs across both sides of the air-blood barrier. A, alveolus; Nu, nucleus of the capillary endothelial cell. (Human lung specimen, transmission electron microscope. From Berne RM, Levy MN, Koeppen BM, Stanton BA: *Physiology,* ed 5, Philadelphia, 2004, Elsevier.)

The Arteries of the Pulmonary Circulation Are Ideally Configured to Support Their Functions

The functions of the pulmonary circulation are to reoxygenate blood and eliminate CO_2, to aid in lung fluid balance, and to distribute metabolic products of the lung. The arteries of the pulmonary circulation are thin walled, have minimal smooth muscle, are highly compliant, and are easily distensible. This results in a compliant, low-resistance circulatory system that aids in the flow of blood through the pulmonary circulation via the relatively weak pumping action of the right ventricle. The pressure gradient from the pulmonary artery to the left atrium is only 6 mm (14 mm Hg pulmonary artery minus 8 mm Hg left atrium); this is 15 times less than the pressure gradient differential of 87 mm Hg in the systemic circulation. At rest, this network contains about 75 mL of blood but increases to more than 200 mL with exercise. Despite the increase in blood volume, the pressure within the pulmonary circulation remains low. In part, this is because at rest, not all of the capillaries are open, but they are recruited during periods of high flow. In addition, the high compliance and distensibility of the capillary bed accommodate an increase in volume with little or no change in pressure.

The second circulatory system in the lung is the bronchial circulation

Oxygenated blood from the systemic circulation supplies the structures of the lung, including the trachea, upper airways, surface secretory cells, glands, nerves, visceral pleural surface, lymph nodes, and pulmonary arteries and pulmonary veins in the bronchial circulation. The pressure in the main bronchial arteries is essentially the same as in the aorta; hence, the driving pressure is high. The bronchial circulation supplies the upper respiratory tract; it does not reach the terminal or respiratory bronchioles or the alveoli **(Figure 29–4).** Bronchial blood flow is only 1% of the cardiac output in normal individuals but can increase significantly in individuals with bronchiectasis (bronchiectasis is a chronic dilatation of one or more bronchi, usually as a result of infection). Venous blood returns to the heart from the bronchial circulation either through true bronchial

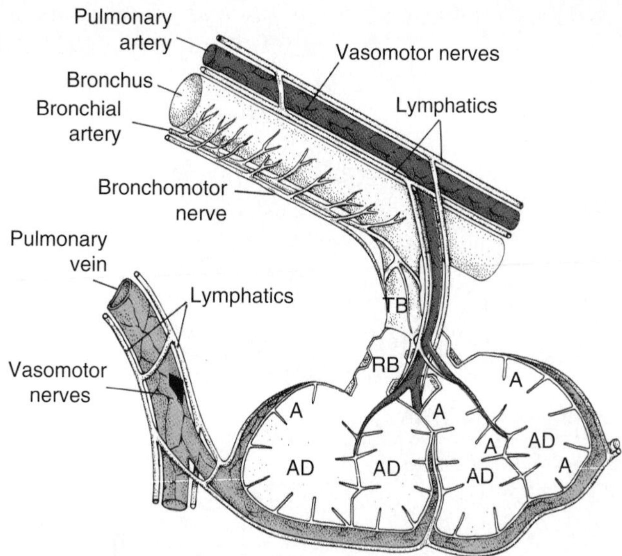

FIGURE 29–4. The anatomical relation between the pulmonary artery, the bronchial artery, the airways, and the lymphatics. TB, terminal bronchioles; RB, respiratory bronchioles; A, alveoli; AD, alveolar ducts. (From Berne RM, Levy MN, Koeppen BM, Stanton BA: *Physiology,* ed 5, Philadelphia, 2004, Elsevier.)

veins or through bronchopulmonary veins. Approximately one third of the bronchial circulation returns to the right side of the heart via the bronchial veins. The remainder flows through small bronchopulmonary anastomoses (connections) into the pulmonary veins and into the left side of the heart. This results in a small amount of deoxygenated, venous blood mixing with oxygenated blood, which contributes to the small, normal venous admixture (right-to-left shunt) in normal individuals and to the Aa gradient of 15 mm Hg in normal individuals.

Blood flow in the lung is affected by gravity

Blood flow in the lung is affected by PVR, gravity, alveolar pressure, and the arterial to venous pressure gradient. Under normal circumstances, the resistance in the pulmonary circulation is about 10 times less than that in the systemic circulation and remains low even during exertion or exercise.

Because it is a low-pressure, low-resistance system, pulmonary blood flow is dramatically influenced by gravity. This results in an uneven distribution of blood in the lung. In upright individuals, blood flow increases from the apex of the lung (lowest flow) to the base of the lung, where it is greatest. During exercise or other times of stress, the difference in blood flow in the apical and basal regions in upright individuals becomes less because of the increase in flow and the increase in arterial pressure.

Lung volume affects PVR through its influence on the alveolar capillaries **(Figure 29–5)**. At end inspiration, the fully distended air-filled alveoli compress the alveolar capillaries and increase PVR. In contrast, pulmonary vessels outside of the alveoli increase in diameter during inspiration because of pulling on their walls, and their PVR decreases.

Mechanical ventilation is used to aid individuals who are unable to adequately oxygenate and remove CO_2 from their blood. In mechanical ventilation, a positive pressure is applied to the airways to force air into the lung. As a result, the pressure inside the alveolus increases. This increase can compress pulmonary capillaries and increase PVR. In individuals with lung disease, this pressure effect may not be uniformly distributed. The positive pressure could improve ventilation to airways that are not being well ventilated, but it could also compress capillaries serving normal alveoli. In individuals being mechanically ventilated, it is important to apply sufficient pressure to improve ventilation to the diseased airways without compromising the ventilation to the normal airways. Overventilation in this instance could make ventilation-perfusion mismatching overall in the lung worse instead of better.

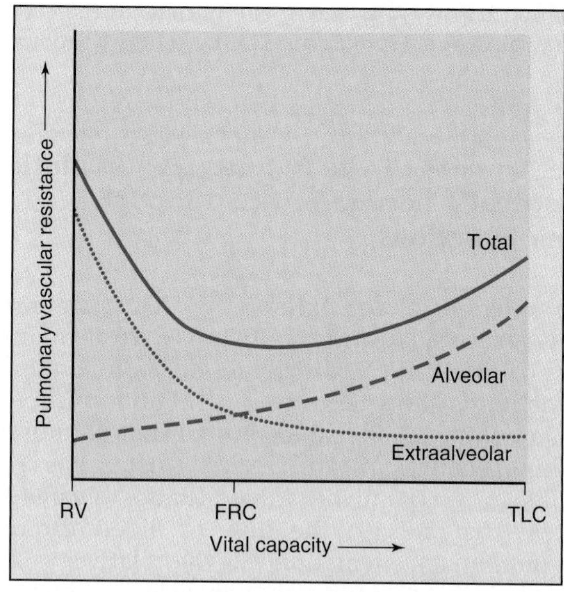

FIGURE 29–5. Schematic representation of the effects of changes in vital capacity on total pulmonary vascular resistance and the contributions to the total afforded by alveolar and extraalveolar vessels. During inflation from residual volume (RV) to total lung capacity (TLC), resistance to blood flow through alveolar vessels increases, whereas resistance through extraalveolar vessels decreases. Thus, changes in total pulmonary vascular resistance form a U-shaped curve during lung inflation, with the nadir at functional residual capacity (FRC). (From Berne RM, Levy MN, Koeppen BM, Stanton BA: *Physiology,* ed 5, Philadelphia, 2004, Elsevier.)

The arterial to venous pressure gradient also affects pulmonary blood flow. Blood must travel up to the apex of the lung from the pulmonary artery. This upward flow is associated with a decrease in hydrostatic pressure, which results in a further decrease in flow in upright individuals to the apex of the lung.

Pulmonary vessels are surrounded by a thin wall of smooth muscle that is regulated by numerous substances. Some of these substances, including endothelin, leukotrienes, angiotensin, and thromboxane A_2, cause constriction of the smooth muscle. THE MOST POTENT CONSTRICTOR OF PULMONARY VESSEL SMOOTH MUSCLE IS HYPOXIA (LOW LEVELS OF O_2). This response is different from that of the systemic circulation. In the systemic circulation, a low Pa_{O_2} relaxes the arterioles. In the lung, a low P_{AO_2} constricts nearby arterioles. This decreases local blood flow and shifts (shunts) it to other regions of the lung with higher P_{AO_2} values, an important self-control (homeostatic) mechanism to achieve optimal ventilation and oxygenation. In the face of a global reduction in P_{AO_2}, such as that which occurs at high altitude, however, all the resistance vessels constrict, and there is no other region of the lung to shunt the blood to. As a result, there is an increase in PVR.

Primary pulmonary hypertension is a disease of increased pressure in the pulmonary arteries of unknown cause. Patients report progressive shortness of breath beginning with activity and then occurring even at rest. Elevated levels of endothelin have been found in the smooth muscle of pulmonary vessels in these individuals, and antiendothelin drugs offer some promise in the treatment of this disease. Pulmonary hypertension can also develop as a result of other diseases (secondary pulmonary hypertension) and is seen in advanced chronic obstructive lung disease (particularly emphysema), in interstitial lung diseases, after multiple chronic **pulmonary emboli** (blood clots in the lung), and in diseases associated with blood vessel inflammation **(vasculitis).**

Ventilation and Perfusion Are Essential for Normal Gas Exchange

Both ventilation and perfusion are essential elements for gas exchange, but they are insufficient to ensure normal gas exchange. For example, consider the situation in which an area of the lung is perfused but not ventilated. Overall perfusion and ventilation may be normal, but in this area, normal gas exchange cannot occur because ventilation is absent. Thus, the incoming deoxygenated blood will remain deoxygenated.

The ventilation-perfusion ratio ($\dot{V}/\dot{Q}$) is the ratio of ventilation to blood flow. It can be defined for a single alveolus, for a group of alveoli, or for the entire lung. At the level of the lung, the ratio is defined as the total alveolar ventilation divided by the cardiac output (i.e., $\dot{V}_A/\dot{Q}_T$). When ventilation exceeds perfusion, the ventilation-perfusion ratio is greater than 1 ($\dot{V}/\dot{Q} > 1$), and when perfusion exceeds ventilation, the ventilation-perfusion ratio is less than 1 ($\dot{V}/\dot{Q} < 1$).

In normal individuals at the level of the lung, alveolar ventilation is about 4.0 L/min; pulmonary blood flow is about 5.0 L/min. Thus, in normal individuals at rest, the $\dot{V}/\dot{Q}$ in the lung is 0.8. This *overall* $\dot{V}/\dot{Q}$ ratio (i.e., $\dot{V}_A/\dot{Q}_T$) is composed, however, of a wide range of $\dot{V}/\dot{Q}$ ratios from different individual lung units. From the apex to the base in the upright position, ventilation increases more slowly than perfusion **(Figure 29–6)**. Specifically, at the apex of the lung where both ventilation and perfusion are decreased compared with the base, the decrease in

Ventilation-Perfusion Relationships

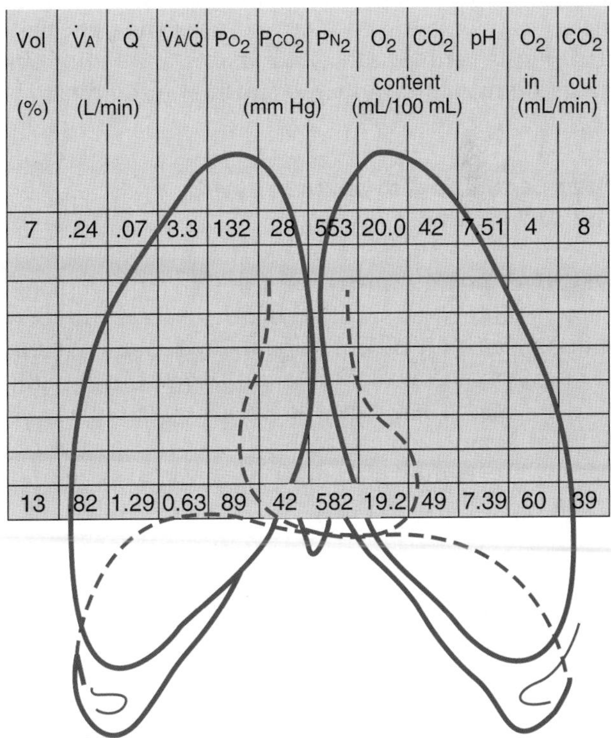

FIGURE 29–6. Regional differences in gas exchange down the normal lung. For clarity, only the values for alveolar ventilation ($\dot{V}_A$) and blood flow ($\dot{Q}$) at the apex and base are shown. (From Berne RM, Levy MN, Koeppen BM, Stanton BA: *Physiology,* ed 5, Philadelphia, 2004, Elsevier.)

perfusion is greater than the decrease in ventilation, and thus normal lung units at the apex of the lung in the upright individual have $\dot{V}/\dot{Q}$ ratios greater than 1. In contrast, perfusion is greater than ventilation at the base, and $\dot{V}/\dot{Q}$ ratios are less than 1.

Venous admixture reduces the efficiency of gas exchange

Venous blood that returns to the heart without passing by air-filled alveoli remains deoxygenated and leads to **venous admixture** because the venous, deoxygenated blood mixes with oxygenated blood from the lung. Venous admixture lowers the $Pa{O_2}$ and causes a decrease in O_2 saturation. There are two major sources of venous admixture. The first is due to venous blood that bypasses the air-filled lung completely because of an anatomical abnormality, usually a defect in the heart (anatomical shunt). The second is due to blood that perfused the lung but did not perfuse an area that was ventilated (ventilation-perfusion mismatch). Normally, approximately 1% of the cardiac output is involved in venous admixture. This occurs from some of the bronchial veins that drain into the left atrium and the thebesian veins of the left ventricular myocardium that drain into the left ventricle rather than into the coronary sinus of the right ventricle. This venous admixture is responsible for the Aa gradient of 15 mm Hg in normal individuals.

Hypoxemia and hypoxia are not the same thing

Arterial hypoxemia is defined as an abnormal $Pa{O_2}$, which in an adult at sea level is a $Pa{O_2}$ less than 80 mm Hg. **Hypoxia** is defined as insufficient O_2 to carry out normal metabolic functions, usually a $Pa{O_2}$ less than 60 mm Hg. **Hypercapnia** is defined as an increase in $Pa{CO_2}$ above the normal range (40 ± 2 mm Hg), and **hypocapnia** is defined as a decrease in $Pa{CO_2}$ below the normal range (usually less than 35 mm Hg).

The two-compartment lung model is a useful way to examine ventilation-perfusion relationships

A useful way to examine the interaction and relationship between ventilation and perfusion is the two–lung unit model **(Figure 29–7)**. Two alveoli are ventilated, each of which is supplied by a part of the cardiac output. When ventilation is uniform, half of the inspired gas goes to each alveolus, and when perfusion is uniform, half of the cardiac output goes to each alveolus. In this normal unit, the ventilation-perfusion ratios in each of the alveoli are the same and are equal to 1. The alveoli are perfused by mixed venous blood that is deoxygenated and contains increased $P{CO_2}$. Alveolar O_2 is higher than mixed venous O_2, and this provides a gradient for the movement of O_2 into the blood. In contrast, mixed venous CO_2 is greater than the alveolar CO_2. This provides a gradient for the movement of CO_2 into the alveolus. Note that in this ideal model, alveolar-arterial O_2 values do not differ (Aa gradient = 0).

There are four major causes of hypoxemia. All of them involve some form of ventilation-perfusion mismatching—perfusion that bypasses the lung (anatomical shunt), absent ventilation to areas being perfused (physiological shunt), low ventilation to areas being perfused ($\dot{V}/\dot{Q}$ mismatching), or hypoventilation (underventilation of lung units).

Cyanotic congenital heart diseases are the most common types of anatomical shunts

If a portion of the cardiac output bypasses the lung completely and mixes with oxygenated blood, an anatomical shunt has been created. In

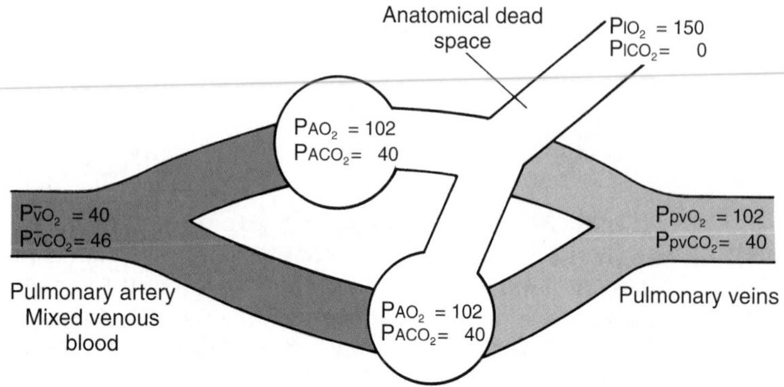

FIGURE 29–7. Simplified lung model showing two normal parallel lung units. Both units receive equal quantities of fresh air and blood flow for their size. The blood and alveolar gas partial pressures, P, are normal values in a resting person. (From Berne RM, Levy MN, Koeppen BM, Stanton BA: *Physiology*, ed 5, Philadelphia, 2004, Elsevier.)

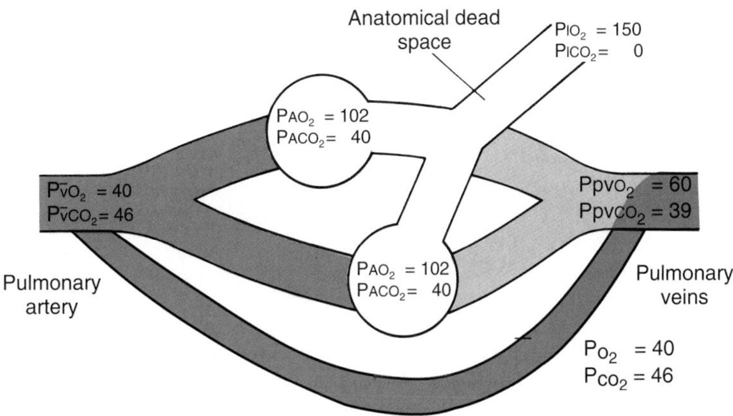

FIGURE 29–8. Right-to-left shunt. Alveolar ventilation is normal, but a portion of the cardiac output bypasses the lung and mixes oxygenated blood. The Pa_{O_2} will vary according to the size of the shunt. (From Berne RM, Levy MN, Koeppen BM, Stanton BA: *Physiology*, ed 5, Philadelphia, 2004, Elsevier.)

an anatomical shunt, alveolar ventilation, the distribution of alveolar gas, and the composition of the alveolar gas are normal. The distribution of the cardiac output has, however, been changed **(Figure 29–8)**. Some of the blood now bypasses the gas-exchanging unit and is said to be "shunted." Because this blood is deoxygenated, the model is called a right-to-left shunt. AN IMPORTANT FEATURE OF AN ANATOMICAL SHUNT IS THAT THE HYPOXEMIA IT CREATES CANNOT BE ABOLISHED BY GIVING THE INDIVIDUAL 100% OXYGEN TO BREATHE. This is because the blood that bypasses the ventilation is never exposed to the enriched oxygen, and thus it continues to be deoxygenated. Most often these anatomical shunts occur within the heart (cyanotic congenital heart disease), and they occur when deoxygenated blood from the right atrium or ventricle crosses the septum and mixes with blood from the left atrium or ventricle.

Physiological shunts occur when there is no ventilation to an alveolus that is being perfused

If an airway is completely blocked, the alveoli supplied by that airway will receive no ventilation. All of the ventilation will go to the other lung units, while the perfusion will be equally distributed to both ventilated and nonventilated lung units **(Figure 29–9)**. The lung unit without ventilation but with perfusion has a $\dot{V}/\dot{Q}$ of 0. Because there is no ventilation, the blood that is perfusing this unit remains deoxygenated. Like in an anatomical shunt, deoxygenated blood bypasses a gas-exchanging unit. The difference is that in the physiological shunt, it is because of underlying airway disease, whereas in the anatomical shunt, it is because of an anatomical abnormality usually involving the heart. **Atelectasis** (obstruction to ventilation of a gas-exchanging unit with subsequent loss of volume) is the most common cause of a physiological shunt and can be due to obstruction to ventilation by mucous plugs, airway edema, foreign bodies, or tumors in the airway.

Low $\dot{V}/\dot{Q}$, also known as $\dot{V}/\dot{Q}$ mismatching, is the most common cause of hypoxemia

Most respiratory diseases produce global changes of varying extent in the lungs. For example, in chronic bronchitis, there will be some airways that appear to be normal; some airways will have a small amount of mucus that will cause an increase in resistance and a small decrease in ventilation to the alveoli supplied by that airway; some airways will have more mucus, and some will have significant obstruction with mucus, cellular (particularly goblet

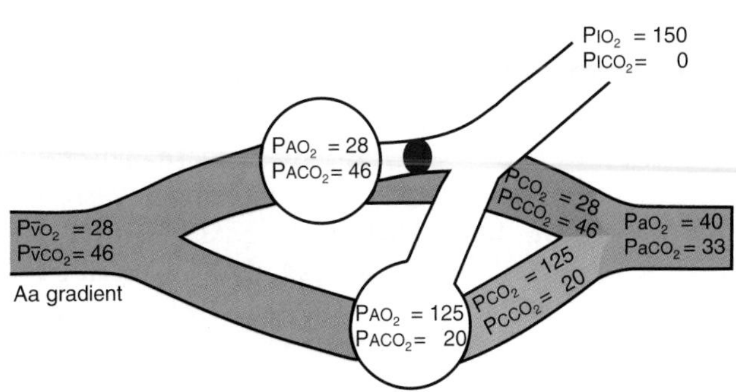

FIGURE 29–9. Schema of a physiological shunt (venous admixture). Notice the marked decrease in arterial P_{O_2} compared with P_{CO_2}. The Aa gradient is 85 mm Hg (Aa gradient = P_{AO_2} – Pa_{O_2}; 125 mm Hg – 40 mm Hg). (From Berne RM, Levy MN, Koeppen BM, Stanton BA: *Physiology*, ed 5, Philadelphia, 2004, Elsevier.)

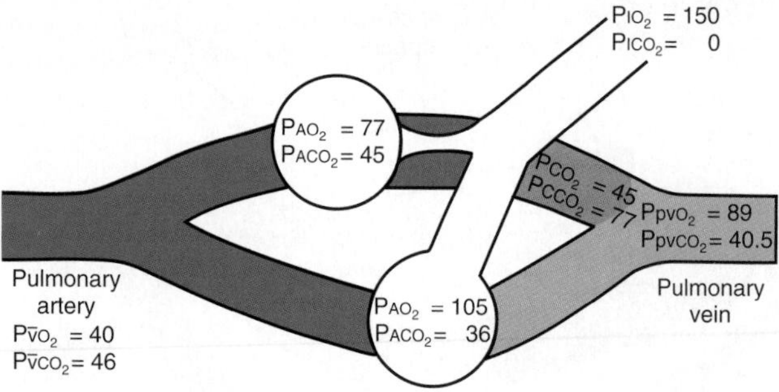

FIGURE 29–10. Effects of ventilation-perfusion mismatching on gas exchange. The decrease in ventilation to the one-lung unit could be due to mucous obstruction, airway edema, bronchospasm, a foreign body, or a tumor. (From Berne RM, Levy MN, Koeppen BM, Stanton BA: *Physiology,* ed 5, Philadelphia, 2004, Elsevier.)

cell) hyperplasia, and airway swelling. As a result, individual airways will have varying degrees of abnormal ventilation, but in all instances in which there is some obstruction, ventilation will be decreased out of proportion to perfusion **(Figure 29–10).** Blood flow, however, will be normally distributed. This results in a situation that is called $\dot{V}/\dot{Q}$ mismatching or, more specifically, low $\dot{V}/\dot{Q}$ (i.e., a $\dot{V}/\dot{Q} < 1$). As a result, the alveolar and end-capillary gas compositions will vary according to the degree of obstruction. Both the arterial O_2 and CO_2 contents will be abnormal in the blood that comes from the units with the decreased ventilation. The measured arterial O_2 and CO_2 levels depend on the extent and number of lung units affected by the disease. An increase in the Aa gradient will be present. Supplemental oxygen, however, will correct the hypoxemia as poorly ventilated lung units will receive enriched oxygen.

Hypoventilation will decrease arterial O_2 and increase arterial CO_2

Underventilation will bring less fresh gas to the alveoli. As a result, the O_2 levels in the alveoli will decrease and the CO_2 levels will increase. The relationship between alveolar ventilation and arterial CO_2 is linear **(alveolar CO_2 gas equation) (Figure 29–11).** If ventilation is halved, arterial CO_2 will double. ONE OF THE HALLMARKS OF HYPOVENTILATION IS A NORMAL AA GRADIENT. This occurs because the airways and capillaries are functioning normally; they are, however, being presented with less fresh gas to exchange. Patients with respiratory muscle weakness, including those with muscular dystrophy or diaphragmatic paralysis, are at risk for hypoventilation. Hypoventilation produces both hypercapnia and hypoxemia.

Abnormalities in diffusion are rare causes of hypoxemia

Although increases in red cell transit time could result in arterial hypoxia, equilibration between the alveolar and capillary O_2 and CO_2 occurs so rapidly that this is a rare cause of hypoxia; it is a problem **(diffusion disequilibrium)** only during exercise at high altitude. Thickening of the air-blood barrier **(alveolar-capillary block)** is also a rare cause of decreased diffusing capacity and hypoxia. Such thickening would result in progressive recruitment of previously unperfused capillaries and restoration of normal flow until the process is severe.

Hypoventilation and wasted ventilation are responsible for hypercapnia

As described previously, alveolar ventilation and alveolar CO_2 are directly related. Hypoventilation always decreases the PaO_2 and increases the $PaCO_2$ except when the individual is breathing an enriched source of oxygen.

Wasted ventilation occurs when pulmonary blood flow decreases markedly in the presence of normal ventilation (i.e., $\dot{V}/\dot{Q} > 1 \rightarrow \infty$). This is most

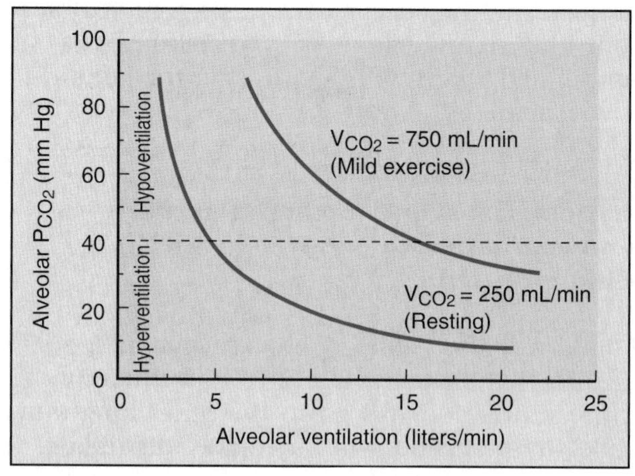

FIGURE 29–11. Alveolar PCO_2 as a function of alveolar ventilation in the lung. Each line corresponds to a given metabolic rate associated with a constant production of CO_2 (VCO_2 isometabolic line). Normally, alveolar ventilation is controlled to maintain an alveolar PCO_2 of about 40 mm Hg. During hypoventilation, the alveolar ventilation is low relative to VCO_2, and alveolar PCO_2 rises. During hyperventilation, the alveolar ventilation is excessive relative to VCO_2, so the alveolar PCO_2 falls. (From Berne RM, Levy MN, Koeppen BM, Stanton BA: *Physiology,* ed 5, Philadelphia, 2004, Elsevier.)

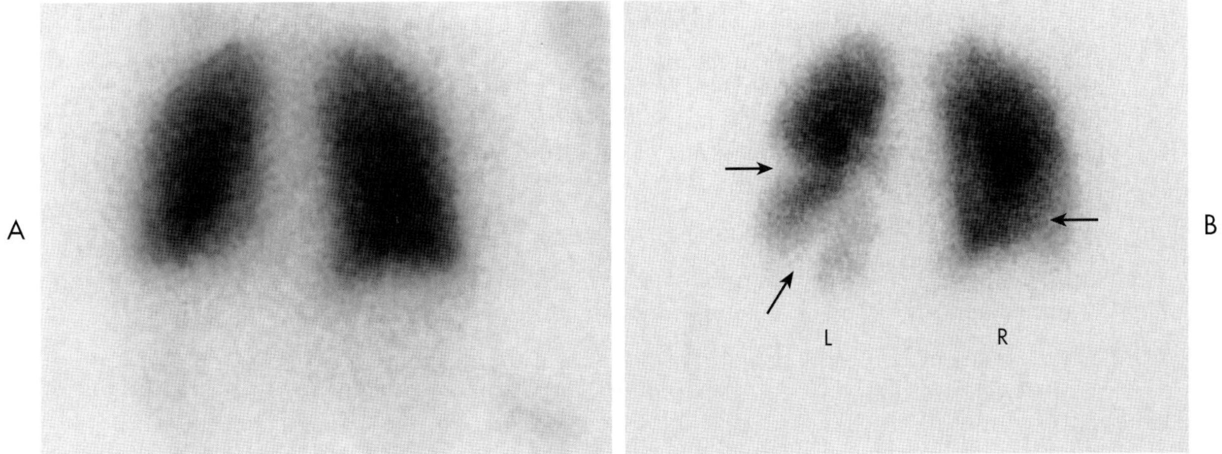

FIGURE 29–12. **A**, Normal perfusion scan (performed by intravenous injection of a radioactive tracer) demonstrates normal blood flow distribution in all lobes of the lung. **B**, Abnormal perfusion scan demonstrates diminished blood flow to the right and left lower lobes as a result of occluding pulmonary emboli *(arrows)*. The ventilation-perfusion mismatching explains this patient's hypoxemia.

often due to a **pulmonary embolus** that obstructs blood flow **(Figure 29–12)**. In this situation, the ventilation is wasted because it fails to oxygenate any blood. The ventilation to the rest of the lung is now abnormal (less ventilation for the perfusion, that is, relative hypoventilation) because more of the blood flow goes through areas with "normal" ventilation. As a result, P_{CO_2} increases and P_{O_2} decreases. Compensation (homeostasis) occurs rapidly after a pulmonary embolus with a decrease in ventilation to the nonperfused lung units and redistribution to the areas of the lung being perfused.

$\dot{V}/\dot{Q}$ abnormalities but not anatomical shunts respond to 100% oxygen

The measurement of the arterial O_2 is one of the ways that an anatomical shunt can be distinguished from other causes of hypoxemia. In the normal lung, the alveolar O_2 content will rapidly increase after exposure to 100% oxygen [$P_{AO_2} = (760 - 47)1.0 - 40/0.8 = 663$ mm Hg], and this is associated with a marked increase in the arterial O_2 content to more than 500 mm Hg at sea level. In contrast, in the individual with an anatomical shunt, exposure to 100% oxygen for 15 minutes will not correct the hypoxemia because mixed venous blood continues to flow through the shunt and to mix with blood that has perfused normal units. The blood that has perfused the normal units will increase in O_2 content, but not the blood through the shunt. As a result, the P_{aO_2} increases only to approximately 150 mm Hg in patients with an anatomical (cyanotic congenital heart disease) shunt after exposure to 100% oxygen.

Changes in cardiac output will also cause hypoxemia

A change in cardiac output is the only nonrespiratory factor that affects gas exchange. The O_2 content will decrease and the CO_2 will increase with decreasing cardiac output, especially in individuals with underlying lung disease.

Summary

- The sum of the partial pressures of a gas must equal the total pressure. The partial pressure of gas (P_{gas}) is equal to the fraction of gas in the gas mixture (F_{gas}) times the total pressure (P_{tot}).
- The conducting airways do not participate in gas exchange. Therefore, the partial pressures of oxygen, nitrogen, and water vapor remain unchanged in the airways until the gas reaches the alveolus.
- The partial pressure of O_2 in the alveolus is given by the alveolar air equation. This equation is used to calculate the Aa gradient, the most useful measurement of abnormal arterial O_2.
- The relationship between CO_2 production and alveolar ventilation is defined by the alveolar CO_2 equation. There is an inverse relationship between the partial pressure of CO_2 in the alveolus ($PACO_2$) and the alveolar ventilation ($\dot{V}A$), irrespective of the exhaled quantity of CO_2. In normal individuals, the $PACO_2$ is tightly regulated to remain constant around 40 mm Hg.
- There are regional differences in ventilation and perfusion, due in large part to the effects of gravity.
- The pulmonary circulation is a low-pressure, low-resistance system with a driving pressure that is almost $^1/_{16}$ that of the systemic circulation.
- The recruitment of new capillaries is a unique feature of the lung and allows stress adjustments, as in the case of exercise. The arteries of the pulmonary circulation are thin walled, and they have minimal smooth muscle. The pulmonary vessels are seven times more compliant than the systemic vessels.
- Pulmonary vascular resistance (PVR) is the change in pressure from the pulmonary artery (PPA) to the left atrium (PLA) divided by the cardiac output (QT). This resistance is about 10 times less than in the systemic circulation.
- In upright, resting subjects, blood flow increases linearly from the apex of the lung to the base of the lung, where the flow is the greatest.
- The ventilation-perfusion ratio (also referred to as $\dot{V}/\dot{Q}$) is the ratio of ventilation to blood flow. In the normal lung, the overall ventilation-perfusion ratio is about 0.8. When ventilation exceeds perfusion, the ventilation-perfusion ratio is greater than 1 ($\dot{V}/\dot{Q} > 1$), and when perfusion exceeds ventilation, the ventilation-perfusion ratio is less than 1 ($\dot{V}/\dot{Q} < 1$).
- The $\dot{V}/\dot{Q}$ at the top of the lung is high in upright individuals (increased ventilation relative to very little blood flow), whereas the $\dot{V}/\dot{Q}$ at the bottom of the lung is very low. In normal individuals breathing room air, the Aa gradient is less than 15 mm Hg.
- There are four mechanisms of hypoxemia: anatomical shunt, physiological shunt, $\dot{V}/\dot{Q}$ mismatching, and hypoventilation.
- There are two mechanisms of hypercapnia: increase in dead space and hypoventilation.
- A change in cardiac output is the only nonrespiratory factor that affects gas exchange.

Bibliography

Bongartz G et al: Pulmonary circulation, *Eur Radiol* 8:698, 1998.

Glenny RW: Blood flow distribution in the lung, *Chest* 114:8S, 1998.

Henig NR, Pierson DJ: Mechanisms of hypoxemia, *Respir Care Clin North Am* 6:501, 2000.

Case Studies

Case 29–1

A 40-year-old mountain climber has the following blood gas values at sea level (760 mm Hg): Pa_{O_2}, 96 mm Hg; Pa_{CO_2}, 40 mm Hg; pH, 7.40 on F_{IO_2} = 0.21. He climbs to the top of Pikes Peak (barometric pressure, 445 mm Hg).

1. **What is his Pa_{O_2} at the top of Pikes Peak? (Assume his Pa_{CO_2} and R are unchanged.)**
   A. 24 mm Hg
   B. 34 mm Hg
   C. 44 mm Hg
   D. 54 mm Hg
   E. 64 mm Hg

Case 29–2

A 79-year-old man is admitted to the hospital in acute respiratory distress resulting from emphysema complicated by pneumonia. He is conscious but confused, disoriented, and slow to respond to questions. He uses accessory muscles to breathe, and there is decreased chest expansion and motion of the diaphragm. His blood pressure is low at 90/65, and he has poor capillary refill, a sign of poor perfusion. The patient is started on oxygen therapy with a 24% Venturi mask (F_{IO_2} 24%). An arterial blood gas analysis reveals the following values: pH, 7.33; Pa_{O_2}, 48 mm Hg; Pa_{CO_2}, 67 mm Hg; HCO_3^-, 34 mEq/L.

1. **Which of the following is the least likely explanation for his hypoxemia (low Pa_{O_2})?**
   A. Ventilation-perfusion mismatch
   B. Right-to-left intrapulmonary shunt
   C. Diffusion barrier to gas transfer
   D. Low cardiac output
   E. Bronchial obstruction

2. **To further evaluate the cause of hypoxemia in this patient, the physician decides to calculate the alveolar to arterial O_2 gradient. Which of the following statements about gas gradients in the lung is false?**
   A. The alveolar to arterial CO_2 gradient in the lung is usually 0.
   B. The alveolar to arterial O_2 gradient in the lung is normally less than 15 mm Hg.
   C. The alveolar to arterial O_2 gradient will help the physician determine whether the hypoxemia is due to hypoventilation or ventilation-perfusion mismatch.
   D. The alveolar to arterial CO_2 gradient is usually greater than 50 mm Hg.
   E. The physician needs to know the barometric pressure to calculate the alveolar O_2 concentration.

3. **What is the $P_{AO_2} - Pa_{O_2}$ gradient (Aa gradient) in this patient? (Assume sea level of 760 mm Hg and R = 0.8.)**
   A. 21 mm Hg
   B. 30 mm Hg
   C. 35 mm Hg
   D. 39 mm Hg
   E. 44 mm Hg

Case 29–3

A 20-year-old man has abrupt onset of muscle weakness. He is unable to walk and is having difficulty swallowing. On physical examination, general muscle weakness is noted. His pulse is 90/min, respirations are 18/min, and blood pressure is 118/60. An arterial blood gas analysis on room air reveals the following values: pH, 7.30; Pa_{CO_2}, 54 mm Hg; Pa_{O_2}, 70 mm Hg.

1. **What is the $P_{AO_2} - Pa_{O_2}$ (Aa gradient) difference? (Assume sea level of 760 mm Hg and R = 0.8.)**
   A. 6 mm Hg
   B. 12 mm Hg
   C. 16 mm Hg
   D. 20 mm Hg
   E. 26 mm Hg

2. **What is the most likely cause of this man's hypoxemia (low Pa_{O_2})?**
   A. Ventilation-perfusion mismatch
   B. Anatomical shunt
   C. Physiological shunt
   D. Hypoventilation
   E. Alveolar-capillary block

Chapter 30: Oxygen and Carbon Dioxide Transport

Objectives

- ❖ Describe the fundamental principles of gas diffusion.
- ❖ Describe the mechanisms of O_2 and CO_2 transport.
- ❖ Explain the importance of hemoglobin in O_2 transport.
- ❖ Describe CO_2 production, metabolism, and transport.

The respiratory and circulatory systems function together to transport sufficient O_2 from the lungs to the tissues to sustain normal cellular activity and to transport CO_2 from the tissues to the lungs. The intracellular metabolism of sugars in mitochondria is the major metabolic process for O_2 use and CO_2 production. THE INTRACELLULAR METABOLISM OF O_2 IN THE MITOCHONDRIAL ELECTRON TRANSPORT SYSTEM PROVIDES THE CELL WITH ITS PRIMARY SOURCE OF ENERGY, ADENOSINE TRIPHOSPHATE (ATP). CO_2, a product of active cellular glucose metabolism, is transported from the tissues via systemic veins to the lungs, where it is expired **(Figure 30–1)**. To enhance uptake and transport of these gases, specialized mechanisms (i.e., oxygen-hemoglobin binding and HCO_3^- transport of CO_2) have evolved that enable O_2 uptake and CO_2 expiration not only to occur simultaneously but also to facilitate each other. To gain an understanding of the mechanisms involved in the transport of these gases, one must consider gas diffusion properties as well as transport and delivery mechanisms.

Gas Movement Throughout the Respiratory System Occurs Predominantly via Diffusion

The respiratory and circulatory systems contain several unique anatomical and physiological features to facilitate gas diffusion: large surface areas for gas exchange (alveolar to capillary and capillary to tissue membrane barriers) with short distances to travel; substantial partial pressure gradient differences; and gases with advantageous diffusion properties. The transport and delivery of O_2 from the lungs to the tissue and vice versa for CO_2 are dependent on basic gas diffusion laws.

Gases in the lung diffuse down a partial pressure gradient from higher to lower pressures

The process of gas diffusion is passive, non–energy dependent, and similar whether diffusion occurs in a gas or liquid state. Gases behave according to the **ideal gas law** and for the most part will maintain their molecular characteristics in the liquid state, where they establish what is referred to as a partial pressure (P_{gas}). Dalton's basic gas law states that the sum of the partial pressures of the various gases is equal to the total pressure. Theoretically, this means that when the partial pressure of one gas drops, the partial pressure of another gas must equally rise, as long as the total pressure remains constant. Thus, pertaining to the partial pressures of O_2 (PO_2) and CO_2 (PCO_2) in blood, the rise in one partial pressure should be accompanied by a fall in the other. Gases diffuse down the partial pressure gradient from higher to lower pressure. The rate of diffusion of a

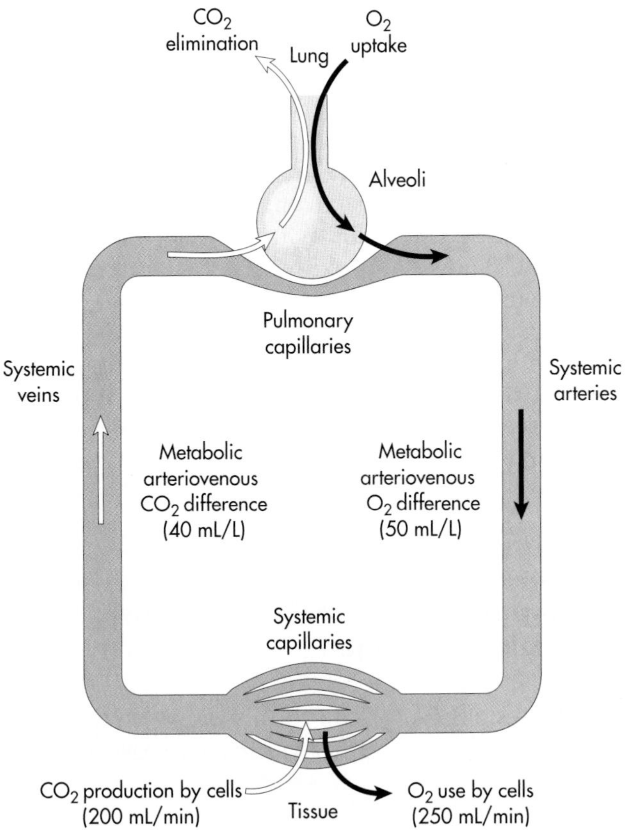

FIGURE 30–1. O_2 and CO_2 transport occurs in both arterial and venous blood. The used O_2 is present in arterial blood, where it is extracted and transferred from arterial capillaries to the tissue. Only about 25% of transported O_2 is actually taken up by the tissue. Aerobic cellular metabolism of glucose and the conversion of carbohydrates to fats are major sources of CO_2, which is transported from the cells to the systemic capillaries. The CO_2 is then transported via systemic veins and expired via diffusion from the pulmonary capillaries to the alveoli. The flow rates for O_2 and CO_2 shown are for 1 liter of blood. Their ratio is the respiratory exchange rate, R, which at rest is ≈0.80.

gas through a liquid is described by **Graham's law,** which states that the rate is directly proportional to the solubility coefficient of the gas and inversely proportional to the square root of its gram molecular weight. Calculation of the diffusion properties for O_2 and CO_2 demonstrates that CO_2 has approximately a 20 times greater rate of diffusion than O_2. **Fick's law** states that the diffusion of a gas ($\dot{V}_{gas}$) across a sheet of tissue is *directly* related to the surface area of the tissue (A), the diffusion constant of the specific gas (D), and the partial pressure difference of the gas on each side of the tissue ($P_1 - P_2$) and *inversely* related to tissue thickness (T) **(Figure 30–2).** That is:

$$\dot{V}_{gas} = \frac{A \cdot D \cdot (P_1 - P_2)}{T}$$

By a derivation of Fick's equation and with use of carbon monoxide (CO) diffusion properties (i.e., low solubility in the capillary membrane and high solubility in blood), a physiological measurement has been developed to assess diffusion abnormalities, referred to as the diffusion capacity of the lung for CO (DLCO): $\dot{V}CO = DL\ (P_1 - P_2)$.

$$DLCO = \frac{\dot{V}CO}{(P_1 - P_2)} = \frac{\dot{V}CO}{PACO}$$

The assessment of DLCO has become a classic measurement of the diffusion capabilities of the alveolar-capillary membrane. It is useful in the differential diagnosis of certain restrictive and obstructive lung diseases.

DLCO MEASUREMENT

DLCO is a classic measurement of the diffusion capabilities of the alveolar-capillary membrane. It is useful in the diagnosis of restrictive lung diseases, such as interstitial pulmonary fibrosis, and in distinguishing between chronic bronchitis and emphysema. For example, a patient with interstitial pulmonary fibrosis (a restrictive lung disease) inhales a single breath of 0.3% CO from residual volume to total lung capacity. He holds his breath for 10 seconds and then exhales. After the exhaled gas is discarded from the dead space, a representative sample of alveolar gas from late in exhalation is obtained. The average alveolar partial pressure of CO is 0.1 mm Hg, and 0.25 mL of CO has been taken up. The diffusion capacity for CO in this patient is

$$DLCO = \frac{\dot{V}CO}{PACO} = \frac{0.25\,\text{mL}/10\text{ sec} \times 60\text{ sec/min}}{0.1\text{ mm Hg}}$$
$$= 15\,\text{mL/min/mm Hg}$$

The normal range for DLCO is 20 to 30 mL/min/mm Hg. In patients with interstitial pulmonary fibrosis, there is an initial alveolar inflammatory response with subsequent scar formation (connective tissue deposition—collagen) within the interstitial space. The inflammation and scar tissue thicken the interstitial space, making it more difficult for gas diffusion to occur, thus resulting in a decreased DLCO. This is a classic characteristic of certain types of restrictive lung diseases; gas readily enters the alveolus but is inhibited in its ability to diffuse into the blood.

O_2 and CO_2 exchange in the lung are perfusion limited

Different gases have different solubility factors. Gases that are relatively insoluble in blood (e.g., anesthetic gases—nitrous oxide and ether) and do not chemically combine with blood equilibrate

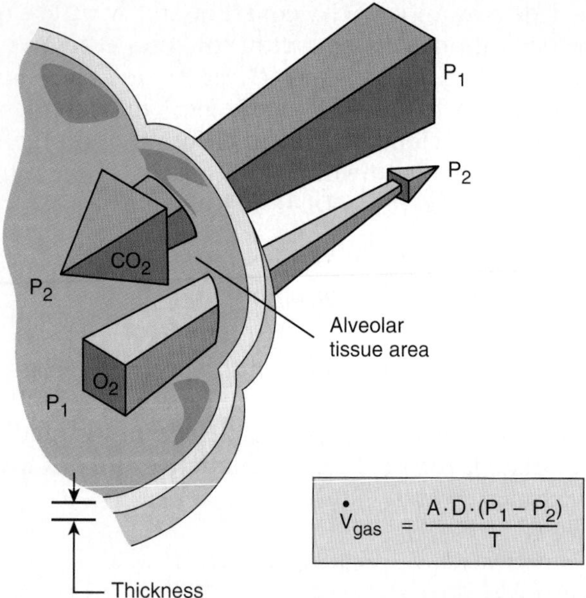

FIGURE 30–2. Fick's law states that the diffusion of a gas across a sheet of tissue is *directly* related to the surface area of the tissue, the diffusion constant of the specific gas, and the partial pressure difference of the gas on each side of the tissue and *inversely* related to tissue thickness. (From Berne RM, Levy MN, Koeppen BM, Stanton BA: *Physiology,* ed 5, Philadelphia, 2004, Elsevier.)

rapidly between alveolar gas and blood. The equilibration occurs in significantly less time than the 0.75 second the red blood cell spends in the capillary bed (capillary transit time). The exchange for these gases is considered **perfusion limited** because the partial pressure of the gas in blood leaving the capillary has reached equilibrium with alveolar gas and is thus only limited by the amount of blood perfusing the alveolus. In contrast, a **diffusion-limited** gas, such as CO, has a low solubility in the alveolar-capillary membrane but a high solubility in blood because of its high affinity for hemoglobin (Hgb). These features prevent the equilibration of CO between alveolar gas and blood during the red blood cell transit time.

The high **affinity** of CO for Hgb enables large amounts of CO to be taken up in blood with little or no appreciable increase in its partial pressure. Gases that are chemically bound to Hgb do not exert a partial pressure in blood. Exchange of CO is still occurring as the red blood cell leaves the capillary because its rate of equilibration is slow relative to the time spent in the capillary (**Figure 30–3**). LIKE CO, BOTH CO_2 AND O_2 HAVE RELATIVELY LOW SOLUBILITY IN THE ALVEOLAR-CAPILLARY MEMBRANE BUT HAVE HIGH EFFECTIVE SOLUBILITY IN BLOOD BECAUSE OF THEIR CHEMICAL BINDING TRANSPORT MECHANISMS. However, their rate of equilibration is sufficiently rapid for complete equilibration to occur during the transit time of the red blood cell within the capillary. Equilibration for O_2 and CO_2 usually occurs within 0.25 second. Thus, O_2 and CO_2 transfer is normally perfusion limited. Although CO_2 has a greater rate of diffusion than O_2 in blood, it has a lower membrane-blood solubility ratio. As a consequence, O_2 and CO_2 take approximately the same amount of time to reach equilibration in blood.

Diffusion limitation for O_2 and CO_2 could occur if the red blood cell spends less than 0.25 second in the capillary bed. On occasion, this can be seen in very fit athletes during vigorous exercise and in healthy subjects who exercise at high altitude.

Hemoglobin Is the Major Transport Molecule for Oxygen

O_2 diffuses passively from the alveolus and dissolves in the plasma while maintaining its gaseous state.

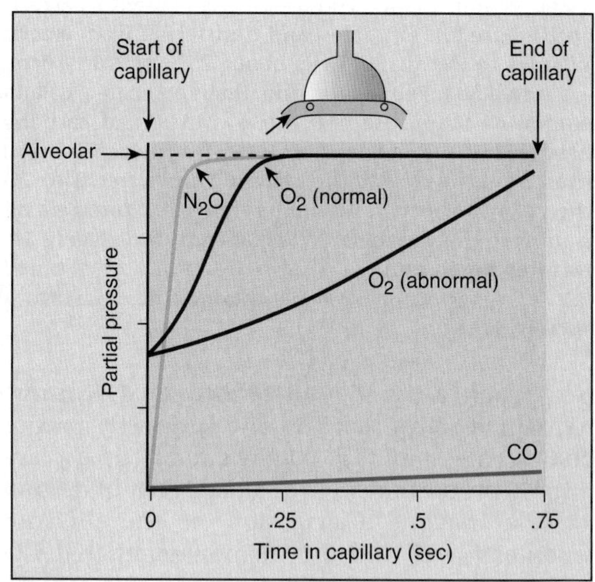

FIGURE 30–3. Uptake of nitrous oxide (N_2O), carbon monoxide (CO), and O_2 in blood relative to their partial pressures and the transit time of the red blood cell in the capillary. For gases that are perfusion limited (N_2O and O_2), their partial pressures have equilibrated with alveolar pressure before they exit the capillary. In contrast, the partial pressure of CO, a gas that is diffusion limited, does not reach equilibrium with alveolar pressure. O_2 in rare conditions can become diffusion limited. (From Berne RM, Levy MN, Koeppen BM, Stanton BA: *Physiology,* ed 5, Philadelphia, 2004, Elsevier.)

It is this form that is measured clinically in an arterial blood gas sample as the PaO_2. Only a small percentage of O_2 is carried in its dissolved form, and its contribution to the total O_2 transport under normal conditions is almost negligible, although it can become a significant factor in conditions of severe hypoxemia.

THE BINDING OF O_2 TO HGB TO FORM OXYHEMOGLOBIN WITHIN RED BLOOD CELLS IS THE PRIMARY TRANSPORT MECHANISM OF O_2. The O_2-carrying capacity of blood is enhanced about 65 times by its ability to bind to Hgb.

The Hgb molecule is a protein (66,500 MW) with two major components: four nonprotein *heme* groups, each containing iron in the reduced ferrous (Fe^{++}) form, which is the site of O_2 binding; and a *globin* portion consisting of four polypeptide chains. Adults have two α chains and two β chains (HgbA), whereas children younger than 1 year have fetal Hgb (HgbF) consisting of two α chains and two γ chains. THIS DIFFERENCE IN THE STRUCTURE OF HGBF INCREASES ITS AFFINITY FOR O_2 AND AIDS IN THE TRANSPORT OF O_2 ACROSS THE PLACENTA. In addition, as will be discussed later in this chapter, HgbF provides advantages in people with sickle cell disease and is not affected or inhibited by the glycolysis product 2,3-diphosphoglycerate in red blood cells, thus further enhancing O_2 uptake. During the first year of life, HgbF is replaced with HgbA.

The binding of O_2 to Hgb alters the light absorption properties of Hgb, which is responsible for the change in color between oxygenated arterial blood and deoxygenated venous blood. The binding and dissociation of O_2 with Hgb occur in milliseconds, which is well suited for the 0.75 second the red blood cell spends in the capillary. There are approximately 280 million Hgb molecules per red blood cell, providing a unique and efficient mechanism to transport O_2. Myoglobin, a protein similar in structure and function to Hgb, has only one subunit of the Hgb molecule. It aids in the transfer of O_2 from blood to muscle cells and in the storage of O_2, which is especially critical under O_2-deprived conditions.

Abnormalities of the Hgb molecule occur with alterations in the sequence (i.e., sickle cell disease) or spatial arrangements of the globin polypeptide chains and result in abnormal function. Compounds such as CO, nitric oxide (NO), and various cyanides (released during the burning of plastics or in the workplace in photographic darkrooms, electroplating, and mining) can oxidize the iron molecule in the heme group, changing it from the reduced ferrous state to the ferric state (Fe^{+++}), and thereby alter the ability of O_2 to bind to Hgb.

SICKLE CELL DISEASE

In an inherited homozygous condition known as **sickle cell disease,** individuals have an amino acid substitution (valine for glutamic acid) on the β chain of the Hgb molecule. This creates a sickle cell Hgb (HgbS), which when it is unbound (deoxyhemoglobin) transforms into a gelatinous material that distorts the normal biconcave shape of the red blood cell to a crescent or "sickle" form. This change in shape increases the tendency of the red blood cell to form thrombi or clots that obstruct small vessels and creates a clinical condition known as acute sickle cell episode. The symptoms of such an episode depend on the site of the obstruction (i.e., stroke, pulmonary infarction) but are commonly associated with intense pain. The spleen is a common site of infarction, and the ensuing tissue damage compromises the immune capabilities of the individual, rendering the person susceptible to recurrent infections. In the homozygous form, this is a life-shortening clinical condition; however, in the heterozygous form (sickle cell trait), individuals have a sixfold reduction in the risk for dying of malaria. The enhanced protection from malaria may be due to impaired growth of the parasite at low O_2 tensions. Thus, there is a survival advantage to the heterozygous individual in regions of the world where malaria is prevalent, which may explain why the sickle cell mutation has been preserved through evolution. The increased affinity of HgbF for O_2 renders advantages to individuals with sickle cell disease in that it has a higher binding affinity for O_2, and the cells do not desaturate as much and are less likely to sickle. Thus, during the first year of life, children are less susceptible than older children are. Sickle cell disease is most prevalent in individuals of African descent but is also observed in Hispanic and other ethnic populations.

The S shape of the oxyhemoglobin dissociation curve illustrates advantages of the binding relationship between O_2 and Hgb

The majority of O_2 in plasma quickly diffuses into red blood cells and chemically binds to the Hgb molecule to facilitate transport. This process is reversible at the tissue level, where Hgb gives up its O_2 to the tissue. The oxyhemoglobin dissociation curve illustrates the relationship between PO_2 in the blood and the number of O_2 molecules bound to Hgb **(Figure 30–4)**. The S shape of the curve demonstrates the dependence of Hgb saturation on the PO_2, especially at partial pressures below 60 mm Hg. THE CLINICAL SIGNIFICANCE OF THE FLAT PORTION OF THE OXYHEMOGLOBIN DISSOCIATION CURVE (>60 MM HG) IS THAT A DROP IN PO_2 OVER A WIDE RANGE OF PARTIAL PRESSURES (100 MM HG TO 60 MM HG) HAS ONLY A MINIMAL EFFECT ON HGB SATURATION,

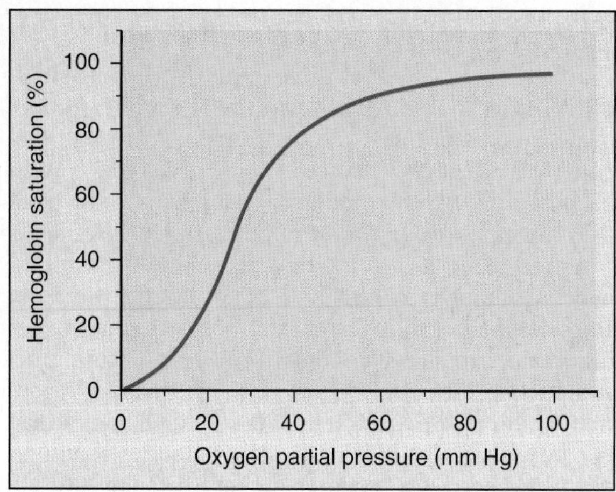

FIGURE 30–4. Oxyhemoglobin dissociation showing the relationship between the O_2 partial pressure in blood and the percentage of Hgb binding sites that are occupied by O_2 molecules (percentage saturation). Adult hemoglobin (HgbA) is about 50% saturated at a Po_2 of 27 mm Hg, 90% saturated at 60 mm Hg, and 98% saturated at 100 mm Hg. (From Berne RM, Levy MN, Koeppen BM, Stanton BA: *Physiology,* ed 5, Philadelphia, 2004, Elsevier.)

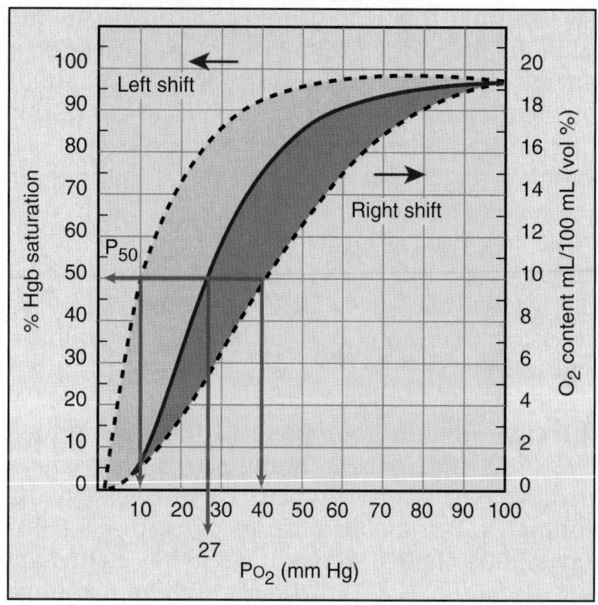

FIGURE 30–5. P_{50} represents the partial pressure at which Hgb is 50% saturated with O_2. When the O_2 dissociation curve shifts to the right, the P_{50} increases. When the curve shifts to the left, the P_{50} decreases. (From Berne RM, Levy MN, Koeppen BM, Stanton BA: *Physiology,* ed 5, Philadelphia, 2004, Elsevier.)

WHICH REMAINS AT 90%, A LEVEL SUFFICIENT FOR NORMAL O_2 TRANSPORT AND DELIVERY. The clinical significance of the steep portion (<60 mm Hg) of the curve is that a large amount of O_2 is released from Hgb with only a small change in Po_2, which facilitates the release and diffusion of O_2 to the tissue. The point on the curve where 50% of the Hgb is saturated with O_2 is called the P_{50} and is 27 mm Hg in normal adults **(Figure 30–5)**.

Physiological factors can shift the oxyhemoglobin dissociation curve

The oxyhemoglobin dissociation curve can be shifted in numerous clinical conditions to either the right or left **(Figure 30–6)**. The curve is shifted to the right when the affinity of Hgb for O_2 decreases, which enhances O_2 dissociation. This results in decreased Hgb binding to O_2 at a given Po_2, thus increasing the P_{50}. When the affinity of Hgb for O_2 increases, the curve is shifted to the left, thereby reducing the P_{50}. In this state, O_2 dissociation and delivery to tissue are inhibited.

Shifts to the right or left of the dissociation curve have little effect when they occur at O_2

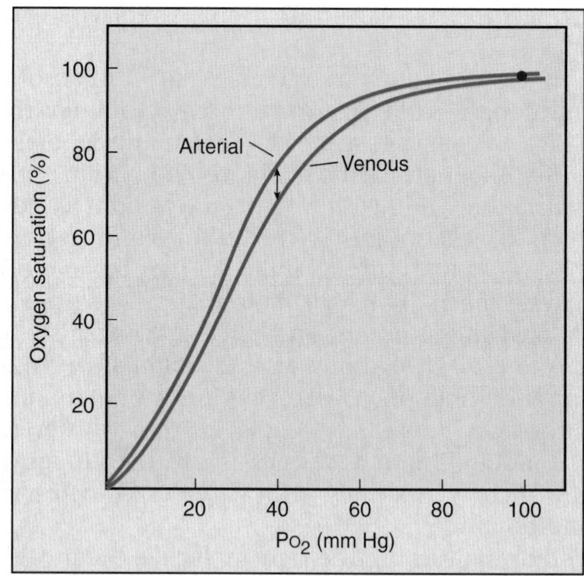

FIGURE 30–6. Normal arterial and venous $HgbO_2$ equilibrium curves. In the lung, the effect of the shift to the left caused by decreased [H^+] enhances O_2 uptake. In the systemic capillaries, significant O_2 unloading begins at about Po_2 = 70 mm Hg. The rising [H^+] caused by the entry of CO_2 shifts the curve to the right, enhancing O_2 dissociation. The P_{50} of the arterial curve is 26 mm Hg; the P_{50} of the venous curve is 29 mm Hg. (From Berne RM, Levy MN, Koeppen BM, Stanton BA: *Physiology,* ed 5, Philadelphia, 2004, Elsevier.)

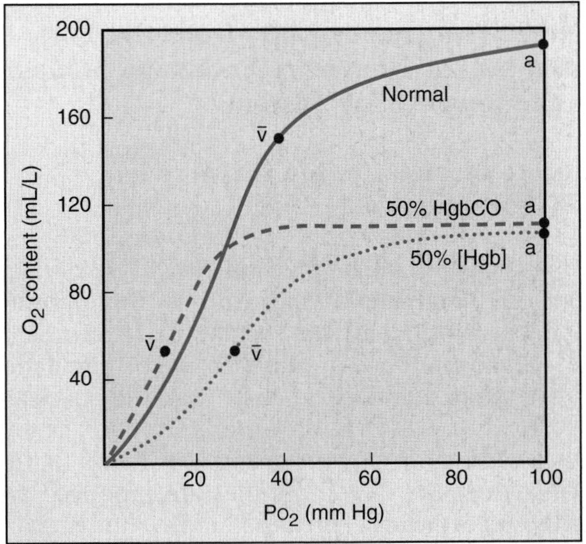

FIGURE 30–7. Comparison of O_2 content curves under three conditions shows why carboxyhemoglobin (HgbCO) is so toxic to the O_2 transport system. The 50% [Hgb] represents a reduction in circulating hemoglobin by half; 50% HgbCO represents binding of half the circulating hemoglobin with CO. The 50% [Hgb] and 50% HgbCO curves show the same decreased O_2 content in arterial blood. However, CO has a profound effect in lowering venous Po_2. The arterial (a) and mixed venous ($\bar{v}$) points of constant cardiac output are indicated. (From Berne RM, Levy MN, Koeppen BM, Stanton BA: *Physiology,* ed 5, Philadelphia, 2004, Elsevier.)

partial pressures within the normal range (80 to 100 mm Hg). However, at O_2 partial pressures below 60 mm Hg (steep part of the curve), shifts in the oxyhemoglobin dissociation curve can dramatically influence O_2 transport. Changes in blood pH will shift the oxyhemoglobin dissociation curve. CO_2 production and release into the blood result in the generation of increased H^+ ions and a decrease in pH. This shifts the dissociation curve to the right, which has a beneficial effect by aiding in the release of O_2 from Hgb for diffusion into the tissue. The shift to the right is due to the decrease in pH and to a direct effect of CO_2 on Hgb. This effect of CO_2 on the affinity of Hgb for O_2 is known as the **Bohr effect** and is due in part both to the change in pH that occurs as CO_2 increases and to the direct effect of CO_2 on Hgb. The Bohr effect enhances O_2 uptake in the lungs and O_2 delivery to the tissue **(Figure 30–7)**. Conversely, as blood passes through the lungs, CO_2 is exhaled, resulting in a decrease in H^+ and an increase in pH, which results in enhanced O_2 binding to Hgb in the lung and a shift to the left in the dissociation curve.

Changes in the levels of a metabolite of red blood cell glycolysis, 2,3-diphosphoglycerate (2,3-DPG), can also shift the oxyhemoglobin dissociation curve. The affinity of 2,3-DPG for Hgb is greater than that of O_2, and thus it directly competes with O_2 for Hgb sites. Conditions such as hypoxia, decreased Hgb concentration, and increased pH cause an elevation in 2,3-DPG levels, which results in a shift to the right in the dissociation curve. Stored blood samples have decreased levels of 2,3-DPG, resulting in a shift to the left in the dissociation curve, and thus have difficulty in unloading the O_2 to tissue.

Blood Hgb content, O_2 saturation, and cardiac output influence O_2 delivery to tissue

Each Hgb molecule can bind up to four O_2 atoms, and each gram of Hgb can bind up to 1.34 mL of O_2. The term O_2 saturation (So_2) refers to the amount of O_2 bound to Hgb relative to the maximal amount of O_2 (100% O_2 capacity) that can bind Hgb. At 100% O_2 capacity, the heme groups of the Hgb molecules are fully saturated with O_2, and at 75% So_2, three of the four heme groups are occupied. The binding of O_2 to each heme group increases the affinity of the Hgb molecule to bind additional O_2. The O_2 content in blood is the sum of the O_2 bound to Hgb and the dissolved O_2. The O_2 content is decreased in the presence of increased CO_2 and CO and in individuals with anemia. So_2 is reduced by the inhalation of environmental air pollutants and is also reduced in infants who sleep facedown (i.e., rebreathing expired breath), which may increase their risk for sudden infant death syndrome.

O_2 DELIVERY FROM THE LUNGS TO THE TISSUES IS DEPENDENT ON SEVERAL FACTORS, INCLUDING CARDIAC OUTPUT, THE HGB CONTENT OF BLOOD, AND THE ABILITY OF THE LUNG TO OXYGENATE THE BLOOD. Not all of the O_2 carried in the blood is unloaded at the tissue level. The actual O_2 extracted from the blood by the tissue is the difference between the arterial O_2 content and the venous O_2 content times the cardiac output. Under normal conditions, Hgb leaves the lung 75% saturated with O_2. Only about 25% of this O_2 is used by tissue. Hypothermia, relaxation of skeletal muscles, and an increase in cardiac output reduce the O_2 consumption. Conversely, a decrease in the cardiac output, anemia, hyperthermia, and exercise increase O_2 consumption.

METHEMOGLOBIN

Gases that have a higher affinity for Hgb than O_2, such as CO (≈200 times greater) and NO (≈200,000 times greater), dramatically affect O_2 uptake and tissue delivery with life-threatening clinical consequences. They bind to Hgb at the same site as O_2 does, thus preventing O_2 uptake. In addition, their binding enhances the affinity of O_2 to Hgb, thus inhibiting the release and delivery of O_2 at the tissue site. Hgb bound to these types of compounds is referred to as **methemoglobin,** and under normal conditions, about 1% to 2% of Hgb is in this state. CO is an odorless and colorless gas that is difficult to detect and can be emitted from cigarette smoke, fires, automobile exhaust, and faulty furnaces. In smokers and in individuals living in high-density traffic areas, methemoglobin levels can reach 10%. Levels above 5% to 7% are considered hazardous. NO, an endogenous hormone synthesized by endothelial cells, has vasodilatation properties and is used clinically in the treatment of pulmonary hypertension. These compounds bind to Hgb rapidly and are extremely difficult to dissociate from Hgb. Clinical strategies to treat exposure to CO or NO involve dissociating the compound from Hgb by administering high concentrations of inhaled O_2 and increasing the barometric pressure by placing the subject in a barometric chamber.

Insufficient O_2 delivery results in tissue hypoxia

TISSUE HYPOXIA REFERS TO A CONDITION IN WHICH THERE IS INSUFFICIENT O_2 AVAILABLE TO THE CELLS TO MAINTAIN ADEQUATE AEROBIC METABOLISM FOR NORMAL CELLULAR ACTIVITIES. Anaerobic metabolism is then stimulated, resulting in the generation of increased levels of lactate and H^+ and the subsequent formation of lactic acid. The net result can lead to a significant decrease in the blood pH. There are four major types of tissue hypoxia that can occur via different mechanisms, the most common of which is **hypoxic hypoxia (Table 30–1).** In cases of severe hypoxia, the extremities, toes, and fingertips may appear blue-gray (cyanotic) because of lack of O_2 and increased deoxyhemoglobin.

Proper Transport of CO_2 from the Body Provides the Necessary Exchange of Gases in the Respiratory System

Glucose metabolism is a major source of CO_2 production

CO_2 is a major factor in regulating H^+ concentrations in blood and tissues and is an important chemical stimulus in the regulation of respiration via chemoreceptors in the peripheral circulation and central nervous system. AEROBIC CELLULAR METABOLISM OF GLUCOSE AND THE CONVERSION OF CARBOHYDRATES TO FATS ARE THE MAJOR SOURCES OF CO_2 PRODUCTION. Six CO_2 molecules are produced and six O_2 molecules are consumed during the metabolism of one glucose molecule. CO_2 is produced at a rate of about 200 mL/min under normal conditions, and 80 molecules of CO_2 will typically be expired via the lung for every 100 molecules of O_2 entering the capillary bed. The ratio of expired CO_2 to O_2 uptake is referred to as the **respiratory exchange ratio** and, under normal conditions, is 0.8 (80 CO_2 to 100 O_2). This ratio is similar at the tissue to blood compartment, where it is referred to as the **respiratory quotient**.

The body has enhanced storage capabilities for CO_2 compared with O_2, and hence Pa_{O_2} is much more affected by changes in ventilation than is Pa_{CO_2}. Whereas Pa_{O_2} is dependent on several factors in addition to alveolar ventilation, Pa_{CO_2} is solely dependent on alveolar ventilation and CO_2 production. There is an inverse relationship between alveolar ventilation and Pa_{CO_2}.

HCO_3^- is the major transport mechanism of CO_2 in blood

The predominant transport mechanism of CO_2 is via HCO_3^- within red blood cells **(Figure 30–8)**, although it is also transported as dissolved CO_2

TABLE 30-1. TISSUE HYPOXIA

Type of Hypoxia	Cause	Pa_{O_2}	Ca_{O_2}	Amount O_2 Delivered	Amount O_2 Used
Hypoxic	Pulmonary disease with: ↓ Pa_{O_2} ↓ $\dot{V}/\dot{Q}$ ratio	Low	Low	Low	Normal
Circulatory	Vascular disease Arterial-venous shunt	Normal	Normal	Low	Normal
Anemic	CO poisoning Anemia	Normal	Low	Normal	Normal
Histotoxic	Cyanide poisoning Sodium azide	Normal	Normal	Normal	Low

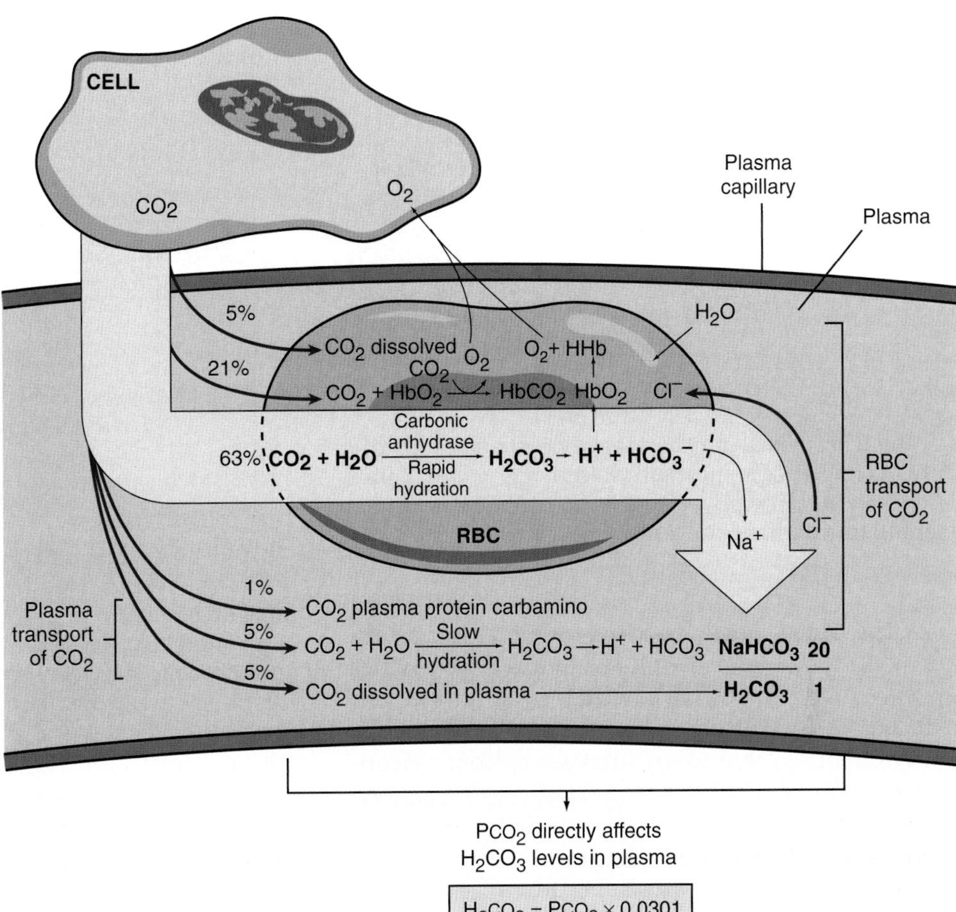

FIGURE 30–8. Mechanisms of CO_2 transport. The predominant mechanism by which CO_2 is transported from tissue cells to lung is in the form of HCO_3^-. (From Berne RM, Levy MN, Koeppen BM, Stanton BA: *Physiology,* ed 5, Philadelphia, 2004, Elsevier.)

and carbamino protein complexes (i.e., CO_2 binds to plasma proteins and to Hgb). Once CO_2 diffuses through the tissue and reaches the plasma, it quickly dissolves and establishes a partial pressure (PCO_2). THE REACTION OF CO_2 WITH H_2O TO FORM CARBONIC ACID (H_2CO_3) PROVIDES THE MAJOR PATHWAY FOR THE GENERATION OF HCO_3^-.

$$CO_2 + H_2O \longleftrightarrow H_2CO_3 \longleftrightarrow H^+ + HCO_3^-$$

This reaction normally proceeds slowly; however, it is catalyzed within red blood cells by the enzyme carbonic anhydrase. The HCO_3^- diffuses out of the red blood cell in exchange for Cl^-, the **chloride shift,** which helps the cell maintain its electrostatic homeostasis and osmotic equilibrium.

The CO_2 to HCO_3^- pathway is reversible; it can be shifted to the right to generate more HCO_3^- in response to CO_2 entering the blood from the tissue or shifted to the left as CO_2 is exhaled in the lungs. The free H^+ ions are quickly buffered within the red blood cell by binding to Hgb. The H^+ ion buffering is critical to keep the reaction moving toward the synthesis of HCO_3^-; high levels of free H^+ will push the reaction back in the opposite direction.

The CO_2 to HCO_3^- pathway plays a critical role in the regulation of H^+ ions and in maintaining the acid-base balance in the body

H^+ ion concentrations have a dramatic effect on many metabolic processes within cells, and their regulation is essential for normal homeostasis. The blood pH value is measured to assess H^+ concentrations. The normal pH range for adults is narrow at 7.35 to 7.45 and must be maintained through various buffer systems throughout the body (i.e., blood, tissue, respiratory, and renal). In the respiratory system, the CO_2 to HCO_3^- pathway provides a major mechanism to buffer and help regulate H^+.

$$\begin{array}{l} CO_2 + H_2O \longleftrightarrow \\ \quad H_2CO_3 \longleftrightarrow H^+ + HCO_3^- \\ \qquad\qquad\qquad \updownarrow \\ \qquad\qquad\qquad H^+ + Hgb \longleftrightarrow H \cdot Hgb \end{array}$$

HENDERSON-HASSELBALCH EQUATION

The Henderson-Hasselbalch equation illustrates the influence of HCO_3^- and H_2CO_3 on blood pH.

For example, under normal conditions, pK = 6.1 derived from a dissociation constant, HCO_3^- = 24 mEq/L, and H_2CO_3 = 1.2 mEq/L. Thus, according to the Henderson-Hasselbalch equation:

$$pH = pK + \log\frac{[HCO_3^-]}{[H_2CO_3]} = 6.1 + \log\frac{24\,mEq/L}{1.2\,mEq/L}$$

$$= 6.1 + \log\frac{20}{1} = 6.1 + 1.3 = 7.4$$

The dependence of pH on the concentration ratio of HCO_3^- and H_2CO_3 is apparent, which under normal conditions is 20:1. The pH will increase or decrease in direct correlation to a rise or fall in the concentration ratio.

As the P_{ACO_2} levels increase or decrease, so do the blood HCO_3^- and H_2CO_3 levels and Pa_{CO_2}. Acute hyperventilation, from exercise or anxiety, can reduce P_{ACO_2}, resulting in an increase in pH (respiratory alkalosis) due to an increase in the concentration ratio of HCO_3^- versus H_2CO_3. Conversely, if P_{ACO_2} is increased by hypoventilation from an overdose of a respiratory depressant, the pH will decrease (respiratory acidosis) because of a decrease in the concentration ratio of HCO_3^- versus H_2CO_3. Acid-base imbalances can also occur from other metabolic problems, such as metabolic acidosis (lactic acidosis, ketoacidosis, renal failure) and metabolic alkalosis (e.g., hypokalemia, hypochloremia, vomiting, high doses of steroids) and are discussed in more detail in the chapters on the renal system.

The CO_2 dissociation curve is linear

In contrast to O_2, the dissociation curve for CO_2 in blood is linear and almost directly related to the P_{CO_2} (**Figure 30–9**). The degree of Hgb saturation with O_2 has a major effect on the CO_2 dissociation curve. Although O_2 and CO_2 bind to Hgb at different sites, deoxygenated Hgb has a greater affinity for CO_2 than oxygenated Hgb. Thus, deoxygenated blood (venous blood) freely takes up and transports more CO_2 than oxygenated arterial blood does. The deoxygenated Hgb more readily forms carbamino compounds and also more readily binds free H^+ ions released during the formation of HCO_3^-. THE EFFECT OF CHANGES IN OXYHEMOGLOBIN SATURATION ON THE RELATIONSHIP OF THE CO_2 CONTENT TO P_{CO_2} IS REFERRED TO AS THE **HALDANE** EFFECT AND IS REVERSED IN THE LUNG WHEN O_2 IS TRANSPORTED FROM THE ALVEOLI TO THE RED BLOOD CELLS. This effect is illustrated by a shift to the left in the CO_2 dissociation curve in venous blood compared with arterial blood.

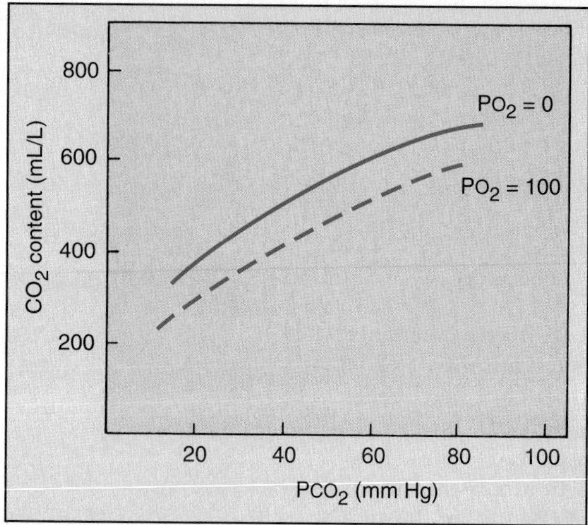

FIGURE 30–9. Blood CO_2 equilibrium curves (arterial and venous). Venous blood can transport more CO_2 than arterial blood can at any given P_{CO_2}. Compared with the $HgbO_2$ equilibrium curve, the CO_2 curves are essentially straight lines between P_{CO_2} of 20 and 80 mm Hg. (From Berne RM, Levy MN, Koeppen BM, Stanton BA: *Physiology,* ed 5, Philadelphia, 2004, Elsevier.)

Summary

- The diffusion and transport of O_2 and CO_2 are determined by basic gas diffusion laws and depend primarily on pressure gradients.
- Gases (nitrous oxide, ether, helium) that have a rapid rate of air to blood equilibration are perfusion limited, and gases (e.g., CO) that have a slow air to blood equilibration rate are diffusion limited. Under normal conditions, O_2 transport is perfusion limited, but it can be diffusion limited in certain conditions.

- DLCO is a classic measurement of the diffusion capabilities of the alveolar-capillary membrane. It is useful in the diagnosis of restrictive lung diseases, such as interstitial pulmonary fibrosis, and in distinguishing between chronic bronchitis and emphysema.
- The major transport mechanism of O_2 in the blood is within the red blood cell bound to Hgb; for CO_2, it is within red blood cells in the form of HCO_3^-.
- Tissue hypoxia occurs when insufficient amounts of O_2 are supplied to the tissue to carry out normal levels of aerobic metabolism.
- The reversible reaction of CO_2 with H_2O to form H_2CO_3 with its subsequent dissociation to HCO_3^- and H^+ is catalyzed by the enzyme carbonic anhydrase within red blood cells and is the major pathway for HCO_3^- generation.
- The CO_2 dissociation curve from blood is linear and directly related to PCO_2. The PCO_2 is solely dependent on alveolar ventilation and CO_2 production.
- The O_2 dissociation curve is S shaped, not linear. In the plateau area (between 60 and 100 mm Hg), increasing or decreasing the PO_2 has only a minimal effect on Hgb saturation. This ensures adequate Hgb saturation over a large range of PO_2.
- The CO_2 to HCO_3^- pathway plays a critical role in the regulation of H^+ ions and in maintaining the acid-base balance in the body.

Bibliography

Benesch R, Benesch RE: Intracellular organic phosphates as regulators of oxygen release by hemoglobin, *Nature* 221:618, 1969.

DeMeo DL et al: Ambient air pollution and oxygen saturation, *Am J Respir Crit Care Med* 170:383, 2004.

Greenough A: Sickle cell disease—pulmonary complications and a proinflammatory state? *Am J Respir Crit Care Med* 169:663, 2004.

Patel AL et al: Occurrence and mechanisms of sudden oxygen desaturation in infants who sleep face down, *Pediatrics* 111:328, 2003.

Perrella M, Bresciani D, Rossi-Bernardi L: The binding of CO_2 to human hemoglobin, *J Biol Chem* 250:5413, 1975.

Perutz MF et al: Identification of residues responsible for the alkaline Bohr effect in hemoglobin, *Nature* 222:1240, 1969.

Roughton FJ: Average time spent by blood in human lung capillaries and its relation to the rates of CO uptake and elimination in man, *Am J Physiol* 143:621, 1945.

Russell JA, Phang PT: The oxygen delivery-consumption controversy, *Am J Respir Crit Care Med* 149:433, 1994.

West JB: Effect of slope and shape of dissociation curve on pulmonary gas exchange, *Respir Physiol* 8:66, 1969.

Case Studies

Case 30–1

On a cold winter morning, your neighbor and her son come over to pick up your children to give them a ride to school. No one answers the door, and all she hears is the old noisy furnace running. She becomes worried and enters your house to find that no one is awake except your teenage son, who is barely conscious, confused, and disoriented. She tries to wake you and your husband with no success, and she notices that you are breathing rapidly. She calls 911 and opens all the windows. Later, on inspection, it was revealed that the furnace was faulty and carbon monoxide was being emitted.

1. **How does carbon monoxide affect the interactions of O_2 to Hgb?**
   A. Prevents binding, increases affinity, inhibits release, shifts dissociation curve to the left
   B. Prevents binding, increases affinity, inhibits release, shifts dissociation curve to the right
   C. Prevents binding, decreases affinity, enhances release, shifts dissociation curve to the left

D. Enhances binding, decreases affinity, enhances release, shifts dissociation curve to the right
E. Enhances binding, increases affinity, inhibits release, shifts dissociation curve to the left

2. **What would you predict the subjects' blood pressure, heart rate, and respiratory rate to be?**
A. Decreased blood pressure, increased heart rate, increased respiratory rate
B. Increased blood pressure, increased heart rate, increased respiratory rate
C. Decreased blood pressure, decreased heart rate, increased respiratory rate
D. Decreased blood pressure, decreased heart rate, decreased respiratory rate
E. Increased blood pressure, increased heart rate, decreased respiratory rate

Case 30–2

A 10-month old African-American infant is brought into the emergency department with a history of crankiness, crying a lot, and at times shortness of breath. The parents state that she has not been eating well and seems to have lost energy. This pattern of behavior has been getting worse during the last few weeks, and they think she has developed a fever again. About 6 weeks ago, the infant had a severe cold and fever. On your examination, she appears somewhat pale, especially in the palms and lips; her fingers and toes are swollen (hand-foot syndrome), and she seems to be sensitive to touch in these areas. At first the parents thought she may have had a cold or the flu, so they did not bring her to the hospital sooner and just treated her at home. There are many considerations for a diagnosis, but on questioning the parents, you find out that one of the parents has sickle cell trait (heterozygous for the sickle cell gene). The other parent has not been tested. You do genetic testing and determine that the other parent also has sickle cell trait and that the infant is homozygous for HgbS and has sickle cell disease.

1. **What types of hemoglobin would you expect to find in her blood?**
A. HgbF only
B. HgbF and HgbA
C. HgbA only
D. HgbF and HgbS
E. HgbS only

2. **What is the underlying cause of the infant's recurrent infections?**
A. Immunosuppression due to liver disease
B. Immunosuppression due to spleen damage
C. Immunosuppression due to lack of thymus development
D. Immunosuppression due to kidney disease
E. Undernourishment

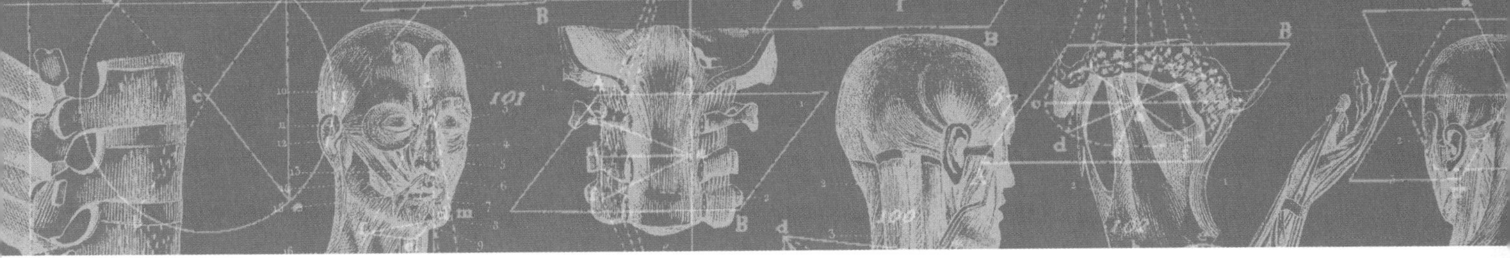

Chapter 31: Control of Respiration

Objectives

- ❖ Describe the central organization of breathing.
- ❖ Explain the role of central and peripheral chemoreceptors and pulmonary mechanoreceptors in regulating respiration.
- ❖ Describe ventilatory control during special circumstances (e.g., exercise and high altitude).
- ❖ Describe the effects of abnormalities in ventilatory control.

We breathe to maintain normal levels of O_2 and CO_2 in the blood in a pattern that minimizes work. Respiration demonstrates both automaticity and self-modulation (voluntary). We really cannot "hold our breath until we turn blue," but we can hold our breath up to the so-called breaking point. Control of ventilation refers to the generation and regulation of rhythmic breathing by the respiratory center in the brainstem and its modification by the input of information from higher brain centers and from systemic receptors (see Figure 27–6). This chapter discusses the neural and chemical controls of respiration that are fundamental to life and the four major sites of ventilatory control: the respiratory control center, the central chemoreceptors, the peripheral chemoreceptors, and the pulmonary mechanoreceptors.

CO_2 Is the Most Important Regulator of Ventilation

Ventilation is regulated by the levels of CO_2, O_2, and pH in the arterial blood, with CO_2 levels being the most important. Both the rate and depth of breathing are controlled to maintain the Pa_{CO_2} close to 40 mm Hg even during times of stress, such as exercise. Central and peripheral chemoreceptors respond to changes in arterial CO_2.

The slope of the relationship between minute ventilation and inspired CO_2 is a test of CO_2 sensitivity and is called the **ventilatory response to CO_2 (Figure 31–1).** THE VENTILATORY RESPONSE TO CO_2 IS MODIFIED BY THE STATE OF WAKEFULNESS, BY ARTERIAL OXYGENATION, AND BY THE ACID-BASE STATUS OF THE BODY. The effects of CO_2 are greater when the individual is awake because of the greater activity in the reticular formation. The ventilatory response to CO_2 is also enhanced by hypoxia **(Figure 31–2)** and by $[H^+]$ **(Figure 31–3).** In a metabolic acidosis, the sensitivity to CO_2 is increased.

Narcotics such as benzodiazepines and alcohol depress respiration by shifting the CO_2–ventilation response curve to the right and by reducing the slope (Figure 31–1). This results in an elevated Pa_{CO_2} and a reduced Pa_{O_2}. However, the Aa gradient (difference between alveolar and arterial O_2) remains normal, as the cause of the hypoxemia is **hypoventilation** (underventilation).

Respiration is controlled primarily by the brainstem

The respiratory control center is located in the reticular formation of the medulla oblongata beneath the floor of the fourth ventricle **(Figure 31–4).** Much of what we know about ventilatory control mechanisms comes from transection and ablation

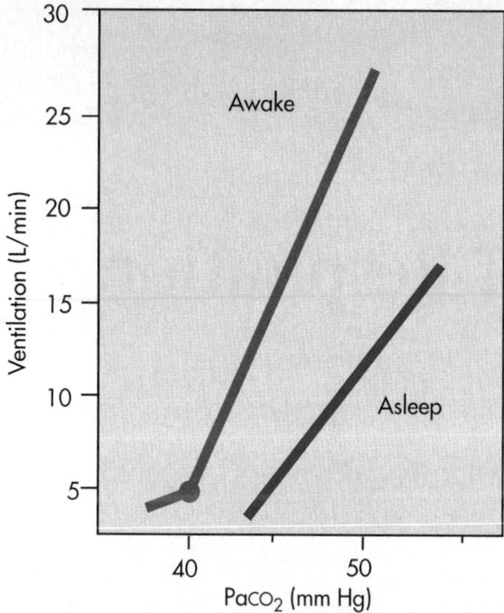

FIGURE 31–1. CO_2–ventilation response curve. Ventilation is sensitive to $Paco_2$, as shown by the red line (awake). In this example from an adult, the normal operating point is 5 L/min at 40 mm Hg *(large dot).* In the awake (alert) state, ventilation becomes insensitive to a decrease in CO_2 below 40 mm Hg. When the reticular activating system is turned off, as during sleep *(blue line),* the CO_2 intercept is increased (shifted to the right), and the slope is decreased (decreased sensitivity).

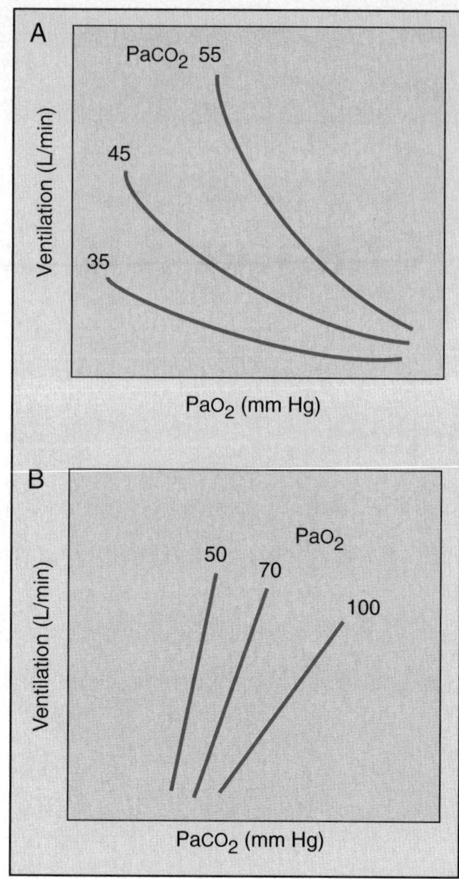

FIGURE 31–2. The effects of hypoxia (A) and hypercapnia (B) on ventilation as the other respiratory gas partial pressure is varied. A, At a given $Paco_2$, ventilation increases as Pao_2 decreases. When the $Paco_2$ decreases during hypoxia, ventilation decreases at lower levels of Pao_2. The hypoxia response is mediated through the carotid body chemoreceptors. B, The sensitivity of the ventilatory response to CO_2 is enhanced by hypoxia. (From Berne RM, Levy MN, Koeppen BM, Stanton BA: *Physiology,* ed 5, Philadelphia, 2004, Elsevier.)

experiments in anesthetized animals (**Figures 31–5 and 31–6**). If the brainstem of an anesthetized animal is transected above the medulla, inspiration and exhalation are unchanged, even if all other afferents to the area including the vagus nerves are severed. If the brainstem is transected below this area, breathing ceases. Within the intervening area, there are two dense, bilateral aggregations of respiratory neurons that are involved in respiratory pattern generation. The first group is the **dorsal respiratory group** (DRG), which is composed of cells in the nucleus tractus solitarius located in the dorsomedial region of the medulla. They consist primarily of inspiratory neurons and project to the contralateral spinal cord, where they serve as the principal initiators of the activity of the phrenic nerves.

The second group of cells is the **ventral respiratory group** (VRG), which is located bilaterally in the ventrolateral region of the medulla and is composed of three cell groups (the rostral nucleus retrofacialis, the caudal nucleus retroambiguus, and the nucleus ambiguus). The VRG contains both inspiratory and expiratory neurons. The neurons in the nucleus ambiguus are both inspiratory and expiratory and contain vagal motor neurons that innervate the laryngeal and pharyngeal muscles. The nucleus retroambiguus contains inspiratory and expiratory neurons; the expiratory neurons drive the contralateral internal intercostal and abdominal muscles, and the inspiratory neurons supply the external intercostals as well as another group of neurons that project within the medulla only. Cells in the nucleus retrofacialis are the only cells in the VRG that have been shown to inhibit inspiratory cells in the DRG.

The apneustic center is located in the pons

If the brainstem is transected in the pons at the level of the pontine respiratory group or pneumotaxic center (level 2), a breathing pattern called **apneusis** results if the vagus nerves are also transected. Apneustic breathing consists of prolonged inspiratory efforts interrupted by occasional exhalations. Apneusis is probably caused by a sustained discharge of medullary inspiratory neurons, which

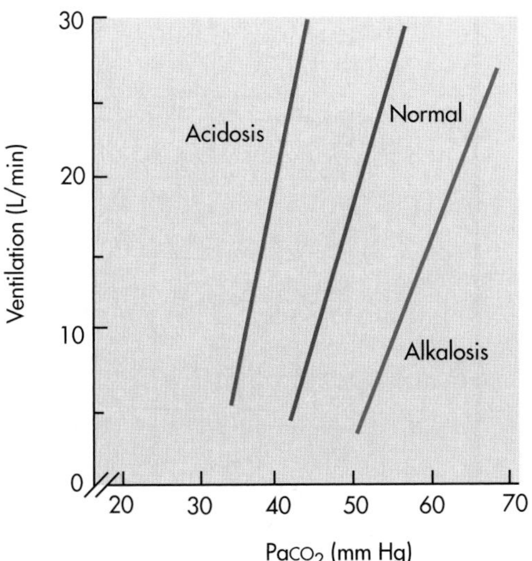

FIGURE 31–3. Effect of [H+] on ventilatory response to CO_2. In chronic metabolic acidosis, the ventilatory sensitivity to CO_2 increases, resulting in greater levels of ventilation than in normal or alkalotic states. (Data from Fencl V et al: *J Appl Physiol* 27:67, 1969.)

may be the site of afferent information that terminates inspiration. Apneusis results when this inspiratory cutoff mechanism is inactivated.

Apneustic breathing can be seen after head trauma that damages the pons. These patients breathe with inspiratory breathholds that last many seconds followed by brief exhalations. The finding of such a breathing pattern helps localize the site of injury.

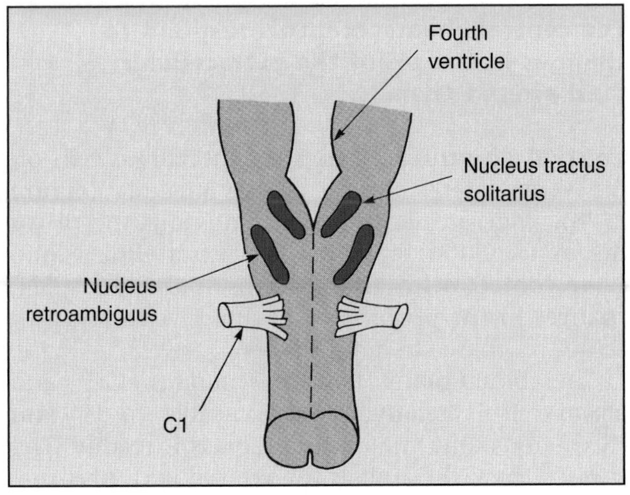

FIGURE 31–4. The respiratory control center is located in the medulla (the most primitive portion of the brain). The neurons are mainly in two areas called the nucleus tractus solitarius and the nucleus retroambiguus. C1, first cervical nerve. (From Berne RM, Levy MN, Koeppen BM, Stanton BA: *Physiology*, ed 5, Philadelphia, 2004, Elsevier.)

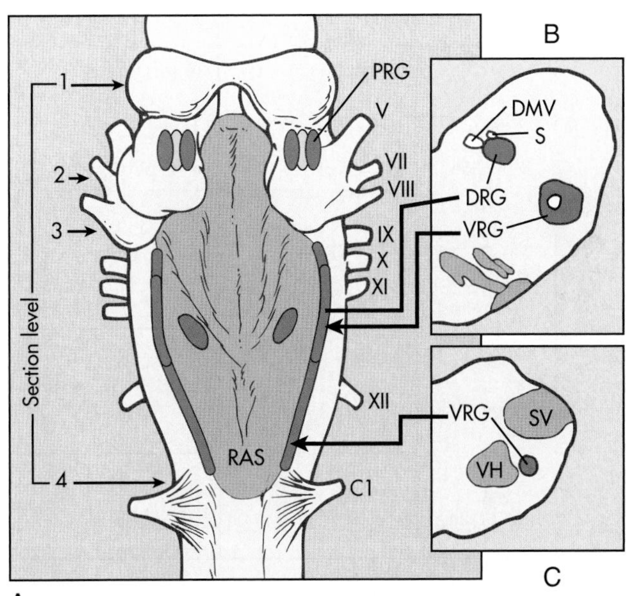

FIGURE 31–5. Dorsal view of the brainstem (**A**) and cross sections at the midmedulla and caudal medulla (**B** and **C**, respectively) illustrating locations of the dorsal (DRG), ventral (VRG), and pontine (PRG) respiratory neuron groups (the metabolic controllers of breathing). The colors roughly indicate the locations of neurons that fire during inspiration *(red)*, expiration *(blue)*, or both *(yellow)*. The reticular activating system (RAS) surrounds and interdigitates with the various neuronal groups. The roman numerals (right side of A) show the corresponding cranial nerves, some of which have both sensory and motor divisions. The arabic numerals (left side of A) show the classic levels of brainstem transections (1 to 4), which helped early physiologists to localize the respiratory neuron groups. Breathing patterns caused by successive ablations from rostral to caudal are shown in Figure 31–6. C1, first cervical nerve; DMV, dorsal motor nucleus of the vagus; S, nucleus of the tractus solitarius; SV, spinal trigeminal nucleus; VH, ventral horn.

Rhythmic breathing requires tonic inspiratory drive and phasic expiratory output

Inspiration begins with an abrupt increase in discharge from the inspiratory neurons. This leads to progressive contraction of the respiratory muscles during automatic breathing. At the end of inspiration, there is an off-switch event that results in a marked decrease in neuron firing, at which point exhalation begins. Inspiration neuron firing decreases and becomes absent during phase II of exhalation.

Thus, rhythmic breathing depends on a continuous (tonic) inspiratory drive from the DRG and on intermittent (phasic) expiratory inputs from the cerebrum, thalamus, cranial nerves, and ascending spinal cord sensory tracts **(Figure 31–7)**.

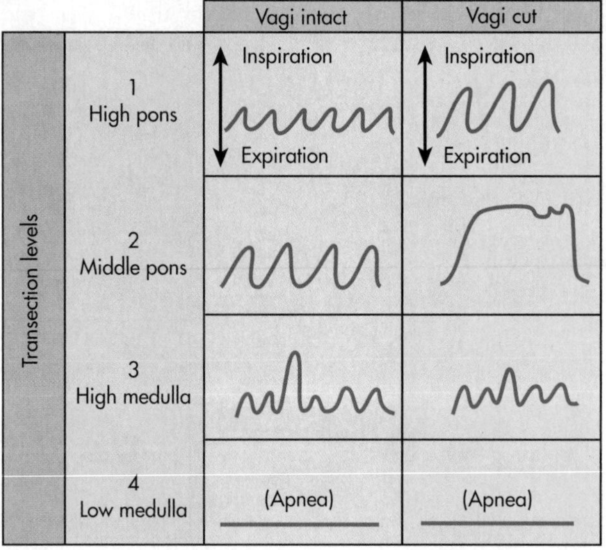

FIGURE 31–6. Different patterns of breathing produced by successive transections of the brainstem in anesthetized animals. These patterns may also occur in humans with selected brainstem lesions. The four levels of transection correspond to the numbers in Figure 31–5, *A*. The importance of the sensory division of the vagus nerve, carrying information about the state of lung inflation, is shown by contrasting the intact to the cut columns. For transection level 1, there is no effect on the basic breathing pattern, showing that the main controller lies caudal. Furthermore, it eliminates all volitional (conscious) changes in breathing (not shown here). When vagal sensory input is eliminated, breathing slows, and tidal volume increases. Skipping down to transection level 4, breathing stops completely, showing that the main controller lies rostral. For transection level 2, as long as sensory input from the vagus nerve continues, ablation of the pontine respiratory group has only a moderate slowing effect on breathing, with tidal volume increased to maintain alveolar ventilation at approximately normal. After vagotomy, apneustic breathing (deep inspiration held for many seconds) appears. For transection level 3, irregular, gasping breathing develops, which is not affected by cutting the vagus nerves. Clearly, medullary controllers are sufficient to sustain life but are not adequate for providing normal modulation of breathing.

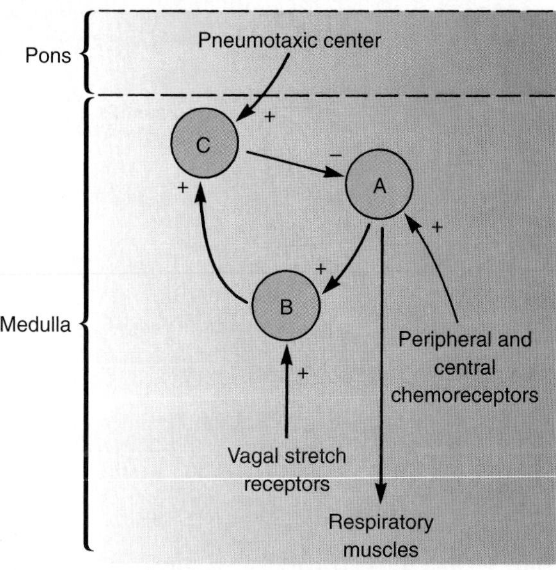

FIGURE 31–7. The basic wiring diagram of the brainstem ventilatory controller. The signs of the main outputs *(arrows)* of the neuron pools indicate whether the outputs are excitatory (+) or inhibitory (–). Pool A provides tonic inspiratory stimuli to the muscles of breathing. Pool B is stimulated by pool A and provides additional stimulation to the muscles of breathing, and pool B stimulates pool C. Other brain centers feed pool C (inspiratory cutoff switch), which sends inhibitory impulses to pool A. Afferent information (feedback) from various sensors acts at different locations: chemoreceptors act on pool A, and intrapulmonary sensory fibers act via the vagus nerves on pool B. A pneumotaxic center in the anterior pons receives input from the cerebral cortex, and it modulates the pool C group. (From Berne RM, Levy MN, Koeppen BM, Stanton BA: *Physiology,* ed 5, Philadelphia, 2004, Elsevier.)

Young infants are capable of breathing and swallowing simultaneously. The large epiglottis of the newborn is capable of directing incoming milk laterally into the oropharynx down and around the glottis. Babies also lack the breathing interrupter reflexes that are activated in older children and adults. This ability to breathe and swallow simultaneously is lost at about 1 year of age.

The central chemoreceptors respond to changes in the pH of the extracellular fluid around them

Central chemoreceptors are specialized cells on the ventrolateral surface of the medulla (**Figure 31–8**). They are sensitive to changes in the pH of the extracellular fluid. Because extracellular fluid is in contact with the cerebrospinal fluid (CSF), changes in the pH of the CSF affect ventilation by acting on these chemoreceptors.

The blood-brain barrier separates CSF and plasma. It is relatively impermeable to H^+ and HCO_3^- ions, but CO_2 diffuses across it readily. The P_{CO_2} in the CSF parallels the arterial P_{CO_2} pressure. Because CO_2 is also produced by the cells of the brain as a product of metabolism, the P_{CO_2} of the CSF is usually higher than that of the arterial blood, and the pH is slightly more acidic (7.33) than in plasma (7.40).

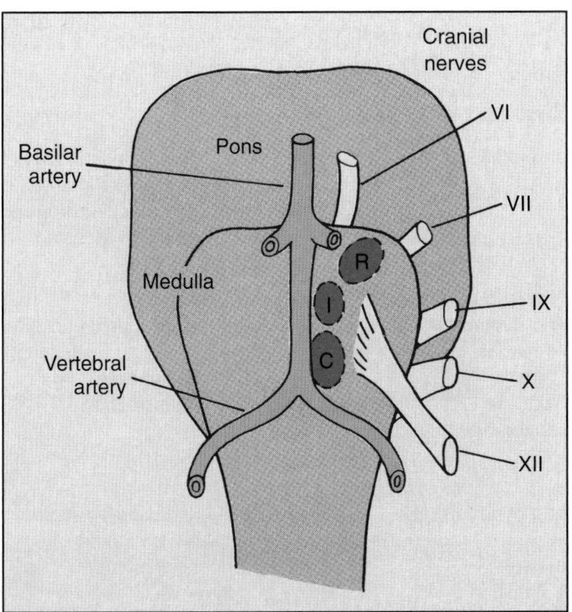

FIGURE 31–8. The locations of the three CO_2 ($[H^+]$)–sensitive areas on the ventrolateral medulla. The receptor cells are not actually at the surface but are close to it. R, I, and C refer to the rostral, intermediate, and caudal receptor areas. (From Berne RM, Levy MN, Koeppen BM, Stanton BA: *Physiology,* ed 5, Philadelphia, 2004, Elsevier.)

In the CSF, at any given $[HCO_3^-]$, increases in PCO_2 will be associated with decreases in pH (Henderson-Hasselbalch equation). Thus, an increase in arterial PCO_2 results in an increase in CSF PCO_2 and a decrease in CSF pH. This decrease in pH stimulates the central chemoreceptors, resulting in an increase in ventilation. The relationship between PCO_2 and ventilation is linear.

The relationship between ventilation and PCO_2 is important clinically. For example, if CO_2 production doubles in a patient on a ventilator because of either fever or infection, the minute ventilation (tidal volume × respiratory frequency) must double to maintain the same level of CO_2 in the arterial blood.

THUS, THE CO_2 IN BLOOD REGULATES VENTILATION BY ITS EFFECT ON THE PH OF THE CSF. Prolonged changes in arterial PCO_2 are associated with homeostatic mechanisms that adjust the ionic composition and $[HCO_3^-]$ of CSF to regulate the change in pH and bring the system back to normal. These changes occur during several hours, in contrast to the changes in CSF PCO_2 that can occur in minutes.

Peripheral chemoreceptors in the carotid and aortic bodies are the only chemoreceptors that respond to changes in PO_2

The carotid and aortic bodies are peripheral chemoreceptors that transmit afferent information to the central respiratory control center. They respond to changes in PO_2 (not O_2 content), PCO_2, and pH. They are the only chemoreceptors that respond to changes in PO_2 and account for approximately 40% of the total ventilatory response to changes in PCO_2. They are exquisitely sensitive. Small increases in chemoreceptor discharge occur even with small decreases in arterial PO_2, but marked increases in chemoreceptor discharge occur when the PO_2 decreases below 60 mm Hg. Afferent nerves synapse with type I cells known as **glomus cells** in the peripheral chemoreceptors and transmit information to the brainstem through the carotid sinus nerve (carotid body) and vagus nerve (aortic body).

Patients with severe obstructive pulmonary disease and hypercapnia can experience dyspnea and worsening hypoxemia. Inadvertently, they may be prescribed O_2 at high doses. Homeostatic mechanisms in the CSF over time have increased HCO_3^- concentrations in the CSF, resulting in a normal pH. As a result, the HCO_3^- buffering capacity modulates the effects of CO_2 changes, and these individuals breathe on a hypoxic basis regulated by the peripheral chemoreceptors. The supplemental O_2 improves their PaO_2 levels and decreases their minute ventilation, resulting in an increase in CO_2 levels. If this is not recognized, these individuals may die. Treatment is reduction of the supplemental O_2 to treat the hypoxemia but not to the level of suppressing ventilatory drive.

Pulmonary Mechanoreceptors Affect Ventilation and Ventilatory Patterns

Ventilation can also be affected by a number of reflexes that arise from the chest wall and lung (**Table 31–1**). The **Hering-Breuer** inspiratory-inhibitory reflex is a stretch reflex mediated by vagal fibers. When this reflex is elicited, it results in cessation of inspiration by stimulating off-switch neurons in the medulla. It is stimulated by tidal volumes in adults greater than 1 L and is especially important in newborns.

The **diving reflex** is initiated by stimulation of nasal or facial receptors with cold water and results in apnea or cessation of breathing and bradycardia.

TABLE 31–1. TRACHEOBRONCHIAL RECEPTOR PROPERTIES

Receptor Type	End-Organ Location	Stimuli	Reflexes
Myelinated vagal fibers			
Slowly adapting receptor	Among airway smooth muscle cells	Lung inflation	Hering-Breuer inflation reflex Hering-Breuer deflation reflex Inspiratory time—shortening Bronchodilation Tachycardia Hyperpnea
Rapidly adapting receptor (irritant receptor)	Among airway epithelial cells	Lung hyperinflation Exogenous and endogenous agents Histamine Prostaglandins	Hering-Breuer deflation reflex Cough Mucus secretion Bronchoconstriction
Unmyelinated vagal fibers			
C-fiber ending (J receptors)	Pulmonary interstitial space Close to pulmonary circulation Close to bronchial circulation	Lung hyperinflation Exogenous and endogenous agents Capsaicin Phenyldiguanide Histamine Bradykinin Serotonin Prostaglandins	Apnea, followed by rapid shallow breathing Bronchoconstriction Bradycardia Hypotension Mucus secretion

From Berne RM, Levy MN, Koeppen BM, Stanton BA: *Physiology,* ed 5, Philadelphia, 2004, Elsevier.

It prevents aspiration in individuals in the initial stages of drowning.

Mechanical stimulation of receptors in the nasopharynx and pharynx produces the **aspiration or sniff reflex.** This reflex brings material from the nasopharynx to the pharynx, where it can be swallowed or expectorated. It is also important in swallowing when it inhibits respiration and causes laryngeal closure.

The larynx has receptors that protect the lower respiratory tract by causing apnea, cough, or vigorous expiratory movements when it is stimulated.

The lower airway has three major types of receptors (Table 31–1). **Irritant receptors,** also known as rapidly adapting pulmonary stretch receptors, are located in the trachea and large airways. These receptors are stimulated by inhaled dust, noxious gases, or cigarette smoke and transmit information through myelinated vagal afferent fibers, resulting in an increase in airway resistance, reflex apnea, and cough. **Slowly adapting pulmonary stretch fibers** respond to mechanical stimulation and are activated by lung inflation. They also transmit information through myelinated vagal fibers. When they are stimulated, such as in individuals with chronic obstructive pulmonary disease, these pulmonary stretch fibers delay the onset of the next inspiratory effort and allow a longer expiratory phase that is essential in individuals with airway obstruction. Finally, specialized receptors in the terminal respiratory units that respond to chemical or mechanical stimulation are known as juxtaalveolar or **J receptors.** Their afferent input uses unmyelinated vagal C fibers. They may be responsible for the dyspnea (shortness of breath) and the altered ventilatory patterns (rapid, shallow) in interstitial lung edema and in some inflammatory lung diseases.

Exercise results in an increase in ventilation that is directly related to the increase in CO_2 production

The cardiovascular changes that occur during exercise have been described previously (see Chapters 24 and 26). Here we briefly discuss the ventilatory changes (**Figure 31–9**). Ventilation increases immediately when exercise begins, and this increase in minute ventilation closely matches the increase in O_2 consumption and CO_2 production in the body that accompanies exercise. Ventilation is linearly related to CO_2 production and O_2 consumption at low to moderate levels of activity. As a result, there is little change in blood gases during exercise until

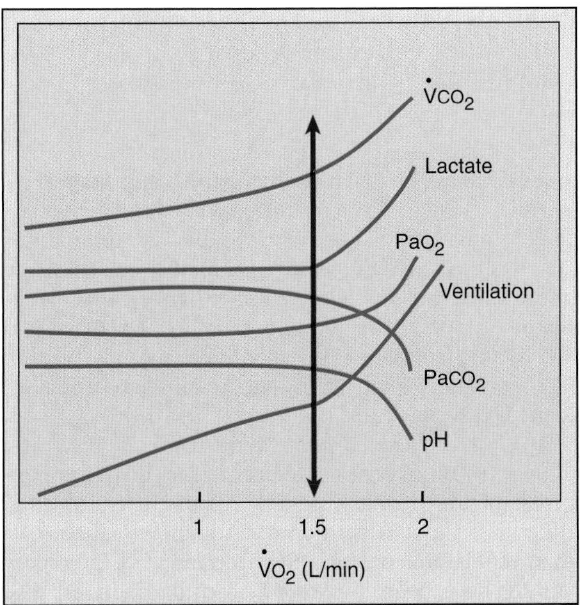

FIGURE 31–9. Some important metabolic changes that occur during exercise. The anaerobic threshold *(arrow)* is marked by a sudden change in the measured variables, which is due mainly to the developing lactic acidosis as anaerobic glycolysis takes over more and more of the muscle energy supply caused by relative failure of the body to supply sufficient O_2 to the muscles at the rate demanded by the level of exercise. (From Berne RM, Levy MN, Koeppen BM, Stanton BA: *Physiology,* ed 5, Philadelphia, 2004, Elsevier.)

maximal levels are achieved, during which arterial PCO_2 decreases slightly and arterial O_2 increases slightly. During heavy exercise, arterial pH falls as lactic acid is being liberated from muscles during anaerobic metabolism (Figure 31–9). What produces the increase in ventilation with exercise, however, is not known since there are no blood gas changes, but afferents from muscles and joint mechanoreceptors may play a role.

High altitude results in arterial hypoxemia

With increasing altitude, barometric pressure falls and inspired O_2 decreases. The resulting arterial hypoxemia stimulates hyperventilation initially by stimulating peripheral chemoreceptors. This increase in ventilation decreases arterial CO_2 and increases pH that in turn decreases stimulation of the central chemoreceptors in a negative feedback mechanism. With time at high altitude, acclimatization occurs through several different mechanisms:

- $NaHCO_3$ excretion by the kidney reduces plasma HCO_3^-, which raises the arterial pH toward normal.
- The ventilatory response to CO_2 steepens (increased sensitivity) as a result of the lower PaO_2, and this decreases the negative feedback mechanism.
- The concentration of 2,3-diphosphoglycerate in the red blood cells increases and more erythropoietin is manufactured, resulting in an increase in hemoglobin and a rightward shift of the oxyhemoglobin dissociation curve.

Intolerance to high altitude, called **chronic mountain sickness,** is relieved by the descent to a lower altitude or by the administration of supplemental O_2. Persons who have experienced chronic mountain sickness should never ascend to high altitude again because they are at risk for a recurrence.

Brief apnea occurs in many normal individuals during sleep

Approximately one third of normal individuals have brief episodes of apnea or hypoventilation during sleep. Most of the time, these episodes last less than 10 seconds, occur in the lighter stages of slow wave and rapid eye movement sleep, and have no effect on arterial PO_2 or PCO_2. Prolonged apnea occurs in a group of diseases known as the **sleep apnea syndromes,** of which there are two major categories **(Figure 31–10)**.

OBSTRUCTIVE SLEEP APNEA IS THE MOST COMMON SLEEP APNEA SYNDROME. It occurs when the upper airway (usually the hypopharynx) closes during inspiration. Similar to snoring, obstructive sleep apnea is more severe, obstructs the airway, and causes cessation of airflow. Hundreds of episodes can occur nightly and are associated with brief periods of self-arousal. This arousal occurs when the arterial hypoxemia and hypercapnia stimulate both peripheral and central chemoreceptors. Respiration is briefly restored until the next event occurs. Sleep deprivation occurs even though the individuals do not awaken fully with each episode. Complications of obstructive sleep apnea include polycythemia, right-sided cardiac failure (cor pulmonale), and pulmonary hypertension secondary to the recurrent, hypoxic events. THE MOST COMMON CAUSE OF OBSTRUCTIVE SLEEP APNEA IS OBESITY.

> Obstructive sleep apnea is underdiagnosed. It causes excessive daytime somnolence that leads to a significant number of motor vehicle accidents. Obstructive sleep apnea can contribute to many other diseases, including hypertension, right-sided heart failure, chronic respiratory failure, cardiac arrhythmias during sleep, and possibly even sudden death.

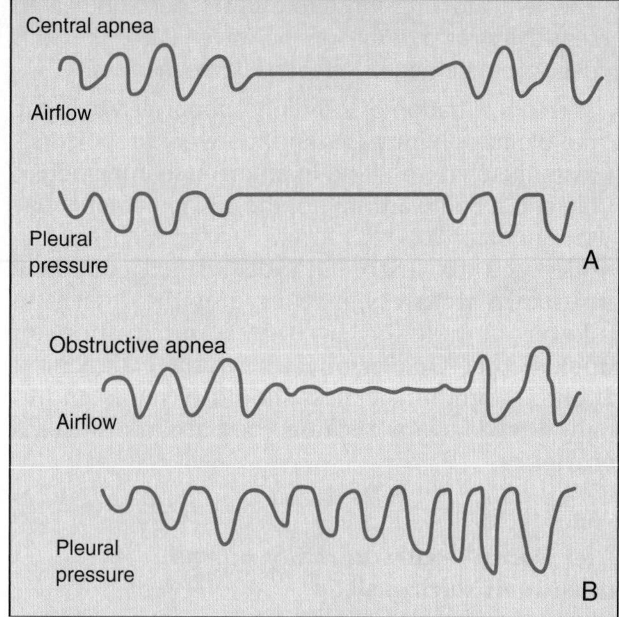

FIGURE 31–10. The two main types of sleep apnea. A, Central apnea is characterized by no attempt to breathe, as demonstrated by no pleural pressure oscillations. B, In obstructive sleep apnea, the pleural pressure oscillations increase as CO_2 rises. This indicates that airflow resistance is very high owing to upper airway obstruction. (From Berne RM, Levy MN, Koeppen BM, Stanton BA: *Physiology*, ed 5, Philadelphia, 2004, Elsevier.)

Central sleep apnea occurs when there is a decrease in ventilatory drive to the respiratory motor neurons. These individuals make no respiratory efforts. Blood gas changes are less severe in individuals with central sleep apnea, but the same complications can occur when the apnea is severe and recurrent.

Central alveolar hypoventilation, also known as Ondine's curse, is a rare disease in which voluntary breathing is intact, but abnormalities in automaticity exist. It is the most severe of the central sleep apneas. As a result, people with central alveolar hypoventilation can breathe as long as they do not fall asleep. For these individuals, mechanical ventilation or, more recently, bilateral diaphragmatic pacing (similar to a cardiac pacemaker) can be lifesaving.

Sudden infant death syndrome is the most common cause of death in infants in the first year of life, outside of the perinatal period. Although the cause of sudden infant death syndrome is not known, abnormalities in ventilatory control, and particularly in CO_2 responsiveness, have been implicated. Placing infants on their back to sleep (reducing the potential for CO_2 rebreathing) has dramatically decreased (but not eliminated) the death rate from this syndrome.

Cheyne-Stokes ventilation is an abnormality in ventilatory control characterized by a varying tidal volume and ventilatory frequency. It is seen in some individuals with central nervous system disease and also in normal individuals during sleep at high altitudes.

Summary

- ❖ Respiratory control is both automatic and voluntary.
- ❖ Ventilatory control is composed of the respiratory control center, central chemoreceptors, peripheral chemoreceptors, and pulmonary mechanoreceptors.
- ❖ The arterial P_{CO_2} is the major factor that influences ventilation.
- ❖ The respiratory control center is composed of the dorsal respiratory group and the ventral respiratory group. Rhythmic breathing depends on a continuous (tonic) inspiratory drive from the dorsal respiratory group and on intermittent (phasic) expiratory inputs from the cerebrum, thalamus, cranial nerves, and ascending spinal cord sensory tracts.
- ❖ The peripheral and central chemoreceptors respond to changes in P_{CO_2} and pH. The peripheral chemoreceptors (carotid and aortic bodies) are the only chemoreceptors that respond to changes in P_{O_2}.
- ❖ Acute hypoxia and chronic hypoxia affect breathing differently because of slow adjustments in cerebrospinal fluid $[H^+]$, which alters CO_2 sensitivity.

- Irritant receptors protect the lower respiratory tract from particles, chemical vapors, and physical factors, primarily by inducing cough.
- C-fiber J receptors in the terminal respiratory units are stimulated by distortion of the alveolar walls (by lung congestion or edema).
- At low to moderate levels of exercise, ventilation is linearly related to both CO_2 production and O_2 consumption.
- The hyperventilation that occurs early at high altitude is the result of peripheral chemoreceptor stimulation secondary to hypoxemia.
- The two most important clinical abnormalities of breathing are obstructive sleep apnea and central sleep apnea.

Bibliography

Coleridge HM, Coleridge JCG: Pulmonary reflexes: neural mechanisms of pulmonary defense, *Annu Rev Physiol* 56:69, 1994.

Cutz E et al: Peripheral chemoreceptors in congenital central hypoventilation syndrome, *Am J Respir Crit Care Med* 155:358, 1997.

Funk GD, Feldman JL: Generation of respiratory rhythm and pattern in mammals: insights from development studies, *Curr Opin Neurobiol* 5:778, 1995.

Jammes Y, Speck DF: Respiratory control by diaphragmatic and respiratory muscle afferents. In Dempsey JA, Pack AI, eds: *Regulation of breathing,* New York, 1995, Marcel Dekker.

Jordan D: Central nervous pathways and control of the airways, *Respir Physiol* 125:67, 2001.

Robin ED et al: Alveolar gas tensions, pulmonary ventilation and blood pH during physiologic sleep in normal subjects, *J Clin Invest* 37:981, 1998.

Schafer T: Variability of vigilance and ventilation: studies on the control of respiration during sleep, *Respir Physiol* 114:37, 1998.

Stradling JR, Davies RJ: Sleep. 1: Obstructive sleep apnoea/hypopnoea syndrome: definitions, epidemiology, and natural history, *Thorax* 59:73, 2004.

Case Studies

Case 31–1

An 18-year-old college student hit a tree while riding his all-terrain vehicle. He was not wearing a helmet. He is initially apneic at the site, but with resuscitation, he begins to breathe at a rate of 25 breaths/minute with paradoxical breathing (outward movement of his abdominal muscles with inspiration). An x-ray examination reveals a fractured cervical vertebra with a spinal transection at C2.

1. **Which of the following structures of respiration have been affected by this injury?**
   A. Pons
   B. Medulla
   C. DRG
   D. VRG
   E. Phrenic nerve

2. **What are the physiological effects of the injury on respiration?**
   A. Reduced vital capacity, mild hypercapnia and hypoxemia, reduced maximal inspiratory pressure
   B. Normal vital capacity, mild hypercapnia and hypoxemia, normal maximal inspiratory pressure
   C. Reduced vital capacity, normal P_{CO_2} and P_{O_2}, normal maximal inspiratory pressure
   D. Periods of apnea during sleep
   E. Apneustic breathing

Case 31–2

An obese 48-year-old physician complains of daytime sleepiness, fatigue, and morning headaches. His wife reports snoring with multiple episodes of abrupt arousal each night. She will not allow him to drive long distances because he frequently falls asleep at the wheel. He was recently hospitalized for a deep vein thrombosis and was found at that time to have evidence of right-sided heart failure. An arterial blood gas analysis on room air revealed a PaO_2 of 59 mm Hg, a $PaCO_2$ of 65 mm Hg, pH of 7.37, and saturation of 89% while awake. His hemoglobin concentration was 16.3 g/dL.

1. **If a polysomnogram (sleep study) were performed, what would it most likely reveal?**
   - **A.** Brief, infrequent episodes of no airflow at the nose or mouth with no attempt to breathe and no change in arterial O_2
   - **B.** Brief, infrequent episodes of no airflow at the nose or mouth with vigorous attempts to breathe, hypoxemia, and hypercapnia
   - **C.** Prolonged, multiple episodes of no airflow at the nose or mouth with no attempt to breathe, hypoxemia, and worsening hypercapnia
   - **D.** Prolonged, multiple episodes of no airflow at the nose or mouth with vigorous attempts to breathe, worsening hypoxemia, and worsening hypercapnia
   - **E.** Prolonged, multiple episodes of no airflow at the nose or mouth with vigorous attempts to breathe, but no change in arterial O_2 or CO_2

Case 31–3

A 27-year-old woman with cystic fibrosis and severe obstructive pulmonary disease is admitted to the hospital with increasing dyspnea, cyanosis, and increased productive cough. Her chest radiograph displays severe hyperinflation with flattened diaphragms and increased markings consistent with airway inflammation and bronchiectasis (dilatation of airways resulting from chronic infection). On physical examination, her respiratory rate (RR) is 24 breaths per minute (NL = 12/min), and her breath sounds are diminished with copious crackles at the bases. Treatment begins with supplemental O_2 therapy by nasal cannula, and a series of arterial blood gas samples are obtained.

	PaO_2	$PaCO_2$	pH	RR
On room air	55 mm Hg	55 mm Hg	7.35	24
On 1 L O_2	62 mm Hg	60 mm Hg	7.31	20
On 2 L O_2	75 mm Hg	69 mm Hg	7.23	16

1. **Which of the following statements is *not* correct?**
   - **A.** The most appropriate supplemental O_2 flow for this patient is 2 L O_2.
   - **B.** The higher arterial PO_2 in this patient while she is receiving supplemental O_2 blunts her respiratory response to CO_2.
   - **C.** On room air, this patient demonstrates a hypoxemia-induced increase in ventilation.
   - **D.** During sleep, this patient is at risk for worsening hypercapnia.
   - **E.** On room air, this patient demonstrates a chronic respiratory acidosis.

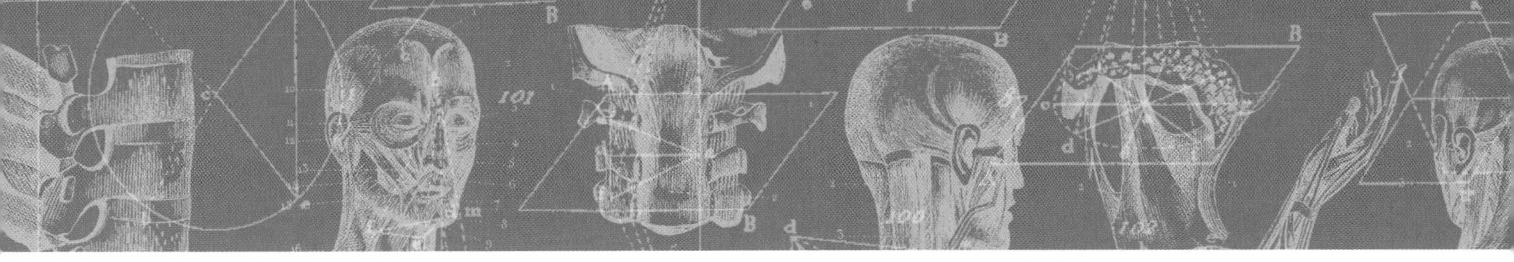

Chapter 32: Nonrespiratory Functions of the Lung

Objectives

- ❖ Explain how the mucociliary transport system clears particulates from the lung.
- ❖ Describe the mucosal immune system in the lung.
- ❖ Describe adaptive and innate immune cells unique to the lung.

In addition to gas exchange, the lung also functions as a primary defense system. To cope with environmental exposure and the constant insult of inhaled foreign agents, the lung has developed unique structural features (e.g., mucociliary transport system) as well as unique adaptive (i.e., intraepithelial T lymphocytes, IgA antibodies) and innate (i.e., alveolar macrophages) immune response mechanisms. These structural features as well as the specialized immune system are integral components of the mucosal immune system in the lung. THE RESPIRATORY, GASTROINTESTINAL, AND URINARY SYSTEMS ARE PART OF THE BODY'S **MUCOSAL IMMUNE SYSTEM,** WHICH CAN FUNCTION INDEPENDENTLY OF THE SYSTEMIC IMMUNE SYSTEM. In this chapter, we first describe the structural features that limit environmental exposure and then address the immune defense system.

The Mucociliary Transport System Is Composed of Periciliary Fluid, a Mucus Layer, and Cilia Functioning Together to Remove Particulates from the Lung

Many irritant and toxic particulates are continuously inhaled with normal respiration, and thus a continuous system for the clearance of this material has evolved. THE MUCOCILIARY TRANSPORT SYSTEM PROTECTS THE LUNG BY TRAPPING AND REMOVING BACTERIAL, VIRAL, AND OTHER INHALED PARTICULATES FROM THE CONDUCTING AIRWAYS. There are three major components of mucociliary transport: two fluid layers, referred to as the **sol** and **gel** phases; and **cilia,** hairlike structures on the surface of bronchial epithelial cells **(Figure 32–1)**.

The sol phase or **periciliary fluid** is composed of nonviscous serous fluid and lies immediately adjacent to the bronchial epithelial cells. Pseudostratified, ciliated columnar epithelial cells, which line the conducting airways to the level of the bronchioles, produce the periciliary fluid layer via active Na^+ and Cl^- ion transport. This active transport process is regulated by intracellular cAMP and Ca^{++} ions and by Cl^- channels. The balance between Cl^- secretion and Na^+ absorption maintains the serous environment and regulates the depth of the periciliary fluid at about 7 μm. Maintenance of the normal depth and ion composition of the periciliary fluid is essential for optimal cilia movement.

Cystic fibrosis is an autosomal, recessive disease that is characterized by thick, tenacious, dehydrated airway secretions. In this disease, the airway epithelium demonstrates decreased Cl^- secretion. In cystic fibrosis, mutations in a Cl^- ion channel, the cystic fibrosis transmembrane conductance regulator (CFTR), results in decreased Cl^- secretion. The result is thick mucus and less water in the airway lumen.

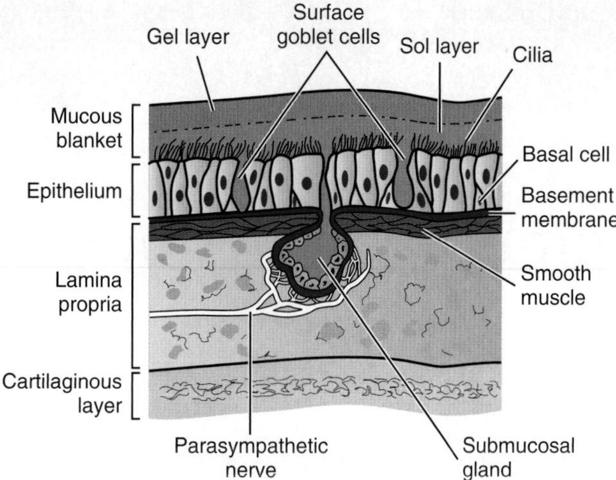

FIGURE 32–1. Epithelial lining of the tracheobronchial tree. The cilia of the epithelial cell reside in the periciliary fluid layer with the mucus on top. Interspersed between the ciliated epithelial cells are surface secretory (goblet) cells and submucosal glands. (From Berne RM, Levy MN, Koeppen BM, Stanton BA: *Physiology,* ed 5, Philadelphia, 2004, Elsevier.)

The gel phase or **mucus layer** is composed of a mixture of macromolecules, with viscosity and elastic properties, and lies on top of the periciliary fluid as a discontinuous blanket. Surface secretory cells **(goblet cells)** in the conducting airways and the **mucous** and **serous** cells in **submucosal tracheobronchial glands** produce and secrete mucus. Also, **Clara** cells located in the epithelium of bronchioles contribute to the composition of mucus with the secretion of a "non-mucinous" material containing carbohydrates and proteins. Airway mucus is a mixture of macromolecules including proteins, glycoproteins, electrolytes, and water, resulting in a complex with a characteristic low viscosity and high elasticity **(Figure 32–2).** This mucus layer is predominantly water (95% to 97%) and is 5 to 10 μm thick. Normal individuals produce approximately 100 mL of mucus per day, most of which is reabsorbed by the epithelial cells. The remainder, approximately 10 mL per day, is propelled up the mucociliary escalator and swallowed. During active stages of lung disease, local inflammatory mediators are released, such as histamine and arachidonic acid metabolites, which stimulate mucus production.

Goblet cells are present approximately every five to six ciliated cells in the respiratory epithelium down to the fifth level of the tracheobronchial division and then decrease in frequency and finally disappear beyond the twelfth tracheobronchial division in normal individuals. In the presence of disease, goblet cells can be found farther down the tracheobronchial tree, thus making these smaller airways more susceptible to obstruction by mucous plugging. They secrete neutral and acidic

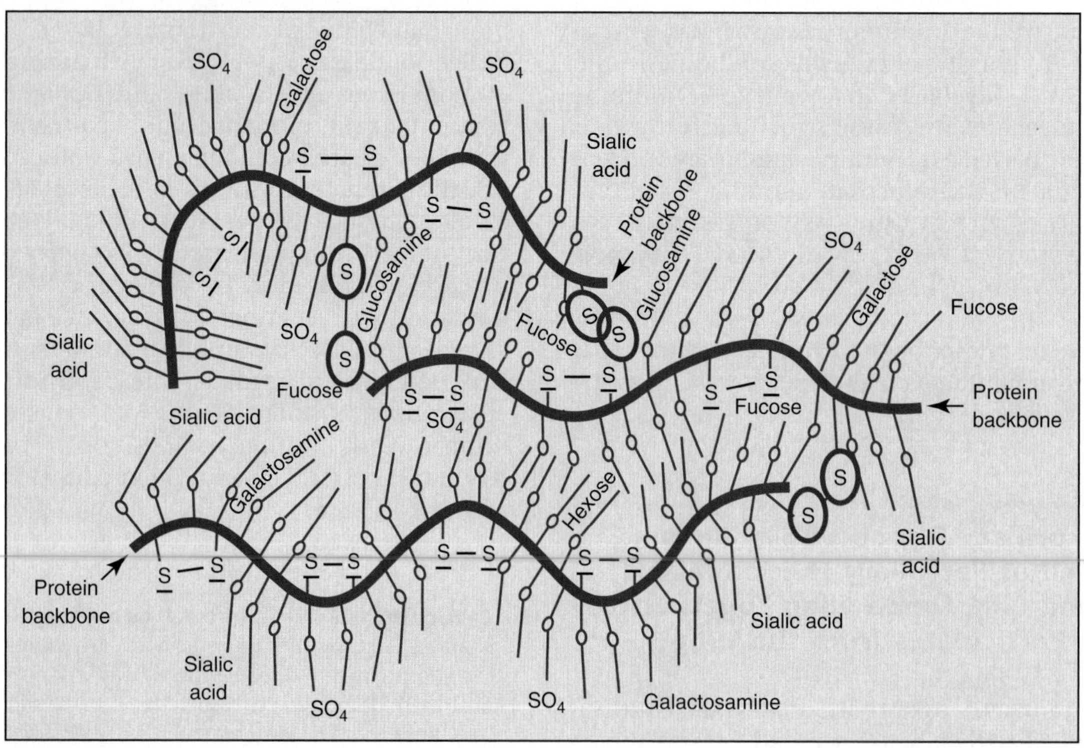

FIGURE 32–2. Schematic drawing of mucus. Note the protein backbone with glycoprotein side chains and the "O" glycosidic and disulfide bonds. (From Berne RM, Levy MN, Koeppen BM, Stanton BA: *Physiology,* ed 5, Philadelphia, 2004, Elsevier.)

glycoproteins rich in sialic acid via exocytosis in response to chemical stimuli. In the presence of infection or cigarette smoke and in patients with chronic bronchitis, goblet cells increase in size and number and secrete more mucus. Often, the mucus also has an increased viscosity and is discolored as observed in a sputum sample.

Sputum is expectorated mucus. However, in addition to mucus, sputum contains serum proteins, lipids, electrolytes, calcium, and DNA from degenerated white blood cell nuclei (collectively known as bronchial secretions) and extrabronchial secretions including nasal, oral, lingual, pharyngeal, and salivary secretions. The color of sputum correlates more closely with the amount of time it has been present in the lower respiratory tract than with the type of infection.

Submucosal tracheobronchial glands are present in the upper regions of the conducting airways, adjacent to cartilage, and empty into the airway lumen via a ciliated duct. Mucus secretion within the gland is under parasympathetic (cholinergic), sympathetic (adrenergic), and peptidergic (vasoactive intestinal polypeptide) neural control. The secretory mucous cells are located near the distal end of the duct; the secretory serous cells are located at the most distal end of the duct. Although both secrete mucus, the morphological features and mucus composition of mucous and serous cells are distinctively different **(Table 32–1).** The glands can be increased in number and size and can extend to the bronchioles in diseases such as chronic bronchitis. The result is increased mucus production and alterations in chemical composition (i.e., increased viscosity and decreased elasticity) manifested clinically as airway obstruction.

TABLE 32–1. PROPERTIES OF SUBMUCOSAL GLAND CELLS

	Serous Cells	Mucous Cells
Granules	Small, electron dense	Large, electron lucent
Glycoproteins	Neutral Lysozyme, lactoferrin	Acidic
Hormone	α- > β-adrenergic	β- > α-adrenergic
Receptors	Muscarinic	Muscarinic
Degranulation	α-adrenergic Cholinergic Substance P	β-adrenergic Cholinergic

Data from Welsh MJ: Production and control of airway secretions. In Fishman AP: *Pulmonary diseases and disorders,* ed 2, New York, 1988, McGraw-Hill.

On the surface of bronchial epithelial cells are **cilia,** hairlike structures that aid in the movement of mucus. Cilia beat at a rate of 900 to 1200 strokes/min with a coordinated oscillation in a characteristic, biphasic, and wavelike rhythm called metachronism. There is a power forward stroke, during which the tips of the cilia extend upward into the viscous gel layer, propelling the mucus forward, and a slow return stroke, when the cilia recede and are contained completely in the nonviscous sol layer. In the respiratory system, cilia are present on epithelial cells in the nasopharynx, trachea, bronchi, and bronchioles; they beat in the direction to propel the mucus into the pharynx, where it is swallowed "downward" in the nasopharynx and "upward" in the case of tracheobronchial cells. It is estimated that there are approximately 200 cilia per cell with an average length of 2 to 5 μm. They are composed of nine microtubular doublets that surround two central microtubules and are held together by dynein arms, nexin links, and spokes **(Figure 32–3).** The central microtubule doublet contains an ATPase enzyme, which is responsible for the ATP-dependent contractile beat of the cilia. Effective clearance requires both normal ciliary activity and normal periciliary fluid and mucus composition. Inhaled material is trapped on

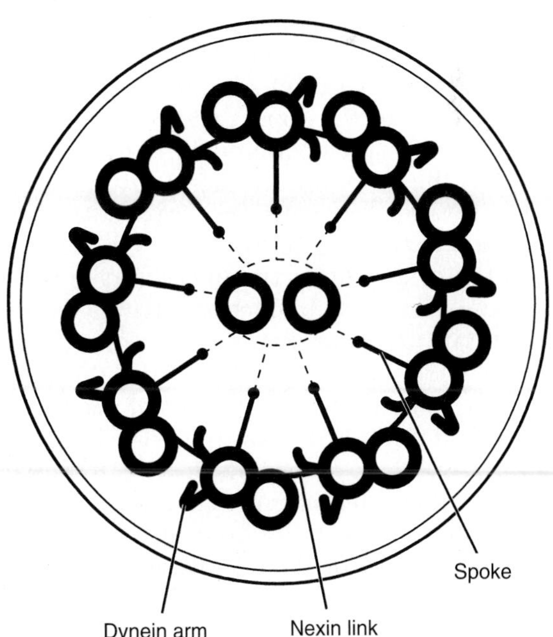

FIGURE 32–3. Schematic cross-sectional diagram of cilium showing its main structural components. (From Palmblad J et al: Ultrastructural, cellular, and clinical features of the immotile-cilia syndrome. *Annu Rev Med* 35:483, 1984. Reprinted with permission from the *Annual Review of Medicine,* Volume 35, ©1984 by Annual Reviews www.annualreviews.org.)

TABLE 32–2. GENERAL CHARACTERIZATION OF PARTICLE DEPOSITION IN THE LUNG ACCORDING TO SIZE

Particle Size (μm)	Deposition Site	Influence
>10	Nasal passages Trachea Nasopharynx	Impaction
2-10	Trachea Bronchi (10-12 generations) Airway bifurcations	Turbulent airflow Airflow changes Inertial impaction
0.2-2	Distal airways—bronchioles	Slower airflow Gravity (sedimentation)
<0.2	Terminal bronchioles Alveoli	Diffusion

the more viscous mucus layer; the watery serous periciliary fluid allows the cilia to move freely with only their tips contacting the mucus and propelling it toward the mouth.

The size, density, and velocity of the particle as well as distance to travel, lung anatomy, and relative humidity within the lung all contribute to **particle deposition** in the lung. In general, particle size, velocity, and lung anatomy (e.g., bifurcations) are the most important factors in particle deposition within the lung **(Table 32–2)**. The mucociliary transport system removes particles from the terminal bronchioles to the upper airways, where they are coughed up and either expectorated or swallowed in a matter of minutes. The rate of clearance is faster in the upper regions of the lung (i.e., trachea and main stem bronchi, 5 to 20 mm/min) than in the lower bronchioles (0.1 mm/min). PARTICLE CLEARANCE FROM THE AREA BELOW THE TERMINAL BRONCHIOLES TO THE ALVEOLUS OCCURS FOR THE MOST PART INDEPENDENTLY OF THE MUCOCILIARY TRANSPORT SYSTEM AND IS THUS CONSIDERABLY SLOWER, OFTEN CONSIDERED THE "ACHILLES HEEL" OF PARTICLE CLEARANCE IN THE LUNG. Particle clearance from this area is dependent on phagocytosis by alveolar macrophages, which can either destroy the particle internally or transport it to regions in the terminal bronchioles, where the macrophage can be picked up by the mucociliary transport system. In individuals with occupational lung diseases, such as pneumoconiosis (the "black lung" disease of coal miners), the highest concentration of particles is usually seen just beyond the terminal bronchioles. In general, the longer inhaled material remains in the airways, the greater the probability that lung damage will occur. Once particles in the terminal airways have entered the interstitium, clearance is even slower and the likelihood of lung damage even greater. The terminal respiratory unit is the most common location of airway damage for all types of occupational lung disease and airborne particles.

DISEASES ASSOCIATED WITH ABNORMALITIES IN MUCOCILIARY CLEARANCE

Immotile cilia syndrome is associated with abnormal ciliary microstructure. **Kartagener's syndrome** is associated with immotile cilia and comprises the triad of situs inversus with bronchiectasis and sinusitis. Any process that interferes with normal ciliary beating will interfere with particle clearance. These types of diseases are usually associated with chronic and persistent infections. Patients with **asthma** have increased mucus production and mucus with increased viscosity. They can experience abnormalities in mucociliary clearance secondary to changes in the character of their mucus in the absence of infection.

The Mucosal Immune System Provides the Major Immune Defense Mechanisms for the Lung

The respiratory tract is continuously exposed to inhaled foreign substances—from inert, nonpathological particles to pathogenic viruses and bacteria. To avoid a continuous inflammatory response in the lung, the immune system must be able to discriminate between what is harmful and what is not. Although inflammation is a protective response to injury or an invading pathogen, its presence impedes organ system function. The lung and other mucosal tissues (respiratory, gastrointestinal, and urinary systems) have evolved a unique mucosal immune system designed to eliminate inhaled foreign agents in a noninflammatory manner. Found in these mucosal tissues are specialized **adaptive** immune cells (i.e., T lymphocytes with γδT-cell receptors and IgA-secreting plasma cells) and specialized **innate** immune cells (i.e., natural killer cells, dendritic cells, and alveolar macrophages) **(Table 32–3)**. This selective recognition system limits the inflammatory response to foreign nonpathological inhaled substances.

The lymphatic system and lymphoid tissues in the lung filter fluids and particulates through organized lymphoid structures (lymph nodes, lymph nodules, and lymph aggregates) and a diffuse submucosal network of scattered lymphocytes and dendritic cells. THE LYMPH NODES ARE PART OF THE SYSTEMIC IMMUNE SYSTEM; THE OTHER LYMPHOID STRUCTURES MAKE UP THE MUCOSAL IMMUNE SYSTEM OR THE **MUCOSA-ASSOCIATED LYMPHOID TISSUE (MALT).** MALT regions in the lung are referred to as bronchus-associated lymphoid tissue (BALT), and

TABLE 32–3. INNATE AND ADAPTIVE IMMUNE CELLS IN THE RESPIRATORY SYSTEM

Cell Type	Location	Function
TCRγδ lymphocytes	Intraepithelial	Selective antigen recognition Immunoregulation (↓ IgE)
TCRαβ lymphocytes	Lamina propria	Specific adaptive immunity Immunoregulation (Th1/Th2 cytokines)
B lymphocytes	Submucosa	IgA antibody synthesis
Dendritic cells	Diffuse in lung interstitium	Antigen presentation Immunoregulation (tolerance)
Alveolar macrophages	Alveoli and alveolar ducts	Phagocytosis Immunoregulation (cytokines)
NK cells	Diffuse in lung interstitium	Targeted cytotoxicity Immunoregulation (tolerance)
NK/T cells	Diffuse in lung interstitium	Immunoregulation (IL-4)

Data from Berne RM, Levy MN, Koeppen BM, Stanton BA: *Physiology,* ed 5, Philadelphia, 2004, Elsevier.

their counterpart in the gastrointestinal tract is gut-associated lymphoid tissue (GALT).

The anatomical structures of lymphoid tissue in the lung become less organized as one transcends the lung from the most upper airways (hilum) to the periphery (alveoli). Mature lymph nodes with germinal centers are common in the hilar region around the main stem bronchi. BALT predominates at the next level of organization with lymph nodules and aggregates in the more upper regions of the conducting airways adjacent to major airway branches and blood vessels. Sporadic lymphoid nodules and isolated lymphocytes are found more commonly in the more peripheral conducting airways down to the alveoli. There are no organized lymphoid structures in the alveolar spaces.

Although the lymph nodules making up BALT are not true lymph nodes, they are still a major processing center for antigens. THE EPITHELIUM ASSOCIATED WITH BALT IS COMPOSED OF A MIXTURE OF EPITHELIAL CELLS AND LYMPHOCYTES AND IS REFERRED TO AS A **LYMPHOEPITHELIUM.** This lymphoepithelium lacks ciliated epithelial cells, creating a break in the mucociliary clearance system, which enhances fluid and particulate flow into BALT. Although it has not yet been observed in BALT, a highly specialized epithelial cell with many microfolds (M cells) has been observed in GALT, which may provide clues as to how antigens are processed in BALT. These M cells appear to form pockets or invaginations for antigen processing where clusters of macrophages and lymphocytes collect **(Figure 32–4).** Areas of BALT are apparent in the histological examination of normal mouse lungs but are observed in the lungs of humans only with pathological conditions, such as upper respiratory tract infections.

In addition to aggregates of cells, MALT contains a substantial number of solitary B and T

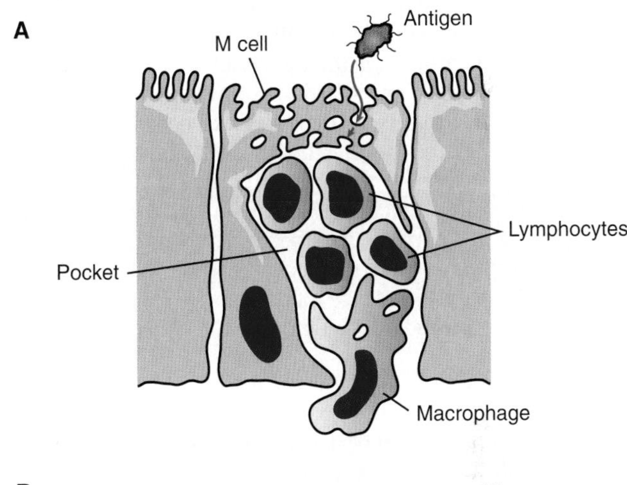

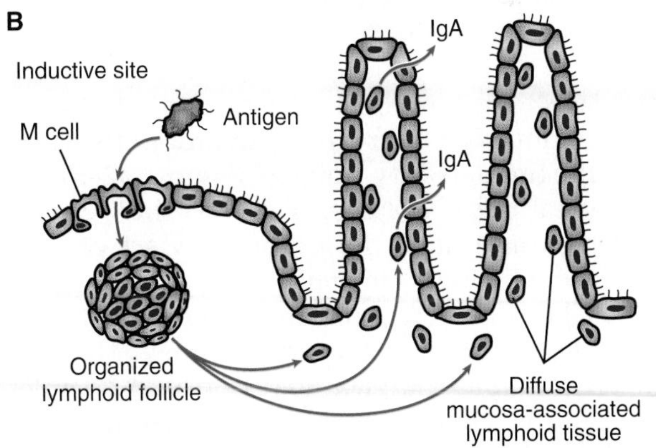

FIGURE 32–4. Representation of MALT, M cells, and IgA synthesis. A, M cells located in mucosal epithelium endocytose antigen in the lumen and transport it for processing to submucosal pockets of immune cells. B, Diagram of mucous membrane showing secretion of IgA antibodies in response to antigen endocytosed by M cells at an inductive site. Activated B cells migrate from the lymphoid follicle to nearby mucosa-associated lymphoid tissue, where they differentiate into IgA-producing plasma cells. (From Berne RM, Levy MN, Koeppen BM, Stanton BA: *Physiology,* ed 5, Philadelphia, 2004, Elsevier.)

lymphocytes, which are scattered regularly throughout the connective tissue. Lymphocytes in the lamina propria (lamina propria lymphocytes) resemble those found in the systemic immune system, $CD4^+$ (helper) T cells with T-cell receptors composed of α and β chains (TCRαβ cells). In contrast, lymphocytes in the epithelial layer (intraepithelial lymphocytes) are predominantly $CD8^+$ (cytotoxic-suppressor) T cells with T-cell receptors composed of γ and δ chains (TCRγδ cells). MALT provides a first line of defense for these highly exposed mucosal surfaces.

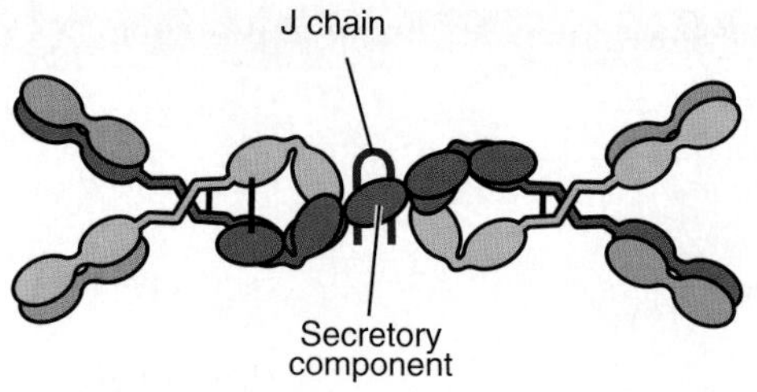

Structure of secretory IgA

A

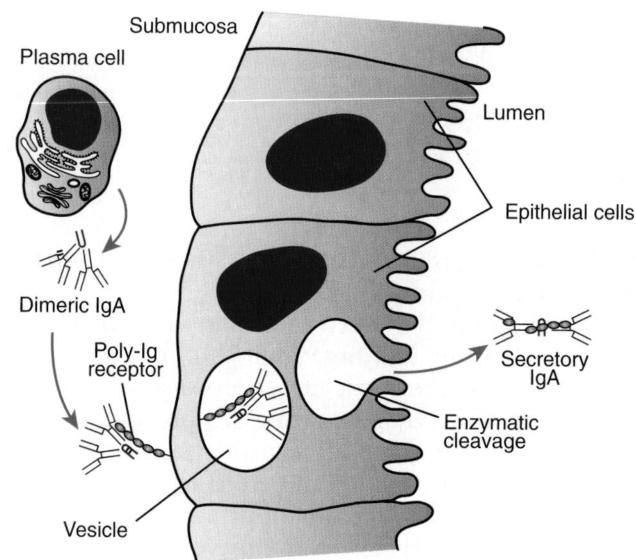

Formation of secretory IgA

B

FIGURE 32–5. Structure and formation of secretory IgA. A, Secretory IgA consists of at least two IgA molecules that are covalently linked by a J chain and covalently associated with the secretory component. The secretory component contains five Ig-like domains and is linked to dimeric IgA *(thick black line)* between its fifth domain and one of the IgA heavy chains. B, Secretory IgA is formed during transport through mucous membrane epithelial cells. Dimeric IgA binds to a poly-Ig receptor on the basolateral membrane of an epithelial cell and is internalized by receptor-mediated endocytosis. After transport of the receptor-IgA complex to the luminal surface, the poly-Ig receptor is enzymatically cleaved, releasing the secretory component bound to the dimeric IgA. (From Berne RM, Levy MN, Koeppen BM, Stanton BA: *Physiology,* ed 5, Philadelphia, 2004, Elsevier.)

An important feature that distinguishes lymph nodes in the systemic immune system from **MALT** is that true lymph nodes are encapsulated and have an afferent (entering) and efferent (leaving) pattern of lymphatic fluid drainage, which is not present in MALT. Once an antigen is processed through a lymph node, it can be assumed that systemic sensitization has occurred or will soon occur. In contrast, although MALT is organized, it is not encapsulated, and there is only afferent lymph drainage. It appears that there is direct communication between organs of MALT and that sensitization via one organ is transposed to all MALT tissues through a "lymphatic-like" drainage network. The systemic immune system and MALT may work independently of each other, and sensitization of one may not transpose to the other. This may serve as a defense mechanism in limiting sensitization only to mucosal tissues.

Plasma cells producing IgA antibodies and TCRγδ T cells are unique adaptive immune cells in MALT

The B cells found in MALT have a selectivity to differentiate into **IgA-secreting plasma cells** when they are stimulated by antigen **(Figure 32–5)**. In submucosal areas, plasma cells synthesize and secrete IgA in a dimer form linked by a **J chain.** The antibody-dimer migrates to the surface of epithelial cells, where it undergoes pinocytosis and eventual secretion into the airway lumen. The IgA-antigen immune complex does not bind complement in the classical manner as other immune complexes do, thus limiting its inflammatory properties. Also, the IgA-antibody system is effective in binding particulates and viruses, creating large complexes, which aids in their removal through the mucociliary clearance system before they invade epithelial cells.

In contrast to the systemic location of TCRαβ cells, **TCRγδ cells** are preferentially localized to the epithelial surfaces (epitheliotropism) of mucosal tissues, suggesting a role in immunosurveillance and maintenance of homeostasis. These TCRγδ cells are the predominant intraepithelial lymphocytes throughout MALT. They exhibit several unique properties for immunosurveillance (i.e., limited antigen recognition capability and low proliferative capacity) that limit the initiation of an inflammatory response. TCRγδ cells have been shown to suppress IgE responses to inhaled antigen in mice and to be increased in various diseases, such as asthma, sarcoidosis, hypersensitivity pneumonitis, allergic rhinitis, and infections (bacterial, viral, and parasitic).

DISEASES ASSOCIATED WITH ABNORMALITIES IN THE IMMUNE RESPONSE

In allergic diseases, such as **asthma,** an antibody synthesis switchover occurs, and IgE becomes the predominant antibody synthesized to the allergen. The IgE binds to tissue mast cells and in the presence of allergen leads to their degranulation and release of proinflammatory and bronchoconstricting mediators **(Figure 32–6).** **Hypersensitivity lung diseases** are associated with an altered immune response to nonpathological organisms. It is not a typical allergic response in that symptoms arise 4 to 6 hours after contact with the inciting agent, and eosinophils are not a prominent component. The pathological process in the lung is more of a granulomatous-like response with ensuing interstitial fibrosis. **Goodpasture's syndrome** is an autoimmune response to the lung basement membrane resulting in hemorrhagic disease. **IgA deficiency** is the most common inherited immunoglobulin deficiency and is commonly associated with chronic lung disease.

Natural killer cells, dendritic cells, and alveolar macrophages are unique innate immune cells in MALT

Natural killer (NK) cells and NK/T cells ($CD3^+$ NK cells) are derived developmentally from a lymphoid lineage in the bone marrow. They are a major component of the body's innate immune defense system against invading pathogens, such as herpes viruses and various bacteria. Although they share many functional activities with lymphocytes, they do not directly fit into the classification of a T or B lymphocyte. NK cells are named for their ability to kill target cells via the release of toxins (i.e., granular enzymes, perforins, and serine esterases) without prior sensitization. In addition to their cytotoxic activity, they produce cytokines similar to those of lymphocytes that can modulate adaptive immune responses. A resident population of functionally active NK cells is present in the lung interstitium, and these NK cells play a role in asthma and allergic diseases.

Whether the inhaled substance stays within the airway lumen or attaches to and penetrates the epithelium determines the fate and type of response

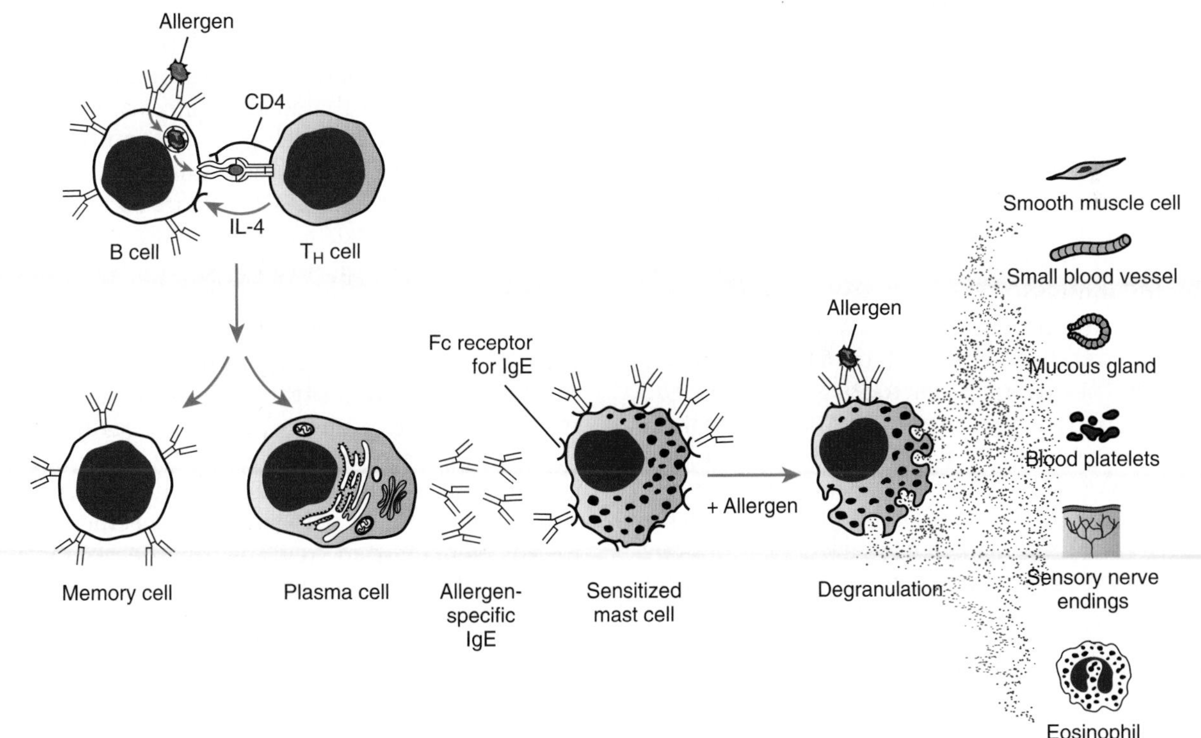

FIGURE 32–6. General mechanism underlying an allergic reaction. Exposure to an allergen activates B cells to form IgE-secreting plasma cells. The secreted IgE molecules bind to IgE-specific Fc receptors on mast cells and blood basophils. On a second exposure to the allergen, the bound IgE is cross-linked, triggering the release of pharmacologically active mediators *(purple)* from mast cells and basophils. The mediators cause smooth muscle contraction, increased vascular permeability, and vasodilation. (From Berne RM, Levy MN, Koeppen BM, Stanton BA: *Physiology,* ed 5, Philadelphia, 2004, Elsevier.)

generated. Differentiated cells of the myeloid lineage, **dendritic cells** and alveolar macrophages, are the first nonepithelial cells within the lung to contact and respond to foreign inhaled substances. Alternatively, if the foreign material travels to the air spaces in the lower respiratory system (alveolar ducts and alveoli), it will most likely be phagocytosed by alveolar macrophages, and if it penetrates and reaches interstitial areas, it will come into contact with dendritic cells. In either case, macrophage-type mononuclear cells play a critical role in host defense in the lung.

The major functions of dendritic cells are to capture, process, and present antigen to T cells, resulting in either activation or suppression of the T-cell response **(Box 32–1).** Dendritic cells are commonly found throughout the respiratory tract in the parenchyma of the lung and are usually associated with the epithelium. The upper airways are more densely populated with dendritic cells than the smaller airways are. The anatomical location of these cells correlates well with particle deposition in the airways.

Alveolar macrophages are found mostly in the alveolus adjacent to the epithelium and less frequently in the terminal airways and interstitial space. They migrate freely throughout the alveolar spaces and serve as a first line of defense in the lower air spaces. They readily phagocytose foreign particles and substances as well as surfactant and cellular debris from dead cells. Once a particle is engulfed, the major mechanisms for killing are typical of phagocytic cells and include O_2 radicals, enzymatic activity, and halogen derivatives within lysosomes. The ability of the alveolar macrophage to kill foreign material rapidly and without mounting an inflammatory response enhances the lung defense system immensely and is a major contributor to the overall defense system. The phagocytic activity of the alveolar macrophage inhibits the binding of particulates to the alveolar epithelium and their subsequent penetration into the interstitium. THE ALVEOLAR MACROPHAGE PROVIDES AN IMPORTANT LINK BETWEEN THE ALVEOLAR SPACES, THE ACHILLES HEEL POST–TERMINAL BRONCHIOLE REGION, AND THE MUCOCILIARY TRANSPORT SYSTEM. The alveolar macrophage can transport engulfed particles to ciliated regions of the mucociliary transport system for elimination. In addition, the alveolar macrophage can suppress T-cell activity by direct contact with the T cell or through the secretion of soluble factors, such as nitric oxide, prostaglandin E_2, and the immunosuppressive cytokines interleukin-10 and transforming growth factor-β.

BOX 32–1: FUNCTIONS OF THE DENDRITIC CELL

- Capture and process antigen
- Migrate to lymphoid tissues
- Present antigen to lymphocytes via major histocompatibility complex
- Activate lymphocytes and enhance stimulatory response
- Express lymphocyte co-stimulatory molecules
- Secrete cytokines
- Induction of tolerance

In certain circumstances, such as the inhalation of silica particles, the alveolar macrophage can phagocytose the particle but is unable to destroy it, and the macrophage eventually dies. The result is that the alveolar macrophage now has localized and concentrated silica particles in the Achilles heel region of the lung. The silica particles are not removed from this region by the mucociliary transport system and thus accumulate there and enter the lung interstitium, which leads to a granulomatous-like inflammatory response, interstitial fibrosis, and restrictive lung disease **(silicosis).** Silica is present in many work environments including foundries, mining, and photography. There is concern that silicosis may become a leading problem in occupational lung disease.

Lung epithelial cells have Toll-like receptors

The inhalation of each breath brings both nonpathogenic and pathogenic substances into the lung. Since most inhaled substances are nonpathogenic, the body has developed a recognition system to identify potentially harmful pathogenic substances. THE SYSTEM IS BASED ON THE RECOGNITION OF PATHOGEN-ASSOCIATED MOLECULAR PATTERNS (PAMPS) ON THE ORGANISM OR SUBSTANCE, WHICH IS THEN RECOGNIZED BY A FAMILY OF RECEPTORS ON HOST CELLS CALLED TOLL-LIKE RECEPTORS (TLRS). Activation of this system initiates inflammatory host defense mechanisms to fight off the pathogen. The TLRs are transmembrane proteins similar in nature to the interleukin-1 receptor. Thus far, 10 TLRs (i.e., TLRs 1 to 10) have been identified with different specificities for various pathogens. The specificity resides in the leucine-rich regions of the extracellular domain of the molecule. TLR-4 has been shown to have specificity for the gram-negative bacterial product lipopolysaccharide, whereas TLR-2 has specificity for lipoproteins associated with gram-positive bacteria. In the lung, both bronchial epithelial cells and alveolar type II epithelial cells have been shown to express TLR-2 and TLR-4. Macrophages and dendritic cells in the lung and other organs also express TLRs. Thus, in addition to classic phagocytic cells, both bronchial and alveolar epithelial cells can play active roles in host defense via the PAMP-TLR recognition system.

Summary

- The respiratory system has developed unique structural (mucociliary transport system) and immunological (mucosal immune system) features to cope with the constant environmental exposure to foreign substances in a manner that inhibits or limits an inflammatory response.
- The three components of the mucociliary transport system are the sol phase (periciliary fluid), gel phase (mucus), and cilia.
- The depth of the periciliary fluid layer is maintained by the balance between Cl^- secretion and Na^+ absorption and is essential for normal ciliary beating.
- Mucus is a complex macromolecule composed of glycoproteins, proteins, electrolytes, and water with low viscous and high elastic mechanical properties.
- Mucus is produced by goblet cells, Clara cells, and the mucous and serous cells residing in the tracheobronchial glands.
- BALT is part of the mucosa-associated lymphoid tissue system and is mainly composed of nonencapsulated aggregates of lymph nodules throughout the conducting airways.
- Specialized innate immune cells that play important roles in host defense in the lung are NK cells, NK/T cells, dendritic cells, and alveolar macrophages.
- TCRγδ cells and IgA-synthesizing plasma cells are highly specialized adaptive immune cells unique to the lung and other mucosal tissues.
- The nonciliated lymphoepithelium of BALT establishes a break in the mucociliary blanket, which acts as a "drain," facilitating the collection and immune processing of foreign particles through BALT.
- Bronchial and alveolar epithelial cells express Toll-like receptors and play an active role in host defense.

Bibliography

Armstrong L et al: Expression of functional toll-like receptor-2 and -4 on alveolar epithelial cells, *Am J Respir Cell Mol Biol* 31:241, 2004.

Banchereau J, Steinman RM: Dendritic cells and the control of immunity, *Nature* 392:245, 1998.

Charkraborty A et al: Stimulatory and inhibitory differentiation of human myeloid dendritic cells, *Clin Immunol* 94:88, 2000.

Hertz CJ et al: Activation of toll-like receptor 2 on human tracheobronchial epithelial cells induces the antimicrobial peptide human beta defensin-2, *J Immunol* 171:6820, 2003.

McMenamin C et al: Regulation of IgE responses to inhaled antigen in mice by antigen-specific γδ T cells, *Science* 265:1869, 1994.

Schramm CM et al: Proinflammatory roles of T-cell receptor (TCR) γδ and TCRαβ lymphocytes in a murine model of asthma, *Am J Respir Cell Mol Biol* 22:218, 2000.

Sheehan JK et al: The structure and heterogeneity of respiratory mucus glycoproteins, *Am Rev Respir Dis Suppl* 144:S4, 1991.

Verdugo P: Goblet cells secretion and mucogenesis, *Annu Rev Physiol* 52:157, 1990.

Wanner A, Salathe M, O'Riordan TG: Mucociliary clearance in the airways, *Am J Respir Crit Care Med* 154:1868, 1996.

Welsh MJ: Electrolyte transport by airway epithelia, *Physiol Rev* 67:1143, 1987.

Case Studies

Case 32–1

A 60-year-old woman complains of shortness of breath and a chronic cough, which have progressively increased during the past 10 years. She worked for 30 years in a metal pouring foundry making molds for sculptures. She has no history of cigarette smoking. On spirometry, her FVC and FEV_1 are reduced with a normal FEV_1/FVC. You perform a bronchoscopy (i.e., bronchoalveolar lavage and a transectional biopsy).

1. **What type of lung disease do you suspect?**
   A. Obstructive lung disease with increased goblet cells
   B. Obstructive lung disease with loss of elastic properties
   C. Restrictive lung disease secondary to infection
   D. Restrictive lung disease secondary to occupational exposure
   E. Obstructive lung disease secondary to genetic deficiency

2. **Which of the following would you expect to see on histological examination?**
   A. Interstitial hemorrhage, edema fluid, and a predominant neutrophil infiltrate
   B. A granulomatous-like lesion with interstitial fibrosis and abnormal large foamy macrophages
   C. Interstitial hemorrhage, edema fluid, and a predominant macrophage infiltrate
   D. A granulomatous-like lesion with interstitial fibrosis and a predominant neutrophil infiltrate
   E. Minimum inflammatory response with extremely large alveoli called bullae

3. **What would you expect her diffusion capacity (DLCO) and lung volume to be?**
   A. Normal
   B. Increased DLCO, normal lung volume
   C. Decreased DLCO, decreased lung volume
   D. Increased DLCO, decreased lung volume
   E. Decreased DLCO, increased lung volume

Case 32–2

A 28-year-old man with immotile cilia is referred to you by a urology clinic for a pulmonary evaluation. He has a history of chronic cough, sinus infections, and chronic ear infections. At the visit, he has no acute respiratory symptoms.

1. **What would you predict his pulmonary function test results to be?**
   A. FEV_1/FVC normal, DLCO normal
   B. FEV_1/FVC increased, DLCO increased
   C. FEV_1/FVC decreased, DLCO normal
   D. FEV_1/FVC decreased, DLCO decreased
   E. FEV_1/FVC increased, DLCO normal

2. **What would you expect to see on chest x-ray examination?**
   A. Normal lung fields, normal heart size
   B. Asymmetrical lung infiltrates, enlarged heart
   C. Symmetrical lung infiltrates, normal heart size
   D. Asymmetrical lung infiltrates, normal heart size
   E. Symmetrical lung infiltrates, enlarged heart

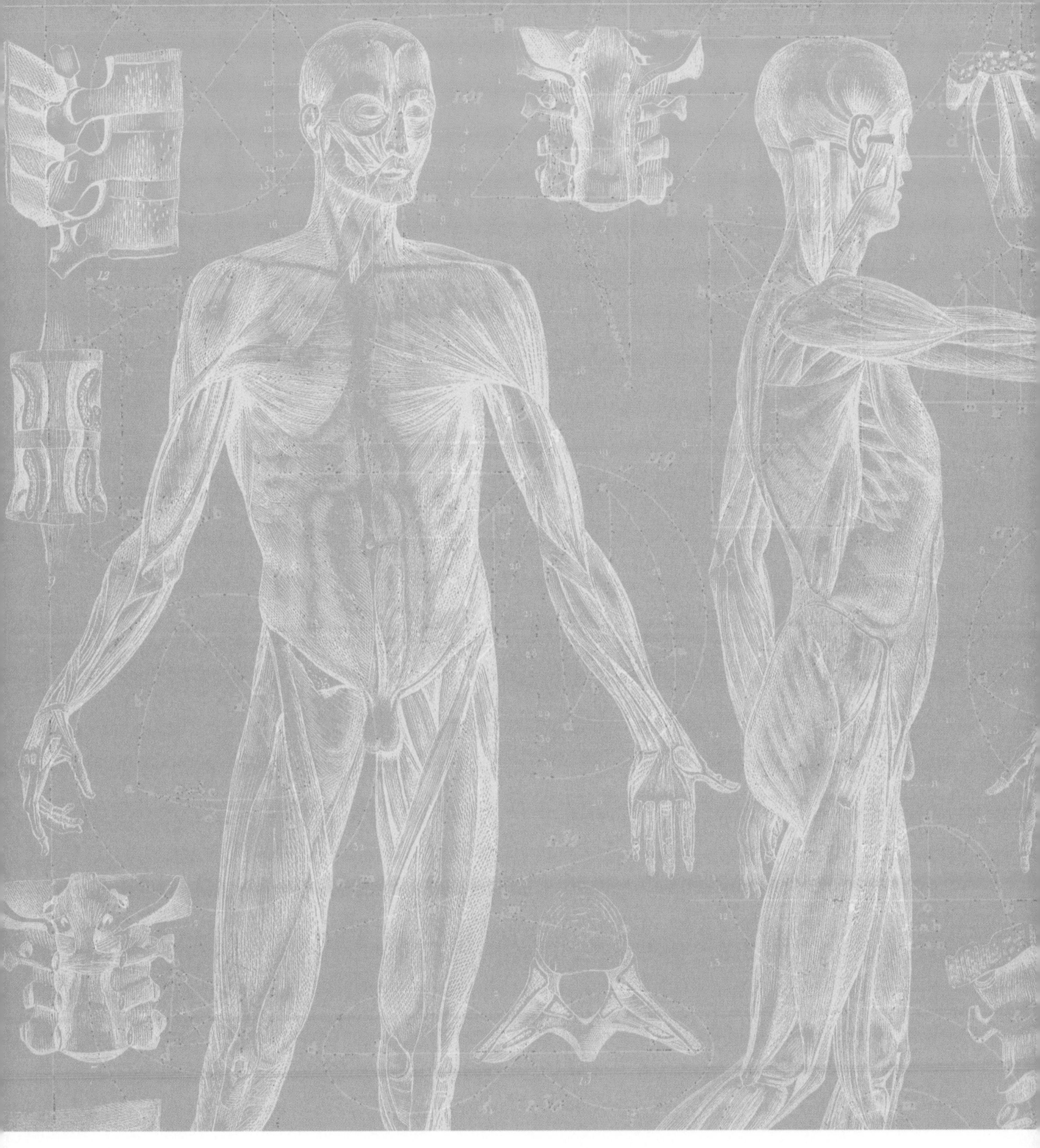

Part Six: Digestive System

Howard C. Kutchai

Chapter 33: Motility of the Gastrointestinal Tract

Objectives

- ❖ Describe the characteristics and functions of the layers of the wall of the gastrointestinal tract.
- ❖ Explain the neural control of gastrointestinal functions.
- ❖ Describe the function of slow waves.
- ❖ Describe the swallowing reflex.
- ❖ Explain the control of gastric emptying.
- ❖ Describe the contractile behavior of the small intestine.
- ❖ Describe the motility of the colon and the defecation reflex.

The digestive system consists of the gastrointestinal tract and certain associated glandular organs producing secretions that function in the gastrointestinal tract. Major subdivisions of the gastrointestinal tract include the mouth, esophagus, stomach, small intestine, and large intestine. Major glands of the digestive system include the salivary glands, the liver and gallbladder, and the pancreas. The digestive system functions to digest foodstuffs and to absorb nutrient molecules into the bloodstream. The activities by which the digestive system carries out these functions may be subdivided into motility (discussed in this chapter), secretion (see Chapter 34), and digestion and absorption (see Chapter 35). **Motility** refers to movements of the gastrointestinal tract that mix and circulate the gastrointestinal contents and propel them along the length of the tract.

The Wall of the Gastrointestinal Tract Has a Layered Structure

The structure of the gastrointestinal tract varies greatly from region to region, but common features exist in the overall organization of the tissue. **Figure 33–1** depicts the general layered structure of the gastrointestinal tract wall.

The **mucosa** consists of the epithelium, the lamina propria, and the muscularis mucosae. The **epithelium** is a single layer of specialized cells that lines the lumen of the gastrointestinal tract. The nature of the epithelium varies greatly from one part of the digestive tract to another. The **lamina propria** consists largely of loose connective tissue containing collagen and elastin fibrils. It is rich in several types of glands and contains lymph nodules and capillaries. The **muscularis mucosae** is the thin, innermost layer of intestinal smooth muscle. Contractions of the muscularis mucosae throw the mucosa into folds and ridges.

The **submucosa** consists largely of loose connective tissue with collagen and elastin fibrils. In some regions, submucosal glands are present. The larger nerve trunks and blood vessels of the intestinal wall travel in the submucosa.

The **muscularis externa** typically consists of two substantial layers of smooth muscle cells: an inner circular layer and an outer longitudinal layer. Contractions of the muscularis externa mix and

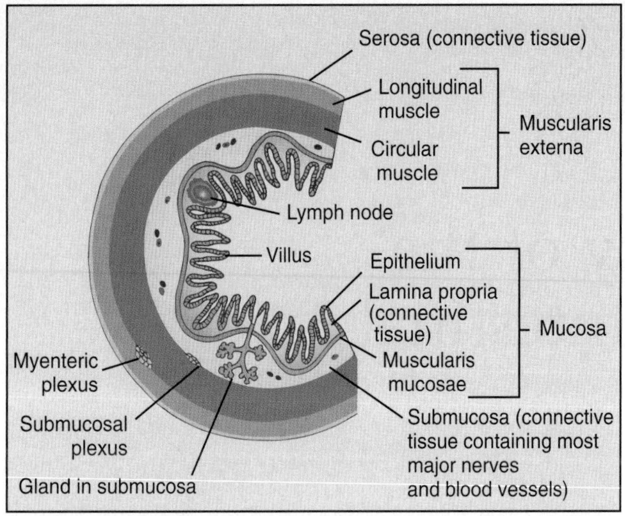

FIGURE 33–1. General organization of the layers of the gastrointestinal tract.

circulate the contents of the lumen and propel them along the gastrointestinal tract.

The wall of the gastrointestinal tract contains many neurons. A dense network of nerve cells in the submucosa is the **submucosal plexus (Meissner's plexus).** The prominent **myenteric plexus (Auerbach's plexus)** is located between the circular and longitudinal smooth muscle layers. The submucosal and myenteric plexuses, together with the other neurons of the gastrointestinal tract, constitute the **intramural plexuses** or the **enteric nervous system,** which helps integrate the motor and secretory activities of the gastrointestinal system. If the sympathetic and parasympathetic nerves to the gut are cut, many motor and secretory activities continue because these processes are controlled by the enteric nervous system.

The **serosa,** or **adventitia,** is the outermost layer. It consists mainly of connective tissue covered with a layer of squamous mesothelial cells.

The Functions of the Gastrointestinal Tract Are Regulated by Hormones, Paracrine Agonists, and Substances Released from Neurons

Hormones are produced by endocrine cells and released into the blood to reach their target cells via the circulation. Paracrine agonists are released by cells in the vicinity of the target cells and reach the target cells by diffusion. Neurocrine substances are released by neurons in the digestive system. Regulation is classified as **endocrine, paracrine,** or **neurocrine,** depending on the cell type that produces the regulatory substance and the substance's route of delivery to the target cell (see Chapter 5).

MUCH HORMONAL AND NEURAL REGULATION IS INTRINSIC TO THE GASTROINTESTINAL TRACT. That is, the cells that regulate and the cells that respond reside in the gastrointestinal tract. However, gastrointestinal functions are also controlled by hormones released by cells outside the gastrointestinal tract and by neurons whose cell bodies lie outside the gastrointestinal tract. The overlapping layers of intrinsic and extrinsic hormonal and neural control allow the subtle and precise control of gastrointestinal functions.

Hormones and paracrine mediators influence gastrointestinal functions

Endocrine cells in the mucosa or submucosa of the stomach and intestine and in the pancreas produce an array of hormones **(Table 33–1)**. Some of these act on secretory cells located in the wall of the gastrointestinal tract, in the pancreas, or in the liver to alter the rate or the composition of their secretions (see Chapter 34). Other hormones act on smooth muscle cells in particular segments of the gastrointestinal tract, on gastrointestinal sphincters, or on the musculature of the gallbladder (see Chapter 34).

Paracrine substances also regulate the secretory and motor functions of the gastrointestinal tract. For example, histamine released from cells in the wall of the stomach is a key physiological agonist of HCl secretion by gastric parietal cells (see Chapter 34).

The gastrointestinal mucosal immune system also regulates motor and secretory activities of the digestive tract

Other paracrine agonists are released by cells of the **gastrointestinal immune system.** The mass of cells with immune function in the gastrointestinal tract is approximately equal to the combined mass of immunocytes in the rest of the body. The mucosal immune system secretes antibodies in response to certain food antigens and mounts an immunological defense against many pathogenic microorganisms. Remarkably, the mucosal immune system is typically **tolerant** of most of the foreign proteins ingested in food.

The components of the gastrointestinal immune system include cells in mesenteric lymph nodes, **Peyer's patches** in the wall of the intestine, and immunocytes in the mucosa and submucosa **(Figure 33–2)**. Among the cells with immune function in the mucosa and submucosa are intraepithelial lymphocytes, B and T cells, plasma cells, mast

TABLE 33–1. GASTROINTESTINAL HORMONES: HORMONES PRODUCED BY CELLS IN THE GASTROINTESTINAL TRACT AND THE PANCREAS

Location of Cells That Produce the Hormone	Hormone	Cells That Produce the Hormone
Stomach	Gastrin	G
	Somatostatin	D
Duodenum or jejunum	Secretin	S
	Cholecystokinin (CCK)	I
	Motilin	M
	*Gastric inhibitory peptide (GIP)	K
	Somatostatin	D
Pancreatic islets	Insulin	β
	Glucagon	α
	Pancreatic polypeptide	PP
	Somatostatin	D
Ileum or colon	Enteroglucagon	L
	Peptide YY	L
	Neurotensin	N
	Somatostatin	D

*GIP is also known as **glucose-dependent insulinotropic peptide** because it stimulates insulin secretion. GIP may be more potent in this action than it is as an inhibitor of gastric motility and secretion. Gastrin, cholecystokinin, secretin, gastric inhibitory peptide, and motilin have physiological roles in the gastrointestinal system. The physiological roles of the other listed hormones remain to be explained.

cells, macrophages, and eosinophils. **Inflammatory mediators** such as histamine, prostaglandins, leukotrienes, cytokines, and others are released by immunocytes in the mucosa and submucosa. These substances diffuse to secretory and smooth muscle cells in the gastrointestinal tract to affect their activities and modulate the function of certain neurons in the gastrointestinal tract.

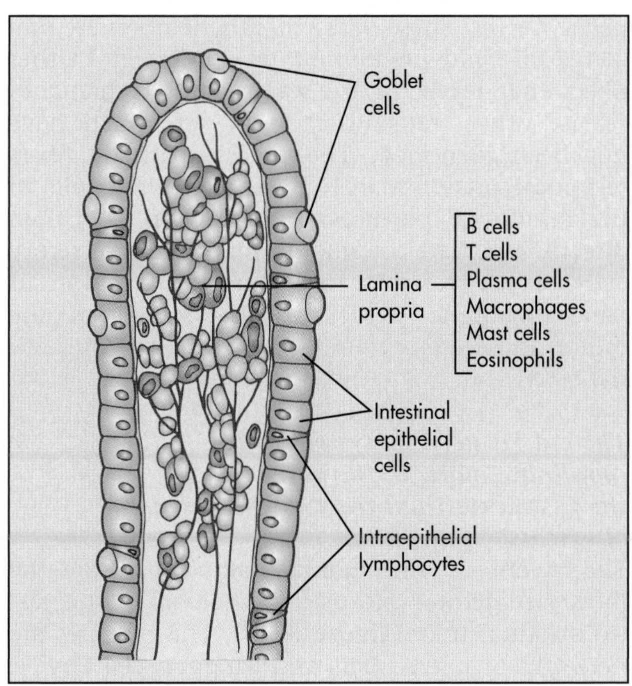

FIGURE 33–2. Small intestinal villus showing intraepithelial lymphocytes and various immunocytes in the lamina propria. (Modified from Kagnoff MF. In Sleisenger MH, Fordtran JS, eds: *Gastrointestinal disease,* ed 5, Philadelphia, 1993, WB Saunders.)

Important diseases involve hyperactivity of the gastrointestinal immune system. Patients with **celiac disease,** also known as **celiac sprue** and **gluten enteropathy,** mount an allergic response to gliadin, a component of gluten in wheat flour. As a consequence, the villi become shortened and microvilli become much less numerous, so that the absorptive surface of the small intestine is markedly decreased, and thus multiple nutrients may be poorly absorbed. Celiac disease is best treated with a diet that excludes gluten. **Inflammatory bowel disease** is characterized by an increased population of lymphocytes and macrophages in the lamina propria, where T lymphocytes are involved in causing inflammation. The chronic inflammation of the intestine in most cases results in diarrhea and abdominal pain. The most common inflammatory bowel diseases are ulcerative colitis and Crohn's disease. Ulcerative colitis is confined to the colon and can usually be cured by surgical removal of the affected section of colon. Crohn's disease, by contrast, can occur in any part of the small or large intestine and sometimes involves both the small intestine and the colon. In Crohn's disease, if the inflamed segment of bowel is removed, the disease is likely to recur elsewhere.

The gastrointestinal tract has both autonomic and intrinsic innervation

The gastrointestinal tract is innervated by the sympathetic and parasympathetic nervous systems (extrinsic innervation) and by the neurons of the enteric nervous system (intrinsic innervation). The interplay between local control by enteric neurons and regulation by the parasympathetic and sympathetic systems, as well as responses by the mucosal immune system, allows fine control of gastrointestinal functions.

Sympathetic innervation of the gastrointestinal tract is mainly via postganglionic adrenergic fibers

Postganglionic sympathetic fibers, whose cell bodies are in prevertebral and paravertebral ganglia **(Figure 33–3)**, innervate the gastrointestinal tract. The celiac, superior and inferior mesenteric, and hypogastric plexuses provide sympathetic innervation to various segments of the gastrointestinal tract. MOST OF THE SYMPATHETIC FIBERS DO NOT DIRECTLY INNERVATE STRUCTURES IN THE GASTROINTESTINAL TRACT BUT RATHER TERMINATE ON NEURONS IN THE INTRAMURAL PLEXUSES. Some vasoconstrictor sympathetic fibers directly innervate the blood vessels of the gastrointestinal tract. Other sympathetic fibers innervate glandular structures in the wall of the gut.

Stimulation of sympathetic input to the gastrointestinal tract inhibits motor activity of the muscularis externa but stimulates contraction of the muscularis mucosae and certain sphincters. The sympathetic nerves do not directly inhibit contractions of the muscularis because few sympathetic nerve endings lie in the muscularis externa. Rather, the sympathetic nerves influence neural circuits in the enteric nervous system, and these circuits provide input to the smooth muscle cells. The sympathetic nerves may reinforce this effect by reducing blood flow to the muscularis externa. Other fibers that travel with the sympathetic nerves may be cholinergic; still others release noncholinergic neurotransmitters. In general, activation of sympathetic nerves also reduces secretory activity of the gastrointestinal tract.

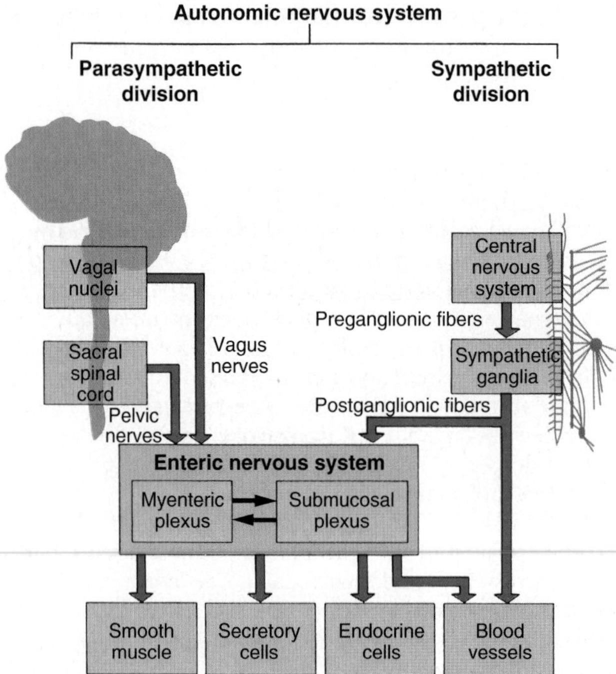

FIGURE 33–3. Major features of the autonomic innervation of the gastrointestinal tract. In most cases, the autonomic nerves influence the functions of the gastrointestinal tract by modulating the activities of the neurons of the enteric nervous system.

Parasympathetic innervation of most of the gastrointestinal tract is via branches of the vagus nerves

Parasympathetic innervation of the gastrointestinal tract down to the level of the transverse colon is provided by branches of the vagus nerves (Figure 33–3). The remainder of the colon, the rectum, and the anus receive parasympathetic fibers from the pelvic nerves. These parasympathetic fibers are preganglionic and predominantly cholinergic. Other fibers that travel in the vagus and its branches release other transmitters, some of which have not been identified. The parasympathetic fibers terminate predominantly on the ganglion cells in the intramural plexuses. The ganglion cells then directly innervate the smooth muscle and secretory cells of the gastrointestinal tract. Excitation of parasympathetic nerves usually stimulates the motor and secretory activities of the gastrointestinal tract.

The enteric nervous system can coordinate many of the activities of the gastrointestinal tract in the absence of extrinsic innervation

The myenteric and submucosal plexuses are the most well-defined plexuses in the wall of the gastrointestinal tract **(Figure 33–4)**. The plexuses are networks of nerve fibers and ganglion cell bodies. Interneurons in the plexuses connect afferent sensory fibers with efferent neurons to smooth muscle and secretory cells to form reflex arcs that are wholly within the wall of the gastrointestinal tract. Consequently, the myenteric and submucosal plexuses can coordinate activity in the absence of extrinsic innervation of the gastrointestinal tract. Axons of plexus neurons innervate gland cells in

TABLE 33–2. TYPES OF NEURONS IN THE ENTERIC NERVOUS SYSTEM*

Type of Neuron	Function
Motor neurons	
Motor neurons to muscle cells	
Excitatory	Promote contraction of smooth muscle
Inhibitory	Inhibit contraction of smooth muscle
Motor neurons to blood vessels	Vasodilator neurons
Motor neurons to epithelial cells	Promote secretion of electrolytes and water
Motor neurons to gland cells	Promote secretion of specific substances
Motor neurons to endocrine cells	Promote secretion of hormones
Sensory neurons	Respond to stretch or to chemical stimuli
Associative neurons	Interneurons in motor, secretomotor, and vasomotor pathways
Intestinofugal neurons	Neurons with cell bodies in enteric ganglia and nerve terminals in sympathetic ganglia

*The cell bodies of these neurons are in submucosal and myenteric ganglia.

the mucosa and submucosa, smooth muscle cells in the muscularis externa and muscularis mucosae, and intramural endocrine and exocrine cells. The major classes of neurons present in the enteric nervous system and their functions are summarized in **Table 33–2.**

The myenteric and submucosal plexuses are interconnected to coordinate motor and secretory or absorptive activity of the gastrointestinal tract. However, in general, the myenteric plexus is primarily involved in the regulation of motility; the submucosal plexus is primarily involved in the regulation of secretion and absorption (see later).

Reflex control of the gastrointestinal tract occurs via local and central reflex pathways

AFFERENT FIBERS IN THE GASTROINTESTINAL TRACT PROVIDE THE AFFERENT LIMBS OF BOTH LOCAL AND CENTRAL REFLEX ARCS **(Figure 33–5). Chemoreceptor** and **mechanoreceptor** endings are present in the mucosa and muscularis externa. The cell bodies of many of these sensory receptors are located in the myenteric and submucosal plexuses. The axons of some of these receptor cells synapse with other cells in the plexuses to mediate local reflex activity. Other sensory receptors send their axons back to the central nervous system. The complex afferent and efferent innervation of the gastrointestinal tract allows fine control of secretory and motor activities.

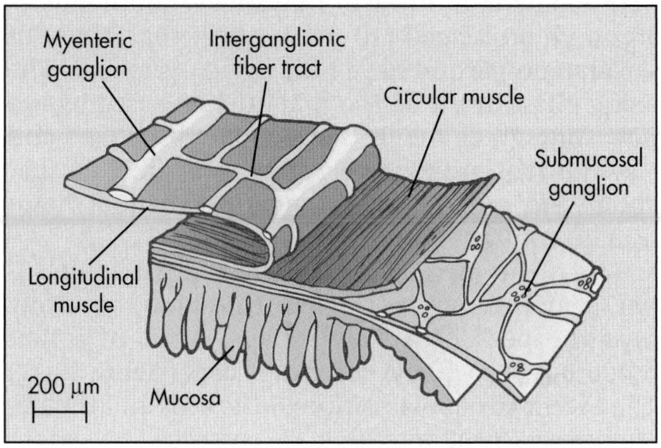

FIGURE 33–4. Enteric neurons of the submucosal and myenteric plexuses in the wall of the gastrointestinal tract. The plexuses consist of ganglia interconnected by fiber tracts. (Modified from Furness JB, Costal M: *Neuroscience* 5:1, 1980.)

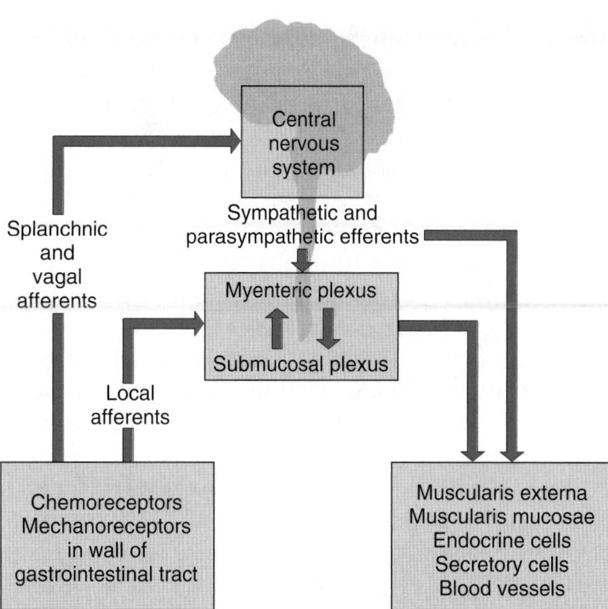

FIGURE 33–5. Local and central reflex pathways in the gastrointestinal system.

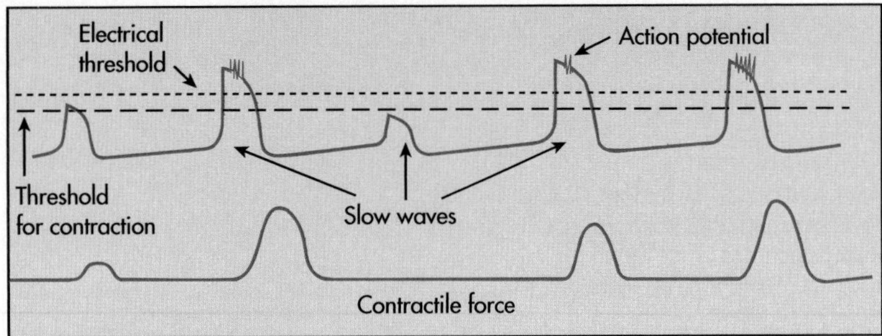

FIGURE 33–6. Contraction of small intestinal smooth muscle occurs when the depolarization caused by the slow wave exceeds a threshold for contraction. When depolarization of a slow wave exceeds the electrical threshold, a burst of action potentials occurs. Action potentials elicit much stronger contractions than occur in the absence of action potentials.

Gastrointestinal Smooth Muscle Cells Have Unique Mechanical and Electrophysiological Properties

The general properties of smooth muscle are discussed in Chapter 14. The smooth muscle cells of the gastrointestinal tract are long (about 500 μm) and slender (5 to 20 μm across). They are arranged in bundles that are separated and defined by connective tissues.

Oscillations of the resting membrane potential of gastrointestinal smooth muscle are called slow waves

The resting membrane potential of gastrointestinal smooth muscle is typically smaller than that of skeletal muscle. The resting membrane potential of gastrointestinal smooth muscle cells ranges from approximately −40 to −80 mV. The electrogenic Na^+,K^+-ATPase (see Chapter 2) contributes significantly to the resting membrane potential in smooth muscle. In guinea pig taenia coli, for example, about one third of the resting membrane potential results from the electrogenicity of Na^+,K^+-ATPase.

In most other excitable tissues, the resting membrane potential is rather constant. In gastrointestinal smooth muscle, the resting membrane potential typically varies over time. Oscillations of the resting membrane potential, called **slow waves** (also known as the **basic electrical rhythm**), are characteristic of gastrointestinal smooth muscle (**Figure 33–6**). The frequency of slow waves varies from about 3 per minute in the stomach to 12 per minute in the duodenum.

Slow waves are generated by **interstitial cells** (also known as interstitial cells of Cajal), which have properties of both fibroblasts and smooth muscle cells. A thin layer of interstitial cells is located between the longitudinal and circular layers of muscularis externa. Processes of the interstitial cells form gap junctions with longitudinal and circular smooth muscle cells. These gap junctions enable the slow waves to be conducted rapidly to both muscle layers. Because the smooth muscle cells of both longitudinal and circular layers are well coupled electrically (the cells of the circular layer are more highly coupled than those of the longitudinal layer), the slow wave spreads throughout the smooth muscle of each segment of the gastrointestinal tract.

The amplitude and, to a lesser extent, the frequency of the slow waves can be modulated by the activity of intrinsic and extrinsic nerves and by circulating hormones. In general, sympathetic nerve activity decreases the amplitude of the slow waves or abolishes them, whereas stimulation of parasympathetic nerves increases the size of the slow waves. IF THE PEAK OF THE SLOW WAVE IS ABOVE THRESHOLD FOR THE CELLS TO FIRE ACTION POTENTIALS, ONE OR MORE ACTION POTENTIALS MAY BE TRIGGERED DURING THE PEAK OF THE SLOW WAVE (Figure 33–6).

Ca^{++} enters smooth muscle cells during action potentials that may occur on the crests of the slow waves

Action potentials in gastrointestinal smooth muscle are more prolonged (10 to 20 msec) than those of skeletal muscle and have little or no overshoot. The rising phase of the action potential is caused by ion flow through channels that conduct both Ca^{++} and Na^+ and that are relatively slow to open. Ca^{++} that enters the cell during the action potential helps initiate contraction.

When the membrane potential of gastrointestinal smooth muscle reaches threshold, typically near the peak of a slow wave, a train of action potentials (1 to 10 per second) occurs (Figure 33–6). The extent of depolarization of the cells and the frequency of action potentials are enhanced by certain hormones and compounds liberated from excitatory nerve endings. Inhibitory hormones and neuroeffector substances hyperpolarize the smooth muscle cells and may abolish action potential spikes.

Action potentials greatly increase the force of contractions of gastrointestinal smooth muscle cells

In the example shown in Figure 33–6, slow waves without action potentials elicit weak contractions of the smooth muscle layers. Much stronger contractions are evoked by the action potentials intermittently triggered near the peaks of the slow waves. THE GREATER THE NUMBER OF ACTION POTENTIALS OCCURRING AT THE PEAK OF A SLOW WAVE, THE MORE INTENSE THE CONTRACTION OF THE SMOOTH MUSCLE. Because smooth muscle cells contract rather slowly (about one tenth as fast as skeletal muscle), the individual contractions caused by each action potential in a burst are not visible as distinct twitches; rather, they sum temporally to produce a smoothly increasing level of tension (Figure 33–6).

Between bursts of action potentials, the tension developed by gastrointestinal smooth muscle falls, but not to zero. This nonzero resting, or baseline, tension developed by the smooth muscle is called **tone.** The tone of gastrointestinal smooth muscle is altered by neuroeffectors, hormones, and drugs.

The Enteric Nervous System Functions as a Semiautonomous "Enteric Brain"

The enteric nervous system directly controls the patterns of muscular and secretory activities, but contraction and secretion are also regulated more indirectly by the autonomic nervous system. The neurons of the intramural plexuses send axons to the smooth muscle layers, and each axon may branch extensively to innervate many smooth muscle cells. Neuromuscular interactions in the gastrointestinal tract do not involve true neuromuscular junctions with specialization of the postjunctional membrane, as occurs at neuromuscular junctions in skeletal muscle. The circular smooth muscle layer of the muscularis externa is heavily innervated by excitatory and inhibitory motor nerve terminals closely associated with the plasma membranes of the smooth muscle cells. Longitudinal smooth muscle cells are much less richly innervated by the neurons of the intrinsic plexuses than the cells of the circular layer, and the neuromuscular contacts are not so intimate.

The enteric nervous system of the large and small intestines alone contains about 10^8 neurons, about as many neurons as in the spinal cord. Figure 33–4 depicts the myenteric and submucosal plexuses and their locations in the wall of the intestine. Both plexuses consist of ganglia that are interconnected by tracts of fine, unmyelinated nerve fibers. The neurons in the ganglia include sensory neurons, with their sensory endings in the wall of the gastrointestinal tract. These sensory endings respond to mechanical deformation, particular chemical stimuli, and temperature. Some of the neurons in the enteric ganglia are effector neurons that send axons to smooth muscle cells of the circular or longitudinal layers, secretory cells of the gastrointestinal tract, or gastrointestinal blood vessels. Many of the neurons in the enteric ganglia are interneurons that are part of the network of neurons integrating the sensory input to the ganglia and formulating the output of the effector neurons.

A large number of neuromodulatory substances are present in enteric neurons. Most of the neuromodulatory substances that function in the central nervous system (see Chapter 4) are also present in the gastrointestinal tract. **Table 33–3** summarizes information about neurotransmitters and neuromodulators in the enteric nervous system.

Many neurons in myenteric ganglia are motor neurons that excite or inhibit the smooth muscle cells of the muscularis externa

Excitatory motor neurons release **acetylcholine** onto muscarinic receptors on the smooth muscle cells; they also release **substance P.** Inhibitory motor neurons release **vasoactive intestinal polypeptide** (VIP) and **nitric oxide** (NO). About one third of neurons in myenteric ganglia are sensory. Other myenteric neurons project to neurons in submucosal ganglia. Most myenteric interneurons release acetylcholine onto nicotinic receptors on motor neurons or on other interneurons.

Many neurons in submucosal ganglia regulate secretion by glandular, endocrine, and epithelial cells

Stimulatory secretomotor neurons release acetylcholine and VIP onto gland cells or epithelial cells. The numerous sensory neurons in submucosal ganglia respond to chemical stimuli or mechanical deformation of the mucosa, and they are the afferent limbs of secretomotor reflexes. Submucosal interneurons release acetylcholine onto other neurons in submucosal ganglia or project to myenteric ganglia. Submucosal ganglia also contain vasodilator neurons that release acetylcholine, VIP, or both products onto submucosal blood vessels.

TABLE 33–3. SUBSTANCES THAT FUNCTION OR MAY FUNCTION AS NEUROTRANSMITTERS IN THE ENTERIC NERVOUS SYSTEM

Substance	Location and Function
Established and probable neurotransmitters	
Acetylcholine (ACh)	Excitatory transmitter to smooth muscle, intestinal epithelial cells, parietal cells, and certain endocrine cells and at neuron-neuron synapses
Adenosine triphosphate (ATP)	Inhibitory transmitter to smooth muscle
Calcitonin gene–related peptide (CGRP)	Released by enteric sensory neurons onto interneurons in enteric ganglia and central ganglia
Gastrin-releasing peptide	Released by secretomotor neurons onto G cells
Nitric oxide (NO)	Inhibitory transmitter to smooth muscle cells
Substance P (and other tachykinins)	Excitatory transmitter to smooth muscle cells
Vasoactive intestinal polypeptide (VIP)	Inhibitory transmitter to smooth muscle cells, excitatory secretomotor transmitter to epithelial and gland cells, vasodilator transmitter
Present in neurons, but transmitter function not established	
Cholecystokinin (CCK)	Present in some secretomotor neurons and interneurons, may contribute to excitation
Dynorphin and related peptides	Present in some secretomotor neurons, interneurons, and motor neurons to muscle
Enkephalins and related peptides	Present in some interneurons and in motor neurons to smooth muscle
Galanin	Present in some secretomotor neurons, interneurons, and inhibitory motor neurons to smooth muscle
Glutamate	May be an excitatory transmitter at synapses between enteric neurons
γ-Aminobutyric acid (GABA)	Present, but transmitter role is not known
Neuropeptide Y	May inhibit secretion of electrolytes and water
Serotonin (5-HT)	May be excitatory transmitter at synapses between enteric neurons
Somatostatin	Present in numerous enteric neurons, but transmitter role is not established

There are apparently no inhibitory secretomotor neurons in the enteric nervous system.

The component cells of intrinsic reflexes are all located in the walls of the gastrointestinal tract

Numerous intrinsic reflexes control the motor and secretory activities of each segment of the gastrointestinal tract. A well-characterized intrinsic reflex is shown in **Figure 33–7.** LOCALIZED MECHANICAL OR CHEMICAL STIMULATION OF THE INTESTINAL MUCOSA ELICITS CONTRACTION ABOVE (ORAL TO) AND RELAXATION BELOW (ANAL TO) THE POINT OF STIMULATION. Many sensory stimuli to the mucosa release **serotonin (5-HT)** from mucosal enterochromaffin cells. 5-HT stimulates the mucosal endings of sensory neurons. The sensory neurons release **CGRP (calcitonin gene–related peptide)** onto interneurons in the submucosal and myenteric plexuses. The interneurons then activate excitatory motor neurons above the point of stimulation and inhibitory neurons below the point of stimulation. The excitatory neurons release acetylcholine and substance P and the inhibitory neurons release VIP and NO onto intestinal smooth muscle cells.

Chewing Is Frequently a Reflex Behavior

Chewing can be carried out voluntarily, but it is more frequently a reflex behavior. Chewing lubricates food by mixing it with salivary mucus, mixes starch-containing food with salivary amylase, and subdivides food so that it can be mixed more readily with the digestive secretions of the stomach and duodenum.

Swallowing Is Accomplished via a Complex Reflex

Swallowing can be initiated voluntarily, but thereafter it is almost entirely under reflex control. THE SWALLOWING REFLEX IS A RIGIDLY ORDERED SEQUENCE OF EVENTS THAT PROPELS FOOD FROM THE MOUTH TO THE STOMACH. During swallowing, respiration is reflexly inhibited, thereby preventing the entrance of food into the trachea. The afferent limb of the swallowing reflex begins with touch receptors, most notably those near the opening of the pharynx. Sensory impulses from these receptors are transmitted to certain areas in the medulla. The central

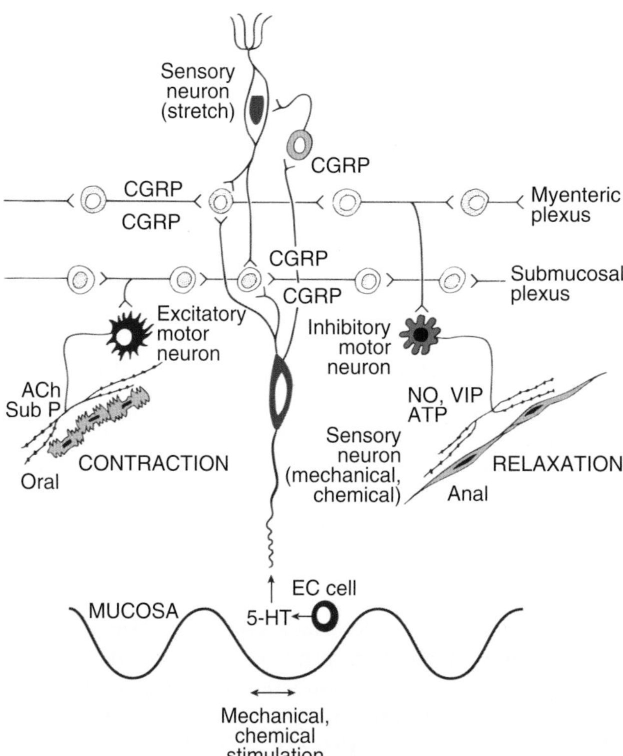

FIGURE 33–7. Localized mechanical or chemical stimulation of the intestinal mucosa or stretch of the muscularis externa typically elicits contraction above and relaxation below the point of stimulation. The figure depicts the neuronal circuitry responsible for this reflex. In the center of the figure are two sensory neurons: a stretch-sensitive neuron with soma in the myenteric plexus (white cytoplasm, colored nucleus) and a chemosensitive or mechanosensitive neuron whose soma is in the submucosal plexus. Stimulation of either of these sensory neurons results in ascending (oral) excitation and descending (anal) inhibition of contraction of the smooth muscle of muscularis externa. Stimuli to the mucosa evoke release of serotonin (5-HT) from enterochromaffin (EC) cells in the mucosa. Sensory neurons are stimulated by 5-HT. The myenteric stretch receptors, by contrast, respond directly to stretch. Sensory neurons release predominantly CGRP (calcitonin gene–related peptide) onto interneurons in the enteric plexuses. ACh, acetylcholine; NO, nitric oxide; Sub P, substance P; VIP, vasoactive intestinal polypeptide.

integrating areas for swallowing lie in the medulla and lower pons; these areas are collectively called the **swallowing center.** Motor impulses travel from the swallowing center to the musculature of the pharynx and upper esophagus via various cranial nerves and to the remainder of the esophagus via vagal motor neurons.

The oral phase of swallowing is voluntary

The **oral phase** of swallowing is initiated when the tip of the tongue separates a bolus of food from the mass in the mouth. The bolus to be swallowed is moved upward and backward in the mouth by pressing first the tip of the tongue and later the more posterior portions of the tongue against the hard palate. This forces the bolus into the pharynx, where the bolus stimulates the tactile receptors that initiate the swallowing reflex.

The pharyngeal phase of swallowing propels food from the pharynx into the esophagus

The **pharyngeal phase** of swallowing involves the following sequence of events, which occurs in less than 1 second:

1. The soft palate is pulled upward, and the palatopharyngeal folds move inward toward one another. This prevents the reflux of food into the nasopharynx and provides a narrow passage through which food moves into the pharynx.
2. The vocal cords are pulled together. The larynx is moved forward and upward against the epiglottis. These actions prevent food from entering the trachea and help open the upper esophageal sphincter.
3. The upper esophageal sphincter relaxes to receive the bolus of food **(Figure 33–8)**. The pharyngeal superior constrictor muscles then contract strongly to force the bolus deeply into the pharynx.
4. A **peristaltic wave** is initiated with contraction of the pharyngeal superior constrictor muscles, and the wave moves toward the esophagus (Figure 33–8). This forces the bolus of food through the relaxed **upper esophageal sphincter.**

DURING THE PHARYNGEAL STAGE OF SWALLOWING, RESPIRATION IS REFLEXLY INHIBITED.

The esophageal phase of swallowing involves the body of the esophagus and both esophageal sphincters

The **esophageal phase** of swallowing is controlled mainly by the swallowing center. After the bolus of food passes the upper esophageal sphincter, the sphincter reflexly constricts. A peristaltic wave then begins just below the upper esophageal sphincter and traverses the entire esophagus in less than 10 seconds (Figure 33–8). This initial wave, called **primary peristalsis,** is controlled by the swallowing center. The peristaltic wave travels down the

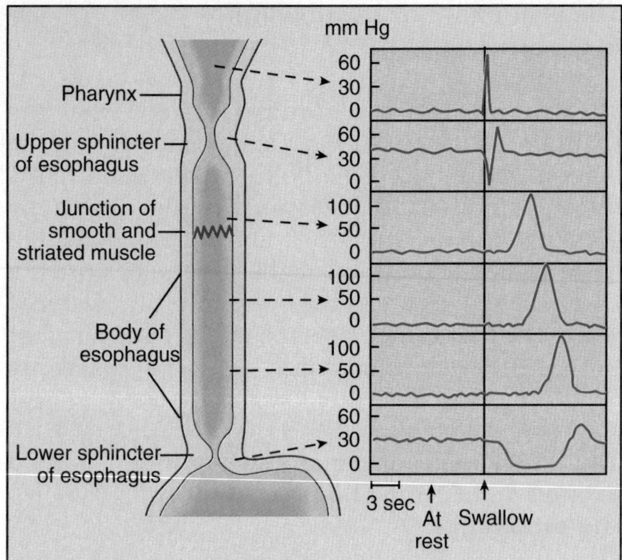

FIGURE 33–8. Pressures in the pharynx, esophagus, and esophageal sphincters during swallowing. Note the reflex relaxation of the upper and lower esophageal sphincters and the timing of the relaxation. (Data from Christensen JL. In Christensen JL, Wingate DL, eds: *A guide to gastrointestinal motility,* Bristol, England, 1983, John Wright & Sons.)

esophagus at 3 to 5 cm/sec. THE **LOWER ESOPHAGEAL SPHINCTER** RELAXES EARLY IN THE ESOPHAGEAL PHASE AND REMAINS RELAXED UNTIL FOOD IS DRIVEN THROUGH IT BY THE ESOPHAGEAL PERISTALTIC WAVE (Figure 33–8).

If primary peristalsis is insufficient to clear the esophagus of food, distention of the esophagus initiates another peristaltic wave, called **secondary peristalsis,** which begins above the site of distention and moves downward. Input from esophageal sensory fibers to the central and enteric nervous systems modulates both primary and secondary esophageal peristalsis.

The Esophagus Moves Food from the Pharynx to the Stomach

In the upper third of the esophagus, both the inner circular and the outer longitudinal muscle layers are striated. In the lower third, the muscle layers are composed entirely of smooth muscle cells. In the middle third, skeletal and smooth muscles coexist, with a gradient from all skeletal muscle above to all smooth muscle below. The esophageal musculature, both striated and smooth, is innervated mainly by branches of the vagus nerve. Somatic motor fibers of the vagus nerves form motor end plates on striated muscle fibers. Visceral motor nerves are preganglionic parasympathetic fibers that synapse primarily on the nerve cells of the myenteric plexus. Neurons of the myenteric plexus directly innervate the smooth muscle cells of the esophagus and communicate with one another.

The upper and lower esophageal sphincters prevent the entry of air and gastric contents, respectively, into the esophagus. The lower esophageal sphincter opens when a wave of esophageal peristalsis begins (Figure 33–8). The opening of the lower esophageal sphincter is mediated by impulses in branches of the vagus nerves. In the absence of esophageal peristalsis, the sphincter must remain tightly closed to prevent reflux of the gastric contents, which would cause esophagitis and the sensation of heartburn.

In individuals with **incompetence of the lower esophageal sphincter,** gastric juice can **reflux** (move back up) into the lower esophagus and cause erosion of the esophageal mucosa. This syndrome is known as **gastroesophageal reflux disease** or **GERD.** Reflux can be a problem because the pressure in the thoracic esophagus is close to intrathoracic pressure, which is usually less than intraabdominal pressure. The difference between intraabdominal and intrathoracic pressures increases during each inspiration (see Chapter 28). The reflux of gastric contents up into the esophagus is opposed by the lower esophageal sphincter. In addition, because the crura of the diaphragm wrap around the esophagus at the level of the lower esophageal sphincter, contraction of the diaphragm increases the pressure in the lower esophageal sphincter with each inspiration. Weakness of the diaphragm or **hiatal hernia** can exacerbate incompetence of the lower esophageal sphincter.

The lower esophageal sphincter is controlled by nerves and hormones

The resting pressure in the lower esophageal sphincter is about 30 mm Hg. The tonic contraction of the circular musculature of the sphincter is regulated by nerves, both intrinsic and extrinsic, and by hormones and neuromodulators. A significant fraction of basal tone in this sphincter is mediated by vagal cholinergic nerves. Stimulation of sympathetic nerves to the sphincter also causes the lower esophageal sphincter to contract.

Vagal inhibitory fibers relax the lower esophageal sphincter. The intrinsic and extrinsic innervation of the lower esophageal sphincter is both excitatory and inhibitory. A major component of the sphincter's relaxation that occurs in response to primary peristalsis in the esophagus is mediated by noncholinergic vagal fibers inhibitory to the circular muscle of the lower esophageal sphincter, perhaps through the release of VIP or NO.

In some individuals, the sphincter fails to relax sufficiently during swallowing, so food may not be able to enter the stomach. This condition is known as **achalasia.** Therapy for achalasia may involve mechanical dilation or surgical weakening of the lower esophageal sphincter or administration of drugs that inhibit the tone of the lower esophageal sphincter. Individuals with **diffuse esophageal spasm** have prolonged and painful contraction of the lower part of the esophagus instead of the normal esophageal peristaltic wave after swallowing.

Contractions of the Stomach Mix and Propel Gastric Contents

Gastric motility allows the stomach to serve as a reservoir for the large volume of food that may be ingested at a single meal, to fragment food into smaller particles and mix the food with gastric secretions so that digestion can begin, and to empty gastric contents into the duodenum at a controlled rate. The **fundus** and the **body** of the stomach (**Figure 33–9**) can accommodate volume increases as large as 1.5 L without a great increase in intragastric pressure; the phenomenon is called **receptive relaxation.** Contractions of the fundus and body are normally weak, so much of the gastric contents remains relatively unmixed for long periods. Thus, the fundus and body of the stomach serve as reservoirs. In the antrum, however, contractions are vigorous and thoroughly mix antral chyme with gastric juice and subdivide food into smaller particles. The antral contractions empty the gastric contents in small squirts into the duodenal bulb. The rate of gastric emptying is adjusted by several mechanisms so that chyme is not delivered to the duodenum too rapidly. The physiological mechanisms that underlie this behavior are discussed later.

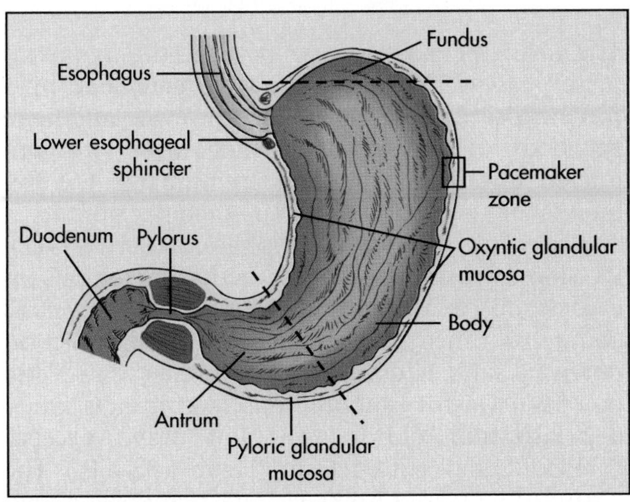

FIGURE 33–9. Major anatomical and functional subdivisions of the stomach.

Structure and extrinsic innervation of the stomach

The basic structure of the gastric wall follows the scheme presented in Figure 33–1. However, the muscularis externa of the stomach has a third, obliquely oriented layer between the circular and longitudinal layers. Also, the circular muscle layer of muscularis externa is more prominent than the longitudinal layer. The muscularis externa of the fundus and body is relatively thin, but that of the antrum is considerably thicker, and the thickness increases toward the pylorus.

The stomach is richly innervated by extrinsic nerves and by the neurons of the enteric nervous system. Axons from the cells of the intramural plexuses innervate the smooth muscle and secretory cells.

Parasympathetic innervation is by the vagus nerves, and sympathetic innervation is from the celiac plexus. In general, parasympathetic nerves stimulate gastric smooth muscle motility and gastric secretions, whereas sympathetic activity inhibits these functions. Numerous sensory afferent fibers leave the stomach in the vagus nerves, and some travel with sympathetic nerves. Other fibers are the afferent links of intrinsic reflex arcs via the intramural plexuses of the stomach. Some of these afferent fibers relay information about intragastric pressure, gastric distention, intragastric pH, or pain.

The body and fundus relax in response to gastric filling

When a wave of esophageal peristalsis begins, the lower esophageal sphincter reflexly relaxes. This is followed by receptive relaxation of the fundus and body of the stomach. The stomach also relaxes if it is directly filled with gas or liquid. The nerve fibers in the vagi are a major efferent pathway for reflex relaxation of the stomach. The vagal fibers that mediate this response release VIP as their transmitter.

Before effective drugs for blocking gastric acid secretion were available, it was common to treat duodenal ulcers by cutting the vagus nerves to the stomach (vagotomy) to diminish the rate of gastric acid secretion. This procedure also eliminates the efferent pathway of the receptive relaxation reflex so that in response to ingestion of a meal, intragastric pressure increases to a much greater level than normal. The accelerated emptying of gastric contents that results is known as the **dumping syndrome.** In this disorder, gastric contents are emptied into the small intestine faster than they can be processed; thus, these patients often develop chronic diarrhea.

The rate of emptying of gastric contents depends on their physical properties

The muscle layers in the fundus and body are thin; weak contractions characterize these parts of the stomach. As a result, the contents of the fundus and the body tend to form layers based on the density of the contents. Gastric contents may remain unmixed for as long as an hour after eating. Fats tend to form an oily layer on top of the other gastric contents. Consequently, fats are emptied later than other gastric contents. Liquids can flow around the mass of food contained in the body of the stomach and are emptied more rapidly into the duodenum **(Figure 33–10)**. Large or indigestible particles are retained in the stomach for a longer period.

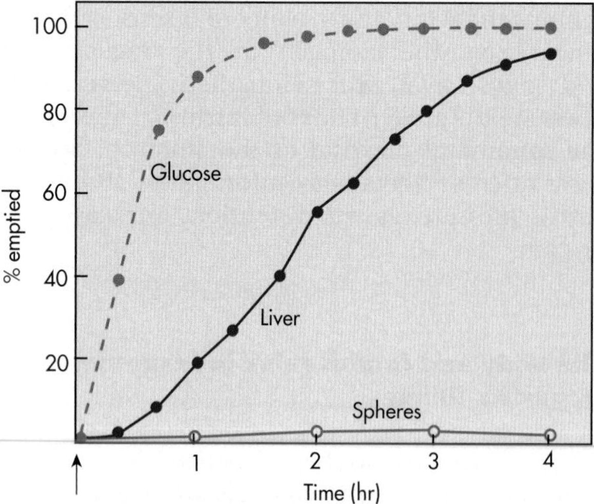

FIGURE 33–10. Rates of emptying of different meals from a dog's stomach. A solution (400 mL of 1% glucose *[green line]*) is emptied faster than a digestible solid (50 g of cubed liver *[blue line]*). The indigestible solid (40 7-mm plastic spheres *[red line]*) remains in the stomach under these conditions. (Data from Hinder RA, Kelly KA: *Am J Physiol* 233:E335, 1977.)

Gastric contractions, with a frequency of about three per minute, usually begin in the middle of the body of the stomach and travel toward the pylorus. The contractions increase in force and velocity as they approach the gastroduodenal junction. As a result, the major mixing activity occurs in the antrum, the contents of which are mixed rapidly and thoroughly with gastric secretions.

The pattern of gastric contractions after eating differs from that during fasting

After an individual eats, regular contractions of the antrum occur at a rate of about three per minute. As discussed later, the rate of gastric emptying is regulated by feedback mechanisms that diminish the force of antral contractions.

IN A FASTED ANIMAL, THE PATTERN OF ANTRAL CONTRACTIONS IS DIFFERENT. The antrum is quiescent for 75 to 90 minutes; then a brief period (5 to 10 minutes) of intense electrical and motor activity occurs. This activity is characterized by strong contractions of the antrum and a relaxed pylorus. During this period, even large chunks of material that remain from the previous meal are emptied from the stomach. The period of intense contractions is followed by another 75 to 90 minutes of quiescence. This cycle of contractions in the stomach is part of a pattern of contractile activity that periodically sweeps from the stomach to the terminal ileum during fasting. This cyclic contractile activity is known as the **migrating myoelectric complex** and is discussed later.

Slow waves and action potentials elicit gastric contractions

The gastric peristaltic waves occur at the frequency of the gastric slow waves that are generated by a **pacemaker zone** (Figure 33–9) near the middle of the body of the stomach. These waves are conducted toward the pylorus. In humans, the frequency of slow waves is about three per minute.

The gastric slow wave is triphasic **(Figure 33–11)**. Its shape resembles that of action potentials in cardiac muscle. However, the gastric slow wave lasts about 10 times longer than the cardiac action potential, and it does not overshoot (i.e., reverse polarity). Gastric smooth muscle contracts when depolarization during the slow wave exceeds threshold for contraction (Figure 33–11). The greater the extent of depolarization and the longer the cell remains depolarized above the threshold, the greater the force of contraction. In the gastric

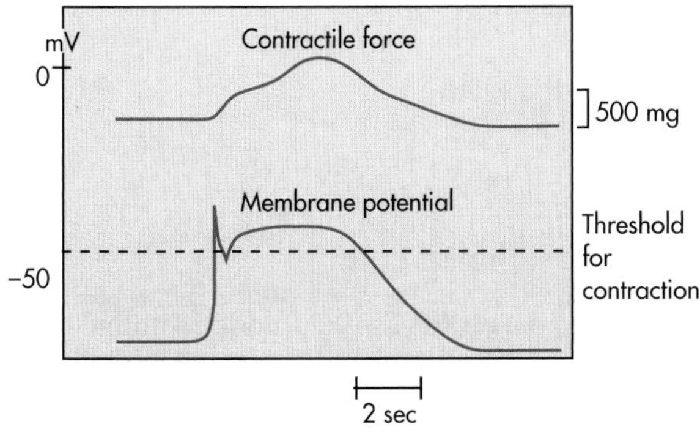

FIGURE 33–11. Relationship between the contraction of the smooth muscle of a dog's stomach *(upper tracing)* and an intracellularly recorded slow wave *(lower tracing)*. Contraction occurs when the depolarizing phase of the slow wave exceeds the threshold for contraction, even though there are no action potential spikes on the plateau of the slow wave. When action potentials occur, a much stronger contraction is elicited. (Data from Szurszewski J. In Johnson LR, ed: *Physiology of the gastrointestinal tract,* New York, 1981, Raven Press.)

antrum, action potential spikes typically occur during the plateau phase; when action potentials occur, the resulting contraction is much stronger than in the absence of action potentials (Figure 33–6). Acetylcholine and the hormone **gastrin** stimulate gastric contractility by increasing the amplitude and duration of the plateau phase of the gastric slow wave. Norepinephrine has the opposite effect.

Passage of gastric contents through the pylorus is highly regulated

The pylorus separates the gastric antrum from the duodenal bulb, the first part of the **duodenum.** The pylorus functions as a sphincter. The circular smooth muscle of the pylorus forms two ringlike thickenings followed by a connective tissue ring that separates the pylorus from the duodenum.

The duodenum has a basic electrical rhythm of 10 to 12 slow waves per minute compared with the 3 per minute of the stomach. The duodenal bulb is influenced by the basic electrical rhythms of both the stomach and the postbulbar duodenum. Thus, the duodenal bulb contracts somewhat irregularly. However, the antrum and duodenum are coordinated; when the antrum contracts, the duodenal bulb relaxes. The essential functions of the gastroduodenal junction are to allow the carefully regulated emptying of gastric contents at a rate consistent with the ability of the duodenum to process the chyme and to prevent regurgitation of duodenal contents back into the stomach.

The gastric mucosa is highly resistant to acid, but it may be damaged by bile. The duodenal mucosa has the opposite properties. Thus, too-rapid gastric emptying may lead to **duodenal ulcers,** whereas regurgitation of duodenal contents may contribute to **gastric ulcers.**

The pylorus is densely innervated by both vagal and sympathetic nerve fibers. Sympathetic fibers increase the constriction of the sphincter. Vagal fibers are either excitatory or inhibitory to pyloric smooth muscle. Excitatory cholinergic vagal fibers stimulate constriction of the sphincter. Inhibitory vagal fibers release another transmitter, probably VIP, that relaxes the sphincter. The hormones cholecystokinin, gastrin, gastric inhibitory peptide, and secretin all elicit constriction of the pyloric sphincter.

Gastric emptying is regulated in response to the nature of duodenal contents

The duodenal mucosa and jejunal mucosa have receptors that sense acidity, osmotic pressure, certain fats, and amino acids and peptides (**Figure 33–12**). The presence of fatty acids or monoglycerides (products of fat digestion) in the duodenum dramatically decreases the rate of gastric emptying. The chyme that leaves the stomach is usually hypertonic, and it becomes more hypertonic because of the action of the digestive enzymes in the duodenum. Gastric emptying is retarded by hypertonic solutions in the duodenum, a duodenal pH below 3.5, and the presence of amino acids and peptides in the duodenum. The results of these mechanisms are as follows:

1. Fat is not emptied into the duodenum at a rate greater than that at which it can be emulsified by the bile acids and lecithin of the bile (see Chapter 35).
2. Acid is not dumped into the duodenum more rapidly than it can be neutralized by pancreatic and duodenal secretions and other mechanisms.
3. The rates at which the other components of chyme are presented to the small intestine do not exceed the rate at which the small intestine can process those components.

Neural and hormonal mechanisms elicited by duodenal contents slow gastric emptying. In response to the acid in the duodenum, the force of gastric contractions promptly decreases, and duodenal motility increases. This response has neural and hormonal components. The presence of acid in the duodenum releases **secretin,** which diminishes the rate of gastric emptying by inhibiting antral

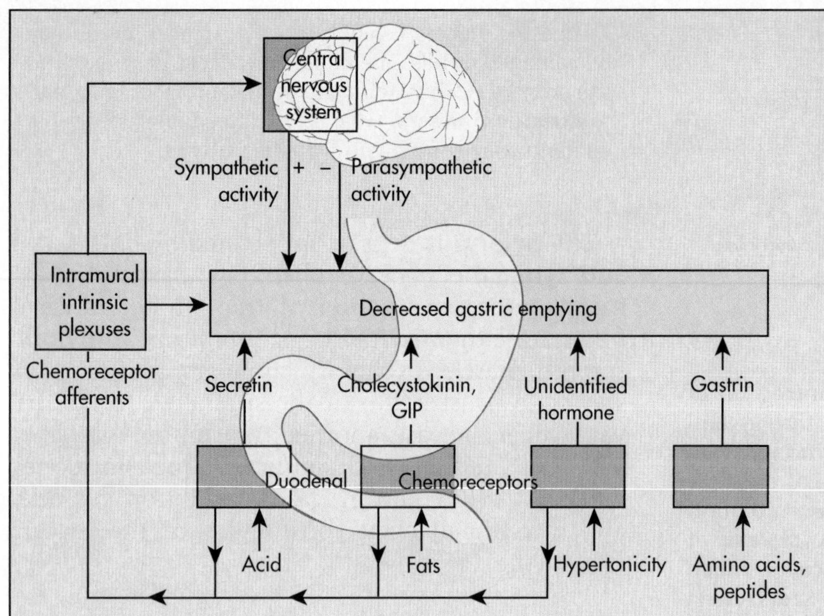

FIGURE 33–12. Duodenal stimuli elicit the neural and hormonal inhibition of gastric emptying. GIP, gastric inhibitory peptide.

contractions and stimulating contraction of the pyloric sphincter (Figure 33–12).

The presence of fat digestion products in the duodenum and jejunum decreases the rate of gastric emptying. This response results partly from the release of **cholecystokinin** from the duodenum and jejunum. Cholecystokinin decreases the rate of gastric emptying by relaxing gastric smooth muscle and contracting the pyloric sphincter. The presence of fatty acids in the duodenum and jejunum releases another hormone, **gastric inhibitory peptide,** that also decreases the rate of gastric emptying, again by relaxing gastric smooth muscle and contracting the pyloric sphincter. Hyperosmotic solutions in the duodenum and jejunum slow the rate of gastric emptying. This response has both neural and hormonal components. The neural component is mediated via the vagus; the hormonal component has not yet been identified.

Peptides and amino acids release **gastrin** from **G cells** located in the antrum of the stomach and the duodenum. Gastrin increases the strength of antral contractions and increases constriction of the pyloric sphincter; the net effect probably diminishes the rate of gastric emptying.

In some patients with **duodenal ulcers,** the underlying physiological malfunction may be diminished effectiveness of the mechanisms by which hormones released from the duodenum decrease the rates of gastric emptying and gastric acid secretion. In normal individuals, experimental instillation of acid into the duodenum via a nasogastric tube dramatically decreases the rate and force of contractions of the gastric antrum. In some patients with duodenal ulcers, this response to acid in the duodenum is markedly diminished.

Vomiting Is the Expulsion of Gastric (and Sometimes Duodenal) Contents from the Gastrointestinal Tract via the Mouth

Vomiting is often preceded by a feeling of nausea, a rapid or irregular heartbeat, dizziness, sweating, pallor, and dilation of the pupils. It is usually preceded by **retching,** in which gastric contents are forced up into the esophagus but do not enter the pharynx.

Vomiting is a reflex behavior controlled and coordinated by a **vomiting center** in the medulla oblongata. Many areas in the body have receptors that provide afferent input to the vomiting center. Distention of the stomach and duodenum is a strong stimulus that elicits vomiting. Tickling the back of the throat, painful injury to the genitourinary system, dizziness, and certain other stimuli can bring about vomiting.

Certain chemicals, called **emetics,** can elicit vomiting. Some emetics do this by stimulating receptors in the stomach or more often in the duodenum. The widely used emetic **ipecac** stimulates duodenal receptors. Certain other emetics (e.g., **apomorphine**) act at the level of the central nervous system on receptors in the floor of the fourth ventricle, in an area known as the **chemoreceptor trigger zone.** The chemoreceptor trigger zone lies on the blood side of the blood-brain barrier and thus can be reached by most blood-borne substances.

When the vomiting reflex is activated, the sequence of events is the same regardless of the stimulus that initiates the reflex. Early events include a wave of **reverse peristalsis** that sweeps from the middle of the small intestine to the duodenum. The pyloric sphincter and the stomach relax to receive the intestinal contents. A forced inspiration then occurs against a closed glottis. This decreases intrathoracic pressure, whereas the lowering of the diaphragm increases intraabdominal pressure. A forceful contraction of abdominal muscles then sharply elevates intraabdominal pressure and drives gastric contents into the esophagus. The lower esophageal sphincter relaxes reflexly to receive gastric contents, and the pylorus and antrum contract reflexly. When a person retches, the upper esophageal sphincter remains closed, which prevents vomiting. When the respiratory and abdominal muscles relax, the esophagus is emptied by secondary peristalsis into the stomach. A series of stronger and stronger retches often precedes vomiting.

When a person vomits, the rapid propulsion of gastric contents into the esophagus is accompanied by a reflex relaxation of the upper esophageal sphincter. **Vomitus** is projected into the pharynx and mouth. Entry of vomitus into the trachea is prevented by approximation of the vocal cords, closure of the glottis, and inhibition of respiration.

The Motility of the Small Intestine Mixes and Propels Intestinal Contents

The small intestine accounts for about three fourths of the length of the human gastrointestinal tract. The small intestine is about 5 m long, and chyme typically takes 2 to 4 hours to traverse it. The first 5% or so of the small intestine is the duodenum, which has no mesentery. The remaining small intestine is divided into the jejunum and the ileum. The **jejunum** is more proximal and occupies about 40% of the length of the small bowel. The **ileum** is the distal part of the small intestine and accounts for its remaining length.

The small intestine, particularly the duodenum and the jejunum, is the site of most digestion and absorption. The movements of the small intestine mix chyme with digestive secretions, bring fresh chyme into contact with the absorptive surface of the microvilli, and propel chyme toward the colon.

The most frequent type of movement of the small intestine is termed **segmentation.** Segmentation (**Figure 33–13**) is characterized by closely spaced contractions of the circular muscle layer. The contractions divide the small intestine into small, neighboring segments. In rhythmic segmentation, the sites of the circular contractions alternate so that a given segment of gut contracts and then

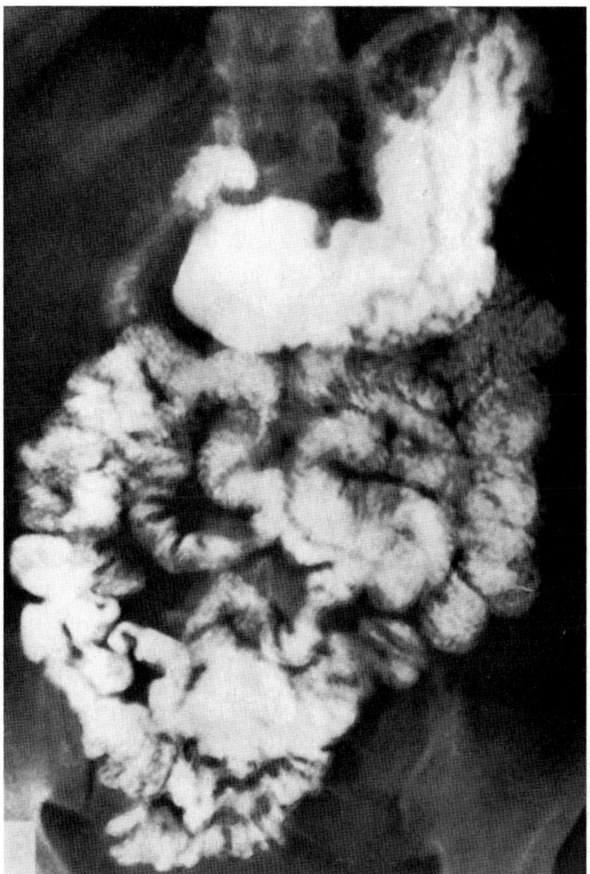

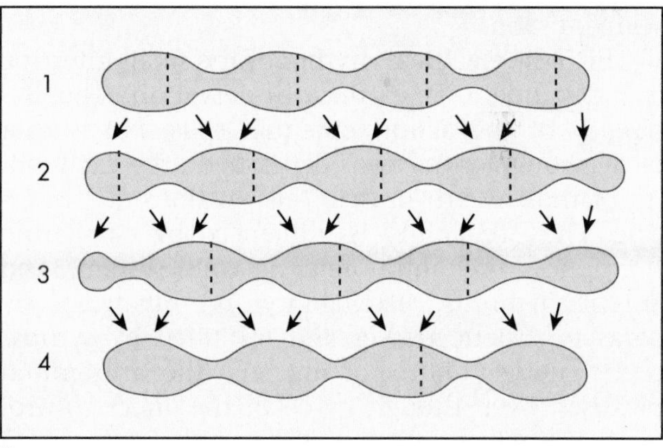

FIGURE 33–13. A, Radiograph showing the stomach and small intestine filled with barium contrast medium in a normal individual. Note that segmentation of the small intestine divides its contents into ovoid segments. B, Sequence of segmental contractions in a portion of a cat's small intestine. Lines 1 through 4 indicate successive patterns in time. The dotted lines indicate where contractions will occur next. The arrows show the direction of chyme movement. (A from Gardner EM et al: *Anatomy: a regional study of human structure,* ed 4, Philadelphia, 1975, WB Saunders; B data from Cannon WB: *Am J Physiol* 6:251, 1902.)

relaxes. Segmentation effectively mixes chyme with digestive secretions and brings fresh chyme into contact with the mucosal surface.

Peristalsis is the progressive contraction of successive sections of circular smooth muscle. The contractions move along the gastrointestinal tract in an orthograde direction. Peristaltic waves occur in the small intestine, but they usually involve only a short length of intestine.

Slow waves and action potentials determine the frequency and force of intestinal contractions

Regular slow waves occur all along the small intestine. The frequency is highest (11 to 13 per minute in humans) in the duodenum and declines along the length of the small bowel (to a minimum of 8 or 9 per minute in humans in the terminal part of the ileum). The slow waves may be accompanied by bursts of action potential spikes. When action potentials occur, they elicit much stronger contractions of the smooth muscle that cause the major mixing and propulsive movements of the small intestine (Figure 33–6). Action potential bursts are localized to short segments of the intestine, and they elicit the highly localized contractions of the circular smooth muscle that cause segmentation.

The basic electrical rhythm of the small intestine is independent of extrinsic innervation. The frequency of the action potential spike bursts that elicit strong contractions depends on the excitability of the smooth muscle cells of the small intestine. The excitability is influenced by circulating hormones, the autonomic nervous system, and enteric neurons. Excitability is enhanced by parasympathetic nerves and inhibited by sympathetic nerves, both acting via the intramural plexuses. Even though much of the direct control of intestinal motility resides in the intramural plexuses, the parasympathetic and sympathetic innervation of the small intestine modulates contractile activity. The extrinsic neural circuits are essential for certain long-range intestinal reflexes, which are discussed later.

Contractions of the duodenum, jejunum, and ileum mix the contents with digestive secretions

Contractions of the duodenal bulb mix chyme with pancreatic and biliary secretions, and they propel the chyme along the duodenum. Contractions of the duodenal bulb typically follow contractions of the gastric antrum. This helps prevent regurgitation of duodenal contents into the stomach.

Segmental contractions occur at about 12 per minute in the duodenum, 10 or 11 per minute in the jejunum, and 8 or 9 per minute in the ileum. Segmentation is more effective at mixing intestinal contents than at propelling them. The low rate of propulsion of chyme in the small intestine allows time for digestion and absorption.

The importance of the slow rate of propulsion in the small intestine can be demonstrated by treatment with agents that alter small intestinal motility. For example, the administration of **codeine** and other **opiates** markedly reduces the frequency and volume of stools. This action results from a decrease in small intestinal motility and a consequent increase in the transit time of jejunal contents. The longer transit time allows more complete absorption of salts and water and certain nutrients in the small intestine so that less than a normal volume enters the colon. **Castor oil,** a potent laxative, contains hydroxy fatty acids that stimulate small intestinal motility and decrease small intestinal transit time. Hence, salts and water are delivered to the colon at a rate that overwhelms the ability of the colon to absorb them; this results in diarrhea.

Intestinal reflexes involve the enteric and autonomic nervous systems

When a bolus of material is placed in the small intestine, the intestine typically contracts behind the bolus and relaxes ahead of it (Figure 33–7), a response known as the **law of the intestine.** This response, which is integrated chiefly in the enteric nervous system, propels the bolus in an orthograde direction, similar to a peristaltic wave.

Certain intestinal reflexes can occur along a considerable length of the gastrointestinal tract. These long-range reflexes depend on the function of both intrinsic and extrinsic nerves. Overdistention of one segment of the intestine relaxes the smooth muscle in the rest of the intestine. This response is known as the **intestinointestinal reflex.**

The stomach and terminal part of the ileum interact reflexly. Elevated secretory and motor functions of the stomach increase the motility of the terminal part of the ileum and accelerate the movement of material through the **ileocecal sphincter.** This response is called the **gastroileal reflex.**

The migrating myoelectric complex occurs during fasting

The contractile behavior of the small intestine previously discussed is characteristic of the period after

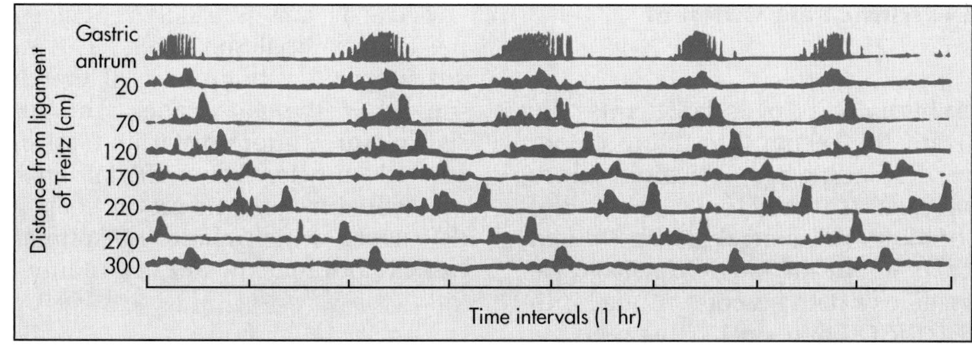

FIGURE 33–14. Contractile activity during the MMC in the stomach and small intestine of a fasting dog. The ligament of Treitz marks the border between the duodenum and the jejunum. (From Itoh Z, Sekiguchi T: *Scand J Gastroenterol Suppl* 82:121, 1983.)

ingestion of a meal. SEVERAL HOURS AFTER PROCESSING OF THE PREVIOUS MEAL, SMALL INTESTINAL MOTILITY FOLLOWS A DIFFERENT PATTERN CHARACTERIZED BY BURSTS OF INTENSE ELECTRICAL AND CONTRACTILE ACTIVITY SEPARATED BY LONGER QUIESCENT PERIODS. This pattern, the **migrating myoelectric complex (MMC),** appears to be propagated from the stomach to the terminal ileum (Figure 33–14). The MMC in the stomach is discussed earlier in this chapter.

The MMC repeats every 75 to 90 minutes in humans **(Figure 33–14)**. About the time that one MMC reaches the distal ileum, the next MMC begins in the stomach. The strongest contractions of the MMC, both in the stomach and in the small intestine, are more vigorous and more propulsive than the contractions that occur in a fed individual. These intense contractions sweep the small bowel clean and empty its contents into the colon. Thus, the MMC has been termed the housekeeper of the small intestine. The MMC inhibits the migration of colonic bacteria into the terminal ileum. Individuals with weak or absent contractions during the active contraction phase of the MMC may be troubled by bacterial overgrowth in the ileum.

The muscularis mucosae contracts irregularly

Irregular contractions of the muscularis mucosae, on average about three per minute, alter the pattern of ridges and folds of the mucosa, mix the luminal contents, and bring different parts of the mucosal surface into contact with freshly mixed chyme. Irregular contractions of intestinal villi, especially in the jejunum, help empty the central lacteals and increase intestinal lymph flow.

Neural mechanisms regulate the passage of material through the ileocecal sphincter

The **ileocecal sphincter** separates the terminal end of the ileum from the **cecum,** the first part of the colon. The sphincter is normally closed, but short-range peristalsis in the terminal part of the ileum relaxes the sphincter and allows a small amount of chyme to squirt into the cecum. The ileocecal sphincter normally allows ileal chyme to enter the colon at a slow enough rate that the colon can absorb most of the salts and water of the chyme. The ileocecal sphincter is coordinated primarily by the neurons of the intramural plexuses, but it is also influenced by autonomic reflexes and hormones.

The Motility of the Colon Facilitates the Absorption of Salts and Water and Permits the Orderly Evacuation of Feces

The colon receives 500 to 1500 mL of chyme per day from the ileum. Most of the salts and water that enter the colon are absorbed; the feces normally contain only about 50 to 100 mL of water each day. Colonic contractions mix the chyme and circulate it across the mucosal surface of the colon. As the chyme becomes semisolid, this mixing resembles a kneading process. The progress of colonic contents is slow, about 5 to 10 cm/hr at most.

One to three times daily, a wave of contraction, called a **mass movement,** occurs. A mass movement resembles a peristaltic wave in which the contracted segments remain contracted for some time. Mass movements push the contents of a significant length of colon in an orthograde direction.

Structure and extrinsic innervation of the colon

The major subdivisions of the large intestine **(Figure 33–15)** are the cecum, ascending colon, transverse colon, descending colon, sigmoid colon, rectum, and anal canal. The structure of the wall of the large bowel follows the general plan presented earlier in this chapter, but the longitudinal muscle layer of the muscularis externa is concentrated into three bands called the **taeniae coli.** In between the taeniae coli, the longitudinal muscle layer is thin. The longitudinal muscle of the rectum and anal canal is substantial and continuous.

Parasympathetic innervation of the cecum and the ascending and transverse colon is via branches of the vagus nerves; that of the descending and sigmoid colon, rectum, and anal canal is via the pelvic nerves from the sacral spinal cord. The parasympathetic fibers end mainly on neurons of the intramural plexuses.

Sympathetic fibers innervate the proximal part of the large intestine via the superior mesenteric plexus, the distal part of the large intestine via the inferior mesenteric and superior hypogastric plexuses, and the rectum and anal canal via the inferior hypogastric plexus. STIMULATION OF THE SYMPATHETIC NERVES STOPS COLONIC MOVEMENTS. VAGAL STIMULATION CAUSES SEGMENTAL CONTRACTIONS OF THE PROXIMAL PART OF THE COLON. STIMULATION OF THE PELVIC NERVES BRINGS ABOUT EXPULSIVE MOVEMENTS OF THE DISTAL COLON AND SUSTAINED CONTRACTION OF SOME SEGMENTS.

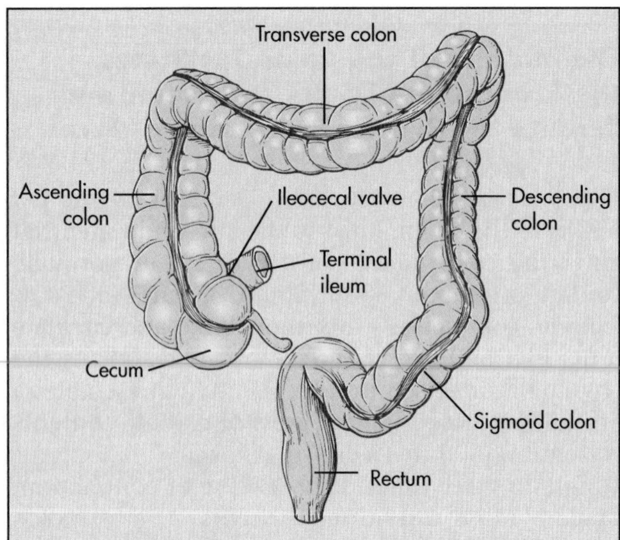

FIGURE 33–15. Major anatomical subdivisions of the colon.

The anal canal is usually kept closed by the internal and external sphincters. The **internal anal sphincter** is a thickening of the circular smooth muscle of the anal canal. The **external anal sphincter** is more distal and consists entirely of striated muscle. The external anal sphincter is innervated by somatic motor fibers via the pudendal nerves, which allow the sphincter to be controlled both reflexly and voluntarily.

The motility of the cecum and proximal colon is minimally propulsive

Most contractions of the cecum and proximal part of the large bowel are segmental and are more effective at mixing and circulating the contents than at propelling them. In the proximal colon, "antipropulsive" patterns occur. Reverse peristalsis and segmental propulsion toward the cecum both take place; consequently, chyme is retained in the proximal colon, and the absorption of salts and water is facilitated.

Because the taeniae coli are shorter than the circular muscle layer of the colon, the colon is divided into neighboring ovoid segments called **haustra (Figure 33–16)**. Localized segmental contractions of colonic circular muscle, called **haustral contractions,** result in back-and-forth mixing of luminal contents.

The distal part of the colon is normally filled with semisolid feces via a mass movement. Segmental contractions knead the feces and thereby facilitate absorption of the remaining salts and water. About one to three times daily, mass movements occur and sweep the feces toward the rectum.

Colonic motility is regulated by intrinsic and extrinsic nerves. As in other segments of the gastrointestinal tract, the intramural plexuses control the contractile behavior of the colon, and the extrinsic autonomic nerves to the colon are modulatory. The **defecation reflex,** discussed later, is an exception to this rule: it requires the function of the sacral spinal cord via the pelvic nerves.

Colonic smooth muscle has both slow waves and myenteric potential oscillations

Two classes of rhythm-generating cells reside in the colon. Interstitial cells near the inner border of the circular muscle produce regular slow waves with a frequency of about six per minute. The slow waves have high amplitude, and their shape resembles that of gastric slow waves. Interstitial cells near

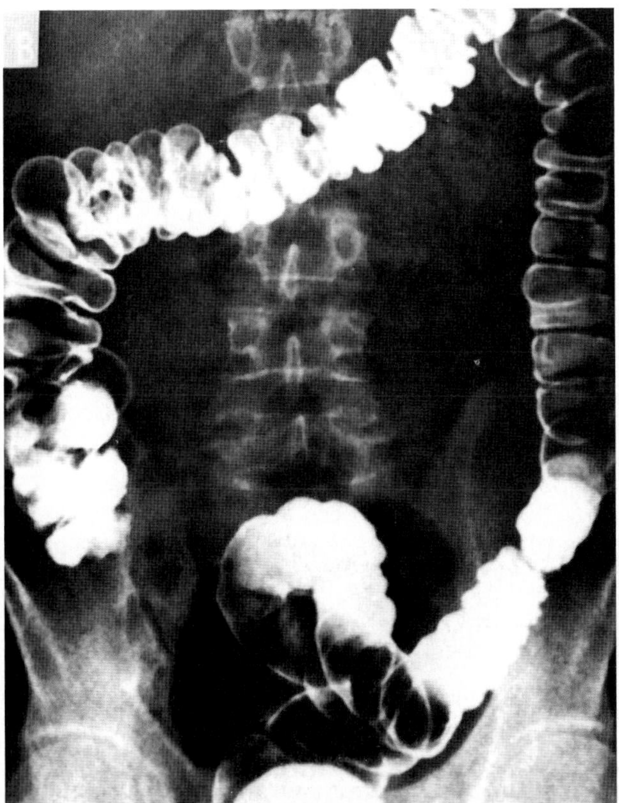

FIGURE 33–16. Radiograph showing a prominent haustral pattern in the colon of a normal individual. (From Keats TE: *An atlas of normal roentgen variants,* ed 2, St. Louis, 1979, Mosby.)

the outer border of the circular muscle produce **myenteric potential oscillations,** which are low in amplitude and much higher in frequency than the slow waves.

The circular muscle does not usually fire action potentials. Contractile agonists, such as acetylcholine released from excitatory enteric motor neurons, enhance contractions by increasing the duration of the slow waves. The longer slow waves elicit contractions of the circular muscle.

Longitudinal colonic muscle displays the myenteric potential oscillations. In contrast with the circular smooth muscle, the longitudinal muscle cells fire occasional action potentials at the peaks of the myenteric potential oscillations. The action potentials elicit contraction of the longitudinal muscle. Contractile agonists increase the frequency of action potentials.

Reflex control of colonic motility involves intrinsic and extrinsic neurons

Distention of one part of the colon reflexly relaxes other parts. This **colonocolonic reflex** is mediated by the enteric nervous system and is modulated by the sympathetic fibers that supply the colon. After a meal enters the stomach, the motility of proximal and distal colon and the frequency of mass movements increase reflexly via the **gastrocolic reflex.**

Coordination of the rectum and the anal canal is important in defecation. The rectum is usually empty or nearly so. The rectum is more active than the sigmoid colon in segmental contractions, so the rectal contents tend to move retrogradely into the sigmoid colon. The anal canal is tightly closed by the anal sphincters. Before defecation, the rectum is filled as a result of a mass movement in the sigmoid colon. Filling of the rectum brings about reflex relaxation of the internal anal sphincter and reflex constriction of the external anal sphincter and causes the urge to defecate. People who lack functional motor nerves to the external anal sphincter defecate involuntarily when the rectum is filled. The reflex reactions of the sphincters to rectal distention are transient. If defecation is postponed, the sphincters regain their normal tone, and the urge to defecate temporarily subsides.

In **Hirschsprung's disease,** also known as **congenital megacolon,** enteric neurons are congenitally absent from part of the colon. Frequently, only a short length of colon proximal to the internal anal sphincter is involved, but larger segments of the colon may also be affected. In a normal person, filling of the rectum by a mass movement leads to reflex relaxation of the distal rectum and the internal anal sphincter. In the absence of enteric neurons, this reflex relaxation cannot occur. This results in functional obstruction of the distal colon and dilation of the colon above the obstruction.

The integrating center for the defecation reflex is in the sacral spinal cord. When circumstances are appropriate, an individual voluntarily relaxes the external anal sphincter to allow defecation to proceed. Defecation is a complex behavior involving both reflex and voluntary actions. The integrating center for the reflex actions is in the sacral spinal cord and is modulated by higher centers. The principal efferent pathways are cholinergic parasympathetic fibers in the pelvic nerves. The sympathetic nervous system does not play a significant role in normal defecation.

Voluntary actions are important in defecation. The external anal sphincter is voluntarily held in the relaxed state. Intraabdominal pressure is elevated to aid in the expulsion of feces. Evacuation is normally preceded by a deep breath, which moves the diaphragm downward. The glottis is then closed, and contraction of the respiratory muscles on full lungs elevates both the intrathoracic and intraabdominal pressures. Contractions of the muscles of the abdominal wall further increase intraabdominal pressure, which may be as great as 200 cm H_2O. This helps force feces through the relaxed sphincters. The muscles of the pelvic floor are relaxed to allow the floor to drop. This helps straighten the rectum and prevent rectal prolapse.

Summary

- ❖ The gastrointestinal tract has a characteristic layered structure consisting of mucosa, submucosa, muscularis externa, and serosa.
- ❖ The gastrointestinal tract receives both sympathetic and parasympathetic innervation.
- ❖ Contractions of the smooth muscle of the muscularis externa mix and propel the contents of the gastrointestinal tract.
- ❖ Gastrointestinal smooth muscle cells are electrically coupled, and their resting membrane potential oscillates with a rhythm characteristic of each segment of the gastrointestinal tract.
- ❖ The membrane potential oscillations, called slow waves, control the timing and force of contractions of gastrointestinal smooth muscle.
- ❖ The nerve plexuses of the gastrointestinal tract, the enteric nervous system, contain about 10^8 neurons, as many as in the spinal cord. The enteric nervous system contains motor neurons, sensory neurons, and interneurons.
- ❖ Enteric sensory neurons function as the afferent arms of enteric reflex arcs by which the enteric nervous system controls most of the motor and secretory activities of the gastrointestinal tract.
- ❖ The autonomic nervous system modulates the activities of the enteric nervous system.
- ❖ Swallowing is a reflex coordinated by a swallowing center in the medulla and pons.
- ❖ Contractions of the stomach mix food with gastric juice and mechanically subdivide the food.
- ❖ Hormonal and neural mechanisms initiated by the presence of acid, fats, amino acids, and peptides, as well as hypertonicity in the duodenum, regulate gastric emptying.
- ❖ Segmentation is the major contractile activity in the small intestine. Segmental contractions mix and circulate intestinal contents but are not very propulsive.
- ❖ In a fasted individual, a different pattern of motility, the MMC, occurs. The MMC sweeps the stomach and small intestine clear of any debris left from the previous meal.
- ❖ In the proximal colon, antipropulsive contractions predominate, which allows time for the absorption of salts and water. In the transverse and descending colon, haustral contractions mix and knead colonic contents to facilitate the extraction of salts and water.
- ❖ Filling of the rectum with feces initiates the defecation reflex. The integrating center for the defecation reflex is in the sacral spinal cord.

Bibliography

Biancani P, Harnett KM, Behar J: Esophageal motor function. In Yamada T, ed: *Textbook of gastroenterology,* ed 4, Philadelphia, 2003, Lippincott Williams & Wilkins.

Bornstein JC, Costa M, Grider JR: Enteric motor and interneuronal circuits controlling motility, *Neurogastroenterol Motil* 16(suppl 1):34, 2004.

Furness JB et al: Intrinsic primary afferent neurons and nerve circuits within the intestine, *Prog Neurobiol* 72:143, 2004.

Furness JB et al: The enteric nervous system and its extrinsic connections. In Yamada T, ed: *Textbook of gastroenterology,* ed 4, Philadelphia, 2003, Lippincott Williams & Wilkins.

Hasler WL: Physiology of gastric motility and gastric emptying. In Yamada T, ed: *Textbook of gastroenterology,* ed 4, Philadelphia, 2003, Lippincott Williams & Wilkins.

Hasler WL: Motility of the small intestine and colon. In Yamada T, ed: *Textbook of gastroenterology,* ed 4, Philadelphia, 2003, Lippincott Williams & Wilkins.

Miller LJ: Gastrointestinal hormones and receptors. In Yamada T, ed: *Textbook of gastroenterology,* ed 4, Philadelphia, 2003, Lippincott Williams & Wilkins.

Plant RL: Anatomy and physiology of swallowing, *Otolaryngol Clin North Am* 31:477, 1998.

Pope CE II: The esophagus for the nonesophagologist, *Am J Med* 103:19S, 1997.

Quigley EM: Gastric and small intestinal motility in health and disease, *Gastroenterol Clin North Am* 25:113, 1996.

Sanders KM, Ordog T, Ward SM: Physiology and pathophysiology of the interstitial cells of Cajal: from bench to bedside. IV. Genetic and animal models of GI motility disorders caused by loss of interstitial cells of Cajal, *Am J Physiol Gastrointest Liver Physiol* 282:G747, 2002.

Smith TK, Kang SH, Vanden Berghe P: Calcium channels in enteric neurons, *Curr Opin Pharmacol* 3:588, 2003.

Wood JD: Neuropathophysiology of irritable bowel syndrome, *J Clin Gastroenterol* 35(suppl 1):S11, 2002.

Case Studies

Case 33–1

A 42-year-old woman reports difficulty in swallowing solid foods; liquids are less difficult to swallow. Chest pain follows eating, and she frequently regurgitates after eating. When the recumbent patient underwent fluoroscopy after a barium swallow, her lower esophagus was somewhat dilated compared with normal, but her upper esophagus was of normal caliber. Subsequent swallows initiated by the patient showed that the barium was cleared from the esophagus very slowly. The acute administration of amyl nitrite caused the barium to be cleared more rapidly. Manometric studies showed a resting pressure in the lower esophageal sphincter of about 60 mm Hg, with a decrease to about 45 mm Hg after a swallow. The patient was treated with forceful dilation of the lower esophageal sphincter by a pneumatic dilating device. The patient's ability to swallow solid food was dramatically improved after the dilation procedure. Some 15 months after the dilation, the patient returned because swallowing had again become difficult.

1. **The slow rate of barium clearance from the esophagus is most likely the result of which of the following mechanisms?**
   - A. Decreased resting pressure of the lower esophageal sphincter
   - B. Increased pressure of the lower esophageal sphincter
   - C. Decreased resting pressure of the upper esophageal sphincter
   - D. Increased pressure of the upper esophageal sphincter
   - E. Reverse peristalsis of the esophagus

2. **Which of the following characterizes the functioning of esophageal musculature of this patient?**
   - A. There is no abnormality of the musculature of the lower esophageal sphincter.
   - B. The innervation of the lower esophageal sphincter is functioning normally.
   - C. Hypertrophy of the lower esophageal sphincter may be present.
   - D. The patient suffers from diffuse esophageal spasm.
   - E. Hypertrophy of the upper esophageal sphincter may be present.

3. **Regarding therapy for this patient's swallowing difficulties:**
   - A. The recurrence of her problems 15 months after dilation is unexpected.
   - B. Pharmacological therapy is unlikely to help the patient.
   - C. Surgical intervention might help alleviate the symptoms.
   - D. Repeating the dilation of the lower esophageal sphincter is unlikely to help relieve the symptoms.
   - E. Swallowing difficulties are likely to improve spontaneously.

Case 33–2

A 5-week-old boy has abdominal distention. His parents report that his bowel movements are infrequent (once every other day, on average) and that he vomits frequently. Digital examination of the baby's rectum reveals that the rectal ampulla is empty; a short squirt of fecal material is expressed when the physician's finger is removed. A lateral x-ray study performed after a barium enema reveals that the distal 7 cm of the rectum has a narrowed lumen and that most of the colon above the narrowed segment is enlarged. When the rectum is distended with a balloon, the internal anal sphincter fails to show the normal transient relaxation. The provisional diagnosis is Hirschsprung's disease.

1. **With regard to diagnosis of this patient's difficulties:**
   - **A.** Failure of the internal anal sphincter to relax on rectal distention clinches the diagnosis of Hirschsprung's disease.
   - **B.** The next step should be a full-thickness biopsy of the rectum.
   - **C.** A suction biopsy of the mucosa would not add useful information.
   - **D.** The presence of enlarged nerve trunks in the mucosa would help confirm the diagnosis.
   - **E.** The barium enema should be repeated after the baby has been fasted for 24 hours.

2. **With regard to management of the baby's illness:**
   - **A.** The disorder is likely to subside once the baby is eating solid food.
   - **B.** The disorder will spontaneously become less severe as the baby grows and develops.
   - **C.** The disorder can be managed with drugs that relax colonic muscle.
   - **D.** The recommended treatment is surgical.
   - **E.** Dilation of the narrowed segment of the colon with a balloon is likely to resolve the malfunction permanently.

3. **What does the recommended surgical treatment of Hirschsprung's disease involve?**
   - **A.** Incision of the circular muscle of the aganglionic segment of colon to weaken it
   - **B.** Removal of most of the colon
   - **C.** Construction of a permanent colostomy
   - **D.** Removal of only the aganglionic segment of the colon
   - **E.** Removal of the entire colon and the last half of the ileum

Chapter 34: Gastrointestinal Secretions

Objectives

- Describe the composition and functions of saliva and explain the cellular processes in acinar and duct cells responsible for the secretion of saliva.
- Describe the regulation of salivary composition and flow rate.
- List the components of gastric juice and their physiological functions.
- Describe the cellular mechanisms responsible for HCl secretion in the stomach.
- Describe the physiological mechanisms that regulate the secretion of HCl in the stomach during the cephalic, gastric, and intestinal phases.
- Explain how mucus and HCO_3^- create a "gastric mucosal barrier" that protects the gastric epithelium from damage by HCl and pepsins.
- List the components of pancreatic juice and their physiological functions.
- Describe the physiological mechanisms in pancreatic acinar and duct cells that are responsible for secretion of pancreatic juice.
- Describe the regulation of pancreatic secretion during the cephalic, gastric, and intestinal phases.
- List the major physiological functions of the liver.
- List the major components of bile and their physiological significance.
- Describe the physiological mechanisms that regulate the secretion of bile.
- Describe the mechanisms responsible for concentration of bile in the gallbladder.
- Describe the regulation of gallbladder emptying during the cephalic, gastric, and intestinal phases.

This chapter deals with the glandular secretion of fluids and compounds that have important functions in the digestive tract. In particular, the secretions of the salivary glands, gastric glands, exocrine pancreas, and liver are considered. The functions of these secretions in digestion are discussed in Chapter 35. In each case, the nature of the secretions and their functions in digestion are discussed, and the regulation of the secretory processes is emphasized. These gastrointestinal secretions are elicited by the action of specific neurocrine, endocrine, and paracrine effector substances on the secretory cells (see Chapter 5). A substance that stimulates secretion is called a **secretagogue.**

Saliva Lubricates Food and Begins the Digestion of Starch

In humans, the salivary glands produce about 1 L of saliva each day. Saliva lubricates food for greater ease of swallowing and also facilitates speaking.

In people who lack functional salivary glands, **xerostomia** (dry mouth), **dental caries,** and infections of the buccal mucosa are prevalent. Saliva contains **secretory immunoglobulins** (antibodies) directed against microorganisms in the mouth. In the absence of these antibodies, organisms that cause buccal infections and dental caries proliferate. The basic pH of saliva also helps prevent dental caries.

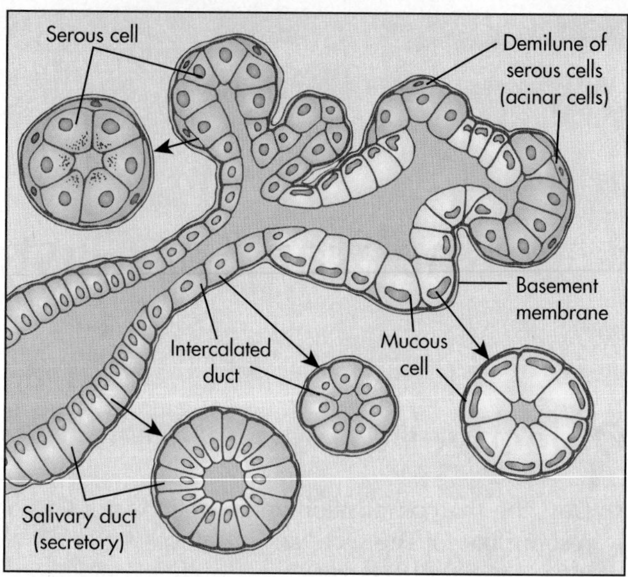

FIGURE 34–1. Structure of the human submandibular gland as seen with the light microscope. (Modified from Braus H: *Anatomie des Menschen,* Berlin, 1934, Julius Springer.)

Saliva contains mucins and an amylase

Mucins, which are glycoproteins produced by the submaxillary and sublingual glands, lubricate food so that it can more readily be swallowed. The major digestive function of saliva is the action of **salivary amylase** on starch. Salivary amylase is an enzyme with the same specificity as the amylase of pancreatic juice; it reduces starch to oligosaccharide molecules (see Chapter 35). The pH optimum of salivary amylase is about 7, but it is active between a pH of 4 and 11. Amylase action continues in the mass of food in the stomach and is terminated only when the contents of the stomach are mixed with enough gastric acid to lower the pH to less than 4. More than half the starch in a well-chewed meal may be reduced to small oligosaccharides by the action of salivary amylase. However, because of the large capacity of the pancreatic amylase to digest starch in the small intestine, starch is well absorbed even in the absence of salivary amylase. Saliva also contains several proline-rich proteins that are heavily glycosylated and have antimicrobial properties.

Secretory end pieces in salivary glands are drained by a system of ducts

In humans, the **parotid glands,** the largest salivary glands, are entirely serous. Their watery secretion lacks mucins. The **submandibular** and **sublingual glands** are mixed mucous and serous glands, and they secrete more viscous saliva that contains mucins. Many smaller salivary glands are present in the oral cavity. The microscopic structure of a mixed salivary gland is depicted in **Figure 34–1**. The **serous acinar cells** located in the **secretory end pieces** (also called **acini**) have apical **zymogen granules** that contain salivary amylase and other salivary proteins. **Mucous acinar cells** secrete mucins into the saliva. **Intercalated ducts** drain the acinar fluid into somewhat larger ducts, the **striated ducts,** which empty into still larger **excretory ducts.** A single large duct brings the secretions of each major gland into the mouth. A **primary secretion** is elaborated in the secretory end pieces. The cells that line the ducts modify the primary secretion.

Actively secreting salivary glands have a high metabolic rate and a high blood flow

The salivary glands produce a prodigious flow of saliva. The maximum rate of production of saliva in humans is about 1 mL/min/g of gland; AT THIS RATE, THE GLAND IS PRODUCING ITS OWN WEIGHT IN SALIVA EACH MINUTE. Salivary glands have a high rate of metabolism and a correspondingly high blood flow; both are proportional to the rate of saliva formation. The blood flow to maximally secreting salivary glands is approximately 10 times that of an equal mass of actively contracting skeletal muscle. Stimulation of the parasympathetic nerves to salivary glands increases blood flow by dilating the vasculature of the glands. **Vasoactive intestinal polypeptide** (VIP) and **acetylcholine** are released from parasympathetic nerve terminals in the salivary glands; both of these compounds contribute to vasodilation during secretory activity.

Both acinar cells and duct cells help determine the composition of saliva

Saliva is hypotonic to plasma

As shown in **Figure 34–2**, saliva is always hypotonic with respect to plasma. Concentrations of Na^+ and Cl^- are significantly less in saliva than in plasma. The greater the secretory flow rate, the higher the tonicity of the saliva; at maximum flow rates, the tonicity of saliva in humans is about 70% that of

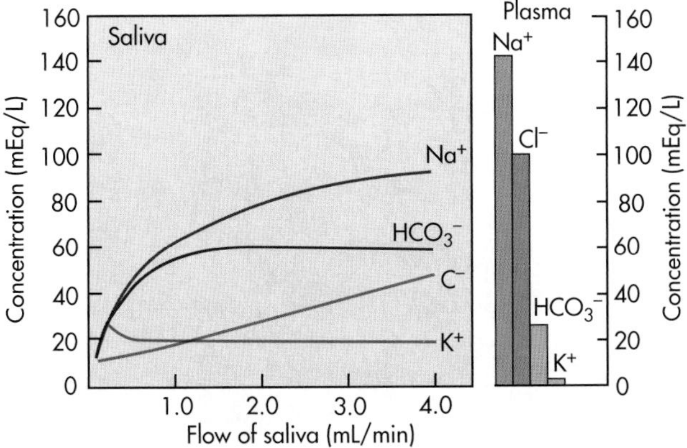

FIGURE 34–2. Average composition of parotid saliva as a function of salivary flow rate. Saliva is hypotonic to plasma at all flow rates. The HCO_3^- level in saliva exceeds that in plasma, except at very low flow rates. (Data from Thaysen JH et al: *Am J Physiol* 178:155, 1954.)

plasma. The pH of saliva from resting glands is slightly acidic. During active secretion, however, the saliva becomes basic, with the pH near 8. The increase in pH with the secretory flow rate is partly caused by the increase in the salivary [HCO_3^-], which can reach levels more than twice the [HCO_3^-] in plasma.

Acinar cells elaborate a primary secretion that is modified by the duct cells

A two-stage model of salivary secretion **(Figure 34–3)** postulates the following:

1. The secretory end pieces, perhaps with the participation of intercalated ducts, produce a primary secretion that is isotonic to plasma. The amylase concentration and the rate of fluid secretion vary with the level and type of stimulation. However, the electrolyte composition of the secretion is fairly constant, and the levels of Na^+ and Cl^- are close to plasma levels. However, the [K^+] is much higher in the fluid in the acini than in plasma.
2. The excretory ducts and probably the striated ducts modify the primary secretion by extracting Na^+ and Cl^- from the saliva and adding K^+ and HCO_3^- to it. The ducts do not add to the volume of saliva.

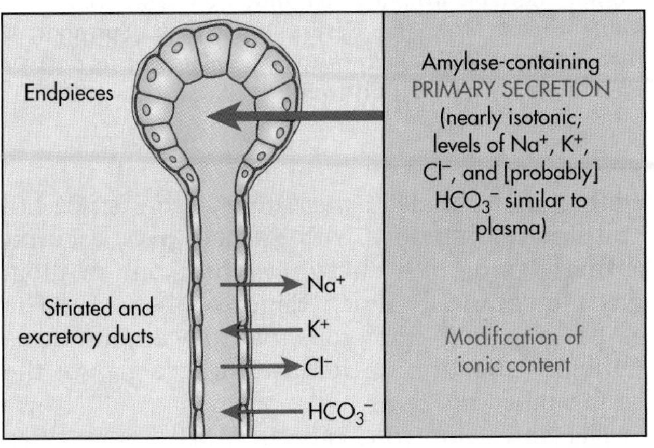

FIGURE 34–3. Two-stage model of salivary secretion. The primary secretion, containing salivary amylase, is secreted by the acinar cells. The striated and excretory ducts modify the composition of saliva.

As saliva flows down the ducts, it becomes progressively more hypotonic. Thus, the ducts remove more ions from saliva than they contribute to it. The faster the flow rate of the saliva down the striated and excretory ducts, the closer is saliva to isotonicity.

In their apical cytoplasm, serous acinar cells have zymogen granules that contain salivary amylase. When the gland is stimulated to secrete, the zymogen granules fuse with the plasma membrane and release their contents into the lumen of an acinus by exocytosis.

Salivary gland functions are regulated principally by parasympathetic nerves

Excitation of either sympathetic or parasympathetic nerves to the salivary glands stimulates salivary secretion, but the effects of the parasympathetic nerves are stronger and last longer. Cutting the sympathetic nerves causes no major defect in the function of the salivary glands. If the parasympathetic supply is interrupted, however, the salivary glands atrophy. THE ESSENTIAL PHYSIOLOGICAL CONTROL OF SALIVARY SECRETIONS IS VIA THE PARASYMPATHETIC NERVOUS SYSTEM.

Sympathetic fibers to the salivary glands come from the superior cervical ganglion. Preganglionic parasympathetic fibers come via branches of the facial and glossopharyngeal nerves (cranial nerves VII and IX, respectively), and they synapse with postganglionic neurons in or near the salivary glands. The acinar cells and ducts are supplied with parasympathetic nerve endings.

Parasympathetic stimulation increases the synthesis and secretion of salivary amylase and mucins, enhances the transport activities of the ductular epithelium, greatly increases blood flow to the glands, and stimulates glandular metabolism and growth. The increase in salivary secretion that results from stimulation of sympathetic nerves is transient. Sympathetic stimulation constricts blood vessels, with consequent reduction in salivary gland blood flow.

Duct cells are stimulated by acetylcholine and norepinephrine

The ducts of salivary glands respond to both cholinergic and adrenergic agonists by increasing their rates of secretion of K^+ and HCO_3^-. Despite the stimulation of both acinar and duct cells by adrenergic agonists, because adrenergic agonists result in greatly diminished blood flow to salivary glands, adrenergic stimulation of salivary flow is transient.

The duct cells secrete more K^+ and HCO_3^- than the Na^+ and Cl^- they reabsorb. In this way, the ducts render saliva hypotonic. The ion transport proteins involved in duct cell secretion include apical membrane Na^+ and CFTR Cl^- channels and Cl^--HCO_3^- antiporters (see Chapter 1).

Acinar cells are stimulated by several neurocrine agonists

Neuroeffector substances that stimulate acinar cell secretions act mainly by elevating intracellular cAMP or by increasing the level of Ca^{++} in the cytosol. Acetylcholine, norepinephrine, substance P, and VIP are released in salivary glands by specific nerve terminals. Each of these neuroeffectors may increase the secretion of salivary amylase and the flow of saliva. Acetylcholine is the major physiological agonist and Ca^{++} is the major physiological second messenger for acinar cell secretion.

Norepinephrine, acting on β receptors, and VIP elevate cAMP in acinar cells. In contrast, acetylcholine, substance P, and the activation of α receptors by norepinephrine increase intracellular [Ca^{++}].

Acinar cells actively take up K^+ and Cl^- across the basolateral membrane via the $1Na^+,1K^+,2Cl^-$ symporter. K^+ leaks back out of the cell via K^+ channels in both apical and basolateral membranes, thereby enhancing the negative membrane potential that helps drive Cl^- across the apical membrane into the acinar lumen. Na^+ enters the lumen partly via the tight junctions between acinar cells. Both Ca^{++} and cAMP stimulate the apical membrane's Cl^- channels. Ca^{++} also stimulates K^+ channels in the basolateral membrane of the acinar cell.

Acetylcholine and other Ca^{++}-mobilizing agonists produce a higher volume of saliva with lower protein concentration than do cAMP-elevating agonists.

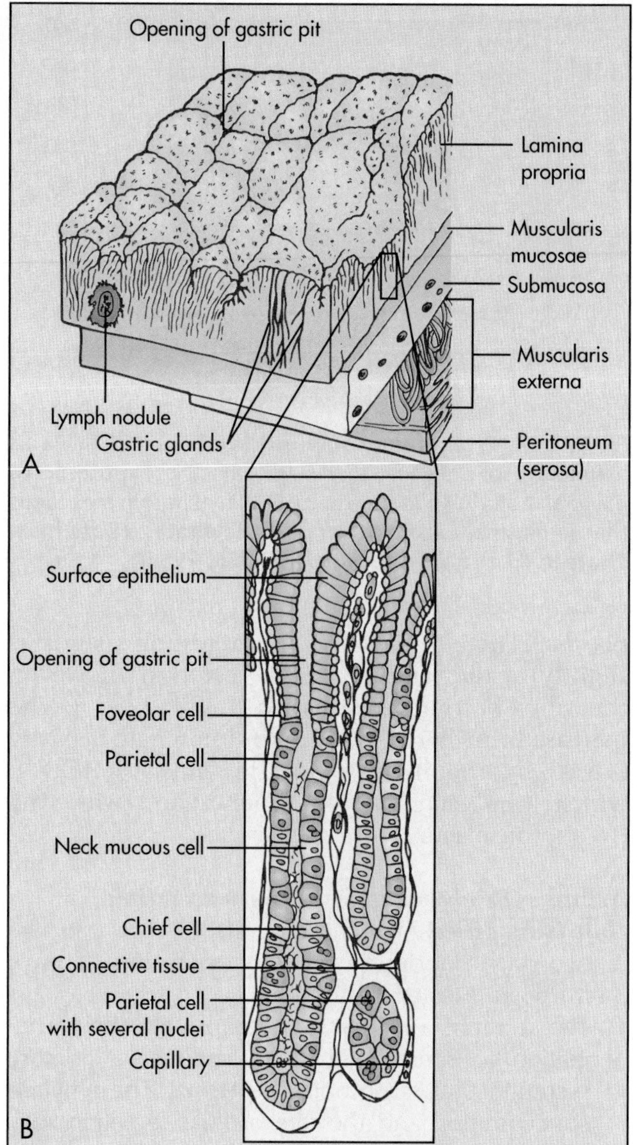

FIGURE 34–4. Structure of the gastric mucosa. A, Reconstruction of part of the gastric wall. B, Two gastric glands from a human stomach. (A modified from Braus H: *Anatomie des Menschen,* Berlin, 1934, Julius Springer; B redrawn from Weis L, ed: *Histology: cell and tissue biology,* ed 5, New York, 1981, Elsevier.)

Gastric Secretions Begin the Digestion of Proteins and Have Other Important Functions

The wall of the stomach contains exocrine glands and endocrine cells

The surface of the gastric mucosa (Figure 34–4) is covered by columnar **epithelial cells** that secrete mucus and an alkaline fluid that protects the epithelium from mechanical injury and gastric acid. The surface is studded with **gastric pits;** each pit is the opening of a duct into which one or more **gastric glands** empty (Figure 34–4, *A*). The gastric pits are so numerous that they account for a significant fraction of the total surface area of the gastric mucosa.

The gastric mucosa can be divided into three regions on the basis of the structures of the glands present. The small **cardiac glandular region,** which is just below the lower esophageal sphincter, contains mainly mucus-secreting gland cells. The remainder of the gastric mucosa is divided into the **oxyntic** (acid-secreting) **glandular region,** which is above the notch, and the **pyloric glandular region,** which is below the notch (see Figure 33–9).

The structure of a gastric gland from the oxyntic glandular region is illustrated in Figure 34–4, *B*. The surface epithelial cells extend slightly into the duct opening. In the narrow neck of the gland are the **mucous neck cells,** which secrete mucus. Deeper in the gland are **parietal** or **oxyntic cells,** which secrete HCl and intrinsic factor, and **chief** or **peptic cells,** which secrete pepsinogens. Oxyntic cells are particularly numerous in glands in the fundus.

Mucus-secreting cells predominate in the glands of the pyloric glandular region. Pyloric glands also contain **G cells,** which secrete the hormone **gastrin,** and **D cells,** which secrete **somatostatin.**

Surface epithelial cells are exfoliated into the lumen at a considerable rate during normal gastric function. They are replaced by mucous neck cells, which differentiate into columnar epithelial cells and migrate up out of the necks of the glands. The capacity of the stomach to repair damage to its epithelial surface in this way is remarkable.

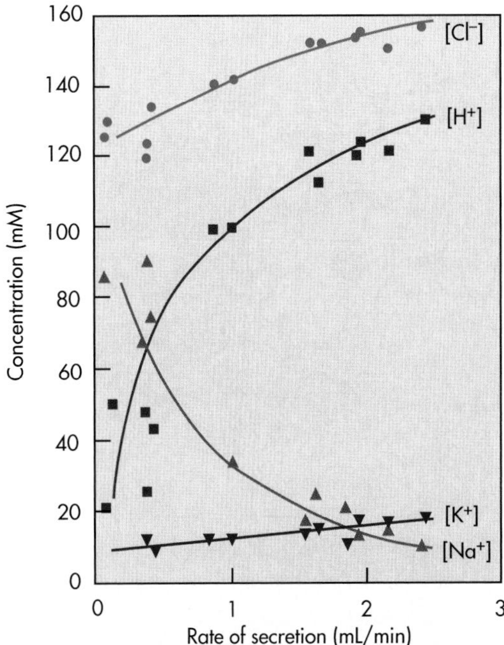

FIGURE 34–5. Concentrations of ions in gastric juice as a function of the rate of secretion in a normal young person. At low flow rates, gastric juice is hypotonic to plasma. At high flow rates, gastric juice approaches isotonicity and contains predominantly H^+ and Cl^-. (Data from Nordgren B: *Acta Physiol Scand* 58[suppl 202]:1, 1963.)

Gastric juice contains salts, water, HCl, pepsins, intrinsic factor, and mucus

The fluid secreted into the stomach is called **gastric juice.** Gastric juice is a mixture of the secretions of the surface epithelial cells, mucous neck cells, and gastric glands. Secretion of all these components increases after a meal.

The ionic composition of gastric juice depends on the rate of secretion. The higher the secretory rate, the higher the [H^+] **(Figure 34–5)**. At lower secretory rates, the [H^+] diminishes and the [Na^+] increases. The [K^+] is always higher in gastric juice than in plasma, and consequently, prolonged vomiting may lead to hypokalemia. At all rates of secretion, Cl^- is the major anion of gastric juice. At high rates of secretion, the composition of gastric juice resembles that of an isotonic solution of HCl. Gastric HCl converts pepsinogens to active pepsins (see later section) and provides an acid pH at which pepsins are active.

Basal (unstimulated) rates of gastric acid production typically range from about 1 to 5 mEq/hr in humans. On maximal stimulation, HCl production rises to 6 to 40 mEq/hr. On average, less HCl is secreted in patients with gastric ulcers, but more than normal is secreted in patients with duodenal ulcers. The reasons for this are discussed later.

> The high acidity of gastric juice kills most ingested microorganisms. Individuals who have low rates of gastric acid secretion, because they either have a disease or are taking medications that suppress HCl secretion, are more susceptible to infection by ingested pathogens.

Dramatic morphological changes in parietal cells accompany gastric acid secretion

Parietal cells have a distinctive ultrastructure **(Figure 34–6)** and an elaborate system of branching **secretory canaliculi,** which course through the cytoplasm and are connected by a common outlet to the cells' luminal surface. Microvilli line the surfaces of the canaliculi. The cytoplasm of unstimulated parietal cells contains numerous tubules and vesicles: the **tubulovesicular system.** The membranes of the tubulovesicles contain the transport proteins responsible for the secretion of H^+ and Cl^- into the lumen of the gland. When parietal cells are stimulated to secrete HCl (Figure 34–6, *B*), tubulovesicular membranes fuse with the plasma membrane of the secretory canaliculi; this extensive membrane fusion greatly increases the number of HCl transporters and Cl^- channels available at the surface of the secretory canaliculi.

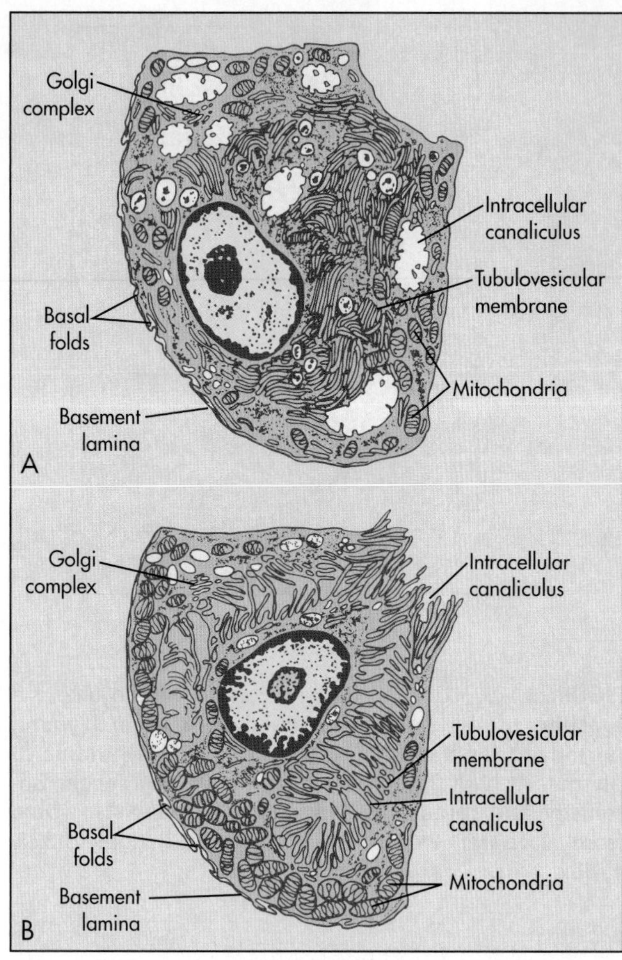

FIGURE 34–6. A, Resting parietal cell with a cytoplasm full of tubulovesicles and an internalized intracellular canaliculus. B, Acid-secreting parietal cell. The tubulovesicles have fused with the membrane of the intracellular canaliculus, which is now open to the lumen of the gland and lined with abundant long microvilli. (From Berne RM, Levy MN, Koeppen BM, Stanton BA: *Physiology,* ed 5, Philadelphia, 2004, Elsevier.)

The prime mover in gastric H^+ secretion is a proton ATPase

At maximal rates of secretion, H^+ is pumped against a concentration gradient that is more than one million to one. Cl^- also enters the gastric lumen against a large electrochemical potential difference. Thus, energy is required for the transport of both H^+ and Cl^-.

The apical membrane of the parietal cell (the membrane that lines the secretory canaliculus) contains H^+,K^+-ATPase, which exchanges H^+ for K^+ **(Figure 34–7)**. This ATPase is the primary H^+ pump. Both H^+ and K^+ are pumped against their electrochemical potential gradients.

When H^+ is pumped out of the parietal cell, an excess of HCO_3^- is left behind. HCO_3^- flows down its electrochemical gradient across the basolateral plasma membrane. The protein that mediates HCO_3^- efflux (a Cl^--HCO_3^- antiporter) transports Cl^- in the opposite direction. Cl^- moves against its electrochemical potential gradient into the cell, and the energy for the active transport of Cl^- comes from the downhill movement of HCO_3^-.

As a result of the combined action of H^+,K^+-ATPase and the Cl^--HCO_3^- antiporter, Cl^- is concentrated in the cytoplasm of the parietal cell. Cl^- leaves the parietal cell at the apical membrane via an anion channel.

The Cl^- channels in the apical membrane of the parietal cell are stimulated by elevated cAMP and by increased intracellular [Ca^{++}]. Elevated cAMP promotes fusion of the tubulovesicular membranes with the secretory canalicular membranes (Figure 34–6). This fusion increases the number of H^+,K^+-ATPase molecules and Cl^- channels available to participate in HCl secretion.

Pepsins begin the digestion of proteins

Pepsins, often collectively called **pepsin,** are a group of proteases secreted by the chief cells of the gastric glands. Pepsins are secreted as inactive proenzymes called **pepsinogens.** The cleavage of acid-labile linkages converts pepsinogens to active pepsins: the lower the pH, the more rapid the conversion. Pepsins also act proteolytically on pepsinogens to form more pepsins.

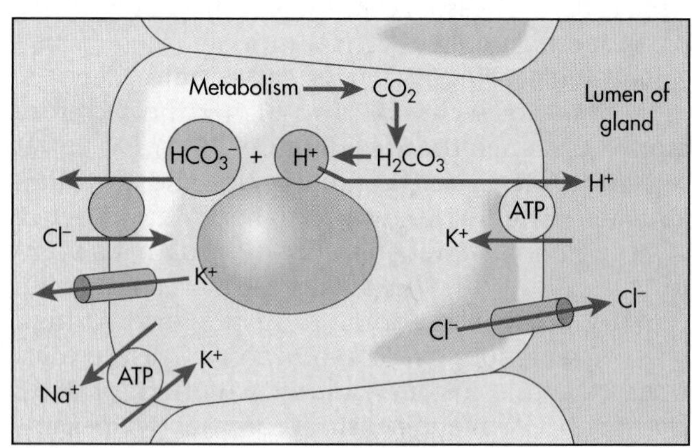

FIGURE 34–7. Simplified view of the major ion transport processes involved in the secretion of H^+ and Cl^- by parietal cells. Cl^- enters the cell across the basolateral membrane against an electrochemical gradient. The downhill efflux of HCO_3^- powers its entry. The high level of HCO_3^- in the cytosol is generated by the active extrusion of H^+ across the luminal membrane. Protons are pumped into the secretory canaliculus by H^+,K^+-ATPase. K^+ recycles across the apical membrane via a K^+ channel. Cl^- enters the canalicular fluid via an ion channel.

The pepsins have their highest proteolytic activity at a pH of 3 and below. Pepsins are endopeptidases that may digest as much as 30% of the protein in a typical meal to oligopeptides. In the absence of pepsins, there is no deficit in protein digestion because there is more than enough protease activity in pancreatic juice to completely digest ingested proteins. When the duodenal contents are neutralized, pepsins are inactivated irreversibly by the neutral pH. Pepsinogens are contained in membrane-bound zymogen granules in the chief cells. The contents of the zymogen granules are released by exocytosis when the chief cells are stimulated to secrete.

Intrinsic factor is required for the normal absorption of vitamin B_{12} by the ileum

Intrinsic factor, a glycoprotein, is secreted by the parietal cells of the stomach. It binds to B_{12} in the small intestine and is required for B_{12} absorption by the ileum. Intrinsic factor is released in response to the same stimuli that evoke the secretion of HCl by parietal cells. THE SECRETION OF INTRINSIC FACTOR IS THE ONLY GASTRIC FUNCTION THAT IS ESSENTIAL FOR HUMAN LIFE.

Mucus and HCO_3^- help protect surface epithelial cells

Secretions that contain glycoprotein mucins are viscous and sticky and are collectively termed **mucus.** Mucins are secreted by mucous neck cells in the necks of gastric glands and by the surface epithelial cells of the stomach. Mucus is stored in large granules in the apical cytoplasm of mucous neck cells and surface epithelial cells; it is released by exocytosis. The secretion of mucus is stimulated by some of the same stimuli that enhance acid and pepsinogen secretion, especially by acetylcholine released from parasympathetic nerve endings near the gastric glands.

The surface epithelial cells also secrete watery fluid with Na^+ and Cl^- concentrations similar to those of plasma but with higher K^+ and HCO_3^- concentrations than in plasma. The high $[HCO_3^-]$ makes the mucus alkaline. Mucus is secreted by the resting mucosa and lines the stomach with a sticky, viscous, alkaline coat. When food is eaten, the rates of secretion of mucus and HCO_3^- increase.

The gastric mucosal barrier requires both mucus and HCO_3^-

Mucus forms a gel on the luminal surface of the mucosa. MUCUS AND THE ALKALINE SECRETIONS ENTRAPPED WITHIN IT CONSTITUTE A GASTRIC MUCOSAL BARRIER THAT PREVENTS DAMAGE TO THE MUCOSA FROM GASTRIC CONTENTS (Figure 34–8). Pepsins cleave certain peptide bonds in the mucin molecules and thereby dissolve the gel. The gel must be replenished via the synthesis of new mucin molecules.

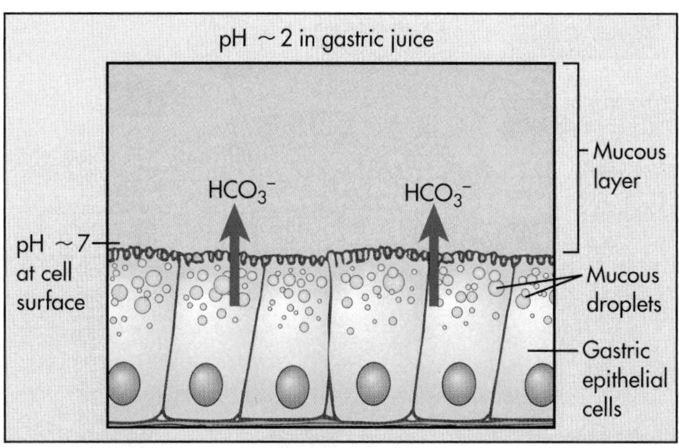

FIGURE 34–8. The protection provided to the mucosal surface of the stomach by the HCO_3^--containing mucus layer is known as the gastric mucosal barrier. Buffering by the HCO_3^--rich secretions of the surface epithelial cells and the restraint to convective mixing caused by the high viscosity of the mucus layer allow the pH at the cell surface to remain near 7, whereas the pH in the gastric juice in the lumen is 1 to 2. Fluid from the glands enters the lumen via 1-μm-diameter channels through the mucus layer.

The mucous gel layer prevents the HCO_3^--rich secretions of the surface epithelial cells from rapidly mixing with the contents of the gastric lumen. Thus, the surface of the epithelial cells can be maintained at a nearly neutral pH despite a luminal pH of about 2.

The gastric mucosal barrier of a normal individual can protect the stomach even when rates of secretion of HCl and pepsins are elevated. If the secretion of either HCO_3^- or mucus is suppressed, however, the gastric mucosal barrier is compromised, and the effects of acid and pepsin on the surface of the stomach may produce **gastric ulcers.** Adrenergic agonists diminish HCO_3^- secretion. This effect may play a role in the pathogenesis of **stress ulcers:** a chronically elevated level of circulating epinephrine may suppress HCO_3^- secretion sufficiently to decrease protection of the epithelial cell surface. Aspirin and other nonsteroidal antiinflammatory agents inhibit the secretion of both mucus and HCO_3^-; prolonged use of these drugs may damage the mucosal surface. Certain prostaglandins inhibit acid secretion and enhance the secretion of mucus and HCO_3^- and thereby help protect the epithelial surface of the stomach.

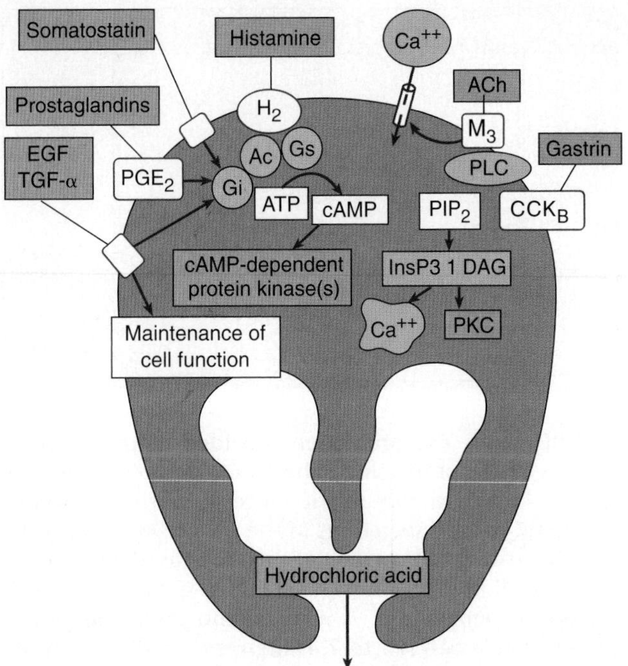

FIGURE 34–9. Signal transduction mechanisms of agonists and antagonists of HCl secretion by parietal cells. Histamine binds to H_2 receptors on the basolateral membranes of parietal cells and activates adenylyl cyclase to bring about elevated cAMP levels. Acetylcholine (ACh) binds to M_3 muscarinic receptors on the basolateral membrane to activate a Ca^{++} channel and to activate phospholipase Cβ to bring about elevation of InsP3 and intracellular Ca^{++}. Gastrin binds to CCK_B/gastrin receptors to mobilize intracellular Ca^{++} stores to increase free cytosolic Ca^{++}. Certain inhibitors of HCl secretion, including somatostatin, prostaglandins (especially of the E class), and certain growth factors, activate G_i and thereby diminish cAMP levels in the cell. Ac, adenylyl cyclase; DAG, diacylglycerol; EGF, epidermal growth factor; PLC, phospholipase C; PKC, protein kinase C; TGF, transforming growth factor. (From Berne RM, Levy MN, Koeppen BM, Stanton BA: *Physiology,* ed 5, Philadelphia, 2004, Elsevier.)

Control of gastric acid secretion

Acetylcholine, histamine, and gastrin are the three physiological agonists of HCl secretion

Each of these secretagogues binds to a distinct class of G protein–coupled receptors on the plasma membrane of the parietal cell and directly stimulates the parietal cell to secrete HCl (**Figure 34–9**). Acetylcholine is released near parietal cells by cholinergic nerve terminals. Gastrin is produced by G cells in the mucosa of the gastric antrum and the duodenum and reaches parietal cells via the bloodstream. Histamine, a paracrine agonist, is released from **enterochromaffin-like (ECL) cells** in the gastric mucosa and diffuses to the parietal cells.

Cellular mechanisms of parietal cell agonists

The receptors for acetylcholine, gastrin, and histamine on the parietal cell basolateral membrane and the intracellular second messengers by which these secretagogues act are shown in Figure 34–9. Histamine elevates cAMP. Acetylcholine and gastrin are Ca^{++}-mobilizing agonists. Acetylcholine also activates a Ca^{++} channel. Somatostatin and prostaglandins, important physiological inhibitors of HCl secretion, inhibit adenylyl cyclase and depress cAMP levels.

Histamine is a major physiological mediator of HCl secretion. **Cimetidine,** a specific antagonist of H_2 receptors, blocks a large portion of the acid secretion elicited by any known secretagogue. ECL cells, present in the gastric mucosa, synthesize and store histamine. When they are stimulated by acetylcholine or gastrin, the ECL cells release histamine, which diffuses to nearby parietal cells to stimulate HCl secretion.

Gastrin is not as potent a direct stimulant of parietal cells as acetylcholine or histamine. The physiological response to elevated levels of gastrin in the blood is greatly attenuated by cimetidine. Thus, a major component of the physiological response to gastrin results from the gastrin-stimulated release of histamine. A large component of acetylcholine's stimulation of HCl secretion is also via its action to promote release of histamine from ECL cells.

Before the discovery of drugs that dramatically diminish the rate of gastric acid secretion, surgery to treat peptic ulcer disease was common. The availability of cimetidine and other H_2 receptor blockers revolutionized therapy for duodenal ulcer disease and other disorders related to the hypersecretion of gastric acid. These drugs usually diminish the secretion of HCl dramatically, and they have few side effects. H_2 receptor blockers are not as effective in patients with **Zollinger-Ellison syndrome.** Such patients have gastrin-secreting tumors and thus have very high serum levels of gastrin. **Omeprazole** (a specific and irreversible inhibitor of H^+,K^+-ATPase) is the current drug of choice for treatment of these patients.

Somatostatin provides an important brake on gastric acid secretion

Somatostatin, released from D cells near the bases of glands in the antrum, is the most important physiological antagonist of HCl secretion. Somatostatin directly inhibits HCl secretion by parietal cells and also suppresses the release of gastrin from G cells and histamine by ECL cells. Somatostatin tonically inhibits HCl secretion, and other inhibitory mechanisms may be mediated largely by somatostatin. Somatostatin secretion is stimulated by gastrin and by H^+ in the lumen of the stomach, so that when HCl secretion is stimulated, the braking action of somatostatin is also increased. **Figure 34–10** summarizes control of HCl secretion by neural, hormonal, and paracrine mechanisms.

The three phases of gastric acid secretion are the cephalic, gastric, and intestinal phases

When the stomach has been empty for several hours, HCl is secreted at a basal rate, which is approximately 10% of the maximal rate. After a meal, the rate of acid secretion by the stomach increases promptly. There are three phases of increased acid secretion in response to food: the **cephalic phase,** elicited before food reaches the stomach; the **gastric phase,** elicited by the presence of food in the stomach; and the **intestinal phase,** elicited by mechanisms that originate in the duodenum and upper jejunum **(Table 34–1).**

THE CEPHALIC PHASE OF GASTRIC SECRETION IS NORMALLY ELICITED BY THE SIGHT, SMELL, AND TASTE OF FOOD. Cholinergic vagal fibers and cholinergic neurons of the intramural plexuses evoke cephalic-phase secretion. Acetylcholine released from these neurons directly stimulates parietal cells to secrete HCl. Acetylcholine also indirectly stimulates acid secretion by releasing gastrin from G cells in the antrum and duodenum and by releasing histamine from ECL cells in the oxyntic gastric mucosa. **Gastrin-releasing peptide,** a peptide released from some cholinergic terminals along with acetylcholine, also enhances the secretion of gastrin by G cells.

In the absence of food in the stomach to buffer the acid secreted, the pH of the antral contents falls rapidly during the cephalic phase. A low pH limits the amount of acid secreted by inhibiting the parietal cells by release of somatostatin and by evoking inhibitory intrinsic neural reflexes.

IN THE GASTRIC PHASE, THE PRINCIPAL STIMULI ARE DISTENTION OF THE STOMACH AND THE PRESENCE OF AMINO

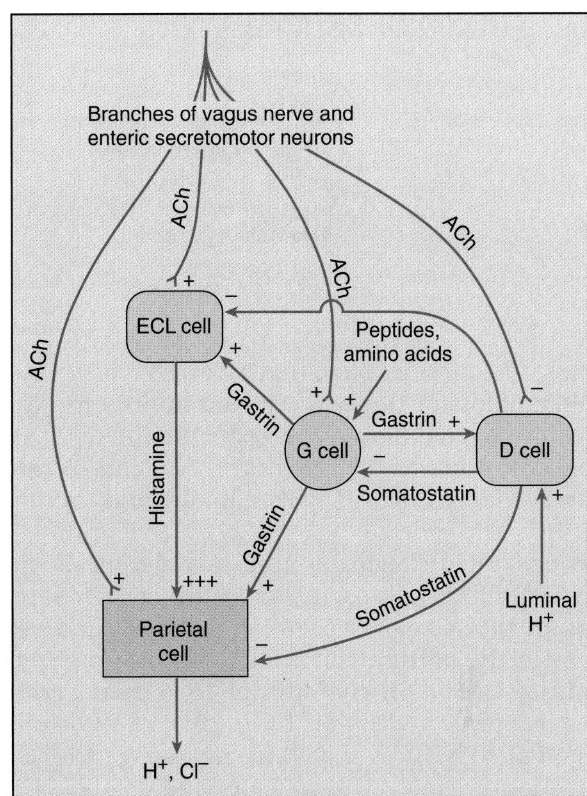

FIGURE 34–10. Control of gastric secretion of HCl. Histamine (the strongest agonist), acetylcholine (ACh), and gastrin evoke HCl secretion by parietal cells. Somatostatin from mucosal D cells tonically suppresses HCl secretion. Vagal impulses stimulate enteric neurons that release acetylcholine to increase secretion of histamine, gastrin, somatostatin, and HCl. Gastrin enhances secretion of histamine by ECL cells. However, gastrin also increases secretion of somatostatin by D cells. Somatostatin acts to inhibit gastrin secretion directly by inhibiting HCl secretion by parietal cells and indirectly by inhibiting gastrin release from G cells and histamine release from ECL cells. (This latter effect is not shown in the figure.) The negative effect on HCl secretion that results from the effects of somatostatin helps prevent the positive feedback loops shown in the figure from evoking uncontrolled high rates of HCl secretion. (From Berne RM, Levy MN, Koeppen BM, Stanton BA: *Physiology,* ed 5, Philadelphia, 2004, Elsevier.)

TABLE 34–1. MECHANISMS FOR STIMULATION OF GASTRIC ACID SECRETION

Phase	Stimuli	Mechanisms of Stimulation of HCl Secretion
Cephalic	Chewing, swallowing, taste, smell of food	Vagal impulses excite enteric secretomotor neurons to parietal, G, and ECL cells
Gastric	Gastric distention Peptides and amino acids in lumen	Local and vagovagal reflexes stimulate parietal cells and release of histamine and gastrin Peptides and amino acids release gastrin from G cells in stomach
Intestinal	Protein digestion products in duodenum Distention of duodenum Amino acids and peptides in blood	Release of gastrin from G cells in intestine and enterooxyntin Enteric and vagovagal reflexes to ECL, G, and parietal cells Release of gastrin from G cells in stomach

TABLE 34–2. MECHANISMS FOR INHIBITION OF GASTRIC ACID SECRETION

Phase	Stimuli	Mechanisms of Inhibition of HCl Secretion
Cephalic and gastric	Vagovagal and enteric neural impulses Low pH in lumen of stomach	Release of gastrin promotes release of somatostatin by D cells Inhibition of parietal and G cells by somatostatin
Intestinal	Low pH in duodenum Digestion products of fats and protein Hypertonicity in duodenum	Vagovagal and enteric reflexes that inhibit HCl secretion Secretin and bulbogastrone inhibit parietal cells CCK and gastric inhibitory peptide inhibit parietal cells Unidentified enterogastrone inhibits HCl secretion

ACIDS AND PEPTIDES RESULTING FROM THE ACTIONS OF PEPSINS. Most of the acid secreted in response to a meal is secreted during the gastric phase. Once the buffering capacity of the gastric contents is saturated, the gastric pH falls rapidly and inhibits further acid release. In this way, the acidity of gastric contents regulates itself. A larger meal, with higher buffering capacity, will elicit greater secretion of HCl. The presence of amino acids and peptides in the antrum elicits HCl secretion partly by causing G cells in the antrum to release gastrin. Intact proteins do not have this effect. Other ingested substances that can enhance gastric acid secretion include Ca^{++}, caffeine, and alcohol. Distention of the stomach evokes local and vagovagal neural reflexes that promote HCl secretion.

DURING THE INTESTINAL PHASE, GASTRIC SECRETION IS MODULATED BY THE DUODENAL CONTENTS. The presence of chyme in the duodenum causes neural and endocrine responses that first stimulate and later inhibit the secretion of acid by the stomach. Early in gastric emptying, when the pH of gastric chyme is greater than 3, the stimulatory influences predominate. Later, when the buffer capacity of gastric chyme is exhausted and the pH of chyme emptied into the duodenum falls to less than 3, inhibitory influences prevail. **Tables 34–1** and **34–2** summarize the major mechanisms that stimulate and inhibit gastric acid secretion.

Gastric secretion is enhanced by distention of the duodenum and by the presence of protein digestion products (peptides and amino acids) in the duodenum. The duodenum and proximal jejunum contain G cells that release gastrin when they are stimulated by peptides and amino acids.

Several mechanisms that operate during the intestinal phase inhibit gastric secretion (Table 34–2). These mechanisms are evoked by the presence of acid, fat digestion products, and hypertonicity in the duodenum and proximal part of the jejunum.

Acid solutions in the duodenum release the hormone **secretin** into the bloodstream. Secretin inhibits gastric acid by inhibiting the release of gastrin by G cells and by decreasing the response of parietal cells to secretagogues. Acid in the duodenum also inhibits gastric acid secretion via a local nervous reflex. Acid in the duodenal bulb releases another hormone, **bulbogastrone,** which inhibits acid secretion by the parietal cells.

The products of triglyceride digestion in the duodenum and proximal part of the jejunum release two hormones, **gastric inhibitory peptide** and **cholecystokinin** (CCK), that inhibit acid secretion by parietal cells. Hyperosmotic solutions in the duodenum release an uncharacterized hormone that inhibits gastric acid secretion.

Patients with gastric ulcers frequently have subnormal rates of HCl secretion. This seems counterintuitive. Gastric ulcers may be caused by a failure of the gastric mucosal barrier to prevent a large decrease in pH at the surface of the gastric mucosa. This suppresses HCl secretion. Duodenal ulcer patients, in contrast, may have elevated rates of HCl secretion. In some cases, hypersecretion of HCl may be caused by diminished sensitivity of the mechanisms that inhibit gastric HCl secretion. As a result, HCl is emptied into the duodenum more rapidly than H^+ can be neutralized, thereby promoting ulceration of the duodenum.

Helicobacter pylori infection is responsible for nearly all cases of gastric and duodenal ulcers not related to medication

Peptic ulcer disease includes both gastric and duodenal ulcers. Among the mechanisms that may contribute to ulcer formation are infection by *Helicobacter pylori* bacteria, diminished effectiveness of the gastric mucosal barrier, and hypersecretion of acid.

Diminished effectiveness of the gastric mucosal barrier and formation of gastric ulcers may result from long-term treatment with nonsteroidal anti-inflammatory agents that diminish the rates of secretion of mucus and HCO_3^-. Hypersecretion of acid may contribute to the formation of duodenal ulcers. In **Zollinger-Ellison syndrome,** a gastrin-secreting tumor results in increased secretion of HCl and the formation of duodenal ulcers.

H. pylori thrives in an acidic environment. These bacteria have high levels of urease, the enzyme that catalyzes the conversion of urea to ammonia and carbon dioxide. Ammonia helps buffer the acid surrounding the bacteria. *H. pylori* colonizes the mucus layer of the stomach and duodenum but does not invade the mucosa. The bacteria secrete proteins that evoke both cellular and humoral immune responses. The invasion of the mucosa by macrophages and other immunocytes results in **chronic superficial gastritis,** which can lead to ulcer disease.

The stomachs of about 40% of the people in the world are infected with *H. pylori.* Most of these people may have chronic superficial gastritis that causes mild symptoms or no symptoms at all. In other individuals, *H. pylori* causes more severe gastritis or ulcerations. Chronic severe gastritis caused by *H. pylori* predisposes the individual to the development of ulcers and ultimately to gastric cancer. Certain strains of *H. pylori* are more likely to cause severe gastritis and cancer than are other strains.

Many duodenal ulcers are associated with *H. pylori* infection of the duodenum. Patients with duodenal ulcers are often hypersecretors of HCl; this may be partly attributed to diminished sensitivity to the inhibition of HCl secretion by secretin released from the duodenum or to other inhibitory mechanisms. The resulting decreased pH of the duodenum is conducive to infection by acid-loving *H. pylori.*

Antibiotic therapy is part of the recommended treatment of gastric or duodenal ulcer disease in *H. pylori*–infected patients. A drug is usually also administered to suppress HCl secretion because such suppression renders *H. pylori* more sensitive to antibiotics. Treatment with omeprazole or H_2 receptor antagonists, but without antibiotics, diminishes the population of *H. pylori* and promotes the healing of ulcers; but when the administration of blockers of acid secretion is discontinued, *H. pylori* again flourish, and in most cases, ulcers recur.

Many of the agonists that stimulate the secretion of HCl also elicit the secretion of pepsinogens

The release rates of acid by parietal cells and of pepsinogens by chief cells are highly correlated. Acetylcholine is a potent stimulus for the chief cells to release pepsinogens. Gastrin also directly stimulates chief cells. Acid in contact with the gastric mucosa stimulates pepsinogen release via a local neural reflex. Secretin and CCK released by the duodenal mucosa stimulate chief cells to secrete pepsinogens. Because of these overlapping mechanisms, when HCl secretion is stimulated, the rate of gastrin secretion is also elevated.

Chief cells increase secretion of pepsinogens in response to agonists that elevate intracellular cAMP (secretin, VIP, and epinephrine and norepinephrine acting on β-adrenergic receptors) and in response to agonists that increase the concentration of intracellular free Ca^{++} (acetylcholine, CCK, and gastrin). Agonists that elevate different intracellular second messengers can potentiate one another's action. Acetylcholine and gastrin appear to be the most physiologically important agonists of pepsinogen secretion. As described in Chapter 35, a low pH is required for the generation of proteolytically active pepsins by spontaneous cleavage of an N-terminal peptide from pepsinogens. Pepsins are unusual in having high proteolytic activity at very low pH (pH 3.5 or less) and in being irreversibly inactivated at neutral pH.

Pancreatic Secretions Include Enzymes That Digest All the Major Foodstuffs

The human pancreas weighs less than 100 g; yet each day, it secretes about 1 L (10 times its mass) of pancreatic juice. The pancreas is unusual in having both endocrine and exocrine secretory functions. The exocrine juice is composed of an **aqueous component** that is rich in HCO_3^-, which helps neutralize HCl in duodenal contents, and an **enzyme component** that contains enzymes for digesting carbohydrates, proteins, and fats (**Table 34–3**). Pancreatic exocrine secretion is controlled by both neural and hormonal signals elicited mainly by the presence of acid and digestion products in the duodenum. Secretin chiefly elicits secretion of the aqueous component, and CCK and acetylcholine are the major secretagogues of pancreatic enzyme secretion.

The structure of the exocrine pancreas resembles that of the salivary glands

Polygonal acinar cells whose primary function is to secrete the enzyme component of pancreatic juice surround the ends of blind-ended, microscopic tubules. The acini are organized into lobules; the tiny ducts that drain the acini are called **intercalated ducts.** These ducts empty into somewhat larger **intralobular ducts.** The intralobular ducts of a particular lobule drain into a single **extralobular duct** that empties the lobule into still larger ducts. The larger ducts converge into a main duct that enters the duodenum with the **common bile duct.**

The endocrine cells of the pancreas reside in the **islets of Langerhans.** Although islet cells account

TABLE 34–3. DIGESTIVE ENZYMES SECRETED BY PANCREATIC ACINAR CELLS

*Secreted as inactive zymogens**	
Trypsinogens	Protein and peptide digestion
Chymotrypsinogen	Protein and peptide digestion
Proelastase	Protein and peptide digestion
Proelastase E	Protein and peptide digestion
Procarboxypeptidases A and B	Protein and peptide digestion
Secreted as active enzymes	
Amylase	Digestion of starch
Glycerol ester hydrolase (also known as pancreatic lipase)	Digestion of triglycerides
Cholesterol ester hydrolase (also known as carboxyl ester lipase)	Digestion of lipid carboxyl esters
Colipase	Enhances action of pancreatic lipase in presence of bile acids
DNase	Digestion of DNA
RNase	Digestion of RNA

*Zymogens are enzymatically inactive. Their enzymatic activity is unmasked in the intestine when an inhibitory peptide sequence is hydrolyzed. The function of the pancreatic enzymes is discussed more fully in Chapter 35.

for less than 2% of the volume of the pancreas, their hormones are essential in regulating metabolism. **Insulin, glucagon, somatostatin,** and **pancreatic polypeptide** are hormones released from cells of the islets of Langerhans (see Chapter 43).

The pancreas is innervated by branches of the vagus nerve and by the enteric nervous system. Vagal fibers synapse with cholinergic neurons that lie within the pancreas and that innervate both acinar and islet cells. Postganglionic sympathetic nerves from the celiac and superior mesenteric plexuses innervate pancreatic blood vessels. Secretion of pancreatic juice is stimulated by parasympathetic activity and inhibited by sympathetic activity. Gastropancreatic and enteropancreatic reflexes are mediated by some continuity of the enteric nervous system of these segments of the gastrointestinal tract with the enteric nervous system in the pancreas that innervates both acinar and duct cells.

The aqueous component of pancreatic juice is elaborated mainly by ductular epithelial cells

Na^+ and K^+ concentrations of pancreatic juice are similar to those in plasma. HCO_3^- (at levels well above those in plasma) and Cl^- are the major anions. The $[HCO_3^-]$ of pancreatic juice varies from approximately 80 mEq/L at low rates of secretion to about 140 mEq/L at high secretory rates **(Figure 34–11)**, and the $[Cl^-]$ varies reciprocally. The aqueous fluid secreted by the intralobular duct cells is slightly hypertonic, and its concentration of HCO_3^- is higher than that of plasma. As the secretion flows down the ducts, water equilibrates across the epithelium so that the pancreatic juice becomes isotonic with plasma.

Under resting (unstimulated) conditions, the aqueous component is produced mainly by the intercalated and other intralobular ducts. When secretion is stimulated by secretin, however, the additional flow comes mostly from the extralobular ducts **(Figure 34–12)**. Secretin is the major physiological stimulus for secretion of the aqueous component. The secretion of the extralobular ducts is

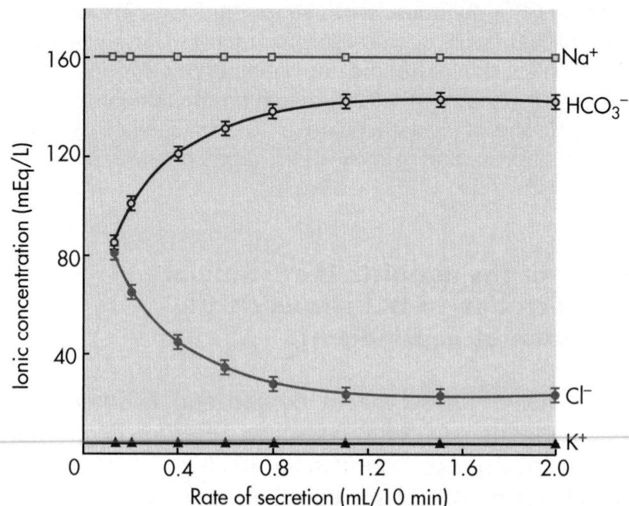

FIGURE 34–11. Concentrations of the major ions in cat pancreatic juice as functions of the secretory flow rate. At all flow rates, the concentration of HCO_3^- in pancreatic juice is well above the plasma level. Secretion was stimulated by the intravenous injection of secretin. (Data from Case RM, Harper AA, Scratcherd T: *J Physiol [Lond]* 201:335, 1969.)

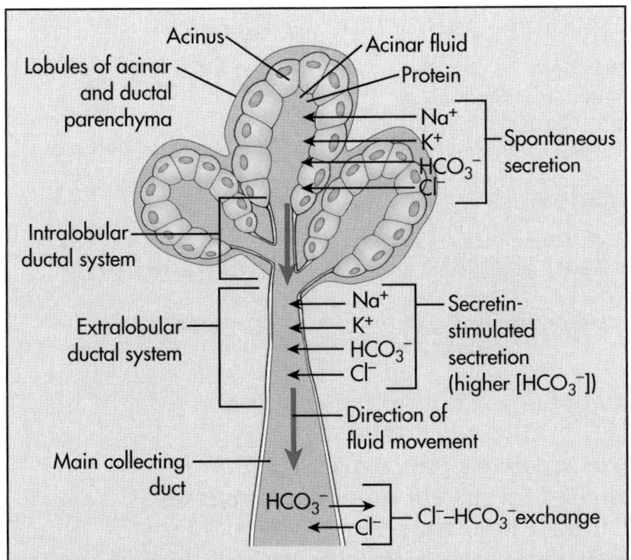

FIGURE 34–12. Locations of important transport processes involved in the elaboration of pancreatic juice. Acinar fluid is isotonic and resembles plasma in its concentrations of Na^+, K^+, Cl^-, and HCO_3^-. CCK and acetylcholine stimulate the secretion of acinar fluid and the proteins secreted by acinar cells. A spontaneous secretion produced by the intralobular ducts has higher concentrations of K^+ and HCO_3^- than in plasma. The hormone secretin stimulates water and electrolyte secretion by the cells lining the extralobular ducts. The secretin-stimulated secretion is still richer in HCO_3^- than the spontaneous secretion. (Modified from Swanson CH, Solomon AK: *J Gen Physiol* 62:407, 1973.)

higher in volume than that of the intralobular ducts and much higher in [HCO_3^-], resembling an isotonic solution of $NaHCO_3$. Thus, the higher the flow rate of pancreatic juice, the higher its [HCO_3^-] and the lower its [Cl^-] (Figure 34–11).

Acinar cells secrete the enzyme component of pancreatic juice

The secretions of the acinar cells constitute the **enzyme component** of pancreatic juice. The fluid secreted by the acinar cells resembles plasma in its tonicity and in its concentrations of various ions. The enzyme component contains enzymes that are important for the digestion of all the major classes of foodstuffs (Table 34–3). If pancreatic enzymes are absent, lipids, proteins, and carbohydrates are malabsorbed.

Proteases of pancreatic juice are secreted in inactive zymogen form. The major pancreatic proteases are **trypsin, chymotrypsin, carboxypeptidase,** and **elastase.** They are secreted as inactive zymogens: **trypsinogen, chymotrypsinogen, procarboxypeptidase,** and **proelastase**. Trypsinogen is specifically activated by **enteropeptidase** (formerly inappropriately called **enterokinase**), which is secreted by the duodenal mucosa. Trypsin then proteolytically activates trypsinogen, chymotrypsinogen, procarboxypeptidase, and proelastase. **Trypsin inhibitor,** a protein present in pancreatic juice, prevents the premature activation of proteolytic enzymes in the pancreatic ducts, which might cause pancreatitis.

Pancreatic juice contains an **amylase** that is secreted in active form. **Pancreatic amylase** cleaves starch molecules into oligosaccharides (see Chapter 35). Pancreatic juice also contains a number of lipid-digesting enzymes, or **lipases.** Among the major pancreatic lipases are **triacylglycerol hydrolase, cholesterol ester hydrolase,** and **phospholipase A_2.**

> Cl^- enters the acinar lumen via electrogenic Cl^- channels in the apical plasma membranes of the acinar cells. The primary molecular defect in **cystic fibrosis** is a mutation in the gene that encodes this Cl^- channel; this mutation results in a dramatic reduction of the number of Cl^- channels present in the apical plasma membranes of certain epithelial cells. The decreased transport of Cl^- into the pancreatic acinar lumen impairs the transport of Na^+ and water. Consequently, in cystic fibrosis, the acini and intercalated ducts of the pancreas and the small airways of the lungs become clogged with mucus. The pancreatic exocrine function of most infants with cystic fibrosis has been irreversibly damaged in utero. For this reason, infants with cystic fibrosis frequently have severe digestive difficulties, especially in the digestion and absorption of fats.

Neural and hormonal stimuli elicit the secretion of pancreatic juice

Stimulation of the vagal branches to the pancreas enhances secretion. The activation of sympathetic fibers inhibits pancreatic secretion, partly by decreasing blood flow to the pancreas. Secretin and CCK, hormones released from the duodenal mucosa, stimulate secretion of the aqueous and enzyme components, respectively. CCK also evokes the release of acetylcholine from nerve endings in the pancreas. Because the aqueous and enzyme components of pancreatic juice are separately controlled (Figure 34–12), the protein content of the juice varies from less than 1% to as much as 10%.

Gastrin is an important agonist during the cephalic phase

Table 34–4 summarizes the physiological regulation of pancreatic secretion during the cephalic,

TABLE 34–4. CONTROL OF EXOCRINE PANCREATIC SECRETION DURING THE CEPHALIC, GASTRIC, AND INTESTINAL PHASES

Phase	Stimuli of Secretion	Mediator or Mechanism
Cephalic	Sight, smell, and taste of food	Vagal and enteric nerve impulses stimulate acinar and duct cells
Gastric	Distention of stomach	Vagovagal and gastropancreatic reflexes stimulate acinar and duct cells
Intestinal	Acid duodenum (pH < 4.5) Amino acids and fatty acids, Ca^{++} Distention of duodenum, hypertonicity in duodenum	Secretin stimulates duct cells CCK stimulates afferent arm of vagovagal reflexes to acinar and duct cells Enteropancreatic reflexes stimulate acinar and duct cells

gastric, and intestinal phases of digestion. Gastrin is released from G cells in the mucosa of the gastric antrum in response to vagal impulses, and gastrin stimulates pancreatic secretion during the cephalic phase. Gastrin is a member of the same class of peptides as CCK, but it is much less potent than CCK as a pancreatic secretagogue. **Figure 34–13** shows the agonists that can elicit secretion from pancreatic acinar cells during the different phases of digestion.

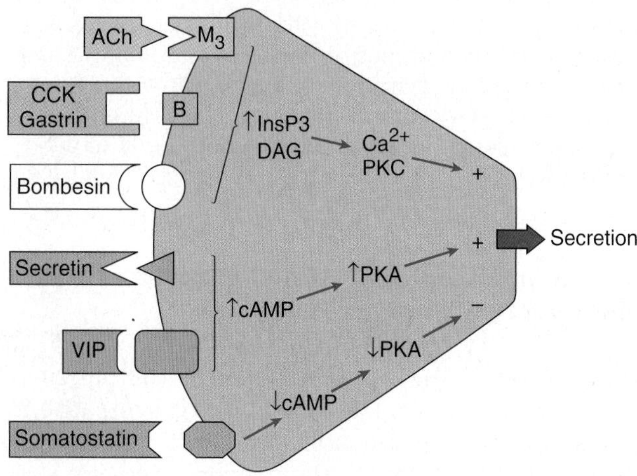

FIGURE 34–13. Agonists that elicit secretion from pancreatic acinar cells and their second-messenger mechanisms. Acetylcholine (ACh) acting on M_3 muscarinic receptors is the major physiological agonist in humans. CCK and gastrin act on CCK-B receptors. Acetylcholine and CCK stimulate secretion by elevating InsP3 and diacylglycerol (DAG), which results in increased cytosolic Ca^{++} and stimulates protein kinase C (PKC). VIP and secretin stimulate secretion by elevating cytosolic cAMP, which enhances the activity of protein kinase A (PKA). Somatostatin inhibits secretion by decreasing cytosolic levels of cAMP. (From Berne RM, Levy MN, Koeppen BM, Stanton BA: *Physiology,* ed 5, Philadelphia, 2004, Elsevier.)

Gastric-phase pancreatic secretion is elicited by gastrin and neural reflexes

During the gastric phase of secretion, gastrin, which is released in response to gastric distention and the presence of amino acids and peptides in the antrum of the stomach, enhances secretion by the pancreas. In addition, an enteric neural reflex (the **gastropancreatic reflex**) and vagovagal reflexes elicited by distention of the stomach evoke pancreatic secretion.

The greatest volume of pancreatic secretion occurs during the intestinal phase

In the intestinal phase of secretion, certain components of the chyme in the duodenum and upper jejunum evoke pancreatic secretion. Acid in the duodenum and upper jejunum elicits the secretion of a large amount of pancreatic juice low in enzyme content. THE HORMONE SECRETIN IS THE MAJOR MEDIATOR OF THIS RESPONSE TO ACID. Secretin is released by S cells in the mucosa of the duodenum and upper jejunum in response to acid in the lumen, and it directly stimulates the epithelial cells of the pancreatic extralobular ducts to secrete the HCO_3^--rich aqueous component of the pancreatic juice. Distention of the duodenum evokes a neural reflex (the **duodenopancreatic reflex**) and vagovagal reflexes that promote pancreatic secretion.

The presence of peptides and certain amino acids in the duodenum elicits the secretion of pancreatic juice rich in enzyme components. Fatty acids and monoglycerides in the duodenum also elicit the secretion of protein-rich pancreatic juice. CCK, A HORMONE RELEASED BY I CELLS IN THE DUODENUM AND UPPER JEJUNUM IN RESPONSE TO THESE DIGESTION PRODUCTS, IS THE MOST IMPORTANT PHYSIOLOGICAL MEDIATOR OF THE ENZYME COMPONENT OF PANCREATIC JUICE. CCK potentiates the stimulatory effect of secretin on the ducts, and secretin potentiates the effect of CCK on acinar cells. It appears that gastrin-releasing peptide released from nerve endings in the pancreas enhances the effects of CCK and secretin.

Functions of the Liver and Gallbladder

The liver is organized into lobules

Each liver **lobule** is organized around a **central vein** (Figure 34–14). At the periphery of the lobule, blood enters the **sinusoids** from branches of the **portal vein** and the **hepatic artery** (see also Chapter 25). In the sinusoids, blood flows toward the center of the lobule between plates of **hepatocytes** one or two cells thick. Because of the large fenestrations between the endothelial cells lining the sinusoids, each hepatocyte is in direct contact with sinusoidal blood. The intimate contact of a large fraction of the hepatocyte surface with blood contributes to the liver's ability to effectively clear the blood of certain classes of compounds. **Biliary canaliculi** lie between adjacent hepatocytes, and the canaliculi drain into bile ducts at the periphery of the lobule.

The metabolic functions of the liver are required for life

The liver is essential in regulating metabolism, synthesizing many proteins and other molecules, storing certain vitamins and iron, degrading certain hormones, and inactivating and excreting many drugs and toxins. It regulates the metabolism of carbohydrates, lipids, and proteins. Liver and skeletal muscles are the two major sites of glycogen storage in the body. When the level of glucose in the blood is high, glycogen is deposited in the liver. When the blood glucose level is low, glycogen is broken down to glucose **(glycogenolysis),** and the glucose is released into the blood. In this way, the liver helps maintain a relatively constant blood glucose level. The liver is also the major site of **gluconeogenesis,** the conversion of amino acids, lipids, or simple carbohydrates (e.g., lactate) into glucose. Several hormones regulate carbohydrate metabolism by the liver (see Chapters 42, 43, and 47).

The liver is also centrally involved in lipid metabolism. As described in Chapter 35, lipids absorbed by the intestine leave the intestine in **chylomicrons** in the lymph. **Lipoprotein lipase** on the endothelial cell surfaces of blood vessels hydrolyzes some of the triglyceride in the chylomicrons and releases glycerol and fatty acids that are taken up by **adipocytes.** This results in the formation of **chylomicron remnants** rich in cholesterol. Chylomicron remnants are taken up by hepatocytes and degraded. Hepatocytes synthesize and secrete **very-low-density lipoproteins,** which are then converted to the other classes of serum lipoproteins. These lipoproteins are the major sources of cholesterol and triglycerides for most other tissues of the body. CHOLESTEROL PRESENT IN BILE REPRESENTS CHOLESTEROL'S ONLY ROUTE OF EXCRETION. Hepatocytes are thus a principal source of cholesterol in the body and the major site of excretion of cholesterol. Thus, HEPATOCYTES PLAY AN IMPORTANT ROLE IN THE REGULATION OF SERUM CHOLESTEROL LEVELS.

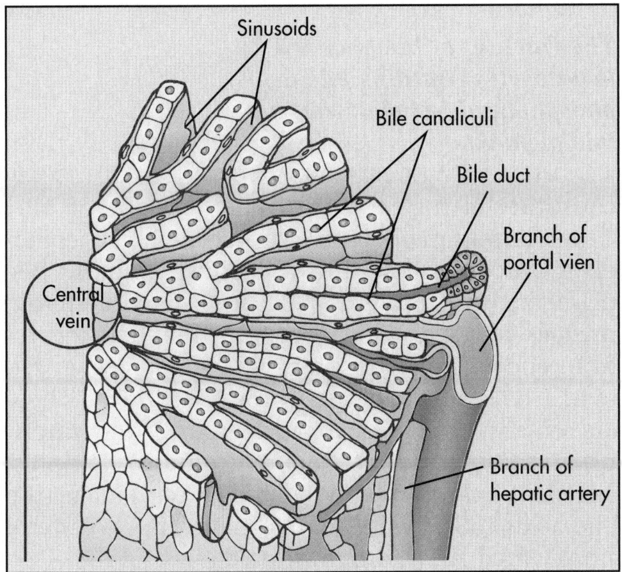

FIGURE 34–14. Classic hepatic lobule. A central vein is located in the center of the lobule, with plates of hepatocytes disposed radially. Branches of the portal vein and hepatic artery are located on the periphery of the lobule, and blood from both perfuses the sinusoids. Peripherally located bile ducts drain the bile canaliculi that run between the hepatocytes. (Modified from Bloom W, Fawcett DW: *A textbook of histology,* ed 10, Philadelphia, 1975, WB Saunders.)

When carbohydrate use is impaired in **diabetes mellitus,** beta oxidation of fatty acids provides a major source of energy for the body (see Chapters 42 and 43). In the liver, the oxidation of fatty acids produces acetoacetate, β-hydroxybutyrate, and acetone. These three compounds are called **ketone bodies.** Ketone bodies are released from hepatocytes and carried via the circulation to other tissues, where they are metabolized. The levels of ketone bodies in the urine and blood can indicate the severity of diabetic acidosis.

The liver is centrally involved in protein metabolism. When proteins are broken down (catabolized), amino acids are deaminated to form ammonia. Ammonia cannot be further metabolized by most tissues and becomes toxic at levels achievable by metabolism. Ammonia is dissipated by conversion to urea, mainly in the liver. The liver also synthesizes all the nonessential amino acids. THE

LIVER SYNTHESIZES ALL THE MAJOR PLASMA PROTEINS, including the plasma lipoproteins, albumins, globulins, fibrinogens, and proteins involved in blood clotting.

The liver stores certain substances that are important in metabolism. Next to hemoglobin in red blood cells, the liver is the most important storage site for iron. Also, certain vitamins, most notably A, D, and B_{12}, are stored in the liver. Hepatic storage protects the body from limited dietary deficiencies of these vitamins.

The liver transforms and excretes many hormones, drugs, and toxins so that they can be excreted. These substances are frequently converted to inactive forms by reactions that occur in hepatocytes. The smooth endoplasmic reticulum of hepatocytes contains systems of enzymes and cofactors that are responsible for the chemical transformations of many substances. Certain other enzymes in the endoplasmic reticulum catalyze the conjugation of many compounds with glucuronic acid, glycine, or glutathione. The transformations that occur in the liver render many compounds more water soluble so that they can more readily be excreted by the kidneys. Some liver metabolites of drugs and hormones are secreted into the bile.

Bile is secreted by hepatocytes and ductular epithelial cells

The hepatic function most important to the digestive tract is the secretion of **bile.** Bile, which is elaborated by hepatocytes, contains bile acids, cholesterol, lecithins, and bile pigments. These constituents, along with an isotonic fluid that resembles plasma in its electrolyte concentrations, are synthesized and secreted by hepatocytes into the bile canaliculi. The bile canaliculi merge into ever-larger ducts and finally into a single large bile duct. The epithelial cells that line the bile ducts secrete a watery fluid that is rich in HCO_3^- and that contributes to the volume of bile leaving the liver.

The secretory function of the liver shares important features with that of the exocrine pancreas. In both organs, the major parenchymal cell type elaborates a primary secretion containing the substances responsible for the major digestive function of the organ. In both the liver and the pancreas, the primary secretion is isotonic to plasma and contains Na^+, K^+, and Cl^- at close to plasma levels, and CCK stimulates the primary secretion. In both the pancreas and the liver, the epithelial cells lining the duct systems modify the primary secretion. When they are stimulated by secretin, the ductular epithelial cells contribute an aqueous secretion with a high [HCO_3^-].

Between meals, bile is diverted into the **gallbladder,** where it is stored and concentrated (see later). From 250 to 1500 mL of bile enters the duodenum each day, and it is a mixture of hepatic and gallbladder bile.

Bile acids emulsify lipids and thereby increase the surface area available to lipolytic enzymes. Bile acids then form **mixed micelles** (see Chapter 35) with the products of lipid digestion. Micelles increase the transport of the products of lipid digestion to the brush border surface; micelles thereby enhance the absorption of lipids by the epithelial cells. Bile acids are actively absorbed, mainly in the terminal ileum. A small fraction of bile acids escapes absorption and is excreted. Bile acids returning to the liver are avidly taken up by hepatocytes and are rapidly resecreted during the course of digestion. The entire bile acid pool is recirculated two or more times in response to a typical meal. The recirculation of the bile acids is known as the **enterohepatic circulation** (see later).

Bile acids lost into the feces are a significant mechanism of cholesterol excretion. Treatment with drugs that inhibit the reabsorption of bile acids in the ileum promotes the synthesis of new bile acids from cholesterol. Such drugs have been used to lower the level of cholesterol in the blood.

The fraction of bile secreted by hepatocytes contains bile acids, phospholipids, cholesterol, and bile pigments

BILE ACIDS ARE THE MAJOR COMPONENT OF BILE. They constitute about 50% of the dry weight of bile. Other important compounds secreted by hepatocytes into the bile include phospholipids, bile pigments, and proteins. Bile acids have a steroid nucleus and are synthesized by the hepatocytes from cholesterol. The major bile acids synthesized by the liver are called **primary bile acids.** These are **cholic acid** (3-hydroxyl groups) and **chenodeoxycholic acid** (2-hydroxyl groups). The presence of the carboxyl and hydroxyl groups makes the bile acids more water soluble than the cholesterol from which they are synthesized.

Bacteria in the digestive tract dehydroxylate some of the bile acids to form **secondary bile acids.** The major secondary bile acids are **deoxycholic acid** (from dehydroxylation of cholic acid) and **lithocholic acid** (from dehydroxylation of chenodeoxycholic acid). Bile contains both primary and secondary bile acids.

Bile acids are normally secreted conjugated with glycine or taurine. In conjugated bile acids, the glycine or taurine is linked by a peptide bond between the carboxyl group of an unconjugated bile acid and the amino group of glycine or taurine. At the near-neutral pH of the gastrointestinal tract, conjugated bile acids are more completely ionized and thus more water soluble than unconjugated bile acids. Conjugated bile acids are present almost entirely as salts of various cations (mostly Na^+) and are often called **bile salts.**

The steroid nucleus of bile acids is almost planar. In solution, bile acids have their polar (hydrophilic) substituents—the hydroxyl groups, the carboxyl moiety of glycine or taurine, and the peptide bond—all on one surface of the molecule. This makes the bile acid molecule amphipathic (i.e., having both hydrophilic and hydrophobic domains). Because they are amphipathic, bile acids tend to form molecular aggregates called **micelles** in which the hydrophobic side of the bile acid faces inside and away from water and the hydrophilic surface faces outward and toward the water (see Chapter 35). When the concentration of bile acids exceeds a certain concentration (called the **critical micelle concentration**), bile acid micelles form. Conjugated bile acids (bile salts) have a lower critical micelle concentration. Above the critical micelle concentration, any additional bile acid goes into the micelles exclusively and not into molecular solution. In bile, the bile acid concentration is normally much greater than the critical micelle concentration.

PHOSPHOLIPIDS IN BILE HELP SOLUBILIZE CHOLESTEROL. Hepatocytes also secrete phospholipids, especially lecithins, into bile. Cholesterol is also secreted into the bile, and this is the major route for cholesterol excretion. Although lecithin and cholesterol are essentially insoluble in water, they dissolve in the interior of bile acid micelles. Lecithin increases the amount of cholesterol that can be solubilized in the micelles.

If more cholesterol is present in the bile than can be solubilized in the micelles, crystals of cholesterol form in the bile. These crystals are important in the formation of **cholesterol gallstones** (the most common gallstones) in the duct system of the liver or more often in the gallbladder.

BILE PIGMENTS ARE END PRODUCTS OF PORPHYRIN CATABOLISM. When senescent red blood cells are degraded in reticuloendothelial cells, the porphyrin moiety of hemoglobin is converted to **bilirubin.** Bilirubin is released into the plasma, where it is bound to albumin. Hepatocytes efficiently remove bilirubin from blood in the sinusoids and conjugate bilirubin with one or two glucuronic acid molecules. Uptake of bilirubin into the hepatocytes occurs via several transporters including OATP. Bilirubin glucuronides are secreted into the bile by MRP2. Bilirubin is yellow and contributes to the yellow color of bile.

Specific transport proteins mediate uptake and secretion of bile acids and bile salts

Enterohepatic circulation of bile acids and salts involves their reabsorption in the terminal ileum (see later and also Chapter 35) into the portal blood, avid uptake as bile salts by hepatocytes, rehydroxylation and reconjugation in the hepatocytes, and rapid resecretion into bile canaliculi. Specific transport proteins are responsible for the uptake and secretion of bile salts. The transporters in the hepatocyte plasma membrane facing sinusoidal blood are different from the transporters in the membrane that bounds the bile canaliculus **(Figure 34–15).**

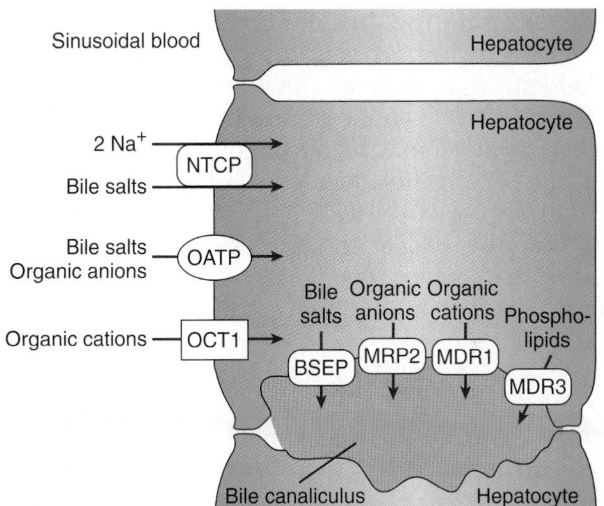

FIGURE 34–15. Transport proteins of hepatocytes. Bile salts are taken up by hepatocytes from sinusoidal blood by two different transporters. NTCP (Na^+-dependent taurocholate transporter) is a secondary active transporter that takes up all of the conjugated bile salts, both primary and secondary. OATP (organic anion transport protein) transports bile salts and bile acids and other organic anions from sinusoidal blood into the hepatocyte. OCT1 (organic cation transporter 1) takes up organic cations from sinusoidal blood. There are four different transport proteins in the canalicular membrane that transport compounds from the hepatocyte cytosol into the bile canaliculus. BSEP (bile salt export protein) transports bile salts into the bile canaliculus. MDR1 (multidrug resistance) protein transports organic cations, and MRP2 (multidrug transporter-related protein) transports organic anions. MDR3 catalyzes the flipping of phosphatidylcholine from the inner leaflet of the plasma membrane to the outer leaflet.

The bile duct epithelium elaborates a HCO_3^--rich aqueous secretion

The epithelial cells that line the bile ducts contribute an aqueous secretion that accounts for about 50% of the total volume of bile. The secretion of the bile duct epithelium is isotonic with plasma and contains Na^+ and K^+ at levels similar to those of plasma. However, the [HCO_3^-] is greater and the [Cl^-] is less than in plasma. The secretory activity of the bile duct epithelium is specifically stimulated by secretin. Acetylcholine released from nerve terminals in the liver and CCK in the blood enhance the stimulatory effects of secretin. The ion transport mechanisms responsible for secretion of the high HCO_3^- isotonic fluid into hepatic ducts are similar to those of extralobular pancreatic ducts.

Bile is concentrated and stored in the gallbladder

Between meals, the tone of the **sphincter of Oddi,** which guards the entrance of the common bile duct into the duodenum, is high. Thus, most bile flow is diverted into the gallbladder. The gallbladder is a small organ, having a capacity of 15 to 60 mL (average, about 35 mL) in humans. Between meals, the liver may secrete many times this volume of bile. The gallbladder concentrates the bile by absorbing Na^+, Cl^-, HCO_3^-, and water from the bile so that the bile acids are concentrated 5 to 20 times. The active transport of Na^+ is the primary active process in the concentrating action of the gallbladder.

Because of its high rate of water absorption, the gallbladder serves as a model for water and electrolyte transport by tight-junctioned epithelia. The **standing osmotic gradient mechanism** for fluid absorption was first proposed for the gallbladder. It was noted that during fluid reabsorption by the gallbladder, the lateral intercellular spaces between the epithelial cells were large and swollen. When fluid transport was blocked, the intercellular spaces almost disappeared. These observations suggested that the intercellular spaces are a major route of fluid flow during absorption.

The primary active transport process is the active transport of Na^+ into the lateral intercellular spaces (**Figure 34–16**). Na^+,K^+-ATPase molecules are especially concentrated in the basolateral membrane near the mucosal (apical) end of the intercellular channels. Cl^- and HCO_3^- are also transported into the intercellular space, probably because of the electrical potential created by electrogenic Na^+ transport. The high NaCl concentration near the apical end of the intercellular space causes the fluid there to be hypertonic. This produces an osmotic flow of water from the lumen, via the tight junctions, and via adjacent cells into the intercellular space. Water distends the intercellular channels because of increased hydrostatic pressure. As a result of water flow from adjacent cells, the fluid becomes less hypertonic as it flows down the intercellular channel, so the fluid is essentially isotonic when it reaches the serosal (basal) end of the channel. Ions and water move across the basement membrane of the epithelium, and the capillaries carry them away.

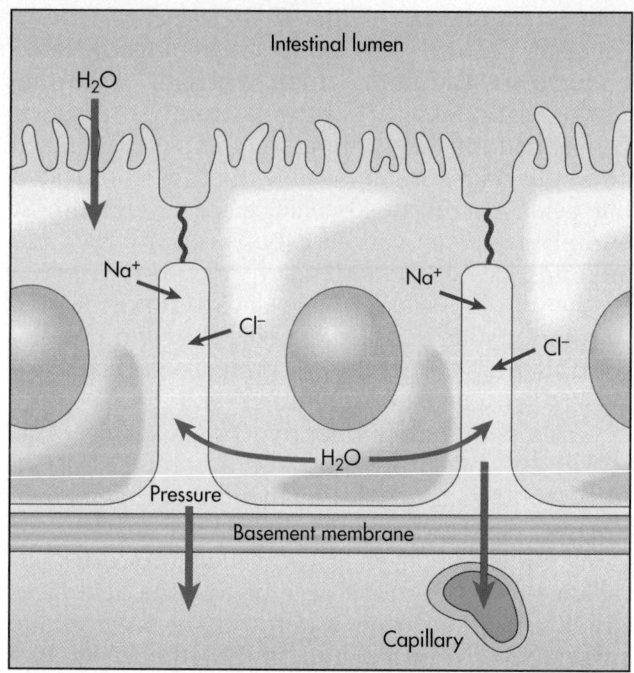

FIGURE 34–16. Water absorption from the gallbladder via the standing gradient osmotic mechanism. Na^+ is actively pumped into the lateral intercellular spaces; Cl^- follows. Water is drawn by osmosis into the intercellular spaces, elevating the intercellular hydrostatic pressure. Water, Na^+, and Cl^- are filtered across the porous basement membrane and enter the capillaries. (From Berne RM, Levy MN, Koeppen BM, Stanton BA: *Physiology,* ed 5, Philadelphia, 2004, Elsevier.)

Emptying of the gallbladder is regulated by nerves and hormones

Emptying of the gallbladder begins several minutes after the start of a meal. Intermittent contractions force bile through the partially relaxed sphincter of Oddi. During the cephalic and gastric phases of digestion, contraction and relaxation of the sphincter are mediated by cholinergic fibers in branches of the vagus nerve and by gastrin released from the stomach. The stimulation of sympathetic nerves to the gallbladder and duodenum inhibits emptying of the gallbladder.

The highest rate of gallbladder emptying occurs during the intestinal phase of digestion; the strongest stimulus for the emptying is CCK. CCK reaches the gallbladder via the circulation and causes strong contractions of the gallbladder and relaxation of the sphincter of Oddi. Substances that mimic the actions of CCK in promoting gallbladder emptying, such as gastrin, are called **cholecystagogues.** Gastrin has the same sequence of five amino acids at its C terminus as CCK does; however, gastrin is not nearly as potent a cholecystagogue as CCK is. Nevertheless, gastrin helps elicit gallbladder contractions during the cephalic and gastric phases of digestion.

Under normal circumstances, the rate of gallbladder emptying is sufficient to keep the concentration of bile acids in the duodenum above the critical micelle concentration.

Bile acids are reabsorbed in the distal ileum and return to the liver in the portal blood

The functions of bile acids in emulsifying dietary lipid and in forming mixed micelles with the products of lipid digestion are discussed in Chapter 35. Normally, by the time chyme reaches the terminal part of the ileum, dietary fat is almost completely absorbed. Bile acids are then absorbed. **Figure 34–17** summarizes the major aspects of the enterohepatic circulation of bile acids and bile salts. Transport mechanisms are present in the brush border of the terminal ileum for uptake of both conjugated and unconjugated bile acids. Conjugated bile acids can be taken up against a large concentration gradient. Because bile acids are also lipid soluble, they can also be taken up by simple diffusion. Bacteria in the terminal part of the ileum and colon deconjugate bile acids and also dehydroxylate them to produce secondary bile acids. Both deconjugation and dehydroxylation lessen the polarity of bile acids and thereby enhance their lipid solubility and their absorption by simple diffusion.

Typically, about 0.2 to 0.6 g of bile acids escapes absorption and is excreted in the feces each day. This quantity is 15% to 35% of the total bile acid pool, and it is normally replenished via the synthesis of new bile acids by the liver. Bile acids, whether they are absorbed by active transport or simple diffusion, are transported away from the intestine in the portal blood, mostly bound to plasma proteins. In the liver, hepatocytes avidly extract the bile acids, as salts, from the portal blood. IN A SINGLE PASS THROUGH THE LIVER, THE PORTAL BLOOD IS ESSENTIALLY CLEARED OF BILE ACIDS. Bile acids in all forms, primary and secondary, both conjugated and deconjugated, are taken up by the

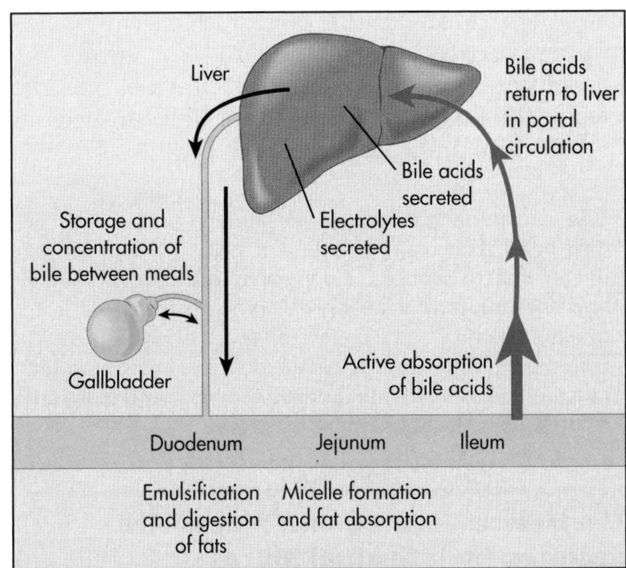

FIGURE 34–17. Overview of the enterohepatic circulation of bile. Bile is dumped into the duodenum as a result of contractions of the gallbladder. In the small intestine, bile acids first emulsify dietary fat and then form mixed micelles with the products of fat digestion. In the terminal ileum, bile acids are reabsorbed. Bile acids return to the liver in the portal blood; they are avidly taken up by hepatocytes and resecreted into bile. Some of the bile acids (15% to 35% of the total pool of bile acids) is excreted each day in the feces.

hepatocytes. The hepatocytes reconjugate almost all the deconjugated bile acids and rehydroxylate some of the secondary bile acids. These bile acids are secreted into the bile along with newly synthesized bile acids (Figure 34–15).

Bile acids in portal blood stimulate hepatocytes to secrete

The rate of return of the bile acids to the liver affects the rate of synthesis and secretion of bile acids. Bile acids in the portal blood stimulate the uptake and resecretion of bile acids by hepatocytes. This is called the **choleretic effect** of bile acids; substances that enhance bile acid secretion are called choleretics. So powerful is the stimulus to resecrete the returning bile acids that the entire pool of bile acids (1.5 to 31.5 g) recirculates twice in response to a typical meal. In response to a meal with a very high fat content, the bile acid pool may recirculate five or more times.

Gallstones have cholesterol or bile pigments as major constituents

Cholesterol is essentially insoluble in water. When bile contains more cholesterol than can be solubilized in the bile acid–lecithin micelles, crystals of cholesterol form in the bile. Such bile is called **supersaturated** with cholesterol. The greater the concentration of bile acids and lecithin in bile, the greater the amount of cholesterol that can be contained in the mixed micelles.

Bile pigment gallstones are another major class of gallstones; their major constituent is the calcium salt of unconjugated bilirubin. Conjugated bilirubin is soluble and does not form insoluble calcium salts in bile. In liver disease, bile may contain elevated levels of unconjugated bilirubin because hepatocytes are deficient in forming the glucuronides of bilirubin. Individuals with liver disease are more likely to form bile pigment stones.

Electrolytes, Water, and Mucus Are Secreted by Intestinal Mucosa

The mucosa of the intestine, from the duodenum through the rectum, elaborates secretions that contain mucus, electrolytes, and water. The total volume of intestinal secretions is about 1500 mL/day. The mucus in the secretions protects the mucosa from mechanical damage. The nature of the secretions and the mechanisms that control secretion vary in different segments of the intestine. The secretions of each segment of the intestine increase during or after a meal. In each intestinal segment, the secretion of water, electrolytes, and mucus is stimulated by parasympathetic nerves and by acetylcholine and VIP released from enteric secretomotor neurons (see Chapter 33). In all segments of the intestine, secretion is stimulated by reflexes evoked by distention and mechanical stimulation of the mucosa.

Duodenal secretions are mostly produced by duodenal glands

The duodenal submucosa contains branching glands that elaborate a secretion rich in mucus. The duodenal epithelial cells also contribute to duodenal secretions, but the glands produce most of the secretion. The duodenal secretion contains mucus and an aqueous component that does not differ significantly from plasma in its concentrations of the major ions.

Small intestinal epithelial cells produce a large volume of isotonic secretion

During normal digestion, an aqueous secretion is elaborated by the epithelial cells at a rate only slightly less than that of fluid absorption by the small intestine (see Chapter 35). Goblet cells, which lie among the columnar epithelial cells of the small intestine, secrete mucus.

Colonic secretions are rich in mucus

The secretions of the colon are smaller in volume but much richer in mucus than the secretions of the small intestine. Mucus is produced by numerous goblet cells in the colonic mucosa. The aqueous component of colonic secretions is enriched in K^+ and HCO_3^- compared with plasma. Colonic secretion is stimulated by mechanical irritation of the mucosa and by activation of cholinergic pathways to the colon. The stimulation of sympathetic nerves to the colon decreases the rate of colonic secretion.

Summary

- The epithelial cells that line the gastrointestinal tract and the cells of various glands associated with the gastrointestinal tract produce secretions that contain water, electrolytes, mucus, and proteins.
- Gastrointestinal secretion is regulated by intrinsic and extrinsic neurons, hormones, and paracrine mediators.
- Salivary glands produce a hypotonic fluid with HCO_3^- concentration greatly in excess of plasma levels. Saliva contains an amylase that begins the digestion of starch.
- The stomach serves as a reservoir for ingested food and empties gastric contents into the duodenum at a regulated rate. Parietal cells secrete HCl and intrinsic factor into the stomach. Chief cells secrete pepsinogens.
- The regulation of HCl secretion in the stomach involves extrinsic and intrinsic nerves, with acetylcholine as the major stimulatory neurotransmitter. Gastrin, a hormone released by G cells in the gastric antrum and in the duodenum, and histamine, a paracrine agonist released by ECL cells in the stomach, are also important physiological agonists of HCl secretion.

- ❖ Acetylcholine stimulates the release of gastrin from G cells in the gastric antrum and histamine from ECL cells in the mucosa of the stomach. Histamine is a potent agonist of parietal cell HCl secretion. Gastrin stimulates the release of somatostatin from D cells in the gastric antrum. Somatostatin is a powerful inhibitor of HCl secretion that serves to prevent uncontrolled HCl secretion.
- ❖ HCl catalyzes the conversion of pepsinogens to active pepsins. Pepsins convert a significant fraction of ingested protein to oligopeptides.
- ❖ Mucus and HCO_3^- secretions form the "gastric mucosal barrier" that protects the epithelial cells of the stomach from the effects of HCl and pepsins.
- ❖ When acid secretion is uncontrolled or when the gastric mucosal barrier is compromised, ulcers can form in the stomach or in the duodenum. Overuse of aspirin and other nonsteroidal antiinflammatory drugs damages the gastric mucosal barrier and may induce ulcers to form. The acid-loving bacterium *Helicobacter pylori* can cause inflammation and ulcers and may lead to gastric cancer.
- ❖ The pancreas produces a HCO_3^--rich fluid that contains enzymes essential for the digestion of carbohydrates, proteins, and fats. Pancreatic acinar cells produce the enzyme component of pancreatic juice; the intralobular and extralobular ducts secrete most of the aqueous component (water and electrolytes) of pancreatic juice.
- ❖ CCK and secretin are hormones released by cells in the duodenum and jejunum in response to the presence of fat digestion products and acid, respectively. CCK is the major physiological agonist of acinar cell secretion of the enzyme component. Secretin is the major stimulus for secretion of HCO_3^--rich fluid by the extralobular ducts of the pancreas. Acetylcholine released from parasympathetic and enteric neurons enhances the effects of CCK and secretin.
- ❖ The liver produces and the gallbladder concentrates bile. Bile is a HCO_3^--rich fluid that contains bile acids, bile pigments, lecithin, cholesterol, and numerous other components. Bile acids play a vital role in the digestion and absorption of lipids.
- ❖ Hepatocytes are responsible for secreting the organic components of bile. The cells of the bile ducts secrete a HCO_3^--rich fluid. CCK is a major secretagogue for secretion by the hepatocytes. Secretin stimulates the bile ducts to produce their HCO_3^--rich fluid. Acetylcholine released from parasympathetic and enteric neurons enhances the effects of CCK and secretin.
- ❖ Bile acids are absorbed in the terminal ileum and return to the liver in the portal vein. Hepatocytes rapidly clear the blood of bile acids and resecrete them. Bile acids in the portal blood are a powerful stimulus that causes the hepatocytes to resecrete bile acids.

Bibliography

Arias IM et al: *The liver: biology and pathobiology,* ed 4, Philadelphia, 2001, Lippincott Williams & Wilkins.

Cancela JM: Specific Ca signaling evoked by cholecystokinin and acetylcholine, *Annu Rev Physiol* 63:99, 2001.

Del Valle J, Todisco A: Gastric secretion. In Yamada T, ed: *Textbook of gastroenterology,* ed 4, Philadelphia, 2003, Lippincott Williams & Wilkins.

Dockray GJ et al: The gastrins: their production and biological activities, *Annu Rev Physiol* 63:119, 2001.

Greger R: Role of CFTR in colon, *Annu Rev Physiol* 62:467, 2000.

Kidd JF, Thorn P: Intracellular Ca and Cl channel activation in secretory cells, *Annu Rev Physiol* 62:493, 2000.

Meier PJ, Stieger B: Bile salt transporters, *Annu Rev Physiol* 64:635, 2002.

Owyang C, Williams JA: Pancreatic secretion. In Yamada T, ed: *Textbook of gastroenterology,* ed 4, Philadelphia, 2003, Lippincott Williams & Wilkins.

Prinz C, Zanner R, Gratzl M: Physiology of gastric enterochromaffin-like cells, *Annu Rev Physiol* 65:371, 2003.

Rozengurt E, Walsh JH: Gastrin, CCK, signaling, and cancer, *Annu Rev Physiol* 63:49, 2001.

Sachs G et al: The gastric biology of *Helicobacter pylori, Annu Rev Physiol* 65:349, 2003.

Samuelson LC, Hinkle KL: Insights into the regulation of gastric acid secretion through analysis of genetically engineered mice, *Annu Rev Physiol* 65:383, 2003.

Weinman SA, Kemmer N: Bile secretion and cholestasis. In Yamada T, ed: *Textbook of gastroenterology,* ed 4, Philadelphia, 2003, Lippincott Williams & Wilkins.

Williams JA: Intracellular signaling mechanisms activated by cholecystokinin regulating synthesis and secretion of digestive enzymes in pancreatic acinar cells, *Annu Rev Physiol* 63:77, 2001.

Yao X, Forte JG: Cell biology of acid secretion by the parietal cell, *Annu Rev Physiol* 65:103, 2003.

Case Studies

Case 34–1

A 25-year-old woman has persistent diarrhea, steatorrhea, and abdominal pain. An upper gastrointestinal radiological series suggests a duodenal ulcer. The presence of the ulcer is confirmed by endoscopy. The patient's basal rate of secretion of gastric HCl is about 12 mmol/hr (the normal range is 1 to 5 mmol/hr). The patient has an elevated serum gastrin level (1145 pg/mL); the normal range is 50 to 150 pg/mL. After a test meal, the patient's serum gastrin level does not increase significantly. The diagnosis is Zollinger-Ellison syndrome, a disorder in which an ectopic tumor secretes high levels of gastrin.

1. **With regard to the patient's disorder:**
   A. The patient is likely to be secreting normal levels of pepsinogens.
   B. Increased pepsin levels and H^+ concentrations in the duodenum did not contribute to her duodenal ulceration.
   C. Her steatorrhea may be a consequence of a low duodenal pH.
   D. Muscarinic antagonists would not partially alleviate the symptoms.

2. **With regard to the etiology and diagnosis of the patient's disorder:**
   A. All patients with elevated gastrin levels have high rates of HCl secretion.
   B. The patient's gastrin level will increase following a meal.
   C. The patient may have an increased number of HCl-secreting glands in her stomach.
   D. The patient has a high probability of gastric ulcers.

3. **With regard to treatment of the patient's disorder:**
   A. Treatment with an antagonist of somatostatin might be useful.
   B. H_2 receptor blockers should be as effective in this woman as in a healthy individual.
   C. Sectioning the vagus nerve branches to the fundus and the body would be ineffective.
   D. Omeprazole should effectively block HCl secretion in this patient.

Case 34–2

A 38-year-old woman complains of pain in the right upper quadrant of her abdomen. The pain usually occurs after eating a heavy meal or a fatty snack. Pain tends to be constant, lasts for about an hour, and is accompanied by nausea. The patient was given 6 g of ipodate calcium (a radiographic contrast agent that is concentrated in the gallbladder) by mouth during 12 hours, and then x-ray studies of her gallbladder, cystic duct, and common bile duct were performed. Several radiolucent stones (5 to 10 mm in diameter) were detected in the gallbladder, but no stones were found in the cystic or common bile duct. The diagnosis is **cholecystitis** probably caused by gallstones in the gallbladder.

1. **With regard to the etiology of the patient's disorder:**
   A. Cholesterol hypersecretion probably contributes to the formation of her cholesterol gallstones.
   B. Abnormalities of gallbladder motility do not usually influence the formation of cholesterol gallstones.
   C. Mucus secretion by gallbladder epithelial cells protects against cholesterol gallstone formation.
   D. If the patient had used nonsteroidal antiinflammatory drugs, this would not have influenced the rate at which cholesterol gallstones formed.

2. **With regard to the diagnosis and treatment of the patient's disorder:**
   A. It is most likely that the patient has cholesterol gallstones.
   B. The fact that the stones are radiolucent indicates that significant calcification of the gallstones has occurred.
   C. Ultrasonography could not confirm the presence of stones in the gallbladder.
   D. The patient does not have bile pigment gallstones.

3. **With regard to treatment of the patient's gallstones:**
   A. If the patient were fed bile salts, the stones would dissolve in a matter of hours.
   B. This patient requires immediate surgery.
   C. Treatment of this patient with an inhibitor of cholesterol synthesis is likely to be effective.
   D. Once the patient's stones are dissolved, additional stones are unlikely to form.

Chapter 35: Digestion and Absorption

Objectives

- Describe digestion and absorption of sucrose, lactose, and branched starch molecules.
- Describe digestion and absorption of proteins.
- Describe digestion and absorption of lipids.
- Describe the transport of water and electrolytes in the small and large intestines.
- Describe the absorption of Ca^{++}.
- Describe the absorption of iron.
- Describe the absorption of water-soluble vitamins, especially vitamin B_{12}.

The cells that line the gastrointestinal tract cannot absorb most nutrients in the forms in which they are ingested. **Digestion** refers to the processes by which ingested molecules are cleaved into smaller ones by enzymes in the gastrointestinal secretions (discussed in Chapter 34) or on the luminal surface of the gastrointestinal tract. As a result of digestion, ingested molecules are converted to smaller molecules that can be absorbed from the lumen of the gastrointestinal tract. **Absorption** refers to the processes by which molecules are transported through the epithelial cells that line the gastrointestinal tract and then enter the blood or lymph draining that region of the gastrointestinal tract.

Digestion and Absorption of Carbohydrates Occur Mainly in the Duodenum and Jejunum

Carbohydrates are the principal source of calories for most people in the world

Plant starch, **amylopectin,** is the major source of carbohydrate in most human diets. Amylopectin is a high-molecular-weight (MW > 10^6), branched polymer of glucose units. A smaller proportion of dietary starch is **amylose,** a lower molecular weight (MW > 10^5), linear α-1,4–linked polymer of glucose. **Cellulose** is a β-1,4–linked glucose polymer. Intestinal enzymes cannot hydrolyze β-glycosidic linkages; thus, cellulose and other molecules with β-glycosidic linkages remain undigested and contribute to **dietary fiber.** The amount of the animal starch **glycogen** ingested varies widely among cultures and among individuals within a given culture. **Sucrose** and **lactose** are the principal dietary disaccharides, and **glucose** and **fructose** are the major monosaccharides.

Saliva and pancreatic juice contain α-amylases that begin the digestion of starch

The structure of a branched starch molecule is depicted in **Figure 35–1**. Starch is a polymer of glucose and consists of chains of glucose units linked by α-1,4 glycosidic bonds. The α-1,4–linked chains of glucoses have branch points formed by α-1,6 glycosidic linkages.

The digestion of starch begins in the mouth with the action of **salivary amylase.** This enzyme catalyzes the hydrolysis of the internal α-1,4 bonds of

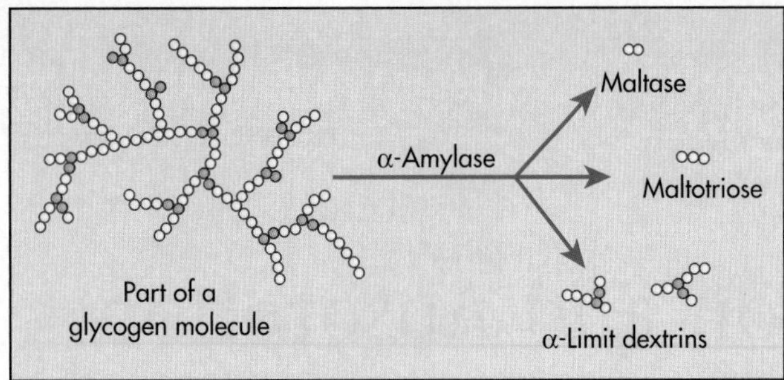

FIGURE 35–1. Structure of a branched starch molecule and the action of α-amylase. The circles represent glucose monomers. The colored circles show glucose units linked by α-1,6 linkages at the branch points. The α-1,6 links and terminal α-1,4 bonds cannot be cleaved by α-amylase.

starch, but it cannot hydrolyze the terminal α-1,4 bonds or the α-1,6 branching bonds. As shown in Figure 35–1, the principal products of α-amylase digestion of starch are maltose, maltotriose, and branched oligosaccharides known as **α-limit dextrins.** Significant digestion of starch by the salivary amylase may occur, but this enzyme is not required for normal digestion and absorption of the starch. After salivary amylase is inactivated by the low pH of gastric contents, no further processing of carbohydrate occurs in the stomach.

Pancreatic juice contains a highly active α-amylase. The products of starch digestion by the pancreatic enzyme are the same as for the salivary amylase, but the total amylase activity in pancreatic juice is considerably greater than that in saliva. Within 10 minutes after entering the duodenum, starch is almost entirely converted to the oligosaccharides shown in Figure 35–1.

The further digestion of these oligosaccharides is accomplished by enzymes that reside in the brush border membrane of the epithelium of the duodenum and jejunum (**Figure 35–2**). The major brush border oligosaccharides are **lactase,** which splits lactose into glucose and galactose; **sucrase,** which splits sucrose into glucose and fructose; **α-dextrinase** (also called **isomaltase**), which "debranches" the α-limit dextrins by cleaving the α-1,6 bonds at the branch points; and **glucoamylase** (also called **maltase**), which cleaves the terminal α-1,4 glycosidic bonds to break maltooligosaccharides down to glucose units. The activities of these four enzymes are highest in the brush border of the upper jejunum, and they gradually decline through the rest of the small intestine.

Glucose, galactose, and fructose are the only monosaccharides that are well absorbed

The duodenum and upper jejunum have the highest capacity to absorb sugars. The capacities of the lower jejunum and ileum are progressively less. Glucose and galactose are actively taken up across the brush border plasma membrane of epithelial cells through a Na^+-monosaccharide symporter called SGLT1 (**Figure 35–3**). Glucose and galactose compete for entry. Na^+ and glucose or galactose are transported into the cell by SGLT1, which has two Na^+ binding sites and one sugar binding site. The presence of Na^+ in the intestinal lumen enhances the absorption of glucose and galactose, and vice versa. The energy released by Na^+ moving down its electrochemical potential gradient is harnessed to transport one glucose or galactose molecule into the

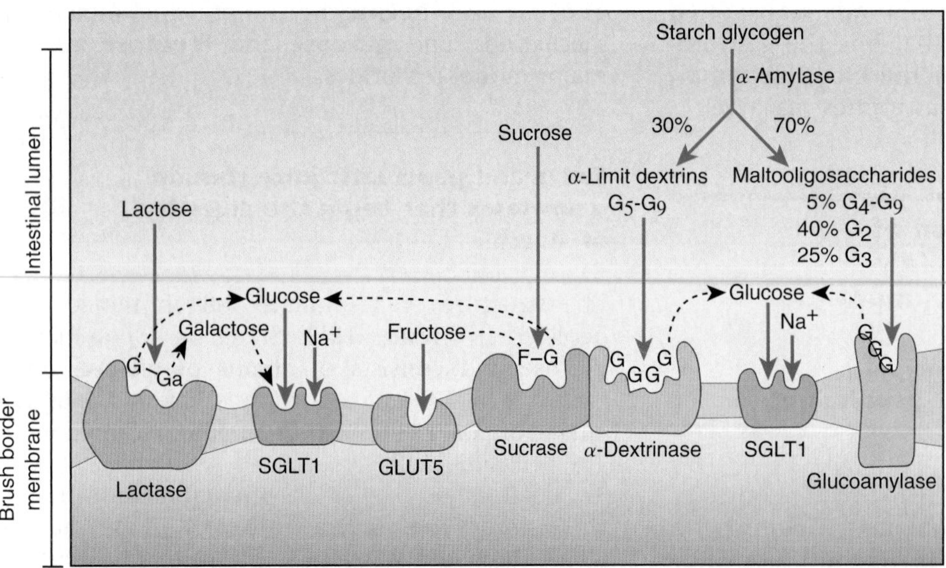

FIGURE 35–2. Functions of the major brush border oligosaccharidases. The glucose, galactose, and fructose molecules released by enzymatic hydrolysis are then transported into the epithelial cells by specific transport proteins in the brush border membrane. F, fructose; G, glucose; Ga, galactose. (Modified from Gray GM: *N Engl J Med* 292:1225, 1975.)

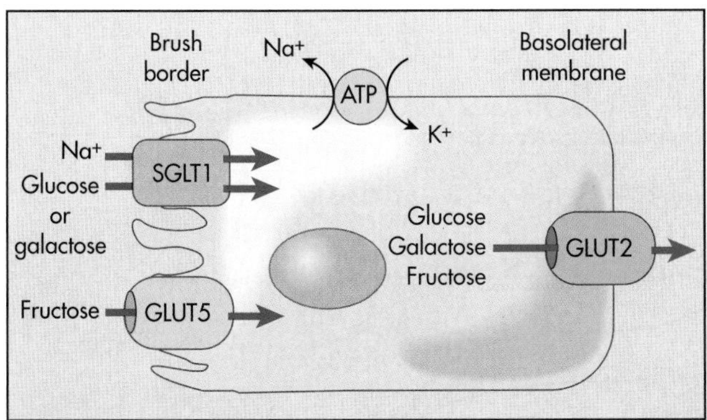

FIGURE 35–3. Glucose and galactose enter the jejunal epithelial cells against a concentration gradient via SGLT1. The gradient of Na^+ provides the energy for sugar entry. Facilitated transport of fructose across the brush border membrane is mediated by GLUT5. All three monosaccharides leave the cell at the basolateral membrane by facilitated transport via GLUT2.

cell against a concentration gradient of the sugar (see Chapter 1). Glucose and galactose leave the intestinal epithelial cell at the basal and lateral plasma membranes via a facilitated transporter (GLUT2), and they diffuse into the mucosal capillaries.

Fructose does not compete well for SGLT1. However, fructose is transported almost as rapidly as glucose and galactose and much more rapidly than other monosaccharides. Fructose is taken up across the brush border membrane by a fructose-specific facilitated transporter (GLUT5). Fructose crosses the basolateral membrane via GLUT2 along with glucose and galactose.

In individuals with low levels of brush border lactase activity, undigested lactose is passed on to the colon. The colonic bacteria rapidly metabolize the lactose, and the bacteria produce gas and release metabolic products that enhance colonic motility and cause diarrhea. This condition is called **lactose intolerance.** Lactose intolerance in the newborn, **congenital lactose intolerance,** is uncommon. Lactose-intolerant infants are usually fed formula with sucrose as the major source of carbohydrate. More than 50% of the world's adults are lactose intolerant. This is genetically determined—most Asian and African adults are lactose intolerant, but most northern European adults tolerate lactose.

About 5% to 15% of ingested carbohydrate escapes digestion and absorption and is passed on to the colon, where it is metabolized by intestinal bacteria to produce short-chain fatty acids and other metabolic products. Short-chain fatty acids—mainly acetate, propionate, and butyrate—are taken up and metabolized by colonic epithelial cells. Short-chain fatty acids (SCFA) are an important fuel for colonic epithelial cells. They are taken up by a Na^+-SCFA symporter in the luminal plasma membrane of colonic epithelial cells.

Digestion and absorption of proteins provide the essential amino acids needed for protein synthesis

The amount of dietary protein varies greatly among cultures and among individuals within a culture. In poor societies, it is difficult for adults to obtain the amount of protein (0.5 to 0.7 g/day/kg of body weight) required to balance the normal catabolism of proteins. It is even more difficult for children to receive the relatively greater amounts of protein required to sustain normal growth. In wealthy societies, a typical individual ingests protein far in excess of the nutritional requirement.

In normal humans, essentially all ingested protein is digested and absorbed by the time intestinal chyme has reached the middle of the jejunum. Most of the protein in digestive secretions and exfoliated cells is also digested and absorbed. The small amount of protein in the feces is derived principally from colonic bacteria, exfoliated colonic cells, and proteins in mucous secretions of the colon.

Digestion of proteins takes place in the stomach and in the upper small intestine

PEPSINS BEGIN THE DIGESTION OF PROTEINS IN THE STOMACH. Pepsinogens are secreted by the chief cells of the stomach and are converted in an acid environment to active **pepsins.** The extent to which pepsins hydrolyze dietary protein is significant but highly variable. At most, about 15% of dietary protein may be reduced to peptides and amino acids by pepsins. The duodenum and small intestine have such a high capacity to digest protein that the total absence of pepsins does not impair the digestion and absorption of dietary protein.

DIGESTION OF PROTEINS IN THE SMALL INTESTINE INVOLVES PANCREATIC PROTEASES AND PEPTIDASES ON THE BRUSH BORDER MEMBRANE SURFACE. Proteases in pancreatic juice play a major role in protein digestion. The most important of these proteases are **trypsin, chymotrypsin, carboxypeptidases A and B,** and **elastase.** Pancreatic juice contains these enzymes in inactive, proenzyme forms (see Chapter 34). The enzyme **enteropeptidase** (formerly known as **enterokinase**), secreted by the mucosa of the duodenum and jejunum, converts trypsino-

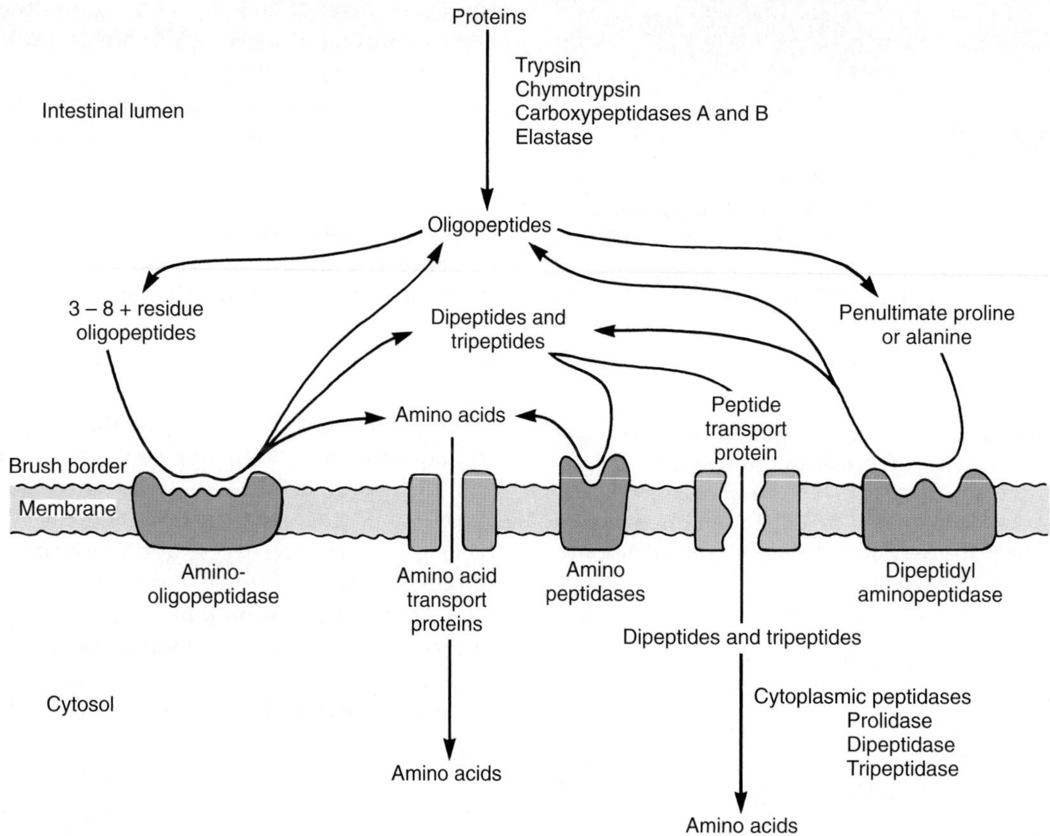

FIGURE 35–4. The hierarchy of proteases and peptidases that function in the small intestine. The pancreatic proteases convert dietary proteins to oligopeptides. Brush border peptidases then convert the oligopeptides to amino acids (about 70%) and dipeptides and tripeptides (about 30%). The amino acids are taken up across the brush border membrane by several amino acid transporters, and dipeptides and tripeptides are taken up by a H^+-peptide symporter. In the enterocyte cytosol, dipeptides and tripeptides are cleaved to single amino acids. (From Berne RM, Levy MN, Koeppen BM, Stanton BA: *Physiology,* ed 5, Philadelphia, 2004, Elsevier.)

gen to active trypsin. Trypsin activates trypsinogen and also converts chymotrypsinogen, procarboxypeptidases A and B, and proelastase to the active enzymes. The pancreatic proteases are very active in the duodenum, and they rapidly convert dietary protein to small peptides. About 50% of ingested protein is digested and absorbed in the duodenum. The brush border of the duodenum and the small intestine contains a number of peptidases **(Figure 35–4)**. These peptidases are integral membrane proteins whose active sites face the intestinal lumen.

The principal products of protein digestion by pancreatic proteases and brush border peptidases are small peptides and single amino acids. The small peptides (mainly dipeptides, tripeptides, and tetrapeptides) are about three or four times more concentrated than single amino acids. Small peptides and amino acids are transported across the brush border plasma membrane into intestinal epithelial cells. In the cytosol of intestinal epithelial cells, small peptides are then hydrolyzed by peptidases; consequently, only single amino acids appear in the portal blood. The cytosolic peptidases are particularly active against dipeptides and tripeptides, which are efficiently transported across the brush border plasma membrane. The brush border peptidases, on the other hand, are mainly active against peptides of four or more amino acids.

Absorption of protein digestion products is accomplished by transporters for amino acids and small peptides

Only minute quantities of intact proteins are absorbed. However, some intact proteins and large peptides are absorbed in sufficient amounts to trigger immunological responses. In ruminants and rodents, but not in humans, the neonatal intestine has a high capacity for the specific absorption of immune globulins present in colostrum. This absorptive process is vital in the development of normal immune competence in ruminants and rodents.

DIPEPTIDES AND TRIPEPTIDES ARE RAPIDLY TRANSPORTED ACROSS THE BRUSH BORDER MEMBRANE. The rate of transport of dipeptides or tripeptides usually exceeds the rate of transport of individual amino acids. For example, glycine is absorbed by the human jejunum less rapidly as the amino acid than it is as glycylglycine or as glycylglycylglycine. A single membrane transporter with broad specificity is responsible for absorption of small peptides. The transporter has high affinity for dipeptides and tripeptides but very low affinities for peptides of four or more amino acid residues. Transport of dipeptides and tripeptides across the brush border plasma membrane is via an H^+-peptide symporter powered by the electrochemical potential difference of H^+ across the membrane.

BRUSH BORDER AND BASOLATERAL PLASMA MEMBRANES DIFFER IN THEIR AMINO ACID TRANSPORT PROTEINS. Amino acids are transported across the brush border plasma membrane into the intestinal epithelial cell by certain specific amino acid transporters. At least seven different transporters have been identified. Some of the transporters depend on the Na^+ gradient, whereas other transport proteins are independent of Na^+.

Hartnup disease is a rare hereditary disorder in which one of the major neutral amino acid transport proteins is deficient in the brush border of the small intestine and the proximal renal tubule. Individuals with Hartnup disease have elevated urinary levels of certain neutral amino acids. However, such patients are not malnourished because the affected neutral amino acids are well absorbed as components of dipeptides and tripeptides in the upper small intestine.

Case 35–1 presented at the end of this chapter deals with niacin deficiency associated with Hartnup disease.

Digestion and Absorption of Lipids Occur Mainly in the Duodenum and Jejunum

The primary lipids of a normal diet are **triglycerides.** The diet contains smaller amounts of **sterols** (such as cholesterol), **sterol esters,** and **phospholipids.** Because lipids are only slightly soluble in water, they pose special problems at every stage of their processing. In the stomach, lipids tend to separate out into an oily phase. In the duodenum and small intestine, lipids are **emulsified** with the aid of bile salts. The emulsion consists of small (micrometer-sized) droplets of lipid coated by bile salts. The large surface area of the emulsion droplets allows access of the water-soluble lipolytic enzymes to their substrates. The digestion products of lipids form tiny molecular aggregates, known as **micelles,** with the bile salts. The micelles are small enough (nanometer scale) to diffuse among the microvilli and to allow absorption of the lipids from molecular solution along the entire surface of the intestinal brush border.

Because fats tend to separate out into an oily phase, they are usually emptied from the stomach later than the other gastric contents. Fat in the duodenum strongly inhibits gastric emptying. This helps ensure that the fat is not emptied from the stomach more rapidly than it can be accommodated by the duodenal mechanisms that provide for emulsification and digestion.

Digestion of lipids occurs in the stomach and the small intestine

Lingual lipase is produced by serous glands in the tongue. **Gastric lipase** is secreted by chief cells. Together, these two lipases constitute **preduodenal lipase.** These enzymes are specific for hydrolysis of triglycerides. In humans, gastric lipase is much more abundant than lingual lipase. The amount of triglyceride hydrolyzed by preduodenal lipases varies considerably among individuals.

Lipases present in pancreatic juice are responsible for hydrolysis of most dietary lipid. The lipolytic enzymes of the pancreatic juice are water-soluble molecules and thus have access to lipids only at the surfaces of the fat droplets. THE SURFACE AVAILABLE FOR DIGESTION IS INCREASED MANY THOUSAND TIMES BY EMULSIFICATION OF THE LIPIDS. Bile salts themselves are rather poor emulsifying agents. However, with the aid of lecithins, which are present in high concentration in bile, the bile salts emulsify dietary fats.

PANCREATIC JUICE CONTAINS THE MAJOR LIPOLYTIC ENZYMES RESPONSIBLE FOR DIGESTION OF LIPIDS. **Glycerol ester hydrolase,** also called **pancreatic lipase,** cleaves the 1 and 1′ fatty acids preferentially from a triglyceride to produce two free fatty acids and one 2-monoglyceride. **Colipase,** a small protein present in pancreatic juice, is essential for the function of glycerol ester hydrolase. Colipase is required for glycerol ester hydrolase to bind to the surface of the emulsion droplets in the presence of bile acids. **Cholesterol esterase** cleaves the ester bond in a cholesterol ester to give one fatty acid and free cholesterol. **Phospholipase A_2** cleaves the ester bond at the 2 position of a glycerophosphatide to yield, in the case of lecithin, one fatty acid and one lysolecithin.

Infants with **cystic fibrosis** (CF) secrete extremely low levels of pancreatic enzymes. This is because the defective Cl^- channels in the apical membranes of pancreatic ductular epithelial cells make the cells unable to secrete Cl^-, Na^+, and water into the acinar lumen. Because little water is secreted, mucus obstructs the small pancreatic ducts, and the pancreatic acinar cells are destroyed. Obstruction by mucus of bronchioles is responsible for the pulmonary problems associated with CF. Because of the deficiency of pancreatic lipases, children with CF have marked difficulties in digesting dietary lipids. Consequently, they may suffer from **steatorrhea** (fatty stool) and malnutrition.

Case 35–2 at the end of the chapter concerns a baby with CF.

Bile salts form mixed micelles with the products of lipid digestion

Triglycerides are not good micelle formers, but 2-monoglycerides are effective in forming mixed micelles with bile salts. The micelles are multimolecular aggregates (about 5 nm in diameter) that contain approximately 20 to 30 molecules **(Figure 35–5)**. Bile salts are flat molecules that have a polar face and a nonpolar face. Much of the surface of the micelles is covered with bile salts, with the nonpolar face of the bile salt toward the lipid interior of the micelle and the polar face toward the outside. Hydrophobic molecules, such as long-chain fatty acids, monoglycerides, phospholipids, cholesterol, and fat-soluble vitamins, tend to partition into the micelles. Bile salts must be present at a certain minimal concentration, called the critical micelle concentration, before micelles will form. Bile salts are normally present in the duodenum at greater than the critical micelle concentration.

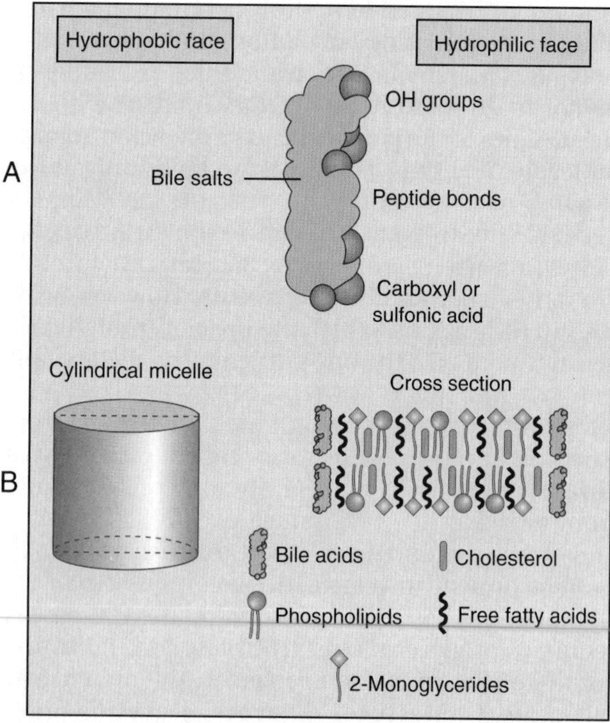

FIGURE 35–5. Structure of bile salts and micelles. A, A bile salt molecule is amphipathic because it has a hydrophobic face and a hydrophilic face. B, Model of the structure of a bile salt–lipid mixed micelle showing the way that bile salts and the major products of lipid digestion pack into the mixed micelle.

Absorption of lipid digestion products takes place in the small intestine

DIFFUSION OF MIXED MICELLES THROUGH THE UNSTIRRED LAYER IS THE RATE-LIMITING STEP IN ABSORPTION OF LIPID DIGESTION PRODUCTS. Micelles are important in the absorption of the products of lipid digestion and in the absorption of most other fat-soluble molecules (e.g., fat-soluble vitamins). The micelles are small enough to diffuse among the microvilli that form the brush border, and this allows the huge surface area of the brush border membrane to participate in lipid absorption **(Figure 35–6)**. The presence of micelles tends to keep the aqueous solution near the brush border plasma membrane saturated with fatty acids, 2-monoglycerides, cholesterol, and other micellar contents.

Because of their high lipid solubility, fatty acids, 2-monoglycerides, cholesterol, and lysolecithin can diffuse across the brush border membrane. In addition, the brush border plasma membrane contains specific transporters that facilitate the transport of particular lipid digestion products. A **Na^+–fatty acid symporter** enhances the movement of long-chain fatty acids across the brush border plasma membrane. Cholesterol can diffuse across the luminal plasma membrane. Cholesterol present in the lumen consists of biliary cholesterol plus cholesterol ingested in food. Only about 50% of the cholesterol is absorbed. The restriction of cholesterol absorption appears to be due mainly to the function of an ABC (ATP-binding cassette) transporter in the brush border membrane. Functioning in a way like the multidrug resistance transporter responsible for multidrug resistance, the cholesterol transporter, a similar ABC transport protein, uses the energy of ATP to remove cholesterol from the membrane and to pump it back into the lumen of the intestine. The cholesterol transporter limits the absorption of plant sterols even more strongly; only about 2% of plant sterols are absorbed.

Because lipids can be taken up across the brush border plasma membrane quite rapidly, the main limitation to the rate of lipid uptake by the

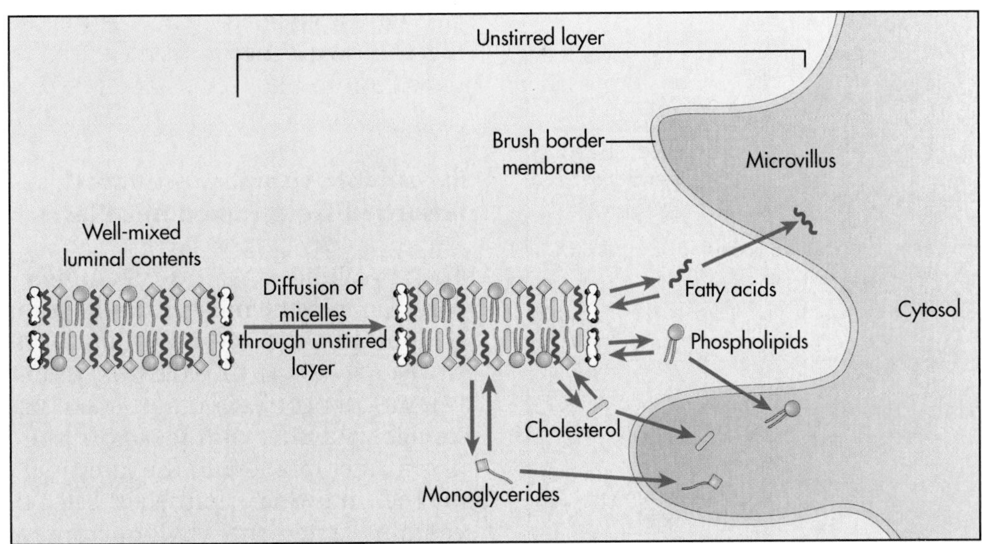

FIGURE 35–6. Lipid absorption in the small intestine. Mixed micelles of bile salts and lipid digestion products diffuse through the unstirred layer. As lipid digestion products are absorbed from free solution, more lipids partition out of the micelles.

epithelial cells of the upper small intestine is the diffusion of the mixed micelles through an unstirred layer on the luminal surface of the brush border plasma membrane (Figure 35–6). Partly because of the convoluted surface of the intestinal mucosa, the fluid in immediate contact with the epithelial cell surface is not readily mixed with the bulk of the luminal contents. This fluid forms an **unstirred layer** with an effective thickness of 200 to 500 μm. Nutrients, including mixed micelles, present in the well-mixed contents of the intestinal lumen must diffuse through the unstirred layer to reach the plasma membrane of the brush border.

The duodenum and jejunum are most active in fat absorption, and most of the ingested fat is absorbed by the time chyme reaches the middle of the jejunum. The fat present in normal stool is not ingested fat (which is completely absorbed), but it is derived from colonic bacteria and from exfoliated intestinal epithelial cells.

THE PRODUCTS OF LIPID DIGESTION ARE REPROCESSED IN THE SMOOTH ENDOPLASMIC RETICULUM OF INTESTINAL EPITHELIAL CELLS. A **cytoplasmic fatty acid–binding protein** transports fatty acids and a **sterol-binding protein** transports cholesterol to the smooth endoplasmic reticulum of intestinal epithelial cells. In the smooth endoplasmic reticulum, which is engorged with lipid after a meal, considerable chemical reprocessing occurs (**Figure 35–7**). The 2-monoglycerides are reesterified with fatty acids at the 1 and 1′ carbons to re-form triglycerides. Lysophospholipids are reconverted to phospholipids. Cholesterol is reesterified to a considerable extent.

CHYLOMICRONS ARE FORMED FROM THE PRODUCTS OF LIPID DIGESTION. The reprocessed lipids accumulate in the vesicles of the smooth endoplasmic reticulum. Phospholipids cover the external surfaces of these lipid droplets. The lipid droplets, approximately 10 nm in diameter at this point, are known as **chylomicrons.** About 10% of their surface is covered by β-lipoprotein, some of which is synthesized in the intestinal epithelial cells. Chylomicrons are ejected from the epithelial cell by exocytosis (Figure 35–7). The chylomicrons leave the cells at the level of the nuclei and enter the lateral intercellular spaces. Chylomicrons are too large to pass through the basement membrane that invests the mucosal capillaries. However, they do enter the lacteals, which have sufficiently large fenestrations for the chylomicrons to pass through. The chylomicrons leave the intestine with the lymph, primarily via the thoracic lymphatic duct, and flow into the venous circulation.

ABSORPTION OF BILE SALTS OCCURS IN THE TERMINAL ILEUM. The absorption of dietary lipids is typically complete by the time chyme reaches the middle of the jejunum. By contrast, bile salts are absorbed largely in the terminal part of the ileum. Bile salts cross the brush border plasma membrane by two routes: by a **Na^+–bile salt symporter** and by simple diffusion (**Figure 35–8**). Conjugated bile salts are the principal substrates for active absorption; deconjugated bile salts have less affinity for the transporter. Deconjugation and dehydroxylation make bile salts less polar and thus better absorbed by simple diffusion.

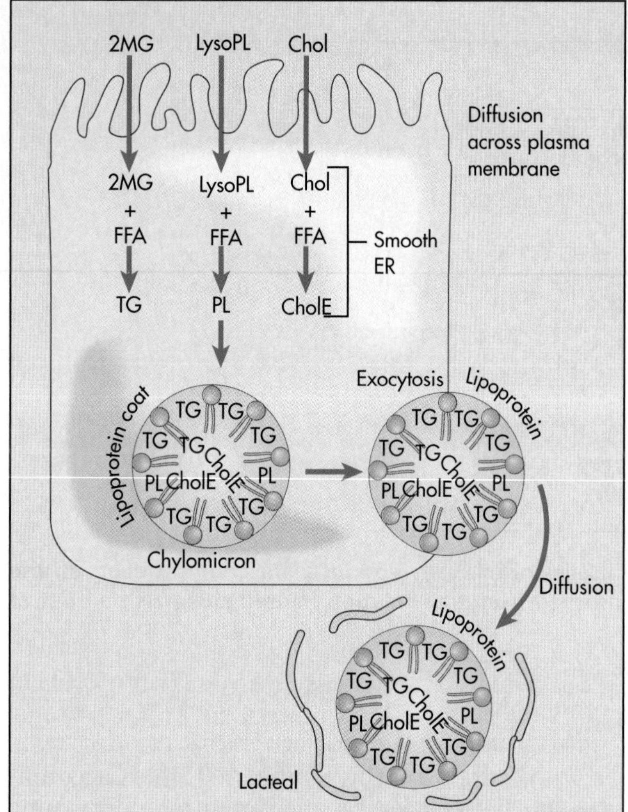

FIGURE 35–7. Resynthesis of lipids in the epithelial cells of the small intestine, formation of chylomicrons, and subsequent transport of chylomicrons into the lymphatic vessels. Chol, cholesterol; CholE, cholesterol ester; ER, endoplasmic reticulum; FFA, free fatty acid; LysoPL, lysophospholipid; 2MG, 2-monoglyceride; PL, phospholipid; TG, triglyceride.

Absorbed bile salts are carried away from the intestine in the portal blood. Hepatocytes avidly extract bile salts, and they essentially clear the bile salts from the blood in a single pass through the liver. Most deconjugated bile salts are reconjugated in the hepatocytes, and some secondary bile salts are rehydroxylated. The reprocessed bile salts, together with newly synthesized bile salts, are secreted into bile (see Chapter 34).

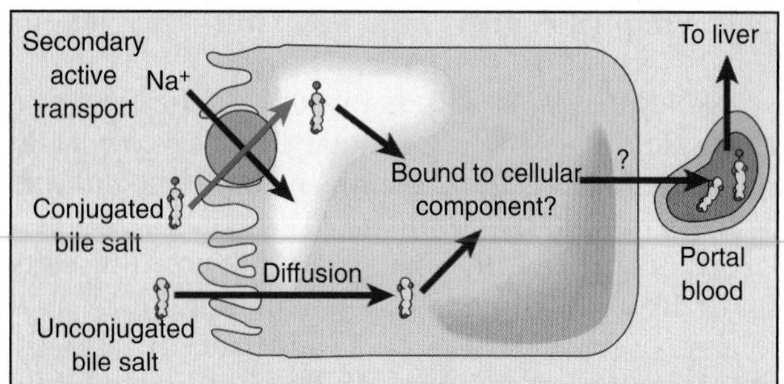

FIGURE 35–8. Absorption of bile salts by epithelial cells of the terminal ileum. Bile salts are absorbed both by simple diffusion and by Na^+–bile salt symporter. Conjugated bile salts are absorbed mainly by this symporter; unconjugated bile salts are absorbed chiefly by diffusion.

Fat-soluble vitamins are mostly absorbed from mixed micelles

The fat-soluble vitamins (vitamins A, D, E, and K) partition into the mixed micelles formed by the bile acids and lipid digestion products. THE PRESENCE OF BILE ACIDS AND LIPID DIGESTION PRODUCTS ENHANCES THE ABSORPTION OF FAT-SOLUBLE VITAMINS. The fat-soluble vitamins diffuse across the brush border plasma membrane into the intestinal epithelial cell. In the intestinal epithelial cell, the fat-soluble vitamins enter the chylomicrons and leave the intestine in the lymph. In addition, a fraction of the ingested load of a fat-soluble vitamin may be absorbed and leave the intestine in the portal blood.

The Gastrointestinal Tract Absorbs and Secretes Water and Electrolytes

Normally, humans absorb about 98% of the water and ions contained in ingested food and gastrointestinal secretions. The *net* movement of water and ions is normally from the lumen to the blood. In most cases, absorption represents the difference between large unidirectional movements from lumen to blood and from blood to lumen.

Net absorption of fluid by the gastrointestinal tract is more than 8 L/day

Typically, about 2 L of water is ingested each day, and approximately 7 L/day is contained in the gastrointestinal secretions (**Figure 35–9**). Only about 100 mL/day of water is lost in the feces. The gastrointestinal tract thus typically absorbs almost 9 L/day. Very little net transport of water occurs in the duodenum. In fact, water is usually added to the chyme to bring it to isotonicity because chyme delivered from the stomach is often hypertonic. The action of digestive enzymes creates still more osmotic activity.

Large net water absorption occurs in the small intestine; the jejunum is more active than the ileum in absorbing water. The net absorption that occurs in the colon is relatively small, about 400 mL/day. However, the colon can absorb water against a larger osmotic pressure difference than can the rest of the gastrointestinal tract.

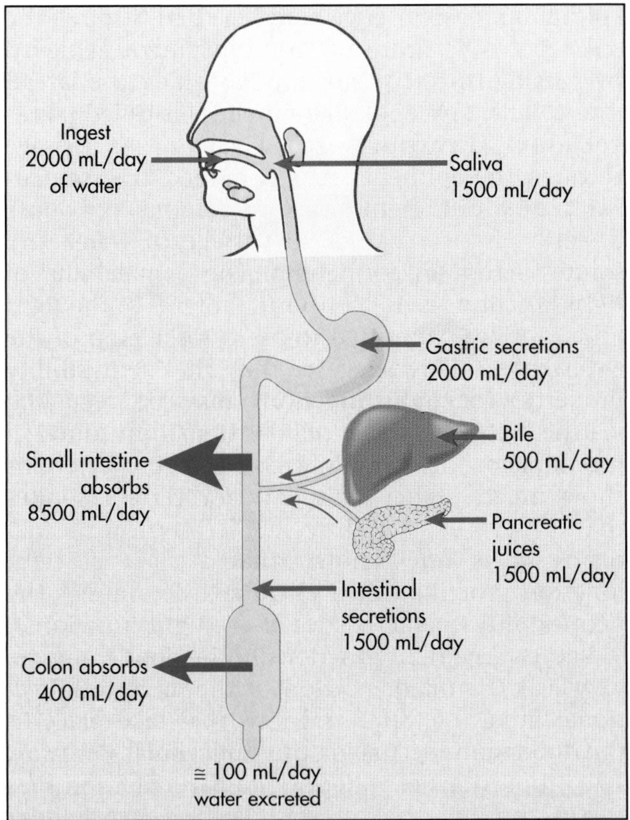

FIGURE 35–9. Overall fluid balance in the human gastrointestinal tract. Approximately 2 L of water is ingested each day, and 7 L of various secretions enter the gastrointestinal tract. Of this total of 9 L, about 8.5 L is absorbed in the small intestine. Approximately 500 mL is passed on to the colon, which normally absorbs 80% to 90% of the water presented to it.

Ion transport processes vary among the segments of the intestine

Table 35–1 summarizes the handling of Na^+, K^+, Cl^-, and HCO_3^- in different intestinal segments. The following sections provide an overview of the transport of these ions by the different intestinal segments. Cellular and molecular mechanisms of transport are discussed in later sections.

Na^+ is absorbed along the entire length of the intestine

Na^+ crosses the brush border membrane down an electrochemical gradient, and it is actively extruded from epithelial cells by the Na^+,K^+-ATPase in the basal and lateral plasma membrane. The contents of the small intestine are isotonic to plasma. Luminal contents have about the same $[Na^+]$ as does plasma, so that Na^+ absorption normally takes place in the absence of a significant concentration gradient. Na^+ absorption is active, however, and can occur against a small electrochemical potential difference for Na^+.

The net rate of absorption of Na^+ is highest in the jejunum. Here, Na^+ absorption is enhanced by the presence of glucose, galactose, and neutral amino acids in the lumen. These substances and Na^+ cross the brush border membrane on the same Na^+-nutrient symporters (e.g., SGLT1). Na^+ moves down its electrochemical potential gradient and provides the energy for moving the sugars (glucose and galactose) and neutral amino acids into the epithelial cells against concentration gradients. Thus, Na^+ enhances the absorption of sugars and amino acids, and vice versa.

The ability of glucose to enhance the absorption of Na^+ and hence of Cl^- and water is exploited in **oral rehydration therapy** for **cholera** and other secretory diarrheas. When patients with cholera drink a solution that contains glucose and NaCl, the absorption of these solutes and water helps counteract the secretory fluxes of water and electrolytes that would otherwise dehydrate the patient. Despite its simplicity, oral rehydration therapy is a major advance because of its great impact on world health.

The net rate of Na^+ absorption in the ileum is smaller. Na^+ absorption in the ileum is only slightly stimulated by sugars and amino acids because the density of Na^+-nutrient symporters is less in the ileum than in the jejunum. The ileum can absorb Na^+ against a larger electrochemical potential than can the jejunum.

TABLE 35–1. TRANSPORT OF NA^+, K^+, CL^-, AND HCO_3^- IN THE INTESTINE

Intestinal Segment	Na^+	K^+	Cl^-	HCO_3^-
Jejunum	Actively absorbed; absorption enhanced by sugars, neutral amino acids	Passively absorbed when $[K^+]$ rises because of absorption of water	Absorbed	Absorbed
Ileum	Actively absorbed	Passively absorbed when $[K^+]$ rises because of absorption of water	Absorbed, some in exchange for HCO_3^-	Secreted, partly in exchange for Cl^-
Colon	Actively absorbed; absorption enhanced by short-chain fatty acids	Net secretion occurs when $[K^+]$ in lumen < 25 mM	Absorbed, some in exchange for HCO_3^-	Secreted, partly in exchange for Cl^-

In the colon, Na^+ is normally absorbed against a large electrochemical potential difference. Na^+ concentrations in the luminal contents can be as low as 25 mM, compared with about 120 mM in the plasma.

Cl^- and HCO_3^- are absorbed in the jejunum

In the duodenum, HCO_3^- is secreted into the lumen, and this HCO_3^- helps neutralize H^+ in chyme from the stomach. In the jejunum, both Cl^- and HCO_3^- are absorbed in large amounts. By the end of the jejunum, most of the HCO_3^- in the hepatic and pancreatic secretions has been absorbed. In the ileum, Cl^- is absorbed, but HCO_3^- is normally secreted. If the $[HCO_3^-]$ in the lumen of the ileum exceeds about 45 mM, the flux from lumen to blood exceeds that from blood to lumen, and net absorption occurs. In the colon, the transport of these ions is qualitatively similar to that in the ileum in that Cl^- is absorbed and HCO_3^- is usually secreted.

K^+ is absorbed from the small intestine but usually secreted into the colon

In the jejunum and in the ileum, the net flux of K^+ is from lumen to blood. As the volume of intestinal contents is reduced by the absorption of water, K^+ is concentrated. This provides a driving force for the movement of K^+ across the intestinal mucosa and into the blood. Evidence for active transport of K^+ in the small intestine is lacking. In the colon, K^+ may be either secreted or absorbed. Net secretion occurs when the luminal $[K^+]$ is less than about 25 mM; above 25 mM, net absorption occurs. Under most circumstances, net secretion of K^+ and HCO_3^- occurs in the colon.

> Most of the absorption of K^+ in the small intestine is caused by the absorption of water, which increases the $[K^+]$ in the lumen. Hence, significant loss of K^+ may occur with diarrhea. If diarrhea is prolonged, $[K^+]$ in the extracellular fluid may decrease. Because maintenance of extracellular $[K^+]$ is important to many body functions, especially those of the heart and other muscles, life-threatening consequences, such as cardiac arrhythmias, may be caused by decreased $[K^+]$. Infants with prolonged diarrhea are particularly susceptible to the development of **hypokalemia** (low plasma $[K^+]$).

Solute and water transport in the intestine is both transcellular and paracellular

Because tight junctions are leaky, some fraction of the water and ions that traverse the intestinal epithelium passes between rather than through the epithelial cells. Transmucosal movement achieved by passing through tight junctions and the lateral intercellular spaces of an epithelium is called **paracellular transport** (see Chapter 1). Passage through the epithelial cells is termed **transcellular transport.** Tight junctions do not simply pose a static physical barrier to passage of water and solutes across an epithelium. The permeability of tight junctions is not constant. Proteins in the tight junctions are connected to the cytoskeleton of the enterocytes. This suggests that the permeability properties of tight junctions may be regulated via the cytoskeleton by cellular signal-transduction mechanisms. In addition, some tight junctions show much higher specificity for certain solutes than can be explained by simple physical mechanisms. It is now known that a class of tight junction proteins called **claudins** determines the permeability characteristics of the tight junction.

Because the tight junctions in the duodenum are very leaky, a major portion of the large unidirectional fluxes of water and ions that take place in the duodenum occurs via the paracellular pathway. The proportions of water or of a particular ion that passes through the transcellular and paracellular routes are determined by the relative permeabilities of the two pathways for a particular substance. Even in the ileum, where the junctions are much tighter than in the duodenum, significant proportions of water and electrolyte flow across the epithelium via the paracellular route.

Transport of Na^+ by intestinal epithelial cells is a central process in every segment of the intestine

The movement of water across the intestinal epithelium is secondary to the movement of ions and other solutes. In all regions of the intestine, the basolateral plasma membrane contains the Na^+,K^+-ATPase. As a result of the active extrusion of Na^+ ions from the cytoplasm by the Na^+,K^+-ATPase, the electrochemical potential of Na^+ in the cytoplasm is much less than that in the luminal fluid. Na^+ enters the epithelial cell by moving down this large electrochemical potential gradient. Membrane transporters in the luminal membrane of epithelial cells couple the influx of Na^+ to the secondary active transport of sugars, amino acids, and other ions.

Na^+ AND Cl^- ARE ABSORBED BY SIMILAR MECHANISMS IN THE JEJUNUM AND ILEUM. Sodium is absorbed across the luminal membrane by a Na^+-glucose symporter (SGLT1) and by a Na^+–amino acid symporter **(Figure 35–10)**. The density of the Na^+-nutrient symporters is less in ileum than in jejunum. In addition, NaCl

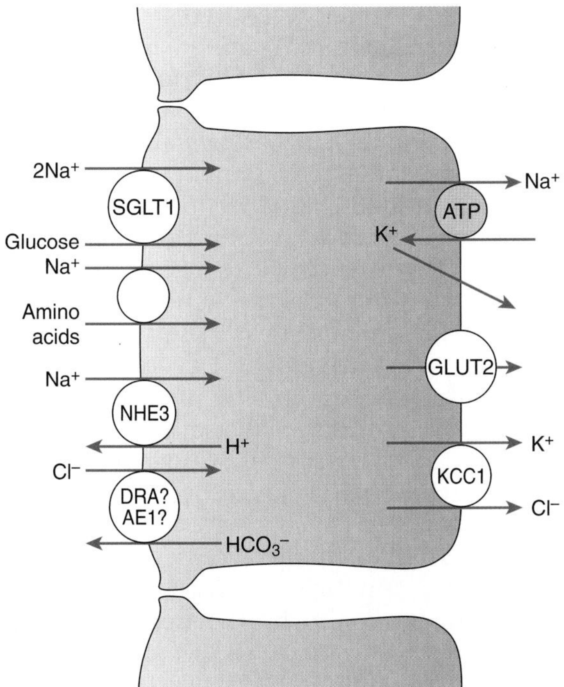

FIGURE 35–10. Major ion transport processes in the jejunum and in the ileum. (From Berne RM, Levy MN, Koeppen BM, Stanton BA: *Physiology,* ed 5, Philadelphia, 2004, Elsevier.)

absorption across the luminal membrane occurs by the parallel operation of Na^+-H^+ antiporters (NHE3) and Cl^--HCO_3^- antiporters (down-regulated in adenoma [DRA] or anion antiporter AE1). The operation of the Na^+-H^+ and Cl^--HCO_3^- antiporters at equal rates results in the net entry of NaCl into the cell. The Na^+ that enters the cell across the luminal membrane is pumped out of the cell into the blood via the Na^+,K^+-ATPase. The glucose that enters the cell is transported across the basolateral membrane into the blood via a glucose transporter, GLUT2. The Cl^- that enters the cell via DRA or AE1 is transported into the blood by a K^+-Cl^- symporter called KCC1.

IN THE COLON, THERE IS NET ABSORPTION OF NaCl. Na^+ is absorbed in the colon by two mechanisms (Figure 35–11). First, as in the ileum and jejunum, it is absorbed by the parallel operation of a Na^+-H^+ antiporter (NHE3) and a Cl^--HCO_3^- antiporter (DRA or AE1) located in the luminal membrane. Second, Na^+ enters the cell across the luminal membrane via a Na^+-selective channel called ENaC, which is an epithelial Na^+ channel. Na^+ absorption by ENaC causes the luminal fluid to be electrically negative relative to the blood and provides the electrochemical driving force for the absorption of Cl^- from the lumen to the blood. Not shown in **Figure 35–11** is the Na^+-SCFA symporter that takes up Na^+ and short-chain fatty acids. Short-chain fatty acids enhance Na^+ absorption.

HCO_3^- IS SECRETED INTO THE DUODENUM. HCO_3^- is secreted into the lumen of the duodenum by the mechanisms depicted in **Figure 35–12**. Some HCO_3^- is produced in the cell from CO_2 and H_2O. In addition, some HCO_3^- also enters the cell across the basolateral membrane by a Na^+-HCO_3^- symporter (NBC1). A Cl^--HCO_3^- antiporter (DRA or AE1) transports HCO_3^- from both sources from the cell into the luminal fluid. The Cl^- that enters the cell in exchange for HCO_3^- recycles back into the luminal fluid across the luminal membrane by the CFTR Cl^- channel. Thus, working together, CFTR and DRA (or AE1) mediate HCO_3^- secretion. The H^+ produced in the cell by the generation of HCO_3^- is transported into the blood across the basolateral membrane by a Na^+-H^+ antiporter (NHE1). The Na^+ that enters the cell in exchange for H^+ is pumped back into the blood by the Na^+,K^+-ATPase.

Absorption of water is powered by the absorption of solutes

The absorption of water depends on the absorption of ions, principally Na^+ and Cl^-. Under normal circumstances, water absorption in the small intestine

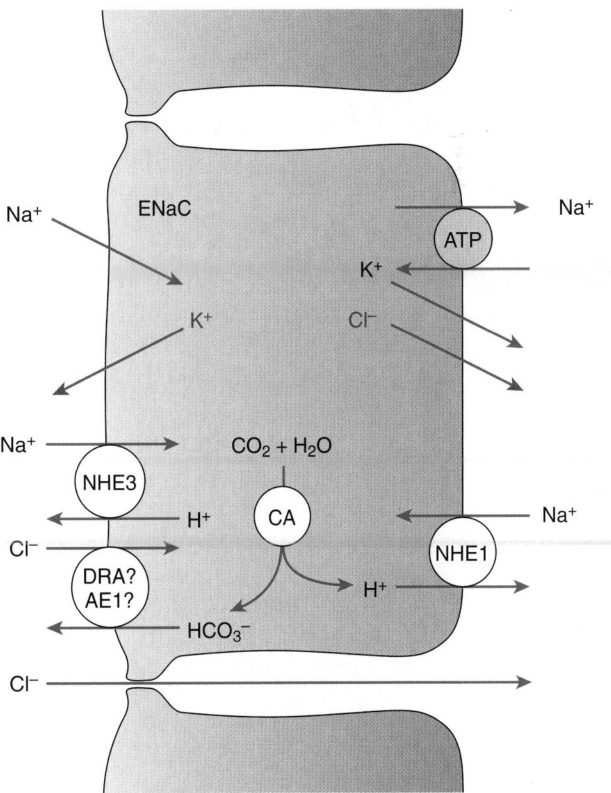

FIGURE 35–11. Mechanisms of NaCl absorption and K^+ secretion in the colon. CA, carbonic anhydrase. (From Berne RM, Levy MN, Koeppen BM, Stanton BA: *Physiology,* ed 5, Philadelphia, 2004, Elsevier.)

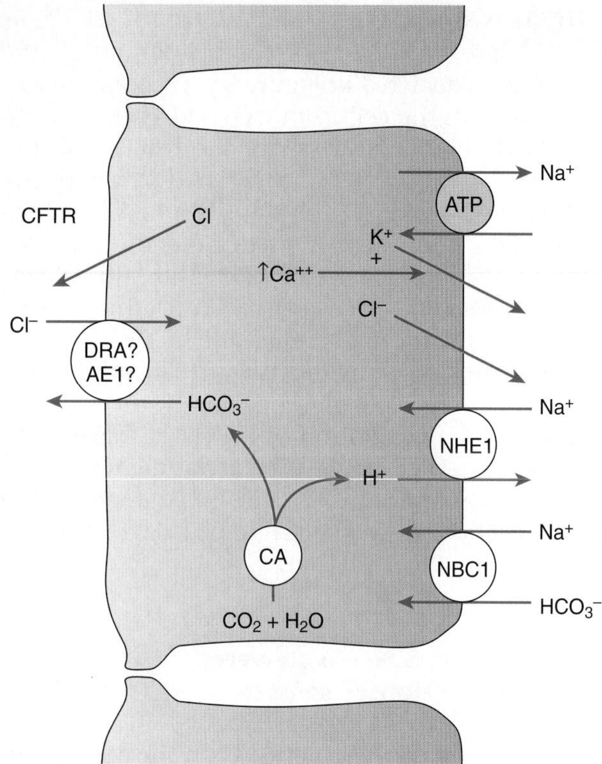

FIGURE 35–12. Mechanisms of HCO_3^- secretion in the duodenum. CA, carbonic anhydrase. (From Berne RM, Levy MN, Koeppen BM, Stanton BA: *Physiology,* ed 5, Philadelphia, 2004, Elsevier.)

occurs in the absence of an osmotic pressure difference between the luminal contents and the blood in the intestinal capillaries. Water absorption by the colon typically proceeds against a transmucosal osmotic pressure gradient. Water is absorbed by a mechanism known as standing gradient osmosis, the features of which are described in Chapter 34.

Because most water absorption takes place in the absence of a transmucosal osmotic pressure difference, the absorption of the end products of digestion, particularly sugars and amino acids, is important in water absorption. The absorption of sugars and amino acids allows more water to be absorbed. The role of aquaporins, water transporters, in intestinal water transport has not been established. It has been proposed that SGLT1, the Na^+-coupled glucose transporter, transports about 250 water molecules from lumen to cytosol for each glucose molecule that passes.

Cells in Lieberkühn's crypts are net secretors of electrolytes and water

Mature epithelial cells near the tips of the villi are usually active in net absorption of water and electrolytes; cells in Lieberkühn's crypts usually function as net secretors. A current view of the ionic transport mechanisms that function in the crypt cells is shown in **Figure 35–13**. In this model, Cl^- is actively taken up at the basolateral plasma membrane by the $1Na^+,1K^+,2Cl^-$ symporter (NKCC1). Cl^- leaves the cell at the luminal membrane via the CFTR Cl^- channel. The membrane potential (cell interior negative) drives Cl^- efflux from the cell. The amount of time that the luminal Cl^- channel remains open is enhanced by cAMP, and basolateral K^+ channels are activated by Ca^{++} or by elevated cAMP. Thus, net secretion by the crypt cells is enhanced by agonists that elevate intracellular cAMP (e.g., prostaglandins and vasoactive intestinal polypeptide) and by Ca^{++}-mobilizing agonists (e.g., acetylcholine). The effects of agonists that elevate cAMP are potentiated by agonists that increase cytosolic Ca^{++}, and vice versa. Na^+ is transported into the lumen, driven by the net luminal electronegativity produced by Cl^- secretion into the lumen.

Agonists that elevate cAMP in the cytosol of enterocytes, in addition to the prosecretory effects just noted, also inhibit the absorption of Na^+ and Cl^- by mature enterocytes.

Agonists that increase cGMP also promote net secretion. Guanylin, a hormone produced by intestinal goblet cells, acts to increase [cGMP].

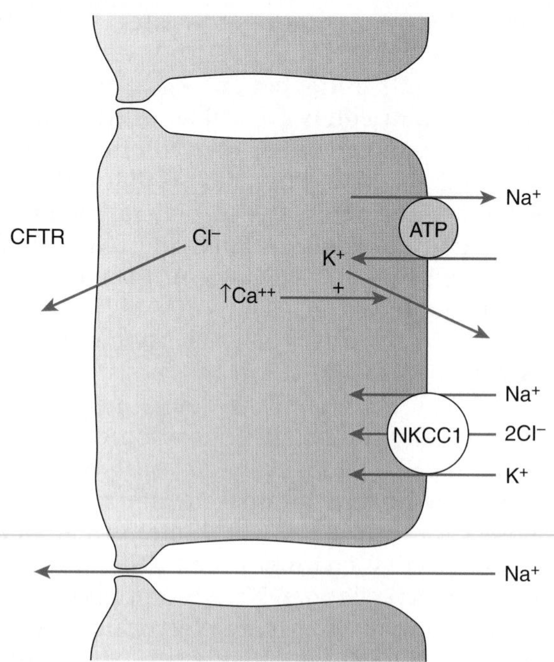

FIGURE 35–13. Ion transport processes involved in secretion of NaCl by cells in crypts of Lieberkühn. CFTR, cystic fibrosis transmembrane regulator. (From Berne RM, Levy MN, Koeppen BM, Stanton BA: *Physiology,* ed 5, Philadelphia, 2004, Elsevier.)

In secretory diarrheal diseases, such as cholera, the secretion of Cl^-, Na^+, and water into the intestinal lumen by the cells in Lieberkühn's crypts is greatly elevated. Cholera is caused by the cholera toxin that is produced by the bacterium *Vibrio cholerae*. Cholera toxin permanently activates adenylyl cyclase and thereby persistently elevates [cAMP] in the crypt cells. cAMP activates the brush border Cl^- channels and thereby increases the secretion of Cl^- (and therefore also of Na^+ and water). Cholera patients may produce as much as 20 L/day of watery stool. Such patients are likely to die unless they are promptly and adequately rehydrated.

The luminal Cl^- channel in the cells in Lieberkühn's crypts is the same protein that is defective in CF. Animal experiments show that CF carriers, who have one normal and one defective copy of the gene for the Cl^- channel, suffer significantly less severe diarrhea in response to cholera than do normal individuals. Resistance of CF carriers to secretory diarrheas may explain the high prevalence of this mutation, with 1 in 20 American adults being CF carriers.

Absorption of electrolytes and water is regulated by nerves, hormones, and paracrine mediators

Rates of absorption and secretion of electrolytes and water are influenced by hormones; sympathetic, parasympathetic, and enteric nervous systems; and cells of the gastrointestinal immune system. Moreover, interactions among these regulatory pathways are also important in the control of secretion and absorption.

Hormones, paracrine agonists, and substances released from neurons in the wall of the gastrointestinal tract regulate the absorption and secretion of water and electrolytes by intestinal epithelial cells. Some of these regulatory substances are listed in **Table 35–2**.

HORMONES CONTROL ABSORPTION AND SECRETION. Some of the hormones that influence absorption and secretion of electrolytes and water are released by cells in the wall of the gastrointestinal tract; others come from endocrine cells located elsewhere in the body. Among the hormones that can influence intestinal absorption and secretion are

TABLE 35–2. ENDOGENOUS COMPOUNDS THAT INFLUENCE INTESTINAL ABSORPTION OF ELECTROLYTES AND WATER

Compounds	Stimulate Net Secretion	Promote Net Absorption
Released by enteric neurons	Acetylcholine Nitric oxide Serotonin Vasoactive intestinal polypeptide* Substance P	Norepinephrine Neuropeptide Y Opioids
Released by enteroendocrine cells or immunocytes in mucosa or submucosa	Histamine Calcitonin Guanylin Bradykinin Platelet-activating factor Reactive oxygen species Prostaglandins Leukotrienes Calcitonin Arachidonic acid Adenosine	Somatostatin
Hormones (reach epithelial cells via blood)	Prostaglandins Atrial natriuretic peptide Gastrin Motilin Bombesin Gastric inhibitory peptide	Epinephrine Enkephalins Aldosterone Glucocorticoids Angiotensin II Peptide YY Prolactin Growth hormone
Present in the lumen	Bile salts Long-chain fatty acids	Short-chain fatty acids

*Note that some compounds may be released by neurons and by enteroendocrine cells or immunocytes. For simplicity, these compounds are listed only once.

mineralocorticoids, glucocorticoids, catecholamines, somatostatin, and enkephalins.

Aldosterone increases net absorption of water and electrolytes in the colon. Aldosterone stimulates the synthesis of the luminal Na^+ channel and the basolateral Na^+,K^+-ATPase.

Glucocorticoids stimulate electrolyte and water absorption in both the small and large intestines. This stimulation is partly due to an increase in the number of Na^+,K^+-ATPase molecules in the basolateral membranes of enterocytes.

Epinephrine acts on α receptors on epithelial cells to increase electroneutral Na^+ absorption in the ileum and to suppress secretory fluxes. Epinephrine also acts on the submucosal ganglia to inhibit secretomotor outflow to epithelial cells.

Somatostatin stimulates electrolyte and water absorption in the ileum and colon and inhibits secretion. In intestinal epithelial cells, somatostatin appears to act by decreasing cellular levels of cAMP. The ability of somatostatin to decrease secretion by crypt cells has led to the use of somatostatin analogues to treat secretory diarrheas. Somatostatin may also act on enteric neurons to suppress secretomotor outflow to enterocytes.

Opioids act on δ receptors in the intestine to stimulate salt and water absorption. Opioids act on other receptor subtypes to inhibit intestinal motility. Both of these effects contribute to the antidiarrheal effects of opioids.

The enteric nervous system regulates absorption and secretion

Most of the direct innervation of intestinal epithelial cells comes from neurons of the enteric nervous system, especially from the submucosal ganglia. The predominant influences of parasympathetic and sympathetic neurons occur via their influences on the activities of enteric neurons. Neural reflexes, both extrinsic and intrinsic to the gastrointestinal tract, regulate the absorptive and secretory activities of intestinal epithelial cells.

Epithelial cells are innervated by secretomotor neurons, predominantly from submucosal ganglia (see Chapter 33) but also from the myenteric ganglia. This innervation stimulates net secretion. Submucosal secretomotor neurons release acetylcholine or vasoactive intestinal polypeptide onto epithelial cells to stimulate secretion. An array of mucosal reflexes controls and coordinates the neural outflow from the enteric nervous system to intestinal epithelial cells. Enteric neurons that inhibit secretion by intestinal epithelial cells have not been found.

Reflexes in the enteric nervous system modulate secretomotor outflow from submucosal ganglia to intestinal epithelial cells. Some of these reflexes are elicited by luminal stimuli, such as distention of the gut lumen; stroking of the mucosal surface; or the presence in the lumen of glucose, acid pH, bile salts, ethanol, or an antigen to which the gastrointestinal immune system has previously been sensitized. All of these stimuli evoke reflex stimulation of secretion. Most of these stimuli also enhance propulsive motility in the stimulated gut segment. These actions demonstrate the interplay between neural control of secretion and motility.

PARASYMPATHETIC FIBERS INFLUENCE THE ENTERIC NERVOUS SYSTEM TO PROMOTE NET SECRETION OF ELECTROLYTES AND WATER. The enteric nervous system is heavily innervated by parasympathetic fibers, to both myenteric and submucosal ganglia. Stimulation of the parasympathetic fibers diminishes absorptive fluxes and enhances secretion. Parasympathetic fibers do not directly innervate epithelial cells to a significant degree. Parasympathetic tone apparently contributes to basal rates of secretion. Cholinergic input to the interneurons and secretomotor neurons, especially in the submucosal plexus, enhances secretomotor outflow to epithelial cells and perhaps to other mucosal effector cells also.

THE SYMPATHETIC NERVOUS SYSTEM ENHANCES NET ABSORPTION OF WATER AND ELECTROLYTES. Chemical ablation of the sympathetic nerves diminishes absorption. In diabetics, autonomic neuropathy may cause decreased sympathetic outflow to the intestine and contribute to **"diabetic diarrhea."** Some adrenergic fibers directly innervate epithelial cells, where norepinephrine acts on α receptors to enhance absorption. Sympathetic input to the enteric nervous system diminishes the secretomotor outflow by enteric neurons, especially in the submucosal ganglia, to epithelial cells. Norepinephrine, acting on α receptors, has multiple effects on neurons of submucosal ganglia. These effects decrease the secretomotor outflow to epithelial cells. Somatostatin, which also stimulates absorption, is co-released with norepinephrine at some nerve terminals. Catecholamines and α-adrenergic agents can strongly inhibit intestinal secretion evoked by cholera toxin and other potent secretagogues.

THE GASTROINTESTINAL IMMUNE SYSTEM INFLUENCES ABSORPTION OF WATER AND ELECTROLYTES. The cells of the gastrointestinal immune system contain numerous mediators that influence gastrointestinal salt and water transport (Table 35–2). Most of these compounds enhance net secretion of water and electrolytes. Inflammatory mediators stimulate secretion of electrolytes and water by crypt cells, inhibit absorption by villus cells, and in some cases enhance proliferation of crypt cells. The mediators include histamine, serotonin, prostaglandins and thromboxanes, leukotrienes, platelet-activating factor, adenosine, reactive oxygen species, nitric oxide, and endothelin. The cells that contain these mediators include mast cells, phagocytes, lymphocytes, basophils, neutrophils, endothelial cells, and fibroblasts.

Primed mast cells play a central role in the gastrointestinal response to an antigen. A primed mast cell carries antibody on its surface. When the antibody recognizes its particular antigen, the mast cell degranulates and releases many different mediators. Several of these mediators induce hypersecretion of electrolytes and water by the epithelial cells as well as induce hypermotility. Mast cells also release cytokines that recruit other mucosal immune cells to the response. These cells may then also release secretagogues.

Mediators released from mast cells and other gastrointestinal immunocytes evoke secretion in two ways: they directly affect intestinal epithelial cells to stimulate secretion or inhibit absorption, and they act on enteric neurons to increase the activity in secretomotor circuits. Histamine and prostaglandins appear to be key mediators of these effects on enteric neurons.

In addition to acting as targets of the immune mediators, enteric neurons modulate the release of these mediators from mast cells and influence the function of other gastrointestinal immunocytes. Neurons release substance P onto mast cells to stimulate degranulation of the mast cells and contribute to neurogenic inflammation and to secretion of water and electrolytes.

Inhibition of absorption and promotion of secretion of water and electrolytes by inflammatory mediators play a key role in inflammatory bowel disease, Crohn's disease, and other immune disorders. Prosecretory neural tone can enhance the responses to secretory mediators.

There are four general causes of pathological alterations of water and electrolyte absorption

General causes of abnormalities in the absorption of salts and water include

- deficiency of a normal ion transport system;
- malabsorption of a nonelectrolyte (nutrient), which results in osmotic diarrhea;
- hypermotility of the intestine, which leads to abnormally rapid flow of intestinal contents past the absorptive epithelium; and
- enhanced rate of net secretion of water and electrolytes by the intestinal mucosa.

Examples of each of these classes of abnormalities follow.

DEFICIENCY OF AN ION TRANSPORT SYSTEM ALTERS FLUID AND ELECTROLYTE ABSORPTION. In congenital chloride diarrhea, the Cl^--HCO_3^- antiporter in the brush border plasma membrane of the ileum and colon is impaired. As a result, Cl^- absorption is severely diminished. Impairment of Cl^- absorption leads to a type of diarrhea in which the stools contain an unusually high $[Cl^-]$; the $[Cl^-]$ in the stool exceeds the sum of the concentrations of Na^+ and K^+. In addition, because the Na^+-H^+ antiporter continues to operate, H^+ is eliminated in the feces without HCO_3^- to neutralize it. The net loss of H^+ with retention of HCO_3^- contributes to metabolic alkalosis. The protein that is mutated in this disease is the anion antiporter DRA.

MALABSORPTION OF A NUTRIENT MAY CAUSE OSMOTIC DIARRHEA. In any of the carbohydrate malabsorption syndromes, the sugar that is retained in the lumen of the small intestine increases the osmotic pressure of the luminal contents. Water is also retained as a result, and consequently an increased volume of chyme is passed on to the colon. When the increased volume flow overwhelms the ability of the colon to absorb electrolytes and water, diarrhea results. In addition, the high level of carbohydrates provides a medium that supports increased growth and metabolism of colonic bacteria. The increased production of CO_2 by colonic bacteria contributes to gaseousness and **borborygmi** (i.e., intestinal rumbling and gurgling), and certain products of bacterial metabolism inhibit absorption of electrolytes by the colonic epithelium.

In some disorders, the surface area of the intestinal mucosa is dramatically decreased, leading to the malabsorption of nutrients, electrolytes, and water. In these disorders, the height of small intestinal villi is markedly reduced and the number of microvilli is diminished. This occurs in **celiac disease** (gluten enteropathy), in response to infection by certain rotaviruses, and in a disease of uncertain etiology called **tropical sprue.** Celiac disease is also known as **celiac sprue.**

HYPERMOTILITY OF THE INTESTINE MAY CONTRIBUTE TO MALABSORPTION. Hypermotility is common in inflammatory bowel disease. The causes of hypermotility of the intestine are not well understood. Hypermotility of the small intestine may deliver electrolytes and water to the colon at rates faster than they can be absorbed by the colonic epithelial cells. Hypermotility of the colon may result in the elimination of feces before the maximal amount of salts and water can be extracted from them. Hypermotility may add to other factors that cause diarrhea. In cases of fat malabsorption, colonic bacteria metabolize lipids and produce certain waste products, such as hydroxylated fatty acids, that enhance the motility of the colon and inhibit salt and water absorption by the colonic epithelium.

ENHANCED SECRETION OF WATER AND ELECTROLYTES MAY RESULT IN SECRETORY DIARRHEA. Increased secretion of water and electrolytes is an important mechanism in serious diarrheal diseases. As mentioned previously, immature epithelial cells in Lieberkühn's crypts normally function to secrete Na^+, Cl^-, and water. When the secretory activities of the crypt cells are elevated, the unidirectional secretory flux may exceed the unidirectional absorptive flux, so that net secretion prevails. Cholera, discussed previously, is the best understood type of secretory diarrhea. Other agents that elevate cAMP in intestinal epithelial cells also lead to secretion of water and electrolytes.

The epithelial cells of the crypts of Lieberkühn of the small intestine are also stimulated to secrete electrolytes and water by elevated intracellular $[Ca^{++}]$ (Figure 35–13). Acetylcholine, serotonin, substance P, and neurotensin elicit intestinal secretion of water and electrolytes by increasing intracellular $[Ca^{++}]$. All these agents are present in intrinsic neurons of the intestinal wall and thus may contribute to diarrhea in certain pathological situations.

Ca^{++} Is Actively Absorbed in All Segments of the Intestine

The duodenum and jejunum are especially active in absorbing Ca^{++}, and they can absorb Ca^{++} against a greater than 10-fold concentration gradient. The ability of the intestine to absorb Ca^{++} is regulated. Animals with a calcium-deficient diet increase their ability to absorb Ca^{++}, but animals receiving high-calcium diets have less capacity to absorb Ca^{++}. Intestinal absorption of Ca^{++} is stimulated by vitamin D (see Chapter 44).

Ca^{++} moves down its electrochemical potential gradient into intestinal epithelial cells through Ca^{++} channels in the brush border plasma membrane **(Figure 35–14)**. An integral protein of the brush border plasma membrane, called the **intestinal membrane calcium-binding protein,** appears to bind Ca^{++} near the inner surface of the brush border membrane.

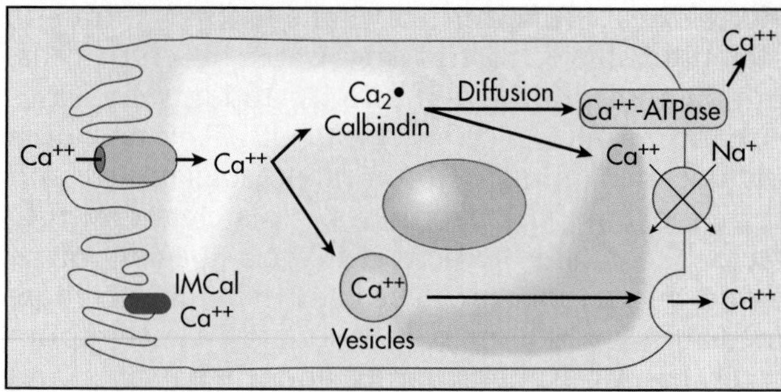

FIGURE 35–14. Cellular mechanisms involved in Ca^{++} absorption in the small intestine. IMCal, intestinal membrane calcium-binding protein.

Ca^{++} is bound to calbindin in the cytosol of epithelial cells

The cytosol of the intestinal epithelial cells contains a calcium-binding protein called **calbindin**. In mammals, calbindin has a molecular weight of about 9000 and binds two Ca^{++} with high affinity. The level of calbindin in the epithelial cells correlates well with the capacity to absorb Ca^{++}. Calbindin allows large amounts of Ca^{++} to traverse the cytosol, but it averts concentrations of free Ca^{++} that are high enough to form insoluble salts with intracellular anions. In addition, Ca^{++} traverses the epithelial cell cytosol in membrane-bound vesicles, with which a fraction of the calbindin is associated.

Ca^{++} is transported across the basolateral membrane by two transporters

The basolateral plasma membrane contains two transport proteins that are capable of ejecting Ca^{++} from the cell against its electrochemical potential gradient. A Ca^{++}-ATPase uses the energy of ATP to extrude Ca^{++} across the basolateral plasma membrane. A smaller amount of Ca^{++} is transported across the basolateral plasma membrane by a Na^+-Ca^{++} antiporter. The Ca^{++}-containing vesicles are believed to extrude Ca^{++} across the basolateral plasma membrane by exocytosis (Figure 35–14).

Vitamin D enhances Ca^{++} absorption

Vitamin D is essential for development of the normal capacity for Ca^{++} absorption by the intestine. The actions of vitamin D are discussed in more detail in Chapter 44.

In **rickets,** a disease caused by vitamin D deficiency, the rate of absorption of Ca^{++} is very low. In children with rickets, the growth of bones is abnormal due to insufficient availability of Ca^{++}. Because of failure to deposit normal levels of Ca^{++} salts in the bone matrix, bones are softer and more flexible than normal. These changes contribute to the characteristic "bowlegged" appearance of children with rickets.

VITAMIN D HAS MULTIPLE EFFECTS THAT ENHANCE THE ABSORPTION OF Ca^{++} by the epithelium of the small intestine. Treatment with vitamin D increases the transport of Ca^{++} across the brush border membrane; the mechanism of this effect is unclear. Vitamin D treatment also enhances the transport of Ca^{++} through the cytosol of the intestinal epithelial cell by dramatically increasing the level of calbindin. Vitamin D increases the rate of extrusion of Ca^{++} across the basolateral membrane of intestinal epithelial cells by increasing the level of Ca^{++}-ATPase in the membrane.

Ca^{++} absorption decreases in elderly people. This may be due to lower levels of vitamin D or to diminished responsiveness to vitamin D in older people. Gastric acid decreases the formation of insoluble Ca^{++} compounds in the lumen. People, particularly elderly individuals, who chronically use drugs that suppress gastric HCl secretion are at increased risk for malabsorption of Ca^{++}. Ca^{++} malabsorption may occur in inflammatory bowel disease and in disorders such as gluten enteropathy and tropical sprue that diminish the surface area of the brush border.

A Small Fraction of Ingested Iron Is Absorbed

A typical adult should ingest approximately 15 to 20 mg of iron daily. Of this amount, only 0.5 to 1 mg is absorbed by normal adult men, and 1 to 1.5 mg is absorbed by premenopausal adult women. Iron depletion (e.g., caused by hemorrhage) will result in an increased capacity of the intestine to absorb iron. Growing children and pregnant women absorb greater amounts of iron than do adult men.

IRON ABSORPTION IS LIMITED BECAUSE IRON TENDS TO FORM INSOLUBLE SALTS with hydroxide, phosphate, bicarbonate, and other anions present in intestinal secretions. Iron also forms insoluble complexes with other substances typically present in food, such as phytate, tannins, and the fiber of cereal grains. These iron complexes are more soluble at low pH. Therefore, HCl secreted by the stomach enhances iron absorption, whereas iron absorption is usually low in individuals deficient in HCl secretion.

Vitamin C effectively promotes iron absorption by forming a soluble complex with iron and by reducing Fe^{+++} to Fe^{++}. Iron complexed with ascorbate or in the form of Fe^{++} has less tendency to form insoluble complexes than does Fe^{+++} and thus is better absorbed. Individuals who take iron supplements are well advised to ingest vitamin C along with their iron tablets.

Heme iron is relatively well absorbed

Iron is present in the diet as inorganic iron salts and as part of the heme prosthetic groups of proteins such as hemoglobin, myoglobin, and cytochromes. About 20% of ingested heme iron is absorbed. Proteolytic enzymes release heme groups from proteins in the intestinal lumen. Heme is taken up by facilitated transport by the epithelial cells that line the upper small intestine. In the epithelial cell, iron is split from the heme **(Figure 35–15)**. No intact heme is transported into the portal blood.

Absorption of Fe^{++} involves a transporter and an iron-binding protein

Duodenal epithelial cells are principally responsible for absorption of nonheme iron. The brush border plasma membrane has transport proteins that bind Fe^{++} and transport it into the duodenal epithelial cells (Figure 35–15); Fe^{+++} is not transported. The brush border plasma membrane has a transport protein **(DCT1)** that cotransports H^+ and Fe^{++} across the luminal membrane. When the pH of the lumen is more acid than that in the cytosol of the enterocyte, DCT1 uses energy from the H^+ gradient to actively take up Fe^{++} into the cells of the duodenum and upper jejunum. DCT1 cannot transport Fe^{+++}, but an **iron reductase** on the brush border surface can reduce Fe^{+++} to Fe^{++} before transport. In the enterocyte, Fe^{++} is rapidly oxidized to Fe^{+++} by a ferroxidase.

Fe^{+++} is transported from the cytosol across the basolateral plasma membrane by another ion transporter **(IREG1).** IREG1 is associated with a copper-containing oxidase **(hephaestin).** In the blood, Fe^{+++} is bound to the iron carrier protein **transferrin.** Cells elsewhere that take up iron from the blood have membrane receptors for the iron-

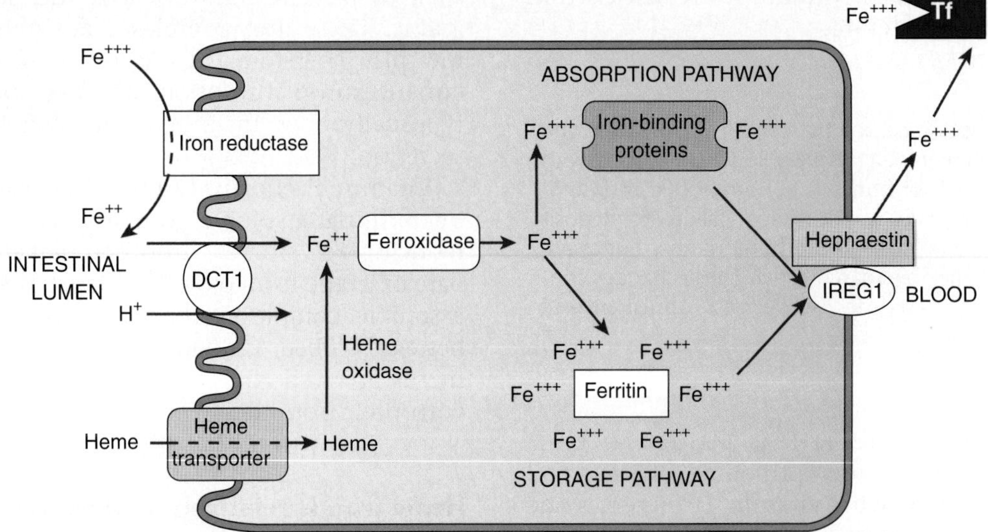

FIGURE 35–15. Iron absorption by the epithelial cells of the small intestine. In the epithelial cells of the small intestine, there are two pools of iron. One pool of iron is bound to ferritin in the epithelial cell. This iron is unavailable for transport across the basolateral membrane. Tf, transferrin. (From Berne RM, Levy MN, Koeppen BM, Stanton BA: *Physiology,* ed 5, Philadelphia, 2004, Elsevier.)

transferrin complex, which is taken up by receptor-mediated endocytosis. Abnormally large amounts of iron are absorbed in a disorder called **idiopathic hemochromatosis.** In some cases of idiopathic hemochromatosis, there are increased levels of the ion transport proteins DCT1 and IREG1.

Iron is stored in enterocytes by ferritin, which is a large complex consisting of 24 apoferritins (MW about 19,000) in the form of a hollow shell with up to 4000 iron atoms bound inside in the form of insoluble iron salts of hydroxide and phosphate.

The iron absorptive capacity of enterocytes is "programmed" when the cells reside in the crypts of Lieberkühn. The crypt cells have basolateral receptors for the transferrin-iron complex. When blood levels of transferrin-iron are high, the cytosolic level of Fe^{++} rises and Fe^{++} binds to an **iron regulatory protein (IRP)** in the cytosol. Bound iron prevents IRP from doing its job, which is regulating the rate of translation or the stability of particular messenger RNAs that encode proteins involved in iron transport. In an iron-depleted individual, less transferrin-iron is taken up, cytosolic levels of Fe^{++} fall, and IRP can then bind to mRNAs. IRP binding to mRNAs results in increased translation of mRNAs encoding the iron transport proteins DCT1 and IREG1 and decreased translation of apoferritin mRNA, thus enhancing the ability of the enterocyte to absorb Fe^{++}. When the level of transferrin-iron in blood is high, Fe^{++} binds to IRP, preventing IRP from having the effects just mentioned on RNA translation. Levels of DCT1 and IREG1 then fall, the level of apoferritin rises, and the enterocytes have lower capacity for absorbing Fe^{++}.

Iron absorption is regulated in accordance with the body's need for iron

IN CHRONIC IRON DEFICIENCY OR AFTER HEMORRHAGE, THE CAPACITY OF THE DUODENUM AND JEJUNUM TO ABSORB IRON IS INCREASED. The intestine also protects the body from the consequences of absorbing too much iron. AN IMPORTANT MECHANISM FOR PREVENTING EXCESS ABSORPTION OF IRON IS THE ALMOST IRREVERSIBLE BINDING OF IRON TO FERRITIN IN THE INTESTINAL EPITHELIAL CELL. Iron bound to ferritin is not available for transport into the plasma (Figure 35–15), and it is lost into the intestinal lumen and excreted in the feces when the intestinal epithelial cell is sloughed off. The amount of apoferritin present in the intestinal cells determines how much iron can be trapped in this nonabsorbable pool. The synthesis of apoferritin is stimulated by iron as described before, and this protects against absorption of excessive amounts of iron.

The capacity of the duodenum and jejunum to absorb iron increases 3 or 4 days after a hemorrhage. The intestinal epithelial cells require this time to migrate from their sites of formation in Lieberkühn's crypts to the tips of the villi, where they absorb. The iron-absorbing capacity of the epithelial cells is programmed when the cells are in Lieberkühn's crypts.

Magnesium, Phosphate, and Copper Are Absorbed in the Small Intestine

Magnesium (Mg^{++}) is absorbed along the entire length of the small intestine. About half the normal dietary intake is absorbed, and the rest is excreted. **Phosphate (Pi)** is absorbed, in part by active transport, all along the small intestine. **Copper (Cu^{++})** is absorbed in the jejunum; approximately 50% of the ingested load is absorbed. Cu^{++} is secreted in the bile bound to certain bile salts; this Cu^{++} is lost in the feces.

Transporters Mediate Absorption of Most of the Water-Soluble Vitamins

Most water-soluble vitamins can be absorbed by simple diffusion if they are taken in sufficiently high doses. Nevertheless, specific transport mechanisms are important in the normal absorption of most water-soluble vitamins (Table 35–3).

Normal absorption of Vitamin B_{12} requires intrinsic factor

A specific active transport process has been implicated in the absorption of vitamin B_{12}. The dietary requirement for B_{12} is fairly close to the maximal absorptive capacity for the vitamin. Enteric bacteria synthesize vitamin B_{12} and other B vitamins, but the colonic epithelium lacks specific mechanisms for their absorption.

When the intestinal absorption of vitamin B_{12} is impaired, the resulting vitamin B_{12} deficiency retards the maturation of red blood cells and causes **pernicious anemia.** Neurologic sensory deficits can also occur. Because of the occurrence of this disorder, much attention has focused on the absorption of vitamin B_{12}. Most patients with pernicious anemia have pronounced atrophy of gastric glands, and their stomachs are defective in secreting HCl and pepsins as well as intrinsic factor. These individuals have circulating antibodies against parietal cells; the antibodies may cause the destruction of parietal cells.

The liver contains a large store (2 to 5 mg) of vitamin B_{12}. Vitamin B_{12} is normally present in the bile (0.5 to 5 μg daily), but approximately 70% of this is normally reabsorbed. Because only about 0.1% of the store is lost daily, even if absorption totally ceases, the store will last for 3 to 6 years.

EVENTS IN THE STOMACH AND IN THE INTESTINE INFLUENCE ABSORPTION OF VITAMIN B_{12}. Most of the vitamin B_{12} present in food is bound to proteins. The low pH in the stomach and the digestion of proteins by pepsins release free vitamin B_{12}, which is then rapidly bound to a class of glycoproteins known as **R proteins.** R proteins are present in saliva and in gastric juice, and they bind vitamin B_{12} tightly over a wide pH range.

Intrinsic factor (IF) is a vitamin B_{12}–binding protein secreted by the gastric parietal cells. IF binds vitamin B_{12} with less affinity than do the R proteins; thus, in the stomach, most of the vitamin B_{12} present in food is bound to R proteins. Pancreatic proteases degrade the complex between R proteins and vitamin B_{12}, which causes vitamin B_{12} to be released. The free vitamin B_{12} is bound by IF. The

TABLE 35–3. INTESTINAL ABSORPTION OF WATER-SOLUBLE VITAMINS

Vitamin	Site of Absorption	Transport Mechanism
Ascorbic acid (C)	Ileum	*Symport with Na^+
Biotin	Duodenum, jejunum	†Facilitated transport?
Choline	Small intestine	Facilitated transport
Folic acid and folate derivatives	Jejunum	Facilitated transport
Inositol	Small intestine	Symport with Na^+?
Nicotinic acid	Jejunum	Diffusion of acid form
Pantothenic acid	Small intestine	Symport with Na^+
Pyridoxine (B_6)	Duodenum, jejunum	Diffusion
Riboflavin (B_2)	Duodenum, jejunum	Facilitated transport
Thiamine (B_1)	Jejunum	Symport with Na^+
Vitamin B_{12}	Distal ileum	Receptor-mediated endocytosis

*Secondary active transport powered by electrochemical gradient of Na^+.
†Via a transporter not linked to energy in any way.

complex of IF and B_{12} is highly resistant to digestion by pancreatic proteases.

RECEPTORS THAT BIND THE IF-B_{12} COMPLEX ARE PRESENT ON THE BRUSH BORDER OF THE DISTAL ILEUM. The normal absorption of vitamin B_{12} depends on the presence of IF (**Figure 35–16**). The brush border plasma membranes of the epithelial cells of the ileum contain receptor proteins that recognize and bind the IF-B_{12} complex. Free IF does not compete for binding, and the receptor does not recognize free vitamin B_{12}. Binding to the receptor is required for normal B_{12} uptake. In the enterocyte, vitamin B_{12} binds to transcobalamin II. The mechanism for vitamin B_{12}–transcobalamin II exit from the cell is unknown. After being absorbed, vitamin B_{12} appears in the portal blood bound to a protein called **transcobalamin II.**

In the complete absence of IF, approximately 1% to 2% of the vitamin B_{12} ingested is absorbed. If large doses of vitamin B_{12} are taken (about 1 mg/day), enough can be absorbed to treat pernicious anemia.

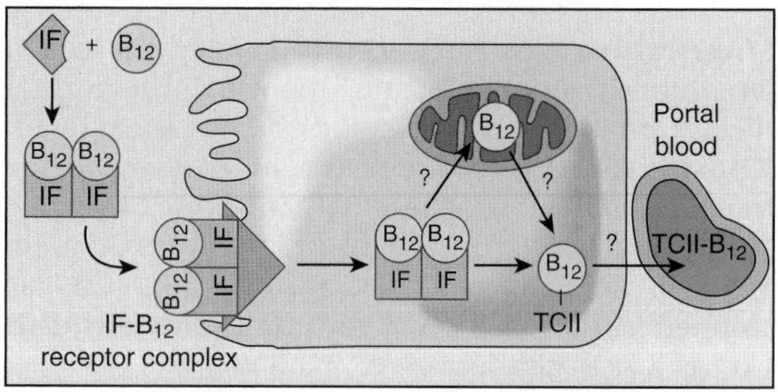

FIGURE 35–16. Mechanism of absorption of vitamin B_{12} by epithelial cells in the ileum. Vitamin B_{12} in portal blood is bound to transcobalamin II (TCII). IF, intrinsic factor.

Summary

- The α-amylases of saliva and pancreatic juice cleave branched starch molecules into maltose, maltotriose, and α-limit dextrins. These digestion products are then reduced to glucose molecules by glucoamylase and α-dextrinase on the brush border membrane.
- Sucrase and lactase on the brush border membrane cleave sucrose and lactose into monosaccharides that can be transported into the intestinal epithelial cells.
- Protein digestion begins in the stomach by pepsins. Pancreatic proteases rapidly cleave proteins in the duodenum and jejunum, primarily to oligopeptides. Peptidases on the brush border membrane reduce oligopeptides to single amino acids and to small peptides.
- Amino acids are transported across the brush border membrane by an array of amino acid transporters. Dipeptides and tripeptides are taken up by a brush border H^+-peptide symporter with broad specificity.
- Triglycerides are the major dietary lipids. Lipids form droplets in the stomach and are emulsified in the duodenum by bile salts. Emulsification greatly increases the surface area available for the action of lipid-digesting enzymes of pancreatic juice.
- The products of triglyceride digestion, 2-monoglycerides and fatty acids, form mixed micelles with bile salts. Cholesterol, fat-soluble vitamins, and other lipids partition into the micelles. Mixed micelles are small enough to diffuse among the microvilli and thus greatly enhance the brush border surface area available for lipid absorption.
- In the epithelial cells, triglycerides and phospholipids are resynthesized and packaged along with other lipids into chylomicrons. Chylomicrons are coated with apolipoproteins and released at the basolateral membrane by exocytosis. Chylomicrons leave the intestine in the lymphatic vessels and the thoracic duct.
- A typical human ingests about 2 L of water daily, and about 7 L enters the gastrointestinal tract in various secretions. About 99% of the water presented to the gastrointestinal tract is absorbed.
- The absorption of water is powered by the absorption of nutrients and electrolytes. The greatest quantity of water is absorbed in the small intestine, especially the jejunum. Mature cells at the tips of the villi are

active in salt, nutrient, and water absorption. Cells in the crypts of Lieberkühn are net secretors of ions and water.

❖ Ca^{++} is actively absorbed in the small intestine. Calbindin, a Ca^{++}-binding protein, facilitates the transport of Ca^{++} through the cytosol of the intestinal epithelial cell. Ca^{++} is transported across the basolateral membrane by the Ca^{++}-ATPase and the Na^{+}-Ca^{++} antiporter.

❖ Vitamin D stimulates the absorption of Ca^{++} by enhancing the synthesis of calbindin and of the Ca^{++}-ATPase of the basolateral membrane.

❖ About 5% of inorganic iron ingested is absorbed by the small intestine; approximately 20% of heme iron is absorbed. Inorganic iron is transported across the brush border plasma membrane by an iron (Fe^{++}) transporter. In the epithelial cells, some iron is bound to ferritin and is unavailable for absorption. The capacity to absorb iron increases in response to hemorrhage.

❖ Most water-soluble vitamins are taken up by specific transporters in the small intestinal brush border plasma membrane.

❖ Vitamin B_{12} is bound to R proteins in saliva and gastric juice. When R proteins are digested, vitamin B_{12} is bound by intrinsic factor (IF). Receptors on the ileal brush border membrane bind the IF-B_{12} complex and allow vitamin B_{12} to be taken up into the ileal epithelial cell. Vitamin B_{12} appears in the plasma bound to transcobalamin II.

Bibliography

Alvarez de la Rosa D et al: Structure and regulation of amiloride-sensitive sodium channels, *Annu Rev Physiol* 62:573, 2000.

Barrett KE, Keely SJ: Chloride secretion by the intestinal epithelium: molecular basis and regulatory aspects, *Annu Rev Physiol* 62:535, 2000.

Davidson NO: Intestinal lipid absorption. In Yamada T, ed: *Textbook of gastroenterology,* ed 4, Philadelphia, 2003, Lippincott Williams & Wilkins.

Farrell JJ: Digestion and absorption of nutrients and vitamins. In Feldman M, Friedman LS, Sleisenger MH, eds: *Gastrointestinal and liver disease,* ed 7, Philadelphia, 2002, WB Saunders.

Field M: Intestinal ion transport and the pathophysiology of diarrhea, *J Clin Invest* 111:931, 2003.

Ganapathy V, Ganapathy ME, Leibach FH: Protein digestion and assimilation. In Yamada T, ed: *Textbook of gastroenterology,* ed 4, Philadelphia, 2003, Lippincott Williams & Wilkins.

Greger R: Role of CFTR in the colon, *Annu Rev Physiol* 62:467, 2000.

Haas M, Forbush III B: The Na-K-Cl cotransporter of secretory epithelia, *Annu Rev Physiol* 62:515, 2000.

Halsted CH, Lönnerdal BL: Vitamin and mineral absorption. In Yamada T, ed: *Textbook of gastroenterology,* ed 4, Philadelphia, 2003, Lippincott Williams & Wilkins.

Hamid MS: Recent advances in carrier-mediated intestinal absorption of water-soluble vitamins, *Annu Rev Physiol* 66:419, 2004.

Kidd JF, Thorn P: Intracellular Ca and Cl channel activation in secretory cells, *Annu Rev Physiol* 62:494, 2000.

Krishnan S, Rajendran VM, Binder HJ: Apical NHE isoforms differentially regulate butyrate-stimulated Na absorption in rat distal colon, *Am J Physiol Cell Physiol* 285:C1246, 2000.

Kunzelmann K, Marcus M: Electrolyte transport in the mammalian colon: mechanisms and implications for disease, *Physiol Rev* 82:245, 2000.

Montrose MH, Keely SJ, Barrett KE: Electrolyte secretion and absorption: small intestine and colon. In Yamada T, ed: *Textbook of gastroenterology,* ed 4, Philadelphia, 2003, Lippincott Williams & Wilkins.

Rothman S, Liebow C, Isenman L: Conservation of digestive enzymes, *Physiol Rev* 82:1, 2002.

Topping DL, Clifton PM: Short-chain fatty acids and human colonic function: roles of resistant starch and nonstarch polysaccharides, *Physiol Rev* 81:1031, 2001.

Sellin JH: Intestinal electrolyte absorption and secretion. In Feldman M, Friedman LS, Sleisenger MH, eds: *Gastrointestinal and liver disease,* ed 7, Philadelphia, 2002, WB Saunders.

Traber PG: Carbohydrate assimilation. In Yamada T, ed: *Textbook of gastroenterology,* ed 4, Philadelphia, 2003, Lippincott Williams & Wilkins.

Case Studies

Case 35–1

A 12-year-old boy presents with a rash reminiscent of pellagra. The rash is reported to occur occasionally and to be exacerbated by exposure to the sun. His diet is judged to contain sufficient niacin and calories but is relatively low in protein. (*Note*: A large fraction of niacin in the body is synthesized from tryptophan.) The patient is not malnourished. The patient's urine contains most of the neutral amino acids in levels 5 to 20 times their normal levels. When the patient is fed a mixture of amino acids, there is only a very small rise (compared with normal individuals) in the plasma levels of those same neutral amino acids that are enriched in the patient's urine. The diagnosis is **Hartnup disease**.

1. **Which of the following statements about this patient is correct?**
   A. Many patients with Hartnup disease are malnourished.
   B. The patient would benefit from being given large oral doses of niacin daily.
   C. The patient probably has very low plasma levels of the neutral amino acids.
   D. High urinary levels of neutral amino acids are not expected in Hartnup disease.

2. **Which of the following statements about this patient is correct?**
   A. A diet richer in protein would be expected to benefit this patient.
   B. If the patient were fed a mixture of all 20 amino acids, the plasma levels of all the neutral amino acids would rise about as much as they would in a normal individual.
   C. None of the patient's five siblings is likely to have a similar disorder.
   D. The patient has pellagra.

3. **Which of the following statements about this patient is correct?**
   A. The patient would benefit from being fed those amino acids that are in high concentration in his urine.
   B. All the neutral amino acids are expected to be at high levels in the patient's urine.
   C. It is unlikely that one of the patient's parents has Hartnup disease.
   D. After the patient is fed partially hydrolyzed protein, his plasma levels of neutral amino acids will rise much less than in a normal individual.

Case 35–2

A 3-month-old infant is brought to the clinic because she does not seem to be growing at a normal rate and she has stools that are bulky, malodorous, and greasy. Examination of a stool smear reveals numerous clear fat droplets. The baby was of normal birth weight, but after the first 3 months of life, she fell below the 10th percentile in body weight. A sweat chloride test shows levels of NaCl in her sweat that are twice the normal levels. The diagnosis is **cystic fibrosis**.

1. **Which of the following statements about this patient is correct?**
   A. Digestive difficulties are unexpected in cystic fibrosis.
   B. Cystic fibrosis is an uncommon disease.
   C. The baby is likely to be deficient in pancreatic proteases as well as pancreatic lipases.
   D. The baby should be put on a low-fat diet immediately.

2. **Which of the following statements about this patient is correct?**
   A. The baby would benefit from taking pancreatic enzymes in enterically coated microspheres that are resistant to acid but release enzymes at pH 5.5 to 6 with each meal.
   B. The baby would not benefit from an inhibitor of gastric acid secretion.
   C. The baby would not benefit from administration of water-soluble forms of fat-soluble vitamins.
   D. The baby would not benefit from a formula enriched in medium-chain triglycerides.

3. **Which of the following statements about the patient is not correct?**
   A. The baby is at no increased risk for abnormalities of the endocrine pancreas.
   B. The baby is likely to have decreased levels of some of the brush border carbohydrate-digesting enzymes.
   C. The baby is likely to have high levels of serum trypsinogen.
   D. The baby is unlikely to have edema.

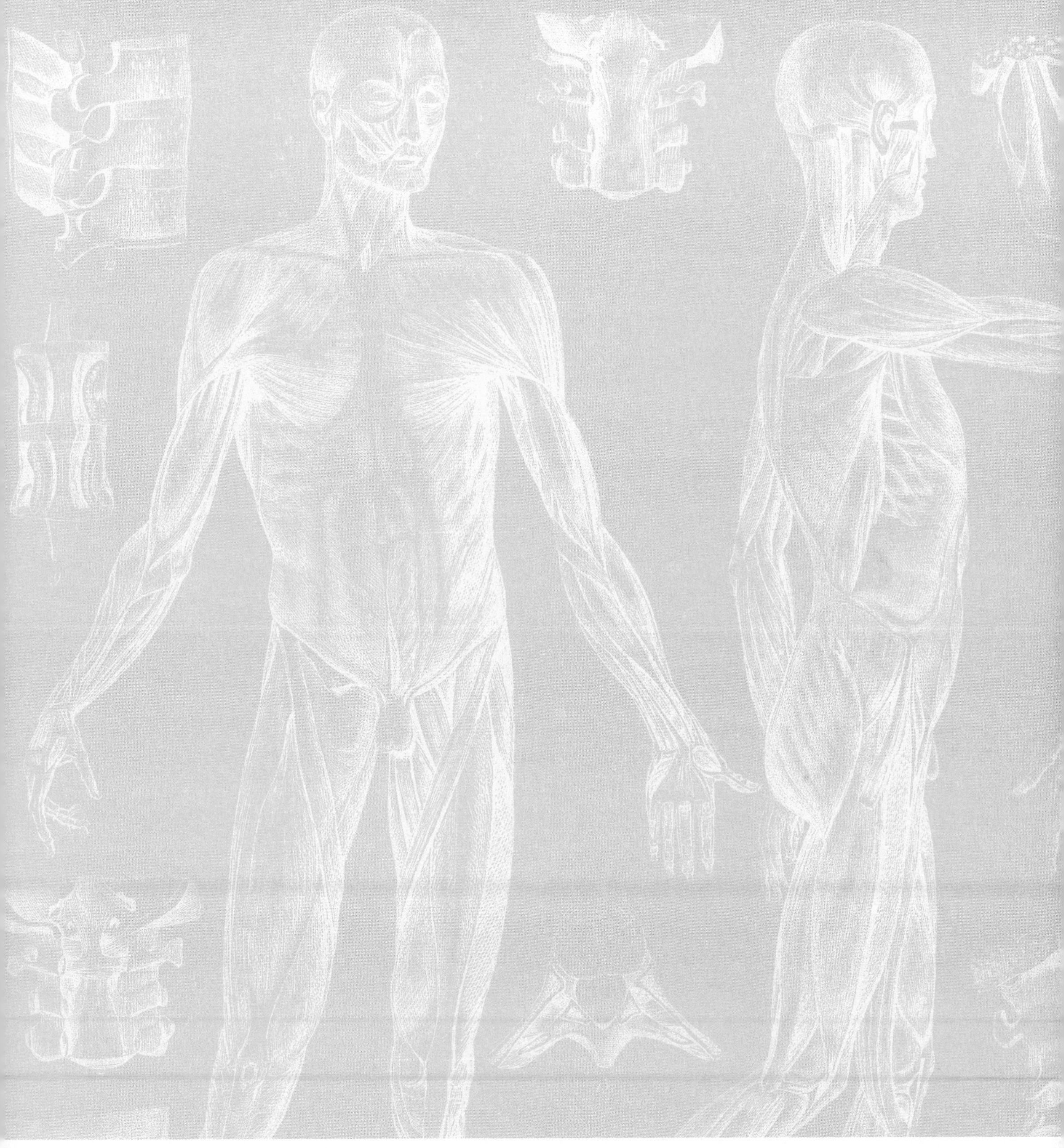

Part Seven: Renal System

Bruce M. Koeppen and Bruce A. Stanton

Chapter 36: Elements of Renal Function

Objectives

- ❖ Describe the anatomy of the kidneys and lower urinary tract.
- ❖ Explain the process of ultrafiltration and the concepts of glomerular filtration rate and renal blood flow.
- ❖ Describe the process of micturition.
- ❖ Explain why knowledge of the glomerular filtration rate is essential in evaluating the severity and course of kidney disease.
- ❖ Describe the concept of autoregulation of the glomerular filtration rate and renal blood flow.
- ❖ Describe the concept of tubuloglomerular feedback.
- ❖ Identify how hormones and the sympathetic nerves affect the glomerular filtration rate and renal blood flow.

The kidneys are excretory and regulatory organs. By excreting water and solutes, the kidneys rid the body of excess water and waste products. In conjunction with the cardiovascular, endocrine, and nervous systems, the kidneys regulate the volume and composition of the body fluids within a narrow range despite wide variations in the intake of food and water. Because of the kidneys' homeostatic role, the tissues and cells of the body can carry out their normal functions in a relatively constant environment.

The Kidneys Have Several Major Functions

The kidneys regulate many things:

- body fluid osmolality and volumes;
- electrolyte balance;
- acid-base balance;
- the excretion of metabolic products and foreign substances; and
- the production and secretion of hormones.

Control of body fluid osmolality is important for the maintenance of normal cell volume in all tissues of the body. Control of body fluid volume is necessary for normal function of the cardiovascular system. The kidneys are also essential in regulating the amount of several important inorganic ions in the body, including Na^+, K^+, Cl^-, HCO_3^-, H^+, Ca^{++}, and $PO_4^=$ (phosphate, Pi). The excretion of these electrolytes must be equal to their daily intake to maintain appropriate balance. If the intake of an electrolyte exceeds its excretion, the amount of this electrolyte in the body increases, and the individual is in **positive balance** for that electrolyte. Conversely, if excretion of an electrolyte exceeds its intake, its amount in the body decreases, and the individual is in **negative balance** for that electrolyte. For many electrolytes, the kidneys are the sole or primary route for excretion from the body.

Another important function of the kidneys is the regulation of acid-base balance. Many of the metabolic functions of the body are exquisitely sensitive to pH. Thus, the pH of the body fluids must be maintained within narrow limits. The pH is maintained by buffers within the body fluids and by the coordinated action of the lungs, liver, and kidneys.

The kidneys excrete a number of the end products of metabolism. These waste products include urea (from amino acids), uric acid (from nucleic acids), creatinine (from muscle creatine), end products of hemoglobin metabolism, and metabolites of hormones. The kidneys eliminate these substances from the body at a rate that matches their production. Thus, the kidneys regulate hormone concentrations within the body fluids. The kidneys also represent an important route for the elimination of foreign substances such as drugs, pesticides, and other chemicals from the body.

Finally, the kidneys are important endocrine organs that produce and secrete renin, calcitriol, and erythropoietin. Renin activates the renin-angiotensin-aldosterone system, which helps regulate blood pressure and Na^+ and K^+ balance. **Calcitriol,** a metabolite of vitamin D_3, is necessary for the normal absorption of Ca^{++} by the gastrointestinal tract and for its deposition in bone (see also Chapter 39). In patients with renal disease, the kidneys' ability to produce calcitriol is impaired and levels of this hormone are reduced. As a result, Ca^{++} absorption by the intestine is decreased. This reduced intestinal Ca^{++} absorption contributes to the bone formation abnormalities seen in patients with chronic renal disease. Another consequence of many kidney diseases is a reduction in erythropoietin production and secretion. Erythropoietin stimulates red blood cell formation by the bone marrow. Decreased erythrocyte production contributes to the anemia that occurs in chronic renal failure. This chapter reviews the anatomy of the kidneys, **glomerular filtration rate** (GFR), and **renal blood flow** (RBF).

A large variety of diseases impair the function of the kidneys, resulting in renal failure. In some instances, the impairment of renal function is transient; but in many cases, renal function progressively declines. Patients in whom the GFR is less than 10% of normal are said to have end-stage renal disease and must undergo renal replacement therapy to survive. Renal replacement therapies include **peritoneal dialysis, hemodialysis,** and **renal transplantation.** Both peritoneal dialysis and hemodialysis, as their names indicate, are based on the process of dialysis, whereby small molecules are removed from the blood by diffusion across a selectively permeable membrane into a solution that lacks these small molecules. In peritoneal dialysis, the peritoneal membrane acts as a dialyzing membrane. Several liters of a solution are introduced into the abdominal cavity and small molecules in blood diffuse across the peritoneal membrane into the solution, which is then removed from the abdominal cavity. In hemodialysis, a patient's blood is pumped through an artificial kidney machine. In the kidney machine, blood is separated from an artificial solution by a dialysis membrane, which allows small molecules to diffuse from blood into the dialysis solution, thereby removing the small molecules from the blood. Patients who are candidates for renal transplantation are treated with dialysis until an appropriate donor kidney can be obtained. Although anemia also used to be a significant problem because of reduced erythropoietin production in end-stage renal disease, patients on chronic dialysis now receive recombinant human erythropoietin (**Box 36–1**).

BOX 36–1: KIDNEY DISEASE IS A MAJOR HEALTH PROBLEM

In the United States:

- Kidney disease affects more than 20 million patients and accounts for more than 80,000 deaths per year.
- Each year, more than 3 million new patients are diagnosed with kidney disease.
- More than 458,000 people are treated for end-stage renal disease (ESRD) every year.
- 275,000 patients with ESRD are receiving either hemodialysis or peritoneal dialysis.
- Diabetes, hypertension, glomerulonephritis, and polycystic kidney disease are the leading causes of ESRD.
- ESRD due to diabetes is increasing at an annual rate of more than 11% per year.
- The health care cost for ESRD is more than $19 billion dollars per year.
- More than 14,000 kidney transplantations are performed each year. Unfortunately, more than 54,000 patients are awaiting kidney transplants.
- Urinary tract infections, kidney stones (i.e., urolithiasis), and interstitial cystitis (i.e., inflammation of the urinary bladder) are also major health care problems. Interstitial cystitis (700,000 patients), urinary stones (1.3 million visits annually at a cost of 1.8 billion dollars), urinary tract infections (8.3 million visits annually), and urinary incontinence (13 million adults affected, mostly older than 65 years, at a cost of $26 billion per year) are serious health concerns.

Structure and Function Are Closely Linked in the Kidneys

The kidneys are paired organs that lie on the posterior wall of the abdomen behind the peritoneum on either side of the vertebral column. The gross anatomical features of the human kidney are illustrated in **Figure 36–1**. The medial side of each kidney contains an indentation through which pass the renal artery and vein, nerves, and pelvis. If a

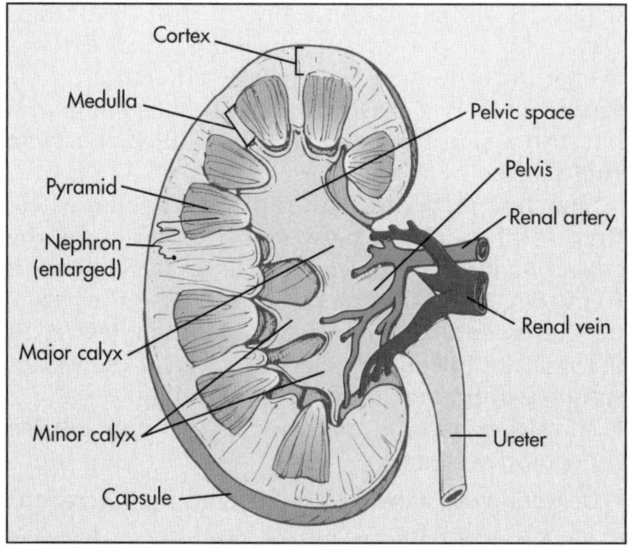

FIGURE 36–1. Structure of a human kidney, cut open to show the internal structures. (Modified from Marsh DJ: *Renal physiology,* New York, 1983, Raven Press.)

kidney were cut in half, two regions would be evident: an outer region called the **cortex** and an inner region called the **medulla.** The cortex and medulla are composed of nephrons (the functional units of the kidney), blood vessels, lymphatics, and nerves. The medulla in the human kidney is divided into conical masses called the **renal pyramids.** The base of each pyramid originates at the corticomedullary border, and the apex terminates in a **papilla,** which lies within a **minor calyx.** Minor calyces collect urine from each papilla. The numerous minor calyces expand into two or three open-ended pouches, the **major calyces.** The major calyces in turn feed into the **pelvis.** The pelvis represents the upper expanded region of the **ureter,** which carries urine from the pelvis to the urinary bladder.

The blood flow to the two kidneys is equal to about 25% (1.25 L/min) of the cardiac output in resting individuals. However, the kidneys constitute less than 0.5% of total body weight. As illustrated in **Figure 36–2** *(left),* the renal artery branches progressively form the **interlobar artery,** the **arcuate artery,** the **interlobular artery,** and

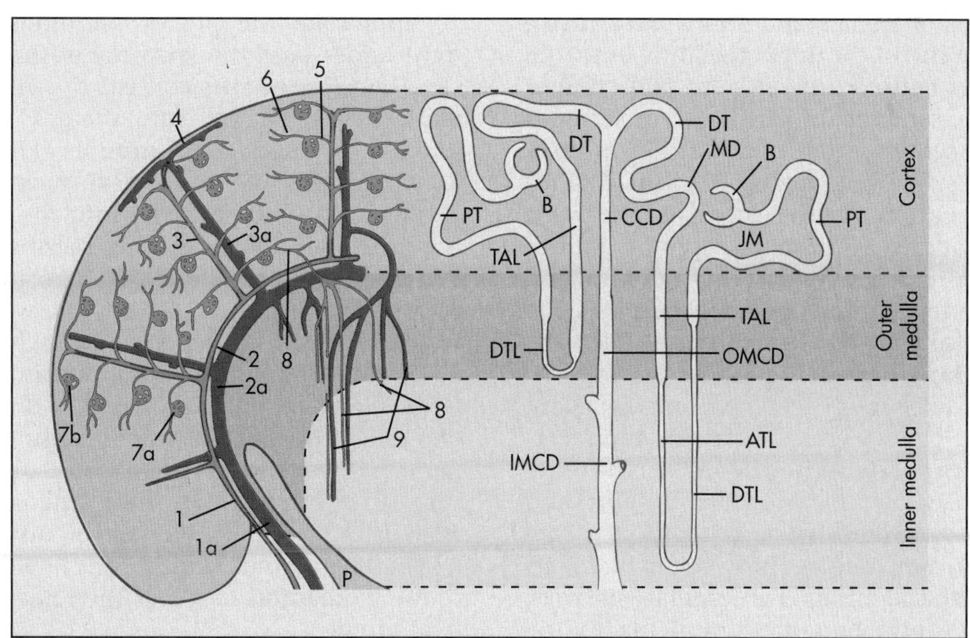

FIGURE 36–2. *Left,* Organization of the vascular system of the human kidney: 1, interlobar arteries; 1a, interlobar veins; 2, arcuate arteries; 2a, arcuate veins; 3, interlobular arteries; 3a, interlobular veins; 4, stellate vein; 5, afferent arterioles; 6, efferent arterioles; 7a, 7b, glomerular capillary networks; 8, descending vasa recta; 9, ascending vasa recta. *Right,* Organization of the human nephron. A superficial nephron is illustrated on the left, and a juxtamedullary (JM) nephron is illustrated on the right. The loop of Henle includes the straight portion of the proximal tubule (PT), descending thin limb (DTL), ascending thin limb (ATL), and thick ascending limb (TAL). B, Bowman's capsule; CCD, cortical collecting duct; DT, distal tubule; IMCD, inner medullary collecting duct; MD, macula densa; OMCD, outer medullary collecting duct; P, pelvis. (Modified from Kriz W, Bankir LA: *Am J Physiol* 254:F1, 1988; and Koushanpour E, Kriz W: *Renal physiology: principles, structure, and function,* ed 2, New York, 1986, Springer-Verlag.)

the **afferent arteriole,** which leads into the **glomerular capillaries** (i.e., glomerulus). The glomerular capillaries come together to form the **efferent arteriole,** which leads into a second capillary network, the peritubular capillaries, which supply blood to the nephron. The vessels of the venous system run parallel to the arterial vessels and progressively form the **interlobular vein, arcuate vein, interlobar vein,** and **renal vein,** which courses beside the ureter.

The functional unit of the kidney is the nephron

Each human kidney contains approximately 1.2 million nephrons, which are hollow tubes composed of a single cell layer. The nephron consists of a **renal corpuscle, proximal tubule, loop of Henle, distal tubule,** and **collecting duct** system (Figure 36–2). The renal corpuscle consists of glomerular capillaries and **Bowman's capsule.** The proximal tubule initially forms several coils, followed by a straight piece that descends toward the medulla. The next segment is the **loop of Henle,** which is composed of the **straight part of the proximal tubule, descending thin limb, ascending thin limb** (only in nephrons with long loops of Henle), and **thick ascending limb.** Near the end of the thick ascending limb, the nephron passes between the afferent and efferent arterioles of the same nephron. This short segment of the thick ascending limb is called the **macula densa.** The distal tubule begins a short distance beyond the macula densa and extends to the point in the cortex where two or more nephrons join to form a **cortical collecting duct.** The cortical collecting duct enters the medulla and becomes the **outer medullary collecting duct** and then the **inner medullary collecting duct.**

Nephrons may be subdivided into superficial and juxtamedullary types (Figure 36–2). The renal corpuscle of each **superficial nephron** is in the outer region of the cortex. Its loop of Henle is short, and its efferent arteriole branches into peritubular capillaries that surround the nephron segments of its own and adjacent nephrons. This capillary network conveys oxygen and important nutrients to the nephron segments, delivers substances to the nephron for secretion (i.e., the movement of a substance from the blood into the tubular fluid), and serves as a pathway for the return of reabsorbed water and solutes to the circulatory system.

The renal corpuscle of each **juxtamedullary nephron** is in the region of the cortex adjacent to the medulla (Figure 36–2, *right*). In comparison with the superficial nephrons, the juxtamedullary nephrons differ anatomically in two important ways: the loop of Henle is longer and extends deeper into the medulla, and the efferent arteriole forms not only a network of peritubular capillaries but also a series of vascular loops called the **vasa recta.**

The vasa recta descend into the medulla, where they form capillary networks that surround the collecting ducts and ascending limbs of the loop of Henle (Figure 36–2). The blood returns to the cortex in the ascending vasa recta. Although less than 0.7% of the RBF enters the vasa recta, these vessels subserve important functions, including

- conveying oxygen and important nutrients to nephron segments;
- delivering substances to the nephron for secretion;
- serving as a pathway for the return of reabsorbed water and solutes to the circulatory system; and
- concentrating and diluting the urine.

The first step in urine formation begins with the passive movement of a plasma ultrafiltrate from the glomerular capillaries into Bowman's space

To appreciate the process of ultrafiltration, one must understand the anatomy of the renal corpuscle. The **glomerulus** consists of a network of capillaries supplied by the afferent arteriole and drained by the efferent arteriole **(Figures 36–3 to 36–5).** During embryological development, the glomerular capillaries press into the closed end of the proximal tubule, forming Bowman's capsule of a renal corpuscle. The capillaries are covered by epithelial cells, called **podocytes,** which form the visceral layer of Bowman's capsule (Figures 36–3 to 36–5). The visceral cells face outward at the vascular pole (i.e., where the afferent and efferent arterioles enter and exit Bowman's capsule) to form the parietal layer of Bowman's capsule. The space between the visceral layer and the parietal layer is **Bowman's space,** which at the urinary pole (i.e., where the proximal tubule joins Bowman's capsule) of the glomerulus becomes the lumen of the proximal tubule.

The endothelial cells of glomerular capillaries are covered by a **basement membrane,** which is surrounded by podocytes (Figures 36–3 to 36–5). The capillary endothelium, basement membrane, and foot processes of podocytes form the so-called **filtration barrier** (Figures 36–3 to 36–5). The endothelium is fenestrated (i.e., contains 700-Å holes; 1Å = 10^{-10} m) and is freely permeable to water, small solutes (such as Na^+, urea, and glucose),

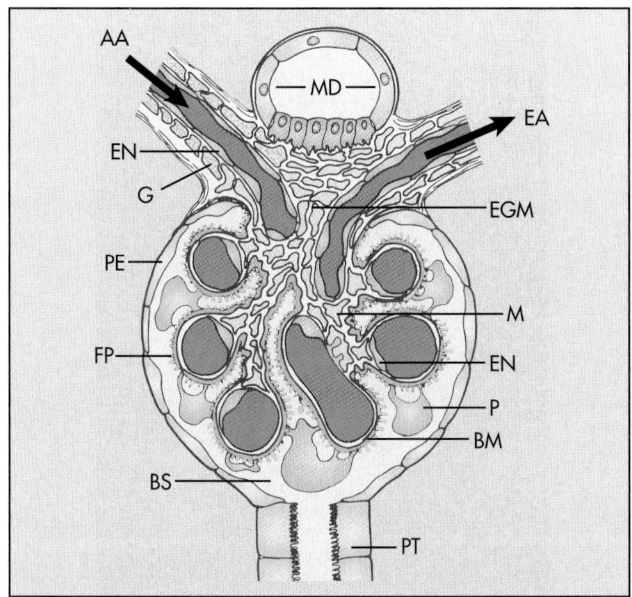

FIGURE 36–3. Anatomy of the renal corpuscle and juxtaglomerular apparatus. The juxtaglomerular apparatus is composed of the macula densa (MD) of the thick ascending limb, extraglomerular mesangial cells (EGM), and renin-producing granular cells (G) of the afferent arterioles (AA). BM, basement membrane; BS, Bowman's space; EA, efferent arteriole; EN, endothelial cell; FP, foot processes of podocyte; M, mesangial cells between capillaries; P, podocyte cell body (visceral cell layer); PE, parietal epithelium; PT, proximal tubule cell. (Modified from Kriz W, Kaissling B. In Seldin DW, Giebisch G, eds: *The kidney: physiology and pathophysiology,* ed 2, New York, 1992, Raven Press.)

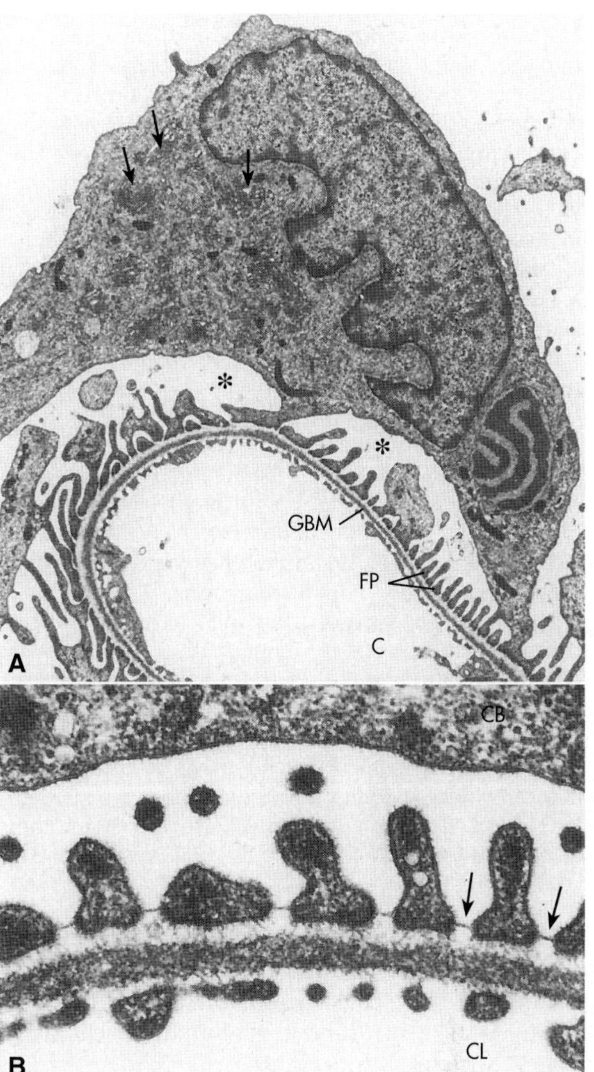

FIGURE 36–4. **A**, Electron micrograph of a podocyte surrounding a glomerular capillary. The cell body of the podocyte contains a large nucleus with three indentations. Cell processes of the podocyte form the interdigitating foot processes (FP). The arrows in the cytoplasm of the podocyte indicate the well-developed Golgi apparatus, and the asterisks indicate Bowman's space. C, capillary lumen; GBM, glomerular basement membrane. **B**, Electron micrograph of the filtration barrier of a glomerular capillary. The filtration barrier is composed of three layers: the endothelium, basement membrane, and foot processes of the podocytes. Note the diaphragm bridging the floor of the filtration slits *(arrows).* CB, cell body of a podocyte; CL, capillary lumen. (From Kriz W, Kaissling B. In Seldin DW, Giebisch G, eds: *The kidney: physiology and pathophysiology,* ed 2, New York, 1992, Raven Press.)

and even many proteins, but it is not permeable to red blood cells, white blood cells, or platelets. Because endothelial cells express negatively charged glycoproteins on their surface, they can retard the filtration of large anionic proteins. The basement membrane, which is a porous matrix of negatively charged proteins, is an important filtration barrier to plasma proteins. The podocytes, which are endocytic, have long finger-like processes that completely encircle the outer surface of the capillaries (Figure 36–5). The processes of the podocytes interdigitate to cover the basement membrane and are separated by gaps called **filtration slits.** Each filtration slit is bridged by a thin diaphragm, which contains pores with dimensions of 40 × 140 Å. The filtration slit diaphragm, which appears as a continuous structure when it is viewed by electron microscopy (Figure 36–4, *B*), is composed of several proteins including nephrin, NEPH1, and podocin **(Figure 36–6)**. The filtration slits retard the filtration of some proteins and macromolecules that cross the basement membrane. BECAUSE THE BASEMENT MEMBRANE AND FILTRATION SLITS CONTAIN NEGATIVELY CHARGED GLYCOPROTEINS, SOME PROTEINS ARE HELD BACK (I.E., NOT FILTERED INTO BOWMAN'S SPACE) ON THE BASIS OF SIZE AND CHARGE. For molecules with an effective molecular radius between 20 and 42 Å, cationic molecules are filtered more readily than anionic molecules.

The **nephrotic syndrome** is produced by a variety of disorders and is characterized by an increase in the permeability of the glomerular capillaries to proteins. The augmented permeability results in an increase in urinary protein excretion **(proteinuria).** Thus, the appearance of proteins in the urine can indicate kidney disease. Individuals with this syndrome may also develop edema and hypoalbuminemia as a result of the proteinuria.

Nephrin and NEPH1 are transmembrane proteins that are major components of the slit diaphragm (Figure 36–6). Mutations in the nephrin gene (*NPHS1*) lead to abnormal or absent slit diaphragms, causing massive proteinuria and renal failure (i.e., congenital nephrotic syndrome). Thus, nephrin plays an essential role in the formation of the normal filtration barrier.

Alport's syndrome is characterized by hematuria (i.e., blood in the urine) and progressive glomerulonephritis (i.e., inflammation of the glomerular capillaries) and accounts for 1% to 2% of all cases of end-stage renal disease. Alport's syndrome is caused by defects in type IV collagen, a major component of the glomerular basement membrane. In about 85% of patients with Alport's syndrome, the disease is X-linked recessive with mutations in the *COL4A5* gene. The remaining 15% of patients also have mutations in type IV collagen genes; six have been identified, but the mode of inheritance is autosomal recessive. In Alport's syndrome, the glomerular basement membrane becomes irregular in thickness and fails to serve as an effective filtration barrier to blood cells and protein.

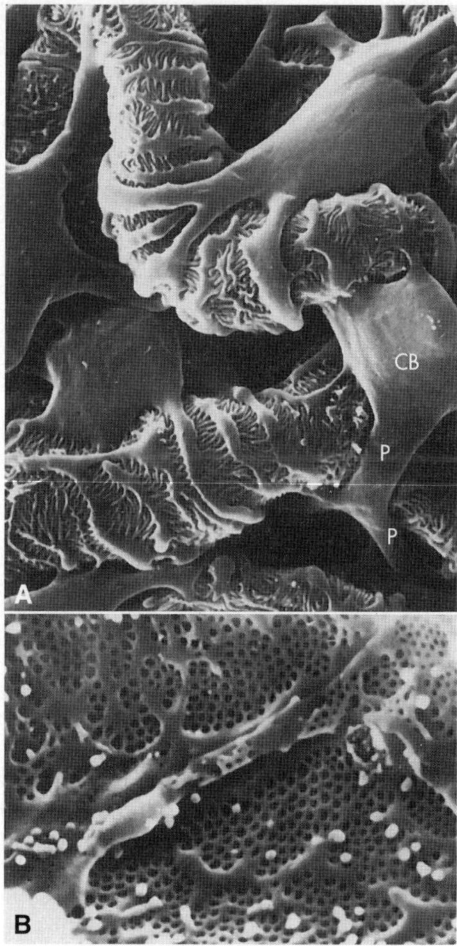

FIGURE 36–5. A, Scanning electron micrograph showing the outer surface of glomerular capillaries. This is the view that would be seen from Bowman's space. Processes (P) of podocytes run from the cell body (CB) toward the capillaries, where they ultimately split into foot processes. Interdigitation of the foot processes creates the filtration slits. B, Scanning electron micrograph of the inner surface (blood side) of a glomerular capillary. This view would be seen from the lumen of the capillary. The fenestrations of the endothelial cells are seen as small 700-Å holes. (From Kriz W, Kaissling B. In Seldin DW, Giebisch G, eds: *The kidney: physiology and pathophysiology,* ed 2, New York, 1992, Raven Press.)

Another important component of the renal corpuscle is the **mesangium,** which consists of **mesangial cells** and the **mesangial matrix** (Figure 36–3). Mesangial cells surround the glomerular capillaries, provide structural support for the glomerular capillaries, secrete the extracellular matrix, exhibit phagocytic activity, and secrete prostaglandins and proinflammatory cytokines. Because they also contract and are adjacent to glomerular capillaries, mesangial cells may influence the GFR by regulating blood flow through the glomerular capillaries or by altering the capillary surface area. Mesangial cells located outside the glomerulus (between the afferent and efferent arterioles) are called **extraglomerular mesangial cells.**

Mesangial cells are involved in the development of immune complex–mediated glomerular disease. Because the glomerular basement membrane does not completely surround all glomerular capillaries (Figure 36–3), some immune complexes can enter the mesangial area without crossing the glomerular basement membrane. Accumulation of immune complexes induces the infiltration of inflammatory cells into the mesangium and promotes the production of proinflammatory cytokines and autocoids by cells in the mesangium. These cytokines and autocoids enhance the inflammatory response. This inflammatory response can lead to cell scarring and eventually obliterates the glomerulus.

The juxtaglomerular apparatus is one component of an important feedback mechanism

The structures that make up the juxtaglomerular apparatus (JGA) include (Figure 36–3)

- the macula densa of the thick ascending limb;
- the extraglomerular mesangial cells; and
- the renin-producing granular cells of the afferent arteriole.

The cells of the macula densa represent a morphologically distinct region of the thick ascending limb.

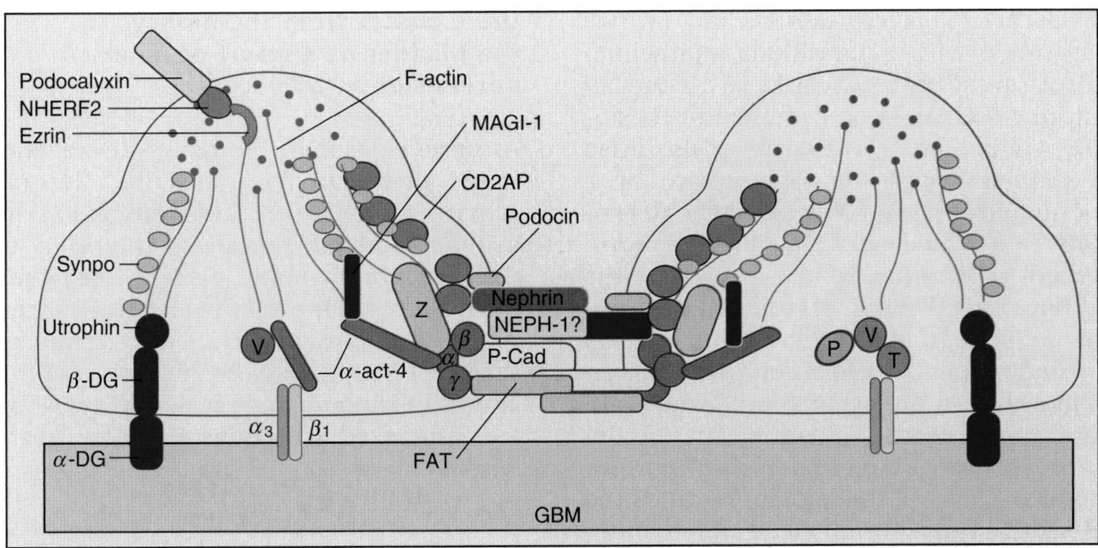

FIGURE 36–6. Anatomy of the podocyte foot process. This figure illustrates the proteins that make up the slit diaphragm between two adjacent foot processes. Many of the proteins that compose the slit diaphragm interact with adapter proteins that bind to the filamentous actin (F-actin) cytoskeleton, which in turn bind to proteins that interact with the glomerular basement membrane (GBM). Abbreviations: α-act-4, α-actinin-4; $\alpha_3\beta_1$, $\alpha_3\beta_1$ integrin; α-DG, α-dystroglycan; CD2AP, an adapter protein that links nephrin and podocin to intracellular proteins; FAT, a protein component of the slit diaphragm; MAGI-1, a membrane-associated guanylate kinase protein; NHERF2, Na^+-H^+ exchanger regulatory factor 2; P, paxillin; P-Cad, P-cadherin; Synpo, synaptopodin; T, talin; V, vinculin; Z, zona occludins. (Modified from Mundel P, Shankland SJ: *J Am Soc Nephrol* 13:3005, 2002.)

This region passes through the angle formed by the afferent and efferent arterioles of the same nephron. The cells of the macula densa contact the extraglomerular mesangial cells and the granular cells of the afferent arterioles. Granular cells of the afferent arterioles are modified smooth muscle cells that manufacture, store, and release renin. **Renin** is involved in the formation of **angiotensin II** and ultimately in the secretion of **aldosterone** (see Chapters 38 and 39). The JGA is one component of the tubuloglomerular feedback mechanism that is involved in the autoregulation of RBF and of GFR (see later section).

Renal nerves help regulate renal blood flow, glomerular filtration rate, and salt and water reabsorption by the nephron

The nerve supply to the kidneys consists of sympathetic nerve fibers that originate in the celiac plexus. There is no parasympathetic innervation. Adrenergic fibers that innervate the kidneys release norepinephrine and dopamine. The adrenergic fibers lie adjacent to the smooth muscle cells of the major branches of the renal artery (interlobar, arcuate, and interlobular arteries) and the afferent and efferent arterioles. Moreover, sympathetic nerves innervate the renin-producing granular cells of the afferent arterioles. Renin secretion is stimulated by increased sympathetic activity. Nerve fibers also innervate the proximal tubule, loop of Henle, distal tubule, and collecting duct; activation of these nerves enhances Na^+ reabsorption by these nephron segments.

Once Urine Leaves the Renal Pelvis, It Flows Through the Ureters and Enters the Urinary Bladder, Where Urine Is Stored

The ureters are muscular tubes about 30 cm long. They enter the **urinary bladder** at its posterior aspect near the base, above the bladder neck. The bladder is composed of two parts: the fundus, or body, which stores urine; and the neck, which is shaped like a funnel and connects with the urethra. The bladder neck, which is 2 to 3 cm long, is also called the posterior urethra. In females, the posterior urethra is the end of the urinary tract and the point of exit of urine from the body. In males, urine flows through the posterior urethra into the anterior urethra, which extends through the penis. Urine leaves the urethra through the external meatus.

The renal calyces, pelvis, ureters, and urinary bladder are lined with a transitional epithelium composed of several layers of cells. A mixture of spiral and longitudinal smooth muscle fibers surrounds this epithelium. The bladder is also lined with a transitional epithelium surrounded by a mixture of smooth muscle fibers called the **detrusor muscle.** Muscle fibers in the bladder neck form the **internal sphincter,** which is not a true sphincter but a thickening of the bladder wall formed by converging muscle fibers. The internal sphincter is not under conscious control. Its inherent tone prevents emptying of the bladder until appropriate stimuli initiate urination. The urethra passes through the **urogenital diaphragm,** which contains a layer of skeletal muscle called the **external sphincter.** This muscle is under voluntary control and can be used to prevent or interrupt urination, especially in males. In females, the external sphincter is poorly developed; thus, it is less important in voluntary bladder control. The smooth muscle cells in the lower urinary tract are electrically coupled, exhibit spontaneous action potentials, contract when stretched, and are under autonomic control.

The walls of the ureters, bladder, and urethra are highly folded and thereby very distensible. In the bladder and urethra, these folds are called **rugae.** As the bladder fills with urine, the rugae flatten, and the volume of the bladder increases with little change in intravesical pressure. The volume of the bladder can increase from a minimal volume of 10 mL after urination to 400 mL with a pressure change of only 5 cm H_2O; this illustrates the highly compliant nature of the bladder.

Innervation of the bladder and urethra controls urination

The smooth muscle of the bladder neck receives sympathetic innervation from the hypogastric nerves. α-Adrenergic receptors, located mainly in the bladder neck and the urethra, cause contraction. Stimulation of these receptors facilitates the storage of urine by inducing closure of the urethra. Sacral parasympathetic fibers (muscarinic) innervate the body of the bladder and cause a sustained bladder contraction. Sensory fibers of the pelvic nerves (visceral afferent pathway) also innervate the fundus. These sensory fibers carry input from receptors that detect bladder fullness, pain, and temperature sensation. The sacral pudendal nerves innervate the skeletal muscle fibers of the external sphincter, and excitatory impulses cause contraction.

Urine passes from the kidneys to the bladder as a result of inherent pacemaker activity

As urine collects in the renal calyces, stretch promotes their pacemaker activity. This pacemaker activity initiates a peristaltic contraction that begins in the calyces and spreads to the pelvis and along the length of the ureter, thereby forcing urine from the renal pelvis toward the bladder. Transmission of the peristaltic wave is caused by action potentials that are generated by the pacemaker and that pass along the smooth muscle syncytium. The ureters are innervated with sensory nerve fibers (pelvic nerves).

Nephrolithiasis (i.e., kidney stones) is a common medical problem. A total of 5% to 10% of Americans develop kidney stones. Most stones (80% to 90%) are composed of calcium salts. The remaining stones are composed of uric acid, magnesium–ammonium acetate, and cysteine. Stones are formed by crystallization in a supersaturated urinary milieu. When the ureter is blocked by a kidney stone, reflex constriction of the ureter around the stone elicits severe flank pain.

Micturition Is the Process of Emptying the Urinary Bladder

Two processes are involved in micturition:

- progressive filling of the bladder until the pressure rises to a critical value; and
- a neuronal reflex called the **micturition reflex,** which empties the bladder.

The micturition reflex is a spinal cord reflex. However, it can be inhibited or facilitated by centers in the brainstem and cerebral cortex.

Filling of the bladder stretches the bladder wall and triggers a reflex initiated by stretch receptors, which causes the bladder wall to contract. Sensory signals from the bladder fundus enter the spinal cord via pelvic nerves and return directly to the bladder through parasympathetic fibers in the same nerves. Stimulation of parasympathetic fibers causes intense contraction of the detrusor muscle. The smooth muscle in the bladder is a syncytium; therefore, stimulation of the detrusor muscle also causes the muscle cells in the neck of the bladder to contract. Because the muscle fibers of the bladder outlet are oriented longitudinally and radially, contraction opens the bladder neck and allows urine to flow through the posterior urethra. Voluntary relaxation of the external sphincter, achieved by cortical inhibition of the pudendal nerve, permits the flow of urine through the external meatus. Voluntary relaxation of the external sphincter is required, and it may be the event that initiates micturition. Interruption of the hypogastric sympathetic nerves and the pudendal nerves to the lower urinary tract does not alter the micturition reflex. In contrast, destruction of the parasympathetic nerves results in complete bladder dysfunction.

The Glomerular Filtration Rate Is Equal to the Sum of the Filtration Rates of All Functioning Nephrons

The GFR is an index of kidney function. A fall generally means that kidney disease is progressing, whereas a recovery generally suggests recuperation. Thus, knowledge of the patient's GFR is essential in evaluating the severity and course of kidney disease.

Creatinine is a byproduct of skeletal muscle creatine metabolism, and it can be used to measure the GFR. Creatinine is freely filtered across the glomerulus into Bowman's space, and to a first approximation, it is not reabsorbed, secreted, or metabolized by the cells of the nephron. Accordingly, the amount of creatinine excreted in the urine per minute equals the amount of creatinine filtered at the glomerulus each minute **(Figure 36–7)**:

$$\text{Amount filtered} = \text{Amount excreted}$$

$$\text{GFR} \times P_{Cr} = U_{Cr} \times \dot{V} \qquad \textbf{36-1}$$

where P_{Cr} is plasma concentration of creatinine, U_{Cr} is urine concentration of creatinine, and $\dot{V}$ is urine flow.

If Equation 36-1 is solved for the GFR:

$$\text{GFR} = C_{Cr} \times \dot{V}/P_{Cr} \qquad \textbf{36-2}$$

THUS, THE CLEARANCE OF CREATININE PROVIDES A MEANS FOR DETERMINING THE GFR. Clearance has the dimensions of volume/time, and it represents a volume of plasma from which all the substance has been removed and excreted into the urine per unit time.

Creatinine is not the only substance that can be used to measure the GFR. Any substance that meets the following criteria can serve as an appropriate marker for the measurement of GFR. The substance must

- be freely filtered across the glomerulus into Bowman's space;
- not be reabsorbed or secreted by the nephron;
- not be metabolized or produced by the kidney; and
- not alter the GFR.

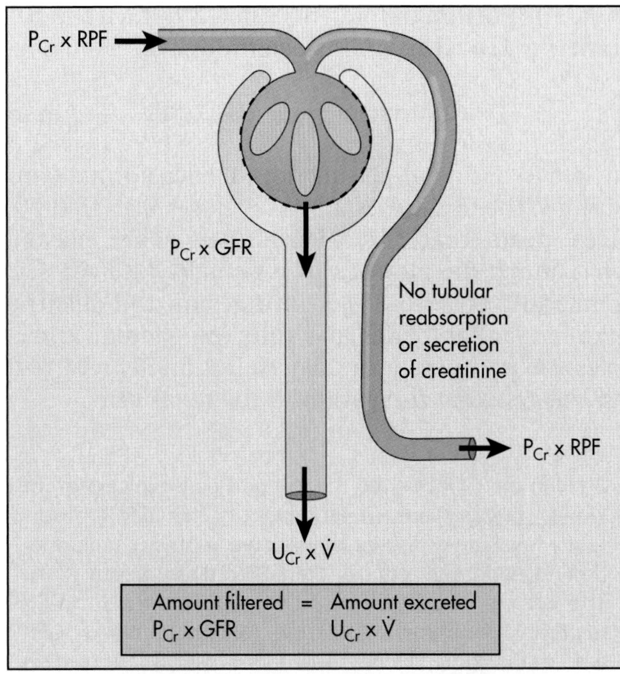

FIGURE 36–7. Renal handling of creatinine. Creatinine is freely filtered across the glomerulus and is, to a first approximation, not reabsorbed, secreted, or metabolized by the nephron. Note that not all the creatinine coming to the kidney in the renal artery gets filtered at the glomerulus (normally, 15% to 20% of plasma creatinine is filtered). The portion that is not filtered is returned to the systemic circulation in the renal vein. GFR, glomerular filtration rate; P_{Cr}, plasma creatinine concentration; RPF, renal plasma flow; U_{Cr}, urinary concentration of creatinine; $\dot{V}$, urine flow rate.

Creatinine is used to estimate the GFR in clinical practice. It is synthesized at a relatively constant rate, and the amount produced is proportional to the muscle mass. However, creatinine is not a perfect substance for measuring GFR because it is secreted to a small extent by the organic cation secretory system in the proximal tubule (see Chapter 37). The error introduced by this secretory component is approximately 10%. Thus, the amount of creatinine excreted in the urine exceeds the amount expected from filtration alone by 10%. However, the method used to measure the plasma creatinine concentration (P_{Cr}) overestimates the true value by 10%. Consequently, the two errors cancel, and in most clinical situations, creatinine clearance provides a reasonably accurate measure of the GFR.

Not all the creatinine (or other substances used to measure the GFR) that enters the kidney in the renal arterial plasma is filtered at the glomerulus. Likewise, not all of the plasma coming into the kidney is filtered. Although nearly all of the plasma that enters the kidney in the renal artery passes through the glomerulus, approximately 10% does not. The portion of filtered plasma is termed the **filtration fraction** and is determined as

$$\text{Filtration fraction} = \text{GFR/RPF} \qquad \textbf{36-3}$$

where RPF is renal plasma flow. Under normal conditions, the filtration fraction averages 0.15 to 0.20. This means that only 15% to 20% of the plasma that enters the glomerulus is actually filtered. The remaining 80% to 85% continues on through the glomerular capillaries and into the efferent arterioles and peritubular capillaries. It is finally returned to the systemic circulation in the renal vein.

A fall in the GFR may be the first and only clinical sign of kidney disease. Thus, measurement of the GFR is important when kidney disease is suspected. A 50% loss of functioning nephrons reduces the GFR only by about 25%. The decline in GFR is not 50% because the remaining nephrons compensate. Because measurements of GFR are cumbersome, kidney function is usually assessed in the clinical setting by measurement of the P_{Cr}, which is inversely related to the GFR **(Figure 36–8)**. However, as Figure 36–8 shows, the GFR must decline substantially before an increase in the P_{Cr} can be detected in a clinical setting. For example, a fall in GFR from 120 to 100 mL/min is accompanied by an increase in the P_{Cr} from 1.0 to 1.2 mg/dL. This does not appear to be a significant change in the P_{Cr}, but the GFR has actually fallen by almost 20%.

The first step in the formation of urine is ultrafiltration of the plasma by the glomerulus

In normal adults, the GFR ranges from 90 to 140 mL/min for men and from 80 to 125 mL/min for women. Thus, in 24 hours, as much as 180 L of plasma is filtered by the glomeruli. The plasma ultrafiltrate is devoid of cellular elements (i.e., red and white blood cells and platelets) and is essentially protein free. The concentrations of salts and of organic molecules, such as glucose and amino acids, are similar in the plasma and ultrafiltrate. Starling forces drive ultrafiltration across the glomerular capillaries, and changes in these forces alter the GFR (see Chapter 22). The GFR and renal plasma flow are normally held within narrow ranges by a phenomenon called **autoregulation** (see Chapter 23).

The next sections of this chapter review the composition of the glomerular filtrate, the dynamics of its formation, and the relationship between renal plasma flow and GFR. In addition, the factors that contribute to the autoregulation of GFR and RBF are discussed.

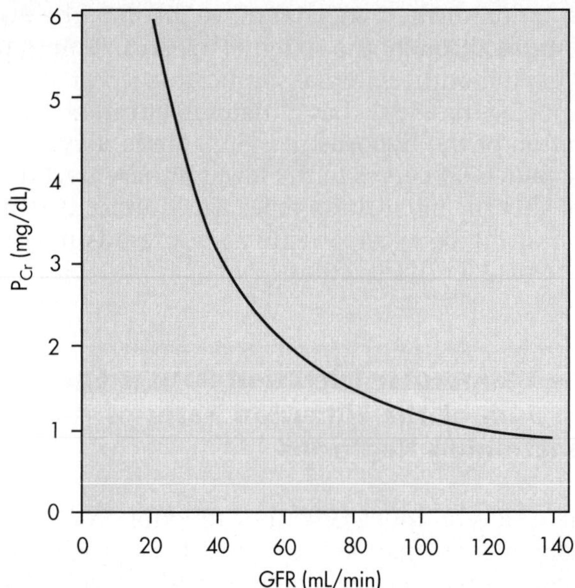

FIGURE 36–8. Relationship between GFR and P_{Cr}. The amount of creatinine filtered is essentially equal to the amount excreted; thus, GFR × P_{Cr} = U_{Cr} × $\dot{V}$. Because the production of creatinine is constant, excretion must be constant to maintain creatinine balance. Therefore, if the GFR falls from 120 to 60 mL/min, the P_{Cr} must increase from 1 to 2 mg/dL to keep the filtration of creatinine and thus its excretion equal to the production rate.

The glomerular filtration barrier determines the composition of the plasma ultrafiltrate

THE GLOMERULAR FILTRATION BARRIER RESTRICTS THE FILTRATION OF MOLECULES ON THE BASIS OF SIZE AND ELECTRICAL CHARGE **(Figure 36–9)**. In general, neutral molecules with a radius smaller than 20 Å are filtered freely, molecules larger than 42 Å are not filtered, and molecules between 20 and 42 Å are filtered to various degrees. For example, serum albumin, an anionic protein that has an effective molecular radius of 35.5 Å, is filtered poorly. Because the filtered albumin is reabsorbed avidly by the proximal tubule, almost no albumin appears in the urine.

Figure 36–9 shows how electrical charge affects the filtration of macromolecules (e.g., dextrans) by the glomerulus. Dextrans are a family of exogenous polysaccharides manufactured in various molecular weights. They can be electrically neutral or have either negative charges (polyanionic) or positive charges (polycationic). As the size (i.e., effective molecular radius) of a dextran increases, the rate at which it is filtered decreases. For any given molecular radius, cationic molecules are more readily filtered than anionic molecules. The reduced filtration rate for anionic molecules is explained by the presence of negatively charged glycoproteins on the

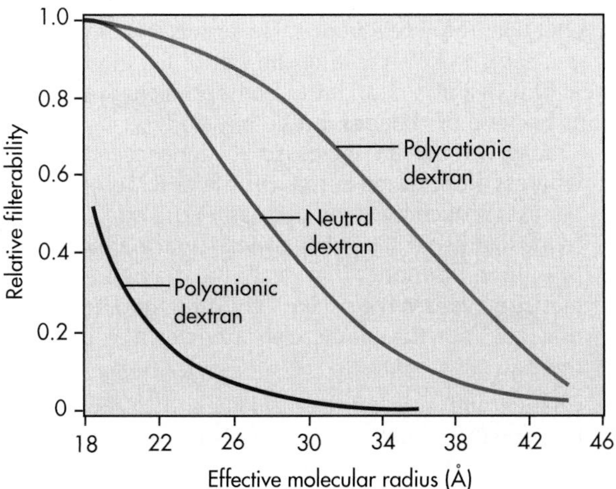

FIGURE 36–9. Influence of size and electrical charge of dextran on its filterability. A value of 1 indicates that it is filtered freely, whereas a value of 0 indicates that it is not filtered. The filterability of dextrans between approximately 20 and 42 Å depends on charge. Dextrans larger than 42 Å are not filtered regardless of charge, and polycationic dextrans and neutral dextrans smaller than 20 Å are freely filtered.

surface of all components of the glomerular filtration barrier. These charged glycoproteins repel similarly charged molecules. Because most plasma proteins are negatively charged, the negative charge on the filtration barrier restricts the filtration of proteins that have a molecular radius of 20 to 42 Å or more.

The importance of the negative charges on the filtration barrier in restricting the filtration of plasma proteins is shown in **Figure 36–10**. The removal of negative charges from the filtration barrier causes proteins to be filtered solely on the basis of their effective molecular radius. Hence, at any molecular radius between approximately 20 and 42 Å, the filtration of polyanionic proteins will exceed the filtration that prevails in the normal state (in which the filtration barrier has anionic charges). In a number of glomerular diseases, the negative charge on the filtration barrier is reduced because of immunological damage and inflammation. As a result, the filtration of proteins is increased, and proteins appear in the urine **(proteinuria).**

The forces responsible for the glomerular filtration of plasma are the same as those in all capillary beds

Ultrafiltration occurs because the Starling forces (i.e., hydrostatic and oncotic pressures) drive fluid from the lumen of glomerular capillaries, across the filtration barrier, and into Bowman's space **(Figure 36–11)**. The hydrostatic pressure in the glomerular capillary (P_{GC}) is oriented to promote the movement of fluid from the glomerular capillary into Bowman's space. Because the reflection coefficient (σ) for proteins across the glomerular capillary is essentially 1, the glomerular ultrafiltrate is protein free, and the oncotic pressure in Bowman's space (π_{BS}) is near 0. Therefore, P_{GC} is the only force that favors filtration. The hydrostatic pressure in Bowman's space (P_{BS}) and the oncotic pressure in the glomerular capillary (π_{GC}) oppose filtration.

As shown in Figure 36–11, a net ultrafiltration pressure (P_{UF}) of 17 mm Hg exists at the afferent end of the glomerulus, whereas at the efferent end, it is 8 mm Hg (where $P_{UF} = P_{GC} - P_{BS} - \pi_{GC}$). Two additional points concerning Starling forces and this pressure change are important. First, P_{GC} decreases slightly along the length of the capillary because of the resistance to flow along the length of the capillary. Second, π_{GC} increases along the length of the glomerular capillary. Because water is filtered and protein is retained in the glomerular capillary, the protein concentration in the capillary rises, and π_{GC} increases.

The GFR is proportional to the sum of the Starling forces that exist across the capillaries $[(P_{GC} - P_{BS}) - \sigma(\pi_{GC} - \pi_{BS})]$ multiplied by the ultrafiltration coefficient (K_f). That is:

$$GFR = K_f[(P_{GC} - P_{BS}) - \sigma(\pi_{GC} - \pi_{BS})] \qquad \textbf{36-4}$$

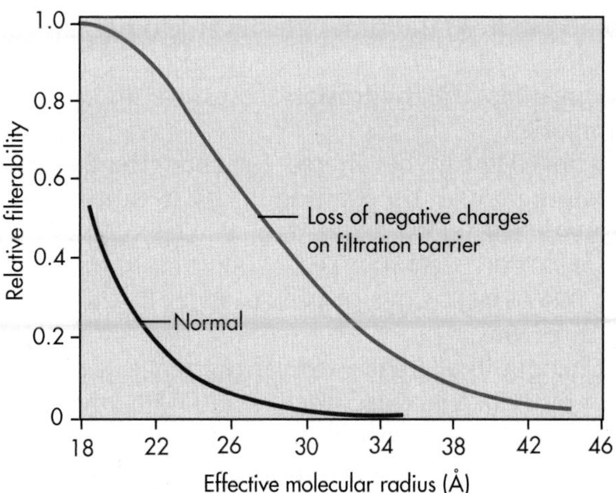

FIGURE 36–10. Reduction of the negative charges on the glomerular wall results in the filtration of proteins on the basis of size only. In this situation, the relative filterability of proteins depends only on the molecular radius. Accordingly, the excretion of polyanionic proteins (20 to 42 Å) in the urine increases because more proteins of this size are filtered.

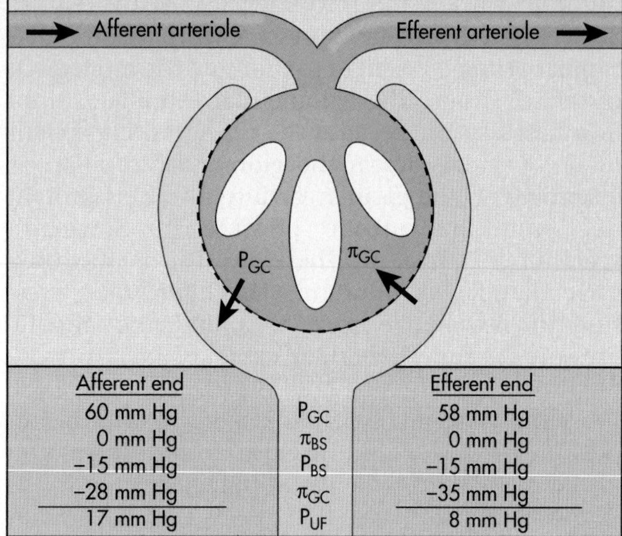

FIGURE 36–11. Idealized glomerular capillary and the Starling forces across it. The reflection coefficient (σ) for protein across the glomerular capillary is 1. P_{BS}, hydrostatic pressure in Bowman's space; P_{GC}, hydrostatic pressure in the glomerular capillary; P_{UF}, net ultrafiltration pressure; π_{GC}, oncotic pressure in the glomerular capillary; π_{BS}, oncotic pressure in Bowman's space. (Because π_{GC} and P_{BS} oppose filtration, they are denoted with minus signs.)

A reduction in the GFR in disease states is most often due to decreases in K_f because of the loss of filtration surface area. The GFR also changes in pathophysiological conditions because of changes in P_{GC}, π_{GC}, and P_{BS}.

- Changes in K_f: an increased K_f enhances the GFR, whereas a decreased K_f reduces the GFR. Some kidney diseases reduce the K_f by decreasing the number of filtering glomeruli (i.e., diminished surface area). Some drugs and hormones that dilate the glomerular arterioles also increase the K_f. Similarly, drugs and hormones that constrict the glomerular arterioles also decrease the K_f.
- Changes in P_{GC}: in acute renal failure, the GFR declines because the P_{GC} falls. As previously discussed, a reduction in the P_{GC} is caused by a decline in renal arterial pressure, an increase in afferent arteriolar resistance, or a decrease in efferent arteriolar resistance.
- Changes in π_{GC}: an inverse relationship exists between the π_{GC} and the GFR. Alterations in the π_{GC} result from changes in protein synthesis outside the kidneys. In addition, protein loss in the urine caused by some renal diseases can lead to a decrease in the plasma protein concentration and thus in the π_{GC}.
- Changes in P_{BS}: an increased P_{BS} reduces the GFR, whereas a decreased P_{BS} enhances the GFR. Acute obstruction of the urinary tract (e.g., a kidney stone occluding the ureter) increases the P_{BS}.

K_f is the product of the intrinsic permeability of the glomerular capillary and the glomerular surface area available for filtration. The rate of glomerular filtration is considerably greater in glomerular capillaries than in systemic capillaries, mainly because K_f is approximately 100 times greater in glomerular capillaries. Furthermore, the P_{GC} is approximately twice as great as the hydrostatic pressure in systemic capillaries.

The GFR can be altered by changing K_f or by changing any of the Starling forces. IN NORMAL INDIVIDUALS, THE GFR IS REGULATED BY ALTERATIONS IN THE P_{GC} THAT ARE MEDIATED MAINLY BY CHANGES IN AFFERENT OR EFFERENT ARTERIOLAR RESISTANCE. P_{GC} is affected in three ways:

- Changes in afferent arteriolar resistance: a decrease in resistance increases the P_{GC} and GFR, whereas an increase in resistance decreases them.
- Changes in efferent arteriolar resistance: a decrease in resistance reduces the P_{GC} and GFR, whereas an increase in resistance elevates them.
- Changes in renal arteriolar pressure: an increase in blood pressure transiently increases the P_{GC} (which enhances the GFR), whereas a decrease in blood pressure transiently decreases the P_{GC} (which reduces the GFR).

Blood Flow Through the Kidneys Serves Several Important Functions

Blood flow through the kidneys

- indirectly determines the GFR;
- modifies the rate of solute and water reabsorption by the proximal tubule;
- participates in the concentration and dilution of urine;
- delivers oxygen, nutrients, and hormones to the cells of the nephron and returns carbon dioxide and reabsorbed fluid and solutes to the general circulation; and
- delivers substrates for excretion in the urine.

Blood flow through any organ may be represented by the following equation:

$$Q = \Delta P / R \qquad \text{36-5}$$

where

Q = blood flow

ΔP = mean arterial pressure minus venous pressure for that organ

R = resistance to flow through that organ (see Chapter 20)

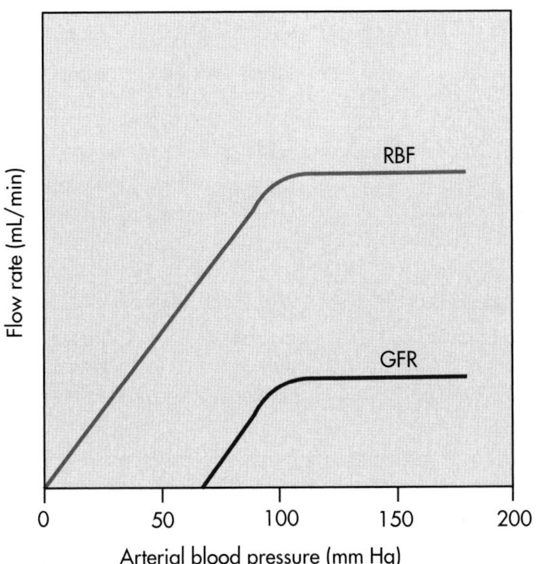

FIGURE 36–12. Relationship between arterial blood pressure and RBF and between arterial blood pressure and GFR. Autoregulation maintains the GFR and RBF relatively constant as blood pressure changes from 90 to 180 mm Hg.

Accordingly, RBF is equal to the pressure difference between the renal artery and the renal vein divided by the renal vascular resistance:

$$\text{RBF} = \text{Aortic pressure} - \text{Renal venous pressure/Renal vascular resistance} \quad \text{36-6}$$

The afferent arteriole, efferent arteriole, and interlobular artery are the major resistance vessels in the kidneys and thereby determine renal vascular resistance. Like most other organs, the kidneys regulate their blood flow by adjusting the vascular resistance in response to changes in arterial pressure (see Chapter 23). As shown in **Figure 36–12**, these adjustments are so precise that blood flow remains relatively constant as arterial blood pressure changes between 90 and 180 mm Hg. The GFR is also regulated over the same range of arterial pressures. The phenomenon whereby RBF and GFR are maintained relatively constant, namely, autoregulation, is achieved by changes in vascular resistance, mainly through the afferent arterioles of the kidneys. Because both the GFR and RBF are regulated over the same range of pressures and because RBF is an important determinant of GFR, it is not surprising that the same mechanisms regulate both flows.

TWO MECHANISMS ARE RESPONSIBLE FOR THE AUTOREGULATION OF RBF AND GFR: ONE MECHANISM THAT RESPONDS TO CHANGES IN ARTERIAL PRESSURE AND ANOTHER THAT RESPONDS TO CHANGES IN THE [NACL] OF TUBULAR FLUID. Both regulate the tone of the afferent arteriole. The pressure-sensitive mechanism, the so-called myogenic mechanism, is related to an intrinsic property of vascular smooth muscle: the tendency to contract when it is stretched (see Chapter 23). Accordingly, when the arterial pressure rises and the renal afferent arteriole is stretched, the smooth muscle contracts. Because the increase in the resistance of the arteriole offsets the increase in pressure, RBF and therefore GFR remain constant; that is, RBF is constant if $\Delta P/R$ is kept constant (see Equation 36-5.)

The second mechanism responsible for the autoregulation of GFR and RBF is the [NaCl]-dependent mechanism known as **tubuloglomerular feedback** (Figure 36–13). This mechanism involves a feedback loop in which the [NaCl] of tubular fluid (or some other factors, such as changes in the cytosolic composition of macula densa cells, changes in interstitial fluid composition surrounding macula densa cells, or changes in

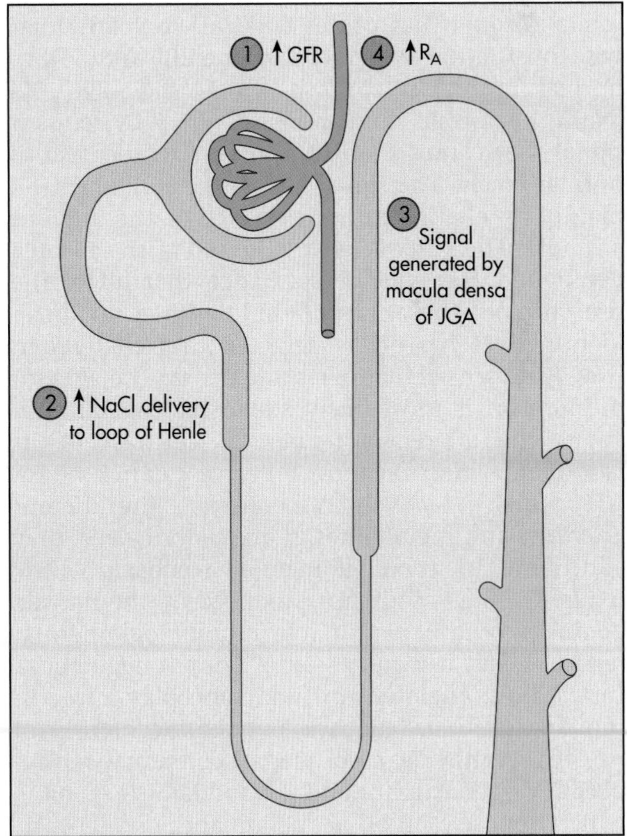

FIGURE 36–13. Tubuloglomerular feedback. An increase in the GFR (1) increases [NaCl] in tubule fluid in the loop of Henle (2), which is sensed by the macula densa of the juxtaglomerular apparatus (JGA) and converted into a signal (3) that increases the resistance of the afferent arteriole (R_A) (4), which decreases the GFR. (Modified from Cogan MG: *Fluid and electrolytes: physiology and pathophysiology,* Norwalk, Conn, 1991, Appleton & Lange.)

TABLE 36–1. MAJOR HORMONES THAT INFLUENCE GLOMERULAR FILTRATION RATE AND RENAL BLOOD FLOW

	Stimulus	Effect on GFR	Effect on RBF
Vasoconstrictors			
Sympathetic nerves	Decreased ECFV	Decrease	Decrease
Angiotensin II	Decreased ECFV	Decrease	Decrease
Endothelin	Increased stretch, angiotensin II, bradykinin, epinephrine; decreased ECFV	Decrease	Decrease
Vasodilators			
Prostaglandins	Decreased ECFV; increased shear stress, angiotensin II	No change	Increase
Nitric oxide	Increased shear stress, acetylcholine, histamine, bradykinin, ATP	Increase	Increase
Bradykinin	Prostaglandins, decreased angiotensin-converting enzyme	Increase	Increase
Atrial natriuretic peptide, brain natriuretic peptide	Increased ECFV	Increase	Increase

ECFV, extracellular fluid volume.

cellular metabolism) is sensed by the macula densa of the JGA and converted into a signal that affects afferent arteriolar resistance and thus the GFR. When the GFR increases and causes the [NaCl] of tubular fluid at the macula densa to rise, the JGA sends a signal that causes renal afferent arteriolar vasoconstriction, which returns the RBF and GFR to normal levels. In contrast, when the GFR and [NaCl] of tubule fluid decrease, the JGA sends a signal that causes the RBF and GFR to increase to normal levels. The signal affects the RBF and GFR mainly by changing the resistance of the afferent arteriole. The variable that is sensed at the macula densa and the effector substance that alters the resistance of the afferent arteriole have not been identified. It has been suggested that changes in [NaCl] are sensed by the macula densa. The effector mechanism is most likely adenosine, which constricts the afferent arteriole (in contrast to its vasodilator effect on most other vasculature beds). ATP, which selectively vasoconstricts the afferent arteriole, and metabolites of arachidonic acid may contribute to tubuloglomerular feedback. Nitric oxide (NO), a vasodilator produced by the macula densa, may also play a role in tubuloglomerular feedback, but it is not essential for autoregulation. In addition, angiotensin II may also play a role in tubuloglomerular feedback, but the mechanism of this effect is not clear. The macula densa may release both a vasoconstrictor and a vasodilator (e.g., NO), which oppose each other's action at the level of the afferent arteriole.

Because animals engage in many activities that can change arterial blood pressure, mechanisms that maintain RBF and GFR relatively constant despite changes in arterial pressure are highly desirable. If the GFR and RBF were to rise or fall suddenly in proportion to changes in blood pressure, urinary excretion of fluid and solute would also change suddenly. Such changes in water and solute excretion without comparable changes in intake would alter the fluid and electrolyte balance. Accordingly, autoregulation of the GFR and RBF provides an effective means for uncoupling renal function from arterial pressure, and it ensures that fluid and solute excretion remains constant.

Three points concerning autoregulation should be noted:

- Autoregulation is absent when arterial pressure is less than 90 mm Hg.
- Autoregulation is not perfect; the RBF and GFR do change slightly as the arterial blood pressure varies.
- Despite autoregulation, the RBF and GFR can be changed by certain hormones and by changes in sympathetic nerve activity (**Table 36–1**).

Individuals with **renal artery stenosis** (narrowing of the artery lumen) caused by atherosclerosis, for example, can have an elevated systemic arterial blood pressure mediated by stimulation of the renin-angiotensin system (see Chapter 38). Pressure in the renal artery proximal to the stenosis is increased, but pressure distal to the stenosis is normal or reduced. Autoregulation is important in maintaining RBF, P_{GC}, and GFR in the presence of this stenosis. The administration of drugs to lower the systemic blood pressure also lowers the pressure distal to the stenosis; accordingly, the RBF, P_{GC}, and GFR fall.

Hormones and Sympathetic Nerves Regulate the Glomerular Filtration Rate and Renal Blood Flow

Several factors and hormones affect the GFR and RBF (Table 36–1). The myogenic mechanism and tubuloglomerular feedback play a key role in maintaining GFR and RBF constant. Sympathetic nerves, angiotensin II, prostaglandins, NO, endothelin, bradykinin, and perhaps adenosine exert major

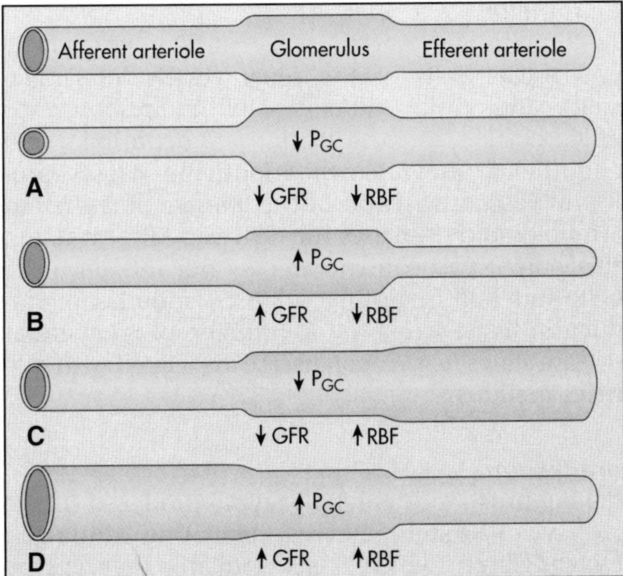

FIGURE 36–14. Relationship between selective changes in the resistance of either the afferent arteriole or the efferent arteriole on RBF and GFR. Constriction of either the afferent or efferent arteriole increases resistance, and according to Equation 36–5 ($Q = \Delta P/R$), an increase in resistance (R) decreases flow (Q) (i.e., RBF). Dilation of either the afferent or efferent arteriole increases flow (i.e., RBF). Constriction of the afferent arteriole (A) decreases the P_{GC} because less of the arterial pressure is transmitted to the glomerulus, thereby reducing the GFR. In contrast, constriction of the efferent arteriole (B) elevates the P_{GC} and thus increases the GFR. Dilation of the efferent arteriole (C) decreases the P_{GC} and thus decreases the GFR. Dilation of the afferent arteriole (D) increases the P_{GC} because more of the arterial pressure is transmitted to the glomerulus, thereby increasing the GFR. (Modified from Rose BD, Rennke KG: *Renal pathophysiology: the essentials,* Baltimore, 1994, Williams & Wilkins.)

control over RBF and GFR. **Figure 36–14** shows how changes in afferent and efferent arteriolar resistance modulate the GFR and RBF.

Sympathetic nerves

The afferent and efferent arterioles are innervated by sympathetic neurons; however, sympathetic tone is minimal when the volume of extracellular fluid is normal (see Chapter 37). Sympathetic nerves release norepinephrine, and circulating epinephrine is secreted by the adrenal medulla. These hormones cause vasoconstriction by binding to α_1-adrenoceptors, which are located mainly on the afferent arterioles. Activation of α_1-adrenoceptors decreases the GFR and RBF. Dehydration and strong emotional stimuli, such as fear and pain, activate sympathetic nerves and reduce the GFR and RBF.

Angiotensin II

Angiotensin II is produced systemically and locally within the kidneys. It constricts the afferent and efferent arterioles and decreases the RBF and GFR (see Chapter 38). **Figure 36–15** shows how norepinephrine, epinephrine, and angiotensin II act together to decrease the RBF and GFR, as would occur, for example, with hemorrhage.

Hemorrhage decreases arterial blood pressure and therefore activates the sympathetic nerves to the kidneys via the baroreceptor reflex (Figure 36–15). Norepinephrine causes intense vasoconstriction of the afferent and efferent arterioles and thereby decreases the GFR and RBF. The rise in sympathetic activity also increases the release of epinephrine and angiotensin II, which cause further vasoconstriction and a fall in RBF. The rise in the vascular resistance of the kidneys and other vascular beds increases the total peripheral resistance. The resulting tendency for blood pressure to increase (blood pressure = cardiac output × total peripheral resistance) offsets the tendency of blood pressure to decrease in response to hemorrhage. Hence, this system works to preserve the arterial pressure at the expense of maintaining a normal GFR and RBF.

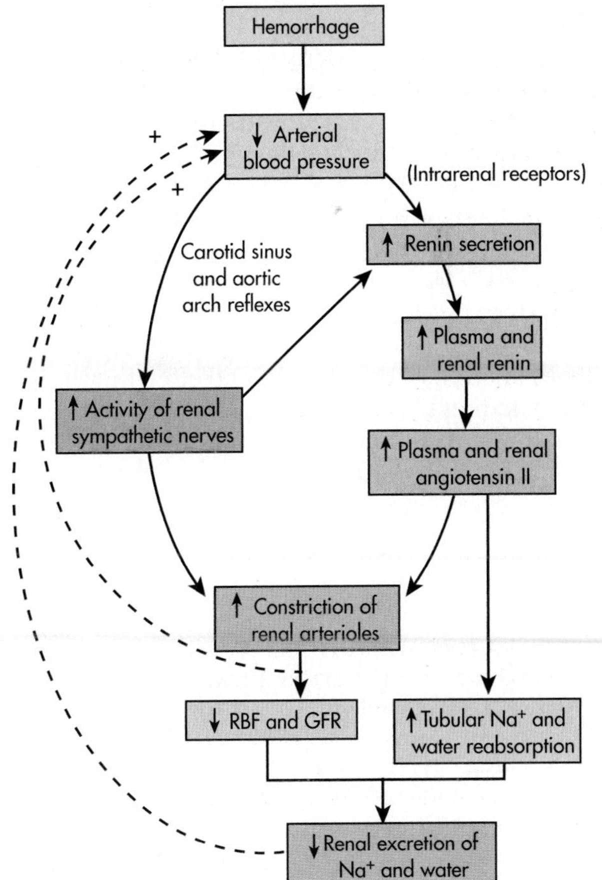

FIGURE 36–15. Pathway by which hemorrhage activates renal sympathetic nerve activity and stimulates the production of angiotensin II. (Modified from Vander AJ: *Renal physiology,* ed 2, New York, 1980, McGraw-Hill.)

Prostaglandins

Prostaglandins may not regulate the RBF or GFR in healthy, resting people. However, during pathophysiological conditions such as hemorrhage, prostaglandins (PGI_2, PGE_1, and PGE_2) are produced locally within the kidneys, and they increase RBF without changing the GFR. Prostaglandins increase RBF by dampening the vasoconstrictor effects of sympathetic nerves and angiotensin II. This effect is important because it prevents severe and potentially harmful vasoconstriction and renal ischemia. Prostaglandin synthesis is stimulated by dehydration and stress (e.g., surgery, anesthesia), angiotensin II, and sympathetic nerves. Nonsteroidal antiinflammatory drugs, such as aspirin and ibuprofen, inhibit the synthesis of prostaglandins. Thus, administration of these drugs during renal ischemia is contraindicated; by blocking the production of prostaglandins, they decrease RBF and increase renal ischemia. Prostaglandins play an increasingly important role in maintaining RBF and GFR as individuals age. Accordingly, nonsteroidal antiinflammatory drugs can significantly reduce RBF and GFR in the elderly.

Nitric oxide

NO, an endothelium-derived relaxing factor, is an important vasodilator under basal conditions, and it counteracts the vasoconstriction produced by angiotensin II and catecholamines. When blood flow increases, a greater shear force acts on the endothelial cells in the arterioles and increases the production of NO. Also, a number of vasoactive hormones, including acetylcholine, histamine, bradykinin, and ATP, cause the release of NO from endothelial cells. Increased production of NO causes dilation of the afferent and efferent arterioles in the kidneys. NO decreases the total peripheral resistance. Inhibition of NO production increases the total peripheral resistance.

Abnormal production of NO is observed in individuals with **diabetes mellitus** and **hypertension.** Excess renal NO production in diabetes may be responsible for glomerular hyperfiltration and damage of the glomerulus, problems characteristic of this disease. Elevated NO levels increase the glomerular capillary pressure secondary to a fall in the resistance of the afferent arteriole. The ensuing hyperfiltration is thought to cause glomerular damage. The normal response to an increase in dietary salt intake includes the stimulation of renal NO production, which maintains blood pressure. In some individuals, NO production may not increase appropriately in response to an elevation in salt intake, so blood pressure rises.

Endothelin

Endothelin is a potent vasoconstrictor secreted by endothelial cells of the renal vessels, mesangial cells, and distal tubular cells in response to angiotensin II, bradykinin, epinephrine, and endothelial shear stress. Endothelin causes profound vasoconstriction of the afferent and efferent arterioles and decreases the GFR and RBF. Although this potent vasoconstrictor may not influence the GFR and RBF in resting subjects, endothelin production is elevated in a number of glomerular disease states (e.g., renal disease associated with diabetes mellitus).

Bradykinin

Kallikrein is a proteolytic enzyme produced in the kidneys. Kallikrein cleaves circulating kininogen to bradykinin, which is a vasodilator that acts by stimulating the release of NO and prostaglandins. Bradykinin increases the GFR and RBF.

Adenosine

Adenosine is produced within the kidneys and causes vasoconstriction of the afferent arteriole, thereby reducing the GFR and RBF. Adenosine may play a role in tubuloglomerular feedback.

Natriuretic peptides

Secretion of atrial natriuretic peptide (ANP) by the cardiac atria and brain natriuretic peptide (BNP) from the cardiac ventricles increases when the volume of extracellular fluid is expanded. Both ANP and BNP dilate the afferent arteriole and constrict the efferent arteriole. Therefore, ANP and BNP produce a modest increase in the GFR with little change in RBF.

ATP

Cells release ATP into the renal interstitial fluid. ATP has dual effects on the GFR and RBF. Under some conditions, ATP constricts the afferent arteriole, reduces RBF and GFR, and may play a role in tubuloglomerular feedback. In contrast, ATP may stimulate NO production and increase the GFR and RBF.

Glucocorticoids

Administration of therapeutic doses of glucocorticoids increases the GFR and RBF.

Histamine

The local release of histamine modulates RBF during the resting state and during inflammation and injury. Histamine decreases the resistance of the afferent and efferent arterioles and thereby increases RBF without elevating the GFR.

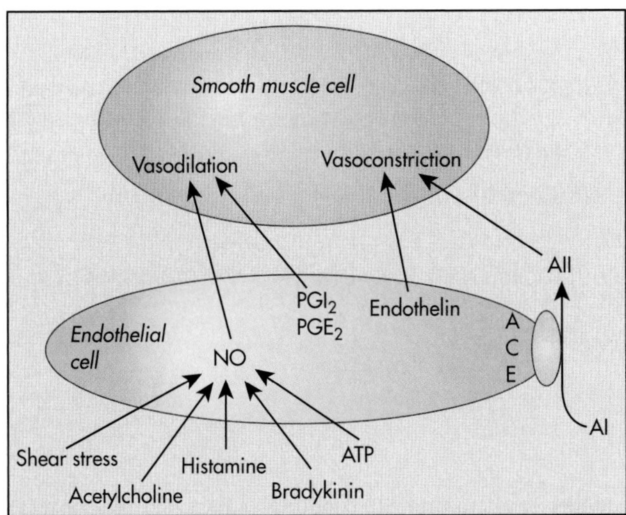

FIGURE 36–16. Examples of the interactions of endothelial cells with smooth muscle or mesangial cells. ACE, angiotensin-converting enzyme; AI, angiotensin I; AII, angiotensin II. (Modified from Navar LG et al: *Physiol Rev* 76:425, 1996.)

Dopamine

The proximal tubule produces the vasodilator substance dopamine. Dopamine has several actions within the kidney, such as increasing RBF and inhibiting renin secretion.

As illustrated in **Figure 36–16,** ENDOTHELIAL CELLS PLAY AN IMPORTANT ROLE IN REGULATING THE RESISTANCE OF THE AFFERENT AND EFFERENT ARTERIOLES BY PRODUCING A NUMBER OF PARACRINE HORMONES, including NO, prostacyclins (PGI_2), endothelin, and angiotensin II. These hormones regulate contraction or relaxation of smooth muscle cells in afferent and efferent arterioles and mesangial cells. Shear stress, acetylcholine, histamine, bradykinin, and ATP stimulate the production of NO, which increases the GFR and RBF. **Angiotensin-converting enzyme** (ACE), located on the surface of endothelial cells lining the afferent arteriole and glomerular capillaries, converts angiotensin I to angiotensin II, which decreases the GFR and RBF. Angiotensin II is also produced locally in juxtaglomerular cells and proximal tubular cells. PGI_2 and PGE_2 secretion by endothelial cells, stimulated by sympathetic nerve activity and angiotensin II, increases the GFR and RBF. Finally, the release of endothelin from endothelial cells decreases the GFR and RBF.

ACE degrades and thereby inactivates bradykinin, and it converts angiotensin I, an inactive hormone, to angiotensin II, an active hormone. Thus, ACE increases angiotensin II levels and decreases bradykinin levels. Drugs called **ACE inhibitors,** which reduce systemic blood pressure in patients with hypertension, decrease angiotensin II levels and elevate bradykinin levels. Both effects lower systemic vascular resistance, reduce blood pressure, and decrease renal vascular resistance, thereby increasing the GFR and RBF (see Chapter 38).

Summary

- The functional unit of the kidney is the nephron. Each nephron consists of a renal corpuscle, proximal tubule, loop of Henle, distal tubule, and collecting duct.
- The renal corpuscle is composed of glomerular capillaries and Bowman's capsule.
- The JGA consists of the macula densa, extraglomerular mesangial cells, and renin-producing granular cells in the afferent arteriole.
- The JGA is one component of an important feedback mechanism that regulates the GFR and RBF.
- The micturition reflex is an automatic spinal cord reflex that can be inhibited or facilitated by centers in the brainstem and cortex.
- The GFR is calculated by measuring creatinine clearance.
- Starling forces across the glomerular capillaries provide the driving force for the ultrafiltration of plasma from the glomerular capillaries into Bowman's space.
- The glomerular ultrafiltrate is devoid of cellular elements, including red and white blood cells and platelets, and contains very little protein but is otherwise identical to plasma.

- ❖ RBF (1.25 L/min) is about 25% of the cardiac output. RBF determines the GFR; modifies solute and water reabsorption by the proximal tubule; participates in concentration and dilution of the urine; delivers oxygen, nutrients, and hormones to the cells of the nephron; returns carbon dioxide and reabsorbed fluid and solutes to the general circulation; and delivers substrates for excretion in the urine.
- ❖ Autoregulation allows the GFR and RBF to remain constant despite changes in arterial blood pressure between 90 and 180 mm Hg.
- ❖ Sympathetic nerves, angiotensin II, prostaglandins, NO, endothelin, ANP, BNP, bradykinin, and adenosine exert substantial control over the GFR and RBF.

Bibliography

Arendshorst WJ, Navar LG: Renal circulation and glomerular hemodynamics. In Schrier RW, Gottschalk CW, eds: *Diseases of the kidney,* ed 6, Boston, 1997, Little, Brown.

Bradley WE: Physiology of the urinary bladder. In Walsh PC et al, eds: *Campbell's urology,* ed 7, Philadelphia, 1988, WB Saunders.

Dupont MC, Steers WD: Disorders of micturition. In Schrier RW, Gottschalk CW: *Diseases of the kidney,* ed 6, Boston, 1997, Little, Brown.

Dworkin LD, Brenner BM: The renal circulations. In Brenner BM, ed: *Brenner and Rector's the kidney,* ed 7, Philadelphia, 2004, WB Saunders.

Kriz W, Kaissling B: Structural organization of the mammalian kidney. In Seldin DW, Giebisch G, eds: *The kidney: physiology and pathophysiology,* ed 3, New York, 2000, Raven Press.

Layfayette RA, Perrone RD, Levy AS: Laboratory evaluation of renal function. In Schrier RW, Gottschalk WR, eds: *Diseases of the kidney,* ed 6, Boston, 1997, Little, Brown.

Maddox DA, Brenner BM: Glomerular ultrafiltration. In Brenner BM, ed: *Brenner and Rector's the kidney,* ed 7, Philadelphia, 2004, WB Saunders.

Mundel P, Shankland SJ: Podocyte biology and response to injury, *J Am Soc Nephrol* 13:3005, 2002.

Pirson Y: Making the diagnosis in Alport's syndrome, *Kidney Int* 56:760, 1999.

Schnerman J: The juxtaglomerular apparatus: from anatomical peculiarity to physiological relevance, *J Am Soc Nephrol* 14:1681, 2003.

Sun D et al: Mediation of tubuloglomerular feedback by adenosine: evidence from mice lacking adenosine A1 receptors, *Proc Natl Acad Sci USA* 98:9983, 2001.

Tanagho EA: Anatomy of the genitourinary tract. In Tanagho EA, Mcanich JW, eds: *Smith's general urology,* ed 14, Norwalk, Conn, 1995, Appleton & Lange.

Tisher CC, Madsen KM: Anatomy of the kidney. In Brenner BM, ed: *Brenner and Rector's the kidney,* ed 7, Philadelphia, 2004, WB Saunders.

Tryggvason K: Unraveling the mechanisms of glomerular ultrafiltration: nephrin, a key component of the slit diaphragm, *J Am Soc Nephrol* 10:2440, 1999.

Vallon V: Tubuloglomerular feedback and the control of glomerular filtration rate, *News Physiol Sci* 18:169, 2003.

Case Studies

Case 36–1

A 75-year-old woman (body weight = 60 kg) was admitted to the intensive care unit after falling at home 2 days earlier. For the first 4 days in the hospital, her urine output was approximately 400 mL/day. On physical examination, she had orthostatic changes in blood pressure (fall in blood pressure on standing), tachycardia, and poor skin turgor. Her serum creatinine level increased progressively from 1.0 mg/dL on the day of admission to 5.9 mg/dL on day 4. After 2 weeks in the intensive care unit, she was transferred to a medical ward, where her urine output was noted to be approximately 1 L/day and her serum creatinine concentration was stable at 1.0 mg/dL. She also had signs and symptoms of congestive heart failure with decreased cardiac output. She fractured several ribs, and she requested medication to relieve the pain. A nonsteroidal antiinflammatory pain reliever was prescribed. By morning, the patient's rib pain was better. Because some edema had developed secondary to the congestive heart failure, she was treated with a diuretic. Her condition responded well to the diuretic, and the edema disappeared. Her serum creatinine level was stabilized at 1.0 mg/dL. A 24-hour urine collection was performed to determine her GFR:

Urine (creatinine)	64.8 mg/dL
Urine volume	1 L
Serum (creatinine)	1.0 mg/dL

1. **Why did the serum creatinine level increase during the first 4 days of this patient's hospitalization?**
   A. The RBF decreased.
   B. Her urine output was low.
   C. Her creatinine metabolism decreased.
   D. Her GFR decreased.
   E. Her blood volume decreased.

2. **The nonsteroidal antiinflammatory pain reliever inhibits prostaglandin synthesis. What is an adverse effect of this pain reliever on renal function?**
   A. It increases RBF.
   B. It decreases the GFR.
   C. It increases urine output.
   D. It increases urinary protein excretion.
   E. It increases creatinine excretion.

Case 36–2

The urine of a 13-year-old boy turned dark brown several weeks after a bout of "strep throat." The diagnosis is glomerulonephritis (i.e., inflammation of the glomerular capillaries). The urine is dark brown because red blood cells are in the urine.

1. **Which of the following will also be found in high concentration in this boy's urine? (Hint: think of the glomerular filtration barrier.)**
   A. Na^+
   B. K^+
   C. Serum albumin
   D. Creatinine
   E. Urea

Chapter 37: Solute and Water Transport Along the Nephron: Tubular Function

Objectives

- ❖ Describe how the components of the nephron determine the composition and volume of urine.
- ❖ Explain how Na^+, Cl^-, other anions, and organic solutes are reabsorbed in the nephron.
- ❖ Explain how the composition and volume of urine are adjusted.
- ❖ Describe how various byproducts of metabolism and organic anions and bases (e.g., drugs) are secreted into the tubular fluid.
- ❖ Describe how hormones, sympathetic nerves, dopamine, and Starling forces regulate NaCl reabsorption by the kidneys.
- ❖ Explain how ADH regulates water reabsorption.

The formation of urine involves three basic processes:

- **ultrafiltration** of plasma by the glomerulus;
- **reabsorption** of water and solutes from the ultrafiltrate; and
- **secretion** of selected solutes into the tubular fluid.

Although an average of 180 L of essentially protein-free fluid is filtered by the human glomeruli each day, less than 1% of the filtered water and NaCl and variable amounts of other solutes are excreted in the urine (**Table 37–1**). By the processes of reabsorption and secretion, the renal tubules modulate the volume and composition of urine (**Table 37–2**). Consequently, the tubules precisely control the volume, osmolality, composition, and pH of the intracellular and extracellular fluid compartments. Transport proteins in cell membranes of the nephron mediate the reabsorption and secretion of solutes and water in the kidneys. Approximately 5% to 10% of all human genes code for transport proteins, and genetic and acquired defects in transport proteins are the cause of many kidney diseases (**Table 37–3**). In addition, numerous transport proteins are important drug targets. This chapter discusses NaCl and water reabsorption, the transport proteins involved in solute and water transport, and some of the factors and hormones that regulate transport. Details on acid-base transport and on K^+, Ca^{++}, and inorganic phosphate (Pi) transport and their regulation are provided in Chapters 39 and 40.

Quantitatively, the Reabsorption of NaCl and Water Represents the Major Function of Nephrons

Approximately 25,000 mEq/day of Na^+ and 179 L/day of water are reabsorbed by the renal tubules (Table 37–1). In addition, renal transport of many

TABLE 37–1. FILTRATION, EXCRETION, AND REABSORPTION OF WATER, ELECTROLYTES, AND SOLUTES BY THE KIDNEYS

Substance	Measure	Filtered*	Excreted	Reabsorbed	Filtered Load Reabsorbed (%)
Water	L/day	180	1.5	178.5	99.2
Na^+	mEq/day	25,200	150	25,050	99.4
K^+	mEq/day	720	100	620	86.1
Ca^{++}	mEq/day	540	10	530	98.2
HCO_3^-	mEq/day	4320	2	4318	99.9+
Cl^-	mEq/day	18,000	150	17,850	99.2
Glucose	mmol/day	800	0	800	100.0
Urea	g/day	56	28	28	50.0

*The filtered amount of any substance is calculated by multiplying the concentration of that substance in the ultrafiltrate by the glomerular filtration rate (GFR); for example, the filtered load of Na^+ is calculated as $[Na^+]_{ultrafiltrate}$ (140 mEq/L) × GFR (180 L/day) = 25,200 mEq/day.

other important solutes is linked either directly or indirectly to Na^+ reabsorption.

THE PROXIMAL TUBULE REABSORBS APPROXIMATELY 67% OF FILTERED WATER, Na^+, Cl^-, K^+, AND OTHER SOLUTES. In addition, the proximal tubule reabsorbs virtually all the glucose and amino acids filtered by the glomerulus. The key element in proximal tubule reabsorption is the Na^+,K^+-ATPase in the basolateral membrane. The reabsorption of every substance, including water, is linked in some manner to the operation of the Na^+,K^+-ATPase.

TABLE 37–2. COMPOSITION OF URINE

Substance	Concentration
Na^+	50-130 mEq/L
K^+	20-70 mEq/L
Ammonium	30-50 mEq/L
Ca^{++}	5-12 mEq/L
Mg^{++}	2-18 mEq/L
Cl^-	50-130 mEq/L
Inorganic phosphate	20-40 mEq/L
Urea	200-400 mM
Creatinine	6-20 mM
pH	5.0-7.0
Osmolality	500-800 mOsm/kg H_2O
Glucose	0
Amino acids	0
Protein	0
Blood	0
Ketones	0
Leukocytes	0
Bilirubin	0

The composition and volume of the urine can vary widely in the healthy state. These values represent average ranges. Water excretion ranges between 0.5 and 1.5 L/day.

Data from Valtin HV: *Renal physiology,* ed 2, Boston, 1983, Little, Brown.

Na^+ is reabsorbed by different mechanisms in the first and the second halves of the proximal tubule

In the first half of the proximal tubule, Na^+ is reabsorbed primarily with HCO_3^- and a number of other solutes (e.g., glucose, amino acids, Pi, lactate). In contrast, in the second half, Na^+ is reabsorbed mainly with Cl^-. This disparity is mediated by differences in the Na^+ transport systems in the first and second halves of the proximal tubule and by differences in the composition of tubular fluid at these sites.

IN THE FIRST HALF OF THE PROXIMAL TUBULE, Na^+ UPTAKE INTO THE CELL IS COUPLED WITH EITHER H^+ OR ORGANIC SOLUTES (**Figure 37–1**). Specific transport proteins mediate Na^+ entry into the cell across the apical membrane. For example, the Na^+-H^+ antiporter (Figure 37–1, *A*) couples Na^+ entry with H^+ extrusion from the cell. H^+ secretion results in sodium bicarbonate ($NaHCO_3$) reabsorption (see also Chapter 40). Na^+ also enters proximal cells via several symporter mechanisms, including Na^+-glucose, Na^+–amino acid, Na^+-Pi, and Na^+-lactate (Figure 37–1, *B*). The glucose and other organic solutes that enter the cell with Na^+ leave the cell across the basolateral membrane via passive transport mechanisms. Any Na^+ that enters the cell across the apical membrane leaves the cell and enters the blood via the Na^+,K^+-ATPase. In brief, the reabsorption of Na^+ in the first half of the proximal tubule is coupled to that of HCO_3^- and a number of organic molecules. The reabsorption of many organic molecules is so avid that they are almost completely removed from the tubular fluid in the first half of the proximal tubule. The reabsorption of $NaHCO_3$ and Na^+–organic solutes across the proximal tubule establishes a transtubular osmotic gradient that provides the driving force for the passive

TABLE 37–3. SOME MONOGENIC RENAL DISEASES INVOLVING TRANSPORT PROTEINS

Diseases	Mode of Inheritance	Gene	Transport Protein	Nephron Segment	Phenotype
Cystinuria, type I	AR	*SLC3A1,* also known as D2/rBAT	Basic amino acid transporter	Proximal tubule	Increased excretion of basic amino acids, nephrolithiasis
Cystinuria, types II and III	IAR	*SLC7A9,* also known as $b^{0,+}$AT	$B^{0,+}$AT	Proximal tubule	Increased excretion of basic amino acids, nephrolithiasis
Proximal renal tubular acidosis	AR	*SLC4A4,* also known as NBC1	Na^+-HCO_3^- symporter	Proximal tubule	Hyperchloremic metabolic acidosis
X-linked nephrolithiasis (Dent's disease)	XLR	*CLC5,* also known as ClC-5	Cl^- channel	Distal tubule	Hypercalciuria, nephrolithiasis
Bartter's syndrome	AR, type I	*SLC12A1,* also known as NKCC2	$1Na^+,1K^+,2Cl^-$ symporter (furosemide sensitive)	TAL	Hypokalemia, metabolic alkalosis, hyperaldosteronism
	AR, type II	*KCNJ1,* also known as ROMK	K^+ channel	TAL	Hypokalemia, metabolic alkalosis, hyperaldosteronism
	AR, type III	*CLCNKB*	Cl^- channel	TAL	Hypokalemia, metabolic alkalosis, hyperaldosteronism
Hypomagnesemia-hypercalciuria syndrome	AR	*PCLN1*	Claudin-16, also known as paracellin	TAL	Hypomagnesemia, hypercalciuria, nephrolithiasis
Gitelman's syndrome	AR	*SLC12A3,* also known as NCC/TSC	Thiazide-sensitive symporter	Distal tubule	Hypomagnesemia, hypokalemic metabolic alkalosis, hypocalciuria, hypotension
Pseudohypoaldosteronism	AR	*SCNN1A, SCNN1B,* and *SCNN1G,* also known as α-ENaC, β-ENaC, and γ-ENaC	α, β, and γ subunit of amiloride-sensitive Na^+ channel	Collecting duct	Increased excretion of Na^+, hyperkalemia, hypotension
Pseudohypoaldosteronism	AD	*MLR*	Mineralocorticoid receptor	Collecting duct	Increased excretion of Na^+, hyperkalemia, hypotension
Liddle's syndrome	AD	*SCNN1B* and *SCNN1G,* also known as β-ENaC and γ-ENaC	β and γ subunit of amiloride-sensitive Na^+ channel	Collecting duct	Decreased excretion of Na^+, hypertension
Nephrogenic diabetes insipidus	AR	*AQP2*	Aquaporin 2 water channel	Collecting duct	Polyuria, polydipsia, plasma hyperosmolality
Distal renal tubular acidosis	AD	*SLC4A1,* also known as AE1	Cl^--HCO_3^- antiporter	Collecting duct	Metabolic acidosis, hypokalemia, hypercalciuria, nephrolithiasis
Distal renal tubular acidosis	AR	*ATP6B1*	Subunit of H^+-ATPase	Collecting duct	Metabolic acidosis, hypokalemia, hypercalciuria, nephrolithiasis
Distal renal tubular acidosis	AR	*ATP6N1A*	Accessory subunit of H^+-ATPase	Collecting duct	Metabolic acidosis, hypokalemia, hypercalciuria, nephrolithiasis

AD, autosomal dominant; AR, autosomal recessive; IAR, incomplete autosomal recessive; TAL, thick ascending limb of Henle's loop; XLR, X-linked recessive. There are 40 different solute transporter families, which form the so-called solute carrier (SLC) series.
Data from Guay-Woodford LM: *Semin Nephrol* 19:312, 1999.

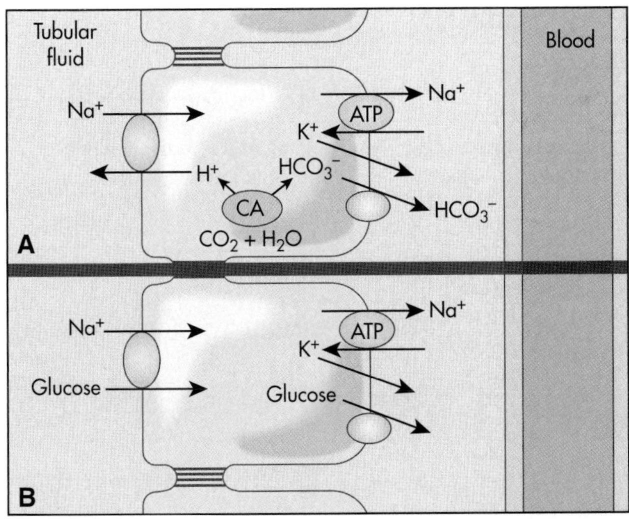

FIGURE 37–1. Na^+ transport processes in the first half of the proximal tubule. These transport mechanisms are present in all cells in the first half of the proximal tubule but are separated into different cells to simplify the discussion. **A,** Operation of the Na^+-H^+ antiporter in the apical membrane and of the Na^+,K^+-ATPase and HCO_3^- transporters including the Cl^--HCO_3^- antiporter and the $1Na^+$-$3HCO_3^-$ symporter (see also Chapter 40) in the basolateral membrane mediates $NaHCO_3$ reabsorption. Note that a single HCO_3^- transporter is illustrated for simplicity. Carbon dioxide and water combine inside the cells to form H^+ and HCO_3^- in a reaction facilitated by the enzyme carbonic anhydrase (CA). **B,** Operation of the Na^+-glucose transporter (SGLT2) in the apical membrane in conjunction with the Na^+,K^+-ATPase and glucose transporter (GLUT2) in the basolateral membrane mediates Na^+-glucose reabsorption. Inactivating mutations in the gene encoding GLUT2 lead to decreased glucose reabsorption in the proximal tubule and glucosuria (i.e., glucose in the urine). Na^+ reabsorption is also coupled with other solutes, including amino acids, Pi, and lactate. Reabsorption of these solutes is mediated by the Na^+-amino acid, Na^+-Pi, and Na^+-lactate symporters located in the apical membrane and the Na^+,K^+-ATPase, amino acid, Pi, and lactate transporters located in the basolateral membrane. Three classes of amino acid transporters have been identified in the proximal tubule: two transport Na^+ in conjunction with either acidic or basic amino acids; one does not require Na^+ and transports basic amino acids. Pi and lactate transporters are also located in the basolateral membrane.

reabsorption of water by osmosis. Because more water than Cl^- is reabsorbed in the first half of the proximal tubule, the $[Cl^-]$ in tubular fluid rises along the length of the proximal tubule.

IN THE SECOND HALF OF THE PROXIMAL TUBULE, Na^+ IS MAINLY REABSORBED WITH Cl^- ACROSS BOTH THE TRANSCELLULAR AND PARACELLULAR PATHWAYS **(Figure 37–2)**. Na^+ is primarily reabsorbed with Cl^- rather than organic solutes or HCO_3^- as the accompanying anion because the Na^+ transport mechanisms in the

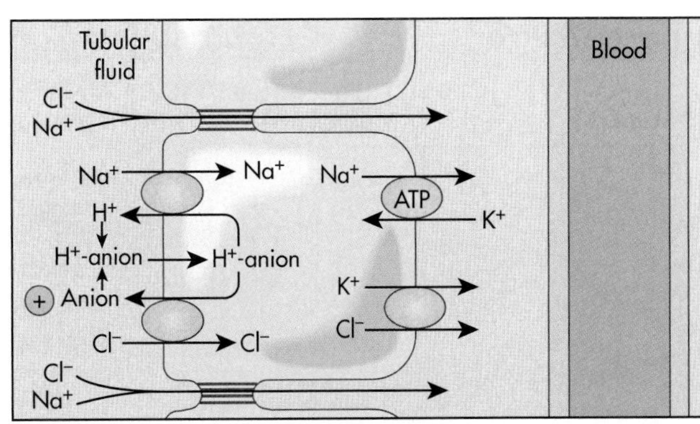

FIGURE 37–2. Na^+ transport processes in the second half of the proximal tubule. Na^+ and Cl^- enter the cell across the apical membrane via the operation of parallel Na^+-H^+ and Cl^--anion antiporters. More than one Cl^--anion antiporter may be involved in this process, but only one is depicted. The secreted H^+ and anion combine in the tubular fluid to form an H^+-anion complex that can recycle across the plasma membrane. Accumulation of the H^+-anion complex in tubular fluid establishes an H^+-anion concentration gradient that favors H^+-anion recycling across the apical plasma membrane into the cell. Inside the cell, H^+ and the anion dissociate and recycle back across the apical plasma membrane. The net result is NaCl uptake across the apical membrane. The anion may be hydroxide ions (OH^-), formate (HCO_2^-), oxalate$^-$, HCO_3^-, or sulfate. The lumen-positive transepithelial voltage, indicated by the plus sign inside the green circle in the tubular lumen, is generated by the diffusion of Cl^- (lumen to blood) across the tight junction. The high $[Cl^-]$ of tubular fluid provides the driving force for Cl^- diffusion. Some glucose is also reabsorbed in the second half of the proximal tubule by a mechanism similar to that described in the first half of the proximal tubule, except the Na^+-glucose symporter (SGLT1) has a higher affinity and lower capacity than the Na^+-glucose symporter in the first part of the proximal tubule (i.e., SGLT2).

second half of the proximal tubule differ from those in the first half. Furthermore, the tubular fluid that enters the second half contains very little glucose and amino acids, but the high concentration of Cl^- (140 mEq/L) in tubule fluid exceeds that in the first half (105 mEq/L). The high $[Cl^-]$ is due to the preferential reabsorption of Na^+ with HCO_3^- and organic solutes in the first half of the proximal tubule.

The mechanism of transcellular Na^+ reabsorption in the second half of the proximal tubule is shown in Figure 37–2. Na^+ enters the cell across the luminal membrane primarily via the parallel operation of an Na^+-H^+ antiporter and one or more Cl^--anion antiporters. Because the secreted H^+ and anion combine in the tubular fluid and reenter the cell, the operation of the Na^+-H^+ and Cl^--anion antiporters is equivalent to NaCl uptake from tubular fluid into the cell. Na^+ leaves the cell via

TABLE 37–4. NaCl TRANSPORT ALONG THE NEPHRON

Segment	Filtered Load Reabsorbed (%)	Mechanism of Na^+ Entry Across Apical Membrane	Major Regulatory Hormones
Proximal tubule	67	Na^+-H^+ exchange, Na^+ cotransport with amino acids and organic solutes, Na^+-H^+/Cl^--anion exchange, paracellular	Angiotensin II, norepinephrine, epinephrine, dopamine
Loop of Henle	25	1Na^+,1K^+,2Cl^- symport	Aldosterone
Distal tubule	≈4	NaCl symport	Aldosterone
Late distal tubule and collecting duct	≈3	Na^+ channels	Aldosterone, ANP, BNP, urodilatin

ANP, atrial natriuretic peptide; BNP, brain natriuretic peptide.

Na^+,K^+-ATPase, and Cl^- leaves the cell and enters the blood via a K^+-Cl^- symporter in the basolateral membrane.

NaCl is also reabsorbed across the second half of the proximal tubule via a **paracellular route.** Paracellular NaCl reabsorption occurs because the rise in the [Cl^-] in the tubule fluid in the first half of the proximal tubule creates a Cl^- concentration gradient (140 mEq/L in the tubule lumen and 105 mEq/L in the interstitium). This concentration gradient favors the diffusion of Cl^- from the tubular lumen across the tight junctions into the lateral intercellular space. Movement of the negatively charged Cl^- causes the tubular fluid to become positively charged relative to the blood. This positive transepithelial voltage causes the diffusion of positively charged Na^+ out of the tubular fluid across the tight junction into the blood. Thus, in the second half of the proximal tubule, some Na^+ and Cl^- is reabsorbed across the tight junctions via passive diffusion. The reabsorption of NaCl establishes a transtubular osmotic gradient that provides the driving force for the passive reabsorption of water by osmosis.

In summary, the reabsorption of Na^+ and Cl^- in the proximal tubule occurs across paracellular and transcellular pathways. Approximately 67% of the NaCl filtered each day is reabsorbed in the proximal tubule. Of this, two thirds moves across the transcellular pathway; the remaining one third moves across the paracellular pathway **(Tables 37–4 and 37–5)**.

Fanconi's syndrome, a renal disease that is either hereditary or acquired, is often associated with glucosuria, osteomalacia, acidosis, and hypokalemia. It results from an impaired ability of the proximal tubule to reabsorb HCO_3^-, amino acids, glucose, and low-molecular-weight proteins. Because other segments of the nephron cannot reabsorb these solutes and protein, Fanconi's syndrome results in increased urinary excretion of HCO_3^-, amino acids, glucose, Pi, and low-molecular-weight proteins.

The proximal tubule reabsorbs 67% of the filtered water

The driving force for water reabsorption is a transtubular osmotic gradient established by solute reabsorption (e.g., NaCl, Na^+-glucose). The reabsorption of Na^+ along with organic solutes, HCO_3^-, and Cl^- from the tubular fluid into the lateral intercellular spaces reduces the osmolality of the tubular

TABLE 37–5. WATER TRANSPORT ALONG THE NEPHRON

Segment	Filtered Load Reabsorbed (%)	Mechanism of Water Reabsorption	Hormones That Regulate Water Permeability
Proximal tubule	67	Passive	None
Loop of Henle	15	Descending thin limb only; passive	None
Distal tubule	0	No water reabsorption	None
Late distal tubule and collecting duct	≈8-17	Passive	ADH, ANP, BNP*

*Atrial natriuretic peptide (ANP) and brain natriuretic peptide (BNP) inhibit ADH-stimulated water permeability.

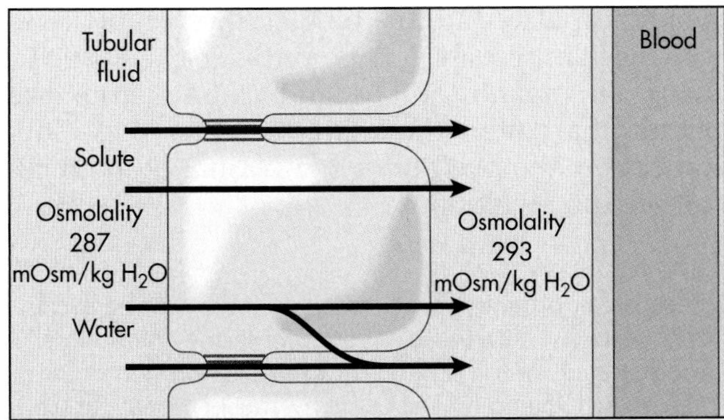

FIGURE 37–3. Routes of water and solute reabsorption across the proximal tubule. The transport of solutes, including Na^+, Cl^-, and organic solutes, into the lateral intercellular space increases the osmolality of this compartment, which establishes the driving force for osmotic water reabsorption across the proximal tubule. This occurs because some Na^+,K^+-ATPase and some transporters of organic solutes, HCO_3^-, and Cl^- are located on the lateral cell membranes and deposit these solutes between cells. Furthermore, some NaCl also enters the lateral intercellular space via diffusion across the tight junction (i.e., paracellular pathway). An important consequence of osmotic water flow across the transcellular and paracellular pathways in the proximal tubule is that some solutes, especially K^+ and Ca^{++}, are entrained in the reabsorbed fluid and are thereby reabsorbed by the process of solvent drag.

fluid and increases the osmolality of the lateral intercellular space **(Figure 37–3)**. Because the proximal tubule is highly permeable to water, water flows via osmosis primarily across the tight junctions. However, some water is reabsorbed across proximal tubular cells. The accumulation of fluid and solutes within the lateral intercellular space increases the hydrostatic pressure in this compartment. This increased hydrostatic pressure forces fluid and solutes into the capillaries. Thus, water reabsorption follows solute reabsorption in the proximal tubule. The reabsorbed fluid is slightly hyperosmotic to plasma. However, this difference in osmolality is so small that it is commonly said that proximal tubule reabsorption is isoosmotic (i.e., 67% of the filtered load of solute and water is reabsorbed). Indeed, there is little difference in the osmolality of tubular fluid at the start and end of the proximal tubule. An important consequence of osmotic water flow across the proximal tubule is that some solutes, especially K^+ and Ca^{++}, are entrained in the reabsorbed fluid and are thereby reabsorbed by the process of solvent drag (Figure 37–3). THE REABSORPTION OF VIRTUALLY ALL ORGANIC SOLUTES, Cl^- AND OTHER IONS, AND WATER IS COUPLED TO Na^+ REABSORPTION. THEREFORE, CHANGES IN Na^+ REABSORPTION INFLUENCE THE REABSORPTION OF WATER AND OTHER SOLUTES BY THE PROXIMAL TUBULE.

Water channels called **aquaporins (AQPs)** mediate the transcellular reabsorption of water across proximal tubule cells. In 2003, Peter Agre received the Nobel Prize in Chemistry for his discovery that AQPs regulate and facilitate water transport across cell membranes, a process essential to all living organisms. The importance of AQPs in renal water reabsorption is underscored by studies in which *AQP1*, a gene expressed in the kidney proximal tubule, was "knocked out" in mice. The rate of water reabsorption by the proximal tubule was 50% less in mice lacking *AQP1* compared with normal mice.

Proteins filtered by the glomerulus are reabsorbed in the proximal tubule

Peptide hormones, small proteins, and small amounts of large proteins such as albumin are filtered by the glomerulus. Overall, only a small percentage of proteins cross the glomerulus and enter Bowman's space (i.e., the concentration of proteins in the glomerular ultrafiltrate is only 40 mg/L). However, the amount of protein filtered per day is significant because the glomerular filtration rate (GFR) is so high:

$$\text{Filtered protein} = \text{GFR} \times [\text{protein}] \text{ in the ultrafiltrate}$$

$$\text{Filtered protein} = 180\ \text{L/day} \times 40\ \text{mg/L} = 7200\ \text{mg/day, or } 7\ \text{g/day}$$

Protein reabsorption in the proximal tubule begins when the proteins are partially degraded by enzymes on the surface of the proximal tubule cells. These partially degraded proteins are taken into cells via endocytosis. Once they are inside the cell, enzymes digest the proteins and peptides into their constituent amino acids, which then leave the cell across the basolateral membrane by transport proteins and are returned to the blood. Normally, this mechanism reabsorbs virtually all of the proteins filtered, and hence the urine is essentially protein free. However, because the mechanism is easily saturated, an increase in filtered proteins causes **proteinuria** (appearance of protein in the urine). Disruption of the glomerular filtration barrier to proteins increases the filtration of proteins and results in proteinuria. Proteinuria is frequently seen with kidney disease.

During routine urinalysis, the presence of traces of protein in the urine is normal. Protein in the urine can be derived from two sources: (1) filtration and incomplete reabsorption by the proximal tubule and (2) synthesis by the thick ascending limb of the loop of Henle. Cells in the thick ascending limb produce **Tamm-Horsfall glycoprotein** and secrete it into the tubular fluid. Because the mechanism for protein reabsorption is "upstream" of the thick ascending limb (i.e., proximal tubule), the secreted Tamm-Horsfall glycoprotein appears in the urine.

Cells of the proximal tubule also secrete organic cations and organic anions

Many of the organic anions and cations (**Boxes 37–1 and 37–2**) secreted by the proximal tubule are end products of metabolism that circulate in the plasma. The proximal tubule also secretes numerous exogenous organic compounds, including *p*-aminohippuric acid (PAH), penicillin, and toxic chemicals. Many of these organic compounds can be bound to plasma proteins and are not readily filtered. Therefore, only a small portion of these potentially toxic substances are eliminated from the body via excretion resulting from filtration alone. Such substances are also secreted from the peritubular capillary into the tubular fluid. These secretory mechanisms are very powerful and remove virtually all organic anions and cations from the plasma that enters the kidneys. Hence, these substances are removed from the plasma by both filtration and secretion.

BOX 37–1: SOME ORGANIC ANIONS SECRETED BY THE PROXIMAL TUBULE

Endogenous Anions	Drugs
cAMP, cGMP	Acetazolamide
Bile salts	Chlorothiazide
Hippurates	Furosemide
Oxalate	Penicillin
Prostaglandins: PGE_2, $PGF_{2\alpha}$	Probenecid
Urate	Salicylate (aspirin)
Vitamins: ascorbate, folate	Hydrochlorothiazide
	Bumetanide
	Nonsteroidal antiinflammatory drugs: indomethacin

BOX 37–2: SOME ORGANIC CATIONS SECRETED BY THE PROXIMAL TUBULE

Endogenous Cations	Drugs
Creatinine	Atropine
Dopamine	Isoproterenol
Epinephrine	Cimetidine
Norepinephrine	Morphine
	Quinine
	Amiloride
	Procainamide

Because all organic anions compete for the same secretory pathway, elevated plasma levels of one anion inhibit the secretion of the others. For example, infusion of PAH can reduce penicillin secretion by the proximal tubule. Because the kidneys are responsible for eliminating penicillin, the infusion of PAH into individuals who receive penicillin reduces penicillin excretion and thereby extends the biological half-life of the drug. In World War II, when penicillin was in short supply, hippurates were given with the penicillin to extend the drug's therapeutic effect.

The histamine H_2 antagonist cimetidine is used to treat gastric ulcers. The organic cation pathway in the proximal tubule secretes cimetidine. It reduces the urinary excretion of procainamide (also an organic cation) by competing with this antiarrhythmic drug for the secretory pathway. The coadministration of organic cations can increase the plasma concentration of both drugs to levels much higher than those seen when the drugs are given alone. This increase can lead to drug toxicity.

Henle's loop reabsorbs approximately 25% of the filtered NaCl and 15% of the filtered water

The reabsorption of NaCl in the loop of Henle occurs in both the thin ascending and thick ascending limb. The descending thin limb does not reabsorb NaCl. The loop of Henle also reabsorbs approximately 15% of the filtered water. Water reabsorption occurs exclusively in the descending thin limb via AQP1 water channels. The ascending limb is impermeable to water. In addition, Ca^{++} and HCO_3^- are also reabsorbed in the loop of Henle (see Chapters 39 and 40 for more details).

The thin ascending limb reabsorbs NaCl by a passive mechanism. The reabsorption of water but not NaCl in the descending thin limb increases the [NaCl] in tubule fluid entering the ascending thin limb. As the NaCl-rich fluid moves toward the cortex, NaCl diffuses out of tubule fluid across the ascending thin limb into the medullary interstitial fluid, down a concentration gradient directed from tubule fluid to interstitium.

The key element in solute reabsorption by the thick ascending limb is the Na^+,K^+-ATPase in the basolateral membrane (**Figure 37–4**). As with reabsorption in the proximal tubule, the reabsorption of every solute by the thick ascending limb is linked to Na^+,K^+-ATPase. This pump maintains a low concentration of cell Na^+, which provides a favorable

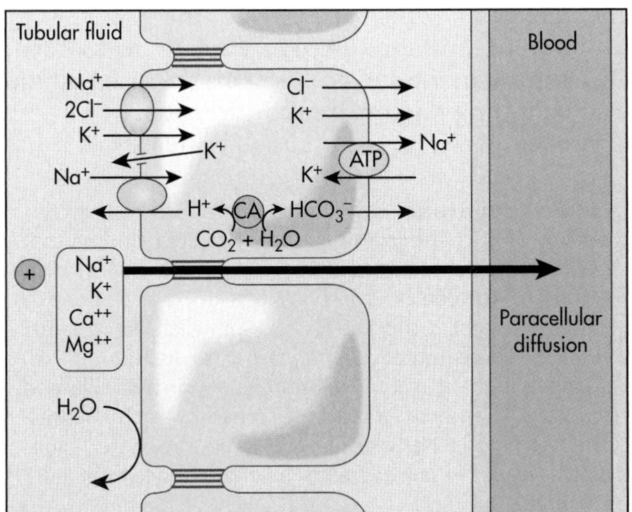

FIGURE 37–4. Transport mechanisms for NaCl reabsorption in the thick ascending limb of the loop of Henle. The positive charge in the lumen plays a major role in driving the passive paracellular reabsorption of cations. Mutations in the apical membrane K^+ channel (ROMK), the apical membrane $1Na^+,1K^+,2Cl^-$ symporter (NKCC1), or the basolateral Cl^- channel (ClC-KB) cause Bartter's syndrome (see the clinical box on Bartter's syndrome). CA, carbonic anhydrase.

chemical gradient for the movement of Na^+ from the tubular fluid into the cell. The movement of Na^+ across the apical membrane into the cell is mediated by the $1Na^+,1K^+,2Cl^-$ symporter (NKCC1), which couples the movement of $1Na^+$ with $1K^+$ and $2Cl^-$. Using the potential energy released by the downhill movement of Na^+ and Cl^-, this symport drives the uphill movement of K^+ into the cell. An Na^+-H^+ antiporter in the apical cell membrane also mediates Na^+ reabsorption as well as H^+ secretion (HCO_3^- reabsorption) in the thick ascending limb (see also Chapter 40). Na^+ leaves the cell across the basolateral membrane via Na^+,K^+-ATPase; K^+, Cl^-, and HCO_3^- leave the cell across the basolateral membrane via separate pathways.

The voltage across the thick ascending limb is important for the reabsorption of several cations. The tubular fluid is positively charged relative to blood because of the unique location of transport proteins in the apical and basolateral membranes. Two points are important:

- Increased salt transport by the thick ascending limb increases the magnitude of the positive charge in the lumen.
- This voltage is an important driving force for the reabsorption of several cations, including Na^+, K^+, Mg^{++}, and Ca^{++}, across the paracellular pathway (Figure 37–4).

The importance of the paracellular pathway to solute reabsorption is underscored by the observation that inactivating mutations of the tight junction protein claudin-16 reduce Mg^{++} and Ca^{++} reabsorption by the ascending thick limb even when the transepithelial voltage is lumen positive.

In summary, salt reabsorption across the thick ascending limb occurs via the transcellular and paracellular pathways. A total of 50% of NaCl reabsorption is transcellular, and 50% is paracellular. Because the thick ascending limb does not reabsorb water, the reabsorption of NaCl and other solutes reduces the osmolality of tubular fluid to less than 150 mOsm/kg H_2O. THUS, BECAUSE THE THICK ASCENDING LIMB PRODUCES A FLUID THAT IS DILUTE RELATIVE TO PLASMA, THE ASCENDING LIMB OF HENLE'S LOOP IS CALLED THE DILUTING SEGMENT.

Bartter's syndrome is a set of autosomal recessive genetic diseases characterized by hypokalemia, metabolic alkalosis, and hyperaldosteronism (Table 37–3). Inactivating mutations in the gene coding for the $1Na^+,1K^+,2Cl^-$ symporter, the apical K^+ channel, or the basolateral Cl^- channel decrease both NaCl reabsorption and K^+ reabsorption by the ascending thick limb, which in turn causes hypokalemia and a decrease in the extracellular fluid volume. The fall in extracellular fluid volume stimulates aldosterone secretion, which in turn stimulates NaCl reabsorption and H^+ secretion by the distal tubule and collecting duct (see later).

Inhibition of the $1Na^+,1K^+,2Cl^-$ symporter in the thick ascending limb by "loop diuretics" such as **furosemide** inhibits NaCl reabsorption by the thick ascending limb and thereby increases urinary NaCl excretion. Furosemide also inhibits K^+ and Ca^{++} reabsorption by reducing the positive lumen voltage that drives the paracellular reabsorption of these ions. Thus, furosemide increases urinary K^+ and Ca^{++} excretion. Furosemide also increases water excretion by reducing the osmolality of the interstitial fluid in the medulla. Water reabsorption by the descending thin limb of the loop of Henle is passive and driven by the osmotic gradient between the tubular fluid in the descending thin limb and the interstitial fluid in the medulla. (Under normal conditions, the osmolality is approximately 290 mOsm/kg H_2O at the beginning of the descending thin limb and approximately 1200 mOsm/kg H_2O in the medulla.) Thus, a reduction of the osmolality of the interstitial fluid reduces water reabsorption by the descending thin limb and thereby increases water excretion.

The distal tubule and collecting duct reabsorb approximately 7% of the filtered NaCl, secrete variable amounts of K^+ and H^+, and reabsorb a variable amount of water (≈8% to 17%)

The initial segment of the distal tubule (early distal tubule) reabsorbs Na^+, Cl^-, and Ca^{++} and is impermeable to water (**Figure 37–5**). NaCl entry into the

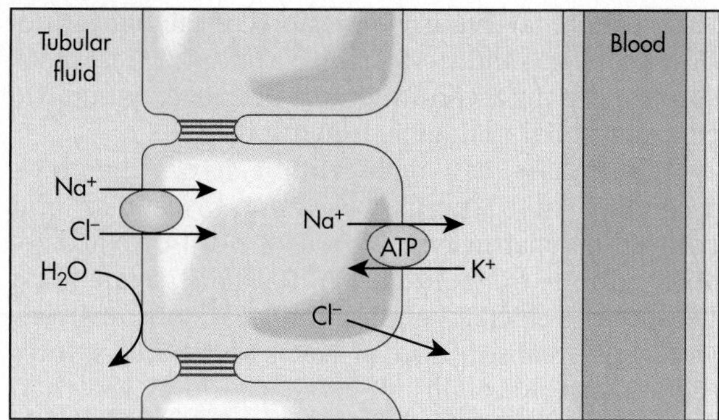

FIGURE 37–5. Transport mechanism for Na^+ and Cl^- reabsorption in the early segment of the distal tubule. This segment is impermeable to water.

cell across the apical membrane is mediated by an Na^+-Cl^- symporter (Figure 37–5). Na^+ leaves the cell via the action of Na^+,K^+-ATPase, and Cl^- leaves the cell via diffusion through Cl^- channels. NaCl reabsorption is reduced by **thiazide diuretics,** which inhibit the Na^+-Cl^- symporter. THUS, DILUTION OF THE TUBULAR FLUID BEGINS IN THE THICK ASCENDING LIMB AND CONTINUES IN THE EARLY SEGMENT OF THE DISTAL TUBULE.

The last segment of the distal tubule (late distal tubule) and the collecting duct are composed of two cell types: **principal cells** and **intercalated cells.** As illustrated in **Figure 37–6**, principal cells reabsorb NaCl and water and secrete K^+. Intercalated cells secrete either H^+ or HCO_3^- and are thus important in regulating acid-base balance (see Chapter 40). Intercalated cells also reabsorb K^+ by the operation of an H^+,K^+-ATPase located in the apical plasma membrane. Both Na^+ reabsorption and K^+ secretion by principal cells depend on the activity of Na^+,K^+-ATPase in the basolateral membrane (Figure 37–6). By maintaining a low concentration of cell Na^+, this pump provides a favorable chemical gradient for the movement of Na^+ from the tubular fluid into the cell. Because Na^+ enters the cell across the apical membrane via diffusion through Na^+-selective channels (ENaC) in the apical membrane, the negative charge inside the cell facilitates Na^+ entry. Na^+ leaves the cell across the basolateral membrane and enters the blood via the action of Na^+,K^+-ATPase. Na^+ reabsorption generates a lumen-negative charge across the late distal tubule and collecting duct, which provides the driving force for Cl^- reabsorption across the paracellular pathway. A variable amount of water is reabsorbed across principal cells in the late distal tubule and collecting duct. Water reabsorption is mediated by the AQP2 water channel located in the apical plasma membrane and AQP3 and AQP4 located in the basolateral membrane of principal cells. In the presence of antidiuretic hormone (ADH), water is reabsorbed. By contrast, in the absence of ADH, the distal tubule and collecting duct reabsorb little water.

Liddle's syndrome is a rare genetic disorder characterized by an increase in the extracellular fluid volume that causes an increase in blood pressure (i.e., hypertension). Liddle's syndrome is caused by activating mutations in either the β or γ subunit of the epithelial Na^+ channel (ENaC). These mutations increase the number of Na^+ channels in the apical cell membrane of principal cells and thereby the amount of Na^+ reabsorbed by each channel. The rate of renal Na^+ reabsorption is inappropriately high, which leads to an increase in the extracellular fluid volume.

There are two different forms of **pseudohypoaldosteronism.** The **autosomal recessive form** is caused by inactivating mutations in the α, β, or γ subunit of the epithelial Na^+ channel (ENaC). The cause of the **autosomal dominant form** is an inactivating mutation in the mineralocorticoid receptor. Pseudohypoaldosteronism is characterized by an increase in Na^+ excretion, a reduction in the extracellular fluid volume, hyperkalemia, and hypotension.

K^+ is secreted from the blood into the tubular fluid by principal cells in two steps (Figure 37–6). First, K^+ uptake across the basolateral membrane is mediated via the action of Na^+,K^+-ATPase. Second, K^+ leaves the cell via passive diffusion. Because the $[K^+]$ inside the cells is high (≈150 mEq/L) and the $[K^+]$ in tubular fluid is low (≈10 mEq/L), K^+ diffuses down its concentration gradient through apical cell

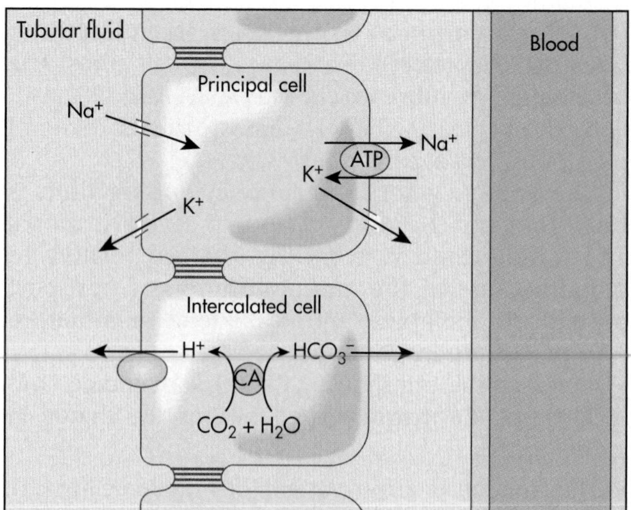

FIGURE 37–6. Transport pathways in principal cells and intercalated cells of the distal tubule and collecting duct. CA, carbonic anhydrase.

membrane K^+ channels into the tubular fluid. Although the negative potential inside the cells tends to retain K^+ within the cell, the electrochemical gradient across the apical membrane favors K^+ secretion from the cell into the tubular fluid (see Chapter 39). The mechanism of K^+ reabsorption by intercalated cells is mediated by an H^+,K^+-ATPase located in the apical cell membrane.

Amiloride is a diuretic drug that inhibits Na^+ reabsorption by the distal tubule and collecting duct by directly inhibiting Na^+ channels in the luminal cell membrane. Amiloride also indirectly inhibits Cl^- reabsorption. The inhibition of Na^+ reabsorption reduces the negative charge in the lumen; this diminishes the driving force for paracellular Cl^- reabsorption and also inhibits K^+ secretion. Consequently, amiloride is frequently referred to as a **K^+-sparing diuretic.** It is most often used in patients who excrete too much K^+ in their urine.

Several Hormones Regulate NaCl Reabsorption

QUANTITATIVELY, ANGIOTENSIN II AND ALDOSTERONE, AS WELL AS URODILATIN, EPINEPHRINE, AND NOREPINEPHRINE RELEASED BY SYMPATHETIC NERVES, ARE THE MOST IMPORTANT HORMONES THAT REGULATE NaCl REABSORPTION AND THEREBY URINARY NaCl EXCRETION **(Table 37–6)**. However, other hormones (including dopamine and glucocorticoids), Starling forces, and the phenomenon of glomerulotubular balance influence NaCl reabsorption. ADH IS THE ONLY MAJOR HORMONE THAT DIRECTLY REGULATES THE AMOUNT OF WATER EXCRETED BY THE KIDNEYS.

Angiotensin II has a potent stimulatory effect on NaCl and water reabsorption in the proximal tubule

Angiotensin II is one of the most potent hormones that stimulates NaCl and water reabsorption in the proximal tubule. A decrease in the extracellular fluid volume activates the renin-angiotensin-aldosterone system (see Chapter 38), thereby increasing the plasma concentration of angiotensin II.

Aldosterone is synthesized by the glomerulosa cells of the adrenal cortex, and it stimulates NaCl reabsorption. It acts on the thick ascending limb of the loop of Henle, distal tubule, and collecting duct. Most of aldosterone's effect on NaCl reabsorption reflects its action on the distal tubule and collecting duct. Aldosterone also stimulates K^+ secretion by the distal tubule and collecting duct (see Chapter 39). Aldosterone enhances NaCl reabsorption across principal cells in the distal tubule and collecting duct by four mechanisms:

- increasing the amount of Na^+,K^+-ATPase in the basolateral membrane;
- increasing the expression of the Na^+ channel (ENaC) in the apical cell membrane;
- elevating serum glucocorticoid-stimulated kinase (SGK) levels, which also increases the expression of ENaC in the apical cell membrane; and
- stimulating channel-activating protease (CAP1, also called prostatin), which directly activates ENaC channels.

Taken together, these actions increase the uptake of Na^+ across the apical cell membrane and facilitate the exit of Na^+ from the cell interior into the blood. The increase in the reabsorption of Na^+ generates a lumen-negative transepithelial voltage

TABLE 37–6. HORMONES THAT REGULATE NaCl AND WATER REABSORPTION

Hormone*	Major Stimulus	Nephron Site of Action	Effect on Transport
Angiotensin II	↑Renin	PT	↑NaCl and H_2O reabsorption
Aldosterone	↑Angiotensin II, $↑[K^+]_p$	TAL, DT/CD	↑NaCl and H_2O reabsorption†
ANP, BNP	↑ECFV	CD	↓H_2O and NaCl reabsorption
Urodilatin	↑ECFV	CD	↓H_2O and NaCl reabsorption
Sympathetic nerves	↓ECFV	PT, TAL, DT/CD	↑NaCl and H_2O reabsorption†
Dopamine	↑ECFV	PT	↓H_2O and NaCl reabsorption
ADH	$↑P_{osm}$, ↓ECFV	DT/CD	↑H_2O reabsorption†

*All of these hormones act within minutes, except aldosterone, which exerts its action on NaCl reabsorption with a delay of 1 hour.
†The effect on H_2O reabsorption does not include the thick ascending limb.
ANP, atrial natriuretic peptide; BNP, brain natriuretic peptide; CD, collecting duct; DT, distal tubule; ECFV, extracellular fluid volume; $[K^+]_p$, plasma K^+ concentration; P_{osm}, plasma osmolality; PT, proximal tubule; TAL, thick ascending limb; ↑, increase; ↓, decrease.

across the distal tubule and collecting duct. This lumen-negative voltage provides the electrochemical driving force for Cl^- reabsorption across the tight junctions (i.e., paracellular pathway) in the distal tubule and collecting duct. Aldosterone secretion is increased by hyperkalemia and by angiotensin II (after activation of the renin-angiotensin system). Aldosterone secretion is decreased by hypokalemia and natriuretic peptides (see later section). Through its stimulation of NaCl reabsorption in the collecting duct, aldosterone also indirectly increases water reabsorption by this nephron segment.

Some individuals with expanded extracellular fluid volume and elevated blood pressure are treated with drugs that inhibit **angiotensin-converting enzyme (ACE inhibitors, e.g., captopril, enalapril, lisinopril)** and thereby lower fluid volume and blood pressure. The inhibition of ACE blocks the degradation of angiotensin I to angiotensin II and thereby lowers plasma angiotensin II levels (see Chapter 38). The decline in plasma angiotensin II concentration has three effects. First, NaCl and water reabsorption by the proximal tubule falls. Second, aldosterone secretion decreases, thus reducing NaCl reabsorption in the thick ascending limb, distal tubule, and collecting duct. Third, because angiotensin is a potent vasoconstrictor, a reduction in its concentration permits the systemic arterioles to dilate and thereby lower arterial blood pressure. ACE also degrades the vasodilator hormone bradykinin; ACE inhibitors therefore increase the concentration of bradykinin. Thus, ACE inhibitors decrease the extracellular fluid volume and the arterial blood pressure by promoting renal NaCl and water excretion and by depressing total peripheral resistance.

Atrial natriuretic peptide, brain natriuretic peptide, and urodilatin inhibit NaCl and water reabsorption

The secretion of **atrial natriuretic peptide** (ANP) by the cardiac atria and **brain natriuretic peptide** (BNP) by the cardiac ventricles is stimulated by a rise in blood pressure and an increase in the extracellular fluid volume. ANP and BNP reduce the blood pressure by decreasing the total peripheral resistance and by enhancing urinary NaCl and water excretion. These hormones also inhibit NaCl reabsorption by the medullary portion of the collecting duct and inhibit ADH-stimulated water reabsorption across the collecting duct. Moreover, ANP and BNP also reduce the secretion of ADH from the posterior pituitary.

Urodilatin and ANP are encoded by the same gene and have similar amino acid sequences. Urodilatin is a 32–amino acid hormone that differs from ANP by the addition of four amino acids to the amino terminus. Urodilatin is secreted by the distal tubule and collecting duct, and it is not present in the systemic circulation; thus, urodilatin influences only the function of the kidneys. Urodilatin secretion is stimulated by a rise in the blood pressure and an increase in the extracellular fluid volume. It inhibits NaCl and water reabsorption across the medullary portion of the collecting duct. Urodilatin is a more potent natriuretic and diuretic hormone than ANP because the ANP that enters the kidneys in the blood is degraded by a neutral endopeptidase that has no effect on urodilatin.

Catecholamines stimulate NaCl reabsorption

Catecholamines released from the sympathetic nerves (norepinephrine) and the adrenal medulla (epinephrine) stimulate NaCl and water reabsorption by the proximal tubule, thick ascending limb of the loop of Henle, distal tubule, and collecting duct. Although sympathetic nerves are not active when the extracellular fluid volume is normal, when extracellular fluid volume declines (e.g., after hemorrhage), sympathetic nerve activity rises and stimulates NaCl and water reabsorption by these four nephron segments.

Dopamine, a catecholamine, is released from dopaminergic nerves in the kidneys and is also synthesized by cells of the proximal tubule. The action of dopamine is opposite to that of norepinephrine and epinephrine. Dopamine secretion is stimulated by an increase in extracellular fluid volume, and its secretion directly inhibits NaCl and water reabsorption in the proximal tubule.

ADH Regulates Water Reabsorption

ADH is the most important hormone that regulates water reabsorption in the kidneys (see Chapter 38). This hormone is secreted by the posterior pituitary gland in response to an increase in plasma osmolality (1% or more) or a decrease in the extracellular fluid volume (>5% to 10% of normal). ADH increases the permeability of the collecting duct to water. It increases water reabsorption by the collecting duct because of the osmotic gradient that exists across the wall of the collecting duct (see Chapters 38 and 45). ADH HAS LITTLE EFFECT ON URINARY NaCl EXCRETION.

Starling forces regulate NaCl and water reabsorption across the proximal tubule

As previously described, Na^+, Cl^-, HCO_3^-, amino acids, glucose, and water are transported into the intercellular space of the proximal tubule. Starling forces between this space and the peritubular capillaries facilitate the movement of the reabsorbed fluid into the capillaries. Starling forces across the wall of the peritubular capillaries are the hydrostatic pressures in the peritubular capillary (P_c) and lateral intercellular space (P_{ic}) and the oncotic pressures in the peritubular capillary (π_c) and lateral intercellular space (π_{ic}). Thus, the reabsorption of water, resulting from Na^+ transport from tubular fluid into the lateral intercellular space, is modified by the Starling forces. Thus:

$$Q = K_f[(P_{ic} - P_c) + \sigma(\pi_c - \pi_{ic})]$$

where Q is flow (positive numbers indicate flow from the intercellular space into blood). Starling forces that favor movement from the interstitium into the peritubular capillaries are the π_c and P_{ic} (**Figure 37–7**). The opposing Starling forces are the π_{ic} and P_c. Normally, the sum of the Starling forces favors the movement of solute and water from the interstitial space into the capillary (see also Chapter 22). However, some of the solutes and fluid that enter the lateral intercellular space leak back into the proximal tubular fluid. Starling forces do not affect transport by the loop of Henle, distal tubule, and collecting duct because these segments are less permeable to water than the proximal tubule is.

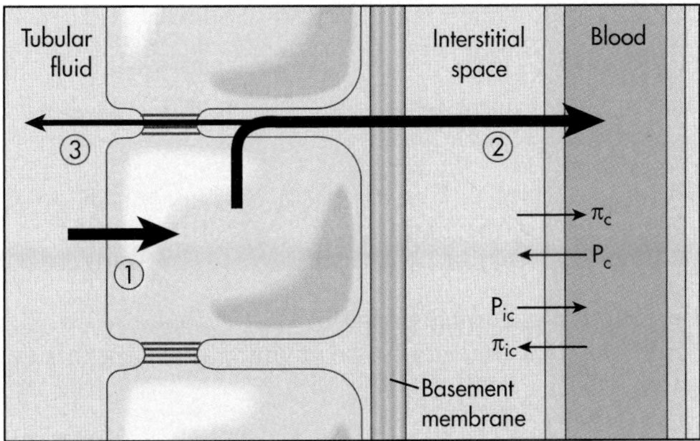

FIGURE 37–7. Routes of solute and water transport across the proximal tubule and the Starling forces that modify reabsorption. Solute and water are reabsorbed across the apical membrane (1). This solute and water then cross the lateral cell membrane. Some of the solute and water reenters the tubule fluid (3), and the remainder enters the interstitial space and then flows into the capillary (2). The width of the arrows is directly proportional to the amount of solute and water moving via the three pathways. Starling forces across the capillary wall determine the amount of fluid flowing through pathway 2 versus pathway 3. Transport mechanisms in the apical cell membranes determine the amount of solute and water entering the cell (1). Thin arrows across the capillary wall indicate the direction of water movement in response to each force.

A number of factors can alter the Starling forces across the peritubular capillaries surrounding the proximal tubule. For example, dilation of the efferent arteriole increases the P_c, whereas constriction of the efferent arteriole decreases it. An increase in the P_c inhibits solute and water reabsorption by increasing the back-leak of NaCl and water across the tight junction, whereas a decrease stimulates reabsorption by decreasing back-leak across the tight junction.

The π_c is partially determined by the rate of formation of the glomerular ultrafiltrate. For example, if one assumes a constant plasma flow in the afferent arteriole, the plasma proteins become less concentrated in the plasma that enters the efferent arteriole and peritubular capillary as less ultrafiltrate is formed (i.e., as GFR decreases). Hence, the π_c decreases. The π_c is directly related to the **filtration fraction:**

$$FF = GFR/RPF$$

where FF is filtration fraction and RPF is renal plasma flow. A fall in the FF resulting from a decrease in GFR at constant RPF decreases the π_c. This in turn increases the backflow of NaCl and water from the lateral intercellular space into the tubular fluid and thereby decreases net solute and water reabsorption across the proximal tubule. An increase in the FF has the opposite effect.

The importance of Starling forces in regulating solute and water reabsorption by the proximal tubule is underscored by the phenomenon of **glomerulotubular (G-T) balance.** Spontaneous changes in GFR markedly alter the filtered load of Na^+ (filtered load = GFR × [Na^+] in the filtered fluid). Without rapid adjustments in Na^+ reabsorption to counter the changes, urine Na^+ excretion would fluctuate widely and disturb the Na^+ balance of the body. However, spontaneous changes in GFR do not alter the Na^+ balance because of the phenomenon of G-T balance. When body Na^+ balance is normal, G-T balance refers to the fact that reabsorption of Na^+ and water increases in proportion to the increase in GFR and filtered load of Na^+. Thus, a constant fraction of the filtered Na^+ and water is reabsorbed from the proximal tubule despite variations in GFR. THE NET RESULT OF G-T BALANCE IS TO

REDUCE THE IMPACT OF GFR CHANGES ON THE AMOUNT OF Na^+ AND WATER EXCRETED IN THE URINE.

Two mechanisms are responsible for G-T balance. One is related to the oncotic and hydrostatic pressure differences between the peritubular capillaries and the lateral intercellular space (i.e., Starling forces). For example, an increase in the GFR (at constant RPF) raises the protein concentration in the glomerular capillary plasma above normal. This protein-rich plasma leaves the glomerular capillaries, flows through the efferent arteriole, and enters the peritubular capillaries. The increased π_c augments the movement of solute and fluid from the lateral intercellular space into the peritubular capillaries. This action increases net solute and water reabsorption by the proximal tubule.

The second mechanism responsible for G-T balance is initiated by an increase in the filtered load of glucose and amino acids. As discussed earlier, the reabsorption of Na^+ in the first half of the proximal tubule is coupled to that of glucose and amino acids. The rate of Na^+ reabsorption therefore partially depends on the filtered load of glucose and amino acids. As the GFR and filtered load of glucose and amino acids increase, Na^+ and water reabsorption also rises.

In addition to G-T balance, another mechanism minimizes changes in the filtered load of Na^+. As discussed in Chapter 36, an increase in the GFR (and thus in the amount of Na^+ filtered by the glomerulus) activates the tubuloglomerular feedback mechanism. This action returns the GFR and filtration of Na^+ to normal values. Thus, spontaneous changes in the GFR (e.g., caused by changes in posture and blood pressure) increase the amount of Na^+ filtered for only a few minutes. The mechanisms that underlie G-T balance maintain urinary Na^+ excretion constant and thereby maintain Na^+ homeostasis until the GFR returns to normal.

Summary

- The four major segments of the nephron—proximal tubule, loop of Henle, distal tubule, and collecting duct—determine the composition and volume of the urine via the selective reabsorption of solutes and water and the selective secretion of solutes.
- Tubular reabsorption allows the kidneys to retain the substances that are essential and to regulate their levels in the plasma.
- The reabsorption of Na^+, Cl^-, other anions, organic solutes, and water constitutes one of the major functions of the nephron. The proximal tubule cells reabsorb 67% of the glomerular ultrafiltrate; cells of the loop of Henle reabsorb about 25% of the NaCl that was filtered and about 15% of the water that was filtered.
- The distal segments of the nephron have a more limited reabsorptive capacity. However, the final adjustments in the composition and volume of the urine and most of the regulation by hormones and other factors occur in distal segments.
- The secretion of substances into tubular fluid is a means of excreting various byproducts of metabolism and of eliminating exogenous organic anions and bases (e.g., drugs) and toxicants from the body.
- Various hormones (including angiotensin II, aldosterone, ADH, ANP, BNP, and urodilatin), sympathetic nerves, catecholamines, and Starling forces regulate NaCl reabsorption by the kidneys. ADH is the major hormone that regulates water reabsorption. ADH has no effect on solute excretion.

Bibliography

Agre P, Kozono D: Aquaporin water channels: molecular mechanisms for human diseases, *FEBS Lett* 555:72, 2003.

Aronson PS: Role of ion exchanges in mediating NaCl transport in the proximal tubule, *Kidney Int* 49:1665, 1996.

Burckhardt G, Bahn A, Wolff NA: Molecular physiology of renal *p*-aminohippurate secretion, *News Physiol Sci* 16:114, 2001.

Burckhardt G, Pritchard JB: Organic anion and cation antiporters. In Seldin DW, Giebisch G, eds: *The kidney: physiology and pathophysiology,* ed 3, Philadelphia, 2000, Lippincott Williams & Wilkins.

De la Rosa A et al: Structure and regulation of amiloride-sensitive sodium channels, *Annu Rev Physiol* 62:573, 2000.

Guay-Woodford LM: Overview: the genetics of renal disease, *Semin Nephrol* 19:312, 1999.

Hebert SC: Molecular mechanisms, *Semin Nephrol* 19:504, 1999.

Hediger MA et al: The molecular basis of solute transport. In Brenner BM, ed: *Brenner and Rector's the kidney,* ed 7, Philadelphia, 2004, WB Saunders.

Ibrahim HN, Rosenberg ME, Hostetter TH: Proteinuria. In Seldin DW, Giebisch G, eds: *The kidney: physiology and pathophysiology,* ed 3, Philadelphia, 2000, Lippincott Williams & Wilkins.

Inui K-I, Masuda S, Saito H: Cellular and molecular aspects of drug transport in the kidney, *Kidney Int* 58:944, 2000.

Knepper MA, Brooks HL: Regulation of the sodium transporters NHE3, NKCC2 and NCC in the kidney, *Curr Opin Nephrol Hypertens* 10:655, 2001.

Lifton RP: Inherited disorders of renal salt homeostasis: insights from molecular genetics studies. In Seldin DW, Giebisch G, eds: *The kidney: physiology and pathophysiology,* ed 3, Philadelphia, 2000, Lippincott Williams & Wilkins.

Meyer M, Forssmann K: The renal urodilatin system: clinical implications, *Cardiovasc Res* 51:450, 2001.

Moe OW et al: Renal transport of glucose, amino acids, sodium, chloride and water. In Brenner BM, ed: *Brenner and Rector's the kidney,* ed 7, Philadelphia, 2004, WB Saunders.

Murer H et al: Proximal tubular phosphate reabsorption: molecular mechanisms, *Physiol Rev* 80:1373, 2000.

Oh YS, Warnock DG: Disorders of the epithelial Na^+ channel in Liddle's syndrome and autosomal recessive pseudohypoaldosteronism type 1, *Exp Nephrol* 8:320, 2000.

Preston GM et al: Appearance of water channels in *Xenopus* oocytes expressing red cell CHIP28 protein, *Science* 256:385, 1992.

Reeves WB, Andreoli TE: Sodium chloride transport in the loop of Henle, distal tubule, and collecting duct. In Seldin DW, Giebisch G, eds: *The kidney: physiology and pathophysiology,* ed 3, Philadelphia, 2000, Lippincott Williams & Wilkins.

Sica DA, Schoolworth AC: Renal handling of organic anions and cations: excretion of uric acid. In Brenner BM, ed: *Brenner and Rector's the kidney,* ed 7, Philadelphia, 2004, WB Saunders.

Silbernagel S, Gekle M: Amino acids and oligopeptides. In Seldin DW, Giebisch G, eds: *The kidney: physiology and pathophysiology,* ed 3, Philadelphia, 2000, Lippincott Williams & Wilkins.

Zelikovic I: Molecular pathophysiology of tubular transport disorders, *Pediatr Nephrol* 16:919, 2001.

Case Studies

Case 37–1

A 45-year-old woman with breast cancer is enrolled in a clinical research trial to evaluate the effectiveness of a new chemotherapeutic drug. She has no other medical problems. After the second dose of the drug, she reports feeling lightheaded when standing. Her blood pressure falls from 145/80 to 110/70 mm Hg when she goes from a supine to a standing position (orthostatic hypotension). In addition, a routine urinalysis shows that her urine contains large quantities of glucose, HCO_3^-, amino acids, phosphate, and organic anions.

1. **On the basis of the urinalysis results, the physician suspects that the chemotherapeutic drug has damaged this woman's kidneys. Which portion of the nephron is mostly likely damaged?**
   - **A.** The glomerulus
   - **B.** The proximal tubule
   - **C.** The thick ascending limb of the loop of Henle
   - **D.** The distal tubule
   - **E.** The collecting duct

2. **The physician attributes the patient's orthostatic hypotension to a decrease in the volume of the extracellular fluid secondary to increased renal Na^+ loss. In response to the decrease in extracellular fluid volume, there will be an increase in which of the following factors that regulate NaCl and water reabsorption by the nephron?**
   - **A.** Aldosterone
   - **B.** ANP
   - **C.** Urodilatin
   - **D.** Dopamine
   - **E.** P_c

Case 37–2

A new diuretic agent is developed, and its effect on healthy volunteers is evaluated. After a single dose of this new diuretic, the urine flow rate increased threefold, the fractional excretion of Na^+ increased from 1% to 20%, the excretion of K^+ and Ca^{++} increased, but neither glucose nor amino acids were found in the urine.

1. **On the basis of the urinalysis results, which portion of the nephron is the site of action of this new diuretic agent?**
   A. The glomerulus
   B. The proximal tubule
   C. The thick ascending limb of the loop of Henle
   D. The distal tubule
   E. The collecting duct

2. **Which of the following membrane transport proteins is inhibited by the new diuretic agent?**
   A. Na^+-glucose symporter
   B. Na^+-H^+ antiporter
   C. $1Na^+,1K^+,2Cl^-$ symporter
   D. Na^+-Cl^- symporter
   E. Na^+ channel

Chapter 38: Control of Body Fluid Osmolality and Extracellular Fluid Volume

Objectives

- ❖ Identify the volume and composition of the various body fluid compartments.
- ❖ Distinguish among the factors that regulate thirst and cause the secretion of ADH (i.e., body fluid osmolality, extracellular fluid volume, blood pressure).
- ❖ Describe the handling of water by the various portions of the nephron, especially how ADH regulates the excretion of water by the kidneys.
- ❖ Explain the relationship among extracellular fluid volume, Na^+ balance, and renal Na^+ excretion.
- ❖ Describe the handling of Na^+ by the various portions of the nephron and the factors that regulate its excretion.
- ❖ Explain the response of the kidneys to both an increase and a decrease in the extracellular fluid volume.

The kidneys play a critical role in maintaining the volume and composition of the body fluids constant despite daily fluctuations in the intake of water and solutes. Water balance involves the regulation of water intake (thirst) and the excretion of water by the kidneys and serves to maintain the osmolality of the body fluids constant. The volume of the extracellular fluid, which includes the vascular system, is determined in large part by the amount of NaCl in this body fluid compartment. By regulating the excretion of NaCl, the kidneys maintain extracellular fluid volume within a narrow range. In this chapter, the regulation of renal water excretion (urine concentration and dilution) and renal NaCl excretion is discussed. A brief overview of the volumes and composition of the various body fluid compartments is also presented.

Body Fluid Compartments

Water within the body is divided into several compartments that have different compositions

Water accounts for approximately 60% of body weight. The water content of different individuals varies with the amount of adipose tissue; the greater the amount of adipose tissue, the smaller the fraction of body weight attributable to water.

As illustrated in **Figure 38–1**, the **total body water** is distributed between two major compartments that are separated by the cell membrane. The **intracellular fluid** (ICF) compartment is the larger compartment; it contains approximately two

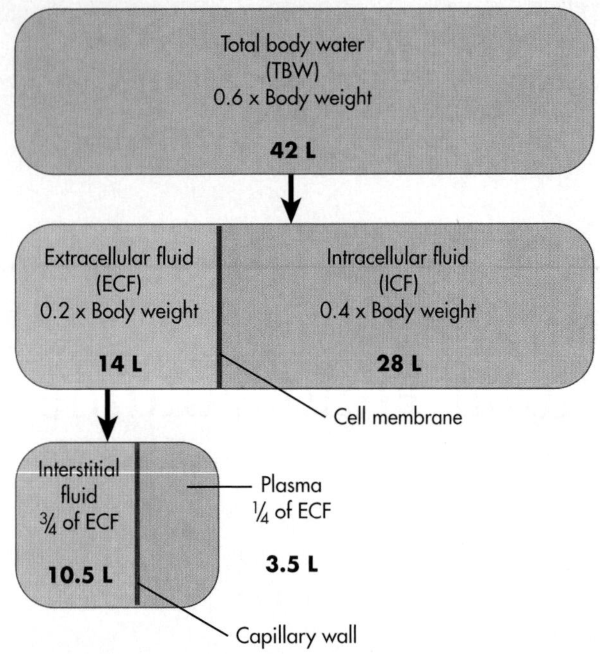

FIGURE 38–1. Relationship among the volumes of the major body fluid compartments. The values shown are calculated for a 70-kg individual.

TABLE 38–1. DISTRIBUTION OF SOME CATIONS AND ANIONS IN EXTRACELLULAR AND INTRACELLULAR FLUID

	ECF	ICF*
Na^+ (mEq/L)	145	12
K^+ (mEq/L)	4	150
Ca^{++} (mEq/L)	5	0.001
Cl^- (mEq/L)	105	5
HCO_3^- (mEq/L)	25	12
Inorganic phosphate (Pi)† (mEq/L)	2	100†
pH	7.4	7.1

*The ICF concentrations are estimates from skeletal muscle and include amounts bound to intracellular proteins and free within the cytosol.
†Intracellular phosphate is primarily in the form of organic molecules (e.g., ATP).

thirds of the total body water. The remaining one third is contained in the **extracellular fluid** (ECF) compartment. The ECF compartment is subdivided into **interstitial fluid** and **plasma;** these compartments are separated by the capillary wall. The interstitial fluid, which represents the fluid surrounding the cells in the various tissues of the body, comprises three fourths of the ECF volume. Included in this compartment is water contained within the bone and dense connective tissue. The plasma volume represents the remaining one fourth of the ECF.

The concentrations of the major cations and anions in the ECF and ICF are summarized in **Table 38–1**. The ionic compositions of the two major compartments of the ECF (interstitial fluid and plasma) are similar because they are separated only by the capillary wall, which is freely permeable to small ions. THE MAJOR DIFFERENCE IN COMPOSITION BETWEEN THE INTERSTITIAL FLUID AND THE PLASMA IS THAT THE PLASMA CONTAINS SIGNIFICANTLY MORE PROTEIN. Although the presence of protein in the plasma can affect the distribution of cations and anions across the capillary wall by the Gibbs-Donnan equation (see Chapter 2), this effect is normally small, and the ionic compositions of the interstitial fluid and plasma can be considered identical.

Because of its abundance, Na^+ (and its attendant anions Cl^- and HCO_3^-) is the major determinant of the osmolality of the ECF. Accordingly, a rough estimate of ECF osmolality can be obtained by simply doubling the [Na^+]. Although the ECF contains many other constituents (e.g., K^+, Ca^{++}, proteins, glucose, urea), these normally contribute only minimally to the total osmolality. Moreover, some of these constituents are permeable across cell membrane (e.g., glucose and urea) and therefore are **ineffective osmoles** that do not cause water to move into or out of cells (see Chapter 1). In contrast, Na^+ and its anions are **effective osmoles.** Thus, multiplying the ECF [Na^+] by 2 provides the best estimate of the effective osmolality. It is the effective osmolality that is most important in determining the impact of changes in body fluid osmolality on ECF and ICF volumes. The normal ECF osmolality ranges from approximately 280 to 295 mOsm/kg H_2O. Because water is in osmotic equilibrium across the capillary wall and across the plasma membrane of cells, measurement of the plasma osmolality also provides an estimate of the osmolality of the ECF, ICF, and interstitial fluid.

In contrast to the ECF, the [Na^+] of ICF is extremely low. K^+ is the predominant cation of the ICF. This asymmetrical distribution of Na^+ and K^+ across the plasma membrane is maintained by the activity of the ubiquitous Na^+,K^+-ATPase (see Chapter 1). The anion composition of the ICF also differs markedly from that of the ECF, with the [Cl^-] and [HCO_3^-] of the ICF being lower in comparison. The major ICF anions are phosphates, organic anions, and protein.

Fluid can shift between body fluid compartments

WATER MOVES FREELY BETWEEN THE VARIOUS BODY FLUID COMPARTMENTS. TWO FORCES DETERMINE THIS MOVE-

MENT: HYDROSTATIC PRESSURE AND OSMOTIC PRESSURE. Hydrostatic pressure, generated by the pumping of the heart (and the effect of gravity on the column of blood in the vessels), and the osmotic pressure of the plasma proteins (oncotic pressure) are important determinants of fluid movement across the capillary wall (see Chapter 22); osmotic pressure differences between the ICF and ECF are responsible for fluid movement across cell membranes. Because the plasma membranes of cells are highly permeable to water, a change in the osmolality of either the ICF or ECF moves water rapidly between these compartments. Thus, EXCEPT FOR TRANSIENT CHANGES, THE ICF AND ECF COMPARTMENTS ARE IN OSMOTIC EQUILIBRIUM.

In contrast to the movement of water, the movement of ions across cell membranes is more variable and depends on the presence of specific membrane transporters (see Chapter 1). Consequently, as a first approximation, fluid exchange between the ICF and ECF under pathophysiological conditions can be analyzed by assuming that appreciable shifts of ions between the compartments do not occur. Thus, fluid shifts between the ICF and the ECF primarily by the movement of water and not ions.

Because body fluids and solutions administered intravenously to patients contain effective and ineffective osmoles, it is preferable to refer to the tonicity of body fluids or intravenous solutions. **Isotonic** solutions (e.g., 0.9% NaCl: osmolality ≈290 mOsm/kg H_2O) do not cause fluid shifts between the ECF and ICF because the effective osmolality of the solution is the same as that of both the ECF and ICF. **Hypotonic** solutions contain fewer effective osmoles than normal ECF and ICF and cause water to move into cells (i.e., cell swelling) when they are infused intravenously. **Hypertonic** solutions have more effective osmoles than normal ECF and ICF and cause water to move out of cells (i.e., cell shrinking) when they are infused intravenously.

Control of Body Fluid Osmolality: Urine Concentration and Dilution

The kidneys are responsible for regulating water balance and under most conditions are the major route for the elimination of water from the body (**Table 38–2**). Another route of water loss from the body is evaporation from the cells of the skin and the respiratory passages. Collectively, water loss by these routes is termed **insensible water loss** because the individual is unaware of its occurrence. Additional water can be lost through sweat. Water loss through this mechanism can increase dramatically in a hot environment, with exercise, or in the presence of fever (**Table 38–3**). Finally, water can be lost from the gastrointestinal tract. Fecal water loss is normally small but increases with diarrhea. Gastrointestinal water losses can also occur with vomiting.

TABLE 38–2. NORMAL ROUTES OF WATER GAIN AND LOSS IN ADULTS AT ROOM TEMPERATURE (23°C)

Route	mL/day
Water intake	
Fluid*	1200
In food	1000
Metabolically produced from food	300
Total	2500
Water output	
Insensible	700
Sweat	100
Feces	200
Urine	1500
Total	2500

*Fluid intake varies widely for both social and cultural reasons.

Renal excretion of water is regulated to maintain water balance

Water loss through sweating, defecation, and evaporation from the lungs and skin is not regulated. In

TABLE 38–3. EFFECT OF ENVIRONMENTAL TEMPERATURE AND EXERCISE ON WATER LOSS AND INTAKE IN ADULTS

	Normal Temperature	Hot Weather*	Prolonged Heavy Exercise*
Water loss			
Insensible loss			
Skin	350	350	350
Lungs	350	250	650
Sweat	100	1400	5000
Feces	200	200	200
Urine†	1500	1200	500
Total loss	2500	3400	6700
Intake	2500	3400	6700

*In hot weather and during prolonged heavy exercise, water balance is maintained only if the individual increases water intake to match the increased loss of water in sweat.

†Decreased water excretion by the kidneys alone is insufficient to maintain water balance.

contrast, RENAL EXCRETION OF WATER IS TIGHTLY REGULATED TO MAINTAIN WATER BALANCE. The maintenance of water balance requires that water intake precisely match water loss from the body. If intake exceeds losses, water balance is positive, and the osmolality of the body fluids decreases. Conversely, when intake is less than losses, water balance is negative, and the osmolality of the body fluids increases.

When water intake is low or when water losses increase, the kidneys conserve water by producing a small volume of urine that is hyperosmotic with respect to plasma (concentrated urine). When water intake is high, a large volume of hypoosmotic urine is produced (dilute urine). In a normal individual, the urine osmolality can vary from approximately 50 to 1200 mOsm/kg H_2O, and the corresponding urine volume can vary from near 18 to 0.5 L/day.

Disorders of water balance alter the plasma [Na^+]

Disorders of water balance alter the body fluid osmolality, which is usually monitored by measuring plasma osmolality. BECAUSE THE MAJOR DETERMINANT OF PLASMA OSMOLALITY IS Na^+ (WITH ITS ANIONS Cl^- AND HCO_3^-), DISORDERS OF WATER BALANCE ALTER THE PLASMA [Na^+]. When an abnormal plasma [Na^+] is evaluated in an individual, it is tempting to suspect a problem in Na^+ balance. However, the problem most often relates to water balance, not Na^+ balance. CHANGES IN Na^+ BALANCE RESULT IN ALTERATIONS IN THE VOLUME OF THE ECF COMPARTMENT, NOT ITS OSMOLALITY (see later section).

> **Hypoosmolality** (a reduction in plasma osmolality) shifts water into cells, and this process results in cell swelling. Symptoms associated with hypoosmolality are related mainly to the swelling of brain cells. For example, a rapid fall in plasma osmolality can alter neurological function and thereby cause nausea, malaise, headache, confusion, lethargy, seizures, and coma. When plasma osmolality is increased (i.e., **hyperosmolality**), water is lost from cells. The symptoms of increased plasma osmolality are also mainly neurological, and they include lethargy, weakness, seizures, and coma.

The kidneys control water excretion independently of their ability to control the excretion of a number of other physiologically important substances (e.g., Na^+, K^+, H^+, urea). Indeed, this ability is necessary for survival because it allows water balance to be achieved without upsetting the other homeostatic functions of the kidneys.

Antidiuretic hormone regulates renal water excretion

Antidiuretic hormone (ADH), or **vasopressin,** acts on the kidneys to regulate the volume and osmolality of the urine. When plasma ADH levels are low, a large volume of urine is excreted **(water diuresis),** and the urine is dilute. When plasma ADH levels are elevated, a small volume of urine is excreted **(antidiuresis),** and the urine is concentrated.

ADH is a small peptide that is 9 amino acids in length. It is synthesized in neuroendocrine cells located within the **supraoptic** and **paraventricular nuclei** of the hypothalamus (see Chapter 45). The synthesized hormone is packaged in neurosecretory vesicles, which are transported down the axon of the cell and stored in the nerve terminals located in the **neurohypophysis (posterior pituitary).** The anatomy of the hypothalamus and pituitary gland is shown in **Figure 38–2.**

The secretion of ADH is regulated by osmotic and hemodynamic factors

The secretion of ADH by the posterior pituitary is influenced by several factors. THE TWO PHYSIOLOGICAL REGULATORS OF ADH SECRETION ARE THE OSMOLALITY OF THE BODY FLUIDS (OSMOTIC) AND VOLUME AND PRESSURE OF THE VASCULAR SYSTEM (HEMODYNAMIC). Of these stimuli, a change in body fluid osmolality is the primary regulator of ADH secretion. Other factors that can alter the secretion of this hormone include nausea (stimulates), natriuretic peptides (inhibit), and angiotensin II (stimulates). A number of drugs also affect ADH secretion. For example, nicotine stimulates secretion, whereas ethanol inhibits it (see also Chapter 45).

Osmotic control of ADH secretion

A CHANGE IN THE BODY FLUID OSMOLALITY IS THE PRIMARY REGULATOR OF ADH SECRETION. Changes in osmolality as small as 1% are sufficient to significantly alter ADH secretion. Cells located in the hypothalamus but distinct from those that synthesize ADH sense changes in body fluid osmolality. These cells, termed **osmoreceptors,** appear to sense changes in body fluid osmolality by either shrinking or swelling. The osmoreceptors respond only to solutes that are effective osmoles (e.g., NaCl). Urea, which is an ineffective osmole, has little effect on ADH secretion.

When the effective osmolality of the body fluids increases, the osmoreceptors send signals to the ADH-synthesizing cells located in the supraoptic and paraventricular nuclei of the hypothalamus,

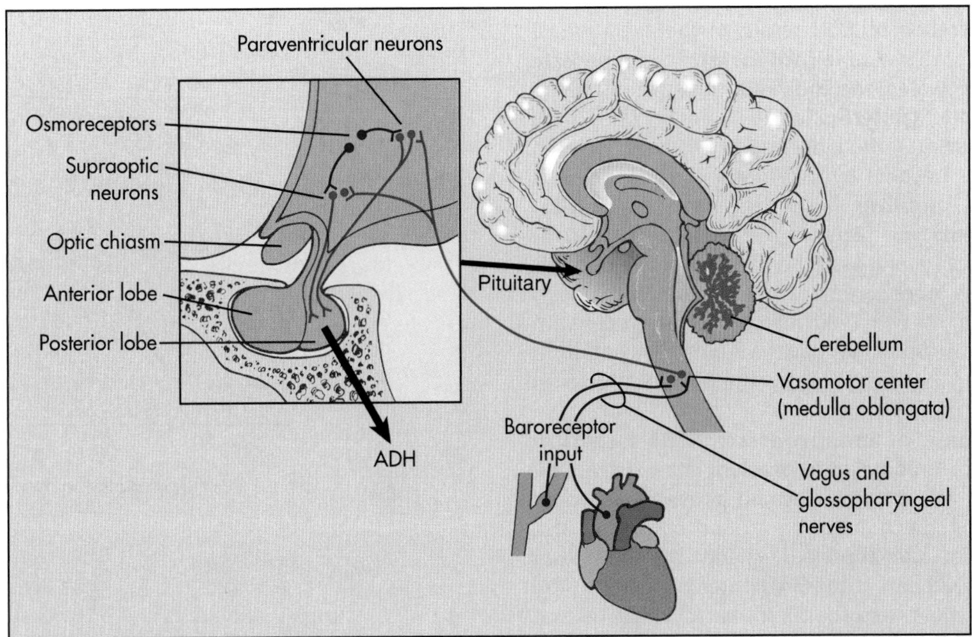

FIGURE 38–2. Anatomical structures of the hypothalamus and pituitary gland (midsagittal section) depicting the pathways for ADH secretion. Also shown are the pathways involved in regulating ADH secretion. Afferent fibers from the baroreceptors are carried in the vagus and glossopharyngeal nerves. The closed box illustrates an expanded view of the hypothalamus and pituitary gland.

stimulating ADH secretion. Conversely, when the effective osmolality of the body fluids is reduced, secretion is inhibited. Because ADH is rapidly degraded in the plasma, circulating levels can be reduced to zero within minutes after secretion is inhibited. As a result, the ADH system can respond rapidly to fluctuations in body fluid osmolality.

Figure 38–3, *A,* illustrates the effect of changes in body fluid osmolality (measured as plasma osmolality) on circulating ADH levels. The **set point** of the system is the plasma osmolality value at which ADH secretion begins to increase. Below this set point, virtually no ADH is released. Above the set point, the slope of the relationship is steep, reflecting the sensitivity of this system. The set point varies among individuals and is genetically determined. In healthy adults, it varies from 280 to 295 mOsm/kg H_2O.

Hemodynamic control of ADH secretion

A DECREASE IN THE BLOOD VOLUME OR ARTERIAL PRESSURE ALSO STIMULATES ADH SECRETION. The receptors activated by this response are located in both the low-pressure side (left atrium and pulmonary vessels) and the high-pressure side (aortic arch and carotid sinus) of the circulatory system (see also Chapter 23). Because the low-pressure receptors are located in the high-compliance side of the circulatory system (i.e., venous), and because the majority of blood is in the venous side of the circulatory system, these low-pressure receptors can be viewed as responding to overall vascular volume. The high-pressure receptors respond to arterial pressure. Both groups of receptors are sensitive to stretch of the wall of the structure in which they are located (e.g., cardiac atrial wall, wall of aortic arch) and are termed **baroreceptors** (see also Chapter 19). Signals from these receptors are carried in afferent fibers of the **vagus** and **glossopharyngeal** nerves to the centers in the brainstem that regulate heart rate and blood pressure. Signals are then relayed from the brainstem to the ADH secretory cells of the supraoptic and paraventricular hypothalamic nuclei. The sensitivity of the baroreceptor system is less than that of the osmoreceptors; a 5% to 10% decrease in blood volume or arterial pressure is required before ADH secretion is stimulated (Figure 38–3, *B*).

Alterations in blood volume or arterial pressure also affect the response to changes in body fluid osmolality. With a decrease in blood volume or arterial pressure, the set point is shifted to lower osmolality values, and the slope of the relationship is steeper. With an increase in blood volume or arterial pressure, the opposite occurs; the set point is shifted to higher osmolality values, and the slope is decreased.

Inadequate secretion of ADH results in the excretion of large volumes of dilute urine **(polyuria).** To compensate for this loss of water, the individual must ingest large volumes of water **(polydipsia)** to maintain body fluid osmolality constant. If the individual is deprived of water, the body fluids become hyperosmotic. This condition is called **central diabetes insipidus, neurogenic diabetes insipidus,** or **pituitary diabetes insipidus.** Central diabetes insipidus can be inherited, although this is rare. It occurs more commonly after head trauma, with brain neoplasms, or with brain infections. Individuals with central diabetes insipidus have a urine-concentrating defect that can be corrected by the administration of exogenous ADH.

The **syndrome of inappropriate ADH secretion (SIADH)** is a common clinical problem characterized by plasma ADH levels that are elevated above what would be expected on the basis of body fluid osmolality and blood volume or arterial pressure (hence the term *inappropriate*). Individuals with SIADH retain water (i.e., reduce renal water excretion). If water intake is not reduced in parallel, their body fluids become progressively hypoosmotic. On the basis of the low body fluid osmolality, the urine of these individuals is characteristically more concentrated than is expected. SIADH can be caused by infections and neoplasms of the brain, drugs (e.g., antitumor drugs), pulmonary diseases, and some carcinomas.

Many different mutations in the gene encoding the ADH molecule have been shown to cause the autosomal dominant form of central diabetes insipidus. The ADH gene is located on chromosome 20 and encodes a preprohormone, which is ultimately processed into three peptides: ADH, a glycoprotein, and neurophysin. In these patients, mutations have been found in all regions of the gene; however, the most common mutation occurs in the portion of the gene that encodes neurophysin. With these mutations, there is defective trafficking of the preprohormone, which accumulates in the endoplasmic reticulum. It is thought that this abnormal accumulation of the preprohormone ultimately leads to the death of the ADH secretory cells in the supraoptic and paraventricular nuclei.

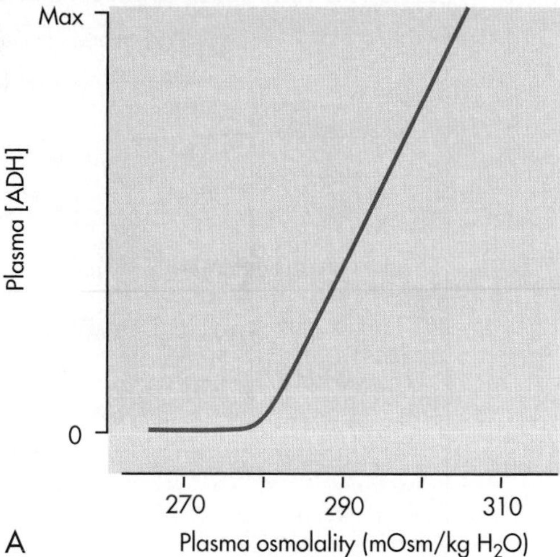

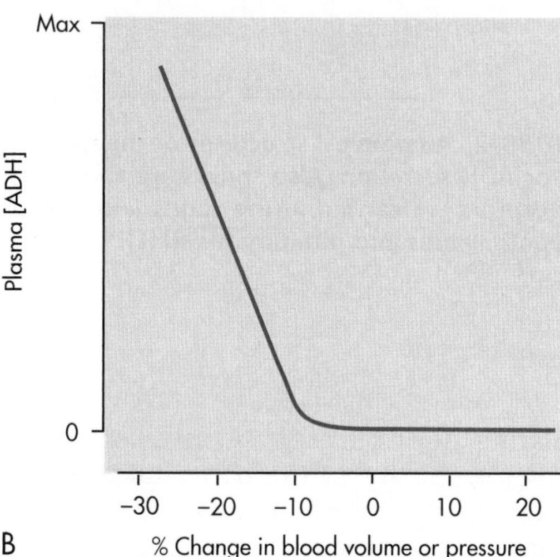

FIGURE 38–3. Osmotic and hemodynamic control of ADH secretion. A, Effect of changes in plasma osmolality (constant blood volume and pressure) on plasma ADH levels. B, Effect of changes in blood volume or pressure (constant plasma osmolality) on plasma ADH levels.

ADH increases the permeability of the collecting duct to water

THE PRIMARY ACTION OF ADH ON THE KIDNEYS IS TO INCREASE THE PERMEABILITY OF THE COLLECTING DUCT TO WATER. In addition, it increases the permeability of the medullary portion of the collecting duct to urea.

The actions of ADH on water permeability of the collecting duct have been extensively studied. ADH binds to a receptor on the basolateral membrane of the principal cell. This receptor, called the V_2 receptor, is coupled to adenylyl cyclase via a stimulatory G protein (see Chapter 5). In response to ADH-receptor binding, intracellular levels of cyclic adenosine monophosphate (cAMP) increase and protein kinase A is activated. Ultimately, intracellular vesicles containing **water channels (aquaporin 2)** are inserted into the apical membrane of the cell via exocytosis.* The apical membrane of the cell, which does not contain water channels in the absence of ADH, is thus transformed from a water-impermeable barrier to a highly water permeable membrane. With the removal of ADH, the water channels are retrieved from the apical membrane via endocytosis, and the membrane is once again impermeable to water. This shuttling of water channels into and out of the apical membrane

* In 2003, the Nobel Prize in Chemistry was awarded to Peter Agre for cloning aquaporin water channels.

provides a mechanism for rapid control of membrane water permeability. The basolateral membrane contains aquaporin 3 and aquaporin 4 and is always permeable to water. Thus, any water that enters the cell through apical membrane water channels exits across the basolateral membrane. This transcellular flow of water results in the net absorption of water from the tubule lumen into the peritubular blood.

The collecting ducts of some individuals do not respond normally to ADH. This lack of response can result from defects in the ADH receptor, failure to insert water channels into the apical membrane, or defective water channels. Regardless of the mechanism, these individuals cannot maximally concentrate their urine. Consequently, they suffer from polyuria and polydipsia. This entity is termed **nephrogenic diabetes insipidus** to distinguish it from central diabetes insipidus. Although nephrogenic diabetes insipidus can be inherited, most cases are secondary to other factors, such as metabolic disorders (e.g., hypercalcemia) or certain drugs. For example, approximately 35% of individuals who take lithium for bipolar disorder develop nephrogenic diabetes insipidus.

The inherited forms of nephrogenic diabetes insipidus result from mutations in either the ADH receptor (V_2) or aquaporin 2. The gene for the V_2 receptor is located on the X chromosome. Thus, this inherited form is X-linked. Most of the mutations in the V_2 receptor result in defective trafficking and trapping of the receptor in the endoplasmic reticulum. The gene coding for aquaporin 2 is located on chromosome 12 and is inherited as an autosomal recessive defect. This is a much less common form of nephrogenic diabetes insipidus. Like mutations in the V_2 receptor, mutations of aquaporin 2 often result in trapping of the protein in the endoplasmic reticulum.

Many of the acquired forms of nephrogenic diabetes insipidus are a result of decreased expression of aquaporin 2 in the cells of the collecting duct. Decreased expression of aquaporin 2 has been documented in the urine-concentrating defects associated with hypokalemia, lithium ingestion, ureteral obstruction, and hypercalcemia. Conversely, increased expression of aquaporin 2 is seen in states of renal water retention (e.g., congestive heart failure and pregnancy).

ADH also increases the permeability of the terminal portion of the inner medullary collecting duct to urea. Urea enters the cell across the apical membrane via a specific urea transporter (UT-A1). Acting through adenylyl cyclase, ADH phosphorylates UT-A1, which leads to increased urea permeability of the apical membrane of the cell. Increased osmolality of the interstitial fluid of the renal medulla also increases the urea permeability of the inner medullary collecting duct. This effect is separate from and additive to that of ADH.

Factors that influence ADH secretion also influence the perception of thirst

WHEN BODY FLUID OSMOLALITY IS INCREASED OR THE BLOOD VOLUME OR PRESSURE IS REDUCED, THE INDIVIDUAL PERCEIVES THIRST. Of these stimuli, hyperosmolality is the more potent. An increase of only 2% to 3% in the plasma osmolality produces a strong desire to drink, whereas decreases of 10% or more in blood volume or arterial pressure are required to produce the same response.

The neural center that regulates water intake (thirst center) is located in the same region of the hypothalamus as the osmoreceptors. Whether the cells of the thirst center are the same as the osmoreceptors or separate and distinct cells is not known. However, like the osmoreceptors, the cells of the thirst center also respond only to effective osmoles (e.g., NaCl). Even less is known about the pathways involved in the thirst response to decreased blood volume or arterial pressure, but it is believed that the pathways are the same as those involved in the regulation of ADH secretion. Angiotensin II, acting on cells of the thirst center, also evokes the sensation of thirst.

The ADH and thirst systems work in concert to maintain water balance. An increase in the plasma osmolality invokes drinking and, via ADH action on the kidneys, the conservation of water. Conversely, when the plasma osmolality is decreased, thirst is suppressed, and in the absence of ADH, renal water excretion is enhanced.

The dilution and concentration of urine require the separation of solute and water excretion

UNDER NORMAL CIRCUMSTANCES, THE EXCRETION OF WATER IS REGULATED SEPARATELY FROM THE EXCRETION OF SOLUTES (e.g., NaCl). For this to occur, the kidneys must be able to excrete urine that is either hypoosmotic or hyperosmotic with respect to the body fluids. This ability to excrete urine of varying osmolality in turn requires that solute be separated from water at some point along the nephron. As discussed in Chapter 37, the reabsorption of solute in the proximal tubule results in the reabsorption of a proportional amount of water. Hence, solute and water are not separated in this portion of the nephron. Moreover, this proportionality between proximal tubule water and solute reabsorption occurs regardless of whether the kidneys excrete dilute or concentrated urine. Thus, the proximal tubule reabsorbs a large portion of the filtered load of solute and water, but it does not produce dilute or concentrated tubular fluid.

Solute and water are separated in the loop of Henle

The loop of Henle, in particular the thick ascending limb, is the major site where solute and water are separated. Thus, the excretion of both dilute and concentrated urine requires normal function of the loop of Henle.

Figure 38–4 summarizes the essential features of the mechanisms whereby the kidneys excrete either a dilute or a concentrated urine. **Table 38–4** also summarizes the transport and passive permeability properties of the nephron segments involved in these processes.

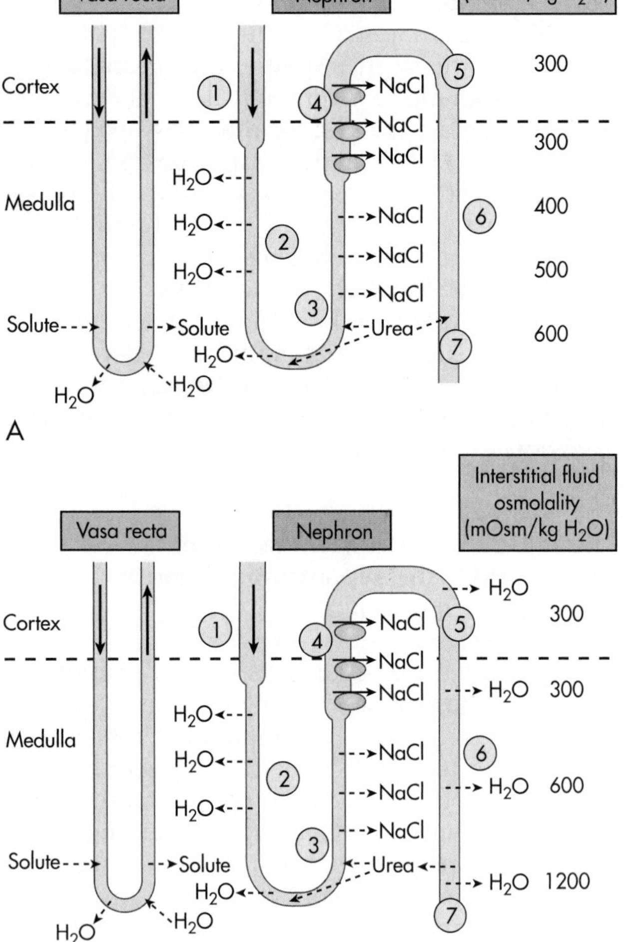

FIGURE 38–4. **A,** Mechanism for the excretion of dilute urine (water diuresis). ADH is absent, and the collecting duct is essentially impermeable to water. Note that the osmolality of the medullary interstitium is reduced during water diuresis. **B,** Mechanism for the excretion of a concentrated urine (antidiuresis). Plasma ADH levels are maximal, and the collecting duct is highly permeable to water. Under this condition, the medullary interstitial gradient is maximal. See text for details.

First, how the kidneys excrete dilute urine (water diuresis) when ADH levels are low or zero is considered. The following numbers refer to those encircled in Figure 38–4, *A*.

1. Fluid entering the descending thin limb of the loop of Henle from the proximal tubule is isoosmotic with respect to plasma. This reflects the essentially isoosmotic nature of solute and water reabsorption in the proximal tubule (see Chapter 37).
2. The descending thin limb is highly permeable to water and much less so to solutes such as NaCl and urea. (Note: urea is an ineffective osmole in many tissues, but it is an effective osmole in many portions of the nephron.) Consequently, as the fluid descends deeper into the hyperosmotic medulla, water is reabsorbed owing to the osmotic gradient set up across the descending thin limb by both NaCl and urea, which are present at high concentration in the medullary interstitium (see later section). Via this process, fluid at the bend of the loop has an osmolality equal to that of the surrounding interstitial fluid. However, although the tubular and interstitial fluids have similar osmolality at the bend of the loop, their compositions differ. The NaCl concentration of the tubular fluid is greater than that of the surrounding interstitial fluid. However, the urea concentration of the tubular fluid is less than that of the interstitial fluid (see later section).
3. The ascending thin limb is impermeable to water but permeable to NaCl and urea. Consequently, as tubular fluid moves up the ascending limb, NaCl is passively reabsorbed (because the luminal NaCl concentration is higher than the interstitial NaCl concentration), whereas urea passively diffuses into the tubular fluid (because the luminal urea concentration is lower than the interstitial urea concentration). The net effect is that the volume of the tubular fluid remains unchanged along the length of the thin ascending limb, but the NaCl concentration decreases and the urea concentration increases. Overall, the movement of NaCl out of the lumen of the thin ascending limb exceeds the movement of urea into the lumen, and the tubular fluid becomes diluted.
4. The thick ascending limb of the loop of Henle is impermeable to water and urea. This portion of the nephron actively reabsorbs NaCl from the tubular fluid and thereby dilutes it. Dilution occurs to such a degree that this segment is often referred to as the **diluting segment** of the kidney. Fluid leaving the thick ascending limb is hypoosmotic with respect to plasma (approximately 150 mOsm/kg H_2O).

TABLE 38–4. TRANSPORT AND PERMEABILITY PROPERTIES OF NEPHRON SEGMENTS INVOLVED IN URINE CONCENTRATION AND DILUTION

Tubule Segment	Active Transport	Passive Permeability*			Effect of ADH
		NaCl	Urea	H_2O	
Loop of Henle					
Descending thin limb	0	+	+	+++	
Ascending thin limb	0	+++	+	0	
Thick ascending limb	+++	+	0	0	
Distal tubule	+	+	0	0	
Collecting duct					
Cortex	+	+	0	0	↑H_2O permeability
Medulla	+	+	++	+	↑H_2O and urea permeability

*Permeability is proportional to the number of plus signs indicated: +, low permeability; +++, high permeability; 0, impermeable.

5. The distal tubule and cortical portion of the collecting duct actively reabsorb NaCl and are impermeable to urea. In the absence of ADH, these segments are not permeable to water. Thus, when ADH is absent or present at low levels (i.e., decreased plasma osmolality), the osmolality of tubule fluid in these segments is reduced further because NaCl is reabsorbed without water. Under this condition, fluid leaving the cortical portion of the collecting duct is hypoosmotic with respect to plasma (approximately 100 mOsm/kg H_2O).
6. The medullary collecting duct actively reabsorbs NaCl. Even in the absence of ADH, this segment is slightly permeable to water and urea. Consequently, some urea enters the collecting duct from the medullary interstitium, and a small volume of water is reabsorbed.
7. The urine has an osmolality as low as approximately 50 mOsm/kg H_2O and contains low concentrations of NaCl and urea. The volume of urine excreted can be as much as 18 L/day, or approximately 10% of the glomerular filtration rate.

Second, how the kidneys excrete concentrated urine **(antidiuresis)** when plasma osmolality and plasma ADH levels are high is considered. The following numbers refer to those encircled in Figure 38–4, *B*.

1-4. These steps are similar to those for production of a dilute urine. In understanding how a concentrated urine is produced, an important point to recognize is that although reabsorption of NaCl by the ascending thin and thick limbs of the loop of Henle dilutes the tubular fluid, the reabsorbed NaCl accumulates in the medullary interstitium and raises the osmolality of this compartment. The accumulation of NaCl in the medullary interstitium is crucial for the production of urine hyperosmotic to plasma because it provides the osmotic driving force for water resorption by the medullary collecting duct. The overall process by which the loop of Henle, in particular the thick ascending limb, generates the hyperosmotic medullary interstitial gradient is termed **countercurrent multiplication.** This term derives from both the form and function of the loop of Henle. The loop of Henle consists of two parallel limbs with tubular fluid flowing in opposite directions (countercurrent flow). Fluid flows into the medulla in the descending limb and out of the medulla in the ascending limb. The ascending limb is impermeable to water and reabsorbs solute from the tubular fluid. Thus, fluid within the ascending limb becomes diluted. This separation of solute and water by the ascending limb is termed the **single effect** of the countercurrent multiplication process. The solute removed from the ascending limb tubular fluid accumulates in the surrounding interstitial fluid and raises its osmolality. Because the descending limb is highly permeable to water, the increased osmolality of the medullary interstitium causes water to be absorbed and thereby concentrates the tubular fluid. The countercurrent flow within the descending and ascending limbs of the loop of Henle magnifies or "multiplies" the osmotic gradient between the tubule fluid in the descending and ascending limbs of the loop of Henle, such that an increasing osmotic gradient is generated throughout the medulla (Figure 38–4).

5. Because of NaCl reabsorption by the thick ascending limb of the loop of Henle, the fluid reaching the collecting duct is hypoosmotic with respect to the surrounding interstitial fluid. Thus, an osmotic gradient is established across the collecting duct. In the presence of ADH, which increases the water permeability of the collecting duct, water diffuses out of the tubule lumen, and the tubule fluid osmolality increases. This diffusion of water out of the

lumen of the collecting duct begins the process of urine concentration. The maximum osmolality that the fluid in the cortical collecting duct can attain is approximately 290 mOsm/kg H_2O (i.e., the same as plasma), which is the osmolality of the surrounding interstitial fluid and plasma. Although the fluid at this point has the same osmolality as the fluid that entered the descending thin limb, its composition has been altered dramatically. Because of NaCl reabsorption by the preceding nephron segments, NaCl accounts for a much smaller portion of the total tubular fluid osmolality. Instead, the tubule fluid osmolality reflects the presence of urea (filtered urea plus urea added in the descending thin and ascending thin limbs of the loop of Henle) and other solutes (e.g., K^+, NH_4^+, creatinine).

6. The osmolality of the interstitial fluid in the medulla progressively increases from the junction between the renal cortex and medulla, where it is approximately 300 mOsm/kg H_2O, to the papilla, where it approximates 1200 mOsm/kg H_2O. Thus, an osmotic gradient exists between tubule fluid and the interstitial fluid along the entire medullary collecting duct. In the presence of ADH, which renders the medullary collecting duct permeable to water, the osmolality of tubule fluid increases as water is reabsorbed. Because the initial portion of the collecting duct is impermeable to urea, it remains in the tubular fluid, and its concentration increases. In the presence of ADH, the urea permeability of the last portion of the medullary collecting duct is increased. Because the urea concentration of the tubular fluid has been increased by water reabsorption in the cortex and outer medulla, its concentration in the tubular fluid is greater than its concentration in the interstitial fluid, and some urea diffuses out of the tubule lumen into the medullary interstitium. The maximal osmolality that the fluid in the medullary collecting duct can attain is equal to that of the surrounding interstitial fluid. The major components of the tubular fluid within the medullary collecting ducts are substances that either have escaped reabsorption or have been secreted into the tubular fluid. Of these, urea is the most abundant.
7. The urine produced when ADH levels are elevated has an osmolality of 1200 mOsm/kg H_2O and contains high concentrations of urea and other nonreabsorbed solutes. Because urea in the tubular fluid equilibrates with urea in the medullary interstitial fluid, its concentration in the urine is similar to that of the interstitium. The urine volume under this condition can be as low as 0.5 L/day.

As just described, water reabsorption by the proximal tubule (67% of the filtered load) and the thin descending limb of the loop of Henle (15% of the filtered load) is essentially the same regardless of whether the urine is dilute or concentrated. As a result, a relatively constant volume of water is delivered to the distal tubule and collecting duct each day. Depending on the plasma ADH concentration, a variable portion of this water is then reabsorbed (8% to 17% of the filtered load), with water excretion ranging from less than 1% to 10% of the filtered load. During antidiuresis, most of the water is reabsorbed in the distal tubule and cortical and outer medullary portions of the collecting duct. Thus, a relatively small volume of fluid reaches the inner medullary collecting duct, where it is then reabsorbed. This distribution of water reabsorption along the length of the collecting duct (the cortex more than the outer medulla more than the inner medulla) allows the maintenance of a hyperosmotic interstitial environment in the inner medulla by minimizing the amount of water entering this compartment.

Medullary interstitial fluid osmolality determines the maximal osmolality of urine

The interstitial fluid of the renal medulla is critically important in concentrating the urine. The osmotic pressure of the interstitial fluid provides the driving force for reabsorbing water from both the descending thin limb of the loop of Henle and the collecting duct. The principal solutes of the medullary interstitial fluid are NaCl and urea, but the concentration of these solutes is not uniform throughout the medulla (i.e., a gradient exists from cortex to papilla). Other solutes also accumulate in the medullary interstitium (e.g., NH_4^+ and K^+), but the most abundant solutes are NaCl and urea. For simplicity, this discussion assumes that NaCl and urea are the only solutes.

At the junction of the medulla with the cortex, the interstitial fluid has an osmolality of approximately 300 mOsm/kg H_2O, with virtually all osmoles attributable to NaCl. The concentrations of both NaCl and urea increase progressively with increasing depth into the medulla. When a maximally concentrated urine is excreted, the medullary interstitial fluid osmolality is approximately 1200 mOsm/kg H_2O at the papilla (Figure 38–4, *B*). Of this value, approximately 600 mOsm/kg H_2O is attributed to NaCl and 600 mOsm/kg H_2O to urea. As described later, NaCl is an effective osmole in the inner medulla and thus is responsible for driving water reabsorption from the medullary collecting duct.

The medullary gradient for NaCl results from the accumulation of NaCl reabsorbed by the nephron segments in the medulla during countercurrent multiplication. The most important segment in this regard is the ascending limb (the thick limb more than the thin limb) of the loop of Henle. Urea accumulation within the medullary interstitium is more complex and occurs most effectively when a hyperosmotic urine is excreted (i.e., antidiuresis). When a dilute urine is produced, especially during extended periods, the osmolality of the medullary interstitium declines (compare Figure 38–4, *A* and *B*). This reduced osmolality is almost entirely caused by a decrease in the concentration of urea. This decrease reflects washout by the vasa recta (see later section) and diffusion of urea from the interstitium into the tubular fluid within the medullary portion of the collecting duct. (Recall that the medullary collecting duct is significantly permeable to urea even in the absence of ADH; see Table 38–4.)

Urea is not synthesized in the kidney but is generated by the liver as a product of protein metabolism. It enters the tubular fluid via glomerular filtration. As indicated in Table 38–4, the permeability of most nephron segments involved in urinary concentration and dilution to urea is relatively low. The important exception is the medullary collecting duct, which has a relatively high urea permeability that is further increased by ADH. As fluid moves along the nephron and as water is reabsorbed in the collecting duct, the urea concentration in the tubular fluid increases. When this urea-rich tubular fluid reaches the medullary collecting duct, where the permeability to urea not only is high but also is increased by ADH, urea diffuses down its concentration gradient into the medullary interstitial fluid, where it accumulates. When ADH levels are elevated, the urea within the lumen of the collecting duct and the interstitium equilibrates. The resultant urea concentration of the urine is equal to that of the medullary interstitium at the papilla, or approximately 600 mOsm/kg H_2O.

Some of the urea within the interstitium enters the descending and ascending thin limbs of the loop of Henle. This urea is then trapped in the nephron until it again reaches the medullary collecting duct, where it can reenter the medullary interstitium. Thus, UREA RECYCLES FROM THE INTERSTITIUM TO THE NEPHRON AND BACK INTO THE INTERSTITIUM. THIS PROCESS OF RECYCLING FACILITATES THE ACCUMULATION OF UREA IN THE MEDULLARY INTERSTITIUM.

As described, the hyperosmotic medullary interstitium is essential for concentrating the tubular fluid within the collecting duct. Because a hyperosmotic medullary interstitium is essential for urine concentration, any condition that reduces this gradient impairs the ability of the kidneys to maximally concentrate the urine. Urea within the medullary interstitium contributes to the total osmolality of the urine. However, because the inner medullary collecting duct is highly permeable to urea, especially in the presence of ADH, urea cannot drive water reabsorption across this nephron segment (i.e., urea is an ineffective osmole). Instead, the urea in the tubular fluid and that in the medullary interstitium equilibrate, and urine with a high concentration of urea is excreted. IT IS THE MEDULLARY INTERSTITIAL NaCl CONCENTRATION THAT IS RESPONSIBLE FOR REABSORBING WATER FROM THE MEDULLARY COLLECTING DUCT AND THEREBY CONCENTRATING THE NONUREA SOLUTES (e.g., NH_4^+ SALTS, K^+ SALTS, CREATININE) IN THE URINE.

The vasa recta function as countercurrent exchangers

The **vasa recta,** the capillary networks that supply blood to the medulla, are highly permeable to solute and water. Like the loop of Henle, the vasa recta form a parallel set of hairpin loops within the medulla (see Chapter 36). Not only do the vasa recta bring nutrients and oxygen to the medullary nephron segments, but, more important, they also remove excess water and solute that is continuously added to the medullary interstitium by these nephron segments. The ability of the vasa recta to maintain the medullary interstitial gradient is flow dependent. A substantial increase in vasa recta blood flow dissipates the medullary gradient (i.e., washout of the medullary interstitial gradient). Alternatively, reduced blood flow reduces oxygen delivery to the nephron segments within the medulla and impairs tubular transport. As a result, the medullary interstitial osmotic gradient cannot be maintained.

Renal water handling is assessed by measuring solute-free water excretion

Assessment of renal water handling includes measurements of urine osmolality and the volume of urine excreted. The range of urine osmolality is 50 to 1200 mOsm/kg H_2O. The corresponding range in urine volume is 18 L to as little as 0.5 L/day. These ranges are not fixed, but they vary from individual to individual.

The maximum amount of water that can be excreted by the kidneys depends on the amount of solute excreted, which in turn depends on food intake. For example, with maximally dilute urine (U_{osm} = 50 mOsm/kg H_2O), the maximum urine output of 18 L/day will be achieved only if the solute excretion rate is 900 mmol/day.

$$U_{osm} = \text{solute excretion/volume excretion} = 900 \text{ mmol/18 L} = 50 \text{ mOsm/kg } H_2O$$

If solute excretion is reduced, as commonly occurs in the elderly with reduced food intake, the maximum urine output will decrease. For example, if solute excretion is only 400 mmol/day, then the maximum urine output (at U_{osm} = 50 mOsm/kg H_2O) of only 8 L/day can be achieved. Thus, individuals with reduced food intake have a reduced capacity to excrete water.

As already discussed, total urine osmolality does not accurately reflect the impact of renal water handling on the maintenance of whole-body water balance because urea (which can account for half of the total urine osmolality) is not an effective osmole. As a result, it is often more appropriate to consider the ability of the kidneys to excrete or to reabsorb **solute-free water.** Solute-free water is an abstract term referring to water that does not contain any solute. When a dilute urine is produced, the kidneys excrete solute-free water. When a concentrated urine is produced, solute-free water is reabsorbed by the kidneys.

THE ABILITY OF THE KIDNEYS EITHER TO EXCRETE OR TO REABSORB SOLUTE-FREE WATER DEPENDS ON ADH. When no ADH is present or levels are low, solute-free water is excreted. When ADH levels are high, solute-free water is reabsorbed. Other factors are also important in determining the ability of the kidneys to excrete or to reabsorb solute-free water.

For the kidneys to excrete solute-free water maximally, the following conditions must exist:

1. ADH must be absent. This prevents water reabsorption by the distal tubule and collecting duct.
2. The tubular structures that separate solute from water (i.e., dilute the luminal fluid) must function normally. In the absence of ADH, the following nephron segments can dilute the luminal fluid: thin ascending limb of the loop of Henle, thick ascending limb of the loop of Henle, distal tubule, and collecting duct. Because of its high transport rate, the thick ascending limb is quantitatively the most important of these segments that separate solute from water.
3. Adequate delivery of tubular fluid to the nephron sites that dilute tubular fluid is required for maximal separation of solute and water. Factors that reduce delivery (e.g., decreased glomerular filtration rate or enhanced proximal tubule reabsorption) impair the ability of the kidneys to maximally excrete solute-free water.

Similar requirements also apply to the reabsorption of solute-free water by the kidneys. For the kidneys to reabsorb solute-free water maximally, the following conditions must exist:

1. Maximum levels of ADH must be present, and the distal tubule and collecting duct must respond to ADH.
2. Reabsorption of NaCl by the nephron segments must be normal. Again, the most important segment is the thick ascending limb of the loop of Henle.
3. Adequate delivery of tubular fluid to the nephron segments that separate solute from water is required. Most important in this regard is the thick ascending limb of the loop of Henle. Delivery of tubular fluid to the loop of Henle in turn depends on the glomerular filtration rate and proximal tubule reabsorption.
4. A hyperosmotic medullary interstitium must be present. The effective interstitial osmolality is maintained by NaCl reabsorption by the loop of Henle (see 2 and 3).

Control of Extracellular Fluid Volume and Regulation of Renal NaCl Excretion

The major solutes of the ECF are the salts of Na^+. Of these, NaCl is the most abundant. Because NaCl is also the major determinant of ECF osmolality, alterations in Na^+ balance are commonly assumed to disturb ECF osmolality. However, under normal circumstances, this is not the case because the ADH and thirst systems maintain body fluid osmolality within a narrow range. For example, the addition of NaCl to the ECF (without water) increases the [Na^+] and osmolality of this compartment. (ICF osmolality also increases because of osmotic equilibration with the ECF.) This increase in osmolality in turn stimulates thirst and the release of ADH from the posterior pituitary. The increased ingestion of water in response to thirst, together with the ADH-induced decrease in water excretion by the kidneys, quickly restores ECF osmolality to normal. However, the volume of the ECF increases in proportion to the amount of water ingested, which in turn depends on the amount of NaCl added to the ECF. Thus, in the new steady state, the addition of NaCl to the ECF is equivalent to adding an isoosmotic solution, and the volume of this compartment increases. Conversely, a decrease in the NaCl content of the ECF lowers the volume of this compartment.

The kidneys adjust NaCl excretion to match daily intake

The kidneys are the major route for excretion of NaCl from the body. As such, the kidneys are important in regulating the volume of the ECF. UNDER NORMAL CONDITIONS, THE KIDNEYS KEEP THE VOLUME OF THE ECF CONSTANT BY ADJUSTING THE EXCRETION OF NaCl TO MATCH THE AMOUNT INGESTED IN THE DIET. If ingestion exceeds excretion, ECF volume increases above normal, whereas the opposite occurs if excretion exceeds ingestion.

The typical diet contains approximately 140 mEq/day of Na^+ (8 g of NaCl), and thus daily Na^+ excretion is also about 140 mEq/day. However, the kidneys can vary the excretion of Na^+ over a wide range. Excretion rates as low as 10 mEq/day can be attained when individuals are prescribed a low-salt diet. Conversely, the kidneys can increase their excretion rate to more than 1000 mEq/day when challenged by the ingestion of a high-salt diet. These changes in Na^+ excretion occur with only modest changes in the steady-state Na^+ content of the body.

The response of the kidneys to abrupt changes in NaCl intake typically takes several hours to several days, depending on the magnitude of the change. During this transition period, the intake and excretion of Na^+ are not matched as they are in the steady state. Thus, the individual experiences either **positive Na^+ balance** (intake higher than excretion) or **negative Na^+ balance** (intake less than excretion). However, by the end of the transition period, a new steady state is established, and intake once again equals excretion. Provided that the ADH and thirst systems are intact and normal, alterations in Na^+ balance change the volume but not the $[Na^+]$ of the ECF. Changes in ECF volume can be monitored by measuring body weight because 1 L of ECF equals 1 kg of body weight.

Renal NaCl excretion is regulated to maintain a constant ECF volume

The ECF is subdivided into two compartments: blood plasma and interstitial fluid. Plasma volume is a determinant of vascular volume and thus of blood pressure and cardiac output. The maintenance of Na^+ balance, and thus of ECF volume, involves a complex system of sensors and effector signals that act primarily on the kidneys to regulate the excretion of NaCl. As can be appreciated from the dependency of vascular volume, blood pressure, and cardiac output on ECF volume, this complex system is designed to ensure adequate tissue perfusion. Because the primary sensors of this system are located in the large vessels of the vascular system, changes in vascular volume, blood pressure, and cardiac output are the principal factors regulating renal NaCl excretion. In a normal individual, changes in ECF volume result in parallel changes in vascular volume, blood pressure, and cardiac output. Thus, a decrease in ECF volume, a situation termed **volume contraction,** results in reduced vascular volume, blood pressure, and cardiac output. Conversely, an increase in ECF volume, a situation termed **volume expansion,** results in increased vascular volume, blood pressure, and cardiac output. The degree to which these cardiovascular parameters change depends on the degree of volume contraction or expansion and the effectiveness of cardiovascular reflex mechanisms. When ECF volume is decreased, renal NaCl excretion is reduced. Conversely, an increase in ECF volume results in enhanced renal NaCl excretion, termed **natriuresis.**

In some pathological conditions (e.g., congestive heart failure, hepatic cirrhosis), the renal excretion of NaCl does not reflect the ECF volume. In both of these situations, the volume of the ECF is increased. However, instead of increased NaCl excretion, as would be expected, there is a reduction in the renal excretion of NaCl. This paradoxical response can be understood by recognizing that the sensors, because of their location in the vascular system, appear to detect a reduced ECF volume in these situations.

Patients with congestive heart failure frequently have an increase in the volume of the ECF, which is manifested as accumulation of fluid in the lungs **(pulmonary edema)** and peripheral tissues **(generalized edema).** This excess fluid is the result of NaCl and water retention by the kidneys. The kidneys' response (i.e., retention of NaCl and water) is paradoxical because the ECF volume is increased. However, this fluid is not in the vascular system but in the interstitial fluid compartment. In addition, blood pressure and cardiac output may be reduced because of poor cardiac performance. Therefore, the sensors located in the vascular system respond as they do in ECF volume contraction and cause NaCl and water retention by the kidneys.

Large volumes of fluid accumulate in the peritoneal cavity **(ascites)** of patients with advanced hepatic cirrhosis. This fluid is a component of the ECF and results from NaCl and water retention by the kidneys. Again, the response of the kidneys in this situation seems paradoxical if only ECF volume is considered. With advanced hepatic cirrhosis, blood pools in the splanchnic circulation. (The damaged liver impedes the drainage of blood from the splanchnic circulation via the portal vein.) Thus, volume and pressure are reduced in the portions of the vascular system where the sensors are found, but venous pressure in the portal system increases, which enhances fluid transudation into the peritoneal cavity. Hence, the kidneys respond as they would during ECF volume contraction, which results in NaCl and water retention and the accumulation of ascites fluid.

The remaining portions of this section examine the relationship between ECF volume and renal NaCl excretion in normal adults, in whom changes in ECF volume result in parallel changes of vascular volume, blood pressure, and cardiac output. The maintenance of a normal volume **(euvolemia)** is reviewed, followed by consideration of the renal response to ECF volume expansion and contraction.

The primary ECF volume sensors are located in the vascular system

The ECF volume is monitored by multiple sensors **(Box 38–1)**. A number of the sensors are located in the vascular system, and they monitor its fullness and blood pressure. These receptors are typically called **volume receptors;** because they respond to stretch, they are also referred to as **baroreceptors.** The sensors within the liver and central nervous system are less well understood and do not seem to be as important as the vascular sensors in monitoring the ECF volume. The hepatic and central nervous system sensors are not considered further.

Low-pressure baroreceptors respond mainly to vascular volume

Baroreceptors are located within the walls of the cardiac atria and pulmonary vessels, and they respond to distention of these structures (see also Chapters 19 and 23). Because the low-pressure side of the circulatory system has a high compliance, the atrial and pulmonary vascular sensors respond mainly to the "fullness" of the vascular system. These baroreceptors send signals to the brainstem via afferent fibers in the vagus nerve. The activity of these sensors modulates both sympathetic nerve outflow and ADH secretion. For example, a decrease in filling of the pulmonary vessels and cardiac atria increases sympathetic nerve activity and stimulates ADH secretion. Conversely, distention of these structures decreases sympathetic nerve activity. In general, 5% to 10% changes in blood volume and pressure are necessary to evoke a response.

The cardiac atria possess an additional mechanism related to the control of renal NaCl excretion. The myocytes of the atria synthesize and store a peptide hormone. This hormone, termed **atrial natriuretic peptide** (ANP), is released when the atria are distended, which reduces blood pressure and increases the excretion of NaCl and water by the kidneys via mechanisms outlined later in this chapter (see also Chapters 19 and 45). The ventricles of the heart also produce a natriuretic peptide termed **brain natriuretic peptide** (BNP), so named because it was first isolated from the brain. Like ANP, BNP is released from the ventricular myocytes by distention of the ventricles. Its actions are similar to those of ANP.

High-pressure baroreceptors respond primarily to arterial blood pressure

Baroreceptors are also present in the arterial side of the circulatory system, located in the wall of the aortic arch, carotid sinus (see also Chapter 23), and afferent arterioles of the kidneys. The aortic arch and carotid baroreceptors send input to the brainstem via afferent fibers in the vagus and glossopharyngeal nerves. The response to this input alters sympathetic outflow and ADH secretion. Thus, a decrease in blood pressure increases sympathetic nerve activity and ADH secretion. An increase in pressure tends to reduce sympathetic nerve activity. The sensitivity of the high-pressure baroreceptors is similar to that in the low-pressure side of the vascular system; 5% to 10% changes in pressure are needed to evoke a response.

The **juxtaglomerular apparatus** of the kidneys (see Chapter 36), particularly the afferent arteriole, responds directly to changes in pressure. If perfusion pressure in the afferent arteriole is reduced, renin is released from the myocytes. Renin secretion is suppressed when perfusion pressure is increased. As described later in this chapter, renin determines blood levels of angiotensin II and aldosterone, both of which play an important role in regulating renal NaCl excretion.

BOX 38–1: VOLUME SENSORS

- Vascular sensors
  - Low pressure
    - Cardiac atria
    - Pulmonary vasculature
  - High pressure
    - Carotid sinus
    - Aortic arch
    - Juxtaglomerular apparatus of kidneys
- Hepatic sensors
- Central nervous system sensors

Constriction of a renal artery by an atherosclerotic plaque, for example, reduces perfusion pressure to that kidney. This reduced perfusion pressure is sensed by the afferent arterioles and results in the secretion of renin. The elevated renin levels increase the production of angiotensin II, which in turn increases systemic blood pressure via its vasoconstrictor effect on arterioles throughout the vascular system. The increased systemic blood pressure is sensed by the afferent arterioles of the contralateral kidney (i.e., the kidney without stenosis of its renal artery), and renin secretion from that kidney is suppressed. In addition, the high levels of angiotensin II act to inhibit renin secretion by the contralateral kidney (negative feedback). The treatment of patients with constricted renal arteries includes surgical repair of the stenotic artery, administration of angiotensin II receptor blockers, or administration of an inhibitor of angiotensin-converting enzyme (ACE). The ACE inhibitor blocks the conversion of angiotensin I to angiotensin II.

Of the two classes of baroreceptors, those on the high-pressure side of the vascular system appear to be more important in influencing sympathetic tone and ADH secretion. For example, patients with congestive heart failure often have an increased vascular volume and dilation of the atria and ventricles. This would be expected to decrease sympathetic tone and inhibit ADH secretion via the low-pressure baroreceptors. However, sympathetic tone is often increased and ADH secretion stimulated in these patients (the renin-angiotensin-aldosterone system is also activated). This reflects the activity of the high-pressure baroreceptors in response to reduced blood pressure and cardiac output secondary to the failing heart.

ECF volume sensors send hormonal and neural signals to the kidneys

The volume sensors elicit signals that act on the kidneys to modulate the excretion of NaCl. Both neural and hormonal signals have been identified. These are summarized in **Box 38–2**, as are their effects on renal NaCl and water excretion.

Renal sympathetic nerves

As described in Chapter 36, sympathetic nerve fibers innervate the afferent and efferent arterioles of the glomerulus as well as the nephron cells. With negative Na^+ balance (i.e., ECF volume depletion), the low- and high-pressure vascular baroreceptors stimulate sympathetic nerve activity, including those fibers innervating the kidneys. This has the following effects:

1. The afferent and efferent arterioles are constricted (mediated by α-adrenergic receptors). This vasoconstriction (the effect appears to be greater on the afferent arteriole) decreases the hydrostatic pressure within the glomerular capillary lumen, which results in a decreased glomerular filtration rate. With this decrease in glomerular filtration, the filtered load of Na^+ to the nephrons is reduced.
2. Renin secretion is stimulated by the cells of the afferent arterioles (mediated by β-adrenergic receptors). As described later, renin ultimately increases the circulating levels of angiotensin II and aldosterone.
3. NaCl reabsorption along the nephron is directly stimulated (mediated by α-adrenergic receptors). Quantitatively, the most important segment influenced by sympathetic nerve activity is the proximal tubule.

BOX 38–2: SIGNALS INVOLVED IN THE CONTROL OF RENAL NaCl AND WATER EXCRETION

Renal Sympathetic Nerves (↑Activity: ↓NaCl Excretion)

↓Glomerular filtration rate

↑Renin secretion

↑Proximal tubule, thick ascending limb of the loop of Henle, distal tubule, and collecting duct NaCl reabsorption

Renin-Angiotensin-Aldosterone (↑Secretion: ↓NaCl Excretion)

↑Angiotensin II levels stimulate proximal tubule NaCl reabsorption

↑Aldosterone levels stimulate the thick ascending limb of the loop of Henle, distal tubule, and collecting duct NaCl reabsorption

↑ADH secretion

Natriuretic Peptides (↑Secretion: ↑NaCl Excretion)

↑Glomerular filtration rate

↓Renin secretion

↓Aldosterone secretion

↓NaCl and water reabsorption by the collecting duct*

↓ADH secretion

ADH (↑Secretion: ↓H_2O Excretion)

↑H_2O absorption by the collecting duct

*Urodilatin may contribute to this effect.

As a result of these actions, INCREASED RENAL SYMPATHETIC NERVE ACTIVITY DECREASES NaCl EXCRETION, an adaptive response that works to restore euvolemia. With positive Na^+ balance (i.e., ECF volume expansion), renal sympathetic nerve activity is reduced. This generally reverses the effects just described.

Renin-angiotensin-aldosterone system

Smooth muscle cells in the afferent arterioles are the site of synthesis, storage, and release of **renin.**

Three factors are important in stimulating renin secretion:

1. **Perfusion pressure.** The afferent arteriole behaves like a high-pressure baroreceptor. When perfusion pressure to the kidneys is reduced, renin secretion is stimulated. Conversely, an increase in perfusion pressure inhibits renin release.
2. **Sympathetic nerve activity.** Activation of the sympathetic nerve fibers that innervate the afferent arterioles increases renin secretion (mediated by β-adrenergic receptors). Renin secretion is decreased as renal sympathetic nerve activity is decreased.
3. **Delivery of NaCl to the macula densa.** Delivery of NaCl to the macula densa regulates the glomerular filtration rate by a process termed **tubuloglomerular feedback** (see Chapter 37). In addition, the macula densa plays a role in renin secretion. When NaCl delivery to the macula densa is decreased, renin secretion is enhanced. Conversely, an increase in NaCl delivery inhibits renin secretion. It is likely that macula densa–mediated renin secretion helps maintain systemic arterial pressure under conditions of a reduced vascular volume. For example, when vascular volume is reduced, perfusion of body tissues (including the kidneys) decreases. This in turn decreases the glomerular filtration rate and the filtered load of NaCl. The reduced delivery of NaCl to the macula densa then stimulates renin secretion, which acts through angiotensin II (a potent vasoconstrictor) to increase the blood pressure and thereby maintain tissue perfusion.

Figure 38–5 summarizes the essential components of the renin-angiotensin-aldosterone system. Renin alone does not have a physiological function; it functions solely as a proteolytic enzyme. Its substrate is a circulating protein, **angiotensinogen,** which is produced by the liver. Angiotensinogen is cleaved by renin to yield a 10–amino acid peptide, **angiotensin I.** Angiotensin I also has no known physiological function, and it is further cleaved to an 8–amino acid peptide, **angiotensin II,** by a converting enzyme **(ACE)** found on the surface of vascular endothelial cells. (Pulmonary and renal endothelial cells are important sites for the conversion of angiotensin I to angiotensin II.) ACE also degrades bradykinin, a potent vasodilator. Angiotensin II has several important physiological functions, including

- stimulation of aldosterone secretion by the adrenal cortex;
- arteriolar vasoconstriction, which increases blood pressure;
- stimulation of ADH secretion and thirst; and
- enhancement of NaCl reabsorption by the proximal tubule.

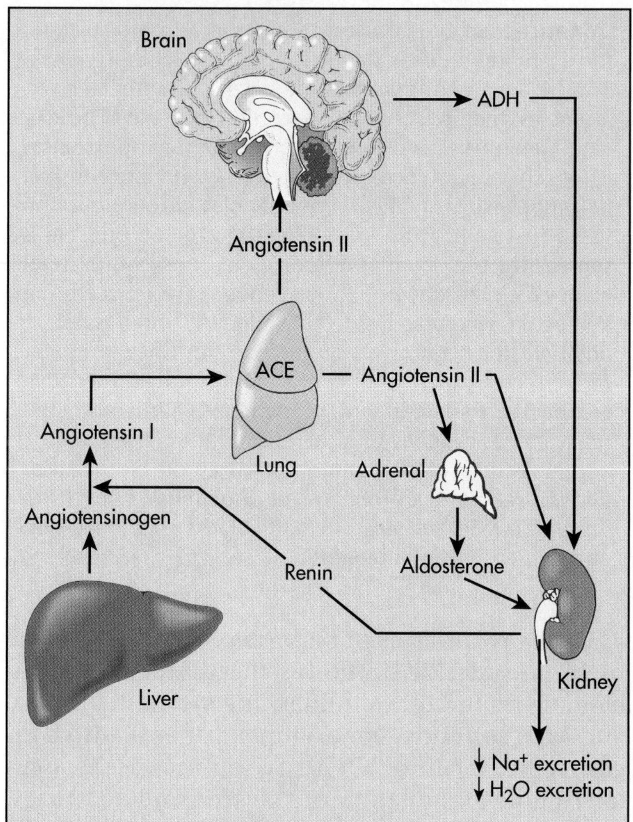

FIGURE 38–5. Essential components of the renin-angiotensin-aldosterone system. Activation of this system results in decreased excretion of Na^+ and water by the kidneys. Angiotensin I is converted to angiotensin II by angiotensin-converting enzyme (ACE), which is present on all vascular endothelial cells. Endothelial cells, especially those within the lungs and kidneys, play a significant role in this conversion process. See text for details.

Angiotensin II is an important secretagogue for **aldosterone** (an increase in the plasma [K^+] is the other important stimulus for aldosterone secretion; see Chapters 39 and 47). Aldosterone is a steroid hormone produced by the glomerulosa cells of the adrenal cortex. Aldosterone acts in a number of ways on the kidneys (see also Chapters 39 and 40). With regard to the regulation of the ECF volume, aldosterone reduces NaCl excretion by stimulating its reabsorption by the thick ascending limb of the loop of Henle, distal tubule, and collecting duct. The effect of aldosterone on renal NaCl excretion depends mainly on its ability to stimulate Na^+ reabsorption in the distal tubule and collecting duct.

Aldosterone stimulates Na^+ reabsorption by the principal cells of the late portion of the distal tubule and collecting duct by increasing Na^+ entry into the cell across the apical membrane as well as increasing the exit of Na^+ from the cell across the basolateral membrane. The increase in apical membrane Na^+

entry occurs via Na^+-selective channels. In the early phase of aldosterone's action (minutes to hours), these Na^+ channels are activated (i.e., increased opening of existing channels); this is followed by a late-phase effect (hours to days) that reflects increased expression of channels in the apical membrane. The increased extrusion of Na^+ from the cell across the basolateral membrane occurs by Na^+,K^+-ATPase, the synthesis of which is increased by aldosterone. Thus, aldosterone increases the reabsorption of Na^+ from the tubular fluid; reduced levels of aldosterone decrease the amount of Na^+ reabsorbed.

Aldosterone also enhances Na^+ reabsorption by cells of the thick ascending limb of the loop of Henle. This action likely reflects an increased entry of Na^+ into the cell across the apical membrane (probably by the apical membrane $1Na^+,1K^+,2Cl^-$ symporter) and an increased extrusion from the cell by the basolateral membrane Na^+,K^+-ATPase.

Diseases of the adrenal cortex can alter aldosterone levels and thereby impair the ability of the kidneys to maintain Na^+ balance and euvolemia. With decreased secretion of aldosterone **(hypoaldosteronism),** the reabsorption of Na^+, mainly by the distal tubule and collecting duct, is reduced, and NaCl is lost in the urine. Because urinary NaCl loss can exceed the amount of NaCl ingested in the diet, negative Na^+ balance ensues, and the ECF volume decreases. In response to the ECF volume contraction, sympathetic tone is increased, and levels of renin, angiotensin II, and ADH are elevated. With increased aldosterone secretion **(hyperaldosteronism),** the effects are the opposite; Na^+ reabsorption, especially by the distal tubule and collecting duct, is enhanced, and excretion of NaCl is reduced. Consequently, ECF volume is increased; sympathetic tone is decreased; and the levels of renin, angiotensin II, and ADH are decreased. As described later, ANP and BNP levels are also elevated in this setting.

As summarized in Box 38–2, ACTIVATION OF THE RENIN-ANGIOTENSIN-ALDOSTERONE SYSTEM, AS OCCURS WITH ECF VOLUME DEPLETION, DECREASES THE EXCRETION OF NaCl BY THE KIDNEYS. This system is suppressed with ECF volume expansion, and renal NaCl excretion is therefore enhanced.

Natriuretic peptides

The body produces a number of substances that act on the kidneys to increase Na^+ excretion.* Of these, natriuretic peptides produced by the heart and kidneys are best understood and are the focus of the following discussion.

The heart produces two natriuretic peptides. Atrial myocytes produce and store the peptide hormone **atrial natriuretic peptide** (ANP), and ventricular myocytes produce and store **brain natriuretic peptide** (BNP). Both peptides are secreted when the heart dilates (i.e., during volume expansion), and they act to relax vascular smooth muscle and promote NaCl and water excretion by the kidneys. The kidney also produces a related natriuretic peptide termed urodilatin. Its actions are limited to promoting NaCl excretion by the kidneys. In general, the actions of the natriuretic peptides, as they relate to renal NaCl and water excretion, antagonize those of the renin-angiotensin-aldosterone system. These actions include the following:

- Vasodilation of the afferent and vasoconstriction of the efferent arterioles of the glomerulus. This increases the glomerular filtration rate and the filtered load of Na^+.
- Inhibition of renin secretion by the afferent arterioles.
- Inhibition of aldosterone secretion by the glomerulosa cells of the adrenal cortex. This occurs via two mechanisms: (1) inhibition of renin secretion by the juxtaglomerular cells, thereby reducing angiotensin II–induced aldosterone secretion; and (2) inhibition of aldosterone secretion by the glomerulosa cells of the adrenal cortex.
- Inhibition of NaCl reabsorption by the collecting duct, which is also caused in part by reduced levels of aldosterone. However, the natriuretic peptides also act directly on the collecting duct cells. Through the second messenger cGMP, the peptides inhibit Na^+ channels in the apical membrane of the cell and thereby decrease Na^+ reabsorption. This effect occurs predominantly in the medullary portion of the collecting duct.
- Inhibition of ADH secretion by the posterior pituitary and ADH action on the collecting duct. This decreases water reabsorption by the collecting duct and thus increases excretion of water in the urine.

THESE EFFECTS OF THE NATRIURETIC PEPTIDES INCREASE THE EXCRETION OF NaCl AND WATER BY THE KIDNEYS. Hypothetically, a reduction in the circulating levels of these peptides would be expected to decrease NaCl and water excretion, but convincing evidence for this effect has not been reported.

Antidiuretic hormone

A decreased ECF volume stimulates ADH secretion by the posterior pituitary. The elevated levels of ADH decrease water excretion by the kidneys, which serves to reestablish euvolemia.

* Adrenomedullin is an example of one of these substances. It is produced by many tissues including the heart, kidneys, and adrenal medulla (from whence its name is derived). Although it is structurally distinct from the natriuretic peptides, its actions are similar to those of ANP and BNP.

During euvolemia, renal NaCl excretion equals dietary NaCl intake

The maintenance of Na^+ balance and therefore euvolemia requires the precise balance between the amount of NaCl ingested and that excreted from the body. IN A EUVOLEMIC INDIVIDUAL, DAILY URINE NaCl EXCRETION EQUALS DAILY NaCl INTAKE.

The amount of NaCl excreted by the kidneys can vary widely. Under conditions of salt restriction (i.e., low-NaCl diet), virtually no Na^+ appears in the urine. Conversely, in individuals who ingest large quantities of NaCl, renal Na^+ excretion can exceed 1000 mEq/day. The kidneys' response to variations in dietary NaCl intake may take several days. During the transition period, excretion does not match intake, and the individual is in either positive (intake exceeds excretion) or negative (intake is lower than excretion) Na^+ balance. When Na^+ balance is altered during these transition periods, the ECF volume changes in parallel. (Water excretion, regulated via the ADH system, is also adjusted to keep plasma osmolality constant, resulting in an isoosmotic change in ECF volume.) Thus, with positive Na^+ balance, the ECF volume expands (detected as an increase in body weight), whereas with negative Na^+ balance, the ECF volume contracts (detected as a decrease in body weight). Ultimately, renal excretion reaches a new steady state, and euvolemia is reestablished as NaCl excretion once again is matched to intake. The time course for the adjustment of renal NaCl excretion varies and depends on the magnitude of the change in NaCl intake. Adaptation to large changes in NaCl intake requires a longer time than does adaptation to small changes in intake.

The general features of Na^+ handling along the nephron must be understood to comprehend how renal Na^+ excretion is regulated. (See Chapter 37 for the cellular mechanisms of Na^+ transport along the nephron.) Most (67%) of the filtered load of Na^+ is reabsorbed by the proximal tubule. An additional 25% is reabsorbed by the thick ascending limb of the loop of Henle and the remainder by the distal tubule and collecting duct.

In a normal adult, the filtered load of Na^+ is approximately 25,000 mEq/day. With a typical diet, less than 1% of this filtered load is excreted in the urine (approximately 140 mEq/day). Because of the large filtered load of Na^+, small changes in Na^+ reabsorption by the nephron can profoundly affect Na^+ balance and thus the volume of the ECF. For example, an increase in Na^+ excretion from 1% to 3% of the filtered load represents an additional loss of approximately 500 mEq/day of Na^+. Because the ECF [Na^+] is 140 mEq/L, such an Na^+ loss would decrease the ECF volume by more than 3 L. (Water excretion would parallel the loss of Na^+ to maintain body fluid osmolality constant: 500 mEq/day ÷ 140 mEq/L = 3.6 L/day of fluid loss.)

During euvolemia, the reabsorption of Na^+ by the distal tubule collecting duct is regulated to reflect dietary NaCl intake

IN EUVOLEMIC SUBJECTS, THE DISTAL TUBULE AND COLLECTING DUCT ARE THE MAIN NEPHRON SEGMENTS WHERE Na^+ REABSORPTION IS ADJUSTED TO MAINTAIN EXCRETION AT A LEVEL APPROPRIATE FOR DIETARY INTAKE. However, other portions of the nephron are also involved in this process. Because the reabsorptive capacity of the distal tubule and collecting duct is limited, these other portions of the nephron must reabsorb the bulk of the filtered load of Na^+. Thus, during euvolemia, Na^+ handling by the nephron can be explained by two general processes:

1. Na^+ reabsorption by the proximal tubule and loop of Henle is regulated so that a relatively constant portion of the filtered load of Na^+ is delivered to the distal tubule and collecting duct. Approximately 8% of the filtered load is delivered to the distal tubule and the collecting duct.
2. Reabsorption of this remaining portion of the filtered load of Na^+ by the distal tubule and collecting duct is regulated so that the amount of Na^+ excreted in the urine matches the amount ingested in the diet. Thus, the distal tubule and collecting duct make final adjustments in Na^+ excretion to maintain the euvolemic state.

Mechanisms for maintaining constant Na^+ delivery to the distal tubule and collecting duct

A number of mechanisms maintain delivery of a constant fraction of the filtered load of Na^+ to the distal tubule and collecting duct. These processes are autoregulation of the glomerular filtration rate (and thus the filtered load of Na^+), glomerulotubular balance, and load dependency of Na^+ reabsorption by the loop of Henle.

Autoregulation of the glomerular filtration rate (see Chapter 36) allows maintenance of a relatively constant filtration rate over a wide range of perfusion pressures. Because the filtration rate is constant, the filtered load of Na^+ to the nephrons is also kept constant.

Despite the autoregulatory control of the glomerular filtration rate, small variations occur. If these changes were not compensated for by an appropriate adjustment in Na^+ reabsorption by the nephron, Na^+ excretion would change markedly. Fortunately, Na^+ reabsorption in the euvolemic state, especially by the proximal tubule, changes in parallel with changes in glomerular filtration rate. This phenomenon is termed **glomerulotubular (G-T) balance** (see Chapter 37). Thus, if the glomerular filtration rate increases, the amount of Na^+ reabsorbed by the proximal tubule also increases. The opposite occurs if the glomerular filtration rate decreases.

The final mechanism that helps maintain the constant delivery of Na^+ to distal tubule and collecting duct involves the ability of the loop of Henle to increase its reabsorptive rate in response to increased delivery of Na^+. The loop of Henle, particularly the thick ascending limb, has a great capacity to increase reabsorption in response to increased Na^+ delivery.

Regulation of Na^+ reabsorption by the collecting duct

When delivery of Na^+ is constant, small adjustments in distal tubule and collecting duct reabsorption are sufficient to balance excretion with intake. A 2% change in the fractional excretion of Na^+ produces more than a 3-L change in the volume of the ECF. (Water excretion would parallel the loss of Na^+ to maintain body fluid osmolality constant: 500 mEq/day ÷ 140 mEq/L = 3.6 L/day of fluid loss.) Aldosterone is the primary regulator of Na^+ reabsorption by the distal tubule and collecting duct and thus of Na^+ excretion under this condition. When aldosterone levels are elevated, Na^+ reabsorption by the principal cells is increased (excretion decreased). When aldosterone levels are decreased, Na^+ reabsorption is decreased (excretion increased).

In addition to aldosterone, a number of other factors, including natriuretic peptides, prostaglandins, adrenomedullin, and sympathetic nerves, alter Na^+ reabsorption by the distal tubule and collecting duct. However, the relative effects of these other factors on the regulation of Na^+ reabsorption during euvolemia are unclear.

As long as variations in the dietary intake of NaCl are minor, the mechanisms previously described can regulate renal Na^+ excretion appropriately and thereby maintain euvolemia. However, these mechanisms cannot effectively handle significant changes in NaCl intake. When NaCl intake changes significantly, ECF volume expansion or ECF volume contraction occurs. In such cases, additional factors are invoked to act on the kidneys to adjust Na^+ excretion and thereby reestablish the euvolemic state.

Renal NaCl excretion is increased in response to an increase in ECF volume

During ECF volume expansion, the volume sensors send signals to the kidneys. These signals result in increased excretion of NaCl and water. The signals acting on the kidneys include

- decreased activity of the renal sympathetic nerves;
- release of ANP and BNP from the heart and urodilatin in the kidneys;
- inhibition of ADH secretion from the posterior pituitary and decreased ADH action on the collecting duct;
- decreased renin secretion and thus decreased production of angiotensin II; and
- decreased aldosterone secretion, which is caused by reduced angiotensin II levels and elevated natriuretic peptide levels.

The integrated response of the nephron to these signals is illustrated in **Figure 38–6**. Three general responses to ECF volume expansion occur (the numbers correlate with those encircled in Figure 38–6):

1. **The glomerular filtration rate increases.** The glomerular filtration rate increases mainly as a result of the decrease in sympathetic nerve activity. Sympathetic fibers innervate the afferent and efferent arterioles of the glomerulus and control their diameter. Decreased sympathetic nerve activity leads to arteriolar dilation. Because the effect appears to be greater on the afferent arterioles, the hydrostatic pressure within the glomerular capillary is increased, thereby increasing the glomerular filtration rate (because the renal plasma flow increases to a greater degree than the glomerular filtration rate, the filtration fraction decreases). Natriuretic peptides also increase the glomerular filtration rate by dilating the afferent and constricting the efferent arterioles. Thus, the increased natriuretic peptide levels that occur during ECF volume expansion contribute to this response. With the increase in the glomerular filtration rate, the filtered load of Na^+ increases.
2. **The reabsorption of Na^+ decreases in the proximal tubule.** Several mechanisms may act to reduce Na^+ reabsorption by the proximal tubule, but the precise role of each of these mechanisms remains controversial. Because activation of the sympathetic nerve fibers that innervate this nephron segment stimulates Na^+ reabsorption, the decreased sympathetic nerve activity that results from ECF volume expansion decreases Na^+ reabsorption. In addition, angiotensin II directly stimulates Na^+ reabsorption by the proximal tubule. Because angiotensin II levels are also reduced under this condition, proximal tubule Na^+ reabsorption decreases as a result. The increased hydrostatic pressure within the glomerular capillaries also tends to increase the hydrostatic pressure within the peritubular capillaries. In addition, the decrease in filtration fraction reduces the peritubular oncotic

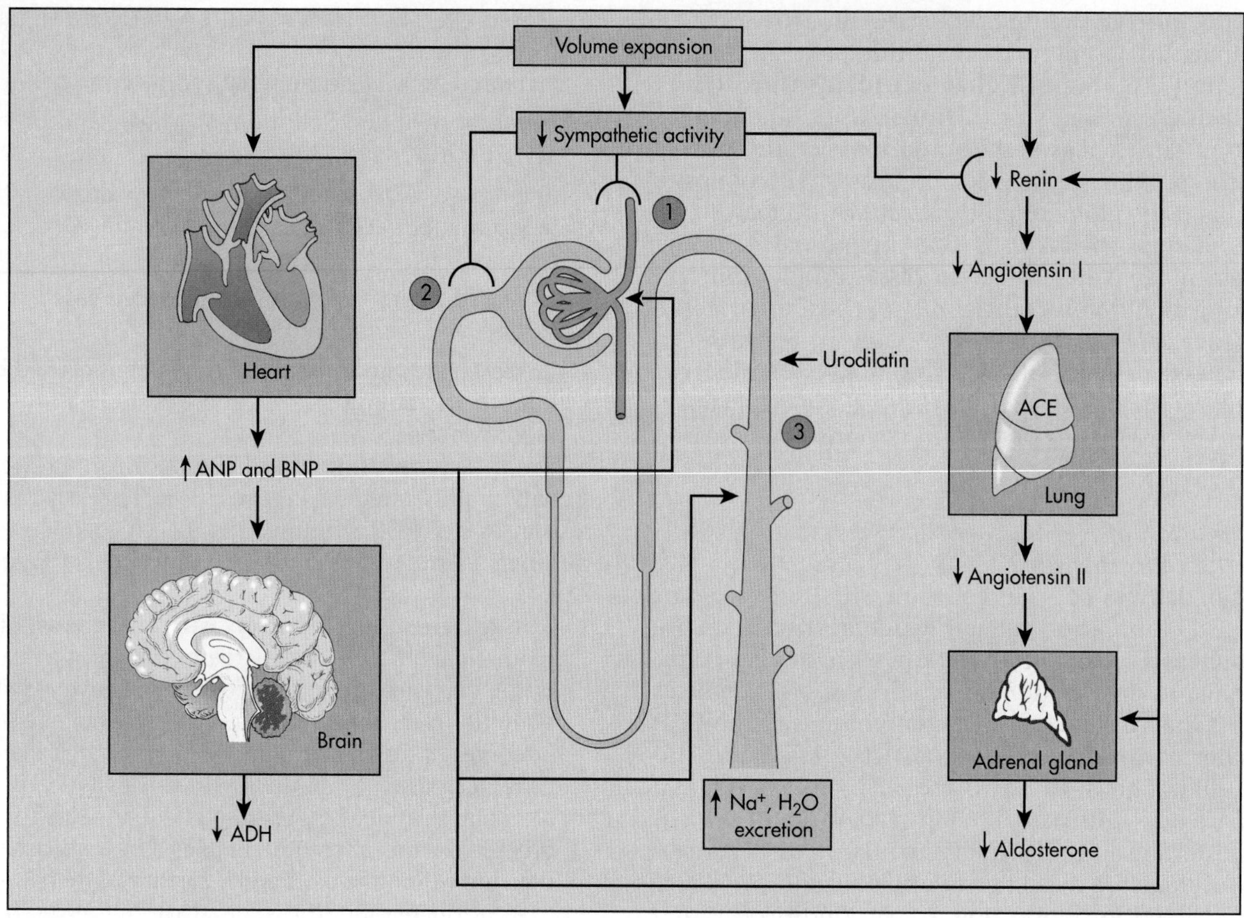

FIGURE 38–6. Integrated response to the expansion of ECF volume. Numbers refer to the description of the response in the text. ACE, angiotensin-converting enzyme; ANP, atrial natriuretic peptide; BNP, brain natriuretic peptide.

pressure. These alterations in the capillary Starling forces reduce the absorption of solute (e.g., NaCl) and water from the lateral intercellular space and thus reduce tubular reabsorption. (See Chapter 37 for a complete description of this mechanism.)

3. **Na^+ reabsorption decreases in the distal tubule and collecting duct.** Both the increase in the filtered load and the decrease in NaCl reabsorption by the proximal tubule result in the delivery of large amounts of NaCl to the loop of Henle. Because activation of the sympathetic nerves and aldosterone stimulate NaCl reabsorption by the loop of Henle, the reduced nerve activity and low aldosterone levels that occur with ECF volume expansion could reduce NaCl reabsorption. However, because reabsorption by the thick ascending limb is load dependent, these effects are offset, and the fraction of the filtered load of Na^+ reabsorbed is actually increased. Nevertheless, the amount of Na^+ delivered to the distal tubule and collecting duct exceeds that observed in the euvolemic state. The amount of Na^+ delivered to the distal tubule and collecting duct varies in proportion to the degree of ECF volume expansion. This increased load of Na^+ overwhelms the reabsorptive capacity of these segments, and this capacity is even further impaired by the actions of natriuretic peptides (on the medullary collecting duct) and by the decrease in the circulating levels of aldosterone.

The final component in the response to ECF volume expansion is the excretion of water. As Na^+ excretion increases, plasma osmolality begins to fall. This decreases the secretion of ADH. ADH secretion is also decreased in response to the elevated levels of natriuretic peptides. In addition, these natriuretic peptides inhibit the action of ADH on the collecting duct. Together, these effects decrease water reabsorption by the collecting duct and thereby increase water excretion by the kidneys. Thus, the excretion of Na^+ and water occurs in concert; euvolemia is restored, and body fluid osmolality remains constant. As already noted, the time course of this response (hours to days) depends on the magnitude of the ECF volume expansion. Thus, if the degree of ECF volume expansion is small, the mechanisms just described generally restore euvolemia within 24 hours. However, with large degrees of ECF volume expansion, the response can take several days.

In summary, the renal response to ECF volume expansion involves the integrated action of all parts of the nephron:

- The filtered load of Na^+ is increased.
- Proximal tubule reabsorption is reduced (the glomerular filtration rate is increased, whereas proximal reabsorption is decreased; thus, G-T balance does not occur under this condition).
- The delivery of Na^+ to the distal tubule and collecting duct is increased. This increased delivery, along with the inhibition of reabsorption, results in the excretion of a larger fraction of the filtered load of Na^+ and thus restores euvolemia.

Renal NaCl excretion is decreased in response to a decrease in ECF volume

During ECF volume contraction, the volume sensors send signals to the kidneys, which reduce NaCl and water excretion. The signals that act on the kidneys include

- increased renal sympathetic nerve activity;
- increased secretion of renin, which results in elevated angiotensin II levels and thus increased secretion of aldosterone by the adrenal cortex;
- inhibition of ANP and BNP secretion by the heart and urodilatin production by the kidneys; and
- stimulation of ADH secretion by the posterior pituitary.

The integrated response of the nephron to these signals is illustrated in **Figure 38–7**. The general response is as follows (the numbers correlate with those encircled in Figure 38–7):

1. **The glomerular filtration rate decreases.** Afferent and efferent arteriolar constriction results from increased renal sympathetic nerve activity. The effect appears to be greater on the afferent than on the efferent arteriole. This causes the hydrostatic pressure in the glomerular capillary to fall and thereby decreases the glomerular filtration rate (because the renal plasma flow decreases more than the glomerular filtration rate, filtration fraction increases). This decrease in the glomerular filtration rate reduces the filtered load of Na^+.

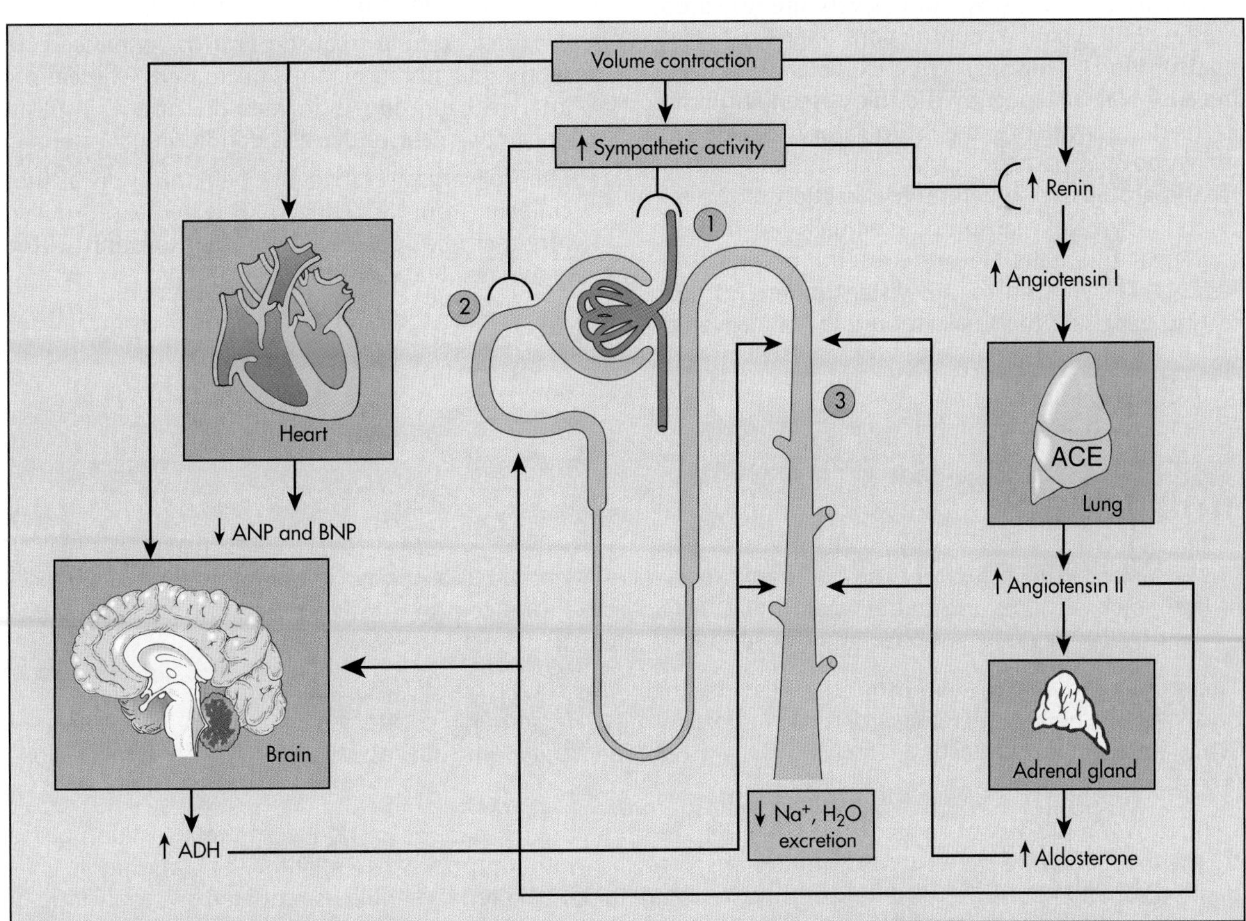

FIGURE 38–7. Integrated response to ECF volume contraction. Numbers refer to the description of the response in the text. Urodilatin levels are also decreased (not depicted). ACE, angiotensin-converting enzyme; ANP, atrial natriuretic peptide; BNP, brain natriuretic peptide.

2. **Na^+ reabsorption by the proximal tubule is increased.** Several mechanisms augment Na^+ reabsorption in this segment. For example, increased sympathetic nerve activity and angiotensin II levels directly stimulate Na^+ reabsorption by the proximal tubule. The decreased hydrostatic pressure within the glomerular capillaries also leads to a decrease in the hydrostatic pressure within the peritubular capillaries. In addition, the increased filtration fraction results in an increase in the peritubular oncotic pressure. These alterations in the capillary Starling forces facilitate the movement of fluid from the lateral intercellular space into the capillary and thereby stimulate the reabsorption of solute (e.g., NaCl) and water by the proximal tubule. (See Chapter 37 for a complete description of this mechanism.)
3. **Na^+ reabsorption by the distal tubule and collecting duct is enhanced.** The reduced filtered load and enhanced proximal tubule reabsorption decrease the delivery of Na^+ to the loop of Henle. Increased sympathetic nerve activity and aldosterone stimulate Na^+ reabsorption by the thick ascending limb. Because sympathetic nerve activity is increased and aldosterone levels are elevated during ECF volume contraction, increased Na^+ reabsorption by this segment is expected. However, because Na^+ transport by the thick ascending limb is load dependent, the stimulatory effects of increased sympathetic nerve activity and aldosterone are offset. Therefore, the fraction of the filtered load of Na^+ reabsorbed is actually less than in the euvolemic state. Nevertheless, the result is that less Na^+ is delivered to the distal tubule and collecting duct, and the small amount of Na^+ delivered is almost completely reabsorbed because transport in these segments is enhanced. This stimulation of Na^+ reabsorption is mainly induced by increased aldosterone levels. In addition, natriuretic peptides, which inhibit collecting duct reabsorption, are not present.

Finally, water reabsorption by the collecting duct is enhanced by ADH, the levels of which are elevated through activation of the low- and high-pressure vascular baroreceptors as well as by the elevated levels of angiotensin II. As a result, water excretion is reduced; with the Na^+ retained by the kidneys, euvolemia is reestablished, and body fluid osmolality remains constant. The time course of this reexpansion of the ECF (hours to days) and the degree to which euvolemia is attained depend on the magnitude of the ECF volume contraction as well as the dietary intake of Na^+. Thus, the kidneys reduce Na^+ excretion, and euvolemia is restored as NaCl is ingested. (That is, increasing the NaCl intake reestablishes euvolemia more quickly.)

In summary, the nephron's response to ECF volume contraction involves the integrated action of all its segments:

- The filtered load of Na^+ is decreased.
- Proximal tubule reabsorption is enhanced (the glomerular filtration rate is decreased, whereas proximal reabsorption is increased; thus, G-T balance does not occur under this condition).
- The delivery of Na^+ to the beginning distal tubule collecting duct is reduced. This decreased delivery, together with enhanced Na^+ reabsorption, virtually eliminates Na^+ from the urine.

Summary

- The osmolality and volume of the body fluids are maintained within a narrow range despite wide variations in the intake of water and solute (mainly NaCl). The kidneys are central to this regulatory process by virtue of their ability to vary the excretion of water and solutes.
- The regulation of body fluid osmolality requires that water intake match water loss from the body. When body fluid osmolality increases, ADH secretion and thirst are stimulated, and renal water excretion decreases. When body fluid osmolality decreases, ADH secretion and thirst are suppressed, and renal water excretion increases.
- Central to the process of concentrating and diluting the urine is the loop of Henle. The reabsorption of NaCl by the loop of Henle allows the separation of solute and water, a process essential for the elaboration of dilute urine. By this same mechanism, the interstitial fluid in the renal medulla is rendered hyperosmotic. This hyperosmotic medullary interstitial fluid in turn provides the osmotic driving force for the reabsorption of water from the lumen of the collecting duct when ADH is present and thus allows the kidney to concentrate the urine.

- Disorders of water balance alter body fluid osmolality. Changes in body fluid osmolality are manifest by a change in the plasma [Na^+]. Positive water balance (intake exceeds excretion) decreases the body fluid osmolality and causes hyponatremia. Negative water balance (intake is lower than excretion) increases the body fluid osmolality and causes hypernatremia.
- Maximal excretion of solute-free water by the kidneys requires the normal function of nephrons (especially the thick ascending limb of the loop of Henle), the adequate delivery of tubular fluid to the nephrons, and the absence of ADH. Maximal reabsorption of solute-free water by the kidneys requires the normal function of nephrons (especially the thick ascending limb of the loop of Henle), the adequate delivery of tubular fluid to the nephrons, a hyperosmotic medullary interstitium, the presence of ADH, and the responsiveness of the collecting duct to ADH.
- The volume of the ECF is determined by Na^+ balance. When Na^+ intake exceeds excretion, positive Na^+ balance exists, and ECF volume expansion occurs. Conversely, when Na^+ excretion exceeds Na^+ intake, negative Na^+ balance exists, and ECF volume contraction occurs. The kidneys are the primary route for Na^+ excretion from the body.
- During euvolemia, Na^+ excretion by the kidneys is matched to the amount of Na^+ ingested in the diet.
- With ECF volume expansion, low- and high-pressure volume sensors initiate a response that ultimately leads to the increased excretion of NaCl and water by the kidneys and the reestablishment of euvolemia. The components of this response include a decrease in sympathetic outflow to the kidneys, suppression of the renin-angiotensin-aldosterone system, and release of natriuretic peptides from the heart and kidneys. At the level of the kidneys, the glomerular filtration rate is enhanced, and therefore the filtered load of Na^+ increases. In addition, Na^+ reabsorption by the proximal tubule, distal tubule, and collecting duct is reduced. Together, these changes in renal Na^+ handling enhance Na^+ excretion. With ECF volume contraction, this sequence of events is reversed.

Bibliography

Abassi ZA et al: Control of extracellular fluid volume and the pathophysiology of edema formation. In Brenner BM, ed: *Brenner and Rector's the kidney,* ed 7, Philadelphia, 2004, WB Saunders.

Agre P et al: Aquaporin water channels—from atomic structure to clinical medicine, *J Physiol* 542:3, 2002.

Agre P et al: Aquaporin water channels in mammalian kidney. In Seldin DW, Giebisch G, eds: *The kidney: physiology and pathophysiology,* ed 3, Philadelphia, 2000, Lippincott Williams & Wilkins.

Berl T, Verbalis J: Pathophysiology of water metabolism. In Brenner BM, ed: *Brenner and Rector's the kidney,* ed 7, Philadelphia, 2004, WB Saunders.

Bichet DG, Mallie J-P: Hypernatremia and polyuric disorders. In DuBose TD Jr, Hamm LL, eds: *Acid-base and electrolyte disorders,* Philadelphia, 2002, WB Saunders.

Bichet DG: Polyuria and diabetes insipidus. In Seldin DW, Giebisch G, eds: *The kidney: physiology and pathophysiology,* ed 3, Philadelphia, 2000, Lippincott Williams & Wilkins.

Blantz RC et al: Renin-angiotensin-aldosterone system. In DuBose TD Jr, Hamm LL, eds: *Acid-base and electrolyte disorders,* Philadelphia, 2002, WB Saunders.

Brown D, Nielsen S: Cell biology of vasopressin action. In Brenner BM, ed: *Brenner and Rector's the kidney,* ed 7, Philadelphia, 2004, WB Saunders.

Chonchol M, Berl T: Hyponatremia. In DuBose TD Jr, Hamm LL, eds: *Acid-base and electrolyte disorders,* Philadelphia, 2002, WB Saunders.

Deen PM et al: Nephrogenic diabetes insipidus, *Curr Opin Nephrol Hypertens* 9:591, 2000.

DiBona GF, Kopp UC: Neural control of renal function. In Seldin DW, Giebisch G, eds: *The kidney: physiology and pathophysiology,* ed 3, Philadelphia, 2000, Lippincott Williams & Wilkins.

Fitzsimmons JT: Physiology and pathophysiology of thirst and sodium appetite. In Seldin DW, Giebisch G, eds: *The kidney: physiology and pathophysiology,* ed 3, Philadelphia, 2000, Lippincott Williams & Wilkins.

Greger R: Physiology of renal sodium transport, *Am J Med Sci* 319:51, 2000.

Humphreys MH, Valentin JP: Natriuretic humoral agents. In Seldin DW, Giebisch G, eds: *The kidney: physiology and pathophysiology,* ed 3, Philadelphia, 2000, Lippincott Williams & Wilkins.

Inoue T et al: Physiological effects of vasopressin and atrial natriuretic peptide in the collecting duct, *Cardiovasc Res* 51:470, 2001.

Knepper MA, Gamba G: Urine concentration and dilution. In Brenner BM, ed: *Brenner and Rector's the kidney,* ed 7, Philadelphia, 2004, WB Saunders.

Morello JP, Bichet DR: Nephrogenic diabetes insipidus, *Annu Rev Physiol* 63:607, 2001.

Palmer BF et al: Physiology and pathophysiology of sodium retention. In Seldin DW, Giebisch G, eds: *The kidney: physiology and pathophysiology,* ed 3, Philadelphia, 2000, Lippincott Williams & Wilkins.

Robertson GL: Vasopressin. In Seldin DW, Giebisch G, eds: *The kidney: physiology and pathophysiology,* ed 3, Philadelphia, 2000, Lippincott Williams & Wilkins.

Sands JM, Layton HE: Urine concentrating mechanism and its regulation. In Seldin DW, Giebisch G, eds: *The kidney: physiology and pathophysiology,* ed 3, Philadelphia, 2000, Lippincott Williams & Wilkins.

Schnermann J, Briggs JP: Function of the juxtaglomerular apparatus: control of glomerular hemodynamics and renin secretion. In Seldin DW, Giebisch G, eds: *The kidney: physiology and pathophysiology,* ed 3, Philadelphia, 2000, Lippincott Williams & Wilkins.

Suzuki T et al: The role of the natriuretic peptides in the cardiovascular system, *Cardiovasc Res* 51:489, 2001.

Case Studies

Case 38–1

A previously healthy 45-year-old man is admitted to the hospital with pneumonia. His blood pressure is 140/75 mm Hg, and his plasma [Na^+] is 142 mEq/L; both are within the normal range. His condition is treated with intravenous antibiotics and fluids. On the third hospital day, his blood pressure is unchanged, but his plasma [Na^+] is 130 mEq/L. His urine osmolality is 450 mOsm/kg H_2O. He has no edema, and his blood pressure does not change when he goes from a reclining to a standing position.

1. What is the most likely cause for the development of hyponatremia in this man?

A. Decreased ingestion of NaCl
B. Increased renal excretion of NaCl
C. Positive water balance
D. Shift of water from the ICF to the ECF
E. Shift of Na^+ from the ECF to the ICF

2. What would be the most appropriate way to return the plasma [Na^+] to its normal value?

A. Administer ADH
B. Restrict water intake
C. Increase water intake
D. Restrict NaCl intake
E. Increase NaCl intake

Case 38–2

A 56-year-old woman has a history of congestive heart failure. Because of poor cardiac output, she is easily fatigued and has developed generalized edema (i.e., increased interstitial fluid volume) with swelling of her ankles and legs. Her plasma [Na^+] has decreased from a normal value of 145 to 130 mEq/L. As part of her therapy, she receives a drug that inhibits ACE.

1. What would be the most appropriate change in this woman's intake of NaCl and water?

	Water intake	NaCl intake
A.	Increase	Increase
B.	Increase	Restrict
C.	Restrict	Increase
D.	Restrict	Restrict
E.	No change	No change

2. Administration of an ACE inhibitor would be expected to have which of the following effects on circulating levels of renin, aldosterone, and bradykinin?

	Renin	Aldosterone	Bradykinin
A.	Decreased	Decreased	Decreased
B.	Decreased	Decreased	Increased
C.	Increased	Increased	Decreased
D.	Increased	Decreased	Increased
E.	Increased	Increased	Increased

Chapter 39: Potassium, Calcium, and Phosphate Homeostasis

Objectives

- ❖ Explain how K^+ is crucial for many cellular functions.
- ❖ Describe how hormones and the kidneys maintain K^+ homeostasis.
- ❖ Describe the regulation of K^+ excretion by the kidneys.
- ❖ Describe how pathophysiological factors alter K^+ homeostasis.
- ❖ Explain how Ca^{++} and Pi subserve many important cellular functions.
- ❖ Describe how the kidneys regulate Ca^{++} and Pi homeostasis.
- ❖ Explain how hormones regulate plasma levels of Ca^{++} and Pi.
- ❖ Describe how the kidneys regulate the excretion of Ca^{++} and Pi.

The kidneys play an essential role in regulating the amount of several important inorganic ions in the body, including K^+, Ca^{++}, and phosphate (Pi). So that appropriate balance, or homeostasis, can be maintained, the excretion of these electrolytes must be equal to their daily intake. If the intake of an electrolyte exceeds its excretion, the amount of this electrolyte in the body increases, and the individual is in positive balance for that electrolyte. Conversely, if excretion of an electrolyte exceeds its intake, its amount in the body decreases, and the individual is in negative balance for that electrolyte. For K^+, Ca^{++}, and Pi, the kidneys are the sole or primary route of excretion from the body. Accordingly, this chapter focuses on how the kidneys maintain K^+, Ca^{++}, and Pi homeostasis.

K^+, One of the Most Abundant Cations in the Body, Is Critical for Many Cell Functions

Despite wide fluctuations in dietary K^+ intake, its concentration in cells and extracellular fluid (ECF) remains remarkably constant. Two sets of regulatory mechanisms safeguard K^+ homeostasis. First, several mechanisms regulate the $[K^+]$ in the ECF. Second, other mechanisms maintain the amount of K^+ in the body constant by adjusting renal K^+ excretion to match dietary K^+ intake. It is the kidneys that regulate K^+ excretion.

Total body K^+ is 50 mEq/kg of body weight, or 3500 mEq for a 70-kg individual. A total of 98% of the K^+ in the body is located within cells, where the average $[K^+]$ is 150 mEq/L. A high intracellular $[K^+]$ is required for many cell functions, including cell growth and division and volume regulation. Only 2% of total body K^+ is located in the ECF, where the normal concentration is approximately 4 mEq/L. A $[K^+]$ in the ECF that exceeds 5.0 mEq/L constitutes **hyperkalemia.** Conversely, a $[K^+]$ in the ECF of less than 3.5 mEq/L constitutes **hypokalemia.**

HYPOKALEMIA IS ONE OF THE MOST COMMON ELECTROLYTE DISORDERS IN CLINICAL PRACTICE AND CAN BE OBSERVED IN AS MANY AS 20% OF HOSPITALIZED PATIENTS. The most common causes of hypokalemia include administration of diuretic drugs, Gitelman's syndrome (a genetic defect in the Na^+-Cl^- symporter in the apical membrane of distal tubule cells), and surreptitious vomiting (i.e., bulimia). HYPERKALEMIA IS ALSO A COMMON ELECTROLYTE DISORDER AND IS SEEN IN 1% TO 10% OF HOSPITALIZED PATIENTS. Hyperkalemia is often seen in patients with renal failure, in patients taking drugs including angiotensin-converting enzyme (ACE) inhibitors and K^+-sparing diuretics, in patients with hyperglycemia (i.e., high blood glucose levels), and in the elderly.

The large concentration difference of K^+ across cell membranes (approximately 146 mEq/L) is maintained by the operation of Na^+,K^+-ATPase. This K^+ gradient is important in maintaining the potential difference across cell membranes (see Chapters 2 and 17). Thus, K^+ is critical for the excitability of nerve and muscle cells as well as for the contractility of cardiac, skeletal, and smooth muscle cells.

Cardiac arrhythmias are produced by both hypokalemia and hyperkalemia. The electrocardiogram (ECG) monitors the electrical activity of the heart and is a fast and easy way to determine whether changes in the plasma $[K^+]$ influence the heart and other excitable cells. In contrast, measurements of the plasma $[K^+]$ by the clinical laboratory require a blood sample, and values are often not immediately available. The first sign of hyperkalemia is the appearance of tall, thin T waves in the ECG. Further increases in the plasma $[K^+]$ prolong the PR interval, depress the ST segment, and lengthen the QRS interval of the ECG. Finally, as the plasma $[K^+]$ approaches 10 mEq/L, the P wave disappears, the QRS interval broadens, the ECG appears as a sine wave, and the ventricles fibrillate (i.e., manifest rapid, uncoordinated contractions of muscle fibers). Hypokalemia prolongs the QT interval, inverts the T wave, and lowers the ST segment of the ECG.

After a meal, the K^+ absorbed by the gastrointestinal tract enters the ECF within minutes **(Figure 39–1)**. If the K^+ ingested during a normal meal (≈33 mEq) were to remain in the ECF compartment, the plasma $[K^+]$ would increase by a potentially lethal 2.4 mEq/L (33 mEq added to 14 L of ECF):

$$33 \text{ mEq}/14 \text{ L} = \Delta 2.4 \text{ mEq/L}$$

This rise in the plasma $[K^+]$ is prevented by the rapid (minutes) uptake of K^+ into cells. Because the excretion of K^+ by the kidneys after a meal is relatively slow (hours), the uptake of K^+ by cells is essential to prevent life-threatening hyperkalemia. Maintaining total body K^+ constant requires that all the K^+ absorbed by the gastrointestinal tract must eventually be excreted by the kidneys. This process requires about 6 hours.

Several Hormones Promote the Uptake of K^+ into Cells After a Rise in Plasma $[K^+]$

Several hormones, including epinephrine, insulin, and aldosterone, increase K^+ uptake into skeletal muscle, liver, bone, and red blood cells by stimulating Na^+,K^+-ATPase, the $1Na^+,1K^+,2Cl^-$ symporter, and the Na^+-Cl^- symporter (Figure 39–1 and **Box 39–1**). Acute stimulation of K^+ uptake (i.e., within minutes) is mediated by an increased turnover rate of existing Na^+,K^+-ATPase, $1Na^+,1K^+,2Cl^-$, and Na^+-Cl^- transporters, whereas the chronic increase in K^+ uptake (i.e., within hours to days) is mediated by an increase in the quantity of Na^+,K^+-ATPase. A rise in the plasma $[K^+]$ that follows K^+ absorption by the gastrointestinal tract stimulates insulin secretion from the pancreas, aldosterone release from the adrenal cortex, and epinephrine secretion from the adrenal medulla. In contrast, a decrease in the plasma $[K^+]$ inhibits the release of these hormones. Whereas insulin and epinephrine act within a few minutes, aldosterone requires about an hour to stimulate K^+ uptake into cells.

Epinephrine can lower plasma $[K^+]$

Catecholamines affect the distribution of K^+ across cell membranes by activating α- and β_2-adrenergic receptors. The stimulation of α adrenoceptors releases K^+ from cells, especially in the liver; the stimulation of β_2 adrenoceptors promotes K^+ uptake by cells.

BOX 39–1: MAJOR FACTORS, HORMONES, AND DRUGS INFLUENCING THE DISTRIBUTION OF K^+ BETWEEN THE INTRACELLULAR AND EXTRACELLULAR FLUID COMPARTMENTS

Physiological: keep plasma $[K^+]$ constant
- Epinephrine
- Insulin
- Aldosterone

Pathophysiological: displace plasma $[K^+]$ from normal
- Acid-base balance
- Plasma osmolality
- Cell lysis
- Exercise

Drugs that induce hyperkalemia
- Dietary potassium supplements
- ACE inhibitors
- K^+-sparing diuretics
- Heparin

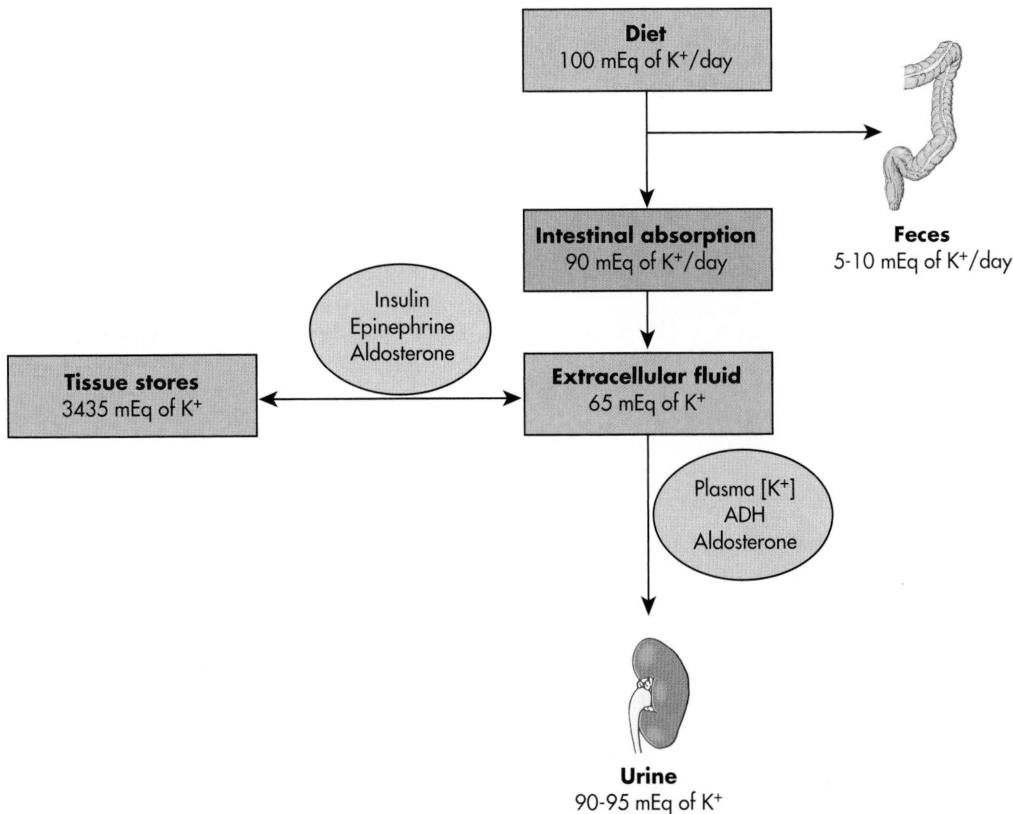

FIGURE 39–1. Overview of K^+ homeostasis. ADH, antidiuretic hormone. See text for details.

For example, the activation of β_2 adrenoceptors after exercise is important in preventing hypokalemia. The rise in plasma [K^+] after a K^+-rich meal is greater if the patient has been pretreated with propranolol, a β_2 adrenoceptor antagonist. Furthermore, the release of epinephrine during stress (e.g., myocardial ischemia) can rapidly lower the plasma [K^+].

Insulin is the most important hormone

Insulin also stimulates K^+ uptake into cells (see also Chapter 43). The importance of insulin is illustrated by two observations. First, the rise in plasma [K^+] after a K^+-rich meal is greater in patients with diabetes mellitus (i.e., insulin deficiency) than in normal people. Second, insulin (and glucose to prevent insulin-induced hypoglycemia) can be infused to correct hyperkalemia. Insulin is the most important hormone that shifts K^+ into cells after the ingestion of K^+ in a meal.

Balanced levels of aldosterone prevent hypokalemia and hyperkalemia

Aldosterone, like catecholamines and insulin, promotes K^+ uptake into cells. A rise in aldosterone levels (e.g., primary aldosteronism) causes hypokalemia, whereas a fall in aldosterone levels (e.g., Addison's disease) causes hyperkalemia. As discussed later, aldosterone also stimulates urinary K^+ excretion. Thus, aldosterone alters the plasma [K^+] by acting on K^+ uptake into cells and by altering urinary K^+ excretion.

Some Hormones, Drugs, and Factors Disturb Normal K^+ Uptake by Cells

The acid-base balance comprises both metabolic acidosis and metabolic alkalosis

In general, metabolic acidosis increases the plasma [K^+], whereas metabolic alkalosis decreases it. In contrast, respiratory acid-base disorders have little or no effect on the plasma [K^+]. Metabolic acidosis produced by the addition of inorganic acids (e.g., HCl, H_2SO_4) increases the plasma [K^+] much more than does an equivalent acidosis produced by the accumulation of organic acids (e.g., lactic acid, acetic acid, keto acids). The reduced pH (i.e., increased [H^+]) promotes the movement of H^+ into

TABLE 39–1. NET EFFECTS OF HORMONES AND OTHER FACTORS ON K^+ SECRETION BY THE DISTAL TUBULE AND COLLECTING DUCT

Condition	Direct or Indirect	Flow	Urinary Excretion
Hyperkalemia	Increase	Increase	Increase
Aldosterone			
Acute	Increase	Decrease	No change
Chronic	Increase	No change	Increase
Glucocorticoids	No change	Increase	Increase
ADH	Increase	Decrease	No change
Acidosis			
Acute	Decrease	No change	Decrease
Chronic	Decrease	Large increase	Increase
Alkalosis	Increase	Increase	Large increase

Data from Field MJ, Berliner RW, Giebisch GH. In Narins R, ed: *Textbook of nephrology: clinical disorders of fluid and electrolyte metabolism*, ed 5, New York, 1994, McGraw-Hill.

cells and the reciprocal movement of K^+ out of cells to maintain electroneutrality.

Metabolic alkalosis has the opposite effect; the plasma [K^+] decreases as K^+ moves into cells and H^+ exits. The mechanism responsible for this shift is not fully understood. The movement of H^+ may occur as the cells buffer changes in the [H^+] of the ECF. As H^+ moves across the cell membranes, K^+ moves in the opposite direction, and thus cations are neither gained nor lost across cell membranes (Table 39–1).

Although organic acids produce a metabolic acidosis, they do not cause significant hyperkalemia. Two explanations have been suggested for the reduced ability of organic acids to cause hyperkalemia. First, the organic anion may enter the cell with H^+ and thereby eliminate the need for K^+-H^+ exchange across the membrane. Second, organic anions may stimulate insulin secretion, which moves K^+ into cells. This movement may counteract the direct effect of the acidosis, which moves K^+ out of cells.

The osmolality of the plasma also influences the distribution of K^+ across cell membranes

An increase in the osmolality of the ECF enhances K^+ release by cells and thus increases extracellular [K^+]. The plasma K^+ level may increase by 0.4 to 0.8 mEq/L for an elevation of 10 mOsm/kg H_2O in plasma osmolality. In patients with diabetes mellitus who do not take insulin, plasma K^+ is often elevated in part because of the lack of insulin and in part because of the increase in plasma [glucose], which increases plasma osmolality. Hypoosmolality has the opposite action. The alterations in plasma [K^+] associated with changes in osmolality are related to changes in cell volume. For example, as plasma osmolality increases, water leaves cells because of the osmotic gradient across the plasma membrane. Water leaves cells until the intracellular osmolality equals that of the ECF. This loss of water shrinks cells and causes the cell [K^+] to rise. The rise in intracellular [K^+] provides a driving force for the exit of K^+ from cells. This sequence increases plasma [K^+]. A fall in plasma osmolality has the opposite effect.

Cell lysis causes hyperkalemia, an abnormally high plasma [K^+]

Cell lysis causes hyperkalemia, which results from the addition of intracellular K^+ to the ECF. Severe trauma (e.g., burns) and some conditions such as **tumor lysis syndrome** (i.e., chemotherapy-induced destruction of tumor cells) and **rhabdomyolysis** (i.e., destruction of skeletal muscle) destroy cells and release K^+ and other cell solutes into the ECF. In addition, gastric ulcers may cause the seepage of red blood cells into the gastrointestinal tract. The blood cells are digested, and the K^+ released from the cells is absorbed and can cause hyperkalemia.

More K^+ is released from skeletal muscle cells during exercise than during rest

The ensuing hyperkalemia depends on the degree of exercise. In people walking slowly, the plasma [K^+] increases by 0.3 mEq/L. The plasma [K^+] may increase by at least 2.0 mEq/L with vigorous exercise.

Exercise-induced changes in the plasma [K^+] usually do not produce symptoms and are reversed after several minutes of rest. However, exercise can lead to life-threatening hyperkalemia in individuals who have endocrine disorders that affect the release of insulin, epinephrine, or aldosterone; in individuals whose ability to excrete K^+ is impaired (e.g., renal failure); or in those who take certain medications, such as β_2-adrenergic blockers. For example, during exercise, the plasma [K^+] may increase by at least 2 to 4 mEq/L in individuals who take ß$_2$-adrenergic receptor antagonists for hypertension.

BECAUSE ACID-BASE BALANCE, PLASMA OSMOLALITY, CELL LYSIS, AND EXERCISE DO NOT MAINTAIN THE PLASMA [K^+] AT A NORMAL VALUE, THEY DO NOT CONTRIBUTE TO K^+ HOMEOSTASIS (Box 39–1). The extent to which these pathophysiological states alter the plasma [K^+] depends on the integrity of the homeostatic mechanisms that regulate plasma [K^+] (e.g., the secretion of epinephrine, insulin, and aldosterone).

The Kidneys Play a Major Role in Maintaining K^+ Balance

The kidneys excrete 90% to 95% of the K^+ ingested in the diet (Figure 39–1). Excretion equals intake even when intake increases by as much as 10-fold. This balance of urinary excretion and dietary intake underscores the importance of the kidneys in maintaining K^+ homeostasis. Although small amounts of K^+ are lost each day in the stool and sweat (approximately 5% to 10% of the K^+ ingested in the diet), this amount is essentially constant, is not regulated, and therefore is relatively less important than the K^+ excreted by the kidneys. K^+ SECRETION FROM THE BLOOD INTO THE TUBULAR FLUID BY THE CELLS OF THE DISTAL TUBULE AND COLLECTING DUCT SYSTEM IS THE KEY FACTOR IN DETERMINING URINARY K^+ EXCRETION **(Figure 39–2)**.

Because K^+ is not bound to plasma proteins, it is freely filtered by the glomerulus. When normal individuals have an average diet, urinary K^+ excretion is about 15% of the amount filtered. Accordingly, K^+ must be reabsorbed along the nephron. When dietary K^+ intake increases, however, K^+ excretion can exceed the amount filtered. Thus, K^+ can also be secreted.

The proximal tubule reabsorbs about 67% of the filtered K^+ under most conditions. Approximately 20% of the filtered K^+ is reabsorbed by the loop of Henle, and as with the proximal tubule, the amount reabsorbed is a constant fraction of the amount filtered. In contrast to these segments, which can only reabsorb K^+, the distal tubule and collecting duct are able to reabsorb or secrete K^+. The rate of K^+ reabsorption or secretion by the distal tubule and collecting duct depends on a variety of hormones and factors. When K^+ intake is normal (100 mEq/day), K^+ is secreted. A rise in dietary K^+ intake increases K^+ secretion. K^+ secretion can increase the amount of K^+ that appears in the urine so that it approaches 80% of the amount filtered (Figure 39–2). In contrast, a low-K^+ diet activates K^+ reabsorption along the distal tubule and collecting duct so that urinary excretion falls to about 1% of the K^+ filtered by the glomerulus (Figure 39–2). The kidneys cannot reduce K^+ excretion to the same low levels as they can for Na^+ (i.e., 0.2%). Therefore, hypokalemia can develop in individuals prescribed a K^+-deficient diet. Because the magnitude and direction of K^+ transport by the distal tubule and collecting duct are variable, the overall rate of urinary K^+ excretion is determined by these tubular segments.

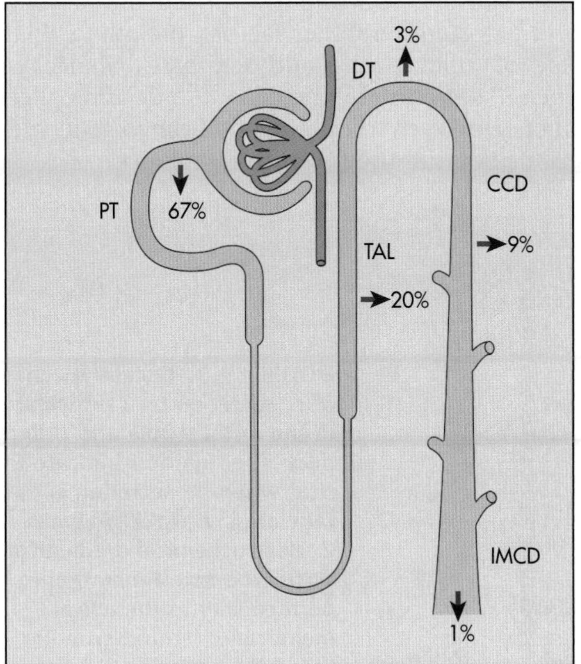

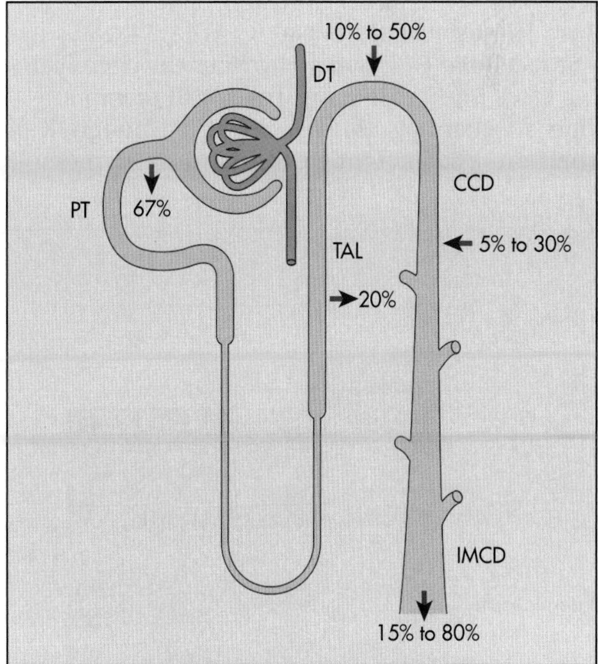

FIGURE 39–2. K^+ transport along the nephron. K^+ excretion depends on the rate and direction of K^+ transport by the distal tubule and collecting duct. Percentages refer to the amount of filtered K^+ reabsorbed or secreted by each nephron segment. *Left,* Dietary K^+ depletion. An amount of K^+ equal to 1% of the filtered load of K^+ is excreted. *Right,* Normal and increased dietary K^+ intake. An amount of K^+ equal to 15% to 80% of the filtered load is excreted. CCD, cortical collecting duct; DT, distal tubule; IMCD, inner medullary collecting duct; PT, proximal tubule; TAL, thick ascending limb.

In individuals with advanced **renal disease,** the kidneys are unable to eliminate K^+ from the body. The plasma [K^+] therefore rises. The resulting hyperkalemia reduces the resting membrane potential (i.e., the voltage becomes less negative), which decreases the excitability of neurons, cardiac cells, and muscle cells by inactivating fast Na^+ channels in the membrane. Severe, rapid increases in the plasma [K^+] can lead to cardiac arrest and death. In contrast, in patients taking diuretic drugs for hypertension, urinary K^+ excretion often exceeds dietary K^+ intake. Accordingly, the K^+ balance is negative, and hypokalemia develops. This decline in the extracellular [K^+] hyperpolarizes the resting cell membrane (i.e., the voltage becomes more negative) and reduces the excitability of neurons, cardiac cells, and muscle cells. Severe hypokalemia can lead to paralysis, cardiac arrhythmias, and death. Hypokalemia can also impair the ability of the kidneys to concentrate the urine and can stimulate the renal production of NH_4^+. Therefore, the maintenance of a high intracellular [K^+], a low extracellular [K^+] , and a high K^+ concentration gradient across cell membranes is essential for a number of cellular functions.

The cellular mechanism of K^+ secretion by principal cells in the distal tubule and collecting duct is a two-step process

The two processes of cellular K^+ secretion are (1) K^+ uptake from blood across the basolateral membrane by Na^+,K^+-ATPase and (2) diffusion of K^+ from the cell into the tubular fluid. Na^+,K^+-ATPase creates a high intracellular [K^+], which provides the chemical driving force for K^+ exit across the apical membrane through K^+ channels **(Figure 39–3)**. Although K^+ channels are also present in the basolateral membrane, K^+ preferentially leaves the cell across the apical membrane and enters the tubular fluid. K^+ transport follows this route for two reasons. First, the electrochemical gradient of K^+ across the apical membrane favors its downhill movement into the tubular fluid. Second, the permeability of the apical membrane to K^+ is greater than that of the basolateral membrane. Therefore, K^+ preferentially diffuses across the apical membrane into the tubular fluid. The three major factors that control the rate of K^+ secretion by the distal tubule and the collecting duct are

1. the activity of Na^+,K^+-ATPase;
2. the driving force (electrochemical gradient) for K^+ movement across the apical membrane; and
3. the permeability of the apical membrane to K^+.

Every change in K^+ secretion results from an alteration in one or more of these factors.

Intercalated cells reabsorb K^+ via an H^+,K^+-ATPase transport mechanism located in the apical membrane. This transporter mediates K^+ uptake in exchange for H^+. The pathway of K^+ exit from intercalated cells into the blood is unknown. The reabsorption of K^+ is activated by a low-K^+ diet.

THE REGULATION OF K^+ EXCRETION IS ACHIEVED MAINLY BY ALTERATIONS IN K^+ SECRETION BY PRINCIPAL CELLS OF THE DISTAL TUBULE AND COLLECTING DUCT. Plasma [K^+] and aldosterone are the major physiological regulators of K^+ secretion. Antidiuretic hormone (ADH) also stimulates K^+ secretion; however, it is less important than the plasma [K^+] and aldosterone. Other factors, including the flow rate of tubular fluid and acid-base balance, influence K^+ secretion by the distal tubule and collecting duct. However, they are not homeostatic mechanisms because they disturb K^+ balance.

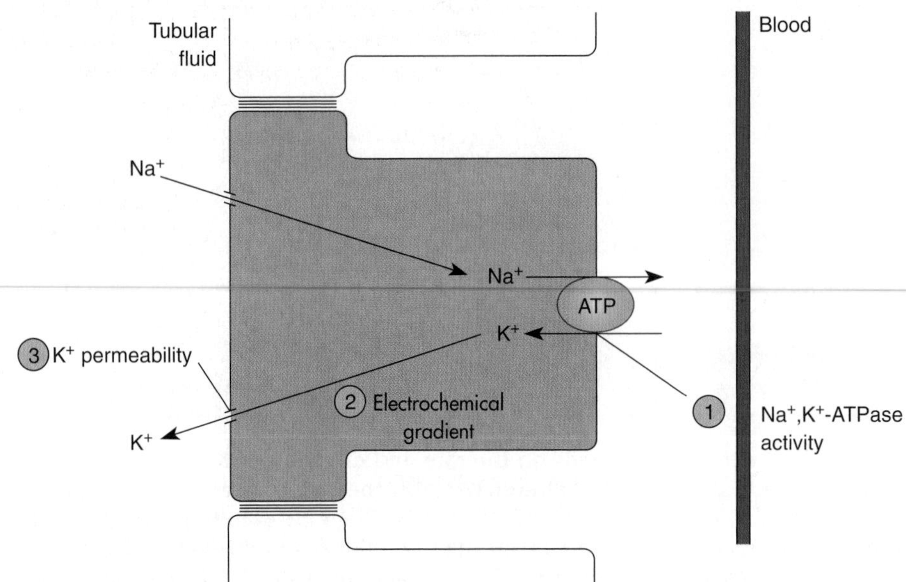

FIGURE 39–3. Cellular mechanism of K^+ secretion by a principal cell in the distal tubule and collecting duct. The numbers indicate the sites where K^+ secretion is regulated. 1, Na^+,K^+-ATPase; 2, electrochemical gradient of K^+ across the apical membrane; 3, K^+ permeability of the apical membrane. (From Berne RM, Levy MN, Koeppen BM, Stanton BA: *Physiology,* ed 5, Philadelphia, 2004, Elsevier.)

Hormones and the plasma [K^+] regulate urinary K^+ excretion

Plasma [K^+]

Plasma [K^+] is an important determinant of K^+ secretion by the distal tubule and collecting duct (**Box 39–2**). Hyperkalemia (e.g., resulting from a high-K^+ diet or from rhabdomyolysis) stimulates secretion within minutes. Several mechanisms are involved.

- Hyperkalemia stimulates Na^+,K^+-ATPase and thereby increases K^+ uptake across the basolateral membrane. This uptake raises the intracellular [K^+] and increases the electrochemical driving force for K^+ exit across the apical membrane.
- Hyperkalemia increases the permeability of the apical membrane to K^+.
- Hyperkalemia stimulates aldosterone secretion by the adrenal cortex, which, as discussed later, acts synergistically with the plasma [K^+] to stimulate K^+ secretion.
- Hyperkalemia increases the flow rate of tubular fluid, which, as discussed later, stimulates K^+ secretion by the distal tubule and collecting duct.

Hypokalemia (e.g., caused by a low-K^+ diet or diarrhea) decreases K^+ secretion via actions opposite to those described for hyperkalemia. Hence, hypokalemia inhibits Na^+,K^+-ATPase, decreases the electrochemical driving force for K^+ efflux across the apical membrane, reduces the permeability of the apical membrane to K^+, and reduces plasma aldosterone levels.

Chronic hypokalemia (plasma [K^+] < 3.5 mEq/L) occurs most often in patients who receive diuretics for hypertension. Hypokalemia also occurs in patients who vomit, have nasogastric suction, have diarrhea, abuse laxatives, or have hyperaldosteronism. Hypokalemia occurs because the excretion of K^+ by the kidneys exceeds the dietary intake of K^+. Vomiting, nasogastric suction, diuretics, and diarrhea can decrease the ECF, which in turn stimulates aldosterone secretion. Because aldosterone stimulates K^+ excretion by the kidneys, its action contributes to the development of hypokalemia.

Chronic hyperkalemia (plasma [K^+] > 5.0 mEq/L) occurs most frequently in individuals with reduced urine flow, low plasma aldosterone levels, and renal disease in which the glomerular filtration rate falls to below 20% of normal. In these individuals, hyperkalemia occurs because the excretion of K^+ by the kidneys is less than the dietary intake of K^+. Less common causes for hyperkalemia occur in people with deficiencies of insulin, epinephrine, and aldosterone secretion or in people with metabolic acidosis caused by inorganic acids.

BOX 39–2: MAJOR FACTORS AND HORMONES INFLUENCING K^+ EXCRETION

Physiological: keep K^+ balance constant
- Plasma [K^+]
- Aldosterone
- ADH

Pathophysiological: displace K^+ balance
- Flow rate of tubule fluid
- Acid-base balance
- Glucocorticoids

Aldosterone

A chronic (i.e., ≥24 hours) elevation in the plasma aldosterone concentration enhances K^+ secretion across principal cells in the distal tubule and collecting duct by five mechanisms:

1. increasing the amount of Na^+,K^+-ATPase in the basolateral membrane;
2. increasing the expression of the Na^+ channel (ENaC) in the apical cell membrane;
3. elevating serum glucocorticoid-stimulated kinase (SGK) levels, which also increases the expression of ENaC;
4. stimulating channel-activating protease (CAP1, also called prostatin), which directly activates ENaC; and
5. stimulating the permeability of the apical membrane to K^+.

Taken together, these actions increase the cell [K^+] and enhance the driving force for K^+ exit across the apical membrane. Aldosterone secretion is increased by hyperkalemia and by angiotensin II (after activation of the renin-angiotensin system). Aldosterone secretion is decreased by hypokalemia and natriuretic peptides released from the heart (see Chapter 37).

Although an acute (i.e., within hours) increase in aldosterone levels enhances the activity of Na^+,K^+-ATPase, K^+ excretion does not increase. The reason for this lack of increase relates to the effect of aldosterone on Na^+ reabsorption and tubular flow. Aldosterone stimulates Na^+ reabsorption and thereby water reabsorption and thus decreases tubular flow. The decrease in flow in turn decreases K^+ secretion (as discussed in more detail later). However, chronic stimulation of Na^+ reabsorption expands the ECF and thereby returns tubular flow to normal. These actions allow the direct stimulatory effect of aldosterone on the distal tubule and collecting duct to enhance K^+ excretion.

Antidiuretic hormone

ADH increases the electrochemical driving force for K^+ exit across the apical membrane of principal cells by stimulating Na^+ uptake across the apical membrane of principal cells. The increased Na^+ uptake reduces the electrical potential difference across the apical membrane (i.e., the interior of the cell becomes less negatively charged). Despite this effect, ADH does not change K^+ secretion by these nephron segments. The reason for this relates to the effect of ADH on tubular fluid flow. ADH decreases tubular fluid flow by stimulating water reabsorption. The decrease in tubular flow in turn decreases K^+ secretion (explained later). The inhibitory effect of a decreased flow of tubular fluid offsets the stimulatory effect of ADH on the electrochemical driving force for K^+ exit across the apical membrane. If ADH did not increase the electrochemical gradient favoring K^+ secretion, urinary K^+ excretion would fall as ADH levels increase and urinary flow rates decrease. Hence, K^+ balance would change in response to alterations in water balance. Thus, the effects of ADH on the electrochemical driving force for K^+ exit across the apical membrane and tubule flow enable urinary K^+ excretion to be maintained constant despite wide fluctuations in water excretion.

K^+ excretion is perturbed by changes in the flow of tubular fluid and disorders of acid-base balance

Although plasma [K^+], aldosterone, and ADH play important roles in regulating K^+ balance, the factors and hormones discussed next perturb K^+ balance (Box 39–2).

Flow of tubular fluid

A rise in the flow of tubular fluid (e.g., with diuretic treatment, ECF volume expansion) stimulates K^+ secretion within minutes, whereas a fall (e.g., ECF volume contraction caused by hemorrhage, severe vomiting, or diarrhea) reduces K^+ secretion by the distal tubule and collecting duct. Increments in tubular fluid flow are more effective in stimulating K^+ secretion as dietary K^+ intake is increased. Alterations in tubular fluid flow influence K^+ secretion by four mechanisms.

1. As flow increases, for example, after the administration of diuretics or as the result of an increase in the ECF volume, so does the [Na^+] of tubule fluid. This increase in [Na^+] facilitates Na^+ entry across the apical membrane of distal tubule and collecting duct cells, thereby decreasing the cell interior negative membrane potential. Depolarization of the cell membrane potential increases the electrochemical driving force that promotes K^+ secretion across the apical cell membrane.
2. Increased Na^+ uptake into cells activates the Na^+,K^+-ATPase in the basolateral membrane, thereby increasing K^+ uptake across the basolateral membrane.
3. An increase in tubule flow enhances the K^+ permeability of the apical plasma membrane by an unknown mechanism. The increase in K^+ uptake across the basolateral membrane and in the K^+ permeability of the apical plasma membrane enhances K^+ secretion.
4. An increase in tubule flow minimizes the rise in tubular fluid [K^+] as the secreted K^+ is washed downstream.

Therefore, because of these four mechanisms, K^+ secretion increases as flow rises. However, an increase in flow rate during a water diuresis does not have a significant effect on K^+ excretion, primarily because during a water diuresis, the [Na^+] of tubule fluid does not increase as flow rises.

Acid-base balance

Another factor that modulates K^+ secretion is the [H^+] of the ECF. Acute alterations (within minutes to hours) in the pH of the plasma influence K^+ secretion by the distal tubule and collecting duct. Alkalosis (i.e., a plasma pH above normal) increases K^+ secretion, whereas acidosis (i.e., a plasma pH below normal) decreases it. An acute acidosis reduces K^+ secretion via two mechanisms: (1) it inhibits Na^+,K^+-ATPase and thereby reduces the cell [K^+] and the electrochemical driving force for K^+ exit across the apical membrane, and (2) it reduces the permeability of the apical membrane to K^+. Alkalosis has the opposite effects.

The effect of metabolic acidosis on K^+ excretion is time dependent. When metabolic acidosis lasts for several days, urinary K^+ excretion is stimulated. This occurs because chronic metabolic acidosis decreases the reabsorption of water and solute (e.g., NaCl) by the proximal tubule by inhibiting Na^+,K^+-ATPase. Hence, the flow of tubular fluid is augmented through the distal tubule and collecting duct. The inhibition of proximal tubular water and NaCl reabsorption also decreases the ECF volume and thereby stimulates aldosterone secretion. In addition, chronic acidosis, caused by inorganic acids, increases the plasma [K^+], which stimulates aldosterone secretion. The rise in tubular fluid flow, plasma [K^+], and aldosterone levels offsets the effects of acidosis on the cell [K^+] and apical membrane permeability, and K^+ secretion rises. Thus, metabolic acidosis may either inhibit or stimulate K^+ excretion, depending on the duration of the disturbance. Renal K^+ excretion remains elevated during chronic metabolic acidosis and may even increase further, depending on the cause of the acidosis.

Glucocorticoids

Glucocorticoids also stimulate K^+ excretion. However, this effect is indirect and is mediated by an increase in the glomerular filtration rate, which increases tubular flow.

As discussed earlier, the rate of urinary K^+ excretion is frequently determined by simultaneous changes in hormone levels, acid-base balance, or flow (Table 39–1). The powerful effect of flow often enhances or opposes the response of the distal tubule and collecting duct to hormones and changes in acid-base balance. This interaction can be beneficial in the case of hyperkalemia, in which the change in flow enhances K^+ excretion and thereby restores K^+ homeostasis. However, this interaction can also be detrimental, as in the case of alkalosis, in which changes in flow and acid-base status alter K^+ homeostasis.

Ca^{++} and Pi Are Multivalent Ions That Have Many Complex and Vital Functions

In a normal adult, the renal excretion of Ca^{++} and Pi is balanced by gastrointestinal absorption. If the plasma concentrations decline substantially, gastrointestinal absorption, bone resorption (i.e., loss of Ca^{++} and Pi from bone), and renal tubular reabsorption increase and return plasma concentrations of Ca^{++} and Pi to normal levels. During growth and during pregnancy, intestinal absorption exceeds urinary excretion, and these ions accumulate in newly formed fetal tissue and bone. In contrast, bone disease (e.g., **osteoporosis**) or a decline in lean body mass increases urinary loss of multivalent ions (i.e., Ca^{++} and Pi) without a change in intestinal absorption. In these conditions, Ca^{++} and Pi are lost from the body. IN CONJUNCTION WITH THE GASTROINTESTINAL TRACT AND BONES, THE KIDNEYS PLAY A MAJOR ROLE IN MAINTAINING PLASMA Ca^{++} AND Pi LEVELS.

Ca^{++} plays a major role in many cellular processes

Cellular processes in which Ca^{++} plays a part include bone formation, cell division and growth, blood coagulation, hormone-response coupling, and electrical stimulus–response coupling (e.g., muscle contraction, neurotransmitter release). A total of 99% of Ca^{++} is stored in bone, approximately 1% is found in the intracellular fluid (ICF), and 0.1% is located in the ECF. The total [Ca^{++}] in plasma is 10 mg/dL (2.5 mM or 5 mEq/L), and the concentration of Ca^{++} is normally maintained within very narrow limits. A low ionized plasma [Ca^{++}] **(hypocalcemia)** increases the excitability of nerve and muscle cells and can lead to hypocalcemic **tetany,** which is characterized by skeletal muscle spasms. An elevated ionized plasma [Ca^{++}] **(hypercalcemia)** may decrease neuromuscular excitability or produce cardiac arrhythmias, lethargy, disorientation, and even death. Within cells, Ca^{++} is sequestered in the endoplasmic reticulum and mitochondria or is bound to proteins. Thus, intracellular [Ca^{++}] is very low (0.1 to 1 μM). The large concentration gradient for Ca^{++} across cell membranes is maintained by a Ca^{++}-ATPase pump in all cells and by a $3Na^+$-$1Ca^{++}$ antiporter in some cells.

Ca^{++} HOMEOSTASIS DEPENDS ON TWO FACTORS: (1) THE TOTAL AMOUNT OF Ca^{++} IN THE BODY AND (2) THE DISTRIBUTION OF Ca^{++} BETWEEN BONE AND THE ECF. The total body Ca^{++} level is determined by the relative amounts of Ca^{++} absorbed by the gastrointestinal tract and excreted by the kidneys **(Figure 39–4).** Ca^{++} is absorbed by the gastrointestinal tract through an active, carrier-mediated transport mechanism that is stimulated by **calcitriol,** a metabolite of vitamin D_3 (see also Chapters 35 and 44). Net Ca^{++} absorption is normally 200 mg/day, but it can increase to 600 mg/day when calcitriol levels rise. In adults, Ca^{++} excretion by the kidneys equals the amount absorbed by the gastrointestinal tract (200 mg/day), and it changes in parallel with the reabsorption of Ca^{++} by the gastrointestinal tract. Thus, in adults, Ca^{++} balance is maintained because the amount of Ca^{++} ingested in an average diet (1500 mg/day) equals the amount lost in the feces (1300 mg/day, the amount that escapes absorption by the gastrointestinal tract) plus the amount excreted in the urine (200 mg/day).

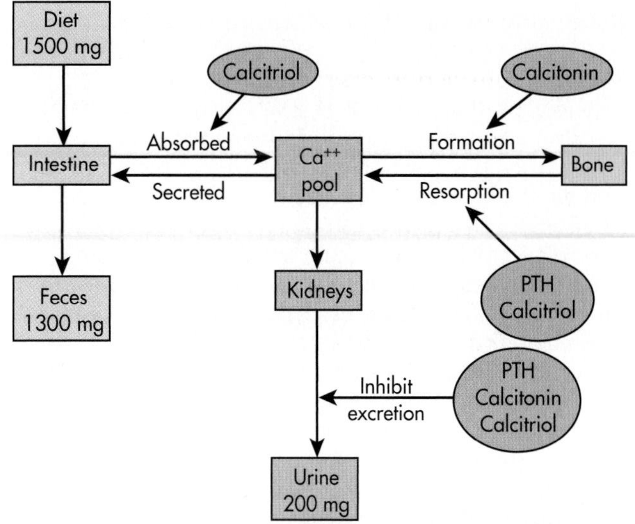

FIGURE 39–4. Overview of Ca^{++} homeostasis. PTH, parathyroid hormone. See text for details.

The second factor that controls Ca^{++} homeostasis is the distribution of Ca^{++} between bone and the ECF. THREE HORMONES (PARATHYROID HORMONE, CALCITRIOL, AND CALCITONIN) REGULATE THE DISTRIBUTION OF Ca^{++} BETWEEN BONE AND THE ECF AND THEREBY REGULATE THE PLASMA [Ca^{++}]. In humans, however, calcitonin may not participate significantly in Ca^{++} homeostasis. Parathyroid hormone (PTH) is secreted by the parathyroid glands, and its secretion is stimulated by a decline in the plasma [Ca^{++}] (i.e., hypocalcemia). Hypocalcemia stimulates the calcium-sensing receptor (CaSR) in the plasma membrane of parathyroid glands, which in turn increases PTH gene expression and release. PTH increases the plasma [Ca^{++}] by stimulating bone resorption, increasing Ca^{++} reabsorption by the kidneys, and stimulating the production of calcitriol, which in turn increases Ca^{++} absorption by the gastrointestinal tract and facilitates PTH-mediated bone resorption. The production of calcitriol, a metabolite of vitamin D_3 produced in the kidney proximal tubule, is stimulated by hypocalcemia and hypophosphatemia. In addition, hypocalcemia stimulates PTH secretion, which also stimulates vitamin D_3 production by the proximal tubule cells. Calcitriol increases the plasma [Ca^{++}] primarily by stimulating Ca^{++} absorption from the gastrointestinal tract. It also facilitates the action of PTH on bone and increases the expression of key Ca^{++} transport and binding proteins in the kidneys. Calcitonin is secreted by thyroid C cells, and its secretion is stimulated by hypercalcemia. Calcitonin decreases the plasma [Ca^{++}] mainly by stimulating bone formation (i.e., deposition of Ca^{++} in bone). **Figure 39–5** illustrates the relationship between the plasma [Ca^{++}] and plasma levels of PTH and calcitonin. As already noted, calcitonin does not play a major role in Ca^{++} homeostasis in humans.

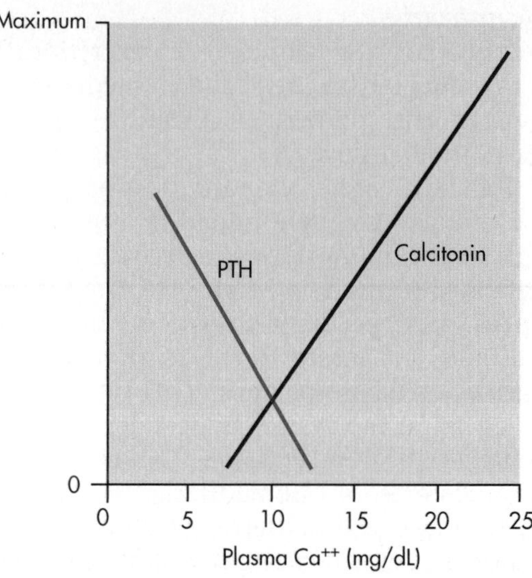

FIGURE 39–5. Effect of the plasma [Ca^{++}] on plasma levels of PTH and calcitonin. (Data from Azria M: *The calcitonins: physiology and pharmacology,* Basel, Switzerland, 1989, Karger.)

Conditions that lower PTH levels (e.g., hypoparathyroidism after parathyroidectomy for an adenoma) reduce the plasma [Ca^{++}], which can cause hypocalcemic tetany (intermittent muscle contractions). In severe cases, **hypocalcemic tetany** can cause death by asphyxiation. Hypercalcemia can also cause lethal cardiac arrhythmias and decreased neuromuscular excitability. Clinically, the most common causes of hypercalcemia are primary hyperparathyroidism and malignancy-associated hypercalcemia. Primary hyperparathyroidism results from the overproduction of PTH caused by a tumor of the parathyroid glands. In contrast, malignancy-associated hypercalcemia, which occurs in 10% to 20% of all patients with cancer, is caused by the secretion of **parathyroid hormone–related peptide** (PTHrP), a PTH-like hormone secreted by carcinomas in various organs. Increased levels of PTH and PTHrP cause hypercalcemia and hypercalciuria.

Approximately 50% of the Ca^{++} in plasma is ionized; 45% is bound to plasma proteins (mainly albumin); and 5% is complexed to several anions, including HCO_3^-, citrate, Pi, and $SO_4^=$. The pH of plasma influences this distribution. Acidosis increases the percentage of ionized Ca^{++} at the expense of Ca^{++} bound to proteins, whereas alkalosis decreases the percentage of ionized Ca^{++}, again by altering the Ca^{++} bound to proteins. Individuals with alkalosis are susceptible to tetany, whereas individuals with acidosis are less susceptible to tetany, even when total plasma Ca^{++} levels are reduced. The increase in the [H^+] in patients with metabolic acidosis causes more H^+ to bind to plasma proteins, HCO_3^-, citrate, Pi, and $SO_4^=$, thereby displacing Ca^{++}. This displacement increases the plasma concentration of ionized Ca^{++}. In alkalosis, the [H^+] of plasma decreases. Some H^+ ions dissociate from plasma proteins, HCO_3^-, citrate, Pi, and $SO_4^=$ in exchange for Ca^{++}, thereby decreasing the plasma concentration of ionized Ca^{++}. In addition, the plasma albumin concentration also affects ionized plasma [Ca^{++}]. Hypoalbuminemia increases the ionized [Ca^{++}], whereas hyperalbuminemia decreases ionized plasma [Ca^{++}]. Under both conditions, the total plasma [Ca^{++}] may not reflect the total ionized [Ca^{++}], which is the physiological relevant measure of Ca^{++} homeostasis. The Ca^{++} available for glomerular filtration consists of the ionized fraction and the amount complexed with anions. Thus, about 55% of the Ca^{++} in the plasma is available for glomerular filtration.

Ca^{++} is reabsorbed along the nephron

Normally, 99% of the filtered Ca^{++} (i.e., ionized and complexed) is reabsorbed by the nephron. The proximal tubule reabsorbs about 70% of the filtered Ca^{++}. Another 20% is reabsorbed in the loop of Henle (mainly the cortical portion of the thick ascending limb), about 9% is reabsorbed by the distal tubule, and less than 1% is reabsorbed by the collecting duct. About 1% (200 mg/day) is excreted in the urine. This fraction is equal to the net amount absorbed daily by the gastrointestinal tract. **Figure 39–6** summarizes the handling of Ca^{++} by the different portions of the nephron.

Ca^{++} reabsorption by the proximal tubule occurs via two pathways: transcellular and paracellular. Ca^{++} reabsorption across the cellular pathway accounts for 20% of proximal reabsorption. Ca^{++} reabsorption through the cell is an active process that occurs in two steps. First, Ca^{++} diffuses down its electrochemical gradient across the apical membrane through Ca^{++} channels and into the cell. Second, Ca^{++} is extruded across the basolateral membrane against its electrochemical gradient. The extrusion of Ca^{++} across the basolateral membrane is thought to occur by a Ca^{++}-ATPase. A total of 80% of Ca^{++} is reabsorbed between cells across the tight junctions (i.e., paracellular pathway). This passive, paracellular reabsorption of Ca^{++} occurs via solvent drag along the entire length of the proximal tubule and is also driven by the positive luminal voltage in the second half of the proximal tubule (i.e., diffusion). Thus, approximately 80% of Ca^{++} reabsorption is paracellular and approximately 20% is transcellular in the proximal tubule.

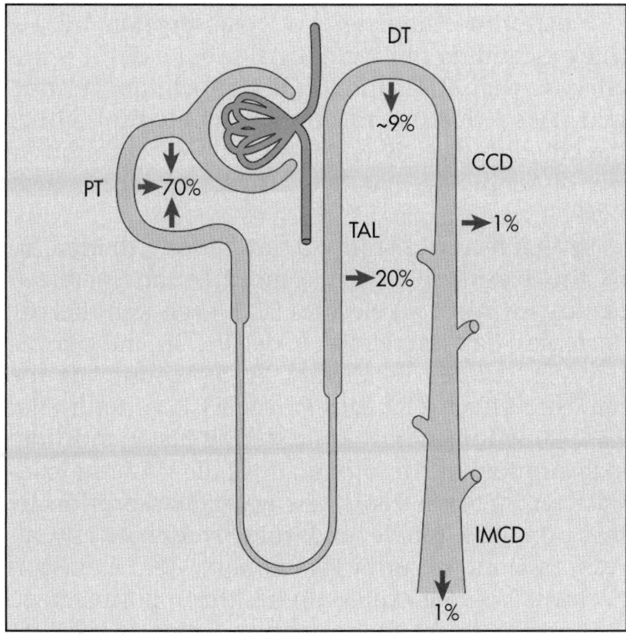

FIGURE 39–6. Ca^{++} transport along the nephron. Percentages refer to the amount of the filtered Ca^{++} reabsorbed by each segment. Approximately 1% of the filtered Ca^{++} is excreted. CCD, cortical collecting duct; DT, distal tubule; IMCD, inner medullary collecting duct; PT, proximal tubule; TAL, thick ascending limb.

Ca^{++} reabsorption by the loop of Henle is restricted to the cortical portion of the thick ascending limb. Ca^{++} is reabsorbed by cellular and paracellular routes via mechanisms similar to those described for the proximal tubule but with one difference. Ca^{++} is not reabsorbed by solvent drag in this segment. (The thick ascending limb is impermeable to water.) In the thick ascending limb, Ca^{++} reabsorption and Na^{+} reabsorption parallel each other. These processes are parallel because of the significant component of Ca^{++} reabsorption that occurs via passive paracellular mechanisms secondary to Na^{+} reabsorption and via the generation of the lumen-positive transepithelial voltage. Loop diuretics inhibit Na^{+} reabsorption by the thick ascending limb of the loop of Henle and in so doing reduce the magnitude of the lumen-positive transepithelial voltage (see Chapter 37). This action in turn inhibits the reabsorption of Ca^{++} via the paracellular pathway. Thus, loop diuretics are used to increase renal Ca^{++} excretion in patients with hypercalcemia. Therefore, Na^{+} reabsorption also changes in parallel with Ca^{++} reabsorption by both the proximal tubule and the thick ascending limb of the loop of Henle. Familial hypomagnesemic hypercalcemia is caused by mutations in claudin-16, a protein that is a component of the tight junctions in thick ascending limb cells. This disorder is characterized by enhanced excretion of Ca^{++} and Mg^{++} due to a fall in the passive reabsorption of these ions across the paracellular pathway in the thick ascending limb. The mutation in the claudin-16 gene reduces the permeability of the paracellular pathway to Ca^{++} and Mg^{++}, thereby reducing passive, paracellular reabsorption of both ions.

In the distal tubule, where the voltage in the tubule lumen is electrically negative with respect to the blood, Ca^{++} reabsorption is entirely active because Ca^{++} is reabsorbed against its electrochemical gradient. Ca^{++} reabsorption by the distal tubule is exclusively transcellular. Calcium enters the cell across the apical membrane by the Ca^{++}-permeable epithelial ion channel (ECaCl) and is extruded across the basolateral membrane by Ca^{++}-ATPase and the $3Na^{+}$-$1Ca^{++}$ antiporter. Na^{+} excretion and Ca^{++} excretion usually change in parallel. However, these processes are not always parallel because the

TABLE 39–2. SUMMARY OF HORMONES AND FACTORS AFFECTING CA^{++} REABSORPTION

	Nephron Location		
Factor or Hormone	PROXIMAL TUBULE	THICK ASCENDING LIMB	DISTAL TUBULE
Volume expansion	Decrease	No change	Decrease
Hypercalcemia	Decrease	Decrease (CaSR)	Decrease (PTH)
Hypocalcemia	Increase	Increase	
Phosphate loading			Increase (PTH)
Phosphate depletion	Decrease		Decrease (PTH)
Acidosis	Decrease		Decrease
Alkalosis	Increase		
PTH	Increase	Increase	Increase
Vitamin D			Increase
Calcitonin		Increase	Increase

CaSR, calcium-sensing receptor.
Data from Yu AS: Renal transport of calcium, magnesium, and phosphate. In Brenner BM, ed: *Brenner and Rector's the kidney,* ed 7, Philadelphia, 2004, WB Saunders.

reabsorption of Ca^{++} and Na^{+} by the distal tubule is independent and is differentially regulated. For example, **thiazide diuretics** inhibit Na^{+} reabsorption by the distal tubule and stimulate Ca^{++} reabsorption by this segment. Accordingly, the net effects of thiazide diuretics are to increase urinary Na^{+} excretion and to reduce urinary Ca^{++} excretion.

PTH is the most important regulator of renal Ca^{++} excretion

Several hormones and factors influence urinary Ca^{++} excretion **(Table 39–2)**. OF THESE, PTH EXERTS THE MOST POWERFUL CONTROL ON RENAL Ca^{++} EXCRETION, AND IT IS RESPONSIBLE FOR MAINTAINING Ca^{++} HOMEOSTASIS. Overall, this hormone stimulates Ca^{++} reabsorption by the kidneys (i.e., reduces Ca^{++} excretion). Although PTH inhibits the reabsorption of NaCl and fluid and therefore of Ca^{++} by the proximal tubule, PTH stimulates Ca^{++} reabsorption by the thick ascending limb of the loop of Henle and the distal tubule. In humans, this effect is greater in the distal tubule. Changes in the ECF $[Ca^{++}]$ also regulate urinary Ca^{++} excretion, with hypercalcemia increasing excretion and hypocalcemia decreasing excretion. Hypercalcemia increases urinary Ca^{++} excretion by reducing proximal tubule Ca^{++} reabsorption (reduced paracellular reabsorption due to increased interstitial fluid $[Ca^{++}]$), inhibiting Ca^{++} reabsorption by the thick ascending limb of the loop of Henle via activation of the CaSR located in the basolateral membrane of these cells (the activity of the $1Na^{+},1K^{+},2Cl^{-}$ symporter is decreased, thereby reducing the magnitude of the lumen-positive transepithelial voltage), and suppressing Ca^{++} reabsorption by the distal tubule by reducing PTH levels. As a result, urinary Ca^{++} excretion declines.

Calcitonin stimulates Ca^{++} reabsorption by the thick ascending limb and distal tubule, but it is less effective than PTH, and it is not known how important this effect is in humans. Calcitriol either directly or indirectly enhances Ca^{++} reabsorption by the distal tubule, but it is also less effective than PTH.

Several factors disturb Ca^{++} excretion. An increase in the plasma [Pi] (e.g., caused by an increased dietary intake of Pi) elevates PTH levels and thereby decreases Ca^{++} excretion. A decline in the plasma [Pi] (e.g., caused by dietary Pi depletion) has the opposite effect. Changes in the ECF volume alter Ca^{++} excretion mainly by affecting NaCl and fluid reabsorption in the proximal tubule. Volume contraction increases NaCl and water reabsorption by the proximal tubule and thereby enhances Ca^{++} reabsorption. Accordingly, urinary Ca^{++} excretion declines. Volume expansion has the opposite effect. Acidosis increases Ca^{++} excretion, whereas alkalosis decreases excretion. The regulation of Ca^{++} reabsorption by pH occurs in the distal tubule. Alkalosis stimulates ECaCl, thereby increasing Ca^{++} reabsorption. By contrast, acidosis inhibits ECaCl, thereby reducing Ca^{++} reabsorption.

Mutations in the gene coding for the CaSR cause disorders in Ca^{++} homeostasis. Familial hypocalciuric hypercalcemia is an autosomal dominant disease caused by an inactivating mutation of CaSR. The hypercalcemia is caused by deranged Ca^{++}-regulated PTH secretion (i.e., PTH levels are elevated at any level of plasma [Ca^{++}]). The hypocalcemia is caused by enhanced Ca^{++} reabsorption in the thick ascending limb and distal tubule due to elevated PTH levels and defective CaSR regulation of Ca^{++} transport in the kidneys. Autosomal dominant hypocalcemia is caused by an activating mutation in CaSR. Activation of CaSRs causes deranged Ca^{++}-regulated PTH secretion (i.e., PTH levels are decreased at any level of plasma [Ca^{++}]). Hypercalciuria results and is caused by decreased PTH levels and defective CaSR-regulated Ca^{++} transport in the kidneys.

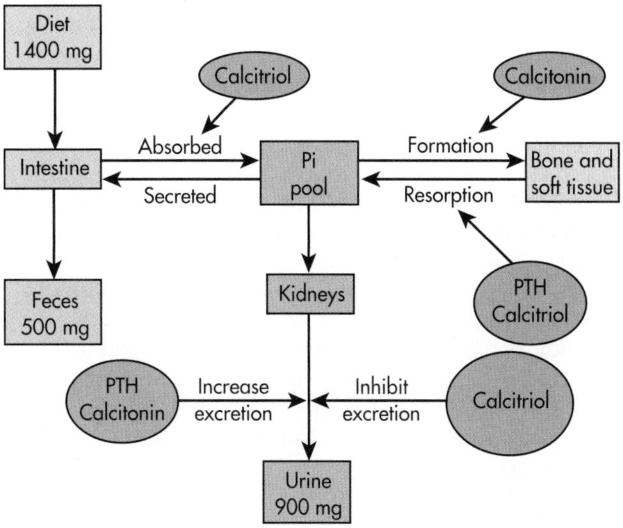

FIGURE 39–7. Overview of Pi homeostasis. See text for details.

Pi is an important component of many organic molecules

Pi is an important component of many organic molecules, including DNA, RNA, ATP, and intermediates of metabolic pathways. It is also a major constituent of bone. Its concentration in plasma is an important determinant of bone formation and resorption. In addition, urinary Pi is an important buffer (titratable acid) for the maintenance of acid-base balance (see Chapter 40). A total of 86% of Pi is located in bone, approximately 14% is located in the ICF, and 0.03% is located in the ECF. The normal plasma [Pi] is 4 mg/dL. Approximately 10% of the Pi in the plasma is protein bound and is therefore unavailable for ultrafiltration by the glomerulus. Accordingly, the [Pi] in the ultrafiltrate is 10% less than that in plasma.

A general scheme of Pi homeostasis is shown in **Figure 39–7**. The maintenance of Pi homeostasis depends on two factors: (1) the amount of Pi in the body and (2) the distribution of Pi between the ICF and ECF compartments. Total body Pi levels are determined by the relative amount of Pi absorbed by the gastrointestinal tract versus the amount excreted by the kidneys. Pi absorption by the gastrointestinal tract occurs via active and passive mechanisms; Pi absorption increases as dietary Pi rises, and it is stimulated by calcitriol. Despite variations in Pi intake between 800 and 1500 mg/day, the kidneys keep the total body Pi balance constant by excreting an amount of Pi in the urine equal to the amount absorbed by the gastrointestinal tract. Thus, renal Pi excretion is the primary mechanism by which the body regulates Pi balance and thereby Pi homeostasis.

The second factor that maintains Pi homeostasis is the distribution of Pi among bone and the ICF and ECF compartments. PTH, calcitriol, and calcitonin regulate the distribution of Pi between bone and the ECF. As with Ca^{++} homeostasis, calcitonin is the least important of the hormones involved in Pi homeostasis in humans. The release of Pi from bone is stimulated by the same hormones (i.e., PTH, calcitriol) that release Ca^{++} from this pool. Thus, the release of Pi is always accompanied by a release of Ca^{++}. In contrast, calcitonin increases bone formation and thereby decreases the plasma [Pi].

THE KIDNEYS ALSO MAKE AN IMPORTANT CONTRIBUTION TO THE REGULATION OF THE PLASMA [Pi]. A small rise in the plasma [Pi] increases the amount of Pi filtered by the glomerulus. Because the kidneys normally reabsorb Pi at a maximum rate, any increase in the amount filtered leads to a rise in urinary Pi excretion. In fact, an increase in the amount of Pi filtered enhances urinary Pi excretion to a value greater than the rate of Pi absorption by the gastrointestinal tract. This process results in a net loss of Pi from the body and decreases plasma [Pi]. In this way, the kidneys regulate the plasma [Pi]. The maximum reabsorptive rate for Pi varies and is regulated by dietary Pi intake. A high-Pi diet decreases the maximum reabsorptive rate of Pi by the kidneys, and a low-Pi diet increases it. This effect is independent of changes in PTH levels.

In patients with **chronic renal failure,** the kidneys cannot excrete Pi. Because of continued Pi absorption by the gastrointestinal tract, Pi accumulates in the body, and the plasma [Pi] rises. The excess Pi forms complexes with Ca^{++} and reduces the plasma [Ca^{++}]. Pi accumulation also decreases the production of calcitriol. This response reduces Ca^{++} absorption by the intestine, an effect that further reduces the plasma [Ca^{++}]. This reduction in plasma [Ca^{++}] increases PTH secretion and Ca^{++} release from bone. These actions result in **osteitis fibrosa cystica** (i.e., increased bone resorption with replacement by fibrous tissue, which renders bone more susceptible to fracture). Chronic hyperparathyroidism (i.e., elevated PTH levels) during chronic renal failure can lead to metastatic calcifications in which Ca^{++} and Pi precipitate in arteries, soft tissues, and viscera (see also Chapter 44). The deposition of Ca^{++} and Pi in heart and lung tissue may cause myocardial failure and pulmonary insufficiency, respectively. The prevention and treatment of hyperparathyroidism and Pi retention include a low-Pi diet or the administration of a "phosphate binder" (i.e., an agent that forms insoluble Pi salts and thereby renders Pi unavailable for absorption by the gastrointestinal tract). Supplemental Ca^{++} and calcitriol are also prescribed.

Figure 39–8 summarizes Pi transport by the various portions of the nephron. The proximal tubule reabsorbs 80% of the Pi filtered by the glomerulus, and the distal tubule reabsorbs 10%. In contrast, the loop of Henle and the collecting duct reabsorb negligible amounts of Pi. Therefore, approximately 10% of the filtered load of Pi is excreted.

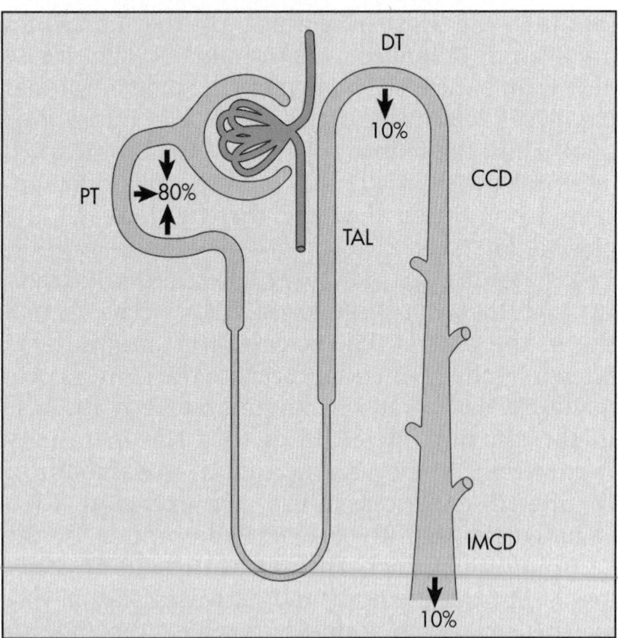

FIGURE 39–8. Pi transport along the nephron. Pi is reabsorbed primarily by the proximal tubule. Percentages refer to the amount of the filtered Pi reabsorbed by each nephron segment. Approximately 10% of the filtered Pi is excreted. CCD, cortical collecting duct; DT, distal tubule; IMCD, inner medullary collecting duct; PT, proximal tubule; TAL, thick ascending limb.

Pi reabsorption by the proximal tubule occurs mainly, if not exclusively, via a transcellular route. Pi uptake across the apical membrane occurs via Na^+-Pi symport mechanisms. Three symporters have been identified; one transports $2Na^+$ with each Pi (type I); the other two transport $3Na^+$ with each Pi (types II and III). The type II symporter is the most important symporter involved in Pi reabsorption by the proximal tubule. Pi exits across the basolateral membrane by a Pi–inorganic anion antiporter. The cellular mechanism of Pi reabsorption by the distal tubule has not been characterized.

PTH is the most important hormone that controls Pi excretion

Several hormones and factors regulate urinary Pi excretion **(Table 39–3)**. PTH, the most important hormone that controls Pi excretion, inhibits Pi reabsorption by the proximal tubule and thereby increases Pi excretion. Dietary Pi intake also regulates Pi excretion by mechanisms unrelated to changes in PTH levels. Pi loading increases excretion, whereas Pi depletion decreases it. Changes in dietary Pi intake modulate Pi transport by altering the transport rate of the type II symporter and by increasing the number of transporters.

ECF volume also affects Pi excretion. Volume expansion increases excretion, and volume contraction decreases it. The effect of ECF volume on Pi excretion is indirect and may involve changes in the levels of hormones other than PTH. Acid-base balance also influences Pi excretion; acidosis increases Pi excretion, and alkalosis decreases it.

TABLE 39–3. SUMMARY OF HORMONES AND FACTORS AFFECTING Pi REABSORPTION BY THE PROXIMAL TUBULE

Factor or Hormone	Proximal Tubule Reabsorption
Volume expansion	Decrease
Hypercalcemia: acute	Increase
Hypercalcemia: chronic	Decrease
Phosphate loading	Decrease
Phosphate depletion	Increase
Metabolic acidosis: chronic	Decrease
Metabolic alkalosis: chronic	Increase
PTH	Decrease
Vitamin D: acute	Increase
Vitamin D: chronic	Decrease

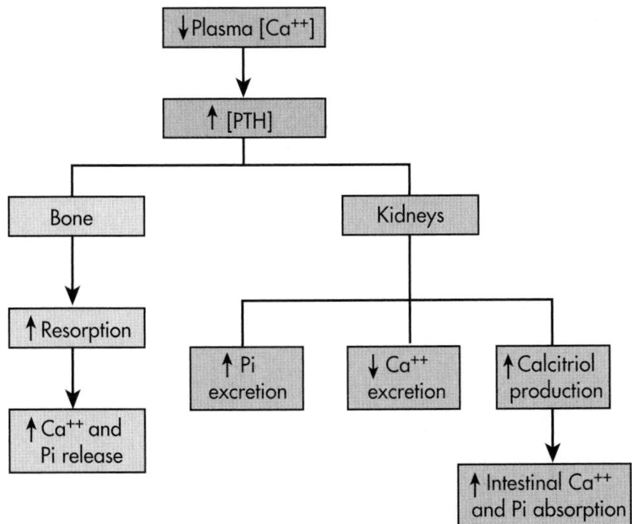

FIGURE 39–9. Effect of PTH on Ca^{++} and Pi homeostasis. The major stimulus of PTH secretion is hypocalcemia. (Data from Rose BD, Rennke HG, eds: *Renal pathophysiology: the essentials,* Baltimore, 1994, Williams & Wilkins.)

Glucocorticoids increase the excretion of Pi. Glucocorticoids increase the delivery of Pi to the distal tubule and collecting duct by inhibiting Pi reabsorption by the proximal tubule. This inhibition enables the distal tubule and collecting duct to secrete more H^+ and to generate more HCO_3^- because Pi is an important urinary buffer (see Chapter 40). Finally, growth hormone decreases Pi excretion. The phosphatonins, including fibroblast growth factor 23 (FGF-23) and frizzled-related protein 4 (FRP-4), are hormones produced by tumors in patients with osteomalacia and inhibit renal Pi reabsorption.

In the absence of glucocorticoids (e.g., in **Addison's disease**), Pi excretion is depressed, as is the ability of the kidneys to excrete titratable acid and to generate new HCO_3^-. Growth hormone also has an important effect on Pi homeostasis. Growth hormone increases the reabsorption of Pi by the proximal tubule. As a result, growing children have a higher plasma [Pi] than adults do, and this elevated [Pi] is important for the formation of bone.

Integrative review of PTH, calcitriol, and calcitonin in Ca^{++} and Pi homeostasis

Hypocalcemia is the major stimulus of PTH secretion. As summarized in **Figure 39–9**, PTH has numerous effects on Ca^{++} and Pi homeostasis. PTH stimulates bone resorption, increases urinary Pi excretion, decreases urinary Ca^{++} excretion, and stimulates the production of calcitriol, which stimulates Ca^{++} and Pi absorption by the intestine. Because changes in Pi handling in bone, the intestines, and the kidneys tend to balance out, PTH increases the plasma [Ca^{++}] while having little effect on the plasma [Pi]. Overall, a rise in the plasma PTH levels increases the plasma [Ca^{++}] and decreases the plasma [Pi]. A decline in plasma PTH levels has the opposite effect.

Calcitriol also plays an important role in Ca^{++} and Pi homeostasis **(Figure 39–10)**. The primary action of calcitriol is to stimulate Ca^{++} and Pi absorption by the intestine. To a lesser degree, it acts with PTH to release Ca^{++} and Pi from the bone and decreases Ca^{++} excretion by the kidneys. The net effect of calcitriol is to increase the plasma [Ca^{++}] and [Pi]. Thus, the major stimuli of calcitriol production are hypocalcemia via PTH and hypophosphatemia (i.e., a low plasma [Pi]).

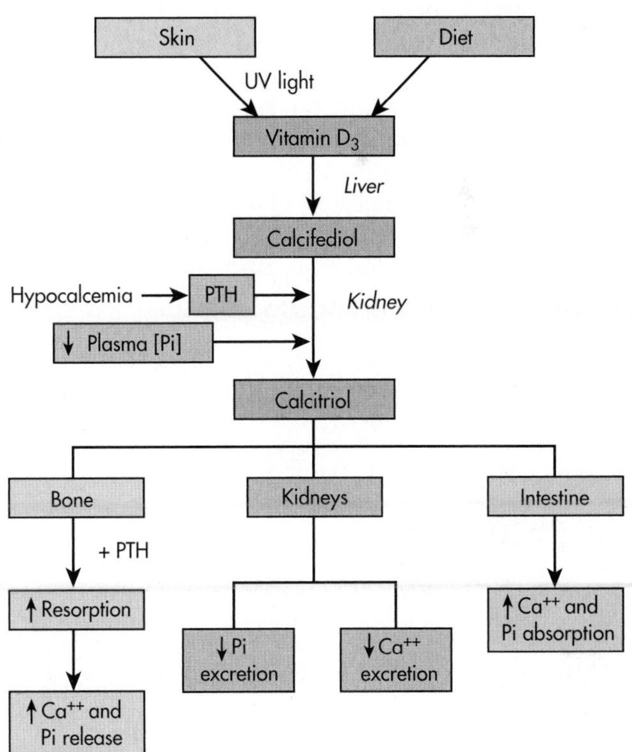

FIGURE 39–10. Activation of vitamin D_3 and its effect on Ca^{++} and Pi metabolism. Hypocalcemia, via PTH, and hypophosphatemia are the major stimuli of the metabolism of calcifediol to calcitriol in the kidneys. The net effect of calcitriol is to increase the plasma [Ca^{++}] and [Pi]. (Data from Rose BD, Rennke HG, eds: *Renal pathophysiology: the essentials,* Baltimore, 1994, Williams & Wilkins.)

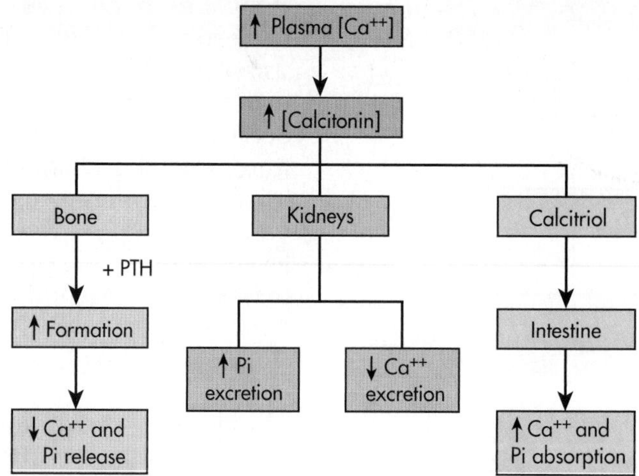

FIGURE 39–11. Effect of calcitonin on Ca^{++} and Pi homeostasis. The major stimulus of calcitonin secretion is hypercalcemia. The net effect of calcitonin is to reduce the plasma [Ca^{++}]. Quantitatively, therefore, the most important effects of calcitonin are to stimulate bone formation and to decrease bone resorption. Although calcitonin reduces urinary Ca^{++} excretion and intestinal Ca^{++} absorption, these effects are relatively minor and have little effect on the plasma [Ca^{++}]. The effects of calcitonin on the kidneys and calcitriol production are relatively minor compared with its effect on bone. (Data from Rose BD, Rennke HG, eds: *Renal pathophysiology: the essentials,* Baltimore, 1994, Williams & Wilkins.)

Although calcitonin does not play a major role in Ca^{++} and Pi homeostasis in humans, it does act, especially in lower mammals, to block bone resorption and stimulate Ca^{++} deposition in bone **(Figure 39–11)**. Also, calcitonin has a modest direct effect to decrease urinary Ca^{++} excretion. The major stimulus of calcitonin secretion is an increase in the plasma [Ca^{++}]. Because changes in Pi handling in bone, the intestines, and the kidneys tend to balance out, calcitonin decreases the plasma [Ca^{++}] while having little effect on the plasma [Pi].

Estrogens defend against PTH-mediated resorption of bone. In estrogen-deficient conditions, most prominently those that follow menopause, the unabated effect of PTH on bone contributes significantly to the development of osteoporosis.

Summary

- K^+ homeostasis is maintained by the kidneys, which adjust K^+ excretion to match dietary K^+ intake, and by the hormones insulin, epinephrine, and aldosterone.
- Other events, such as cell lysis, exercise, and changes in acid-base balance and plasma osmolality, disturb the plasma [K^+].
- K^+ excretion by the kidneys is determined by the rate and direction of K^+ transport by the distal tubule and collecting duct. K^+ secretion by these tubular segments is regulated by the plasma [K^+], aldosterone, and ADH. In contrast, changes in tubular fluid flow and acid-base disturbances perturb K^+ excretion by the kidneys. In K^+-depleted states, K^+ secretion is inhibited, and the distal tubule and collecting duct reabsorb K^+.
- The kidneys, in conjunction with the gastrointestinal tract and bone, play a vital role in regulating the plasma [Ca^{++}] and [Pi].

- Plasma Ca^{++} is regulated by PTH and calcitriol. Calcitonin is not an important regulatory hormone in humans. Ca^{++} excretion by the kidneys is determined by the net rate of intestinal Ca^{++} absorption, the balance between bone formation and resorption, and the net rate of Ca^{++} reabsorption by the distal tubule and thick ascending limb of the loop of Henle.
- Ca^{++} reabsorption by the thick ascending limb is regulated by PTH and calcitriol, both of which stimulate Ca^{++} reabsorption.
- The plasma [Pi] is regulated by the maximal reabsorptive capacity of Pi by the kidneys.
- A fall in the [Pi] stimulates the production of calcitriol, which releases Pi from bone into the ECF and increases Pi absorption by the intestine.

Bibliography

Brown EM, Macleod RJ: Extracellular calcium sensing and extracellular calcium signaling, *Physiol Rev* 81:239, 2001.

Friedman PA: Mechanisms of renal calcium transport, *Exp Nephrol* 8:343, 2000.

Malnic G, Bailey MA, Giebisch G: Control of renal potassium excretion. In Brenner BM, ed: *Brenner and Rector's the kidney,* ed 7, Philadelphia, 2004, WB Saunders.

Mount DB, Zandi-Nejad K: Disorders of potassium balance. In Brenner BM, ed: *Brenner and Rector's the kidney,* ed 7, Philadelphia, 2004, WB Saunders.

Murer H et al: Proximal tubular phosphate reabsorption: molecular mechanisms, *Physiol Rev* 80:1373, 2000.

Yu AS: Renal transport of calcium, magnesium, and phosphate. In Brenner BM, ed: *Brenner and Rector's the kidney,* ed 7, Philadelphia, 2004, WB Saunders.

Case Studies

Case 39–1

An 18-year-old man with insulin-dependent diabetes mellitus was seen in the emergency department. He did not take his insulin during the previous 24 hours because he did not feel well and was not eating. He was weak, nauseated, and thirsty, and he urinated frequently. On physical examination, he had deep and rapid respirations (Kussmaul's respiration). The following laboratory data were obtained:

Plasma [Na^+]	135 mEq/L
Serum [Cl^-]	99 mEq/L
Plasma [K^+]	8 mEq/L
Plasma [HCO_3^-]	7 mEq/L
Blood pH	6.99
Partial pressure of arterial carbon dioxide	30 mm Hg
Plasma [glucose]	1200 mg/dL
Urine	Contains glucose and ketones

The diagnosis of diabetic ketoacidosis was made, and the patient was admitted to the hospital. After insulin was administered, the plasma [K^+] decreased.

1. What caused hyperkalemia in this patient?

A. Frequent urination
B. Ketoacidosis
C. Increased plasma glucose levels
D. Glucose and ketones in the urine
E. Metabolic alkalosis

2. Why did the plasma [K^+] decrease after the administration of insulin?

A. Promotion of K^+ uptake into cells
B. Correction of the ketoacidosis, which allows K^+ to enter cells in exchange for H^+
C. Decrease in polyuria, which stimulates the amount of K^+ excreted in the urine
D. Stimulation of glucose uptake by cells, which increases plasma osmolality and thereby causes K^+ to enter cells
E. Insulin inhibition of Na^+,K^+-ATPase and thereby K^+ uptake into cells

Case 39–2

A 55-year-old woman came to the emergency department with severe flank pain caused by a renal stone lodged in her right ureter. Tests revealed that the renal stone formed because of demineralization of bone and elevated serum levels of PTH. A benign PTH-secreting adenoma of the parathyroid gland was identified.

1. **What values of serum [Ca^{++}] and [Pi] would be predicted for this patient?**
   A. Increased serum [Ca^{++}], decreased serum [Pi]
   B. Increased serum [Ca^{++}], increased serum [Pi]
   C. Unchanged serum [Ca^{++}], unchanged serum [Pi]
   D. Decreased serum [Ca^{++}], decreased serum [Pi]
   E. Decreased serum [Ca^{++}], increased serum [Pi]

2. **The high levels of serum PTH in this woman would be expected to increase Ca^{++} reabsorption in which segment of the nephron?**
   A. The glomerulus
   B. The proximal tubule
   C. The thick ascending limb of the loop of Henle
   D. The distal tubule
   E. The collecting duct

3. **The high levels of serum PTH in this woman would be expected to decrease Pi reabsorption in which segment of the nephron?**
   A. The glomerulus
   B. The proximal tubule
   C. The thick ascending limb of the loop of Henle
   D. The distal tubule
   E. The collecting duct

Chapter 40: Role of the Kidneys in Acid-Base Balance

Objectives

- ❖ Indicate the impact of diet and cellular metabolism on acid-base balance.
- ❖ Distinguish among the roles of the kidneys, lungs, and liver in acid-base balance.
- ❖ Describe the mechanisms for H^+ transport in the various segments of the nephron and ways that these mechanisms are regulated.
- ❖ Distinguish between the reabsorption of the filtered load of HCO_3^- and the generation of new HCO_3^-.
- ❖ Explain the importance of urine buffers, and especially NH_4^+ production and excretion, in the process of new HCO_3^- formation.
- ❖ Identify the defense mechanisms the body uses to minimize the impact of acid and alkali on the pH of body fluids.
- ❖ Distinguish between metabolic and respiratory acid-base disorders.
- ❖ Distinguish between simple and mixed acid-base disorders.

Virtually all cellular, tissue, and organ processes are sensitive to pH. Indeed, life cannot exist outside of a range of body fluid pH from 6.8 to 7.8 (160 to 16 nEq/L of H^+). Each day, acid and alkali are ingested in the diet. Also, cellular metabolism produces a number of substances that have an impact on the pH of body fluids. Without appropriate mechanisms to deal with this daily acid and alkali load and thereby to maintain acid-base balance, many processes necessary for life could not occur. This chapter reviews the maintenance of whole-body acid-base balance. Although the emphasis is on the role of the kidneys in this process, the roles of the lungs and liver are also considered. In addition, the impact of diet and cellular metabolism on acid-base balance is presented. Finally, disorders of acid-base balance are considered, primarily to illustrate the physiological processes involved. Throughout this chapter, **acid** is defined as any substance that adds H^+ to the body fluids; **alkali** is defined as a substance that removes H^+ from the body fluids.

Overview of Acid-Base Balance

The diet of humans contains many constituents that are either acid or alkali. In addition, cellular metabolism produces acid and alkali. Finally, alkali is normally lost each day in the feces. As described later, the net effect of these processes is the addition of acid to the body fluids. For acid-base balance to be maintained, acid must be excreted from the body at a rate equivalent to its addition. If acid addition exceeds excretion, **acidosis** results. Conversely, if acid excretion exceeds addition, **alkalosis** results.

Diet determines metabolically produced acid and alkali

The major constituents of the diet are carbohydrates and fats. When tissue perfusion is adequate, O_2 is available to tissues, and insulin is present at normal levels, carbohydrates and fats are metabolized to CO_2 and H_2O. On a daily basis, 15 to 20 moles of CO_2 are generated through this process. Normally, this large quantity of CO_2 is effectively eliminated from the body by the lungs, so this metabolically derived CO_2 has no impact on acid-base balance. CO_2 is usually termed **volatile acid,** reflecting the fact that it has the potential to generate H^+ after hydration with H_2O (see Equation 40–2). Acid not derived directly from the hydration of CO_2 is termed **nonvolatile acid** (e.g., lactic acid).

The cellular metabolism of other dietary constituents also has an impact on acid-base balance. For example, cysteine and methionine, sulfur-containing amino acids, yield sulfuric acid when they are metabolized, whereas hydrochloric acid results from the metabolism of lysine, arginine, and histidine. A portion of this nonvolatile acid load is offset by the production of bicarbonate (HCO_3^-) through the metabolism of the amino acids aspartate and glutamate. On average, the metabolism of dietary amino acids yields net nonvolatile acid production. Finally, the metabolism of certain organic anions (e.g., citrate) results in the production of HCO_3^-, which offsets nonvolatile acid production to some degree. In balance, in individuals ingesting a meat-containing diet, acid production exceeds HCO_3^- production. In addition to the metabolically derived acids and alkalis, the foods ingested contain acid and alkali. For example, the presence of phosphate ($H_2PO_4^-$) in ingested food increases the dietary acid load. Finally, during digestion, some HCO_3^- is normally lost in the feces (see Chapter 35). This loss is equivalent to the addition of nonvolatile acid to the body. Together, dietary intake, cellular metabolism, and fecal HCO_3^- loss result in the addition of approximately 1 mEq/kg body weight of nonvolatile acid to the body each day (50 to 100 mEq/day for most adults).

When insulin levels are normal, carbohydrates and fats are completely metabolized to $CO_2 + H_2O$. However, if insulin levels are abnormally low (e.g., **diabetes mellitus**), the metabolism of carbohydrates leads to the production of several organic keto acids (e.g., ß-hydroxybutyric acid).

In the absence of adequate levels of O_2 **(hypoxia),** anaerobic metabolism by cells can also lead to the production of organic acids (e.g., lactic acid) rather than $CO_2 + H_2O$. This frequently occurs in normal individuals during vigorous exercise. Poor tissue perfusion, such as that which occurs with reduced cardiac output, can also lead to anaerobic metabolism by cells and thus to acidosis. In these conditions, the organic acids accumulate, and the pH of the body fluids decreases (acidosis). Treatment (e.g., administration of insulin in the case of diabetes) or improved delivery of adequate levels of O_2 to the tissues (e.g., in the case of poor tissue perfusion) results in the metabolism of these organic acids to $CO_2 + H_2O$ and thereby helps correct the acid-base disorder.

Nonvolatile acids are rapidly buffered

Nonvolatile acids do not circulate throughout the body but are immediately buffered. As discussed later, HCO_3^- in the extracellular fluid (ECF) is an important buffer species. Thus, the buffering of nonvolatile acids by HCO_3^- removes HCO_3^- from the ECF. The kidneys must replenish the HCO_3^- that is lost by neutralization of the nonvolatile acids.

Renal Acid Excretion

TO MAINTAIN ACID-BASE BALANCE, THE KIDNEYS MUST EXCRETE AN AMOUNT OF ACID EQUAL TO THE NONVOLATILE ACID PRODUCTION. In addition, they must prevent the loss of HCO_3^- in the urine. This task is quantitatively more important because the filtered load of HCO_3^- is approximately 4320 mEq/day (24 mEq/L × 180 L/day = 4320 mEq/day), compared with only 50 to 100 mEq/day needed to balance nonvolatile acid production.

The reabsorption of filtered HCO_3^- and the excretion of acid occur via H^+ secretion

BOTH THE REABSORPTION OF FILTERED HCO_3^- AND THE EXCRETION OF ACID ARE ACCOMPLISHED VIA H^+ SECRETION BY THE NEPHRONS. Thus, in a single day, the nephrons must secrete approximately 4390 mEq of H^+ into the tubular fluid. Most of the secreted H^+ serves to reabsorb the filtered load of HCO_3^-. Only 50 to 100 mEq of H^+, an amount equivalent to nonvolatile acid production, is excreted in the urine. As a result of this acid excretion, the urine is normally acidic.

The kidneys cannot excrete urine more acidic than pH 4.0 to 4.5. Even at a pH of 4.0, only 0.1 mEq/L of H^+ can be excreted. Therefore, to excrete sufficient acid, the kidneys excrete H^+ with urinary buffers such as phosphate ($HPO_4^=$, $H_2PO_4^-$). Other constituents of the urine can also serve as buffers (e.g., creatinine), although their role is less important than phosphate. Collectively, the various urinary buffers are termed **titratable acids.** This term is derived from the method by which these buffers are quantitated in the laboratory. Typically, alkali (OH^-) is added to a urine sample to titrate its pH to that of plasma (i.e., 7.4). The amount of alkali added is equal to the H^+ titrated by these urine buffers and is termed titratable acid.

The excretion of H^+ as a titratable acid is insufficient to balance the daily nonvolatile acid load. An additional and important mechanism by which the kidneys contribute to the maintenance of acid-base balance is through the synthesis and excretion of **ammonium (NH_4^+).** The mechanisms involved in this process are discussed in more detail later in this chapter. With regard to the renal regulation of acid-base balance, each NH_4^+ excreted in the urine results in the return of one HCO_3^- to the systemic circulation, which replenishes the HCO_3^- lost during neutralization of the nonvolatile acid. Thus, the production and excretion of NH_4^+ are equivalent to the excretion of acid by the kidneys.

Net acid excretion equals nonvolatile acid production

In brief, THE KIDNEYS CONTRIBUTE TO ACID-BASE HOMEOSTASIS BY REABSORBING THE FILTERED LOAD OF HCO_3^- AND EXCRETING AN AMOUNT OF ACID EQUIVALENT TO THE AMOUNT OF NONVOLATILE ACID PRODUCED EACH DAY. This overall process is termed **net acid excretion** (NAE), and it can be quantitated as follows:

$$NAE = [(U_{NH_4^+} \times \dot{V}) + (U_{TA} \times \dot{V})] - (U_{HCO_3^-} \times \dot{V}) \quad \text{40-1}$$

where ($U_{NH_4^+} \times \dot{V}$) and ($U_{TA} \times \dot{V}$) are the rates of excretion (mEq/day) of NH_4^+ and titratable acid (TA) and ($U_{HCO_3^-} \times \dot{V}$) is the amount of HCO_3^- lost in the urine (equivalent to adding H^+ to the body). Again, maintenance of acid-base balance means that the net acid excretion must equal nonvolatile acid production. Under most conditions, very little HCO_3^- is excreted in the urine. Thus, net acid excretion essentially reflects titratable acid and NH_4^+ excretion. Quantitatively, titratable acid accounts for approximately one third and NH_4^+ for two thirds of net acid excretion.

The filtered load of HCO_3^- must be reabsorbed

As indicated by Equation 40–1, net acid excretion is maximized when little or no HCO_3^- is excreted in the urine. Indeed, under most circumstances, very little HCO_3^- appears in the urine. Because HCO_3^- is freely filtered at the glomerulus, approximately 4320 mEq/day is delivered to the nephrons and then reabsorbed. The majority of this HCO_3^- is reabsorbed in the proximal tubule (80% of the filtered load), an additional 15% is reabsorbed by the thick ascending limb of the loop of Henle, and the remainder (5%) is reabsorbed by the distal tubule and collecting duct.

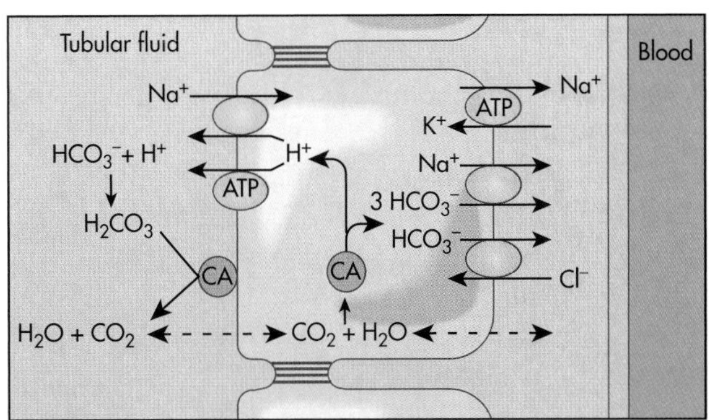

FIGURE 40–1. Cellular mechanism for the reabsorption of filtered HCO_3^- by the cells of the proximal tubule. CA, carbonic anhydrase. See text for details.

The proximal tubule reabsorbs most of the filtered load of HCO_3^-

Figure 40–1 summarizes the primary transport processes responsible for HCO_3^- reabsorption in the proximal tubule. H^+ secretion across the apical membrane of the cell occurs by both an Na^+-H^+ antiporter and an H^+-ATPase. The Na^+-H^+ antiporter (NHE3) is the predominant pathway for H^+ secretion and uses the lumen-to-cell Na^+ gradient to drive this process (i.e., secondary active secretion of H^+). Within the cell, H^+ and HCO_3^- are produced in a reaction catalyzed by **carbonic anhydrase.** The H^+ is secreted into the tubular fluid, whereas the HCO_3^- exits the cell across the basolateral membrane and returns to the peritubular blood. HCO_3^- movement out of the cell across the basolateral membrane is coupled to other ions. The majority of HCO_3^- exits via a symporter that couples the efflux of $1Na^+$ with $3HCO_3^-$. In addition, some of the HCO_3^- exits in exchange for Cl^- (via a Cl^--HCO_3^- antiporter). As noted in Figure 40–1, carbonic anhydrase is also present in the brush border of the proximal tubule cells. This enzyme catalyzes the dehydration of H_2CO_3 in the luminal fluid and thereby facilitates the reabsorption of HCO_3^-.

The cellular mechanism for HCO_3^- reabsorption by the thick ascending limb of the loop of Henle is virtually identical to that in the proximal tubule. The Na^+-H^+ antiporter is the predominant pathway for H^+ secretion.

The distal tubule and collecting duct reabsorb the small amount of HCO_3^- that escapes reabsorption by the proximal tubule and loop of Henle. **Figure 40–2** shows the cellular mechanism of HCO_3^- reabsorption by the collecting duct, where H^+ secretion occurs via the intercalated cell (see Chapter 36). Within the cell, H^+ and HCO_3^- are produced by the hydration of CO_2; this reaction is catalyzed by carbonic anhydrase. H^+ is secreted into the tubular fluid via two mechanisms. The first involves an

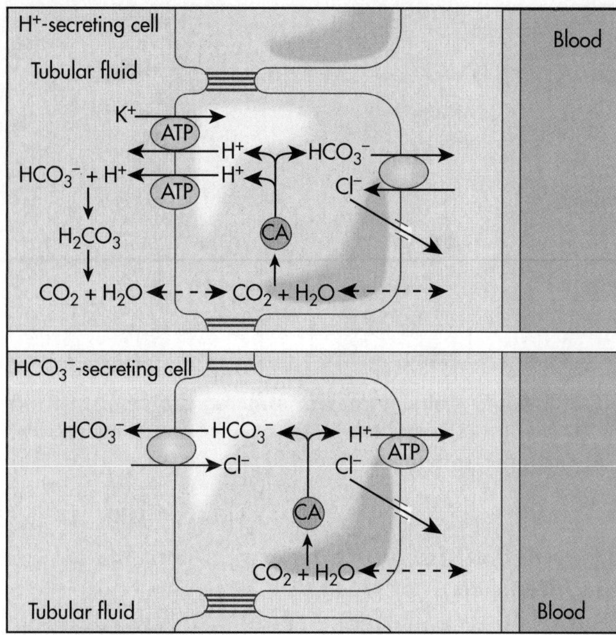

FIGURE 40–2. Cellular mechanisms for the reabsorption and secretion of HCO_3^- by the intercalated cells of the collecting duct. CA, carbonic anhydrase. See text for details.

apical membrane H^+-ATPase. The second couples the secretion of H^+ with the reabsorption of K^+ via an H^+,K^+-ATPase similar to that found in the stomach (see Chapter 34). The HCO_3^- exits the cell across the basolateral membrane in exchange for Cl^- (via a Cl^--HCO_3^- antiporter) and enters the peritubular capillary blood.

A second population of intercalated cells within the collecting duct secrete HCO_3^- rather than H^+ into the tubular fluid. In these intercalated cells, in contrast to the intercalated cells previously described, the H^+-ATPase is located in the basolateral membrane, and a Cl^--HCO_3^- antiporter is located in the apical membrane (Figure 40–2). Their activity can be increased during metabolic alkalosis, when the kidneys must excrete excess HCO_3^-. However, under normal conditions, H^+ secretion predominates in the collecting duct.

The apical membrane of the cells of the collecting duct is not very permeable to H^+, and the pH of the tubular fluid can become quite acidic. Indeed, the most acidic tubular fluid along the nephron (pH = 4.0 to 4.5) is produced there. In comparison, the permeability of the proximal tubule to H^+ and HCO_3^- is much higher, and the tubular fluid pH falls to only 6.5 in this segment. As explained later, the ability of the collecting duct to lower the pH of the tubular fluid is critically important for the excretion of urinary buffers and NH_4^+.

Systemic acid-base balance regulates nephron H^+ secretion

A number of factors regulate the secretion of H^+ by the cells of the nephron **(Table 40–1)**. FROM A PHYSIOLOGICAL PERSPECTIVE, THE PRIMARY FACTOR THAT REGULATES H^+ SECRETION BY THE NEPHRON IS A CHANGE IN THE SYSTEMIC ACID-BASE BALANCE. At the cellular level, this results in changes in the intracellular pH of nephron cells. Whether it is produced by a decrease in the concentration of HCO_3^- in plasma or by an increase in the partial pressure of carbon dioxide (P_{CO_2}), acidosis decreases the pH of the cells of the nephron, creating a more favorable cell–to–tubular fluid H^+ gradient and thereby stimulating H^+ secretion along the entire nephron. Conversely, alkalosis secondary to an increase in the [HCO_3^-] or a decrease in the P_{CO_2} inhibits H^+ secretion secondary to an increase in the intracellular pH of the nephron cells.

Although alterations in the intracellular pH of nephron cells directly influence H^+ secretion across the apical membrane, there is evidence that these changes in pH, perhaps mediated by other intracellular messengers, also alter the activity or expression of key H^+ and HCO_3^- transporters. For example, the intercalated cells of the collecting duct insert more H^+-ATPase into their apical membranes in

TABLE 40–1. FACTORS INFLUENCING H^+ SECRETION BY THE NEPHRON

Factor	Principal Site of Action
Increased H^+ Secretion	
Primary	
Decrease in plasma [HCO_3^-] (↓pH)	Entire nephron
Increase in P_{CO_2}	Entire nephron
Secondary (not directed at maintaining acid-base balance)	
Increase in filtered load of HCO_3^-	Proximal tubule
Decrease in ECF volume	Proximal tubule
Increase in angiotensin II	Proximal tubule
Increase in aldosterone	Collecting duct
Hypokalemia	Proximal tubule, collecting duct
Decreased H^+ Secretion	
Primary	
Increase in plasma [HCO_3^-] (↑pH)	Entire nephron
Decrease in P_{CO_2}	Entire nephron
Secondary (not directed at maintaining acid-base balance)	
Decrease in filtered load of HCO_3^-	Proximal tubule
Increase in ECF volume	Proximal tubule
Decrease in aldosterone	Collecting duct
Hyperkalemia	Proximal tubule
Increase in parathyroid hormone	Proximal tubule

response to acidosis. In the proximal tubule, acidosis also increases the abundance and activity of the apical membrane Na^+-H^+ antiporter. Activity of the $1Na^+$-$3HCO_3^-$ symporter in the basolateral membrane is increased as well with acidosis. It is likely that the effects of inhibited H^+ secretion caused by systemic alkalosis are also mediated in part by the reduced activity or expression of these H^+ and HCO_3^- transporters. Changes in glucocorticoid and endothelin levels may also contribute to the changes seen in H^+ and HCO_3^- transporter activity and expression during changes in systemic acid-base balance. The levels of both are increased during acidosis, and both increase the activity and expression of H^+ and HCO_3^- transporters along the nephron.

Other factors can alter nephron H^+ secretion

Table 40–1 also lists other factors that influence the secretion of H^+ by the cells of the nephron. However, these factors are not directly related to the maintenance of acid-base balance. Because H^+ secretion in the proximal tubule and thick ascending limb of the loop of Henle is linked to the reabsorption of Na^+ (via the Na^+-H^+ antiporter), factors that alter Na^+ reabsorption secondarily affect H^+ secretion. For example, the process of glomerulotubular balance ensures that the resorption rate of the proximal tubule is matched to the glomerular filtration rate (see Chapter 37). Thus, when the glomerular filtration rate is increased, the filtered load to the proximal tubule is increased, and more fluid (including HCO_3^-) is reabsorbed. Conversely, a decrease in the filtered load results in the decreased reabsorption of fluid and thus HCO_3^-.

Alterations in Na^+ balance, through changes in the ECF volume, also have an impact on H^+ secretion. With volume depletion (negative Na^+ balance), H^+ secretion is enhanced. This occurs via several mechanisms. First, the renin-angiotensin-aldosterone system is activated by volume depletion, and Na^+ reabsorption by the nephron is enhanced (see Chapter 38). Angiotensin II acts on the proximal tubule to stimulate the apical membrane Na^+-H^+ antiporter and thereby stimulate H^+ secretion. Aldosterone's primary action on the collecting duct is to stimulate Na^+ reabsorption. However, it also stimulates the intercalated cells to secrete H^+. Second, the peritubular Starling forces across the proximal tubule are altered during volume depletion to enhance overall proximal tubule reabsorption (see Chapter 37). With volume expansion (positive Na^+ balance), H^+ secretion is reduced because of low levels of angiotensin II and aldosterone as well as because of alterations in the peritubular Starling forces (reduced reabsorption by the proximal tubule).

Parathyroid hormone (PTH) also inhibits HCO_3^- reabsorption by the proximal tubule. PTH is mainly involved in the maintenance of Ca^{++} and phosphate balance (see Chapters 39 and 44). However, PTH inhibits the Na^+-H^+ antiporter in the apical membrane of proximal tubule cells. Finally, K^+ balance influences the secretion of H^+ by the proximal tubule, with hypokalemia stimulating and hyperkalemia inhibiting secretion. It is thought that K^+-induced changes in intracellular pH are responsible, at least in part, for this effect, with hypokalemia acidifying and hyperkalemia alkalinizing the cells. Hypokalemia also stimulates H^+ secretion by the collecting duct. This is a result of increased expression of the H^+,K^+-ATPase in the intercalated cells.

NH_4^+ production and excretion form new HCO_3^-

As discussed previously, reabsorption of the filtered load of HCO_3^- is important for maximizing net acid excretion. However, HCO_3^- reabsorption alone does not replenish the HCO_3^- lost during the buffering of the nonvolatile acids produced during metabolism. To maintain acid-base balance, the kidneys must replace this lost HCO_3^- with new HCO_3^-. A portion of the new HCO_3^- is produced while urinary buffers (primarily phosphate) are being excreted. This process is illustrated in **Figure 40–3**. In the collecting duct, when the tubular fluid contains little or no HCO_3^- because HCO_3^- is reabsorbed in "upstream" tubular segments, H^+ secreted into the

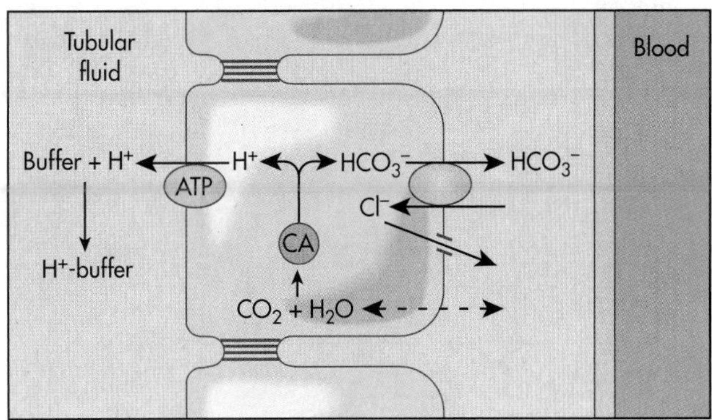

FIGURE 40–3. Excretion of H^+ with non-HCO_3^- urine buffers. The primary urine buffer is phosphate ($HPO_4^=$). Another buffer is creatinine. Collectively, the urine buffers are termed titratable acids. For simplicity, only H^+-ATPase is shown. H^+ secretion by H^+,K^+-ATPase also titrates urine buffers. CA, carbonic anhydrase.

tubular fluid combines with a urinary buffer. Thus, H^+ secretion results in the excretion of H^+ with a buffer, and the HCO_3^- produced in the cell from the hydration of CO_2 is added to the blood. The amount of phosphate excreted each day and therefore available to serve as a urinary buffer is not sufficient to allow adequate generation of new HCO_3^-. Moreover, the amount of phosphate excreted is regulated in response to the need to maintain phosphate balance (see Chapters 39 and 44), not in response to the need to maintain acid-base balance. In contrast, NH_4^+ IS PRODUCED BY THE KIDNEYS, AND ITS SYNTHESIS AND SUBSEQUENT EXCRETION CAN BE REGULATED IN RESPONSE TO THE ACID-BASE REQUIREMENTS OF THE BODY. BECAUSE OF THIS, NH_4^+ EXCRETION IS CRITICALLY INVOLVED IN THE FORMATION OF NEW HCO_3^-.

NH_4^+ is produced in the kidneys via the metabolism of glutamine. Essentially, the kidneys metabolize glutamine, excrete NH_4^+, and add HCO_3^- to the body. However, the formation of new HCO_3^- via this process depends on the kidneys' ability to excrete NH_4^+ in the urine. If NH_4^+ is not excreted in the urine but enters the systemic circulation instead, it is converted into urea by the liver. This conversion process generates H^+, which is then buffered by HCO_3^-. Thus, the production of urea from NH_4^+ consumes HCO_3^- and negates the formation of HCO_3^- through the synthesis and excretion of NH_4^+ by the kidneys.

The process by which the kidneys excrete NH_4^+ is complex. **Figure 40–4** illustrates the essential features of this process. NH_4^+ is produced from glutamine in the cells of the proximal tubule. Each glutamine molecule produces two molecules of NH_4^+ and a divalent anion. The metabolism of this anion ultimately provides two molecules of HCO_3^-. The HCO_3^- exits the cell across the basolateral membrane and enters the peritubular blood as new HCO_3^-. NH_4^+ exits the cell across the apical membrane and enters the tubular fluid. The primary mechanism for the secretion of NH_4^+ into the tubular fluid involves the Na^+-H^+ antiporter, with NH_4^+ substituting for H^+. In addition, NH_3 can diffuse out of the cell into the tubular fluid, where it is protonated to NH_4^+.

A significant portion of the NH_4^+ secreted by the proximal tubule is reabsorbed by the loop of Henle. The thick ascending limb is the primary site of this NH_4^+ reabsorption, with NH_4^+ substituting for K^+ on the $1Na^+,1K^+,2Cl^-$ symporter. In addition, the lumen-positive transepithelial voltage in this segment drives the paracellular reabsorption of NH_4^+.

The NH_4^+ reabsorbed by the thick ascending limb of the loop of Henle accumulates in the medullary interstitium, where it exists in chemical equilibrium with NH_3 ($pK_a = 9.0$). NH_4^+ then reenters the tubular fluid of the collecting duct. The mechanisms by which NH_4^+ is secreted by the collecting duct include (1) transport into cells via the Na^+,K^+-ATPase (NH_4^+ substituting for K^+) and exit from the cell across the apical membrane of intercalated cells via the H^+,K^+-ATPase (NH_4^+ substituting for H^+) and (2) the process of **nonionic diffusion** and **diffusion trapping.** Specific NH_4^+ transport proteins have been localized to cells of the collecting duct (RhBG

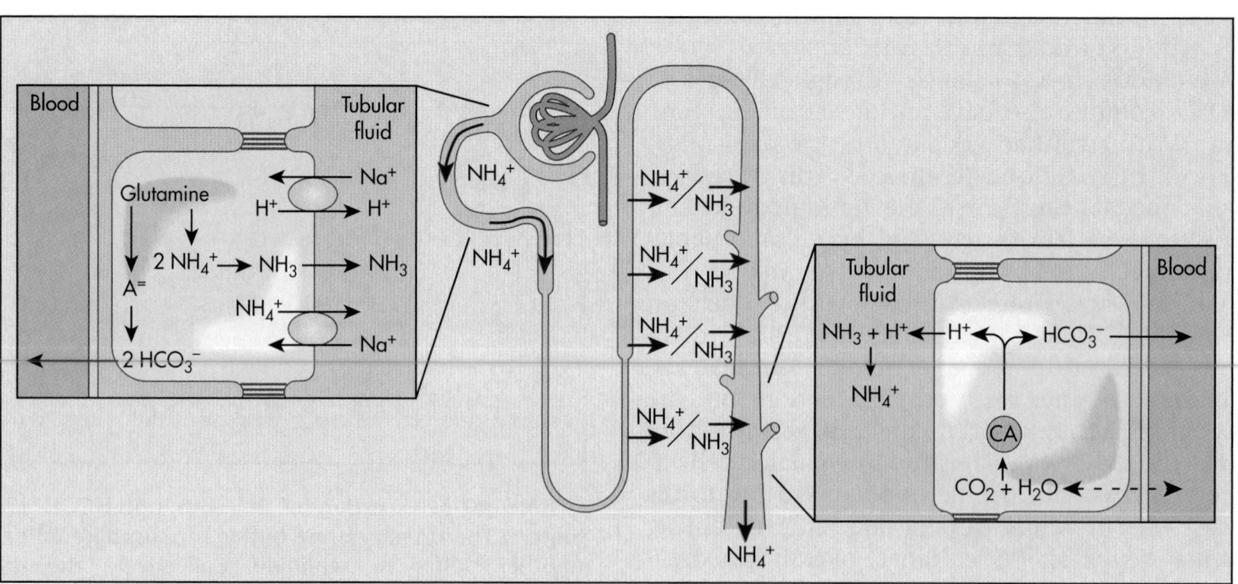

FIGURE 40–4. Production, transport, and excretion of NH_4^+ by the nephron. For every NH_4^+ excreted in the urine, one HCO_3^- is returned to the systemic circulation. See text for details.

and RhCG). However, their role in NH_4^+ secretion has not been elucidated. Of these mechanisms, quantitatively the most important is nonionic diffusion and diffusion trapping. By this mechanism, NH_3 diffuses from the medullary interstitium into the lumen of the collecting duct. As previously described, H^+ secretion by the intercalated cells of the collecting duct acidifies the luminal fluid. (A luminal fluid pH as low as 4.0 to 4.5 can be achieved.) Consequently, NH_3 diffusing from the medullary interstitium into the collecting duct lumen (nonionic diffusion) is protonated to NH_4^+ by the acidic tubular fluid. Because the collecting duct is less permeable to NH_4^+ than to NH_3, NH_4^+ is trapped in the tubule lumen (diffusion trapping) and eliminated from the body in the urine.

H^+ secretion by the collecting duct is critical for the excretion of NH_4^+. If collecting duct H^+ secretion is inhibited, the NH_4^+ reabsorbed by the thick ascending limb will not be excreted in the urine. Instead, it will be returned to the systemic circulation, where, as described previously, it will be converted to urea by the liver and consume HCO_3^- in the process. Thus, new HCO_3^- is produced during the metabolism of glutamine by cells of the proximal tubule. However, the overall process is not complete until the NH_4^+ is excreted (i.e., the production of urea from NH_4^+ by the liver is prevented). Thus, NH_4^+ EXCRETION CAN BE USED AS A "MARKER" OF GLUTAMINE METABOLISM IN THE PROXIMAL TUBULE. IN THE NET, ONE NEW HCO_3^- IS RETURNED TO THE SYSTEMIC CIRCULATION FOR EACH NH_4^+ EXCRETED IN THE URINE.

An important feature of the renal NH_4^+ system is that it can be regulated by systemic acid-base balance. Alterations in the pH of ECF, by affecting the pH of intracellular fluid (ICF), change glutamine metabolism in the cells of the proximal tubule. In addition, as already noted, glucocorticoid levels increase during acidosis, and glucocorticoids stimulate ammoniagenesis (i.e., NH_4^+ production from glutamine). During systemic acidosis, the enzymes in the proximal tubule cell responsible for the metabolism of glutamine are stimulated. This involves the synthesis of new enzyme and requires several days for complete adaptation. With increased levels of this enzyme, NH_4^+ production is increased, allowing enhanced production of new HCO_3^-. Conversely, glutamine metabolism is reduced with alkalosis.

The $[K^+]$ of plasma also alters NH_4^+ production. When hyperkalemia exists, NH_4^+ production is inhibited, whereas hypokalemia stimulates NH_4^+ production. The mechanism by which plasma K^+ alters NH_4^+ production is not fully understood. Alterations in the plasma $[K^+]$ may change the intracellular pH by exchanging H^+ for K^+ (see Chapter 39), and the change in intracellular pH may then control glutamine metabolism. Via this mechanism, the exchange of extracellular K^+ for intracellular H^+ during hyperkalemia would raise intracellular pH and thereby inhibit glutamine metabolism. The opposite would occur during hypokalemia.

Renal tubular acidosis (RTA) refers to conditions in which net acid excretion by the kidneys is impaired. Under these conditions, the kidneys are unable to excrete a sufficient amount of net acid to balance nonvolatile acid production, and acidosis results. RTA can be caused by a defect in H^+ secretion in the proximal tubule **(proximal RTA)** or distal tubule **(distal RTA)** or by inadequate production of NH_4^+.

Proximal RTA can be caused by a variety of hereditary and acquired conditions (e.g., **cystinosis, Fanconi's syndrome,** administration of carbonic anhydrase inhibitors). H^+ secretion by the cells of the proximal tubule is impaired, resulting in decreased reabsorption of the filtered load of HCO_3^-. Consequently, HCO_3^- is lost in the urine, the plasma $[HCO_3^-]$ decreases, and acidosis ensues.

Distal RTA also occurs in a number of hereditary and acquired conditions (e.g., **medullary sponge kidney**), with certain drugs (such as **amphotericin B**), and in conditions secondary to urinary obstruction. Depending on the cause, the secretion of H^+ by the intercalated cells of the collecting duct may be impaired, or the permeability of the collecting duct to H^+ may be increased. In either case, the ability to acidify the tubular fluid is impaired. Consequently, titratable acid excretion is reduced, and nonionic diffusion and diffusion trapping of NH_4^+ are impaired. This in turn decreases net acid excretion, with the subsequent development of acidosis.

Failure to produce and excrete sufficient quantities of NH_4^+ can also reduce net acid excretion by the kidneys. This situation is thought to occur by generalized dysfunction of the collecting ducts with impaired H^+, NH_4^+, and K^+ secretion. This results in the development of hyperkalemia, which in turn impairs ammoniagenesis by the proximal tubule. Because of inadequate NH_4^+ production and excretion, net acid excretion is less than net acid production, and metabolic acidosis develops. If the acidosis that results from any of these forms of RTA is severe, individuals must ingest alkali (e.g., $NaHCO_3$) to maintain acid-base balance. In this way, the HCO_3^- lost each day in the buffering of nonvolatile acid is replenished by new HCO_3^- ingested in the diet.

The Diagnosis of and Approach to Patients with Acid-Base Disorders Frequently Involve the Measurement and Interpretation of Arterial Blood Gases

This analysis, which includes measurements of the partial pressure of oxygen (P_{O_2}), P_{CO_2}, and pH, focuses on the components of the HCO_3^- buffer system and the following reaction:

$$CO_2 + H_2O \leftrightarrow H_2CO_3 \leftrightarrow H^+ + HCO_3^- \quad \textbf{40-2}$$

The first reaction (hydration/dehydration of CO_2) is the rate-limiting step. This reaction, which is normally slow, is greatly accelerated in the presence of the enzyme **carbonic anhydrase.** The second reaction, the ionization of H_2CO_3 to H^+ and HCO_3^-, is virtually instantaneous. From the measurements of P_{CO_2} and pH, the [HCO_3^-] can be calculated by the Henderson-Hasselbalch equation:

$$pH = 6.1 + \log\frac{HCO_3^-}{0.03P_{CO_2}} \quad \textbf{40-3}$$

The pH of the ECF is maintained within a narrow range (7.35 to 7.45). Inspection of Equation 40-3 shows that the pH of the ECF varies when either the [HCO_3^-] or P_{CO_2} is altered. Disturbances of acid-base balance that result from a change in the [HCO_3^-] of ECF are termed **metabolic acid-base disorders;** those resulting from a change in the P_{CO_2} are termed **respiratory acid-base disorders.** These disorders are considered in more detail later in this chapter. The kidneys are primarily responsible for regulating the [HCO_3^-], whereas the lungs regulate the P_{CO_2}.

For simplicity of presentation in this chapter, the value of 7.40 for body fluid pH is used as normal, even though the normal range is 7.35 to 7.45. Similarly, the normal range for P_{CO_2} is 35 to 45 mm Hg. However, a P_{CO_2} of 40 mm Hg is used as the normal value. Finally, a value of 24 mEq/L is considered a normal ECF [HCO_3^-], even though the normal range is 22 to 28 mEq/L.

Defense mechanisms minimize changes in the pH of body fluid

When an acid-base disturbance develops, the body uses a series of mechanisms to defend against the change in the pH of the ECF. THESE DEFENSE MECHANISMS DO NOT CORRECT THE ACID-BASE DISTURBANCE BUT MERELY MINIMIZE THE CHANGE IN pH IMPOSED BY THE DISTURBANCE. RESTORATION OF THE BLOOD pH TO ITS NORMAL VALUE REQUIRES CORRECTION OF THE UNDERLYING PROCESS OR PROCESSES THAT PRODUCED THE ACID-BASE DISORDER. The body has three general mechanisms to defend against changes in body fluid pH produced by acid-base disturbances: (1) extracellular and intracellular buffering, (2) adjustments in blood P_{CO_2} via alterations in the ventilatory rate of the lungs, and (3) adjustments in the renal net acid excretion.

Extracellular and intracellular buffers act quickly to minimize changes in body fluid pH

THE FIRST LINE OF DEFENSE AGAINST ACID-BASE DISORDERS IS EXTRACELLULAR AND INTRACELLULAR BUFFERING. The response of the extracellular buffers is virtually instantaneous, whereas that to intracellular buffering is slower and can take several minutes.

Metabolic disorders that result from the addition of nonvolatile acid or alkali to the body fluids are buffered in both the ECF and ICF. The HCO_3^- buffer system is the principal ECF buffer. When nonvolatile acid is added to the body fluids (or alkali is lost from the body), HCO_3^- is consumed during the process of neutralizing the acid load, and the [HCO_3^-] of the ECF is reduced. Conversely, when nonvolatile alkali is added to the body fluids (or acid is lost from the body), H^+ is consumed, causing more HCO_3^- to be produced from the dissociation of H_2CO_3. Consequently, the [HCO_3^-] increases.

Although the HCO_3^- buffer system is the principal ECF buffer, Pi and plasma proteins provide additional extracellular buffering. The combined action of the buffering processes for HCO_3^-, Pi, and plasma protein accounts for the buffering of approximately 50% of a nonvolatile acid load and 70% of a nonvolatile alkali load. The remainder of the buffering under these two conditions occurs intracellularly. Intracellular buffering involves the movement of H^+ into cells (during buffering of nonvolatile acid) or the movement of H^+ out of cells (during buffering of nonvolatile alkali). H^+ is titrated inside the cell by HCO_3^-, Pi, and the histidine groups on proteins.

Bone represents an additional source of extracellular buffering. With acidosis, buffering by bone results in its demineralization because Ca^{++} is released from bone as Ca^{++}-containing salts bind H^+ in exchange for Ca^{++}.

When respiratory acid-base disorders occur, the pH of body fluid changes as a result of alterations in the P_{CO_2} (see Equation 40-3). Virtually all buffering in respiratory acid-base disorders occurs intracellularly. When the P_{CO_2} rises (respiratory acidosis), CO_2 moves into the cell, where it combines with H_2O to form H_2CO_3. H_2CO_3 then dissociates to H^+ and HCO_3^-. Some of the H^+ is buffered by cellular protein, and HCO_3^- exits the cell and raises the plasma [HCO_3^-]. This process is reversed when the P_{CO_2} is reduced (respiratory alkalosis). Under this condition, the hydration reaction ($H_2O + CO_2 \leftrightarrow H_2CO_3$) is shifted to the left by the decrease in P_{CO_2}. As a result, the dissociation reaction ($H_2CO_3 \leftrightarrow H^+ + HCO_3^-$) also shifts to the left, thereby reducing the plasma [HCO_3^-].

The ventilatory rate of the lungs changes in response to acid-base disorders

THE LUNGS ARE THE SECOND LINE OF DEFENSE AGAINST ACID-BASE DISORDERS. As indicated by the Henderson-Hasselbalch equation (see Equation 40–3), changes in the P_{CO_2} alter the blood pH: a rise decreases the pH, and a reduction increases the pH.

The ventilatory rate determines the P_{CO_2}. Increased ventilation decreases P_{CO_2}, whereas decreased ventilation increases it. The blood P_{CO_2} and pH are important regulators of the ventilatory rate (see Chapter 31). When metabolic acidosis occurs, a rise in the $[H^+]$ (decrease in pH) increases the ventilatory rate. Conversely, during metabolic alkalosis, a decreased $[H^+]$ (increase in pH) leads to a reduced ventilatory rate. With maximal hyperventilation, the P_{CO_2} can be reduced to approximately 10 mm Hg. Because hypoxia, a potent stimulator of ventilation, also develops with hypoventilation, the degree to which the P_{CO_2} can be increased is limited. In an otherwise normal individual, hypoventilation cannot raise the P_{CO_2} above 60 mm Hg. The respiratory response to metabolic acid-base disturbances may be initiated within minutes but may require several hours to be completed.

Renal net acid excretion changes in response to acid-base disorders

THE THIRD AND FINAL LINE OF DEFENSE AGAINST ACID-BASE DISORDERS IS THE KIDNEYS. In response to an alteration in the plasma pH and P_{CO_2}, the kidneys make appropriate adjustments in the excretion of HCO_3^- and net acid. The renal response may require several days to reach completion because it takes hours to days to increase the synthesis and activity of the proximal tubule enzymes involved in NH_4^+ production. In the case of acidosis (increased $[H^+]$ or P_{CO_2}), the secretion of H^+ by the nephron is stimulated, and the entire filtered load of HCO_3^- is reabsorbed. The production and excretion of NH_4^+ are also stimulated, and thus net acid excretion by the kidneys is increased (see Equation 40–1). The new HCO_3^- generated during the process of net acid excretion is added to the body, and the plasma $[HCO_3^-]$ increases.

When alkalosis exists (decreased $[H^+]$ or P_{CO_2}), the secretion of H^+ by the nephron is inhibited. As a result, net acid excretion and HCO_3^- reabsorption are reduced. HCO_3^- appears in the urine. Also, some HCO_3^- is secreted into the urine by the collecting duct. With enhanced excretion of HCO_3^-, the plasma $[HCO_3^-]$ decreases.

The loss of gastric contents from the body (i.e., vomiting, nasogastric suction) produces metabolic alkalosis secondary to the loss of HCl. If the loss of gastric fluid is significant, volume contraction occurs. Under this condition, the kidneys cannot excrete sufficient quantities of HCO_3^- to compensate for the metabolic alkalosis. HCO_3^- is not excreted because the volume contraction enhances Na^+ reabsorption by the proximal tubule and increases aldosterone levels (see Chapter 38). These responses in turn limit HCO_3^- excretion because Na^+ reabsorption in the proximal tubule is coupled to H^+ secretion via the Na^+-H^+ antiporter. As a result, HCO_3^- is reabsorbed because of the need to reduce Na^+ excretion. In addition, the elevated aldosterone levels stimulate H^+ secretion by the collecting duct. Thus, in individuals who lose gastric contents, metabolic alkalosis and paradoxically acidic urine characteristically occur. Correction of the alkalosis occurs only when euvolemia is reestablished. With restoration of euvolemia, HCO_3^- reabsorption by the proximal tubule decreases, as does H^+ secretion by the collecting duct. As a result, HCO_3^- excretion increases, and the plasma $[HCO_3^-]$ returns to normal.

Table 40–2 summarizes the primary alterations and the subsequent defense mechanisms of the various simple acid-base disorders. The defense mechanisms are commonly referred to as **compensatory responses.** In all acid-base disorders, the compensatory response does not correct the underlying disorder but simply reduces the magnitude of the change in pH. Correction of the acid-base disorder requires treatment of its cause.

Metabolic acidosis is characterized by a low plasma $[HCO_3^-]$ and a low pH

Metabolic acidosis can develop via the addition of nonvolatile acid to the body (e.g., diabetic ketoacidosis), the loss of nonvolatile base (e.g., that caused by diarrhea), or the failure of the kidneys to excrete sufficient net acid to replenish the HCO_3^- used to neutralize nonvolatile acids (e.g., renal tubular acidosis, renal failure). As previously described, the buffering of H^+ occurs in both the ECF and the ICF. When the pH falls, the respiratory centers are stimulated and the ventilatory rate is increased (respiratory compensation). This reduces the P_{CO_2}, which further minimizes the fall in plasma pH. Finally, renal net acid excretion is increased. This occurs via the elimination of all HCO_3^- from the urine (enhanced reabsorption of filtered HCO_3^-) and via increased NH_4^+ excretion (enhanced production of new HCO_3^-). If the process that initiated the acid-base disturbance is corrected, the enhanced net acid excretion by the kidneys will ultimately return the pH and $[HCO_3^-]$ to normal. After correction of the pH, the ventilatory rate also returns to normal.

TABLE 40–2. MECHANISMS OF DEFENSE AGAINST ACID-BASE DISORDERS

Disorder	Plasma pH	Primary Alteration	Defense Mechanisms
Metabolic acidosis	↓	↓Plasma [HCO_3^-]	ICF and ECF buffers Hyperventilation (↓PCO_2) ↑Renal NAE
Metabolic alkalosis	↑	↑Plasma [HCO_3^-]	ICF and ECF buffers Hypoventilation (↑PCO_2) ↓Renal NAE
Respiratory acidosis	↓	↑PCO_2	ICF buffers ↑Renal NAE
Respiratory alkalosis	↑	↓PCO_2	ICF buffers ↓Renal NAE

NAE, net acid excretion.

When nonvolatile acid is added to the body fluids, as in **diabetic ketoacidosis,** the [H^+] increases (pH decreases) and the [HCO_3^-] decreases. In addition, the concentration of the anion associated with the nonvolatile acid increases. This change in the anion concentration provides a convenient way of analyzing the cause of a metabolic acidosis by calculating what is termed the **anion gap.** The anion gap represents the difference between the concentration of the major plasma cation (Na^+) and the concentration of the major plasma anions (Cl^- and HCO_3^-):

$$\text{Anion gap} = [Na^+] - ([Cl^-] + [HCO_3^-]) \qquad \textbf{40-4}$$

Under normal conditions, the anion gap ranges from 8 to 16 mEq/L. An anion gap does not actually exist. All cations are balanced by anions. The gap simply reflects the parameters that are measured. In reality:

$$[Na^+] + [\text{Unmeasured cations}] = [Cl^-] + [HCO_3^-] + [\text{Unmeasured anions}] \qquad \textbf{40–5}$$

If the anion of the nonvolatile acid is Cl^-, the anion gap will be normal. (That is, the decrease in the [HCO_3^-] is matched by an increase in the [Cl^-].) The metabolic acidosis associated with diarrhea or renal tubular acidosis has a normal anion gap. In contrast, if the anion of the nonvolatile acid is not Cl^- (e.g., lactate, ß-hydroxybutyrate), the anion gap will increase. (That is, the decrease in the [HCO_3^-] is not matched by an increase in the [Cl^-] but rather by an increase in the concentration of the unmeasured anion.) The anion gap is increased in metabolic acidosis associated with renal failure, diabetes mellitus (ketoacidosis), lactic acidosis, and ingestion of large quantities of aspirin. Thus, CALCULATION OF THE ANION GAP IS A USEFUL WAY OF IDENTIFYING THE ETIOLOGY OF METABOLIC ACIDOSIS.

Metabolic alkalosis is characterized by an elevated plasma [HCO_3^-] and an elevated pH

Metabolic alkalosis can occur via the addition of nonvolatile alkali to the body (e.g., ingestion of antacids), as a result of volume contraction (e.g., hemorrhage), or, more commonly, from the loss of nonvolatile acid (e.g., loss of gastric HCl because of vomiting). Buffering occurs predominantly in the ECF and to a lesser degree in the ICF. The increase in the pH inhibits the respiratory centers, the ventilatory rate is reduced, and thus the PCO_2 is elevated (respiratory compensation). The renal compensatory response to metabolic alkalosis is to increase the excretion of HCO_3^- by reducing its reabsorption along the nephron. Normally, this occurs rapidly and effectively. However, as already noted, when alkalosis occurs with volume depletion (e.g., vomiting in which fluid loss occurs with H^+ loss), HCO_3^- is not excreted. Renal excretion of HCO_3^- is enhanced, and alkalosis is corrected only with restoration of euvolemia. Enhanced renal excretion of HCO_3^- eventually returns the pH and [HCO_3^-] to normal, provided the underlying cause of the initial acid-base disturbance is corrected. When the pH is corrected, the ventilatory rate also returns to normal.

Respiratory acidosis is characterized by an elevated PCO_2 and a reduced pH

Respiratory acidosis results from decreased gas exchange across the alveoli due to either inadequate ventilation (e.g., drug-induced depression of the respiratory centers) or impaired gas diffusion (e.g., pulmonary edema, such as that which occurs in cardiovascular or lung disease). In contrast to the

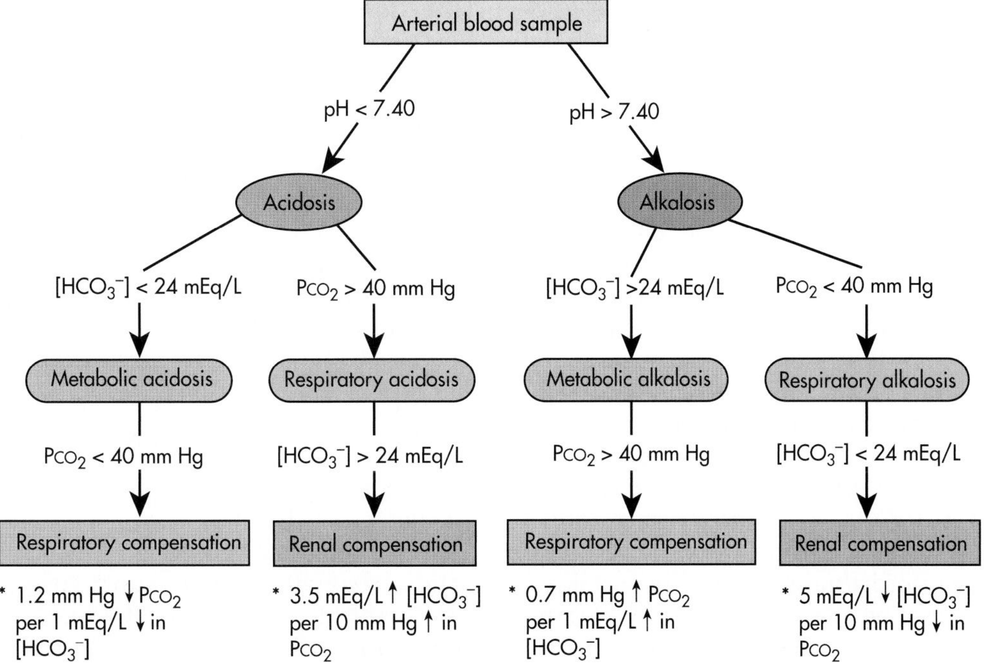

FIGURE 40–5. Approach for the analysis of simple acid-base disorders. (*If the compensatory response is not appropriate, a mixed acid-base disorder should be suspected.)

metabolic disorders, buffering during respiratory acidosis occurs almost entirely in the ICF. The increase in the P_{CO_2} and the decrease in pH stimulate both HCO_3^- reabsorption by the nephron and NH_4^+ excretion (renal compensation). Together, these responses increase net acid excretion and generate new HCO_3^-. The renal compensatory response takes several days to occur. Consequently, respiratory acid-base disorders are commonly divided into acute and chronic phases. In the acute phase, the time for the renal compensatory response is not sufficient, and the body relies on intracellular buffering to minimize the change in pH. Correction of the underlying disorder returns the P_{CO_2} to normal, and renal net acid excretion decreases to its initial level.

Respiratory alkalosis is characterized by a reduced P_{CO_2} and an elevated pH

Respiratory alkalosis results from increased gas exchange in the lungs, usually caused by increased ventilation from stimulation of the respiratory centers (e.g., via drugs or disorders of the central nervous system). Hyperventilation occurs at high altitude and as a result of anxiety, pain, or fear. As noted, buffering is primarily in the ICF. Like respiratory acidosis, respiratory alkalosis has both acute and chronic phases reflecting the time required for renal compensation to occur. With renal compensation, the elevated pH and reduced P_{CO_2} inhibit HCO_3^- reabsorption by the nephron and reduce NH_4^+ production and excretion. As a result of these two effects, net acid excretion is reduced. Correction of the underlying disorder returns the P_{CO_2} to normal, and renal excretion of acid then increases to its initial level.

The Analysis of an Acid-Base Disorder Is Directed at Identifying the Underlying Cause so that Appropriate Therapy Can Be Initiated

The patient's medical history and associated physical findings often provide valuable clues about the nature and origin of an acid-base disorder. In addition, the analysis of an arterial blood sample is frequently required. Such an analysis is straightforward if it is approached systematically. For example, consider the following data:

pH	7.35
$[HCO_3^-]$	16 mEq/L
P_{CO_2}	30 mm Hg

The acid-base disorder represented by these values, or any other set of values, can be determined by the following three-step approach (**Figure 40–5**):

1. Examination of the pH: When the pH is considered first, the underlying disorder can be classified as either an acidosis or an alkalosis. The defense

mechanisms of the body cannot correct an acid-base disorder by themselves. Thus, even if the defense mechanisms are completely operative, the change in pH indicates the acid-base disorder. In the example provided, the pH of 7.35 indicates acidosis.

2. Determination of metabolic versus respiratory disorder: Simple acid-base disorders are either metabolic or respiratory. To determine which disorder is present, the clinician must next examine the $[HCO_3^-]$ and PCO_2. As previously discussed, acidosis could be the result of a decrease in the $[HCO_3^-]$ (metabolic) or an increase in the PCO_2 (respiratory). Alternatively, alkalosis could be the result of an increase in the $[HCO_3^-]$ (metabolic) or a decrease in the PCO_2 (respiratory). For the example provided, the $[HCO_3^-]$ is reduced from normal (normal = 24 mEq/L), as is the PCO_2 (normal = 40 mm Hg). The disorder must therefore be metabolic acidosis; it cannot be a respiratory acidosis because the PCO_2 is reduced.
3. Analysis of a compensatory response: Metabolic disorders result in compensatory changes in ventilation and thus in the PCO_2, whereas respiratory disorders result in compensatory changes in renal net acid excretion and thus in the $[HCO_3^-]$. In an appropriately compensated metabolic acidosis, the PCO_2 is decreased, whereas it is elevated in compensated metabolic alkalosis. With respiratory acidosis, complete compensation results in an elevation of the $[HCO_3^-]$. Conversely, the $[HCO_3^-]$ is reduced in response to respiratory alkalosis. In this example, the PCO_2 is reduced from normal, and the magnitude of this reduction is as expected (Figure 40–5). Therefore, the acid-base disorder is a simple metabolic acidosis with appropriate respiratory compensation.

Multiple acid-base disorders can exist in a patient

If the appropriate compensatory response is not present, a **mixed acid-base disorder** should be suspected. Such a disorder reflects the presence of two or more underlying causes for the acid-base disturbance. A mixed disorder should be suspected when analysis of the arterial blood gas indicates that appropriate compensation has not occurred. For example, consider the following data:

pH	6.96
$[HCO_3^-]$	12 mEq/L
PCO_2	55 mm Hg

When the three-step approach is followed, it is evident that the disturbance is an acidosis that has both a metabolic component ($[HCO_3^-] < 24$ mEq/L) and a respiratory component ($PCO_2 > 40$ mm Hg). Thus, this disorder is mixed. Mixed acid-base disorders can occur, for example, in an individual who has a history of a chronic pulmonary disease, such as emphysema (i.e., chronic respiratory acidosis), and who develops an acute gastrointestinal illness with diarrhea. Because diarrhea fluid contains HCO_3^-, its loss from the body results in the development of metabolic acidosis.

A MIXED ACID-BASE DISORDER IS ALSO INDICATED WHEN A PATIENT HAS ABNORMAL PCO_2 AND $[HCO_3^-]$ VALUES, BUT THE pH IS NORMAL. Such a condition can develop in a patient who has ingested a large quantity of aspirin. The salicylic acid (active ingredient in aspirin) produces metabolic acidosis, and at the same time, it stimulates the respiratory centers, causing hyperventilation and respiratory alkalosis. Thus, the patient has a reduced plasma $[HCO_3^-]$ and a reduced PCO_2.

Summary

- The pH of the body fluids is maintained within a narrow range by the coordinated function of the lungs, liver, and kidneys. These organs maintain acid-base balance by balancing the excretion of acid and alkali with the amounts ingested in the diet and produced by metabolism.
- The kidneys maintain acid-base balance through the excretion of an amount of acid equal to the amount of nonvolatile acid produced by metabolism and the quantity ingested in the diet. The kidneys also prevent the loss of HCO_3^- in the urine by reabsorbing virtually all the HCO_3^- filtered at the glomeruli. Both the reabsorption of filtered HCO_3^- and the excretion of acid are accomplished by the secretion of H^+ by the nephrons.
- Renal net acid excretion (NAE) is quantitated as

$$NAE = [(U_{NH_4^+} \times \dot{V}) + (U_{TA} \times \dot{V})] - (U_{HCO_3^-} \times \dot{V})$$

- Phosphate is the primary urinary buffer (titratable acid). The production (from glutamine metabolism) and excretion of NH_4^+ are critical to the generation of new HCO_3^- by the kidneys and are regulated in response to acid-base disturbances.
- The body uses three lines of defense to minimize the impact of acid-base disorders on body fluid pH: (1) ECF and ICF buffering, (2) respiratory compensation, and (3) renal compensation.
- Metabolic acid-base disorders result from primary alterations in the [HCO_3^-], which in turn result from the addition of acid to or loss of alkali from the body. In response to metabolic acidosis, pulmonary ventilation is increased, which decreases the P_{CO_2}. An increase in the [HCO_3^-] causes alkalosis. This decreases pulmonary ventilation, which elevates the P_{CO_2}. The pulmonary response to metabolic acid-base disorders occurs in a matter of minutes.
- Respiratory acid-base disorders result from primary alterations in the P_{CO_2}. Elevation of the P_{CO_2} produces acidosis, and the kidneys respond with an increase in net acid excretion. Conversely, the reduction of P_{CO_2} produces alkalosis, and renal net acid excretion is reduced. The kidneys respond to respiratory acid-base disorders during several hours to days.

Bibliography

Alpern RJ, Hamm LL: Urinary acidification. In DuBose TD Jr, Hamm LL, eds: *Acid-base and electrolyte disorders,* Philadelphia, 2002, WB Saunders.

Battle D et al: Hereditary distal renal tubular acidosis: new understandings, *Annu Rev Med* 52:471, 2001.

Bidani A et al: Regulation of whole body acid-base balance. In DuBose TD Jr, Hamm LL, eds: *Acid-base and electrolyte disorders,* Philadelphia, 2002, WB Saunders.

Brown D, Breton S: Structure, function and cellular distribution of the vacuolar H^+ATPase (H^+V-ATPase/proton pump). In Seldin DW, Giebisch G, eds: *The kidney: physiology and pathophysiology,* ed 3, Philadelphia, 2000, Lippincott Williams & Wilkins.

Counillon L, Pouyssegur J: The members of the Na^+/H^+ exchanger gene family: their structure, function, expression, and regulation. In Seldin DW, Giebisch G, eds: *The kidney: physiology and pathophysiology,* ed 3, Philadelphia, 2000, Lippincott Williams & Wilkins.

DuBose TD Jr: Acid-base disorders. In Brenner BM, ed: *Brenner and Rector's the kidney,* ed 7, Philadelphia, 2004, WB Saunders.

Emmett M: Diagnosis of simple and mixed disorders. In DuBose TD Jr, Hamm LL, eds: *Acid-base and electrolyte disorders,* Philadelphia, 2002, WB Saunders.

Gennari FJ, Maddox DA: Renal regulation of acid-base homeostasis integrated response. In Seldin DW, Giebisch G, eds: *The kidney: physiology and pathophysiology,* ed 3, Philadelphia, 2000, Lippincott Williams & Wilkins.

Hamm LL: Renal acidification mechanisms. In Brenner BM, ed: *Brenner and Rector's the kidney,* ed 7, Philadelphia, 2004, WB Saunders.

Shayakul C, Alper SL: Inherited renal tubular acidosis, *Curr Opin Nephrol Hypertens* 9:541, 2000.

Silver RB, Soleimani M: H^+-K^+-ATPases: regulation and role in pathophysiological states, *Am J Physiol* 276:F799, 1999.

Soleimani M, Burnham CE: Physiologic and molecular aspects of the Na^+:HCO_3^- cotransporter in health and disease, *Kidney Int* 57:371, 2000.

Wagner CA, Geibel JP: Acid-base transport in the collecting duct, *J Nephrol* 15: S112, 2002.

Case Studies

Case 40–1

A 22-year-old man with insulin-dependent diabetes mellitus is seen in the emergency department. He reports that he "has had the flu for the past couple days." Because he has not felt well and was not eating, he has not taken any insulin during the previous 24 hours. He also reports taking two aspirin tablets before coming to the emergency department because of a headache. On examination, he is found to have rapid and deep respirations. The following laboratory data are obtained:

pH	7.32 (normal: 7.40)
P_{O_2}	100 mm Hg (normal: 100 mm Hg)
P_{CO_2}	30 mm Hg (normal: 40 mm Hg)
[HCO_3^-]	15 mEq/L (normal: 24 mEq/L)

1. What type of acid-base disorder does this man have?
- A. Metabolic acidosis
- B. Metabolic alkalosis
- C. Respiratory acidosis
- D. Respiratory alkalosis
- E. Mixed disorder (metabolic acidosis and respiratory alkalosis)

2. Why are this man's respirations rapid and deep?
- A. The decrease in PCO_2 has stimulated his respiratory center.
- B. Hypoxemia has stimulated his respiratory center.
- C. This is the normal respiratory response to his acid-base disturbance.
- D. There is poor pulmonary gas exchange caused by an infection in his lungs.
- E. Aspirin has stimulated his respiratory center.

3. What is the most important component of the compensatory response of this man's kidneys to his acid-base disorder?
- A. Increased filtered load of HCO_3^-
- B. Decreased secretion of H^+ by the proximal tubule
- C. Increased production and excretion of NH_4^+
- D. Decreased H^+ secretion by the collecting duct
- E. Increased secretion of HCO_3^- by the collecting duct

Case 40–2

A 50-year-old woman with a history of a duodenal ulcer comes to the emergency department because she has had intermittent vomiting for several days. She is admitted to the hospital, and a nasogastric tube is introduced to continuously remove the stomach contents. After 24 hours, the woman has signs of volume depletion. The following laboratory values are obtained:

pH	7.50 (normal: 7.40)
PO_2	100 mm Hg (normal: 100 mm Hg)
PCO_2	47 mm Hg (normal: 40 mm Hg)
$[HCO_3^-]$	35 mEq/L (normal: 24 mEq/L)
Urine pH	6.0

1. What type of acid-base disorder does this woman have?
- A. Metabolic acidosis
- B. Metabolic alkalosis
- C. Respiratory acidosis
- D. Respiratory alkalosis
- E. Mixed disorder (metabolic alkalosis and respiratory acidosis)

2. Why is this woman's urine acidic?
- A. Collecting duct H^+ secretion is stimulated by aldosterone.
- B. H^+ secretion by the proximal tubule is impaired (i.e., proximal renal tubular acidosis).
- C. The filtered load of HCO_3^- is increased.
- D. NH_4^+ production and excretion are increased.
- E. Titratable acid excretion is increased.

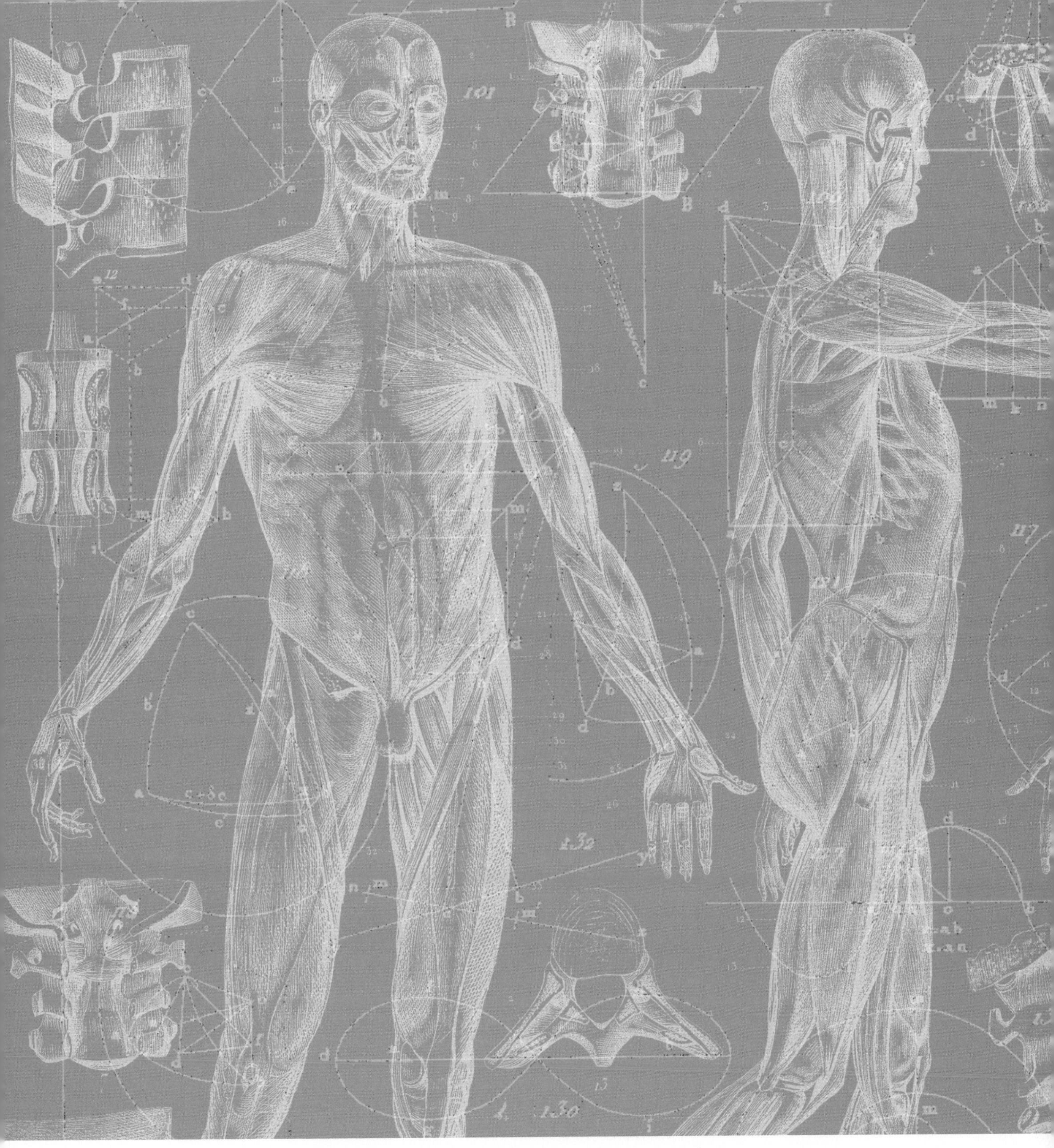

Part Eight: Endocrine System

Saul M. Genuth

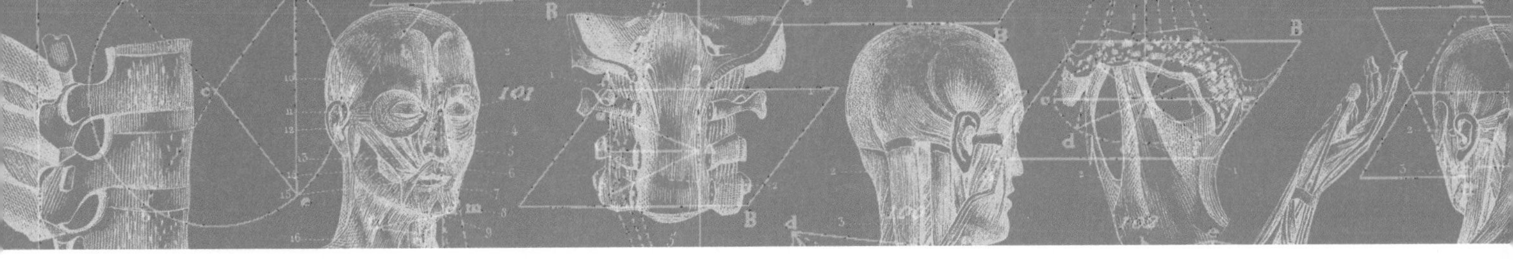

Chapter 41: General Principles of Endocrine Physiology

Objectives

- ❖ Describe the overall workings of the endocrine system.
- ❖ Differentiate various modes of hormone synthesis.
- ❖ Explain the multiple mechanisms of hormone actions.
- ❖ Indicate how hormone production is measured.
- ❖ Explain the factors that determine whole-body responsiveness to hormones.

The endocrine system relates to all of the preceding chapters because it regulates the functioning of every cell, tissue, and organ in the body. Although the endocrine system has numerous components with individual diverse characteristics, this chapter sets forth a set of basic themes that underlie the processes of hormone secretion and action.

The Endocrine System Is a Key Component in Maintenance of Homeostasis

The endocrine system is a key component in the adaptation of the human organism to alterations in the external and internal environment (i.e., maintenance of **homeostasis**). THE ENDOCRINE SYSTEM ACTS TO MAINTAIN A STABLE INTERNAL MILIEU IN THE FACE OF CHANGES IN INFLOW OR OUTFLOW OF SUBSTRATES, MINERALS, WATER, ENVIRONMENTAL SUBSTANCES, HEAT, AND SO ON. Specific endocrine cells, usually grouped in glands, sense the disturbance and respond by secreting chemical substances called **hormones** into the bloodstream. These special molecules are carried via the circulation to various tissues, where they signal and act on their target cells. As a result, the target cells respond in a manner that usually opposes the direction of change that evoked hormone secretion and thereby restores the organism toward its original state. In addition to this fundamental role in maintaining homeostasis, the endocrine system helps initiate, mediate, and regulate the processes of growth, development, maturation, reproduction, and senescence.

A hormone was originally defined as a substance that is elaborated by one type of cell and that carries a signal through the bloodstream to distant target cells. However, this sophisticated method of signaling probably evolved from a more primitive one (**Figure 41–1**). Hormone molecules secreted by endocrine cells can also reach and act on target cells within the same locale simply by diffusing through the interstitial fluid separating them; this process is called **paracrine function.** Secreted hormone molecules can even act back on identical cells to modulate their own secretion or other intracellular processes; this is called **autocrine function.** Moreover, without being secreted, hormone molecules can regulate processes within their own cell of origin; this is called **intracrine function.**

Classic endocrine cells reside in the pituitary, thyroid, adrenal, and parathyroid glands; in the gonads; and in the pancreatic islets. However, hormone-like signaling molecules are also elaborated by other nonclassic endocrine cells, such as

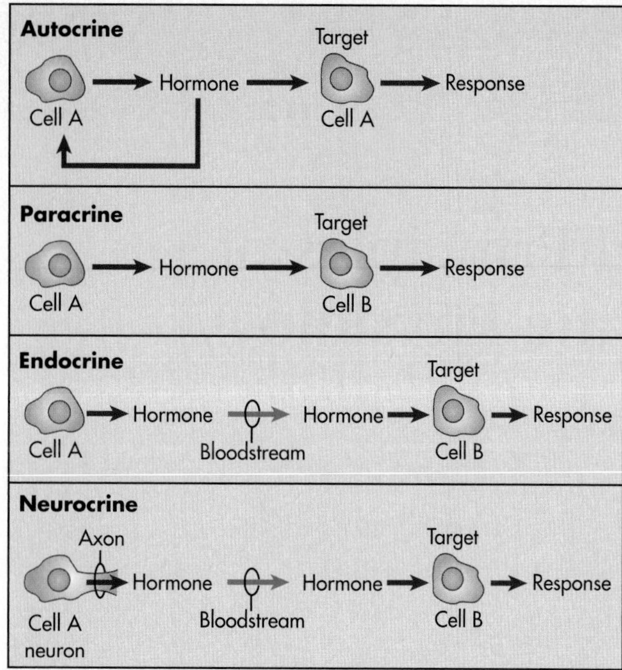

FIGURE 41–1. Mechanisms for cell-to-cell signaling via hormone molecules. In autocrine function, the hormone signal acts back on the cell of origin or adjacent identical cells. In paracrine function, the hormone signal is carried to an adjacent target cell over short distances via the interstitial fluid. In endocrine function, the signal is carried to a distant target cell via the bloodstream. In neurocrine function, the hormone signal originates in a neuron and after axonal transport to the bloodstream is carried to a distant target cell.

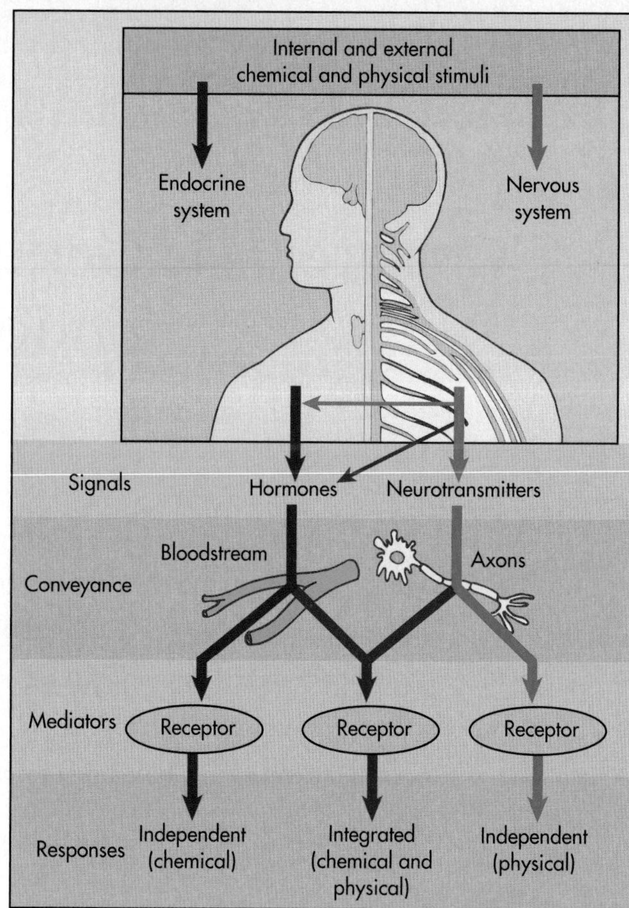

FIGURE 41–2. Overview of the relationship between the endocrine and nervous systems. Similar stimuli may elicit activity of both systems. Hormones secreted by endocrine cells and conveyed via the bloodstream are analogous to neurotransmitters released by neurons after being conveyed by their axons. Neurotransmitters may also stimulate hormone release and themselves act as hormones. Responses are mediated by receptors in each system and may consist of either chemical or physical changes.

neurons, renal cells, cardiac atrial and ventricular cells, endothelial cells, immune system cells (cytokines and lymphokines), adipose cells, mesenchymal cells (growth factors), and platelets.

The endocrine system may act independently of or may be integrated with the nervous system

The endocrine and nervous systems are the major components in the organism's adaptability to change **(Figure 41–2)**. These two signaling systems have several characteristics in common:

- Both neurons and endocrine cells are capable of secreting.
- Both endocrine cells and neurons generate electrical potentials and can be depolarized.
- Some molecules serve as both a neurotransmitter and a hormone.
- The mechanism of action of both hormones and neurotransmitters requires interaction with specific receptors in target cells.
- A similar process and repertory of proteins mediate exocytosis of secretory granules and synaptic vesicles.

Although the endocrine system responds more often to chemical stimuli and the nervous system more often to physical or mechanical stimuli, considerable overlap exists. For example, changes in the quantity of light and changes in plasma substrate concentrations may evoke responses by both systems. Interaction between the two systems takes several forms:

- Some stimuli that cause hormone release are first sensed by the nervous system, which in turn signals an appropriate endocrine cell to respond.
- Some neurons extend their axons in bundles or tracts that terminate adjacent to capillaries.

Stimulation releases their neurotransmitters into the bloodstream. This hybrid form of signal transmission is called **neurocrine function** (Figure 41–1), and the signaling molecules are called **neurohormones** or **neuropeptides.** For example, **antidiuretic hormone** is synthesized in the cell body of a hypothalamic neuron but is released from the end of the neuron's axon into blood bathing the posterior pituitary gland. Antidiuretic hormone then acts on distant cells in the kidney and causes the retention of solute-free water. The stimulus for axonal release of antidiuretic hormone is water deprivation, sensed in the hypothalamus as an increase in plasma osmolality, a decrease in volume, or both reactions.

- Some stimuli evoke integrated endocrine and nervous system responses that augment each other in restoring homeostasis.

The principle of chemical homeostasis and the fundamental relationship of the endocrine system to the nervous system are well illustrated by the response of the organism to a lowered plasma concentration of glucose **(hypoglycemia),** such as that which can occur with strenuous and prolonged exercise (**Figure 41–3**). Because a supply of glucose is absolutely required to sustain brain function, hypoglycemia cannot be tolerated for long. Endocrine cells in the pancreas respond to hypoglycemia by secreting a hormone called **glucagon** that stimulates the release of stored glucose from the liver. Other endocrine cells in the pancreas respond in the opposite way to hypoglycemia by diminishing the secretion of the hormone **insulin,** thereby reducing use of glucose by tissues other than the brain.

Certain cells in the liver and portal vein sense hypoglycemia and signal the nervous system. Certain neurons in the hypothalamus sense hypoglycemia and augment the release of stored hepatic glucose directly by transmitting sympathetic neural impulses to liver cells and indirectly by transmitting sympathetic nervous system impulses to the adrenal medulla. This neuroendocrine gland secretes the hormone **epinephrine,** which acts on the liver to release stored glucose and on other tissues to reduce glucose use. Finally, other neurons in the hypothalamus also sense hypoglycemia and via combined neurocrine and endocrine pathways stimulate the adrenal cortex to secrete the hormone **cortisol.** This hormone augments the synthesis of glucose in the liver to maintain the supply in case initial stores become depleted. Cortisol also inhibits the insulin-stimulated use of glucose by tissues other than the brain. Together these endocrine and neural responses to hypoglycemia promptly raise plasma glucose levels back to normal.

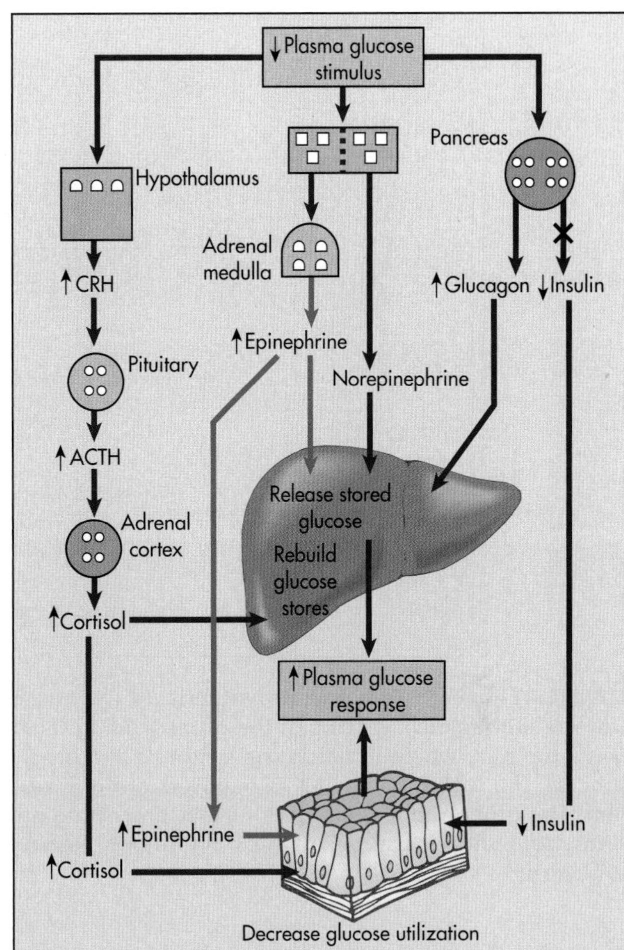

FIGURE 41–3. Integrated endocrine and neural response to hypoglycemia. The anterior pituitary gland, adrenal cortex, adrenal medulla, and pancreatic islets participate in the main endocrine components of the response. The hypothalamus and the sympathetic nervous system participate in the neural components of the response. See text for details on how each component acts to restore the plasma glucose concentration to normal. ACTH, adrenocorticotropic hormone; CRH, corticotropin-releasing hormone.

Hormones Are Synthesized, Stored, and Secreted in a Variety of Ways

Peptide and **protein hormones** are synthesized by a general process that characterizes the synthesis of all secreted proteins (**Figure 41–4**). The gene or DNA molecule that directs hormone synthesis transcribes a messenger RNA molecule. The messenger RNA traverses the nuclear membrane to the cytoplasm, where it translates its message on ribosomes by directing the assembly of the correct sequence of amino acids into a primary gene product. This molecule is larger than the hormone itself and is called a **preprohormone.** At the N

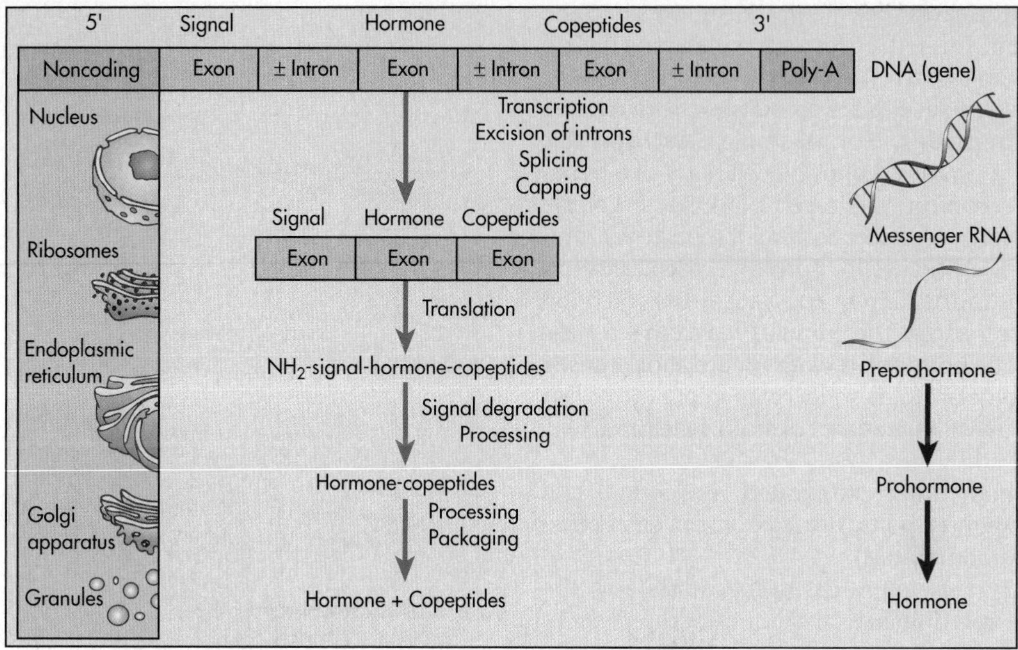

FIGURE 41–4. Peptide hormone synthesis. In the nucleus, the primary gene transcript undergoes excision of introns (noncoding regions), splicing of the exons (coding regions), and capping. The resultant mature messenger RNA enters the cytoplasm, where it directs the synthesis of a precursor peptide sequence (preprohormone) on ribosomes. In this process, the N-terminus signal is removed, and the resultant prohormone is transferred into the endoplasmic reticulum. The prohormone undergoes further processing and is then packaged into secretory granules in the Golgi apparatus. After final cleavage of the prohormone within the granules, the hormone and copeptides are secreted by exocytosis.

terminus, a signal peptide directs the transfer of the preprohormone from the ribosome into the **endoplasmic reticulum.** During this process, the signal peptide is degraded, leaving a **prohormone.** This molecule contains the hormone as well as other peptide sequences.

The prohormone is transferred to the Golgi apparatus, where it undergoes further processing. This may include cleavage; the addition of other chemical units, such as carbohydrate molecules, sialic acid, and sulfonyl groups; or the combination of separate subunits derived from different genes. In the Golgi apparatus, the hormone and its peptide byproducts are packaged together within a secretory granule.

On stimulation of the endocrine cell, the contents of secretory granules are released into the extracellular fluid and then into adjacent bathing capillaries via exocytosis (**Figure 41–5**). By the disaggregation of actin cytoskeleton, contraction of microfilaments, and guidance by microtubules, the secretory granules move to docking sites in the plasma membrane of the cell, tether to the membrane, and fuse with it. This process requires Ca^{++} and ATP, and a **GTP-binding protein** helps attach the granules to specific sites. A small GTPase known as **Raf** is also involved. The mechanisms of granule release require an increase in the

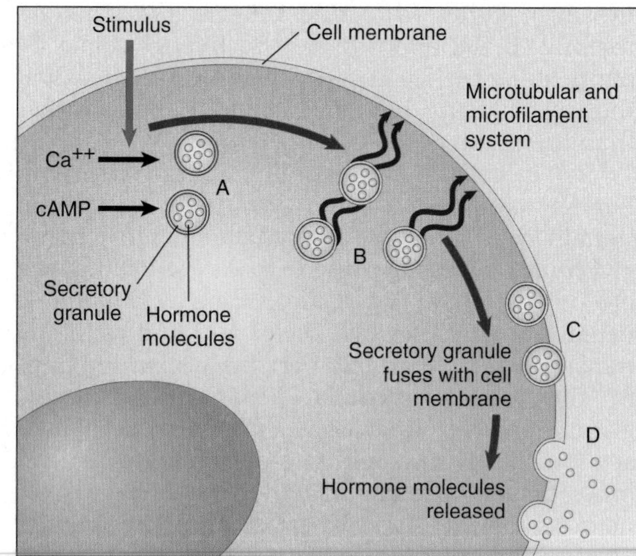

FIGURE 41–5. Secretion of peptide hormones via exocytosis. A, Secretion is initiated by the application of a stimulus that raises the cytosolic Ca^{++} level and also usually raises the intracellular level of cAMP. B, The secretory granules are lined up and translocated to the plasma membrane via activation of a microtubular and microfilament system. C, The membrane of the secretory granule fuses with that of the cell. D, The common membrane is lysed, releasing the hormone into the interstitial space.

intracytoplasmic [Ca^{++}]; the Ca^{++} is derived from both extracellular fluid and intracellular stores within the endoplasmic reticulum and other organelles. Exocytosis is also often preceded by increases in **cAMP** concentration.

Catecholamine hormones (epinephrine, norepinephrine, dopamine) are synthesized from the amino acid tyrosine through a series of enzymatic reactions. However, they are stored in secretory granules and secreted in a manner similar to that of peptide hormones.

Thyroid hormones (thyroxine, triiodothyronine) are synthesized from tyrosine and iodide in a series of reactions that occur with the amino acid already incorporated via peptide linkage into a large protein molecule. The hormones are then sequestered within the protein molecule in a storage space (follicle) shared by a group of surrounding endocrine cells. The secretion of thyroid hormone requires retrieval from the follicle and enzymatic release from its protein storage form.

Steroid hormones (cortisol, aldosterone, androgens, estrogens, progestins, vitamin D) are synthesized from cholesterol by a series of enzymatic reactions. However, they are not stored to any appreciable extent within the gland of origin. Thus, increases in the secretion of a steroid hormone are accomplished by the activation of the entire biosynthetic sequence from cholesterol. In effect, the storage form of all steroid hormones is the intracellular depot of cholesterol.

Prostaglandins are hormones with largely paracrine actions that are synthesized from the unsaturated essential fatty acid **arachidonic acid.** Oxygenation and cyclization are the main processes involved. There is no unique cell of origin of prostaglandins, which are synthesized and act ubiquitously. Arachidonic acid is also the source for epoxyeicosatrienoic acid and derivatives in endothelial, smooth muscle, and renal tubular cells. These paracrine modulators influence vasomotor actions and Na^+ transport.

Genetic diseases causing deficient or abnormal synthesis of peptide or protein hormones are rare and usually involve the hormone gene itself (e.g., insulin). In the case of thyroid or steroid hormones, the product of the mutant gene is usually an enzyme that catalyzes one of the many separate reactions in the biosynthetic sequence for the affected hormone (e.g., adrenal steroid hydroxylases).

The Dominant Mechanism of Regulating Hormone Secretion Is Negative Feedback

The secretion of hormones is related to their roles in maintaining homeostasis. The dominant mechanism of regulation is **negative feedback (Figure 41–6).** If hormone A acts to raise the plasma concentration of substrate B, a decrease in substrate B will stimulate the secretion of hormone A, whereas an increase in substrate B will suppress the secretion of hormone A. In essence, PHYSIOLOGICAL CONDITIONS THAT REQUIRE THE ACTION OF A HORMONE ALSO STIMULATE ITS RELEASE; CONDITIONS OR PRODUCTS RESULTING FROM PRIOR HORMONE ACTION SUPPRESS FURTHER HORMONE RELEASE. This homeostatic partnership may exist between a hormone and one or more substrates, minerals, other hormones, or even physical factors such as fluid volume.

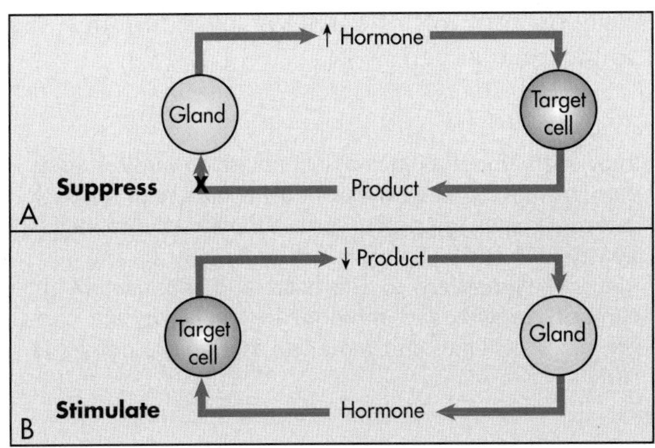

FIGURE 41–6. Negative feedback principle. A, If an increase in hormone secretion stimulates a greater output of product from the target cell, the product feeds back on the gland to suppress further hormone secretion. In this way, hormone excess is limited or prevented. B, If a decrease in the output of product from the target cell stimulates hormone secretion, the hormone in turn stimulates the output of product by the target cell. In this way, product deficiency is limited or corrected.

Positive feedback is occasionally observed. In such circumstances, a product of initial hormone action stimulates further hormone secretion. When the product eventually reaches appropriate concentrations, it may then exert negative feedback on hormone secretion. This mechanism of regulation occurs when a biological process begins at a very low level yet must reach rather high levels in the course of normal physiological function. Feedback regulation may be exerted at all levels of endocrine cell function (i.e., at transcription of the hormone gene, at translation of the gene message, and at release of stored hormone) and cell growth.

Engrafted on homeostatic feedback are patterns of hormone release dictated by diurnal (daily) or ultradian (within a day) rhythms, stages of sleep, seasonal variation, and stages of development (fetal, neonatal, pubertal, senescent). In addition, pain, emotion, fright, injury, and sexual arousal may evoke or shut off the release of hormones via complex neural pathways.

Individuals undergoing major medical or surgical stress demonstrate a pattern of hormonal release (e.g., cortisol, catecholamines, glucagon) that stimulates the mobilization of fuels such as glucose or free fatty acids and augments their delivery to the heart and musculature. In contrast, growth and reproductive processes are suppressed. Hormones also modulate immune responses to stress.

Hormone Turnover Is the Rate at Which Hormones Are Released and Replaced

The binding of hormones by plasma proteins greatly influences hormonal rates of turnover

After secretion into the blood, catecholamine, peptide, and some protein hormones circulate unbound to other plasma constituents. In other instances, they are bound partly to circulating portions of their normal cell receptors or to specific binding proteins. In contrast, thyroid and steroid hormones circulate largely bound to specific globulins as well as to albumin. The extent of protein binding greatly influences the rates at which hormones exit from plasma into interstitial fluid and gain access to target cells. A hormone's plasma half-life (the time required for a 50% decrease in concentration) is increased by strong protein binding.

Larger protein hormones with carbohydrate or sialic acid components have longer half-lives than smaller protein and peptide hormones. After exiting from plasma, hormone molecules may return from other compartments via lymphatic channels, sometimes after dissociation from target cells.

The sum of a hormone's removal processes is expressed as its metabolic clearance rate

Irreversible removal of a hormone from the body results from target cell uptake, metabolic degradation, and urinary or biliary excretion. The sum of all removal processes is expressed in the concept of **metabolic clearance rate** (MCR), or the volume of plasma cleared of hormone per unit of time. In a steady state, this equals the mass of hormone removed per unit of time divided by its plasma concentration:

$$\text{MCR} = \frac{\text{mg/min (removed)}}{\text{mg/mL (plasma)}} = \frac{\text{mL plasma (cleared)}}{\text{min}} \qquad \textbf{41-1}$$

MCR is an expression of the overall efficiency with which a hormone is removed from plasma irrespective of the mechanism. Its derivation is conceptually analogous to that of **renal clearance,** which is explained in Chapter 36. In the case of renal clearance, milligram per minute (mg/min) removed, the measured numerator in Equation 41-1, is the urinary excretion of the substance.

The kidney and liver are the major sites of the metabolic degradation of hormones. Renal clearance of a hormone (e.g., thyroid hormone) is extremely low if it is bound to specific plasma globulins. Although peptide and smaller protein hormones are filtered to some degree by the renal glomeruli, they usually undergo tubular reabsorption and subsequent degradation within the kidney so that only a minute amount appears in the urine.

Metabolic degradation of hormones occurs via enzymatic processes that include proteolysis, oxidation, reduction, hydroxylation, decarboxylation, and methylation. Hormones or their metabolites may also be conjugated to water-soluble molecules, yielding glucuronides and sulfates, which are then excreted in the bile or urine.

The amount of hormone secreted can be estimated from plasma and urine measurements

With the use of isotopic techniques, the total amount of hormone secreted into the bloodstream per unit time can be measured. For clinical purposes, the measurement of hormone in plasma or urine must usually suffice. However, these measurements are valid indices of hormone production if certain conditions exist. In a steady state, the amount of hormone entering the plasma is equal to the amount of hormone exiting the plasma.

$$\text{Secretion rate} = \text{Disposal rate} = \text{Metabolic clearance} \times \text{Plasma concentration} \qquad \textbf{41-2}$$

If the MCR can be taken as a constant (i.e., MCR is assumed to be normal), then the secretion rate is proportional to the plasma level. This is the theoretical basis for using only the plasma hormone measurement as an index of secretory rate. However, the secretion of many hormones is characterized by diurnal variation and episodic spurts.

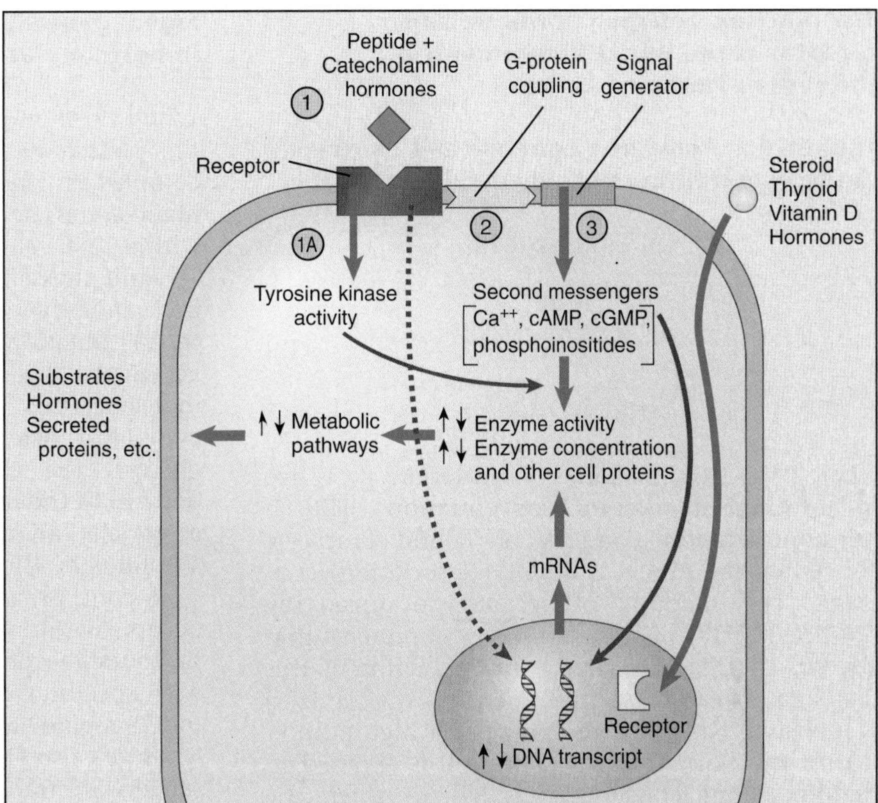

FIGURE 41–7. Hormone actions on target cells. Hormones interact with either the plasma membrane or intracellular receptors. Hormones may generate second messengers within the receptor (e.g., tyrosine kinase activity), cytoplasm (e.g., cAMP), or nucleus (e.g., transcription factors). Metabolic pathways can be regulated by altering the activities or the concentrations of enzymes. Cell growth and architecture may also be modulated.

In such instances, a specifically timed sample or multiple plasma samples may be necessary for a valid estimate.

Similarly, hormone secretion can sometimes be assessed by measuring its urinary excretion in accurately timed collections. This serves to average plasma fluctuations over the collection interval. Urinary excretion is a valid index of secretion rate when kidney function and kidney handling of the hormone are normal.

Hormone Responses Require Recognition by the Target Cell, Generation of Second Messengers, and Various Intracellular Effector Mechanisms

Three major sequential steps are involved in eliciting responses to hormones **(Figure 41–7)**:

1. The hormone must be recognized by the target cell.
2. An intracellular signal must then be generated.
3. One or more intracellular processes (e.g., enzyme reactions, ion movements, cytoskeletal rearrangements, gene transcription) must be increased or decreased.

The binding of hormones to specific receptors causes hormone recognition

Recognition takes place via binding of the hormone to a specific receptor that may be located within the plasma membrane, cytoplasm, nucleus, or possibly other organelles of the target cell. The receptor has a specific binding site with a high affinity for the hormone. The two molecules associate in reversible fashion to form a hormone-receptor complex. The receptor confers specificity to the interaction of a hormone with its target cells. Only cells that have the receptor can respond to the hormone; only hormones for which the cell possesses receptors can affect the cell.

Certain individuals susceptible to **autoimmune diseases** develop antibodies to some of their own hormone receptors. When such antibodies react with the receptor molecules, they may simply block access of the hormone to the receptor and cause biological deficiency (e.g., **hypothyroidism** caused by chronic **autoimmune thyroiditis**). Alternatively, the antibody-receptor combination mimics the hormone-receptor interaction and causes hyperfunction of the gland (e.g., **hyperthyroidism** caused by **Graves' disease**). These conditions are described in Chapter 46.

The reaction between hormone and receptor is the initial determinant of the rate of hormone action

The reaction between a hormone and its receptor can be expressed in classic chemical terms:

$$[H] + [R] \leftrightarrow [HR] \quad \textbf{41-3}$$

$$K = \frac{[HR]}{[H][R]} \quad \textbf{41-4}$$

$$[HR] = K[H][R] \quad \textbf{41-5}$$

where [H] is free hormone concentration, [R] is free or unoccupied receptor concentration, [HR] is hormone-receptor complex or bound hormone concentration, and K is affinity (association) constant. The amount of receptor occupied by hormone ([HR]) is the critical component that governs the magnitude of hormone action at this first step. As can be seen from Equation 41-5, [HR] is increased when the receptor has a high affinity (K) for the hormone, when the cell is exposed to high hormone concentrations [H], or when the receptor number [R] is high.

In some cases, [HR] is the rate-limiting step in the whole sequence of hormone action; therefore, the maximal biological response to these hormones is directly proportional to the number of receptors. In cases in which [HR] is not rate limiting, the biological response can sometimes be maximal when only a small proportion of the available receptors is occupied by hormone.

Receptor molecules undergo continual, regulated turnover

Receptor molecules are continually synthesized, translocated to and inserted into sites of association with hormone molecules, and degraded. These processes can be influenced by their respective hormone partners. Most hormones decrease or "down-regulate" the number of their own receptors; this helps prevent excess hormone action on the cell. Other hormones recruit their own receptors and thereby amplify hormone action on the cell.

Receptors are large protein molecules that may also contain carbohydrate units. The receptors incorporated into plasma membranes have extracellular portions that bind their hormones; transmembrane and intracellular portions interact with signal-generating mechanisms that initiate intracellular actions (see Chapter 5).

Signal generation is the next step in hormone action

When hormone-receptor association occurs within the plasma membrane of the cell, the resultant complex is often coupled to other plasma membrane components (see Chapter 5). These generate within the cell a variety of signal molecules or "second messengers," which then regulate metabolic and other processes (see Figures 5–1 and 41–7). In this situation, the essential information for triggering the cell's response resides in the receptor molecule; this information is transmitted to the cytoplasm when the hormone occupies and changes the conformation of the extracellular domain of the membrane receptor. The hormone is essentially an extracellular signal that is greatly amplified by the second messengers.

In contrast, when hormone-receptor association occurs within the cytoplasm or nucleus, the hormone-receptor complex ultimately interacts with specific DNA molecules, often with the promoter region, and alters gene expression (**Figure 41–8**; see also Figure 41–7). There, the second messengers are transcribed RNA molecules that direct the synthesis of protein molecules. In this situation, essential information for triggering the cell's response resides in the hormone molecule itself as well as in the receptor. The hormone is an intracellular signal.

Plasma membrane–generated second messengers

A variety of mechanisms are used to transduce initial hormone-receptor signals arising within the plasma membrane. These signals lead to the generation of a variety of second messengers within the cytoplasm. They include cAMP, cGMP, Ca^{++}, inositol 1,4,5-trisphosphate (InsP3), diacylglycerol, tyrosine kinases, protein-tyrosine phosphatases, signal transducer and activator of transcription (STAT) proteins, and nitric oxide. These mechanisms are presented in detail in Chapter 5 and should be reviewed before proceeding.

None of the membrane-generated second messengers is unique to any particular hormone, and a single hormone may operate through multiple messengers. In addition, a messenger such as cAMP can also modulate gene expression by binding to a specific protein transcription factor. The combination then binds a regulatory element on target DNA molecules. Thus, peptide and protein hormones can also increase or decrease the synthesis of target enzymes and other proteins.

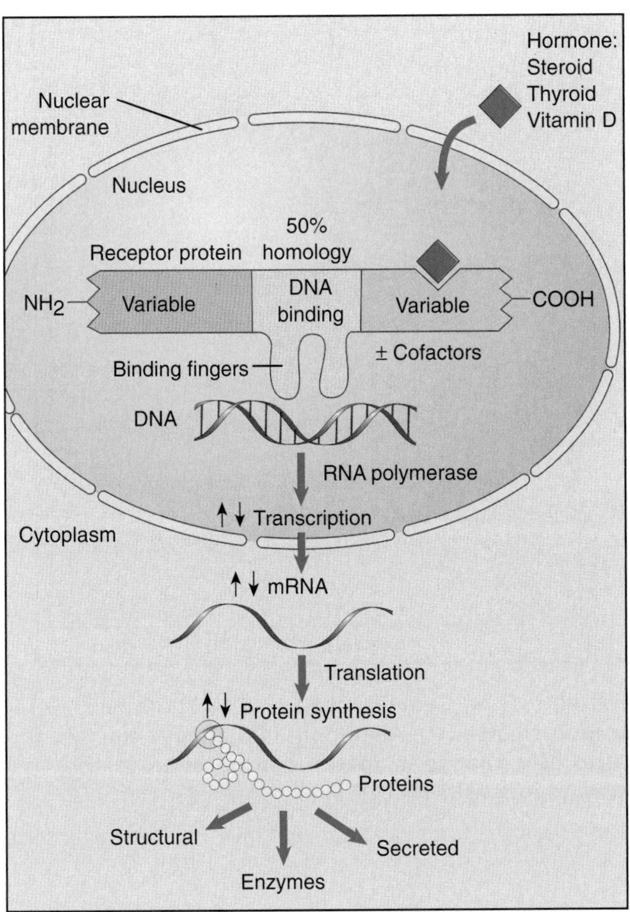

FIGURE 41–8. Mechanism of action of vitamin D, steroid, and thyroid hormones. The hormone combines with a nuclear protein receptor. The carboxyl terminal portion of the receptor varies for each hormone. The midportion of the receptor molecule has considerable similarity among hormones and contains DNA-binding fingers. Binding of the hormone-receptor complex to hormone regulatory elements in DNA molecules, often abetted by nuclear transcription cofactors, either stimulates or suppresses the transcription of target genes. The result is increased or decreased synthesis of cell proteins.

Nuclear second messengers modulate gene expression

Hormones that directly enter the cell (steroids, vitamin D, thyroid hormones) combine with receptor proteins in the cytoplasm and nucleus (Figure 41–8). These receptor proteins, although belonging to several classes, are similarly organized into distinct functional domains. A specific C-terminus domain of the receptor molecule binds the hormone. Another domain in the middle portion of the receptor binds to DNA. This second domain exhibits considerable homology among the various receptors and is encoded by a super-family of genes related to oncogenes (growth-regulating genes). The N-terminus domain has transactivating effects on a gene that may be independent of hormone binding. After binding, the hormone-receptor complex undergoes an activation process, during which the hormone ligand displaces an inactivating or blocking protein from the receptor. After this transformation, the complex can then enter the nucleus or, if it is already there, associate with regulatory elements on target DNA molecules.

The DNA site with which the hormone-receptor complex interacts is termed the **hormone regulatory element;** it is usually "upstream" from the basal promoter site at the 5′ end of the gene. Binding of the hormone-receptor complex to the regulatory element may be modulated by cofactors. Transcription of the primary gene message by RNA polymerase is then either induced or repressed. Thus, by raising or lowering the levels of specific RNA molecules and thereby the rate of translation of the gene message, the hormone increases or decreases the concentration of specific cell proteins. When these are enzymes, the rates of specific metabolic reactions are likewise increased or decreased by the hormone.

There are also several classes of nuclear transcription factors for which the ligands are not hormones but substrates such as fatty acids and cholesterol, inflammatory cytokines, retinoic acid, or even foreign substances and drugs (xenobiotics). These nuclear transcription factors can form dimers with hormone receptors and help mediate hormone actions on target genes, or they can act individually downstream along the pathway of hormone action where the transcription factor binds to its own regulatory element on a gene.

The onset of hormone actions mediated by nuclear second messengers is generally slower than that mediated by cytoplasmic second messengers. There is also a more graded response to increasing the hormone concentration, rather than amplification, because each hormone-receptor unit engages a single DNA molecule. The magnitude of action may be influenced by the concentrations of RNA polymerase, enzymes of protein synthesis or processing, transfer RNA, or amino acids and by the number and activity of ribosomes.

Steroids, thyroid hormone, and vitamin D also have more rapid effects that cannot be accounted for by genomic actions. It is still uncertain whether effects resembling those of extracellular peptide and protein hormones are mediated by an undiscovered class of receptors or by the known receptors docked in unusual locations, such as the plasma membrane or organelles.

Although rare, diseases caused by mutant genes for receptors or G proteins have provided much insight into the mechanisms of hormone action. For example, the reduced activity of a mutant α subunit of a stimulatory G protein leads to diminished cAMP levels, resulting in **deficient action of parathyroid hormone** and then **hypocalcemia** (see Chapter 44). Another mutant G protein, which is constitutively overactive, is associated with continuous **hypersecretion of growth hormone,** or **acromegaly** (see Chapter 45). Loss of function mutant nuclear receptors for thyroid hormone leads to **hypothyroidism** caused by the inability of thyroid target cells to respond normally to the hormone (see Chapter 46). Mutant plasma membrane receptors for insulin cause **diabetes mellitus** (see Chapter 43).

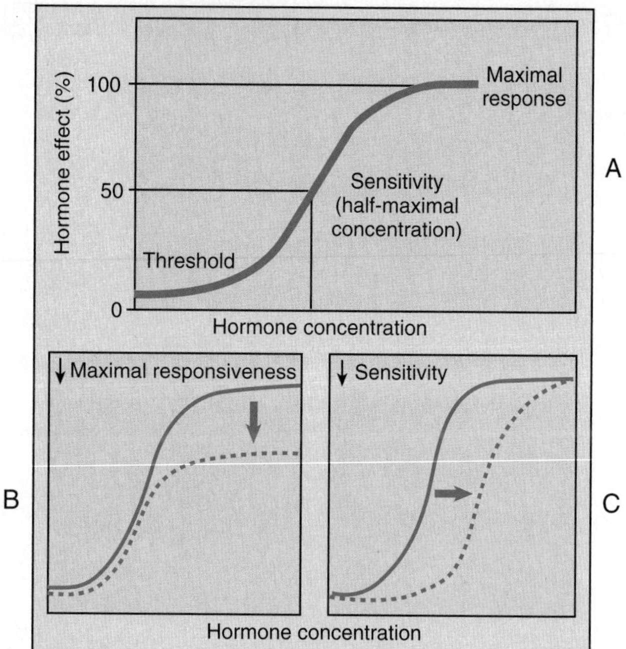

FIGURE 41–9. General shape of a hormone dose-response curve (A). Alterations in this curve can take the form of a change in maximal responsiveness (B) or a change in sensitivity (C).

The outcome of hormone action depends on many factors

The final quantitative outcome of the interaction of a hormone with its target cells depends on several factors. These include hormone concentration; receptor number; duration of exposure to hormone; intervals between consecutive exposures; intracellular conditions, such as concentrations of rate-limiting enzymes, cofactors, or substrates; and concurrent effects of antagonistic or synergistic hormones.

The dose-response curve for the action of a hormone is often sigmoidal (**Figure 41–9**). An intrinsic basal level of cell activity may be observed independent of the hormone. A certain minimal threshold concentration of hormone is required to elicit a measurable response. The effect produced by saturating doses of hormone is defined as the **maximal responsiveness** of the target cells. The concentration of hormone required to elicit a half-maximal response is an index of the **sensitivity** of the target cells to that hormone.

Alterations in the dose-response curve in vivo can take two general forms (Figure 41–9):

1. A decrease in maximal responsiveness may be caused (a) by a decrease in the number of functional target cells, in the total number of receptors per cell, or in the concentration of an enzyme activated by the hormone or (b) by an increase in the concentration of a noncompetitive inhibitor.
2. A decrease in hormone sensitivity may be caused (a) by a decrease in hormone-receptor affinity or number, (b) by an increase in the rate of hormone degradation, or (c) by an increase in the concentration of antagonistic and competitive hormones.

A class of Ca^{++}-activated proteases called **calpains** also influence hormone action. Calpains degrade protein kinases, protein-tyrosine phosphatases, receptors and ion channel proteins, transcription factors, and cytoskeletal proteins. By reducing these mediators of hormone action, the response to some hormones is blunted.

Obesity is a good example of a condition in which sensitivity to a hormone, insulin, is considerably diminished. In **type 2 diabetes** (non–insulin-dependent diabetes), both sensitivity and maximal responsiveness to insulin are reduced, factors that play a major role in causing high plasma glucose levels. A mutation in one of the calpain genes is associated with diabetes in some populations.

Summary

- The function of the endocrine system is to regulate metabolism, fluid status, growth, and sexual development. The endocrine and nervous systems work together to maintain homeostasis.
- Hormones are signaling molecules conveyed by the bloodstream (endocrine), by neural axons and the bloodstream (neurocrine), or by local diffusion (paracrine, autocrine). Hormones may be proteins, peptides, catecholamines, steroids, or iodinated tyrosine derivatives.
- Protein or peptide hormone synthesis begins with the generation of a primary gene product called a prohormone. The prohormone undergoes processing via proteolytic cleavage and glycosylation to yield the hormone.
- Thyroid hormone and catecholamines are synthesized from tyrosine and steroid hormones from cholesterol, both via multiple enzyme reactions.
- Peptide and protein hormones and catecholamines are stored in granules and secreted by exocytosis. Thyroid hormone is stored within protein molecules in large quantities; steroid hormones are not stored at all. Both are released by diffusion.
- Protein, peptide, and catecholamine hormones act on target cells via specific protein receptors located in the plasma membranes. Stimulatory or inhibitory G proteins link the hormone-receptor complex to membrane mechanisms that generate cAMP, cGMP, Ca^{++}, diacylglycerol, InsP3, tyrosine kinases, and protein-tyrosine phosphatases that act as second messengers.
- Thyroid and steroid hormones act via protein receptors located in the nucleus. The hormone-receptor complex interacts with hormone regulatory units in DNA molecules to alter the expression of target genes.
- Plasma levels and urinary excretion rates of a hormone are used clinically as indirect indices of the hormone secretion rate; these indices are valid as long as metabolic and renal clearance of the hormone is normal. The binding of some hormones to plasma proteins also influences their availability to target cells.
- The sensitivity of an organism to hormone action can be influenced by changes in receptor number or affinity, the hormone degradation rate, or competitive antagonists.
- The maximal effect produced by saturating concentrations of hormone can be influenced by the number of target cells, number of receptors, concentration of target enzymes, or noncompetitive antagonists.

Bibliography

Aranda A, Pascual A: Nuclear hormone receptors and gene expression, *Physiol Rev* 81:1269, 2001.

Burgoyne RD, Morgan A: Secretory granule exocytosis, *Physiol Rev* 83:581, 2003.

Chen JD: Steroid/nuclear receptor coactivators. *Vitam Horm* 58:391, 2000.

Combarnous Y: Molecular basis of the specificity of binding of glycoprotein hormones to their receptors, *Endocr Rev* 13:670, 1992.

Freedman LP: Anatomy of the steroid receptor zinc finger region, *Endocr Rev* 13:129, 1992.

Gether U: Uncovering molecular mechanisms involved in activation of G protein–coupled receptors, *Endocr Rev* 21:90, 2000.

Gillette MU, Tischkau SA: Suprachiasmatic nucleus: the brain's circadian clock, *Recent Prog Horm Res* 54:33, 1999.

Habener JF: Genetic control of hormone formation. In Wilson JD, Foster DF, eds: *Textbook of endocrinology,* ed 9, Philadelphia, 1998, WB Saunders.

Kahn CR, Smith RJ, Chin WW: Mechanism of action of hormones that act at the cell surface. In Wilson JD, Foster DF, eds: *Textbook of endocrinology,* ed 9, Philadelphia, 1998, WB Saunders.

Lacy PE: Beta cell secretion: from the standpoint of a pathobiologist, *Diabetes* 19:895, 1970.

Lösel RM et al: Nongenomic steroid action: controversies, questions, and answers, *Physiol Rev* 83:965, 2003.

Morris AJ, Malbon CC: Physiological regulation of G protein–linked signaling, *Physiol Rev* 79:1373, 1999.

Mountz JD et al: Apoptosis and cell death in the endocrine system, *Recent Prog Horm Res* 54:235, 1999.

Strott CA: Sulfonation and molecular action, *Endocr Rev* 23:703, 2002.

Taskén K, Aandahl EM: Localized effects of cAMP mediated by distinct routes of protein kinase A, *Physiol Rev* 84:137, 2003.

Case Study

Case 41–1

A patient comes to a physician with symptoms suggesting deficiency of protein hormone X. However, the measurement of hormone X in the plasma demonstrates an elevated level. When hormone X is administered to the patient, a normal maximal biological response is elicited but only with a higher than normal dose.

1. **Which of the following is *not* a likely explanation for this patient's symptoms?**
   A. A mutant receptor for hormone X
   B. A 50% deficiency of receptors for hormone X
   C. Excessive secretion of a competitive antagonist to hormone X
   D. A 95% deficiency of an enzyme that generates the key second messenger involved in the action of hormone X
   E. The secretion of a mutant hormone X

2. **For which of the following possible causes of the patient's hormone resistance syndrome would the administration of an inhibitor of hormone X secretion be helpful?**
   A. A mutant receptor for hormone X
   B. A 50% deficiency of receptors for hormone X
   C. Excessive secretion of a competitive antagonist to hormone X
   D. A 95% deficiency of an enzyme that generates the key second messenger involved in the action of hormone X
   E. The secretion of a mutant hormone X

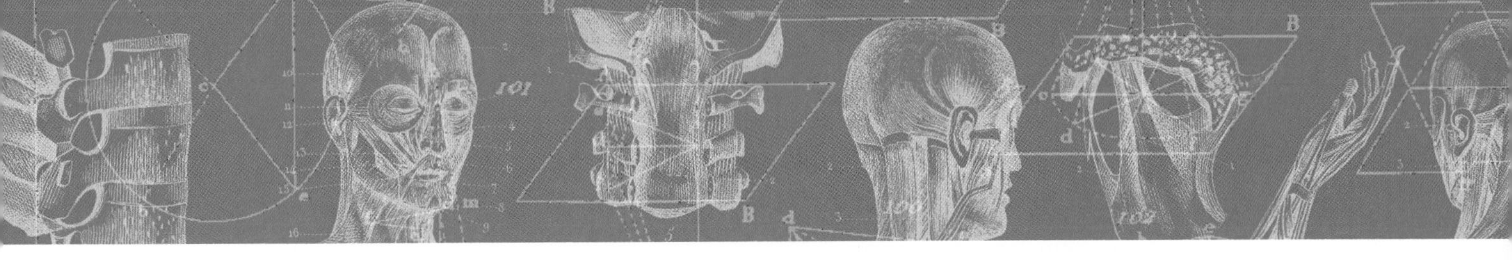

Chapter 42: Whole-Body Metabolism

Objectives

- ❖ Indicate the sources of energy and the forms in which energy is expended in humans.
- ❖ Explain the basic metabolic pathways of energy production and expenditure.
- ❖ Explain the principles of carbohydrate, protein, and fat metabolism and their interrelationships.
- ❖ Describe the patterns of metabolic responses and adaptations to fasting and exercise.
- ❖ Explain the concepts of how energy storage and body weight are regulated.

Metabolism may be broadly defined as the sum of all the chemical and physical processes involved in producing and expending energy from exogenous and endogenous sources, in synthesizing and degrading structural and functional tissue components, and in disposing of resultant waste products. These processes are of fundamental importance to all cells, tissues, organs, and systems discussed throughout this book. REGULATING THE RATE AND DIRECTION OF THE VARIOUS COMPONENTS OF METABOLISM IS ONE OF THE MAJOR FUNCTIONS OF THE ENDOCRINE SYSTEM. Therefore, a firm grasp of the basic elements of metabolism is essential for understanding the important influence of hormones on body functions.

Energy Metabolism Considers Obtaining, Storing, and Expending Sources of Energy

Energy input equals energy output

The laws of thermodynamics require that total energy balance be constantly maintained in living organisms. However, energy may be obtained in various forms, stored in other forms, and expended in many different ways. Therefore, numerous interconversions of chemical, mechanical, and thermal energy are possible. The basic rule is that IN THE STEADY STATE, WHEN BODY WEIGHT AND BODY COMPOSITION ARE STABLE, ENERGY INPUT MUST ALWAYS EQUAL ENERGY OUTPUT. **Figure 42–1** illustrates this overall flow of energy through the human organism.

Energy is derived from the oxidation of carbon and hydrogen in dietary molecules

Energy input consists of foodstuffs, which are classified into three major chemical categories: carbohydrate, fat, and protein. The complete combustion of each chemical type to CO_2 and water yields characteristic amounts of energy, expressed as joules or kilocalories per gram (1 kcal = 4184 J). The combustion of each type also requires characteristic amounts of O_2 per gram, depending on the proportions of carbon, hydrogen, and O_2 in the substance. However, for each class of foodstuff, the energy yield per liter of O_2 used is similar because the ratio of carbon to hydrogen atoms is similar in each class. WITHIN THE BODY, THE CARBON SKELETONS OF CARBOHYDRATE AND PROTEIN CAN BE CONVERTED TO FAT, AND THEIR POTENTIAL ENERGY CAN BE STORED MORE EFFICIENTLY IN THAT MANNER. THE CARBON SKELETONS OF PROTEIN CAN ALSO BE CONVERTED TO CARBOHYDRATE WHEN THAT ENERGY SOURCE IS SPECIFICALLY NEEDED. HOWEVER, IN THE HUMAN, CARBON ATOMS FROM FAT ARE

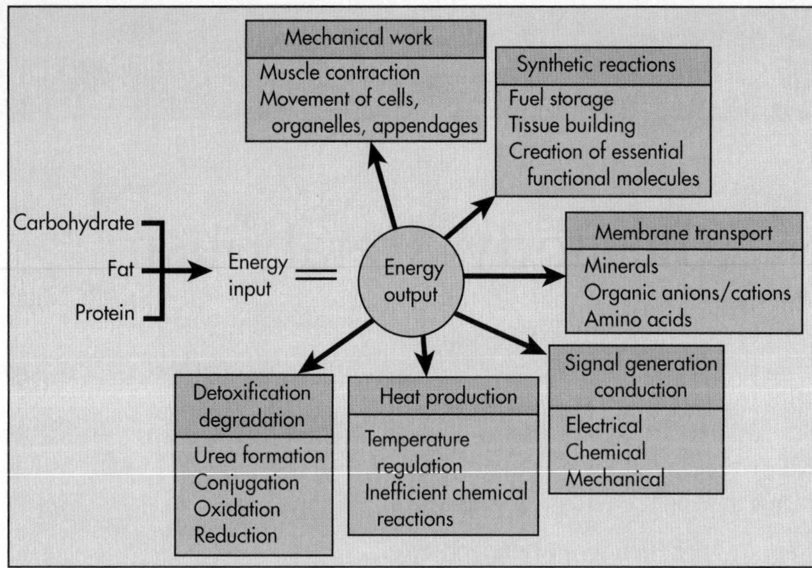

FIGURE 42–1. Energy balance. In a steady state, input as calorie equivalents of food equals output as calorie equivalents of various forms of mechanical and chemical work and heat.

NOT CONVERTED TO CARBOHYDRATE TO ANY SIGNIFICANT EXTENT.

There are several distinct components of energy output

Energy output can be divided into several distinct, measurable components.

First, in individuals at rest, energy is expended in myriad synthetic and degradative chemical reactions; in the generation and maintenance of chemical and electrical gradients of ions and other molecules across cell and organelle membranes; in the creation and conduction of signals, particularly in the nervous system; in the mechanical work of respiration and circulation of the blood; and in obligate heat loss to the environment. This absolute minimal energy expenditure is called the **basal** or **resting metabolic rate** (**BMR** or **RMR**). In the adult human, the BMR amounts to an average daily expenditure of 20 to 25 kcal (84 to 105 kJ)/kg of body weight (1.0 to 1.2 kcal/min), and this uses approximately 200 to 250 mL O_2 per minute.

The BMR is linearly related to lean body mass and body surface area. The central nervous system and muscle mass together account for 60% to 70% of the BMR. The BMR declines in the elderly, partly because lean body mass declines with age. The BMR increases when environmental temperature rises. During sleep, it falls 10% to 15%. Part of the interindividual variation in the BMR is genetically determined. Women have slightly lower BMRs than men do.

Second, the ingestion of food causes a small obligate increase in energy expenditure referred to as **diet-induced thermogenesis.** This is explained by the disposition of the ingested calories, such as the storage of glucose in the large molecule glycogen, or by enhanced protein synthesis from amino acids.

Third, **nonshivering thermogenesis** refers to energy expended specifically to produce heat and maintain the core temperature of the body. Some of this is **obligatory;** essentially all tissues contribute to obligatory thermogenesis, but it is only able to maintain a core temperature of 37°C in an external range of 26°C to 28°C. It is **facultative** when it is evoked by acute exposure to a cold environment. Impulses from the sympathetic nervous system are important mediators of this response to a fall in temperature (see Chapter 10). Facultative thermogenesis may also be used to adjust for prolonged excesses or deficits of energy intake.

Fourth, energy is also expended by sedentary individuals in unconscious and seemingly purposeless activity, such as fidgeting.

Fifth, the additional energy expended in occupational labor and purposeful exercise varies greatly among individuals and from day to day. This component generates the greatest variation in daily calorie intake and underscores the importance of energy stores for buffering temporary discrepancies between energy output and intake.

Of a total average daily expenditure of 2300 kcal (9700 kJ) in a typical sedentary adult, basal metabolism accounts for 60% to 70%, dietary thermogenesis for 5% to 15%, and spontaneous physical activity for 20% to 30%. As many as 3000 additional kilocalories may be used in daily physical work. During short periods of high-intensity exercise, energy expenditure can increase more than 10-fold.

Energy Generation Is Dependent on Chemical and Gaseous Sources

Nucleotides, carbohydrates, and fatty acids compose the chemical pathways

ATP is the major molecular intermediary of usable chemical energy

The basic chemical currency of energy in all living cells consists of the two high-energy phosphate bonds contained in adenosine triphosphate **(ATP).** To a much lesser extent, guanosine triphosphate, cytosine triphosphate, uridine triphosphate, and inosine triphosphate also serve as energy sources after energy from ATP is transferred to them.

Each of the two terminal P—O bonds of ATP contains about 12 kcal of potential energy per mole under physiological conditions of temperature and pH. These bonds are in constant flux. They are generated by substrate oxidation and are consumed as the energy is transferred into other high-energy bonds such as creatine phosphate in muscle, expended in creating lower energy phosphorylated metabolic intermediates such as glucose 6-phosphate, or converted to mechanical work such as the propulsion of spermatozoa. Because the production and transfer of energy is only 65% efficient, about 18 kcal worth of substrate is required to generate each terminal P—O bond of ATP. If 2300 kcal is turned over in a typical day, about 128 moles, or 63 kg, of ATP (a mass approximating body weight) is generated and expended.

The combustion of carbohydrates, chiefly as glucose, includes two major phases

At the end of a cytoplasmic anaerobic phase known as **glycolysis** (Embden-Meyerhof pathway), each glucose molecule has been degraded to two molecules of pyruvate **(Figure 42–2)** but has yielded only 8% of its potential energy content. Glycolysis can serve as a sole source of energy only briefly because the supply of glucose is limited and the pyruvate must be siphoned off via reduction to lactate, which is ultimately noxious if the lactate accumulates.

During the mitochondrial aerobic phase, the two pyruvate molecules are degraded to CO_2 via the **citric acid cycle** (Krebs cycle), and the remaining energy is liberated. In this pathway, **acetyl coenzyme A (acetyl CoA),** initially formed by oxidative decarboxylation of pyruvate, is condensed with oxaloacetate to form citrate. Through a cyclic series of reactions, the carbons of acetyl CoA appear as CO_2, oxaloacetate is regenerated, and much more ATP is formed.

Fatty acids are oxidized, two carbons at a time

The combustion of fat as fatty acids first requires their transfer from the cytoplasm to the mitochondria, where as fatty acyl CoAs they are oxidized via the biochemical sequence known as **beta oxidation.** This process yields two carbons at a time as acetyl CoA until the entire fatty acid molecule is broken down. The resulting acetyl CoA is disposed of via the citric acid cycle. A variable portion of fatty acid oxidation in the liver stops at the last four carbons and yields **acetoacetic** and **β-hydroxybutyric acids.** When the rate of fatty acid delivery to the liver exceeds the capacity of the citric acid cycle, more of these water-soluble keto acids are generated and released by the liver to be oxidized in other tissues.

> The condition known as **ketosis** occurs when fasting is prolonged beyond the usual overnight period or when carbohydrate intake is low and keto acids accumulate. It develops to an extreme degree in **diabetes mellitus** when the hormone insulin is deficient.

The combustion of protein first requires its hydrolysis to yield the component amino acids. Each of these amino acids undergoes degradation by individual pathways, which ultimately lead to intermediate compounds of the citric acid cycle and then to acetyl CoA and CO_2.

The oxidation of all substrates yields large numbers of hydrogen atoms. These atoms are oxidized to water in the mitochondrion in link with phosphorylation of ADP to ATP. In this process, three high-energy P—O bonds are formed for each atom of O_2 used. This usually yields an overall efficiency of 60% to 65% for the recovery of usable chemical energy. The oxidation of substrates can be "uncoupled" from formation of ATP, thereby reducing this efficiency and generating more heat instead, when that is needed. An excess of fatty acids can cause uncoupling by disturbing the flow of protons across the mitochondrial membrane.

Respiratory quotient refers to the ratio of CO_2 exhaled to O_2 inhaled

Substrates yield various amounts of CO_2 for each unit of O_2 consumed

In oxidation, the proportion of CO_2 produced and exhaled ($\dot{V}CO_2$) to O_2 used and inhaled ($\dot{V}O_2$) is characteristic of each major substrate. The ratio of $\dot{V}CO_2$ to $\dot{V}O_2$ is known as the **respiratory quotient (RQ).** As indicated by the following equations, the RQ equals 1.0 for the oxidation of carbohydrate

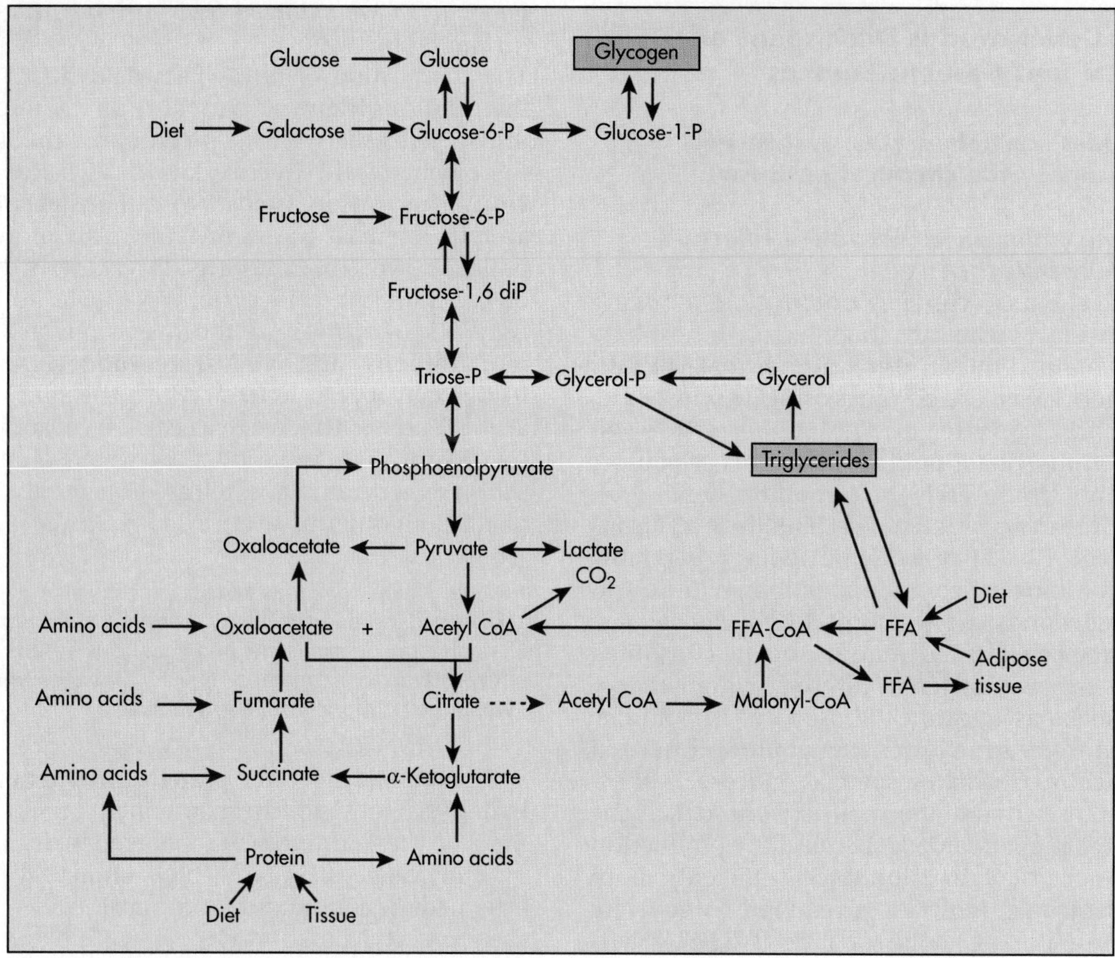

FIGURE 42–2. Chemical pathways of energy transfer and storage. Carbohydrates funnel through glucose 6-phosphate to be stored as glycogen. Alternatively, they can undergo glycolysis to pyruvate and are used for the synthesis of fatty acids. The fatty acids, regardless of source, are esterified with glycerol phosphate and stored as triglycerides. Amino acids from endogenous or exogenous proteins are converted to glucose via oxaloacetate or pyruvate. CoA, coenzyme A; diP, diphosphate; FFA, free fatty acid; P, phosphate.

(e.g., glucose), whereas it equals 0.70 for the oxidation of fat (e.g., palmitic acid).

For carbohydrates:

$$C_6H_{12}O_6 + 6O_2 \rightarrow 6CO_2 + 6H_2O \qquad \textbf{42-1}$$

Glucose:

$$RQ = 6CO_2/6O_2 = 1.0$$

For fats:

$$C_{15}H_{31}COOH + 23O_2 \rightarrow 16CO_2 + 16H_2O \qquad \textbf{42-2}$$

Palmitic acid:

$$RQ = 16CO_2/23O_2 = 0.70$$

The RQ for protein reflects that of the individual RQs of the amino acids and averages 0.80. Ordinarily, however, protein is only a minor energy source.

Normal humans can vary their fuel mix and RQ from 0.7 to 1.0 without difficulty. Patients with poor pulmonary function who cannot excrete CO_2 efficiently benefit from a low RQ. They are therefore given a higher proportion of fat calories as an energy source so that the least amount of CO_2 is produced for the quantity of O_2 used.

Energy Is Stored and Transferred

Energy can be transformed from one chemical type to another and transferred from site to site

The intake of energy in the form of food is periodic. Its time course does not match either the constant rate of energy expenditure in the basal state or the variable rate during intermittent muscle work. Therefore, the organism must have mechanisms for storing ingested energy for future needs. The greatest part of these energy reserves (75%) is in the form of fat, stored as triglycerides, in adipose tissue. In humans of normal weight, fat constitutes 10% to 30% of body weight, but it can reach 80% in very obese individuals. Fat is a particularly efficient storage fuel because it has a high calorie density (i.e., 9 kcal/g) and engenders little additional weight as intracellular water.

Triglycerides are formed by the esterification of free fatty acids with α-glycerol phosphate. Free fatty acids arise largely from the digestion of dietary fat, but they can also be synthesized from acetyl CoA derived from the oxidation of glucose (Figure 42–2). Thus, dietary carbohydrate can be converted to fat in the liver and transferred to adipose tissue for storage in that more efficient form.

Protein (4 kcal/g) constitutes almost 25% of the potential energy reserves, and the component amino acids can contribute to the glucose supply. However, because proteins have vital structural and functional roles, their use as a major source of energy is not desirable.

Carbohydrate (4 kcal/g) in the form of the glucose polymer **glycogen** forms less than 1% of total energy reserves. However, this portion is critical for the support of metabolism of the central nervous system and for short bursts of intense muscle work. Approximately one fourth of the glycogen stores (75 to 100 g) is in the liver, and about three fourths (300 to 400 g) is in the muscle mass. Liver glycogen can be made available to other tissues via the process of **glycogenolysis** and glucose release. Muscle glycogen can be used only by muscle because this tissue lacks the enzyme glucose-6-phosphatase, which is required for the dephosphorylation of glucose before its entrance into the bloodstream (Figure 42–2).

Glycogen can be formed from all three major dietary sugars: glucose, galactose, and fructose. In addition, in the liver (and to a much lesser extent in the kidney), glucose itself can also be synthesized de novo from the three carbon precursors pyruvate, lactate, and glycerol and from parts of the carbon skeleton of the 20 amino acids in protein, except leucine. This process, known as **gluconeogenesis,** converts two pyruvate molecules to glucose.

Gluconeogenesis is not a simple reversal of all the reactions of glycolysis

The chemical free energy change is too large to permit an efficient backward flow of the glycolytic reactions at three steps (Figure 42–2): (1) pyruvate to phosphoenolpyruvate, (2) fructose 1,6-diphosphate to fructose 6-phosphate, and (3) glucose 6-phosphate to glucose. The first step requires energy input in the form of ATP and GTP. Simple phosphatase reactions reverse the last two steps.

Net glucose synthesis cannot occur from acetyl CoA formed from the beta oxidation of fat, even though carbon atoms from acetyl CoA can become part of glucose molecules via oxaloacetate and the citric acid cycle. Thus, fat can contribute to carbohydrate stores only via conversion of the 3-carbon glycerol moiety of triglycerides (via glycerol phosphate) to glucose.

The processes of energy storage and transfer themselves expend energy

The assimilation of dietary sources of energy partly accounts for the stimulation of O_2 use after a meal (i.e., diet-induced thermogenesis). Storing dietary fatty acids as triglycerides in adipose tissue costs only 3% of the original calories, and storing glucose as glycogen costs only 7% of the original calories. In contrast, the conversion of carbohydrate to fat uses 23% of the original calories, and a similar amount is expended in storing dietary amino acids as protein or in converting them to glycogen.

The metabolism of glucose and fatty acids is interrelated

Because glucose and fatty acids are alternative and in effect competing energy substrates, some relationship between their use and their synthesis and storage within cells could be expected. For example, when dietary glucose is plentiful, glycolysis is augmented, more acetyl CoA is generated from pyruvate, and more citrate is formed (Figure 42–2). Citrate then activates the first step in the synthesis of fatty acids (acetyl CoA → malonyl CoA). In addition, glycolysis produces more glycerol phosphate from triose phosphates (Figure 42–2). The combination of increased fatty acid synthesis and glycerol phosphate availability results in the accentuated synthesis of triglycerides and the reduced oxidation of fat. Thus, INCREASED CARBOHYDRATE USE SHIFTS FAT METABOLISM FROM OXIDATION TO STORAGE. Conversely, under circumstances in which the fatty acid supply is augmented, beta oxidation increases. Several of its products (e.g., acyl CoA) then retard glycolysis and enhance gluconeogenesis and glycogen synthesis. Thus, THE INCREASED USE OF FAT AS FUEL SHIFTS CARBOHYDRATE METABOLISM FROM OXIDATION TO STORAGE. Many of these intrinsic chemical checks and balances are reinforced by hormonal signals.

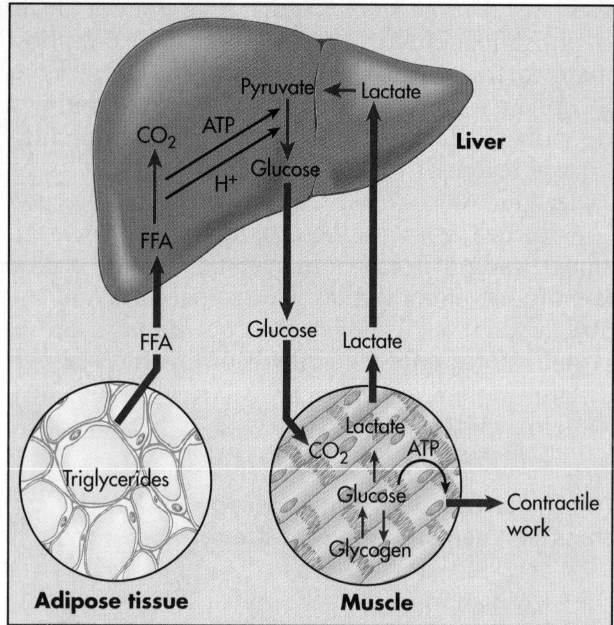

FIGURE 42–3. Interorgan energy transfers. Energy contained in free fatty acid (FFA) can be transferred to energy contained in glucose in the liver. Lactate released from muscle glycogen by glycolysis can carry energy back to the liver, where the lactate is built back into new glucose molecules (and glycogen).

The transfer of energy between organs also occurs (**Figure 42–3**). The stored energy contained within adipose tissue triglycerides is transported as free fatty acids to the liver. There, part of the energy (not the carbon atoms) is effectively transferred to glucose molecules. This is because as fatty acids are oxidized and yield ATP, gluconeogenesis is stimulated concurrently and uses the ATP that was generated. The newly synthesized glucose molecules can then be transported to muscle tissue, where their energy is released during glycolysis and applied to muscle contraction. Furthermore, if the lactate produced exceeds the ability of the muscle to oxidize it rapidly enough in the citric acid cycle, the lactate can be returned to the liver, where it may again be built back up into glucose molecules. From this viewpoint, THE LIVER IS A FLEXIBLE AND VERSATILE ORGAN THAT CAN TRANSMUTE AND TRANSFER ENERGY FROM FUEL DEPOTS TO WORKING TISSUES. Hormones help regulate this process.

When liver disease causes severe hepatic insufficiency (e.g., **alcoholic hepatitis, cirrhosis**), energy metabolism can be markedly distorted. An inability to store glucose as glycogen leads to hypoglycemia during fasting. Inability to take up lactate produced by peripheral anaerobic glycolysis can cause high plasma levels of lactic acid and serious metabolic acidosis.

Carbohydrate Metabolism Is the Body's Method of Processing of Sugars

In addition to providing energy, sugar components of glycoproteins, glycopeptides, and glycolipids have structural and functional roles. Examples include basement membrane collagen, mucopolysaccharides, nerve cell myelin, hormones, and hormone receptors.

Glucose is the central molecule in carbohydrate metabolism

Postabsorptive plasma glucose concentration averages 80 mg/dL (4.5 mM), with a range of 60 to 100 mg/dL.

When the plasma glucose level falls below 60 mg/dL, as may occur with an overdose of insulin taken by a patient with diabetes, the uptake of the sugar and use of O_2 by the brain decrease in parallel. Central nervous system function becomes progressively impaired, leading to convulsions, coma, and even death.

The major products of glycolysis, lactate and pyruvate, circulate at average plasma concentrations of 0.7 and 0.07 mM, respectively. However, when tissues are deprived of O_2, the equilibrium between the two shifts further toward lactate, the reduced molecule. Plasma concentration ratios rise from 10:1 to as high as 30:1. Ischemia may produce very high concentrations of lactate that cause metabolic acidosis (see Chapters 30 and 40).

In the basal state, glucose turnover is about 225 g/day in adults. Approximately 55% of glucose use results in terminal oxidation to CO_2, of which the brain accounts for the greatest part. Another 20% stops at lactate, which then returns to the liver for resynthesis into glucose (Cori cycle) (Figure 42–3). Reuptake by the liver and other splanchnic tissues accounts for the remaining 20% of glucose use. Most of the glucose used (≈70%) in the basal state is independent of insulin, a hormone with otherwise important regulatory effects on glucose metabolism.

The circulating pool of glucose (11 g), which is only slightly larger than the liver output in 1 hour (9 g), can maintain brain oxidation for only 3 hours. This is why the continuous hepatic production of glucose is critical in the fasting state. About 80% of this production results from glycogenolysis and 20% from gluconeogenesis. Lactate is the source of more than half the glucose supplied by gluconeogenesis. The remainder is accounted for by amino acids and glycerol. The supply of lactate comes from glycolysis largely in muscle, red blood cells, and white blood cells. The amino acid precursors come from proteolysis of muscle, and the glycerol comes from adipose tissue lipolysis.

The fate of ingested glucose is largely storage as glycogen

When an individual ingests glucose after overnight fasting, approximately 70% of the load is assimilated by peripheral tissues, mainly muscle, and about 30% by splanchnic tissues, mainly liver. Only 25% is oxidized during the 3 to 5 hours required for complete glucose absorption from the gastrointestinal tract. The remainder is stored as glycogen in muscle and liver. Glucose initially stored as muscle glycogen can later be transferred to the liver by undergoing glycolysis to lactate, which is released into the circulation; the lactate is then taken up by the liver, rebuilt into glucose, and stored as glycogen (Figure 42–3). During absorption of exogenous glucose, hepatic output of the sugar is largely unnecessary and is greatly reduced from basal levels.

Intake of Proteins, Especially Those Containing Amino Acids That Cannot Be Synthesized in the Body, Is Vital to Health

The average adult body contains 10 kg of protein, of which about 6 kg is metabolically active. Amino acids are released daily by proteolysis from muscle, the main endogenous repository. A portion of each amino acid quantity is reused for protein synthesis, and the rest is degraded. A daily dietary protein intake of 0.8 g/kg is ordinarily sufficient for an adult human to remain in balance. When accretion of lean body mass is taking place (e.g., in growing children, pregnant women, and persons recovering from prior illness-induced weight loss), daily protein requirements increase to 1.5 to 2.0 g/kg.

All proteins are composed of the same 20 amino acids. Half of these are called **essential amino acids** because their carbon skeletons, the corresponding α-keto acids, cannot be synthesized by humans. Once present, however, these keto acids can be converted to the essential amino acids by transamination. The other half, the **nonessential amino acids,** can be synthesized endogenously because the appropriate carbon skeletons can be built from glucose metabolites in the citric acid cycle. The essential amino acids must be supplied in the diet in amounts that range from 0.5 to 1.5 g/day. A deficiency of even one essential amino acid disrupts normal protein synthesis.

Milk and egg proteins are particularly rich in essential amino acids, but properly combined vegetable sources can also provide all of them. About 40% of the protein intake of infants and children should consist of essential amino acids to support growth. In adults, this requirement falls to 20%. Many amino acids, including the essential ones, are also precursors for important molecules such as purines, pyrimidines, polyamines, phospholipids, creatine, carnitine, methyl donors, thyroid and catecholamine hormones, and neurotransmitters. Some of these neurotransmitters are amino acids.

A deficiency of protein intake is a worldwide problem. When people are chronically deprived of both protein and calories, marked loss of muscle mass and adipose tissue results. When calories are sufficient but protein is deficient over relatively short periods, a syndrome known as **kwashiorkor** occurs. This is characterized by low plasma albumin levels, edema caused by low plasma oncotic pressure, fragile hair, depressed immune function, deficiency of lymphocytes, reduced wound healing, increased infections, and fatty infiltration of the liver.

Amino acids can be converted to glucose, can be completely oxidized, or can give rise to keto acids

After the removal of the amino group, all 20 amino acids are completely oxidized to CO_2 and water. Each amino acid traverses a specific degradative pathway. (Refer to standard biochemistry textbooks for details.) However, all these pathways converge into three general metabolic processes: gluconeogenesis, ketogenesis, and ureagenesis. Except for leucine, all the amino acids can contribute carbon atoms for the synthesis of glucose. Five ketogenic amino acids give rise to acetoacetate. In the degradation of all amino acids, ammonia is released. Ammonia, incorporated mainly into glutamine and alanine molecules, is then transported to the liver. In the liver, ammonia is "detoxified" through incorporation into urea, a metabolically inert molecule. The urea that results from protein degradation is excreted by the kidney (see Chapter 38).

Protein balance is reflected by nitrogen balance

In the healthy adult under steady-state conditions, the total daily level of nitrogen excreted in the urine as urea plus ammonia, along with minor losses of nitrogen in the feces (0.4 g/day) and skin (0.3 g/day), is equal to that released during the metabolism of exogenous and endogenous protein.

Such an individual is said to be in **nitrogen balance.** When no protein is ingested, the sum of urea plus ammonia nitrogen in the urine reflects almost quantitatively the rate of endogenous protein degradation. When protein breakdown is greatly accelerated by tissue trauma or disease (e.g., after major gastrointestinal surgery or with sepsis), the urea plus ammonia nitrogen in the urine may exceed the protein nitrogen intake. In these cases, the individual is said to be in **negative nitrogen balance.** In a growing child or a previously malnourished individual undergoing protein repletion and a gain in lean body mass, urea plus ammonia nitrogen excretion in the urine is less than the intake of protein nitrogen. This individual is said to be in **positive nitrogen balance.**

Fat Metabolism Occurs in Several Ways

Body fat has multiple components and functions

Fat represents almost half the total daily substrate for oxidation (≈100 g, or 900 kcal). The usual daily intake of fat in the United States is approximately 100 g, or about 40% of total calories. The major component of both dietary and storage fat is triglycerides. These consist largely of long-chain saturated and monounsaturated fatty acids (chiefly palmitic, stearic, and oleic acids) esterified to glycerol. ABOUT 3% TO 5% OF FATTY ACIDS ARE POLYUNSATURATED AND CANNOT BE SYNTHESIZED IN THE BODY. These are termed **essential fatty acids** (linoleic, linolenic, and arachidonic) because they are required as precursors for certain membrane phospholipid and glycolipid substances as well as for important intracellular mediators such as **prostaglandins.** Another component of fat is the steroid molecule **cholesterol,** which serves a variety of functions in membranes and is the precursor for bile acids and steroid hormones. Cholesterol is both ingested and synthesized by most cells.

The typical fat intake previously cited is now deemed excessive for good health, particularly because it promotes **atherosclerosis.** In this common condition, plaques laden with lipid form in the walls of the arteries and are often the sites of thrombosis, which obstructs the flow of blood and causes necrosis of vital tissue such as heart muscle or cerebral cortex. Current nutritional recommendations are for the intake of fat not to exceed 30% and of saturated fat (usually animal fat) not to exceed 10% of total calories. The intake of monounsaturated fat should modestly exceed that of polyunsaturated fat. Cholesterol intake should be less than 600 mg/day and reduced to below 300 mg/day if the plasma cholesterol level is elevated.

The transport of water-insoluble lipids in plasma requires that they be incorporated into complex lipoprotein particles. The protein portion of each particle is derived from several **apoproteins** synthesized in the liver and intestine. These apoproteins serve catalytic functions and interact with specific cell LDL receptors. **Figure 42–4** summarizes the metabolic pathways and interactions of the lipoprotein particles.

Plasma lipid components are associated with specific proteins and have various functions and rates of turnover

Chylomicrons, formed from dietary fat (see Chapter 35), are the lowest density lipoproteins. After their absorption from the gastrointestinal tract, they disappear from plasma rapidly. Their major component is triglycerides, which are partly hydrolyzed by the key enzyme **lipoprotein lipase** on capillary endothelial surfaces. This enzyme is activated by apoprotein C-II and transferred to the chylomicron by **high-density lipoprotein (HDL)** particles (see later section). The resulting free fatty acids are taken up by adipose cells for resynthesis into triglycerides and storage and by other cells for oxidation. The residual lipoprotein particles, which are higher in cholesterol content and are known as **chylomicron remnants,** are taken up by the liver for further degradation. This uptake is directed by apoproteins E and B-48, which react with specific hepatic receptors.

In contrast, **very-low-density lipoprotein (VLDL)** particles are formed in the postabsorptive state by endogenous synthesis in the liver and to a lesser extent in the intestine. They are denser, contain somewhat more cholesterol than chylomicrons, and have a longer plasma half-life. The initial metabolism of VLDL is the same as that of chylomicrons. The product of lipoprotein lipase action consists of particles called **intermediate-density lipoprotein (IDL).** About half the IDLs return to the liver and are taken up, like chylomicron remnants. The other half of the IDLs are further enriched with cholesterol to form **low-density lipoprotein (LDL)** particles. Circulating LDL is responsible for transferring cholesterol into other cells. The uptake of LDL, IDL, and remnant particles takes place through initial interaction between apoproteins E and B-100 and specific cell LDL receptors; this process is then followed by endocytosis.

The uptake of LDL cholesterol by cells has important regulatory actions on intracellular cholesterol metabolism. Cholesterol uptake from plasma down-regulates the LDL receptor and thereby reduces further entrance of the sterol. The uptake of cholesterol also suppresses its own intracellular synthesis.

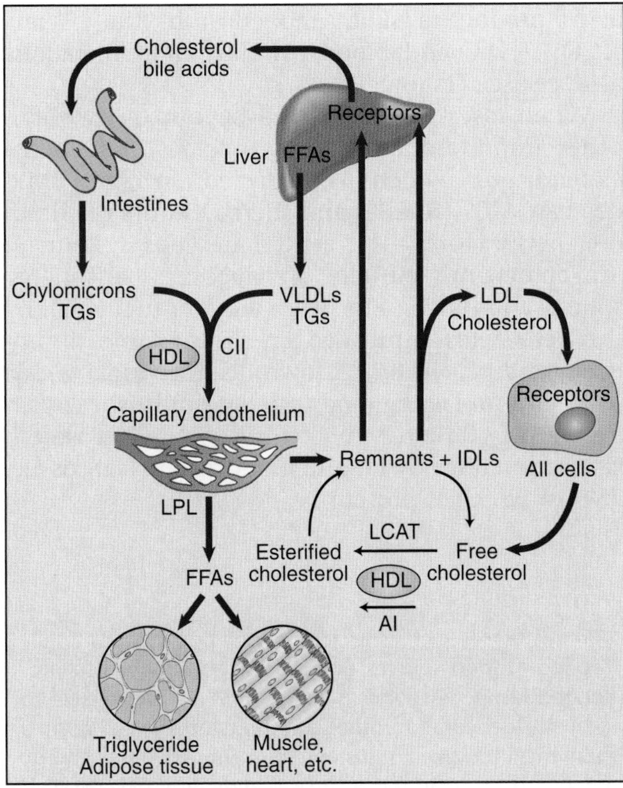

FIGURE 42–4. Lipoprotein metabolism and major aspects of lipid turnover in humans. Exogenous triglycerides (TGs) in the form of chylomicrons absorbed from the intestine and endogenous triglycerides (very-low-density lipoproteins [VLDLs]) produced in the liver both give rise to free fatty acids (FFAs) for storage in adipose tissue and oxidation in muscle. High-density lipoprotein (HDL) particles facilitate the liberation of free fatty acids from triglycerides, and the enzyme lipoprotein lipase (LPL) directly catalyzes this process. The resultant particles, called remnants from chylomicrons and intermediate-density lipoproteins (IDLs) from very-low-density lipoproteins, undergo further change in the circulation, which also is facilitated by high-density lipoprotein. The ratio of esterified cholesterol to free cholesterol is increased in the remnant and IDL particles by the enzyme lecithin–cholesterol acyltransferase (LCAT). The remnant particles are then taken up by the liver for further metabolism. The IDL particles are partly taken up by the liver and partly converted to cholesterol-rich, low-density lipoprotein (LDL) particles. The LDL particles are then taken up by virtually all cells after interaction with specific LDL receptors. Cholesterol, either synthesized in the liver or extracted from remnant and IDL particles, is also excreted into the intestine, partly as bile acids. AI, apoprotein A-I; CII, apoprotein C-II.

HDL particles play key roles in fat metabolism

HDL particles are synthesized in the liver and intestine and have a long half-life. Different types facilitate the major steps in fat metabolism just described. HDL facilitates return of cholesterol released from peripheral tissues to the liver (reverse cholesterol transport), where the cholesterol is used for synthesis of bile acids and new lipoprotein particles. By a direct pathway, HDL particles bind to a class of scavenger receptors (SR-B1) in the liver plasma membrane. By an indirect pathway, HDL particles exchange key apoproteins with the other lipoprotein particles. The smaller, denser HDL_3 particles accept free cholesterol molecules from chylomicrons; from VLDL, IDL, and remnant particles; and from peripheral cells (Figure 42–4). The cholesterol is esterified via the enzyme lecithin–cholesterol acyltransferase; the esterification is activated by apoprotein A-I. The resulting cholesterol esters are then exchanged for triglycerides on other particles via a **cholesterol-ester transfer protein.** The HDL_3 is transformed to the larger, more buoyant HDL_2 particle. The triglycerides are later removed from the HDL_2 particle by the action of **hepatic lipase,** and this restores the denser HDL_3. The net effect of such HDL cycling is to accelerate the clearance of triglycerides from plasma and to regulate the ratios of free to esterified cholesterol.

The plasma concentration of total cholesterol (average, 185 mg/dL) and especially of LDL cholesterol (average, 120 mg/dL) is an important risk factor for atherosclerosis and death from cardiovascular events. On the other hand, a higher plasma level of HDL cholesterol (average, 50 mg/dL) exerts a protective effect against cardiovascular disease. Free fatty acids circulate in an average concentration of 400 μmol/L bound to albumin molecules and with a plasma half-life of only 2 minutes. Half of the turnover of free fatty acids represents oxidation, and the other half represents reesterification to triglycerides.

A nuclear transcription factor, **sterol regulatory element–binding protein,** for which the ligand is cholesterol or other steroid molecules, binds to a sterol regulatory element on target genes. In this way, cholesterol and bile acids help regulate their own production through negative feedback. Other transcription factors help regulate genes required for fatty acid and triglyceride synthesis in an analogous manner.

Genetic abnormalities in apoprotein and lipid receptor particles account for a substantial number of **dyslipidemias.** The premature development of coronary artery disease is often the consequence. For example, mutant apoprotein E molecules cause familial forms of **hyperlipidemia,** which is characterized by elevations of both triglyceride and cholesterol levels caused by the accumulation of IDL and remnant particles. An excessive apoprotein B-100 content of VLDL and LDL particles characterizes **familial combined hyperlipidemia,** in which cholesterol and often triglyceride levels are high. In **familial hypercholesterolemia,** mutant LDL receptors prevent the normal cellular uptake of cholesterol; this diminished uptake results in extremely high plasma cholesterol concentrations (>700 mg/dL) in homozygotes, visible and palpable deposits of cholesterol in skin and tendons, and even coronary thrombosis in children.

Metabolic Adaptations Include Fasting and Exercise

Fasting requires increased glucose production and fat oxidation

In the fasting state, the individual totally depends on endogenous substrates for energy. The mobilization of glucose provides essential fuel for the central nervous system; the release of free fatty acids provides for the oxidative needs of the other tissues. An increase in protein degradation to amino acids is also a fundamental feature of this response.

THE FASTING INDIVIDUAL IS SAID TO BE IN A STATE OF CATABOLISM BECAUSE CARBOHYDRATE, FAT, AND PROTEIN STORES ARE ALL DECREASING.

The liver supplies glucose to the circulation initially by augmenting glycogenolysis. After 12 to 15 hours of fasting, however, hepatic glycogen stores are almost depleted, and a rapid enhancement of gluconeogenesis fills the void. To supply glucose precursors, 75 to 100 g of muscle protein is broken down daily during the first few days. This is reflected in a rising excretion of urea nitrogen in the urine. Gluconeogenesis is also supported by the daily provision of 15 to 20 g of glycerol, which is released by the accelerated lipolysis of triglycerides in adipose tissue. Glucose oxidation in muscle and liver is spared as increasing quantities of free fatty acids become available. Their oxidation in the liver yields keto acids, which can also be oxidized by muscle cells, and further spares the use of glucose. The net shift away from glucose and toward fatty acid oxidation lowers the RQ (see previous section).

These adaptations are also reflected in changing plasma concentrations of substrates. Levels of glucose and alanine, a major gluconeogenic amino acid, decrease, whereas the levels of free fatty acids, glycerol, and branched-chain amino acids, such as leucine, increase. Increased levels of the strong keto acids produce a slight reduction in the plasma HCO_3^- levels and blood pH (i.e., mild metabolic acidosis; see Chapter 40).

When fasting is prolonged beyond a few days, other important adaptations occur. Total energy expenditure, which is reflected in the BMR, decreases 10% to 20% and thereby limits the drain on energy stores. The central nervous system no longer depends entirely on glucose as an energy source, and much of its needs are eventually met by the keto acids. Gluconeogenesis therefore diminishes, and protein breakdown declines to 25 g/day. In long-term fasting, body weight diminishes by an average of 300 g/day; two thirds of the lost weight is accounted for by fat and one third by lean tissue, 25% of which is protein.

Circumstances such as accidental isolation in areas totally lacking in food sources evoke these adaptations to prolonged fasting. As long as sufficient water is available to prevent dehydration, the adipose stores of a normal human (≈10 kg) can sustain the reduced basal energy needs and greatly limited physical activity (≈1400 kcal/day) for up to 60 days. Likewise, the mobilizable protein stores (≈6 kg) can supply the diminished requirements for glucose oxidation. However, the loss of protein leads to progressive muscle weakness, apathy, organ dysfunction, and ultimately death.

Exercise stimulates the production of glucose and the oxidation of fuels

The metabolic response to exercise resembles the response to fasting in that the mobilization and generation of fuels for oxidation are dominant factors. The types and amounts of substrate vary with the intensity and duration of the exercise **(Figure 42–5)**. For very intense, short-term exercise (e.g., a 10- to 15-second sprint), stored creatine phosphate and ATP provide the energy at a rate of approximately 50 kcal/min. When these stores are depleted, additional intensive exercise for up to 2 minutes can be sustained via the breakdown of muscle glycogen to glucose 6-phosphate, and glycolysis yields the necessary energy (at a rate of 30 kcal/min). This anaerobic phase is limited by the accumulation of lactic acid in the exercising muscles and circulation.

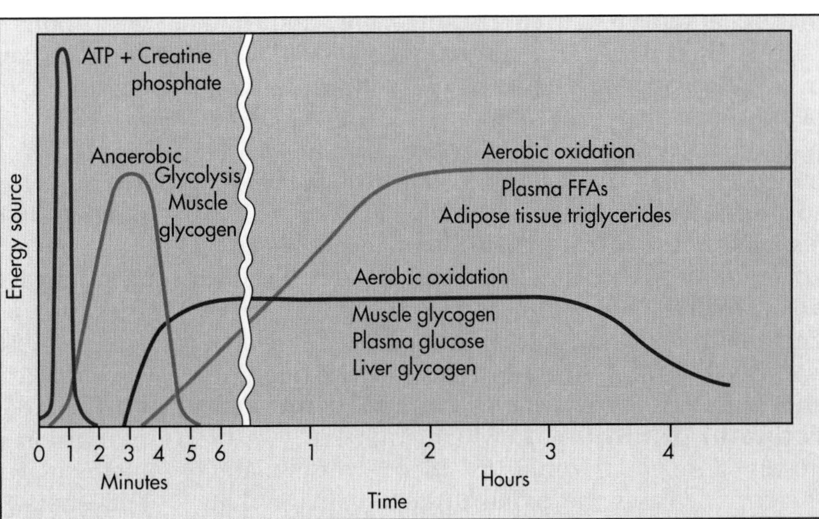

FIGURE 42–5. Energy sources during exercise. Note the sequential use of stored high-energy phosphate bonds as creatine phosphate and glycogen for short-term intensive exercise. Circulating glucose and free fatty acids (FFAs) become increasingly important with time, and the free fatty acids dominate in sustained exercise.

Several muscle diseases resulting from defects in energy generation are caused by a deficiency of an enzyme in the pathway from glycogen to pyruvate and lactate. An example is **McArdle's disease,** or **muscle phosphorylase deficiency.** Such patients experience pain and weakness after exercise. The defect in glycogen mobilization is evidenced by a failure of lactate levels to increase in the antecubital vein after brief forearm muscle anaerobic exercise during which the arterial inflow and blood-borne oxygen are excluded by a cuff.

After several minutes of exhaustive anaerobic exercise, an O_2 debt of 10 to 12 L can be built up. This must be repaid in the following ways before the exercise can be repeated: the accumulated lactic acid must be oxidized or rebuilt into glucose; muscle ATP and creatine phosphate contents must be restored; and the O_2 normally present in the lungs, body fluids, myoglobin, and hemoglobin must be replenished.

For less intense but longer periods of exercise, the aerobic oxidation of substrates is required to produce the necessary energy (at ≈12 kcal/min). Substrates from the blood circulation are added to muscle glycogen. Glucose uptake from plasma increases manyfold in some muscle groups. Adenosine monophosphate (AMP) resulting from ATP breakdown activates a kinase, AMPK, that phosphorylates enzymes whose actions result in increased glucose uptake. Hepatic glucose production increases, initially largely because of glycogenolysis, to meet this need, but gluconeogenesis becomes increasingly important as liver glycogen stores are depleted. However, endurance can be improved by high-carbohydrate feedings for several days before prolonged exercise (e.g., a marathon run) because this increases stores of both liver and muscle glycogen. To support gluconeogenesis, amino acids are increasingly released by muscle proteolysis. Eventually, fatty acids, liberated from adipose tissue triglycerides, form the predominant substrate, which supplies two thirds of the energy needs during sustained exercise. AMPK also phosphorylates enzymes whose actions result in increased fatty acid oxidation. Except for the increases in circulating pyruvate and lactate that result from enhanced glycolysis, the pattern of change in plasma substrates is similar to that of fasting, only occurring more quickly.

Genetic defects in the oxidation of fatty acids lead to reduced exercise capacity and muscle pain or even progressive muscle weakness. Cardiac muscle dysfunction may occur. Deficiencies of **carnitine** or the enzyme **carnitine palmityltransferase** impair the transfer of fatty acids from the cytoplasm into the mitochondria. Deficiencies of beta oxidation enzymes cause even more severe consequences in infants, who cannot tolerate even short fasts because an overdependence on glucose for fuel leads to hypoglycemia.

Energy Stores Are Regulated

The preponderance of stored energy consists of fat, and individuals vary greatly in the amounts and percentages of body weight that are accounted for by adipose tissue. Obesity is a risk factor for type 2 diabetes and cardiovascular disease, but abdominal visceral (omental) fat poses a particularly high risk.

Adipose tissue is not an inert repository of triglycerides. Adipose cells are metabolically active, and their number is not fixed. Preadipocytes in the stromal tissue can be induced to differentiate into mature adipocytes, even in adult life, and this process itself is under hormonal regulation. Moreover, adipocytes synthesize and secrete numerous peptide-signaling molecules that affect metabolism or that function in distant tissues. Among these molecules are the cytokines **tumor necrosis factor-α** and **resistin,** both of which reduce the responsiveness of target tissues to insulin, a key hormonal regulator of glucose and fat metabolism; **adiponectin,** which decreases hepatic glucose production by repressing transcription of the genes coding for phosphoenolpyruvate carboxykinase and glucose-6-phosphatase; and **plasminogen activator inhibitor 1,** which impedes lysis of freshly formed thrombi in blood vessels and thereby increases the hypoxic tissue damage that such clots can cause.

The nuclear transcription factors peroxisome proliferator–activated receptors α and γ (PPARα and PPARγ) are important transducers of metabolic signals in adipose tissue and elsewhere. PPARα-responsive genes are influenced by fatty acid–liganded PPARα, resulting in enhanced fatty acid oxidation in skeletal muscle, heart, and liver. PPARγ-responsive genes are influenced by the liganded receptor in adipose tissue to induce differentiation of preadipocytes to adipocytes, to enhance fatty acid oxidation and synthesis, and to increase secretion of products such as adiponectin that improve sensitivity to insulin in skeletal muscle, heart, and liver.

Pharmacological ligands for PPARα are fibric acid derivatives that are used to lower serum triglycerides in patients with dyslipidemias. Glucose metabolism is enhanced and responsiveness to the hormone insulin is increased by thiazolidinedione drugs, which activate PPARγ. These drugs are used to lower plasma glucose concentration in patients with type 2 diabetes.

The amounts and percentages of body weight accounted for by energy stored as fat in adipose tissue vary greatly among individuals. Studies of human monozygotic twins and animal models of obesity have provided indisputable evidence for a genetic influence that accounts for up to 35% of the variance in human fat mass. Certain mutant genes inexorably cause obesity in animal models. Analogues of the normal animal regulatory genes have been found in the normal human genome. Mutations of these genes, a rare occurrence in humans, are associated with and probably cause obesity.

Environmental and cultural influences, specifically the quality and quantity of the food available and the amount of exercise habitually engaged in, also modulate fat mass. Another factor that may contribute to the propensity for obesity is that humans have more energy-storage adipose cells per unit body mass than most other species do.

Energy stores are held close to particular levels in human adults

Some data suggest the existence of a particular set point for energy stores in each individual. Once adult weight is reached, it tends to be constant until middle age, at which point most humans incur at least a modest weight gain that leads to a higher proportion of body fat. Abdominal fat particularly increases with age and more so in men. Normal and obese individuals subjected to overfeeding or underfeeding experiments return to their approximate starting weight and degree of fatness when they are again allowed free access to food. This compensatory control of appetite (calorie and nutrient intake) resides in the hypothalamus, which contains a hunger center and a satiety center.

Humans who suffer damage to the hypothalamus from neoplasms or infiltrative disorders, such as **sarcoidosis,** sometimes gain large amounts of weight, which they maintain. Conversely, in the hypothalamic dysfunction of **anorexia nervosa,** weight is maintained at low, even life-threatening levels.

The hypothalamic hunger and satiety centers must respond to acute deficits and surfeits of essential substrates, such as glucose and fatty acids, but in addition, these neurons act to regulate energy reserves in the form of adipose tissue over the long term.

Many signals to the hypothalamus, including the sight, smell, taste, sweetness, and palatability of food and a reduction in plasma glucose levels, contribute to the stimulation of appetite. Studies have suggested that a particular pattern of plasma glucose change initiates food seeking. A **transient** rapid decline of 10% in plasma glucose level followed by an equally rapid recovery virtually to baseline preceded the request for a meal in human studies. The transient decline was interpreted by the investigators as a signal probing the ability of glucose stores to maintain homeostasis.

A variety of neuropeptides in the brain and in the gastrointestinal tract and a variety of neurotransmitters carry appetite-regulating signals to and within the central nervous system. Some are nutrient specific, such as serotonin for glucose and enterostatin for fat. Some are under hormonal regulation. For example, insulin strongly inhibits the synthesis of neuropeptide Y, a potent hypothalamic stimulator of food intake; loss of this action in insulin deficiency states is associated with an excessive appetite (polyphagia). Cortisol inhibits the synthesis of corticotropin-releasing hormone, an appetite suppressor; a corticol excess stimulates appetite and weight gain.

Energy expenditure is adjusted to a long continuation of a change in energy intake

Homeostatic setting of energy stores and body weight also occurs via the regulation of energy expenditure. Thus, experimental weight gain and loss evoke an increase and a decrease, respectively, of energy expenditure. In animals, **brown adipose tissue** seems specifically designed for such purposes. The large mitochondria in brown adipose tissue are stimulated by an **uncoupling protein (UCP),** also called **thermogenin,** that disassociates ATP production from O_2 use by causing a mitochondrial H^+ leak and thereby generates heat without producing useful chemical or mechanical work. UCP production is regulated by sympathetic nervous system signals (i.e., norepinephrine interacting with β-adrenergic receptors) and also by thyroid hormone. Brown adipose tissue is clearly present and probably functional in human newborns, who must adapt to a sudden lowering of environmental temperature from that in utero to that outside the mother by increasing heat production. However, this type of adipose tissue is difficult to detect and even more difficult to quantitate in adult humans. Homologous UCPs have been found in white adipose tissue and in the muscles of humans, but their importance in mediating obligatory and facultative thermogenesis remains unproven.

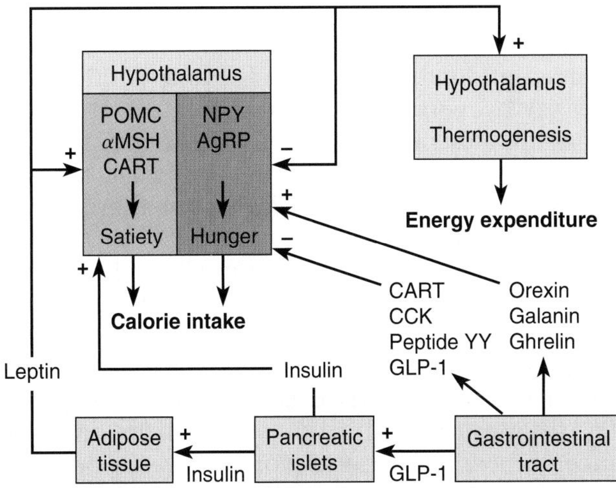

FIGURE 42–6. An overview of major components of the system that regulates energy stores and turnover. Specialized areas of the hypothalamus process incoming afferent signals and through diverse efferent pathways coordinate food seeking and thermogenesis to maintain appropriate long-term energy stores and to provide short-term balancing of energy and substrate needs with their voluntary and involuntary expenditure. An expansion of adipose tissue mass increases leptin secretion, and leptin decreases calorie intake by inhibiting hunger neurons and stimulating satiety neurons. Leptin also increases thermogenesis and energy expenditure. These actions of leptin restore adipose tissue mass to its appropriate set point. Insulin from the pancreatic islets reinforces this process directly by stimulating satiety centrally and indirectly by supporting leptin secretion in adipose tissue. A number of neuropeptides released by enteric neurons in the gastrointestinal tract also signal the hypothalamus. GLP-1 (glucagon-like peptide 1), peptide YY, CCK (cholecystokinin), and CART (cocaine- and amphetamine-regulated transcript) decrease hunger and food seeking; orexins, galanin, and ghrelin (growth hormone–releasing hormone) increase hunger and calorie intake. These signals arise in response to the presence or absence of food in the gut. AgRP, agouti-related peptide; αMSH, α-melanocyte-stimulating hormone; NPY, neuropeptide Y; POMC, proopiomelanocortin; – inhibits; + stimulates.

Energy stores are regulated by multiple mechanisms

Given the ever expanding number of molecules found to be involved in regulating energy intake, output, and stores, it is impossible to give a final definitive description of the system. It is possible, however, to see important relationships among the brain (particularly areas of the hypothalamus), the gastrointestinal tract (particularly the "enteric nervous system"), the pancreatic islets, and adipose tissue (**Figure 42–6**). Both the central sensing point and the command center appear to lie in the hypothalamus. The size of the adipose stores is signaled by its product **leptin,** the secretion and plasma levels of which are proportional to the body mass index. In the brain, leptin receptors are present in vascular cells, hypothalamic cells, and other cells. In response to increases and decreases in adipose stores, higher and lower levels of leptin, respectively, inhibit or stimulate food intake and increase or decrease energy expenditure. Leptin acts on at least two parallel sets of neurons to carry out this function (Figure 42–6). Sympathetic nervous system outflow mediates the leptin-dictated rises and falls in energy expenditure. Insulin from the pancreatic islets reinforces the satiety effects of leptin, as insulin levels increase in response to adiposity. As previously noted, glucose (and possibly fatty acid) levels are sensed by hypothalamic neurons and enteric neurons in the gastrointestinal tract and portal vein to provide short-term control. Numerous peptides, such as ghrelin and peptide YY, released by enteric neurons (Figure 42–6) report either the presence or prolonged absence of food in various levels of the gastrointestinal tract, accordingly signaling the hypothalamus for the need of food seeking or food avoidance.

Many of the molecules listed in Figure 42–6 have other, possibly related functions. Orexins, for example, stimulate hunger but also wakefulness. Their suppression by ingestion of a meal might account for the common occurrence of postprandial sleepiness. Leptin plays a role in the onset of puberty, possibly because reproductive capacity in females is inappropriate until leptin signals that there are sufficient maternal stores of energy. Ghrelin stimulates appetite and growth hormone secretion, possibly coordinating anabolism with the availability of dietary protein. Corticotropin-releasing hormone suppresses food intake and is evoked principally during stressful periods when seeking food may have a low priority. This association may contribute to the common experience of loss of appetite during major illnesses.

Plasma leptin levels do not increase acutely after food intake; thus, leptin probably does not act as an immediate regulator of energy turnover. Fasting for several days decreases leptin levels, whereas continuous hyperinsulinemia stimulated by glucose or food increases leptin levels. These responses may be the result of subtle changes in adipose mass as well as insulin's direct stimulatory effect on leptin production.

The pathological accumulation of energy stores as fat (i.e., obesity) is a major health problem growing to epidemic proportions in many countries with an excess of calories available and a declining need for exercise in essential life activities. A body weight 20% above desirable or a **body mass index (BMI)** of 25 to 27 increases the risk of diabetes, hypertension, and cardiovascular disease; a body weight 40% to 50% above the desirable level or a BMI above 30 increases the risk of death.

The accumulation of fat in abdominal and particularly visceral depots confers especially high risk.

$$\text{BMI} = \text{Weight (kg)} \div \text{Height (m)}^2$$

The exact cause or causes of human obesity are not known. Some obese individuals overeat and recognize an inability to control it, but most believe that their calorie intakes are less than they are actually ingesting.

Many obese individuals also behave as if they have an elevated set point for energy stores. These individuals appear to tenaciously "defend" this set point by decreasing energy expenditure when calorie intake is reduced and significant amounts of weight are lost. Nonobese infants or adults with lower BMRs are at greater risk for future weight gain. However, once obesity is present and static, the BMR and diet-induced thermogenesis (both adjusted for body weight) and the energy cost of exercise are generally equal to the respective values in individuals of normal weight.

In obese animals and humans, the profile of certain hormones involved in the regulation of fat metabolism (increased insulin and cortisol levels, decreased growth hormone levels) generally favors the deposition rather than the mobilization of fat. Endorphin levels are elevated, which may reflect abnormal central appetite stimulation. In addition, the adipose tissue of obese humans contains elevated levels of lipoprotein lipase, the key enzyme that transfers circulating triglycerides into cells. None of these abnormalities has proved to be the primary cause of the common form of human obesity.

Studies of leptin in obese humans suggest that absolute leptin deficiency is an extremely rare cause of obesity. In obese humans, the plasma leptin levels and leptin messenger RNA levels in adipose cells are usually increased and correlate with fat mass. Hence, the peripheral signal indicating that energy stores are too large is usually being generated, but it is not being received or acted on normally in the hypothalamus. However, only rarely has a mutant leptin receptor been found as a cause for obesity. Thus, human obesity is likely to result from defects in the generation of a leptin second-messenger or effector mechanism within the leptin target cells or in effector cell pathways farther "downstream." Rare cases of obesity are caused by mutations in the genes encoding proopiomelanocortin (*POMC*) and melanocortin 4 receptor (*MC4R*) in the satiety limb of leptin action (Figure 42–6). Whether partial resistance to leptin action can be overcome by sufficient exogenous leptin therapy is still under study. The present therapy for fighting obesity—dieting, disciplined exercise, behavior modification, and drugs that may act favorably at some point in the complex system that sets energy stores—is palliative but not curative. Gastric reduction or bypass surgery gives the best long-term results in people with BMI above 35 and associated medical conditions such as diabetes and hypertension. Its popularity is growing despite surgical complications and a low but definite mortality rate.

Summary

- Energy input as carbohydrate, fat, and protein calories must equal energy expenditure. Energy expenditure is composed of basal, diet-induced, and nonshivering thermogenesis and sedentary activity components plus exercise.
- Fatty acids are the major fuel in most tissues except for the central nervous system and red blood cells, where glucose is the major and obligatory oxidative substrate.
- The metabolism of glucose to pyruvate (anaerobic glycolysis), beta oxidation of fatty acids, and the disposal of acetyl CoA by the citric acid cycle lead to the mitochondrial generation of ATP via oxidative phosphorylation.
- Energy is stored mainly as adipose tissue triglycerides, with lesser amounts as protein. Carbohydrate stores as glycogen are very small.
- During long-term fasting, gluconeogenesis from amino acids and glycerol is required to sustain central nervous system metabolism and its critical functions. The pathway of gluconeogenesis is partly a reversal of glycolysis, but it requires special steps from pyruvate to fructose 6-phosphate. Increased use of fatty acids during fasting greatly increases the production of the keto acids β-hydroxybutyrate and acetoacetate.
- Endogenous protein turnover obligates a daily ingestion of proteins, in particular those containing essential amino acids, such as leucine.
- Fat metabolism involves a variety of circulating lipoprotein particles, apoproteins, and their receptors. These transfer triglycerides and cholesterol, originating in the diet or from hepatic synthesis, to and from various tissues.
- Energy needs during exercise are met in sequence by stored muscle creatine phosphate plus ATP, stored muscle glycogen, anaerobic glycolysis, and finally aerobic oxidation of glucose and fatty acids taken up from the plasma.
- The regulation of energy stores at individual set points is complex. Leptin, a secreted adipose tissue product, interacts with hypothalamic receptors to down-regulate appetite and to up-regulate energy expenditure and thereby prevents excessive accumulation of fat.

Bibliography

Barsh GS, Farooqi IS, O'Rahilly S: Genetics of body-weight regulation, *Nature* 404:644, 2000.

Batterham RL et al: Gut hormone PYY_{3-36} physiologically inhibits food intake, *Nature* 418:650, 2002.

Bouchard C, Despres JP, Mauriege P: Genetic and nongenetic determinants of regional fat distribution, *Endocr Rev* 14:72, 1993.

Campfield LA, Smith FJ: Blood glucose dynamics and control of meal initiation: a pattern detection and recognition theory, *Physiol Rev* 83:25, 2003.

Cummings DE et al: A preprandial rise in plasma ghrelin levels suggests a role in meal initiation in humans, *Diabetes* 50:1714, 2001.

DeFronzo RA, Ferrannini E: Regulation of intermediary metabolism during fasting and feeding. In DeGroot LJ, Jameson JL, eds: *Endocrinology,* ed 4, Philadelphia, 2001, WB Saunders.

Desvergne B, Wahli W: Peroxisome proliferator–activated receptors: nuclear control of metabolism, *Endocr Rev* 20:649, 1999.

Foster D: From glycogen to ketones—and back (Banting Lecture 1984), *Diabetes* 33:1188, 1984.

Francis GA et al: Nuclear receptors and the control of metabolism, *Annu Rev Physiol* 65:261, 2003.

Hardie DG, Carling D, Carlson M: The AMP-activated/SNF1 protein kinase subfamily: metabolic sensors of the eukaryotic cell? *Annu Rev Biochem* 67:821, 1998.

Harris RBS: Role of set-point theory in regulation of body weight, *FASEB J* 4:3310, 1990.

Jansky L: Humoral thermogenesis and its role in maintaining energy balance, *Physiol Rev* 75:237, 1995.

Kimball SR et al: Protein metabolism. In Rifkin H, Porte D, eds: *Diabetes mellitus,* ed 4, New York, 1990, Elsevier.

Kirchgessner AL: Orexins in the brain-gut axis, *Endocr Rev* 23:1, 2002.

Leibel RL, Rosenbaum M, Hirsch J: Changes in energy expenditure resulting from altered body weight, *N Engl J Med* 332:621, 1995.

McGarry JD, Foster DW: Ketogenesis. In Porte D Jr, Sherwin RS, eds: *Ellenberg & Rifkin's diabetes mellitus,* ed 5, Stamford, Conn, 1997, Appleton & Lange.

Rigotti A, Miettinen HE, Krieger M: The role of the high-density lipoprotein receptor SR-BI in the lipid metabolism of endocrine and other tissues, *Endocr Rev* 24:357, 2003.

Roberts SB et al: Dietary energy requirements of young adult men, determined by using the doubly labeled water method, *Am J Clin Nutr* 54:499, 1991.

Schwartz MW et al: Central nervous system control of food intake, *Nature* 404:661, 2000.

Shimano H: Sterol regulatory element–binding protein family as global regulators of lipid synthetic genes in energy metabolism, *Vitam Horm* 65:167, 2002.

Shulman GI, Barrett EJ, Sherwin RS: Integrated fuel metabolism. In Porte D Jr, Sherwin RS, eds: *Ellenberg & Rifkin's diabetes mellitus,* ed 5, Stamford, Conn, 1997, Appleton & Lange.

Sims EAH, Danforth E Jr: Expenditure and storage of energy in man, *J Clin Invest* 79:1019, 1987.

Spiegelman BM, Flier JS: Obesity and the regulation of energy balance, *Cell* 104:531, 2001.

Stefan N et al: Plasma adiponectin and endogenous glucose production in humans, *Diabetes Care* 26:3315, 2003.

Unger RH: The physiology of cellular liporegulation, *Annu Rev Physiol* 65:333, 2003.

Wasserman DH: Regulation of glucose fluxes during exercise in the postabsorptive state, *Annu Rev Physiol* 57:191, 1995.

Woods SC et al: Food intake and energy balance. In Porte D Jr, Sherwin RS, eds: *Ellenberg & Rifkin's diabetes mellitus,* ed 5, Stamford, Conn, 1997, Appleton & Lange.

Case Studies

Case 42–1

A 25-year-old man weighing 70 kg and in fit condition embarks on a solo mountain climb in winter. He is injured in an avalanche and fractures both legs. This immobilized person survives for 15 days without calories by drinking melted snow. He is then rescued. On examination, his body temperature is 34°C.

1. **At the time of rescue, which of the following findings would be expected?**
   A. Decreased plasma alanine level
   B. Increased urine nitrogen level
   C. Decreased plasma free fatty acids
   D. Decreased plasma keto acid levels
   E. Increased plasma glucose level

2. **Approximately how many grams of adipose tissue fat might he have lost?**
   A. 2550 g
   B. 1550 g
   C. 1450 g
   D. 3500 g
   E. 5750 g

Case 42–2

A 28-year-old woman sees a physician for obesity, which has been present since early infancy. Of her 10 siblings, 2 have a similar history of obesity. Neither parent is obese, but one grandparent on each side of the family was obese. The patient's height is 5 feet 2 inches, and her weight is 242 pounds. Her body mass index is $110/1.58^2 = 44$. The family history suggests a genetic form of obesity with an autosomal recessive pattern of inheritance.

1. **Which of the following is a candidate gene for causing this syndrome?**
   A. An inactivating mutant gene for neuropeptide Y synthesis
   B. An inactivating mutant gene for a β-adrenergic receptor in adipose tissue
   C. A hyperactivating mutant gene for the leptin receptor
   D. A hyperactivating mutant gene for UCP
   E. An inactivating mutant gene for lipoprotein lipase

2. **With great effort, the patient loses 50 pounds in 6 months on a low-calorie diet and regular exercise. However, she gradually slips back into ad lib eating and her former sedentary ways; during 3 years, her weight restabilizes at 250 pounds. Which of the following is correct?**
   A. She has an abnormal appetite setting.
   B. She has an abnormal low set point for leptin secretion.
   C. She has an abnormal low set point for energy expenditure.
   D. She has an abnormal low set point for UCP production.
   E. She has an abnormal set point for energy stores.

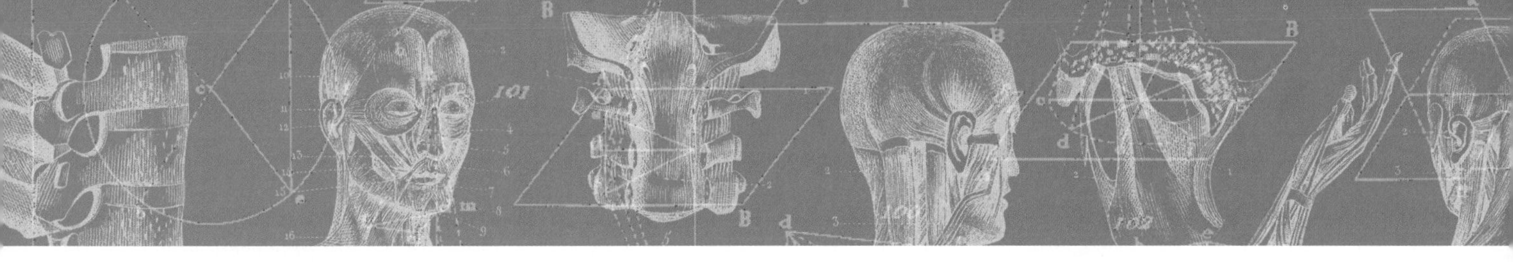

Chapter 43: Hormones of the Pancreatic Islets

Objectives

- ❖ Describe the synthesis and secretion of the two major pancreatic islet hormones: insulin and glucagon.
- ❖ Explain the powerful effects of insulin and glucagon on glucose, fatty acid, and amino acid metabolism and the feedback effects of these substrates on insulin and glucagon secretion.
- ❖ Identify the mechanisms of action of insulin and glucagon on their target cells.
- ❖ Explain the interrelationships between insulin and glucagon, particularly their mutually antagonistic effects on substrate flow in the liver.
- ❖ Describe the respective roles of insulin and glucagon in metabolic adaptations to fasting and exercise.

The major pancreatic islet hormones, **insulin** and **glucagon,** are rapid and powerful regulators of metabolism. Their secretion is determined primarily by plasma substrate levels. TOGETHER, GLUCAGON AND INSULIN COORDINATE THE DISPOSITION OF NUTRIENT INPUT FROM MEALS AS WELL AS THE FLOW OF ENDOGENOUS SUBSTRATES DURING FASTING VIA ACTIONS ON THE LIVER, ADIPOSE TISSUE, AND MUSCLE MASS. In turn, these hormones form regulatory feedback loops with critical substrates. Insulin and glucagon directly or indirectly influence the metabolism and hence the function of all the organ systems described earlier in this book.

The Cells of Origin of Insulin and Glucagon Are Interspersed in Small Islets Scattered Throughout the Pancreas

The proximity of the islets permits each hormone to influence the other's secretion. The islets are composed of 60% β cells, the source of insulin, and 25% α cells, the source of glucagon. The remaining islet cells secrete various neuropeptides with gastrointestinal functions. The islet endocrine cells arise from endoderm in the foregut and differentiate into β cells under the influence of a transcription factor, insulin promoter factor 1 (IPF-1), which also induces insulin secretion. By the tenth week of human gestation, islets secrete insulin.

The strategic location of the islets reflects their functional role

Insulin and glucagon are secreted in response to nutrient inflow and gastrointestinal secretagogues, as are the enzymes of the acinar pancreas (see Chapter 34). The islet hormones may have paracrine effects on nearby acinar cells as well as on each other through tight junctions and gap junctions between the endocrine cells. The location of the islets (**Figure 43–1**) leads to the secretion of insulin and glucagon into the pancreatic veins and then into the portal vein, where they join the influx of nutrients from meals in the splanchnic circulation. This arrangement permits the liver, the central organ in nutrient traffic, to be exposed to higher concentrations of these pancreatic islet hormones than peripheral tissues are. It also permits the liver to modulate the availability of insulin and glucagon

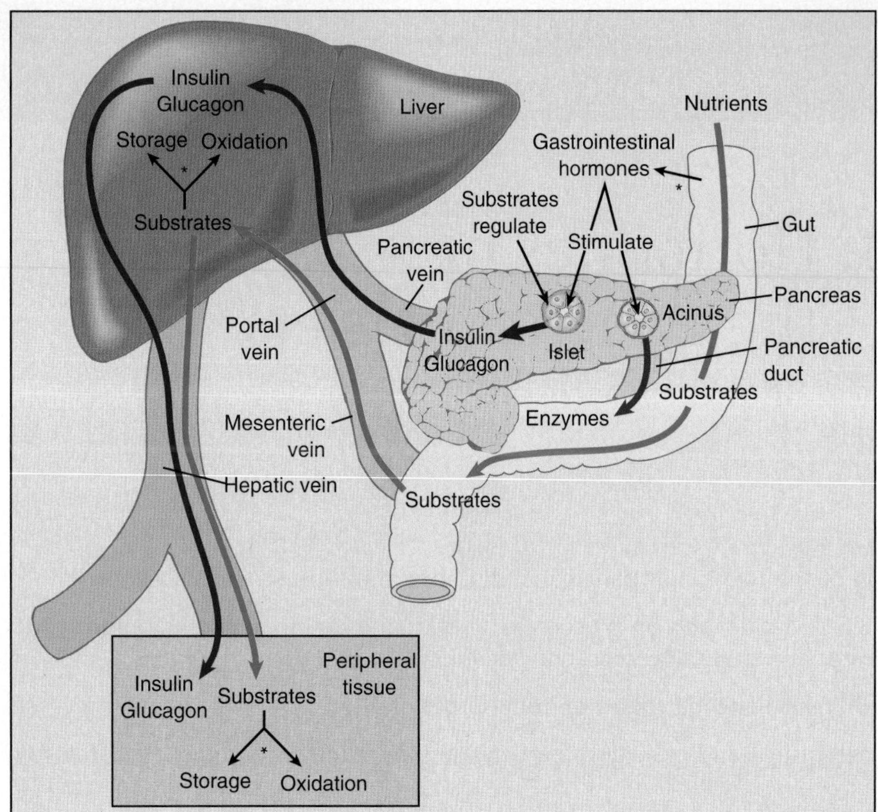

FIGURE 43–1. View of the pivotal location of the pancreatic islets. Secretion of the islet hormones insulin and glucagon is coordinated with the secretion of exocrine pancreatic enzymes. Both are stimulated by the entry of nutrients into the gastrointestinal tract and by gastrointestinal hormones. Pancreatic enzymes reach the intestinal lumen via the pancreatic duct. Islet hormones are secreted into the portal vein and thereby reach the liver with the substrates resulting from nutrient digestion. Within the liver, these hormones direct the storage or oxidation of the ingested substrates. Islet hormones that pass through the liver with substrates similarly affect the metabolism of these substrates by peripheral tissues. Asterisks indicate the action sites.

to peripheral tissues by extracting variable amounts of these hormones during first passage through that organ.

INSULIN AND GLUCAGON ARE OFTEN SECRETED RECIPROCALLY AND ACT RECIPROCALLY. WHEN ONE IS NEEDED, THE OTHER USUALLY IS NOT. The consequences of isolated insulin deficiency—the common disease **type 1 diabetes mellitus**—are so devastating that insulin has dominated physiological thinking. In contrast, isolated glucagon deficiency is virtually unknown in medicine; moreover, it can be compensated for by other mechanisms.

Insulin is synthesized from a prohormone and secreted by exocytosis

Insulin is a peptide hormone with a molecular weight of 6000. It is composed of two straight chains linked by disulfide bridges. The B chain contains the core of biological activity, whereas the A chain contains most of the species-specific sites. Human insulin and molecular variants produced by recombinant DNA techniques have virtually replaced animal insulins for the treatment of diabetes.

The synthesis of insulin by the β cell follows the same general pattern as that for peptide hormones described in Chapter 41. The gene directs the synthesis of a preprohormone, from which the signal peptide is cleaved to yield the single-chain **proinsulin.** Establishment of the disulfide links is followed by the excision of a connecting peptide known as **C peptide.** The Golgi apparatus packages insulin and C peptide together in the secretory granules. These granules also contain zinc, which acts to join six insulin molecules into hexamers.

Insulin is secreted via exocytosis (see Figure 41–5) of its granules, which are arrayed in parallel with microtubules in the β-cell cytoplasm. The microtubules are associated with a web of microfilaments that contain myosin and actin near the plasma membrane. On application of a stimulus, contraction of microfilaments draws the granules to the plasma membrane, where they fuse with it, rupture, and release equimolar amounts of insulin and C peptide. The insulin hexamers ultimately dissociate to monomers that are biologically active.

The metabolism of glucose in the β cell stimulates insulin secretion

The single most important stimulator of insulin release is glucose (**Figure 43–2**). The mechanism involves the following sequence:

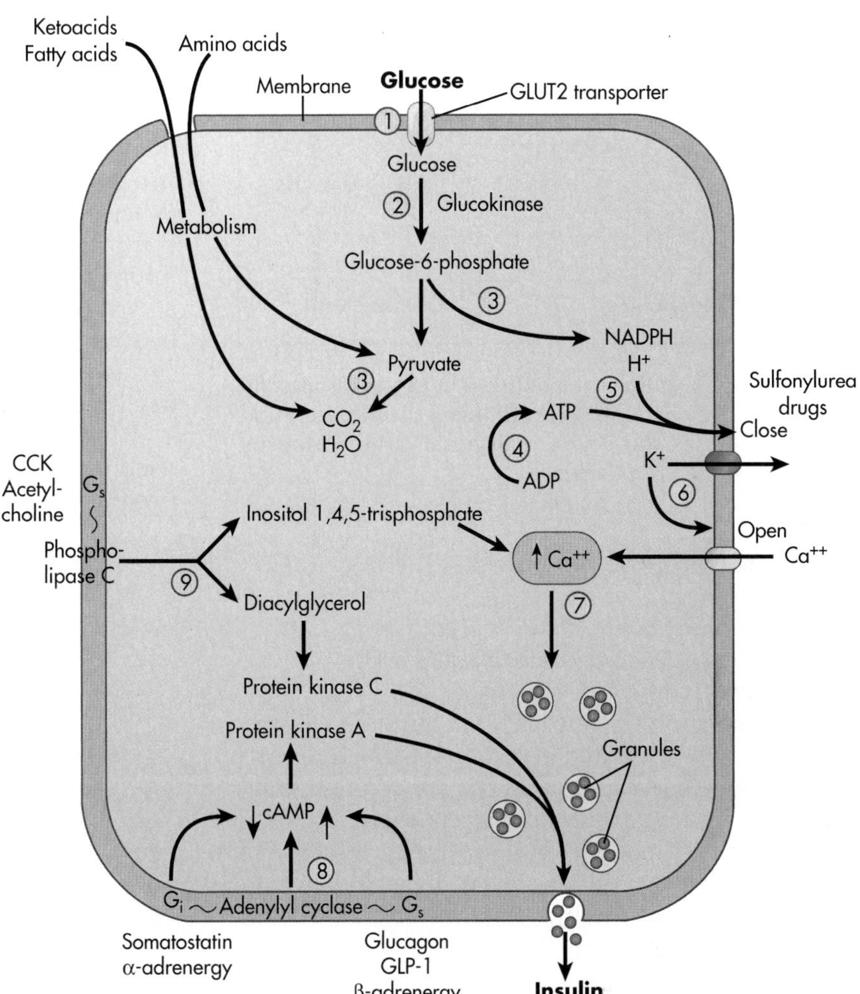

FIGURE 43–2. Regulation of insulin secretion by the β cell. Glucose transport (1) and glucokinase-catalyzed phosphorylation (2) raise glucose 6-phosphate levels. The metabolism of glucose 6-phosphate (3) subsequently leads to increased levels of ATP (4) and NADPH (5) that inhibit or close a K^+ channel (6) and open a Ca^{++} channel (6). Increased Ca^{++} levels then trigger exocytosis of insulin granules (7). Other modulators of secretion act via the adenylyl cyclase–cAMP–protein kinase pathway (8) and the phospholipase-phosphoinositide pathway (9). CCK, cholecystokinin; GLP-1, glucagon-like peptide 1.

1. A specific glucose transporter (GLUT2) facilitates rapid diffusion into the β cell and maintains an intracellular glucose concentration equal to that of interstitial fluid.
2. The enzyme glucokinase, which has a K_m of 5 mM for glucose (slightly above the average fasting concentration), acts as a glucose sensor that controls the rates of glucose use.
3. The products of glucose metabolism, including ATP, nicotinamide adenine dinucleotide phosphate (NADP), and the reduced form of NADP (NADPH), increase, and an ATP-sensitive K^+ channel closes as the ratio of ATP to ADP increases. The K^+ channel is composed of four inner small subunits called Kir6.2, to which ATP binds, and four outer large subunits called SUR1, to which insulin-releasing sulfonylurea drugs bind (Figure 43–2).
4. Binding to either subunit depolarizes the cell, which then triggers the opening of voltage-regulated Ca^{++} channels. The intracellular Ca^{++} increases and triggers exocytosis (see Figure 41–5).
5. G proteins linked to adenylyl cyclase and to phospholipase C mediate the stimulatory and inhibitory actions of other modulators of insulin release via alterations in the levels of cAMP, phosphatidylinositol products (e.g., inositol 1,4,5-trisphosphate [InsP3]), and diacylglycerols (Figure 43–2). In addition to causing insulin release, glucose stimulates the synthesis of hormone by increasing the transcription rate of the insulin gene and the translation rate of its mature messenger RNA.

Type 1 diabetes mellitus results from the complete destruction of β cells and the ultimate loss of all insulin. However, in rare instances, much milder diabetes mellitus is caused by genetic abnormalities in insulin synthesis and secretion; such abnormalities include mutant genes encoding glucokinase, IPF-1, and insulin. In addition, inactivating mutations of the K^+ channel SUR1 subunit can cause neonatal diabetes; hyperactive mutants of SUR1 cause continuous insulin secretion and hypoglycemia.

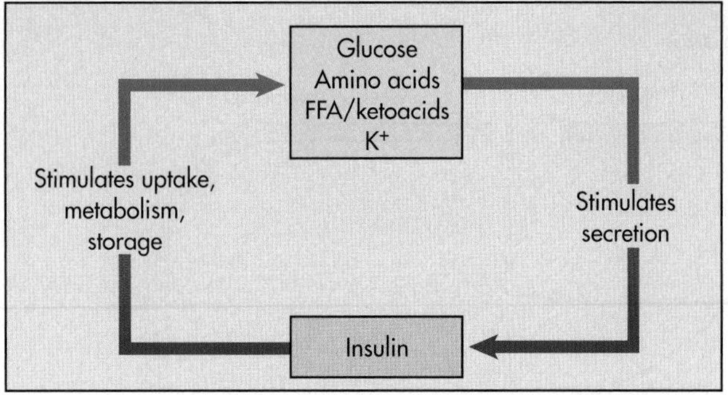

FIGURE 43–3. Feedback relationship between insulin and nutrients. The nutrients that stimulate insulin secretion are the same as those whose disposal is facilitated by insulin. FFA, free fatty acids.

Insulin secretion is regulated

In the broadest sense, insulin secretion is governed by a feedback relationship with the exogenous nutrient supply

When the supply of nutrients is abundant (**Figure 43–3**), insulin is secreted in response to their inflow; the hormone then stimulates the use of these same incoming nutrients and simultaneously inhibits the mobilization of endogenous substrates. When the nutrient supply is low or absent, insulin secretion is dampened, and the mobilization of endogenous fuels is enhanced.

The central regulating molecule is glucose. At plasma glucose levels lower than 50 mg/dL, little or no insulin is secreted, whereas the response is maximal at plasma levels higher than 250 mg/dL. Brief exposure of the β cell to glucose induces a rapid but transient release of insulin. With continuous glucose exposure, this initial response fades, only to be replaced later by a more prolonged second phase.

Glucose entry from the gastrointestinal tract follows digestion of the carbohydrate components of a meal. Under these circumstances, more insulin is released than can be accounted for by the extent to which plasma glucose levels rise. As shown in **Figure 43–4**, the plasma insulin response to an oral glucose load is much greater than the insulin response to the same rise in plasma glucose produced by a variable intravenous glucose infusion. This **incretin effect** accounts for more than half of the insulin secreted in response to oral glucose and for more than half the glucose load that is assimilated into tissues under the influence of insulin. The incretin effect results from secretion of glucagon-like peptide 1 (GLP-1) and glucose-dependent insulinotropic peptide (GIP) by enteric neurons in response to glucose entry into the upper and lower small intestine. GLP-1 and GIP each contribute half of the important incretin effect, but they do not stimulate insulin release in the absence of glucose.

Digestion of the protein in a meal yields amino acids, some of which synergize with glucose in stimulating the β cells. Lipids and their products contribute little directly to the β-cell response to a meal. When the digestion and absorption of nutrients are completed, plasma glucose and amino acid levels return to baseline, and insulin secretion subsides to a rate that is maintained steadily during periods between meals and overnight fasting. An intrinsic cyclic oscillation every 14 minutes characterizes basal secretion.

If fasting is extended for days, insulin secretion declines below the basal rate and then resets at a lower level. In this state, secretion is maintained by

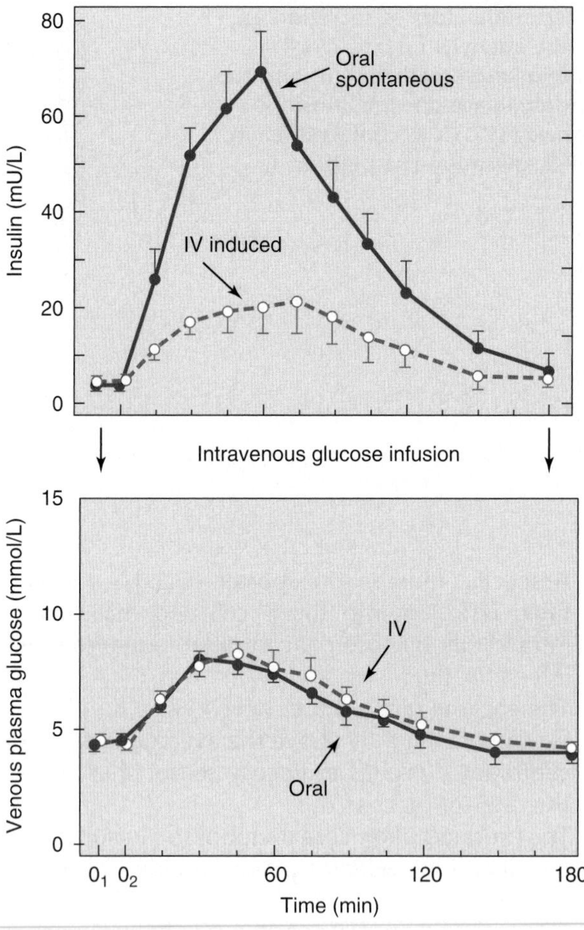

FIGURE 43–4. The incretin effect. The lower panel shows the spontaneous plasma glucose profile produced by the oral administration of a glucose load to normal individuals. Also shown is the deliberate mimicking of this profile by administration of glucose continuously in variable amounts intravenously. Despite the close similarity of the two glucose profiles, the upper panel shows the markedly greater plasma insulin response to the oral glucose load. (Data from Nauck M et al: *Diabetologia* 29:46, 1986.)

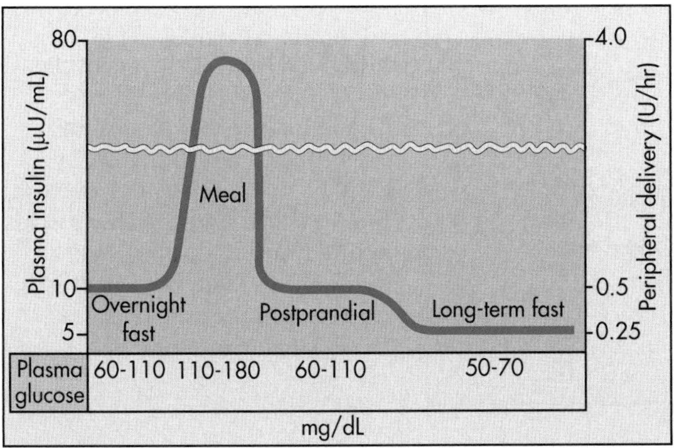

FIGURE 43–5. Pattern of plasma insulin levels and the corresponding insulin delivery rates to the peripheral circulation in various physiological states (10 μU/mL = 7 × 10^{-11} M). The usual prevailing plasma glucose levels are also indicated. Fasting insulin levels regulate the mobilization of endogenous substrates at appropriate rates. Levels after meals stimulate the storage of substrates.

lower but still slightly stimulatory plasma glucose levels, with contributions from greatly elevated levels of keto acids and free fatty acids. Insulin secretion is also modulated by cholinergic and β-adrenergic stimulatory and α-adrenergic inhibitory influences. All these factors cause physiological fluctuations in peripheral plasma insulin levels and in the average equivalent rates of insulin delivery into the peripheral circulation. These changes are summarized in **Figure 43–5**. Chronic exposure to high levels of glucose or lipids is toxic to the β cells.

Type 2 diabetes mellitus is the most common form of the disease. One important factor in this type of diabetes is an early subtle disturbance in the pattern of insulin secretion. This is characterized by altered cyclicity, diminished pulse frequency, and delayed response to rising glucose levels. Eventually, glucose is no longer recognized as a stimulus. The primary cause of such β-cell dysfunction remains unknown.

β-Cell function is quantitated by measurements of C peptide

Peripheral plasma insulin levels are about 7 × 10^{-11} M. Insulin concentration in the portal vein ranges from two to ten times higher than in the peripheral circulation. The liver extracts about half the insulin reaching it, but this varies with the nutritional state. Thus, actual β-cell secretory rates are better estimated by measuring plasma (or even urine) levels of C peptide because this cosecreted molecule is not removed by the liver. Such estimates yield values of 1.0 to 2.5 mg/day (25 to 40 units/day) for insulin secretion. C peptide and the small quantity of proinsulin secreted by β cells as yet have no proven physiological actions.

Insulin has a short plasma half-life (6 to 8 minutes), mainly because of specific degradation in the kidney and liver. However, insulin is also degraded in conjunction with its actions on its target cells after receptor binding and internalization of the hormone. Very little intact insulin is excreted in the urine. C peptide has a much longer half-life and no appreciable hepatic extraction, so its plasma (and urine) levels are a useful indicator of β-cell insulin secretion.

The actions of insulin are varied

Insulin is a strongly anabolic hormone

THE OVERALL THRUST OF INSULIN ACTION IS TO FACILITATE THE STORAGE OF SUBSTRATES AND TO INHIBIT THEIR RELEASE **(Figure 43–6)**. As a result, secreted or administered insulin decreases the plasma concentrations of glucose, of free fatty acids and keto acids, and predominantly of the essential branched-chain amino acids (i.e., leucine, isoleucine, valine). The major sites of insulin action are the liver, muscle, and adipose tissue. In each target tissue, carbohydrate, lipid, and protein metabolism is regulated coordinately.

Under maximal insulin stimulation, the usual rate of glucose use by peripheral tissues increases fivefold to sixfold. Simultaneously, the output of glucose by the liver drops to considerably below half. Most of the extra glucose uptake occurs in muscle, with a small fraction occurring in adipose tissue. Approximately 75% of this glucose is converted to glycogen, and about 25% undergoes glycolysis and terminal oxidation to carbon dioxide. The absolute rate of glucose oxidation, however, is increased threefold by insulin.

The hypersecretion of insulin by a β-cell tumor causes **hypoglycemia.** Hypoglycemia produces central nervous system dysfunction that ranges from mild difficulty in concentrating to severe behavioral disturbances, psychosis, convulsions, and coma. Symptoms are typically worse in the fasting state and are countered by overeating carbohydrates, often with resulting weight gain. The diagnosis is established by demonstrating inappropriately high levels of plasma insulin and C peptide when the plasma glucose concentration is low.

The basal rate of free fatty acid inflow to plasma from adipose tissue is also markedly decreased by insulin. (At the same time, the inflow of glycerol, the other product of triglyceride hydrolysis, is

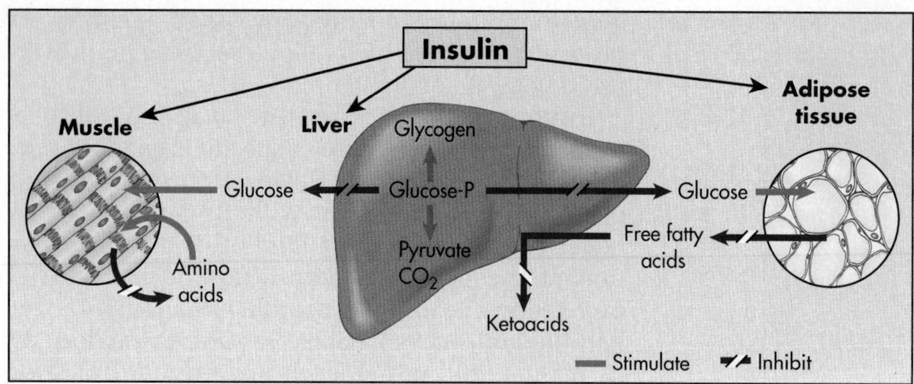

FIGURE 43–6. Effect of insulin on the overall flow of fuels. Tissue uptake of glucose and amino acids is stimulated by insulin; tissue release of glucose, amino acids, and free fatty acids is inhibited by insulin, as is ketogenesis. The net result is a decrease in plasma levels of these substrates.

decreased sharply.) As a result, insulin reduces the basal rate of lipid oxidation more than 90%. Because insulin also stimulates triglyceride synthesis and storage, it facilitates weight gain, despite a central satiety effect on appetite.

The action of insulin on protein turnover can be assessed by determining the hormone's effect on the flux of the essential amino acid leucine. Maximum doses decrease leucine's rate of inflow into plasma to almost half. Because the only source of leucine in the basal state is endogenous protein, insulin must inhibit proteolysis. In addition, insulin decreases leucine's rate of oxidation. The result of such insulin effects is a net gain in body protein.

Insulin stimulates glucose uptake by cells and storage as glycogen

IN MUSCLE AND ADIPOSE TISSUE, INSULIN STIMULATES THE TRANSPORT OF GLUCOSE FROM THE PLASMA INTO THE CYTOPLASM, WHERE IT IS RAPIDLY PHOSPHORYLATED. IN MUSCLE AND LIVER, INSULIN LARGELY STIMULATES GLYCOGEN FORMATION FROM GLUCOSE 6-PHOSPHATE. To a much lesser extent, insulin stimulates the glycolysis and oxidation of glucose. In adipose tissue, insulin's most important carbohydrate effect is to stimulate the production of α-glycerol phosphate from the triose phosphate intermediates of glycolysis. The α-glycerol phosphate is used to esterify free fatty acids and thus store them as triglycerides (see Figure 42–2).

Insulin stimulates the conversion of glucose to glycogen and inhibits the reverse reaction, the breakdown of glycogen to glucose, by increasing the activities or concentrations of glycogen synthase and decreasing those of phosphorylase, respectively (see Figure 42–2). The equilibrium between glucose and glucose 6-phosphate is shifted toward glucose 6-phosphate because the concentration of the phosphorylating enzyme glucokinase is increased by insulin. (In only the liver, the level of the dephosphorylating enzyme glucose-6-phosphatase is decreased by insulin.) Insulin also shifts the balance between glycolysis and gluconeogenesis toward glycolysis and away from gluconeogenesis. Glycolysis is accelerated because insulin increases the key enzymes phosphofructokinase, pyruvate kinase, and pyruvate dehydrogenase; gluconeogenesis is retarded because insulin decreases the enzymes phosphoenolpyruvate carboxykinase, pyruvate carboxylase, and fructose-1,6-diphosphatase (see Figure 42–2).

In the liver, glucose availability reinforces the effects of insulin that lead toward glycogen storage or glycolysis and away from glucose release. Conversely, if plasma glucose levels decline below normal, these effects become attenuated by intrahepatic autoregulatory phenomena as well as by the secretion of hormones whose actions are antagonistic to insulin (e.g., glucagon, epinephrine, cortisol, growth hormone).

Insulin stimulates fat storage

IN ADIPOSE TISSUE, INSULIN FACILITATES TRANSFER OF CIRCULATING FAT INTO THE ADIPOSE CELL BY INDUCING THE ENZYME LIPOPROTEIN LIPASE (see Figure 42–4). More free fatty acid is thereby liberated from circulating triglyceride and is rapidly taken up into the adipose cell, where it is reesterified. Thus, dietary fat not needed for immediate energy generation is stored. OF EQUAL OR GREATER IMPORTANCE, INSULIN PROFOUNDLY INHIBITS THE REVERSE REACTION (i.e., LIPOLYSIS OF STORED TRIGLYCERIDE) BY INHIBITING THE NECESSARY ENZYME HORMONE-SENSITIVE ADIPOSE TISSUE LIPASE. In this manner, the release and delivery of free fatty acids to other tissues are greatly suppressed.

In the liver, insulin favors shunting of incoming free fatty acids away from beta oxidation by inhibiting their transfer into mitochondria and by directing them toward esterification by increasing the production of β-glycerol phosphate. Because beta oxidation is diminished, less β-hydroxybutyrate and acetoacetate are produced. Thus, INSULIN IS POWERFULLY ANTIKETOGENIC.

Virtually complete loss of insulin and its actions causes the striking manifestations of type 1 diabetes mellitus. During a period of weeks, **hyperglycemia** develops to a point exceeding the renal threshold of glucose (see Chapter 37). Large amounts of glucose are lost in the urine; the high urinary glucose concentration creates a continuous osmotic diuresis **(polyuria),** leading to thirst and dehydration. This drain of carbohydrate calories along with catabolic losses of adipose triglyceride stores and lean body mass causes weight loss despite increased food intake **(polyphagia).** Uninhibited lipolysis leads to high plasma levels of free fatty acids, the stimulation of ketogenesis, and very high plasma levels of β-hydroxybutyrate and acetoacetate. The plasma level of HCO_3^- and the pH fall, and a profound metabolic acidosis ensues (see Chapter 40). Coma and death follow unless treatment with insulin, intravenous fluids, and electrolytes is provided.

Insulin also stimulates de novo synthesis of free fatty acids from glucose. Cytoplasmic acetyl coenzyme A (acetyl CoA) derived from pyruvate is shunted toward fatty acid formation because insulin increases the key enzymes acetyl-CoA carboxylase and fatty acid synthase. In addition, insulin stimulates the synthesis of cholesterol from acetyl CoA by activating the key enzyme hydroxymethylglutaryl-CoA reductase. The net effect of insulin is therefore to increase the fat content of the liver and in some circumstances to increase the release of very-low-density lipoprotein from that organ.

Insulin stimulates protein storage

In muscle, insulin stimulates the Na^+-dependent transport of certain amino acids from the plasma, across the cell membrane, and into the cytoplasm, all independently of the transport of glucose. When amino acids are abundant, the overall synthesis of proteins is also increased via the stimulation of transcription and translation. Specific examples are the stimulation by insulin of the synthesis of albumin in the liver and of amylase in the exocrine pancreas. These anabolic effects are reinforced by important anticatabolic effects (i.e., by inhibiting the enzymes of proteolysis and the inhibition of amino acid release from the cell). Moreover, in cartilage and osseous tissue, insulin and structurally related insulin growth factors (see Chapter 45) enhance the general synthesis of proteins as well as of DNA, RNA, and other macromolecules. Thus, INSULIN IS AN IMPORTANT CONTRIBUTOR TO GROWTH, TISSUE REGENERATION, AND BONE REMODELING. Insulin may have autocrine or even intracrine actions (see Chapter 41) on β cells that have insulin receptors and may need insulin's anabolic actions for proliferation.

Insulin regulates plasma cation and anion concentrations

Both glycogen synthesis and protein synthesis require the concurrent cellular uptake of potassium, phosphate, and magnesium. The translocation of all three of these electrolytes from the extracellular space into muscle cells is stimulated by insulin (see Chapter 39). Insulin also stimulates reabsorption of electrolytes by the renal tubules. Preventing the urinary loss of potassium and phosphate also contributes to anabolism, whereas conserving sodium may be related to the need for the additional formation of extracellular fluid to accompany the expansion of lean body mass.

When insulin is administered to patients in **diabetic ketoacidosis,** increased transport into cells can cause profound drops in plasma phosphate, potassium, and magnesium levels. Potassium always, phosphate occasionally, and magnesium rarely must be given intravenously to prevent the serious or even fatal consequences of hypokalemia, hypophosphatemia, or hypomagnesemia.

Insulin has other actions that are relevant to total body energy turnover and stores

Diet-induced thermogenesis, particularly after carbohydrate ingestion, is enhanced by insulin, probably through the stimulation of glycogen formation. Insulin also increases the energy expenditure by stimulating Na^+,K^+-ATPase. Although most parts of the brain are unresponsive to insulin, this hormone probably acts on the hypothalamus. Insulin decreases the synthesis of neuropeptide Y (see Chapter 42). By this action—and by increasing leptin levels—insulin is an appetite suppressant. Since leptin inhibits insulin secretion, leptin and insulin form a negative-feedback loop that regulates energy stores in adipose tissue. If insulin lowers plasma glucose levels to below those needed for normal brain metabolism (i.e., <55 mg/dL), hunger is stimulated by other mechanisms.

Insulin acts through a plasma membrane tyrosine kinase receptor

The initial step in all actions of insulin is binding of the hormone to its plasma membrane receptor **(Figure 43–7)**. This receptor is a glycoprotein composed of two symmetrical units connected by disulfide bonds. Each of these main units is made up of an α subunit that extends externally and binds the hormone and a β subunit that traverses the cell membrane and terminates in an intracytoplasmic tail. Receptor molecules cycle between a cytoplasmic pool and the plasma membrane, and their number is down-regulated by insulin.

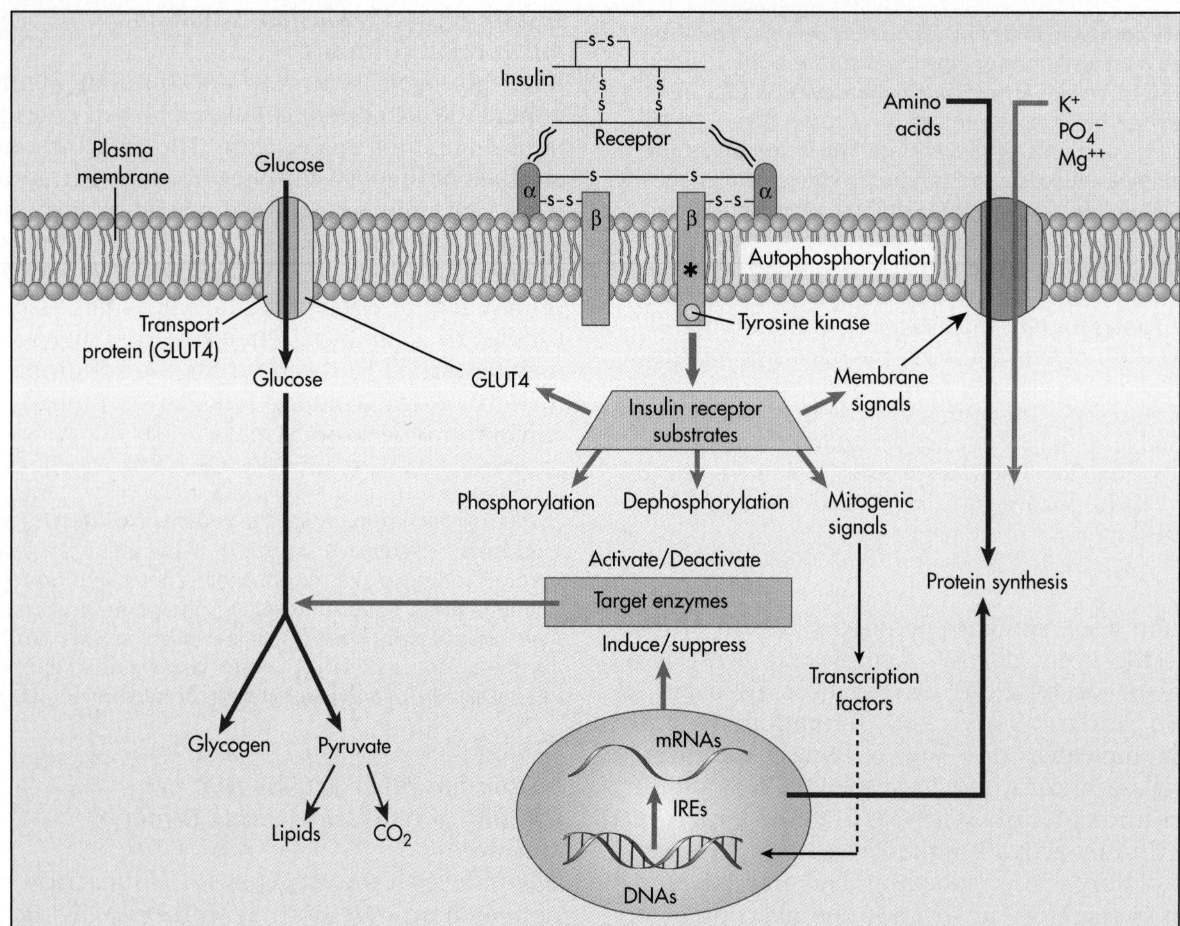

FIGURE 43–7. Insulin action on cells. The binding of insulin to its receptor causes autophosphorylation of the receptor, which then itself acts as a tyrosine kinase that phosphorylates tyrosines in insulin receptor substrates. As a result, these substrates phosphorylate serine and threonine residues in other proteins and enzymes. Numerous target enzymes are ultimately activated or inactivated, and the result is to shift the metabolism of glucose toward glycogen and pyruvate. The glucose transporter GLUT4 is recruited to the plasma membrane, where it facilitates glucose entry into the cell. The transport of amino acids, K^+, Mg^{++}, and PO_4^- into the cell is also facilitated by other mechanisms. The synthesis of various enzymes is induced or suppressed and cell growth is regulated by signal molecules that modulate gene expression. Numerous intermediary molecules are involved. IREs, insulin regulatory elements; mRNA, messenger RNA.

After insulin binds to its receptor, the following steps occur:

1. The β subunit of the receptor undergoes autophosphorylation with ATP at specific tyrosine sites.
2. The phosphorylated receptor itself becomes a tyrosine kinase, which then phosphorylates tyrosines in several large proteins called **insulin receptor substrates.**
3. The activation of insulin receptor substrates initiates a cascade of serine and threonine phosphorylations in multiple intermediary molecules, such as protein kinase B, phosphatidylinositol 3-kinase, growth receptor–binding protein 2, and mitogen-activated protein kinase. The number of mediators of insulin action continues to grow. Metabolic and mitogenic pathways are altered in parallel, although not necessarily synchronously, and they may also cross-react.
4. The target enzymes previously described are rapidly activated or deactivated, by both phosphorylation and dephosphorylation. The same enzymes may be induced or repressed more slowly by modulating gene transcription.
5. Plasma membrane carrier mechanisms are activated.
6. DNA transcription factors related to cell growth are modified.
7. In some target cells (e.g., adipose tissue), cAMP levels are lowered by insulin's stimulation of phosphodiesterase; this contributes to some of the hormone's actions (e.g., the inhibition of lipolysis).

Insulin stimulates a specific glucose carrier system within the plasma membrane of target cells

A particular glucose transporter (GLUT4) facilitates the diffusion (not the active transport) of extracellular glucose into the cytosol of muscle and adipose cells, down an already existing, large concentration gradient. Insulin rapidly increases transfer of GLUT4 from its vesicular cytoplasmic depots to the plasma membrane. Later, insulin increases GLUT4 synthesis. The crucial importance of this action is that at basal physiological insulin concentrations, the transport of glucose into muscle and adipose tissue cells is often the rate-limiting step in glucose metabolism. In comparison, the phosphorylation of glucose is so rapid that intracellular concentrations of free glucose are usually negligible. At the high insulin concentrations that prevail after a meal, the rate-limiting step in glucose metabolism shifts to an intracellular point that also governs insulin actions.

In rare instances, deletions as well as missense and nonsense mutations in the insulin receptor gene cause receptor malfunction and marked resistance to the action of insulin. In affected infants, this can lead to diabetes mellitus, profound disorders of growth, and death. Impaired insulin action (as well as inadequate insulin secretion) is also a major factor, producing hyperglycemia in the common type 2 diabetes mellitus. Because most of these patients are obese and seldom exhibit increased ketogenesis, insulin resistance may be greater in muscle than in adipose tissue.

Insulin secretion is correlated with the appropriate actions of insulin

The major actions of insulin form a hierarchy that is related to successive increases in plasma insulin concentration. The low insulin concentrations that prevail in humans who have fasted overnight are able to partially restrain and thereby regulate the endogenous release rates of free fatty acids and amino acids. Somewhat higher insulin concentrations elicited by incoming dietary nutrients are required to completely shut off unneeded glucose production by the liver. The peak insulin concentrations elicited by a meal greatly stimulate glucose and amino acid uptake by peripheral tissues, especially muscle, and fatty acid uptake by adipose tissue. These actions of insulin ensure that those substrates may be stored for future use.

In addition, the amount of insulin secreted in response to glucose is correlated with the amount of glucose uptake by tissues that can be stimulated by insulin. Put another way and shown in **Figure 43–8**, the more resistant an individual is to insulin action, the more insulin the β cells secrete in compensation. When this physiological linkage is distorted or broken, plasma glucose levels become abnormal.

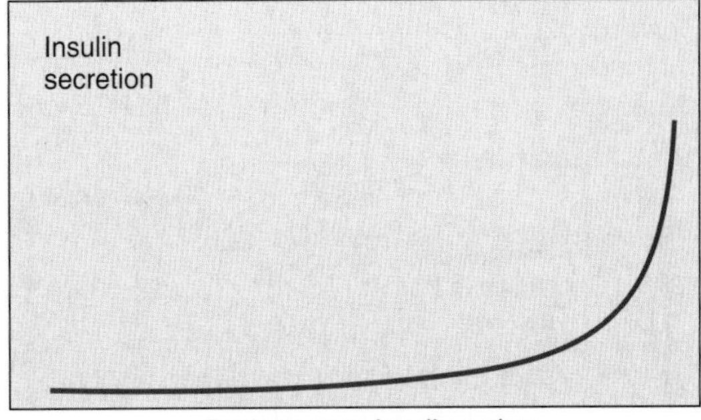

FIGURE 43–8. The relationship between insulin secretion and resistance of tissues to insulin action. The left side of the panel shows that very little insulin is secreted when the tissues are sensitive to insulin—that is, resistance to insulin action is very low. The right side shows that as resistance to insulin increases, insulin secretion is raised exponentially to maintain a normal plasma glucose level.

Amylin Moderates the Glucose-Lowering Effects of Insulin

The β-cell insulin granule contains another peptide product expressed by a different gene but copackaged with insulin. Amylin has 37 amino acids and is released simultaneously with insulin by exocytosis and circulates in plasma at 1% to 2% the concentration of insulin. Its clinical importance lies first in its tendency to polymerize in extracellular fibrils that cause fibrosis in islets of individuals with type 2 diabetes. Additionally, it decreases food intake and the rate of gastric emptying, thereby limiting plasma glucose increase after meals. An amylin analogue is now used in type 2 diabetes therapy.

Glucagon Is Synthesized and Secreted in Response to a Lowering of Plasma Glucose Levels

GLUCAGON IS AN IMPORTANT REGULATOR OF INTRAHEPATIC GLUCOSE AND FREE FATTY ACID METABOLISM. This hormone is a straight-chain peptide with a molecular weight of 3500. The N-terminus residues 1 to 6 are essential for biological activity. The glucagon gene directs the synthesis of a preproglucagon in the α cells of the pancreatic islets. Preproglucagon is processed to a prohormone that subsequently yields glucagon and other peptides of still unknown function. In certain cells of the intestinal tract, the alternative processing of preproglucagon yields glucagon-like peptides with different functions. IN CONTRAST TO INSULIN, GLUCAGON SYNTHESIS IS

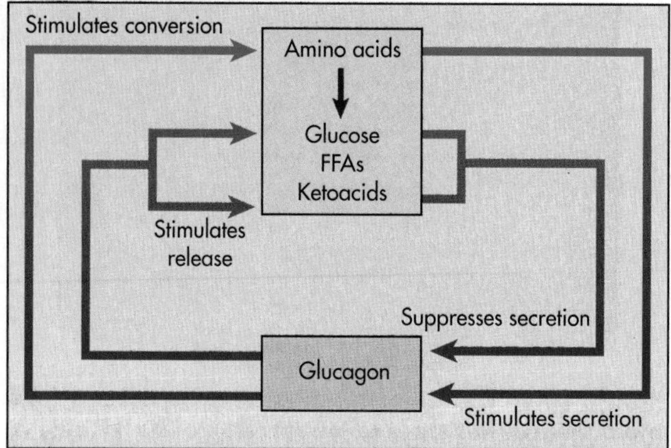

FIGURE 43–9. Feedback relationship between glucagon and nutrients. Glucagon stimulates the production and release of glucose, free fatty acids (FFAs), and keto acids, which in turn suppress glucagon secretion. Amino acids stimulate glucagon secretion, and glucagon in turn stimulates the conversion of amino acids to glucose.

INHIBITED BY HIGH GLUCOSE LEVELS AND STIMULATED BY LOW GLUCOSE LEVELS.

The secretion of glucagon is related in feedback fashion to the principal function of the hormone, namely, the stimulation of glucose output by the liver and the maintenance of plasma glucose levels **(Figure 43–9)**. Thus, hypoglycemia promptly evokes a twofold to fourfold increase in plasma glucagon concentrations from basal levels of about 100 pg/mL (3×10^{-11} M), whereas hyperglycemia suppresses glucagon secretion by more than 50%. These effects of glucose are independently reinforced by insulin, possibly through paracrine action within the islet. Thus, insulin (stimulated by glucose) directly inhibits glucagon secretion; conversely, when insulin is absent, the stimulatory effect of low glucose levels on glucagon secretion is exaggerated.

The other major energy substrate, free fatty acids, also suppresses glucagon release, whereas a sharp decline in plasma levels of free fatty acids is stimulatory. A protein meal and amino acids, which are the substrates for glucose production, stimulate glucagon secretion, but this response is dampened by concurrent glucose or insulin action. As a result, the usual mixed meal produces only small and variable increases in plasma glucagon levels, in contrast to the large and consistent increases in plasma insulin levels (Figure 43–5).

Prolonged fasting and sustained exercise, circumstances that require glucose mobilization, increase glucagon secretion. Under stressful conditions, such as major infection or surgery, glucagon secretion is often greatly augmented. This probably occurs through sympathetic nervous system stimulation of the α cells via α-adrenergic receptors.

Glucagon is extracted by the liver on the first pass, and it has a short half-life in peripheral plasma. The hormone is degraded in the kidney and liver.

In almost all respects, the actions of glucagon are opposite to those of insulin

Glucagon promotes the mobilization rather than the storage of fuels, especially glucose **(Figure 43–10)**. Both glucagon and insulin act at numerous similar control points for glucose metabolism in the liver. Indeed, glucagon can be viewed as the primary hormone that regulates hepatic glucose production and ketogenesis, whereas insulin's main hepatic role may be that of a glucagon antagonist.

GLUCAGON EXERTS AN IMMEDIATE AND PROFOUND GLYCOGENOLYTIC EFFECT THROUGH THE ACTIVATION OF HEPATIC GLYCOGEN PHOSPHORYLASE. Simultaneously, the resynthesis of phosphorylated glucose molecules back to glycogen is prevented by the inhibition of glycogen synthase. Glucagon also stimulates gluconeogenesis via several mechanisms. The hepatic extraction of amino acid precursors is increased. The activities of key gluconeogenic enzymes—pyruvate carboxylase, phosphoenolpyruvate carboxykinase, and fructose-1,6-diphosphatase—are increased, whereas activities of the key glycolytic enzymes—phosphofructokinase and pyruvate kinase—are decreased (see Figure 42–2).

Fructose 2,6-bisphosphate is a mediator of glucagon action

The enzyme pair phosphofructokinase/fructose-1,6-diphosphatase determines the flow between fructose 6-phosphate and fructose 1,6-diphosphate (see

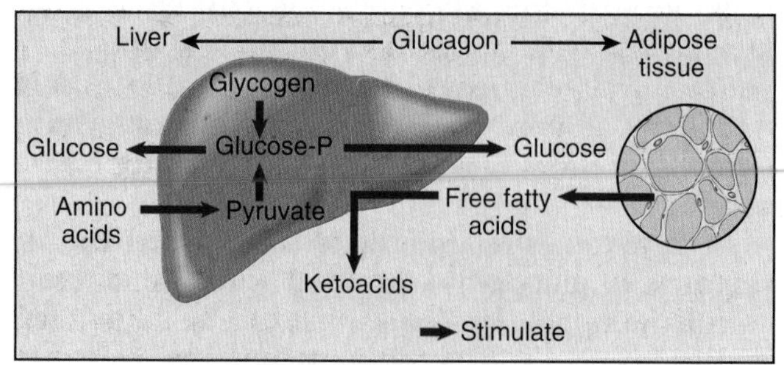

FIGURE 43–10. Effect of glucagon on the overall flow of fuels. The tissue release of glucose, free fatty acids, and keto acids raises the plasma levels of these fuels, whereas the uptake of amino acids by the liver lowers their plasma levels. P, phosphate.

Figure 42–2). Greater phosphofructokinase activity promotes conversion of glucose to lactate; greater fructose-1,6-diphosphatase activity promotes conversion of lactate to glucose. Thus, this enzyme pair determines the relative rates of glycolysis and gluconeogenesis. The activities of these two enzymes in turn are reciprocally regulated by the hepatic level of another metabolite, **fructose 2,6-bisphosphate.** GLUCAGON DECREASES THE CONCENTRATION OF FRUCTOSE 2,6-BISPHOSPHATE, an action that favors the flow from fructose 1,6-diphosphate to fructose 6-phosphate, AND THEREBY STIMULATES GLUCONEOGENESIS. Insulin has the opposite effect, probably by inhibiting the action of glucagon.

The importance of glucagon is shown by the sharp decline in hepatic glucose output that occurs when glucagon secretion is inhibited. Conversely, increasing glucagon concentrations rapidly raise the plasma glucose level. This occurs even in the presence of modestly elevated insulin levels. However, after an initial increase, hepatic glucose production wanes during continuous glucagon administration, probably because rising intracellular glucose levels within the liver feed back to autoregulate glucose synthesis. In addition, insulin release is stimulated by both glucose and glucagon and dampens hepatic glucose output. If glucagon is given in a more physiological fluctuating pattern, however, each increment in the hormone increases hepatic glucose output.

In type 1 diabetes, the loss of α cell responsiveness to a drop in the plasma glucose level (i.e., functional glucagon deficiency) often develops. Patients with such a condition become increasingly vulnerable to the risk of severe hypoglycemia if too large a dose of insulin is administered or if a meal is missed. If hypoglycemia severe enough to impair consciousness occurs, glucagon can be injected to raise plasma glucose levels and restore function of the central nervous system.

Glucagon is a ketogenic hormone

Another key intrahepatic action of glucagon is to direct incoming free fatty acids toward beta oxidation and away from triglyceride synthesis. The mechanism involves the intermediate malonyl CoA, which is an inhibitor of the transfer of free fatty acids into the mitochondria, by decreasing the enzyme carnitine palmitoyltransferase. Glucagon suppresses the synthesis of malonyl CoA by inhibiting the enzyme acetyl-CoA carboxylase. The lower levels of malonyl CoA then allow a greater influx of free fatty acids into the mitochondria for conversion to keto acids.

In diabetic ketoacidosis (see previous section), high plasma glucagon levels provide important contributions to the overproduction of the keto acids. The suppression of glucagon secretion by insulin administration helps restore normal keto acid levels and pH.

Glucagon actions on adipose tissue or muscle are rather insignificant unless insulin is virtually absent. Peripheral glucose use is largely unaffected by glucagon. However, glucagon can activate hormone-sensitive adipose tissue lipase and thereby increase lipolysis, the delivery of free fatty acids to the liver and ketogenesis, and the delivery of glycerol to the liver and gluconeogenesis. Another action of glucagon, opposite to that of insulin, is to inhibit renal tubular Na^+ reabsorption and thus to cause natriuresis.

Glucagon acts through a plasma membrane G protein that stimulates the production of adenylyl cyclase and cAMP

The molecular mechanism of glucagon action begins with hormone binding to a plasma membrane receptor in the liver. The glucagon-receptor complex causes a rapid increase in intracellular cAMP (see Chapter 5). This is followed by a specific enzymatic cascade. Protein kinase A activity increases and converts inactive phosphorylase kinase to active phosphorylase kinase, which then converts inactive phosphorylase to active phosphorylase, and glycogenolysis results. Other enzymes in glucose metabolism whose functional state depends on the addition or removal of covalently bound phosphate are likewise regulated by glucagon.

Substrate Fluxes Are Sensitive to the Relative Availability of Insulin and Glucagon

The usual molar ratio of insulin to glucagon in plasma is about 2.0. Under circumstances that require the mobilization and increased use of endogenous substrates, the insulin/glucagon ratio drops to 0.5 or less. This occurs in fasting, in prolonged exercise (see Chapter 42), and in the neonatal period when the infant is abruptly cut off from maternal fuel supplies but is not yet able to efficiently assimilate exogenous fuel. The ratio usually drops because of both decreased insulin secretion and increased glucagon secretion. Conversely, when substrate storage is advantageous, such as after a pure carbohydrate load or a mixed meal, this ratio rises to 10 or more, mainly because of increased insulin secretion.

Glucagon-like peptide 1 stimulates insulin secretion and reduces the secretion of glucagon

GLP-1 is a 37–amino acid product of the pre-proglucagon gene that is expressed predominantly in intestinal L cells, particularly in the ileum and colon, and is secreted by those cells into the bloodstream. Posttranslation processing leads to the major circulating forms, which are the N-terminal peptides 7-37 and 7-36 amide. GLP-1 is secreted in response to intake of nutrients, oral but not intravenous glucose and galactose, amino acids, and cholinergic and β-adrenergic stimuli. Fasting plasma values are 7×10^{-12} M, and they rise 100% with meals. GLP-1 is cleaved quickly by the plasma enzyme dipeptidyl peptidase, and thus the plasma half-life is less than 2 minutes.

GLP-1 acts on its plasma membrane receptor, and cAMP levels then increase. Important actions of GLP-1 include stimulation of insulin release by augmenting the amplitude of β-cell responses to glucose, stimulation of insulin synthesis, and stimulation of β-cell neogenesis by increasing expression of IPF-1. Other actions of GLP-1 are to decrease glucagon secretion and to slow gastric emptying. Together, all these actions tend to lower the plasma glucose concentration, particularly after meals.

GLP-1 is also expressed in the hypothalamus and brainstem. Its central nervous system actions are to decrease food intake, to decrease water intake, and to increase diuresis.

Because of the array of its actions, GLP-1 has potential for treatment of diabetes, especially type 2. It lowers plasma glucose in patients, but its very short half-life limits its usefulness. Synthesis of GLP-1 analogues resistant to dipeptidyl peptidase action and the administration of inhibitors of the peptidase are currently being explored to enhance the therapeutic effectiveness of GLP-1.

Summary

- The pancreatic islets contain insulin-secreting β cells and glucagon-secreting α cells. The microarchitecture and circulation permit paracrine and neurocrine functioning as well as direct cell-to-cell communication.
- Insulin is the major glucoregulatory, antilipolytic, antiketogenic, and anabolic hormone. It consists of two straight-chain peptides held together by disulfide bonds.
- Insulin secretion is stimulated by glucose (enhanced by oral administration), gastrointestinal peptides (incretins), protein, and cholinergic and β-adrenergic stimuli. Its release is inhibited by α-adrenergic stimuli and by circumstances that require fuel mobilization, such as fasting and exercise.
- Insulin promotes fuel storage. It stimulates muscle glucose uptake and storage as glycogen, lipogenesis in adipose tissue, and protein synthesis. It inhibits adipose tissue lipolysis, ketogenesis, hepatic glycogenolysis, gluconeogenesis, glucose release, and muscle proteolysis.
- Insulin acts through a plasma membrane receptor with tyrosine kinase activity. This leads to modulation of the activities of the enzymes involved in glucose and fatty acid metabolism. Insulin also affects gene expression of numerous enzymes and proteins.
- Insulin decreases plasma levels of glucose, free fatty acids, keto acids, and branched-chain amino acids. Insulin deficiency leads to hyperglycemia, loss of lean body and adipose tissue mass, growth retardation, and ultimately metabolic ketoacidosis.
- Glucagon is a single-chain peptide released in response to hypoglycemia and to amino acids. Glucagon secretion increases during prolonged fasting and exercise.
- Glucagon promotes the mobilization of glucose by stimulating hepatic glycogenolysis and gluconeogenesis. It also increases fatty acid oxidation and ketogenesis. Glucagon increases the plasma levels of glucose, free fatty acids, and keto acids, but it decreases amino acid levels.

- ❖ cAMP is the second messenger for glucagon, and the modification of enzyme activities by phosphorylation is the main mechanism of action.
- ❖ The insulin/glucagon ratio controls the relative rates of glycolysis and gluconeogenesis by altering hepatic fructose 2,6-bisphosphate levels. The two hormones have antagonistic effects at numerous steps in hepatic glucose and fatty acid metabolism.

Bibliography

Adkins A et al: Higher insulin concentrations are required to suppress gluconeogenesis than glycogenolysis in nondiabetic humans, *Diabetes* 52:2213, 2003.

Cook DL, Taborsky GJ: β-Cell function and insulin secretion. In Rifkin H, Porte D, eds: *Diabetes mellitus,* ed 5, New York, 1997, Elsevier Scientific.

Drucker DJ: Glucagon secretion, α cell metabolism, and glucagon action. In DeGroot LJ, Jameson JL, eds: *Endocrinology,* ed 4, Philadelphia, 2001, WB Saunders.

Fehmann H-C, Göke R, Göke B: Cell and molecular biology of the incretin hormones glucagon-like peptide-I and glucose-dependent insulin releasing polypeptide, *Endocr Rev* 16:390, 1995.

Flakoll PJ, Carlson MG, Cherrington AD: Physiologic action of insulin. In LeRoith D, Taylor SI, Olefsky JM, eds: *Diabetes mellitus,* Philadelphia, 2000, Lippincott Williams & Wilkins.

Geng X et al: The insulin secretory granule is the major site of K_{ATP} channels of the endocrine pancreas, *Diabetes* 52:767, 2003.

Gribble FM, Reimann F: Open to control—new hope for patients with neonatal diabetes, *N Engl J Med* 350:1817, 2004.

Kahn SE: Regulation of β-cell function in vivo, *Diabetes Metab Rev* 4:372, 1996.

Kimball SR, Vary TC, Jefferson LS: Regulation of protein synthesis by insulin, *Annu Rev Physiol* 56:321, 1994.

Matschinsky FM, Sweet IR: Annotated questions and answers about glucose metabolism and insulin secretion of β-cells, *Diabetes Metab Rev* 4:130, 1996.

Niswender KD et al: Insulin activation of phosphatidylinositol 3-kinase in the hypothalamic arcuate nucleus: a key mediator of insulin-induced anorexia, *Diabetes* 52:227, 2003.

O'Brien RM, Granner DK: Insulin action: gene regulation. In LeRoith D, Taylor SI, Olefsky JM, eds: *Diabetes mellitus,* Philadelphia, 2000, Lippincott Williams & Wilkins.

Philippe J: Structure and pancreatic expression of the insulin and glucagon genes, *Endocr Rev* 12:252, 1991.

Pirola L, Johnston AM, Van Obberghen E: Modulation of insulin action, *Diabetologia* 47:170, 2004.

Polonsky KS, Given BD, Van Cauter E: Twenty-four-hour profiles and pulsatile patterns of insulin secretion in normal and obese subjects, *J Clin Invest* 81:442, 1988.

Polonsky KS, O'Meara NM: Secretion and metabolism of insulin, proinsulin and C peptide. In DeGroot LJ, Jameson JL, eds: *Endocrinology,* ed 4, Philadelphia, 2001, WB Saunders.

Saad MF et al: Physiological insulinemia acutely modulates plasma leptin, *Diabetes* 47:544, 1998.

Schwartz MW et al: Insulin in the brain: a hormonal regulator of energy balance, *Endocr Rev* 13:387, 1992.

Steiner DF et al: Chemistry and biosynthesis of the islet hormones: insulin, islet amyloid polypeptide (amylin), glucagon, somatostatin, and pancreatic polypeptide. In DeGroot LJ, Jameson JL, eds: *Endocrinology,* ed 4, Philadelphia, 2001, WB Saunders.

Ueki K, Kahn CR: The biochemistry of insulin action. In LeRoith D, Taylor SI, Olefsky JM, eds: *Diabetes mellitus,* Philadelphia, 2000, Lippincott Williams & Wilkins.

Vilsbøll T et al: Both GLP-1 and GIP are insulinotropic at basal and postprandial glucose levels and contribute nearly equally to the incretin effect of a meal in healthy subjects, *Regul Pept* 114:115, 2003.

Weir GC, Bonner-Weir S: Islets of Langerhans: the puzzle of intraislet interactions and their relevance to diabetes, *J Clin Invest* 85:983, 1990.

Case Studies

Case 43–1

A 25-year-old woman with type 1 diabetes comes to the emergency department complaining of thirst, frequent urination, and weakness. She feels "lightheaded" when she stands. Because of nausea and vomiting after a meal in a restaurant the previous day, she stopped eating and taking her insulin. On examination, she is dehydrated and hypotensive. Her breathing is rapid and deep.

1. **Which of the following is likely to be lower than normal?**
   - **A.** Urinary urea levels
   - **B.** Plasma levels of glucagon
   - **C.** Plasma levels of free fatty acids
   - **D.** Blood partial pressure of carbon dioxide
   - **E.** Plasma acetoacetate levels

2. **Which of the following will increase after insulin administration?**
   - **A.** Plasma triglyceride levels
   - **B.** Plasma K^+ levels
   - **C.** Lipoprotein lipase activity
   - **D.** Adipose tissue lipase activity
   - **E.** Plasma phosphate levels

Case 43–2

A 40-year-old woman wins the Boston Marathon in record time.

1. **Which of the following describes her hormone balance as she crosses the finish line?**
   - **A.** Insulin high, glucagon high
   - **B.** Insulin high, glucagon low
   - **C.** Insulin low, glucagon low
   - **D.** Insulin low, glucagon high
   - **E.** Insulin equal to glucagon

2. **Which of the following molecules is decreased in concentration or activity in her liver?**
   - **A.** Fructose 6-phosphate
   - **B.** Phosphoenolpyruvate carboxykinase
   - **C.** Fructose 2,6-bisphosphate
   - **D.** Glucose-6-phosphatase
   - **E.** Phosphorylase

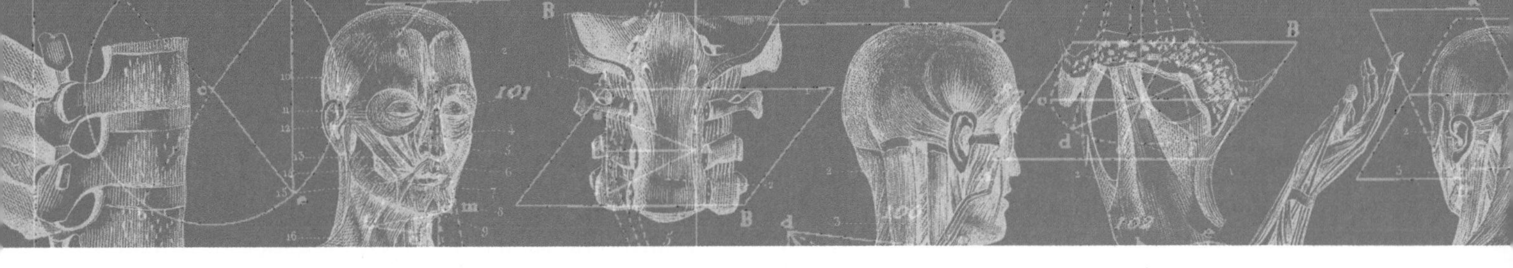

Chapter 44: Endocrine Regulation of the Metabolism of Calcium and Phosphate

Objectives

- ❖ Explain the functions of Ca^{++} and Pi in human biology.
- ❖ Describe the dynamic role of bone in Ca^{++} and Pi metabolism.
- ❖ Describe the sources of vitamin D and its actions on Ca^{++} metabolism.
- ❖ Define the pattern and regulation of PTH synthesis and secretion.
- ❖ Explain the actions of PTH on the kidneys, bones, and gastrointestinal tract.
- ❖ Evaluate the potential roles for PTH-related protein and calcitonin in Ca^{++} metabolism.

Calcium (Ca^{++}) and phosphate (Pi) homeostasis is essential for health and life. The physiological functioning of all other systems described elsewhere in this textbook depends on Ca^{++} and Pi availability. A complex system acts to maintain normal body contents and extracellular fluid levels of these minerals in the face of environmental (e.g., diet) and internal (e.g., pregnancy) changes. The key elements in the regulatory system are **vitamin D** and **parathyroid hormone (PTH),** with subsidiary participation by **calcitonin** and other hormones. THE INTESTINAL TRACT, KIDNEYS, SKELETON, SKIN, AND LIVER ARE ALL INVOLVED IN THE HOMEOSTATIC REGULATION OF Ca^{++} AND Pi METABOLISM (see Chapter 39).

The Calcium Ion Is of Fundamental Importance to All Biological Systems

Intracellular free [Ca^{++}] is maintained by the extracellular [Ca^{++}] and intracellular bound Ca^{++} stores

Calcium, usually complexed to calmodulin (see Chapter 5), participates in numerous important enzymatic reactions. This ion is a vital component in the mechanisms of hormone secretion and hormone action. CALCIUM IS INTIMATELY INVOLVED IN NEUROTRANSMISSION, LEARNING AND MEMORY, MUSCLE CONTRACTION, MITOSIS AND CELL DIVISION, MOBILITY, SECRETION, FERTILIZATION, AND BLOOD CLOTTING. IT IS THE MAJOR CATION IN THE CRYSTALLINE STRUCTURE OF BONE AND TEETH. For these reasons, it is vital that cells be bathed with fluid in which the [Ca^{++}] is kept within narrow limits.

Ca^{++} metabolism may be viewed as having two parts: an intracellular microcomponent and an extracellular macrocomponent. Each is regulated differently and somewhat independently. The crucial intracellular Ca^{++} functions are carried out at an average basal cytosolic free [Ca^{++}] of 10^{-7} M (range, 5×10^{-8} to 3×10^{-7} M). In contrast, the free [Ca^{++}] in extracellular fluid is approximately 10^{-3} M, or 10,000-fold higher. This large extracellular-intracellular gradient is maintained by a low permeability of the plasma cell membrane to Ca^{++} and by the regulated activities of a Ca^{++}-ATPase pump and a Ca^{++}-Na^{+} exchange system (see Chapters 1, 13, 16, and 18). Within the cell, a much larger store of Ca^{++} is bound to various proteins and membranes, to the endoplasmic reticulum, and within the mitochondria. If it were in solution, this Ca^{++} content would be equivalent to an intracellular concentration of 10^{-2} M.

The cytosolic free [Ca^{++}] can be increased as needed, both by augmenting influx from outside the cell and by mobilizing intracellular stores. When Ca^{++} is required to function as a second messenger, the free [Ca^{++}] can rise from 10^{-7} M to as high as 10^{-5} M. In absolute terms, however, this represents the movement of only small amounts of additional Ca^{++} into the cytoplasmic fluid. Such changes are transient (seconds to minutes). The excess cytosolic Ca^{++} is either rapidly extruded from the cell or returned to the intracellular reservoirs. The influx and efflux are so finely balanced that Ca^{++} can serve as an internal cell signal with a large dynamic range of gain and sensitivity.

Extracellular Ca^{++} levels are made up of free, complexed, and protein-bound fractions

The [Ca^{++}] in the extracellular fluid and plasma normally fluctuates little. This helps maintain intracellular Ca^{++} at a proper level. When [Ca^{++}] in plasma and extracellular fluid is either above or below the normal range, intracellular function can be widely and severely affected. Abnormalities in neurotransmission and in the growth and renewal of the skeleton are prominent clinical examples.

The normal range of total [Ca^{++}] in plasma is 8.6 to 10.6 mg/dL, or 2.15 to 2.65 × 10^{-3} M. Because Ca^{++} is a divalent ion, this is equivalent to 4.3 to 5.3 mEq/L. Individual day-to-day variation is less than 10%. Approximately 50% of total plasma Ca^{++} is in the ionized form, Ca^{++}, which is biologically active; 40% is bound to proteins, mainly albumin; and 10% is complexed in nonionic but ultrafilterable forms, such as Ca^{++} bicarbonate (HCO_3^-). The total plasma [Ca^{++}] rises or falls with plasma albumin levels, but this has no biological consequence as long as the ionized [Ca^{++}] remains in the normal range. The equilibrium between ionized and protein-bound Ca^{++} depends on the blood pH. Alkalosis increases the protein-bound concentration and decreases the ionized concentration, whereas acidosis has the opposite effect.

When the [Ca^{++}] drops below normal, neuromuscular irritability develops. This is manifested by numbness and paresthesias ("pins and needles" sensation) and by tetanic contractions of muscles in the hands and feet **(carpopedal spasm)** and, most dangerously, in the larynx, where **airway obstruction** can result. **Epileptic seizures** may also occur. When the [Ca^{++}] is excessive, depressed neurotransmission can cause impaired mentation or consciousness, muscle weakness, and decreased gastrointestinal motility. Individuals who hyperventilate to the point of severe respiratory alkalosis can lower the Ca^{++} level enough (without changing the total concentration) to produce the sensory symptoms described.

Ca^{++} balance reflects dietary intake, gastrointestinal absorption, and renal excretion

The normal turnover of Ca^{++} in the body is complex (see Figure 39–4). Daily dietary Ca^{++} intake may range from 200 to 2000 mg. The percentage of dietary Ca^{++} absorbed from the gut is inversely related to the Ca^{++} intake in a curvilinear manner. Thus, in the face of dietary Ca^{++} deprivation, one important mechanism for maintaining a normal plasma [Ca^{++}] and body Ca^{++} stores is an adaptive increase in the percentage of ingested Ca^{++} that is absorbed. At a daily intake of 1000 mg, about 35% is absorbed. In a steady state, the same amount of Ca^{++}, 350 mg, is excreted. Approximately 150 mg is secreted into intestinal juices and excreted in stools, along with the unabsorbed fraction from the diet. The remaining 200 mg is excreted in the urine. Although the kidney filters about 10,000 mg of non–protein-bound Ca^{++} per day, approximately 98% is reabsorbed by the renal tubules. Therefore, any alteration in renal tubular Ca^{++} transport provides a sensitive means for maintaining Ca^{++} balance.

These control mechanisms are clinically important when Ca^{++} conservation is needed, such as in aged people, whose Ca^{++} intakes typically fall, causing an increase in the danger of **osteoporosis.** These mechanisms protect the mother from hypocalcemia and bone loss during pregnancy, when Ca^{++} stores are drained by the fetus. In contrast, these mechanisms also act to protect against lethal **hypercalcemia** (e.g., hypercalcemia that can occur when metastatic cancer causes the rapid destruction of bone).

Ca^{++} sensing helps control Ca^{++} levels

The homeostatic regulation of Ca^{++} levels in extracellular fluids and in various local cellular environments is under both indirect endocrine control and direct feedback control by the Ca^{++} level itself. Both forms of control are mediated by a Ca^{++}-sensing plasma membrane receptor of the G protein–linked type. The Ca^{++} receptor is located in endocrine and other cells that have principal roles in Ca^{++} homeostasis, including cells secreting PTH and calcitonin, and vitamin D–producing cells, bone-forming and bone-resorbing cells, renal tubular Ca^{++}-reabsorbing cells, and intestinal Ca^{++}-absorbing cells.

The Ca^{++} receptor is coupled via G proteins to adenylyl cyclase; phospholipases A_2, C, and D; and MAP kinase and tyrosine kinases. The overall effect of all these actions mediated by the Ca^{++} receptor is to alter the rates of entry into or the rates of exit from the extracellular fluid to protect against hypercalcemia or hypocalcemia.

Rare clinical syndromes of genetic origin have helped to establish the critical importance of the Ca^{++} receptor. Inactivating mutations in the extracellular portion of the Ca^{++} receptor reduce the affinity of the receptor for Ca^{++}. They reset the system so that hypercalcemia is maintained with inappropriately low urine excretion. By contrast, hyperactivating mutations in the transmembrane domain of the receptor enhance the signal generated by Ca^{++}. This results in maintenance of hypocalcemia by inappropriately high urinary Ca^{++} excretion caused by impaired tubular reabsorption of Ca^{++}.

The Phosphate Ion Is a Component of Many Intermediates in Glucose Metabolism

Pi is of critical importance to all biological systems and is the major intracellular anion

Pi is part of the structure of all high-energy transfer compounds, such as ATP; cofactors, such as nicotinic acid dinucleotide; lipids, such as phosphatidylcholine; and RNA and DNA. Phosphate functions as a covalent modifier of the activity of numerous enzymes. PHOSPHATE IS ALSO AN INTEGRAL PART OF THE CRYSTALLINE STRUCTURE OF BONE. The normal [Pi] in the plasma is 2.4 to 4.5 mg/dL, or 0.81 to 1.45×10^{-3} M. Because the valence of Pi changes with the pH, it is less useful to express normal concentrations in milliequivalents per liter.

Pi balance reflects dietary intake, gastrointestinal absorption, and renal excretion

The daily turnover of Pi is as complex as that of Ca^{++} (see Figure 39–7). In contrast to Ca^{++}, the percentage of Pi absorbed from the diet is relatively constant, and thus the net absorption of Pi from the gut is more linearly related to intake. Therefore, urinary excretion provides the major mechanism for regulation of Pi balance (see Chapter 39). The daily filtered load is approximately 7000 mg, but renal tubular reabsorption can vary from 70% to 100% to compensate for fluctuations in dietary intake. Large stores of Pi (about 100,000 mg) in the soft tissue, as in muscle, are a source for rapid regulation of the plasma concentration. Approximately 200 to 250 mg of Pi enters and leaves the extracellular fluid daily in the course of bone turnover. Severe depletion of Pi can result in serious cardiac and skeletal muscle dysfunction, lysis of red blood cells, and abnormal bone growth.

Bone Turnover Is Regulated

Bone formation and resorption help maintain normal plasma levels of Ca^{++}

The extracellular pool of Ca^{++} is only 1000 mg. The largest store of Ca^{++}, about 1.2 kg, is in the skeleton. Of this, 4000 mg is available for rapid buffering of plasma Ca^{++} without dissolution of bone. Nonetheless, bone is a dynamic tissue that undergoes daily structural turnover. In this process, approximately 500 mg of Ca^{++} is extracted from the extracellular pool as new bone is formed, and a like amount is returned to this pool as old bone is broken down.

Bone formation and resorption are normally coupled to each other in a steady state

Bone is a major and dynamic reservoir for Ca^{++} and Pi (see Figures 39–4 and 39–7). Its composition is 77% inorganic. Therefore, it is essential to understand those aspects of bone structure and function pertinent to the regulation of Ca^{++} and Pi metabolism. Bone is broadly divided into two types: cortical and trabecular. **Cortical** or **compact bone** represents 80% of the total mass and is typified by the thick shafts of the appendicular skeleton (arms and legs). **Trabecular** or **spongy bone** constitutes 20%; it makes up most of the axial skeleton (vertebrae, skull, ribs, pelvis) and bridges the centers of the long bones. Trabecular bone has a fivefold greater surface area than cortical bone, making it more important in the regulation of Ca^{++} metabolism even though it has a lesser mass and is only 25% mineralized, compared with compact cortical bone, which is 80% to 90% mineralized.

Bone formation occurs on the outer surface of cortical bone, whereas bone resorption occurs on its inner surface. Both formation and resorption also take place in specialized nutrient canals within cortical bone and on the surfaces of trabecular bone. Throughout life, the processes of bone formation and resorption are tightly regulated. During growth phases, formation exceeds resorption, and the skeletal mass increases. During childhood and puberty, linear growth occurs between the heads and the ends of the shafts of long bones in specialized areas known as **epiphyseal growth plates.** Chondrocytes (cartilage cells) are recruited from progenitor mesenchymal cells and lay down cartilage in the growth plates. Within the cartilage masses, calcification occurs and bone is formed, replacing the mature chondrocytes and cartilage. The growth plates close off at the end of puberty, when the adult height is reached. Bone width increases by addition of bone to the outer surfaces.

Bone mass varies with stages of life

Total bone mass reaches a peak between the ages of 20 and 30 years. Thereafter, equal rates of formation and resorption prevail until the age of 40 to 50 years, when resorption begins to exceed formation and the total bone mass slowly decreases. The continual process of bone turnover in the adult, known as **remodeling,** involves 10% of the total bone mass per year. Trabecular bone turns over much faster than cortical bone does.

Bone contains several types of cells with different functions

Four major cell types are identified in bone: **osteoblasts; lining cells,** which are descendants of osteoblasts; **osteocytes;** and **osteoclasts** (**Figure 44–1**). Osteocytes compose 90% of all bone cells. Osteoblasts arise from pluripotential mesenchymal cells, some of which differentiate into **osteoprogenitor cells,** within the investing connective tissue. Various **bone morphogenetic proteins** stimulate the development of osteoprogenitor cells, direct their differentiation into osteoblasts, and stimulate their further growth. Osteoclasts arise from the same bone marrow precursor cells as circulating monocytes and tissue macrophages. Together, these bone cell types form the **osteon** and the basic multicellular unit. Osteons have a life span of 6 to 9 months, whereas the basic multicellular unit is responsible for remodeling bone and forming the osteons. Millions of basic multicellular units are active at any one time.

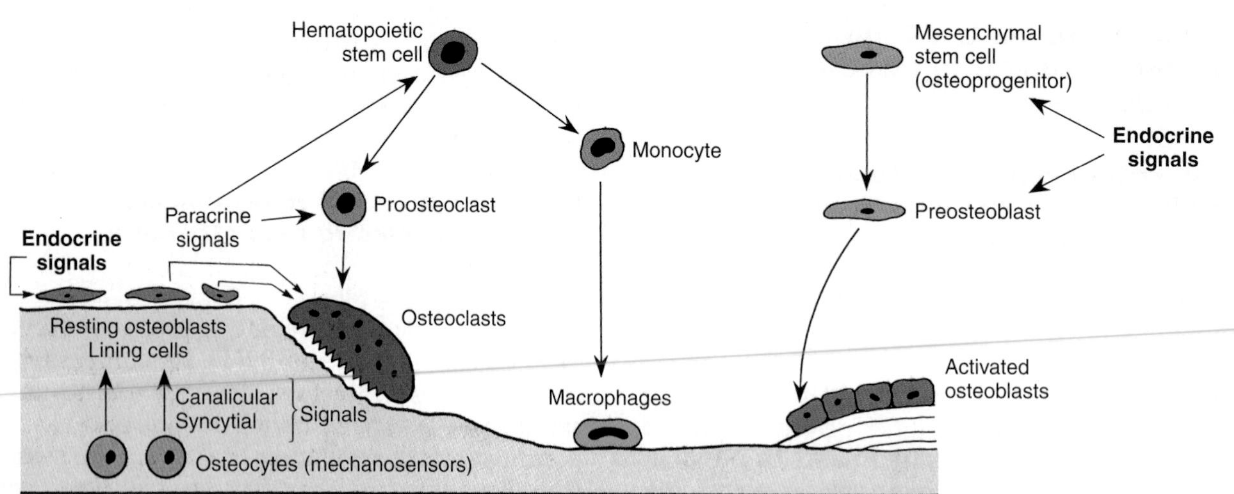

FIGURE 44–1. Bone cells and bone remodeling. Bone remodeling in an osteon is stimulated when mechanosensors in osteocytes entombed in mineralized bone detect structural weakness. Through fluid-filled canaliculi and syncytial processes, they send activating signals to lining cells or resting osteoblasts. Via paracrine cytokine signals, these cells recruit osteoclasts, which uncover and tunnel into the weakened bone. After a suitable amount of bone has been resorbed, another set of osteoblasts is recruited to fill in the resorption cavity with new strong bone. When this mission is completed, the osteoblasts differentiate into osteocytes entombed within the mineralized bone they have just formed.

Women have a smaller bone mass than men do, and during the perimenopausal period, they lose bone rapidly as ovarian function declines. This is caused by estrogen deficiency, but lifelong Ca^{++} intakes that are only marginally adequate also contribute. The resultant **osteoporosis** leads to fractures of the spine and wrist. Later in life, senescent osteoporosis leads to hip fractures in both genders.

Bone formation is carried out by active osteoblasts, which synthesize and secrete type I collagen

The collagen fibrils line up in regular arrays, creating an organic matrix known as **osteoid,** within which Ca^{++} and Pi are deposited in amorphous masses. **Osteocalcin** and **osteonectin,** also secreted by osteoblasts, regulate the final quality and quantity of bone that is formed. The slow addition of OH^- and HCO_3^- ions to the mineral phase produces mature **hydroxyapatite** crystals, which have a molar Ca^{++}-Pi ratio of 1.7. As this completely mineralized bone accumulates and surrounds the osteoblast (life span of 3 months), that now entombed cell loses most of its synthetic activity and becomes an interior osteocyte (life span of 20 years) (Figure 44–1). Osteoblastic activity therefore is observed only on the surfaces of bone, along which resting cells wait to be activated.

THE MINERALIZATION PROCESS CRITICALLY REQUIRES NORMAL PLASMA [Ca^{++}] AND [Pi]. The enzyme **alkaline phosphatase** from the osteoblast also participates. Alkaline phosphatase and osteocalcin circulate in plasma, and their concentrations correlate well with quantitative histological assessments of osteoblastic activity. The entire sequence of bone formation takes 3 months and is under endocrine regulation.

Within each **osteon,** minute fluid-containing channels called **canaliculi** traverse the mineralized bone; through these channels and syncytial processes, the interior osteocytes remain connected with surface lining cells (Figure 44–1). The osteocytes appear to act as mechanosensors that detect weakening of bone and stimulate its repair by removal and replacement.

Osteoclasts are responsible for bone resorption

THE PROCESS OF BONE RESORPTION DOES NOT MERELY EXTRACT Ca^{++}; IT DESTROYS THE ENTIRE ORGANIC MATRIX AS WELL, THEREBY DIMINISHING BONE MASS. The principal cell responsible for bone resorption is the osteoclast, which is a giant multinucleated cell formed by the fusion of several precursors (Figure 44–1). The osteoclast contains large numbers of mitochondria and lysosomes. It attaches to the surface of the bone and creates at this point a ruffled border by infolding its plasma membrane. Within this enclosed zone, the process of dissolution is carried out by collagenase and other enzymes in an acid environment generated by an H^+-ATPase. During this process, the osteoclast literally tunnels its way into the mineralized bone. Ca^{++}, Pi, Mg^{++}, **pyridinolines** and **pyridiniums** (fluorescent products of collagen cross-linkages), **N-telopeptides** of collagen, and the constituent amino acids (including hydroxyproline and hydroxylysine, which are unique to collagen) are all released into the extracellular fluid. Urine levels of the organic products reflect the bone resorption rate. The resorptive phase in an active osteon lasts 2 weeks.

In the bone remodeling process, resorption precedes and initiates formation

The resorption and formation of bone are closely coupled locally. Under conditions of normal mechanical strain, osteocytes produce **osteoprotegerin,** a molecule that restrains bone remodeling by suppressing osteoclast cells. However, when bone becomes weakened or "fatigued," this is sensed by the osteocytes, which then stimulate resting lining osteoblasts to recruit and activate osteoclasts via paracrine signaling. The resultant resorption cavity created by the osteoclasts in weakened bone then becomes the site of subsequent osteoblastic activity, which fills in the recently formed cavity with stronger new bone. Thus, bone resorption by osteoclasts precedes and subsequently triggers replacement bone formation by osteoblasts. However, the entire coupling sequence begins with signals from osteocytes and lining osteoblasts.

The recruitment of osteoblasts and osteoclasts from precursors and the activity of each cell type are regulated by various local factors, including lymphokines, cytokines, tissue growth and transforming factors, prostaglandins, **annexins**, **osteoprotegerin,** and an array of hormones. IN GENERAL, WHETHER THE PRIMARY EFFECT OF A HORMONE IS ON THE FORMATION OR THE RESORPTION OF BONE, THE PHENOMENON OF COUPLING SECONDARILY ALTERS THE OTHER PROCESS IN THE SAME DIRECTION. Therefore, the net effect of a hormone excess or deficiency partly depends on the degree to which the coupling phenomenon defends the total bone mass. As a result of the aging process, the balance shifts toward resorption, and bone mass declines (**Figure 44–2**).

Young, normal **Osteoporotic**

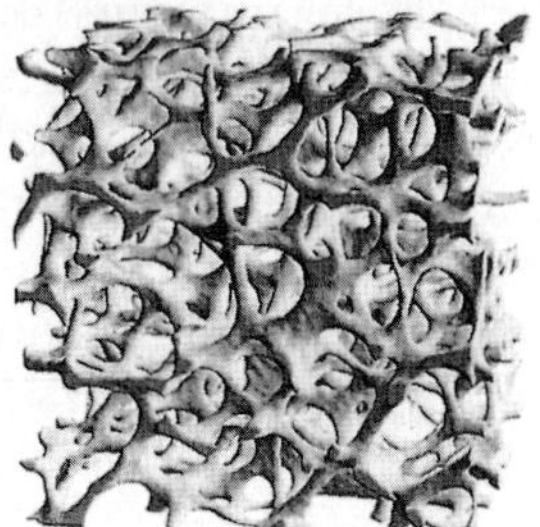
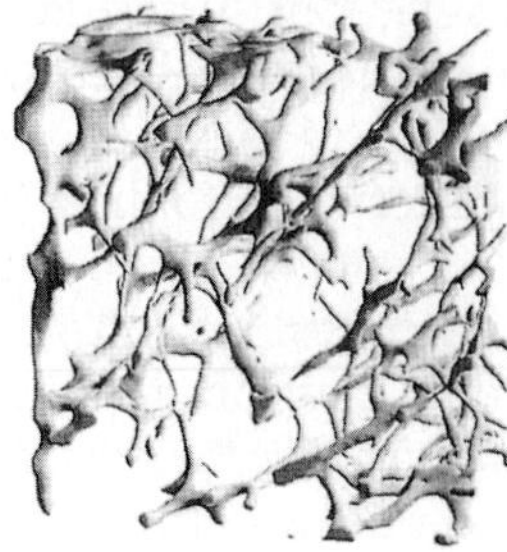

FIGURE 44–2. *Left,* Lumbar spine sample from a young woman. *Right,* An older woman with postmenopausal osteoporosis. Note the marked loss and disorganization of the structure of the trabecular bone from the older woman. (From Riggs L: *Endocr Rev* 23:279, 2002.)

Vitamin D, Through Its Active Metabolites, Is a Major Regulator of Calcium and Phosphate Metabolism

VITAMIN D ACTS TO SUSTAIN NORMAL PLASMA [Ca^{++}] AND [Pi] BY INCREASING THEIR INFLOW FROM THE INTESTINAL TRACT, AND IT ALSO IS REQUIRED FOR NORMAL BONE FORMATION. It is a hormone in the sense that it is synthesized in the body, although not by a classic endocrine gland; after further processing, it is transported through the circulation to act on target cells. It is also a vitamin in the sense that when it cannot be synthesized in sufficient quantities, it must be ingested for health to be maintained.

Vitamin D is synthesized in the skin and ingested largely from animal sources

The sterol structure of the synthesized form of vitamin D (D_3) is shown in **Figure 44–3**. The ingested form (D_2), which is prepared by irradiation of plant or milk ergosterol, differs only slightly. Vitamins D_3 and D_2 are essentially prohormones that undergo metabolic conversion to molecules with identical qualitative and quantitative actions. Henceforth, the term **vitamin D** refers to both.

The minimum daily requirement of vitamin D is approximately 2.5 μg (100 units). Endogenously, it is synthesized in the skin from the precursor **7-dehydrocholesterol** by ultraviolet (UV) irradiation at wavelengths of 290 to 315 nm. The skin pigment melatonin inhibits synthesis by absorbing UV radiation in competition with 7-dehydrocholesterol. Exogenously, the fat-soluble vitamin D is available in fish, liver, and milk, and it is absorbed from the gut, like fats (see Chapter 35). Vitamin D is stored in the body in amounts normally sufficient for several months.

Vitamin D is activated by successive hydroxylations

Once vitamin D enters the circulation from the skin or gut, it is concentrated in the liver. There, it is hydroxylated to 25-hydroxyvitamin D (25-OH-D). This molecule is transported to the kidney, where it undergoes alternative fates **(Figure 44–4)**. Hydroxylation in the 1 position produces the metabolite 1,25-dihydroxyvitamin D (1,25-$(OH)_2$-D), which expresses most if not all of the biological activity of vitamin D. Alternatively, 25-OH-D may be hydroxylated in the 24 position. 24,25-Dihydroxyvitamin D (24,25-$(OH)_2$-D) is only one twentieth as potent as 1,25-$(OH)_2$-D, and it mainly serves to dispose of excess vitamin D.

Vitamin D deficiency can occur in several ways. If individuals who live in sunny climates (e.g., India) and are dependent on vitamin D synthesis move to cloudy countries (e.g., England), they may become deficient in vitamin D if they do not alter their dietary habits or ingest supplementary vitamin D. In urban centers overcast with smog, black infants who are breast-fed are also at risk because less effective UV radiation reaches sites of vitamin D synthesis. When a subject's exposure to sunlight is inadequate, deficiency also results from gastrointestinal diseases that cause malabsorption of fats, such as pancreatic insufficiency. Liver disease leads to diminished rates of 25-hydroxylation and hence to deficient vitamin D action. A common cause of deficient vitamin D action is kidney failure, in which the production of the most active metabolite, 1,25-$(OH)_2$-D, is almost totally lost.

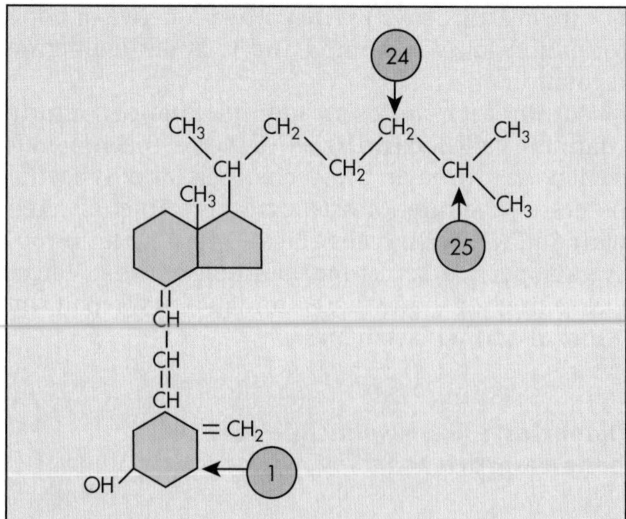

FIGURE 44–3. Structure of vitamin D. Positions 1, 24, and 25 are important sites of hydroxylation that affect biological activity.

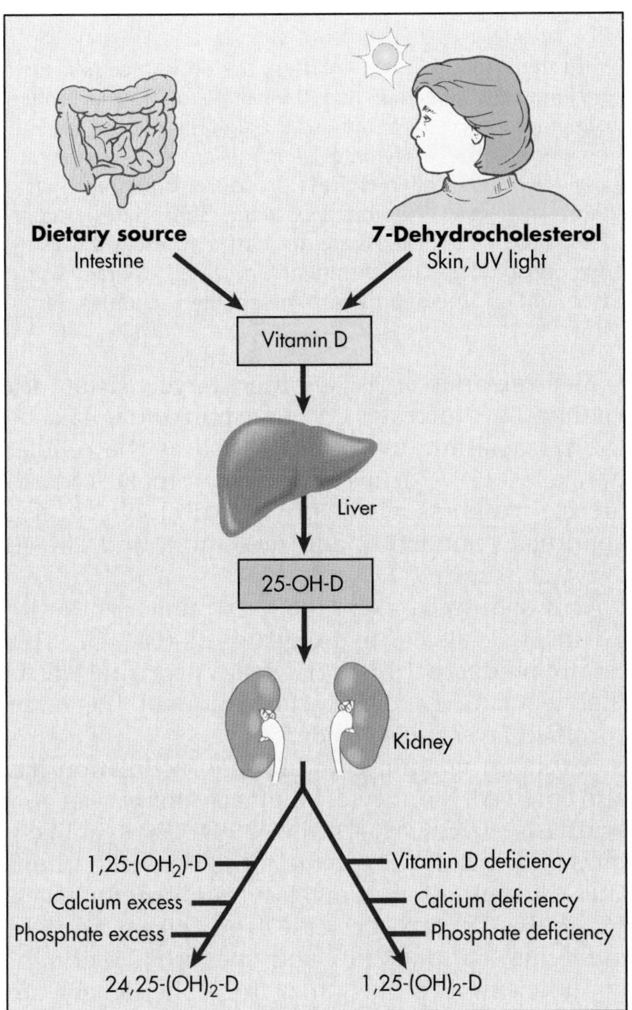

FIGURE 44–4. Vitamin D metabolism. Whether it is synthesized in the skin or absorbed from the diet, vitamin D undergoes hydroxylation of position 25 in the liver. In the kidney, it is further hydroxylated in position 1, when more biological activity is required, or in position 24, when less biological activity is required.

The activation of vitamin D occurs in response to Ca^{++} or Pi deficiency

Feedback control of vitamin D activation occurs through regulation of the renal tubule mitochondrial 1-hydroxylase and 24-hydroxylase enzyme activities (Figure 44–4). 25-OH-D is preferentially directed toward the active metabolite, 1,25-$(OH)_2$-D, whenever Ca^{++}, Pi, or vitamin D itself is lacking. Ca^{++} deprivation leads to a compensatory secretion of **PTH.** This hormone then stimulates 1-hydroxylation. A lowering of plasma Pi and renal Pi content also augments 1-hydroxylase activity. In addition, because 1,25-$(OH)_2$-D is a feedback inhibitor of its own synthesis, in vitamin D deficiency, there is lack of inhibition and compensatory enhancement of 1-hydroxylase activity. In contrast, 24-hydroxylase activity is stimulated by normal to elevated [Ca^{++}] or [Pi] and by 1,25-$(OH)_2$-D. The net result of this regulation is that the supply of active 1,25-$(OH)_2$-D is increased (and that of inactive 24,25-$(OH)_2$-D is decreased) whenever homeostasis requires increasing Ca^{++} and Pi intake from dietary sources or skeletal stores. If an excess of 1,25-$(OH)_2$-D develops, it too can be 24-hydroxylated to 1,24,25-trihydroxyvitamin D (1,24,25-$(OH)_3$-D) and thereby virtually inactivated.

Vitamin D, 25-OH-D, and 1,25-$(OH)_2$-D circulate bound to a protein carrier. 1,25-$(OH)_2$-D has by far the lowest concentration (0.03 μg/L) and the shortest half-life of the three (6 hours). However, regulation of renal synthesis is powerful enough to maintain the appropriate concentration of 1,25-$(OH)_2$-D even when the concentrations of its precursors are quite reduced.

Vitamin D acts on target tissues by modulating gene expression

The active form of vitamin D, 1,25-$(OH)_2$-D, acts through the general mechanism outlined for steroid hormones (see Chapter 41). After binding to a cytosolic receptor, the hormone-receptor complex enters the nucleus, where it stimulates or represses the transcription of messenger RNA for several products. One is **calbindin,** a Ca^{++}-binding protein found in cells of the intestinal mucosa, bone, kidney, and parathyroid glands. Vitamin D increases calbindin levels. Calbindin has significant homology with calmodulin and a high affinity for Ca^{++}. Calbindin is not absolutely essential for vitamin D stimulation of Ca^{++} transport because this process precedes the appearance of the protein in intestinal cells. However, calbindin facilitates transport probably by protecting the cells from the effect of high cytoplasmic [Ca^{++}] during enhanced transport.

Vitamin D increases Ca^{++} absorption from the gut and Ca^{++} availability for bone mineralization

The major action of 1,25-$(OH)_2$-D is to stimulate the absorption of Ca^{++} from the intestinal lumen against a concentration gradient (see Chapter 35). 1,25-$(OH)_2$-D localizes in the nuclei of intestinal villus and crypt cells, where it acts on the brush border. It probably stimulates the production of a plasma membrane Ca^{++} transporter protein. 1,25-$(OH)_2$-D is responsible for the adaptation whereby the intestinal absorption of Ca^{++} increases in response to decreases in dietary intake, as previously described. 1,25-$(OH)_2$-D also augments the active absorption of Pi across the intestinal cell membrane.

Vitamin D has multiple diverse actions in bone. 1,25-$(OH)_2$-D stimulates bone resorption by interacting with its receptor in **osteoblasts.** The osteoblasts then secrete factors such as inflammatory cytokines like interleukins, which drive the resorptive action of the osteoclasts. This effect of 1,25-$(OH)_2$-D is physiologically important in sensitizing the bone to the resorptive effects of PTH.

Vitamin D also regulates growth and differentiation of osteoblasts and chondroblasts by increasing production of transforming growth factor-β. This growth factor increases its target cell size and differentiation but inhibits cell proliferation. The normal mineralization of newly formed osteoid along a regular advancing front is critically dependent on vitamin D. The major mechanism for this action is augmentation of the supply of Ca^{++} and Pi. However, in osteoblasts, 1,25-$(OH)_2$-D represses transcription of the collagen gene and decreases collagen synthesis. In the hormone's absence, unmineralized osteoid accumulates from unregulated collagen synthesis **(Figure 44–5)**, and the bone so formed is weakened.

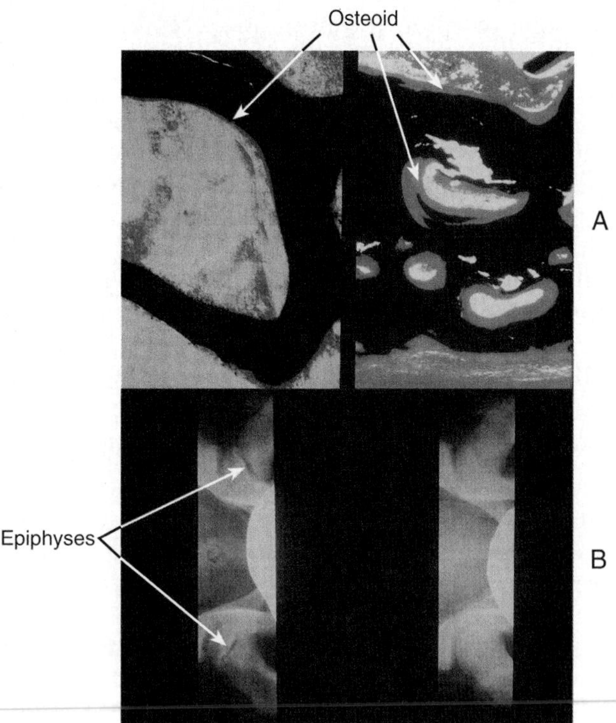

FIGURE 44–5. A, Histological section. *Left,* Normal trabecular bone showing a very low ratio of unmineralized osteoid to mineralized bone. *Right,* Trabecular bone from an individual with vitamin D deficiency showing a much higher proportion of osteoid to mineralized bone (i.e., excess osteoid). B, Radiograph of a child's hip. *Left,* Hip with deficient vitamin D action showing a widened, irregular epiphysis. *Right,* Same hip after effective treatment with vitamin D mineralized the area normally.

The skeletal manifestations of vitamin D deficiency vary with the stage of life. In children, the growth centers are preferentially affected, and the failure of normal bone mineralization leads to abnormal epiphyses (Figure 44–5), bowing of the extremities, and collapse of the chest wall—a disease called **rickets.** In adults, bone pain, vertebral collapse, and fractures along stress lines occur. Plasma Ca^{++} and Pi levels are decreased, whereas the alkaline phosphatase concentration is increased. Therapy with vitamin D or the appropriate metabolite is curative.

Skeletal muscle is another target tissue for vitamin D. It increases Ca^{++} transport and uptake by the sarcoplasmic reticulum as well as the cellular uptake of Pi. A deficiency of vitamin D leads to muscle weakness, electrophysiological evidence of abnormal contraction and relaxation, and altered cytoarchitecture.

The skin cells (keratinocytes) that synthesize vitamin D also 1-hydroxylate 25-(OH)-D. This locally produced 1,25-$(OH)_2$-D has paracrine effects that regulate the orderly formation of the outer cornified layer of the epidermis.

A role for vitamin D in immunomodulation has also emerged. Monocytes and macrophages can also synthesize 1,25-$(OH)_2$-D from 25-OH-D. By a likely intracrine action (Chapter 41), the hormone stimulates differentiation of myelocytes to macrophages. 1,25-$(OH)_2$-D can decrease the production of numerous lymphokines and the proliferation of lymphocytes. It is likely that these phenomena are part of the autocrine or paracrine regulation of immunoactivity engendered by tissue injury or invasion.

In diseases characterized by the formation of granulomas (i.e., **sarcoidosis** or **tuberculosis**), the component macrophages may synthesize excessive amounts of 1,25-$(OH)_2$-D. This can result in hypercalcemia and hypercalciuria.

Interest in vitamin D or analogues as anticancer agents has been awakened by its antiproliferative and prodifferentiation actions. Vitamin D blocks the cell cycle at the G_1/S phase by regulating cyclin-dependent kinases and also induces programmed cell death (apoptosis). 1,25-$(OH)_2$-D suppresses epidermal growth factor and insulin-like growth factor receptors in some common cancer cell lines.

The Function of the Parathyroid Gland Is to Regulate Plasma Calcium and Phosphate Levels

The four parathyroid glands are major regulators of plasma [Ca^{++}] and [Pi] and flux. These four glands develop from branchial pouches at 5 to 14 weeks of fetal life. They descend to lie just posterior to the thyroid gland in the neck. The total weight of adult parathyroid tissue is about 130 mg.

The predominant cell of the parathyroid gland is known as the **chief cell.** These cells are present throughout life and are the source of PTH. A second and related cell type, the **oxyphil cell,** first appears at puberty and increases in number with age. Each active chief cell has a granular endoplasmic reticulum and a large, convoluted Golgi apparatus with vacuoles and vesicles. During hormone secretion, numerous granules undergo exocytosis.

THE PARAMOUNT EFFECT OF PTH IS TO SUSTAIN OR INCREASE THE PLASMA Ca^{++} LEVEL. THIS IS ACCOMPLISHED BY DIRECTLY STIMULATING THE ENTRY OF Ca^{++} INTO PLASMA FROM BONE AND TUBULAR URINE AND INDIRECTLY FROM THE INTESTINAL TRACT (VIA 1,25-$(OH)_2$-D). AN IMPORTANT SECOND EFFECT IS TO DECREASE OR PREVENT AN UNDUE RISE IN THE PLASMA [Pi] LEVEL BY INCREASING THE EXCRETION OF Pi INTO THE URINE.

PTH is synthesized from a prohormone and secreted in response to hypocalcemia

PTH is a single-chain protein (molecular weight, 9600) that contains 84 amino acids. The biological activity of the hormone resides in the N-terminus portion of the molecule within amino acids 1 to 34.

The gene for PTH directs the synthesis of **prepro-PTH.** A total of 25 amino acids are enzymatically cleaved from the N-terminal end, leaving **pro-PTH.** Pro-PTH is then transported to the Golgi apparatus, where another six amino acids are cleaved. The resulting PTH is packaged for storage in secretory granules. The degradation of PTH also occurs within the gland; therefore, not all synthesized molecules reach the circulation.

THE DOMINANT REGULATOR OF PARATHYROID GLAND ACTIVITY IS THE PLASMA Ca^{++} LEVEL. PTH AND IONIZED Ca^{++} FORM A NEGATIVE-FEEDBACK PAIR, AND THE SECRETION OF PTH IS INVERSELY RELATED TO THE PLASMA $[Ca^{++}]$ **(Figure 44–6)**. Maximum secretory rates are achieved when the plasma $[Ca^{++}]$ falls below 3.5 mg/dL. PTH secretion increases within minutes if plasma Ca^{++} is selectively decreased by chelation of total Ca^{++}, even though the plasma total $[Ca^{++}]$ remains unchanged. Conversely, as the $[Ca^{++}]$ increases to 5.5 mg/dL, PTH secretion is progressively diminished. However, secretion reaches a persistent basal rate that is not suppressible by further elevation of the ambient $[Ca^{++}]$.

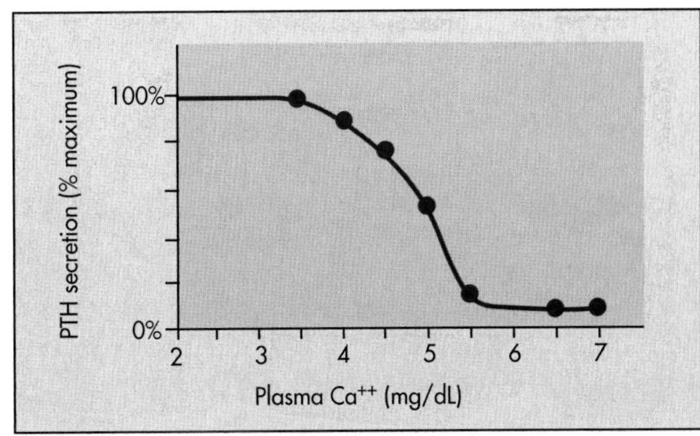

FIGURE 44–6. Inverse relationship between PTH secretion and plasma $[Ca^{++}]$ in humans. Note the maintenance of some PTH secretion even at high Ca^{++} levels. (Data from Brent GA et al: *J Clin Endocrinol Metab* 67:944, 1988.)

A plasma membrane Ca^{++} receptor regulates PTH secretion

The regulation of PTH represents an exception to the general rule that hormone secretion by exocytosis is stimulated by Ca^{++}. A unique **Ca^{++} receptor** within the plasma membrane of the parathyroid cell responds rapidly to alterations in extracellular Ca^{++} levels. A FALL IN THE EXTRACELLULAR Ca^{++} LEVEL ACTIVATES THE RECEPTOR, WHICH VIA G PROTEINS STIMULATES ADENYLYL CYCLASE AND INHIBITS PHOSPHOLIPASE C (see Chapter 5). THE RESULTANT INCREASE IN cAMP AND DECREASE IN CYTOPLASMIC Ca^{++} LEAD TO EXOCYTOSIS OF PTH-CONTAINING GRANULES **(Figure 44–7)**. When the extracellular Ca^{++} level is high, the reverse sequence occurs, and PTH secretion is inhibited (Figure 44–7). The parathyroid cells respond similarly to small variations in plasma $[Mg^{++}]$.

Ca^{++} also modulates PTH turnover within the gland. Prolonged exposure to a high ambient $[Ca^{++}]$ lowers the rate of PTH synthesis and stimulates the intraglandular degradation of PTH. Ca^{++} also regulates the size and number of the parathyroid cells. THE NET EFFECT OF Ca^{++} EXCESS IS A DECREASE IN PARATHYROID CELL MASS AND IN BOTH THE GLANDULAR STORES AND THE RELEASE RATES OF PTH. CONVERSELY, Ca^{++} DEFICIENCY INCREASES PARATHYROID CELL MASS, PTH STORES, SECRETORY RATES, AND ULTIMATELY THE SIZE OF THE GLAND.

Pi increases PTH secretion, even when Ca^{++} is kept constant, via a putative Pi receptor. In addition, by complexing Ca^{++} and decreasing $[Ca^{++}]$, a rise in the plasma [Pi] also indirectly causes a transient increase in PTH secretion. Importantly, 1,25-$(OH)_2$-D directly feeds back on the parathyroid gland to inhibit transcription of the PTH gene, to reduce PTH secretion, and to decrease the proliferation of

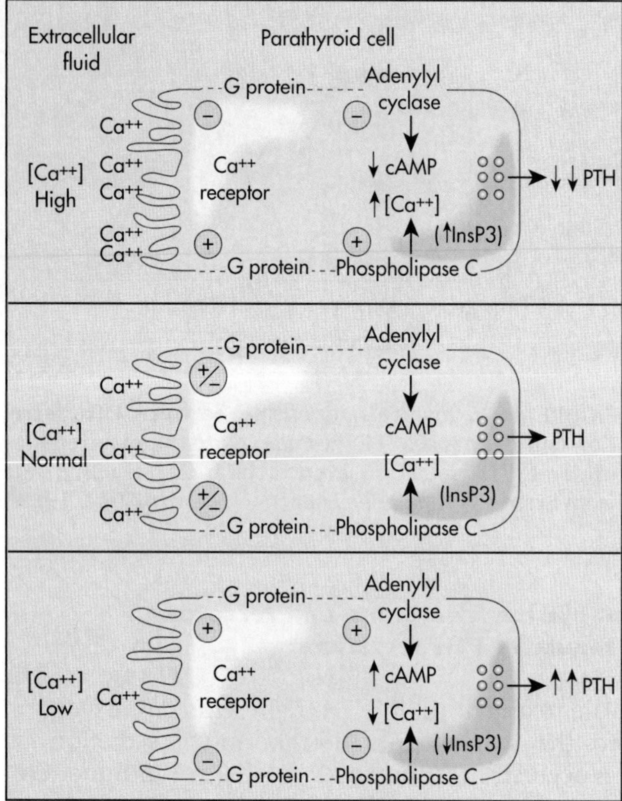

FIGURE 44–7. Mechanism of regulation of PTH secretion by changes in [Ca^{++}] in the extracellular fluid. An increase in the [Ca^{++}] is sensed by a plasma membrane Ca^{++} receptor in the parathyroid cell *(top)*. The activated receptor is linked to an inhibitory G protein, which inhibits adenylyl cyclase. As a result, intracellular levels of cAMP fall. The activated receptor is also linked to a stimulatory G protein that stimulates phospholipase C. As a result, levels of inositol 1,4,5-trisphosphate (InsP3) increase and transduce a rise in the intracellular [Ca^{++}]. Exocytosis of PTH secretory granules and PTH release are *decreased.* The opposite sequence occurs when there is a decrease in the [Ca^{++}] in the extracellular fluid *(bottom);* in that case, exocytosis of PTH secretory granules and PTH release are increased. +, disinhibited or stimulated; –, inhibited or unstimulated; +/–, balanced between stimulated and inhibited.

parathyroid cells. Since PTH stimulates 1,25-$(OH)_2$-D synthesis, PTH and 1,25-$(OH)_2$-D form a direct negative-feedback pair. Severe Mg^{++} depletion also inhibits PTH synthesis and release.

PTH secretion is pulsatile; it increases at night and with aging. The plasma PTH concentration is about 30 pg/mL (3×10^{-12} M). Whereas the hormone itself has a short half-life of minutes, its C-terminus metabolites circulate with half-lives of many hours.

PTH has intracellular effects on the kidneys, the bones, and the gastrointestinal tract

OVERALL, PTH INCREASES PLASMA Ca^{++} LEVELS AND DECREASES PLASMA Pi LEVELS BY ACTING ON THREE MAJOR TARGET ORGANS: THE KIDNEYS, THE BONES, AND, INDIRECTLY, THE GASTROINTESTINAL TRACT. Actions on all three targets ultimately increase Ca^{++} influx into the plasma and raise its concentration **(Figure 44–8)**. In contrast, PTH acts on the kidney to increase the exit of Pi from plasma; this action overwhelms the effect on bone and gut, which increases Pi entry into the plasma; therefore, the plasma [Pi] falls (Figure 44–8).

PTH acts through cAMP as a second messenger

PTH action is initiated by binding to a G protein–linked plasma membrane receptor from a family that includes the glucagon receptor. IN ALL TARGET CELLS, THE ACTIVATION OF ADENYLYL CYCLASE AND AN INCREASE IN cAMP LEVELS FOLLOW. This second messenger then triggers a protein kinase cascade (see Chapter 5), which ultimately leads to the phosphorylation of proteins necessary for the expression of PTH action.

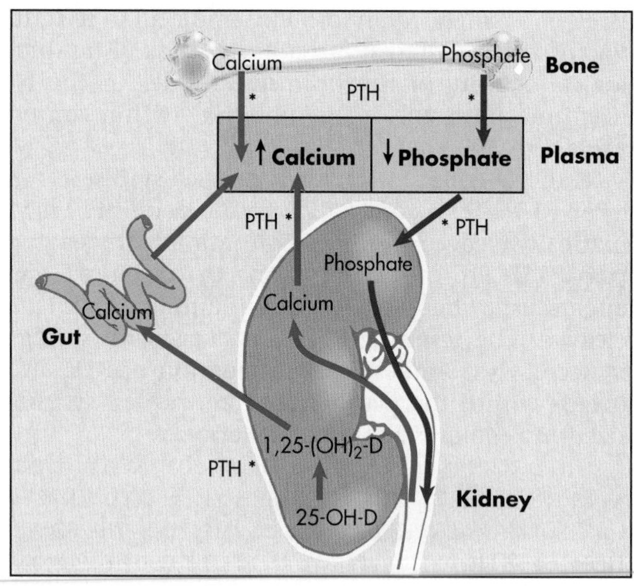

FIGURE 44–8. Overview of PTH actions. PTH acts directly on bone and kidney to increase Ca^{++} influx into plasma. By stimulating 1,25-$(OH)_2$-D synthesis, it also indirectly increases Ca^{++} absorption from the gut. Thus, the plasma Ca^{++} level increases. In contrast, PTH inhibits the renal tubular reabsorption of Pi, thereby increasing urinary Pi excretion. This effect quantitatively offsets the entry of Pi from bone and gut. Therefore, the plasma Pi level decreases.

PTH also stimulates the uptake of Ca^{++} into the cytoplasm of its target cells from intracellular stores and bathing fluid. This may be mediated by increases in phospholipase C and phosphoinositide second messengers (see Chapter 5). The initial uptake of Ca^{++} is reflected in a slight transient hypocalcemia, which immediately follows PTH administration and precedes the classic hypercalcemia. The presence of 1,25-$(OH)_2$-D is required for maximal responsiveness to PTH. A sufficient intracellular [Mg^{++}] is also necessary for PTH to act maximally.

PTH affects the renal system

PTH stimulates Ca^{++} reabsorption and inhibits Pi reabsorption by the renal tubules

PTH increases the reabsorption of Ca^{++} in the distal tubule and ascending loop of Henle. Mg^{++} reabsorption is also increased. In contrast, PTH decreases the reabsorption of Pi in the proximal tubule (see Chapter 39). These effects are mediated by PTH's stimulation of the production of cAMP at the capillary surface of the renal tubular cell. The cAMP is transported to the luminal surface, where it activates protein kinases in the membranes of the brush border that are involved in Ca^{++} and Pi reabsorption. During this process, cAMP is released into the tubular lumen. THEREFORE, THE EARLIEST OBSERVABLE RENAL EFFECT OF PTH IN VIVO IS A DRAMATIC INCREASE IN THE URINARY EXCRETION OF cAMP. The previously described Ca^{++} receptor also modulates Ca^{++} reabsorption by renal tubular cells.

The relationship between urinary Ca^{++} excretion and plasma [Ca^{++}] is altered by PTH (**Figure 44–9**). At any given plasma [Ca^{++}], PTH diminishes the amount of Ca^{++} lost in the urine and thus counters hypocalcemia. Conversely, the suppression of PTH secretion by an excess Ca^{++} load increases Ca^{++} excretion and helps prevent hypercalcemia.

The net effect of prolonged alterations in PTH secretion on urinary Ca^{++} excretion is eventually dominated by the influence of PTH on bone and gut. A continuous excess of PTH eventually elevates the plasma Ca^{++} level and, with it, the load of Ca^{++} filtered by the glomerulus. Therefore, the absolute amount of Ca^{++} excreted in the urine eventually increases despite the stimulation of tubular reabsorption of Ca^{++} by PTH.

In contrast, the relationship between urinary Pi excretion and the plasma Pi level is shifted in the opposite direction by PTH (Figure 44–9). This phosphaturic effect of PTH allows disposal of the extra Pi released when the hormone stimulates bone resorption (see next section). Otherwise, PTH would simultaneously elevate plasma [Ca^{++}] and [Pi] and thereby create the danger of precipitating Ca^{++}-Pi complexes in tissue.

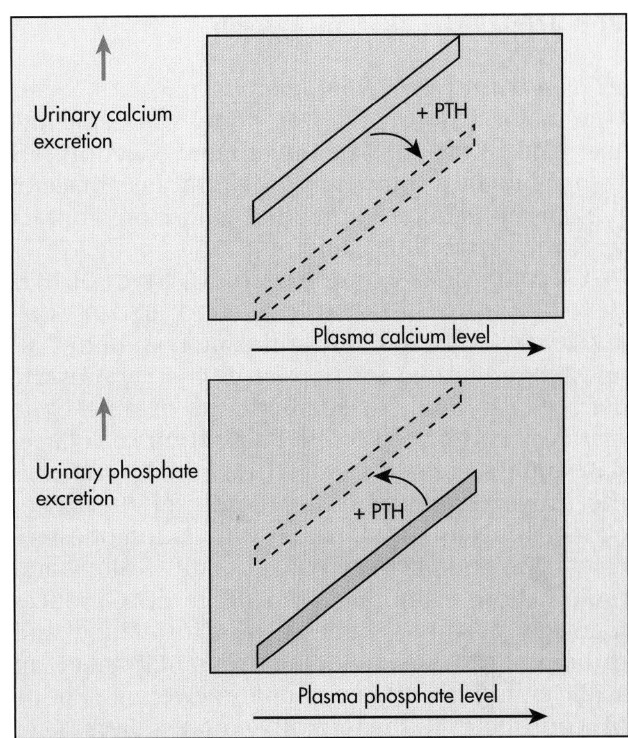

FIGURE 44–9. Renal effects of PTH. At any given level of plasma Ca^{++}, PTH decreases urinary Ca^{++} excretion. At any given level of plasma Pi, PTH increases urinary Pi excretion.

PTH also inhibits the reabsorption of Na^+ and HCO_3^- in the proximal tubule (see Chapter 37). This action may prevent metabolic alkalosis, which could result from the release of HCO_3^- during the dissolution of hydroxyapatite crystals in bone, as discussed later.

PTH directly stimulates the synthesis of 1,25-dihydroxyvitamin D_2 from 25-hydroxyvitamin D

PTH stimulates the synthesis of 1,25-$(OH)_2$-D by increasing cAMP levels and producing a cascade that activates a key cofactor, **renoredoxin,** for the 1-hydroxylase reaction. The decrease in plasma and renal Pi content caused by PTH further augments its direct action on 1-hydroxylase activity. The increase in 1,25-$(OH)_2$-D stimulates Ca^{++} absorption from the gut and raises plasma Ca^{++} levels (Figure 44–8). This important indirect effect of PTH on the intestinal tract again serves the major function of the hormone: to raise plasma Ca^{++}.

PTH affects the skeletal system

PTH mobilizes Ca^{++} from bone

One major action of PTH on bone is to accelerate the removal of Ca^{++}. The initial rapid effect of PTH is to stimulate a transfer of Ca^{++} from the surface of partially mineralized bone that is in close contact with the extracellular fluid.

A SECOND, MORE SLOWLY DEVELOPING EFFECT OF PTH IS TO STIMULATE THE OSTEOCLASTS TO RESORB COMPLETELY MINERALIZED BONE. In this process, both Ca^{++} and Pi are released for transfer ultimately into the extracellular fluid; in addition, the organic bone matrix is hydrolyzed by PTH activation of collagenase and lysosomal enzymes. PTH initially increases the active resorptive ruffled border of the osteoclasts. This is followed by PTH stimulation of osteoclast size, number of nuclei, and fusion and proliferation from precursors. PTH also induces increases in the enzymes acid phosphatase and carbonic anhydrase and the accumulation of an acidic environment. The resultant lowering of bone pH contributes to the resorptive process. Because of collagen degradation, PTH increases the release of hydroxyproline and other bone collagen products into plasma and urine (see section on bone resorption).

The effects of PTH on osteoclasts are partly mediated by osteoblasts

The dramatic effects of PTH on osteoclasts in vitro are not evident in the absence of osteoblasts. Therefore, an initial action of PTH on osteoblasts is required to stimulate release of paracrine factors that secondarily recruit and activate the osteoclasts (e.g., interleukins, macrophage colony-stimulating factor). PTH receptors are present on osteoblasts as well as on osteoclasts. When they are exposed to the hormone, osteoblasts immediately change shape. Later, PTH inhibits the synthesis of collagen by the osteoblasts, probably at the level of transcription. The stimulation of osteoclastic bone resorption and the inhibition of osteoblastic bone formation are achieved by the elevated concentrations of hormone that result from stimulation of the parathyroid glands through hypocalcemia. Thus, these actions of PTH are part of its general mission to restore the plasma [Ca^{++}] level to normal and maintain it there.

PTH also has anabolic actions on bone at lower than bone resorptive concentrations. By stimulating the production of local growth factors, PTH increases the number and activity of osteoblasts. PTH also decreases osteoprotegerin production by osteocytes, thereby relieving the suspension of osteoclastic activity. Thus, PTH can activate a remodeling cycle in osteons. The intermittent administration of PTH to humans in small doses increases trabecular bone mass but still decreases cortical bone. The anabolic effect on bone has proved useful in treatment of osteoporosis with PTH.

> Prolonged excess secretion of PTH occurs in **primary hyperparathyroidism,** usually because of a benign neoplasm in one parathyroid gland. The plasma [Ca^{++}] is high (with attendant symptoms, as previously described), and the [Pi] is often low. The increased renal excretion of Ca^{++} can cause kidney stones. Modest loss of cortical bone may result. In hyperparathyroidism secondary to kidney failure, both 1,25-$(OH)_2$-D and [Ca^{++}] decrease, and the parathyroid glands enlarge. Massive bone resorption by osteoclasts can result, with attendant pain, fractures, and deformities. Cure of hyperparathyroidism requires removal of the excess parathyroid tissue.

PTH-related protein controls bone growth

PTH-related peptide or protein (PTHrP) was originally discovered as a product of human cancers of squamous cell origin that were associated with hypercalcemia. However, bone and cartilage cells, normal skin keratinocytes, lactating mammary epithelium, placenta, and fetal parathyroid glands also synthesize PTHrP.

The gene for PTHrP and the gene for PTH evolved from a common ancestor. Because of the striking homology in their N-terminus amino acids, PTHrP exhibits most of the actions of PTH on bone and kidney by binding to the PTH receptor. PTHrP, however, does not stimulate renal 1-hydroxylase. Hence, patients with hypercalcemia caused by PTHrP do not have elevated plasma 1,25-$(OH)_2$-D levels.

The most important effect of PTHrP is in the epiphyseal growth plate (see earlier). PTHrP produced by later chondrocytes acts on proliferating chondrocytes to stimulate their growth but to inhibit their terminal differentiation. In this fashion, PTHrP regulates and orders the progression of the growth plates at both ends of long bones. Without PTHrP or a functional PTH/PTHrP receptor, bone is abnormal and growth disorganized.

There are also likely to be physiological roles for PTHrP during intrauterine life and early infancy. PTHrP in the placenta and in the fetus may maintain the 30% to 40% increased [Ca^{++}] gradient that exists between fetal and maternal plasma. It may regulate [Ca^{++}] in breast milk and Ca^{++} homeostasis early in neonatal life. PTHrP in skin contributes to regular cellular differentiation.

Calcitonin Is Secreted in Response to an Increased Plasma Calcium Level

Calcitonin (CT) decreases plasma Ca^{++} levels, largely by antagonizing the actions of PTH on bone. CT is secreted by a small population of neuroendocrine cells, known as **C cells** or **parafollicular cells,** in the **thyroid gland.** CT is a straight-chain peptide of 32 amino acids, synthesized from a preprohormone. The hormone is packaged in granules along with N-terminus and C-terminus copeptides of unknown function. Although its role in normal human physiology is uncertain, C-cell neoplasms and other tumors of neural crest origin often secrete great amounts of CT.

The major stimulus of CT secretion is a rise in the plasma [Ca^{++}] of as little as 1 mg/dL. The stimulating effect of Ca^{++} on CT secretion involves the same Ca^{++} receptor as in parathyroid cells and an increase in cAMP. The ingestion of food also increases CT secretion, a response mediated by gastrin and other gastrointestinal hormones. CT circulates in humans at concentrations of 10 to 100 pg/mL (10^{-11} M).

The major effect of CT is to decrease plasma Ca^{++} levels

The binding of CT to its plasma membrane receptors stimulates adenylyl cyclase production and elevates cAMP levels. This second messenger initiates at least a portion of CT action in all target cells. THE HYPOCALCEMIC ACTION OF CT IS CAUSED BY THE INHIBITION OF Ca^{++} TRANSFER INTO THE EXTRACELLULAR FLUID AND OF OSTEOCLASTIC BONE RESORPTION, PARTICULARLY WHEN THEY ARE STIMULATED BY PTH. Continued exposure to CT eventually decreases the number of osteoclasts and alters their morphological features. Since bone formation is also stimulated, denser bone with fewer resorption cavities eventually results.

The importance of CT in humans is controversial. CT deficiency caused by removal of the thyroid gland does not lead to overt hypercalcemia, and extreme CT hypersecretion by tumors rarely produces hypocalcemia. It may be that abnormal CT secretion is easily compensated for by adjustments in PTH and vitamin D levels. A role for CT in fetal bone development and in protection against the declining bone mass of aging has been proposed.

CT is used therapeutically to block bone resorption in situations in which the resorption rate is high (e.g., **Paget's disease**). The hormone is also used to treat **osteoporosis.**

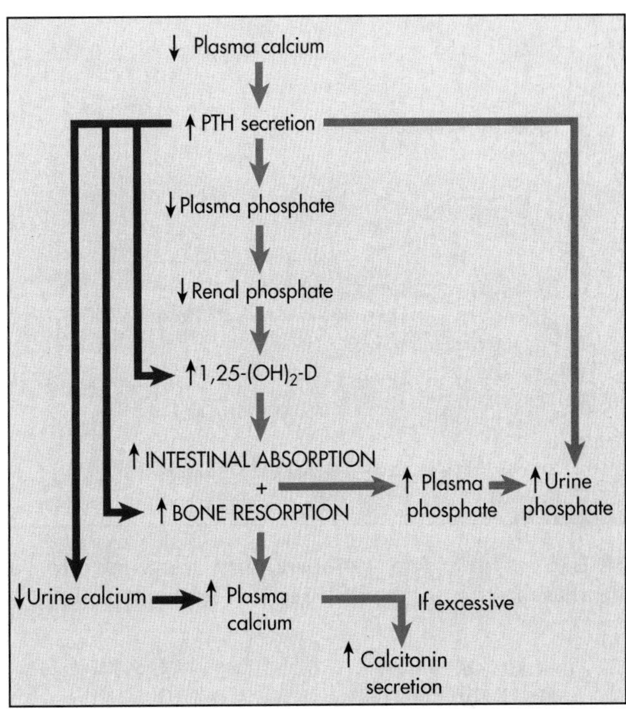

FIGURE 44–10. The compensatory response to a decrease in the plasma [Ca^{++}]. See text for explanation.

An Integrated System Maintains Normal Concentrations of Calcium and Phosphate

Ca^{++} deprivation **(Figure 44–10)** stimulates PTH secretion. PTH increases urinary Pi excretion and thereby decreases the plasma and renal cortical Pi content. Excess PTH secretion, together with the decreased [Pi], stimulates the production of 1,25-$(OH)_2$-D, which raises the plasma [Ca^{++}] back toward normal by increasing the absorption of Ca^{++} from the gut. PTH also increases bone resorption and Ca^{++} reabsorption from the renal tubular urine. TOGETHER THEN, PTH AND 1,25-$(OH)_2$-D RESPOND TO Ca^{++} DEPRIVATION BY INCREASING THE FLUX OF Ca^{++} INTO THE PLASMA. SIMULTANEOUSLY, THE EXTRA Pi THAT ENTERS WITH THE Ca^{++} IS ELIMINATED IN THE URINE VIA PTH ACTION.

Pi deprivation **(Figure 44–11)** directly stimulates 1,25-$(OH)_2$-D production, which increases the flux of Pi into plasma by stimulating bone resorption and Pi absorption from the gut. The extra Ca^{++} that enters simultaneously raises the plasma Ca^{++} level. This suppresses PTH secretion, and the absence of PTH causes urinary Pi excretion to diminish and thus aids in the restoration of plasma [Pi] back to normal. At the same time, the suppression of PTH diminishes renal tubular [Ca^{++}] reabsorption and increases urinary Ca^{++} excretion. THUS, THE EXTRA Ca^{++} THAT WAS MOBILIZED IS ELIMINATED MORE EASILY.

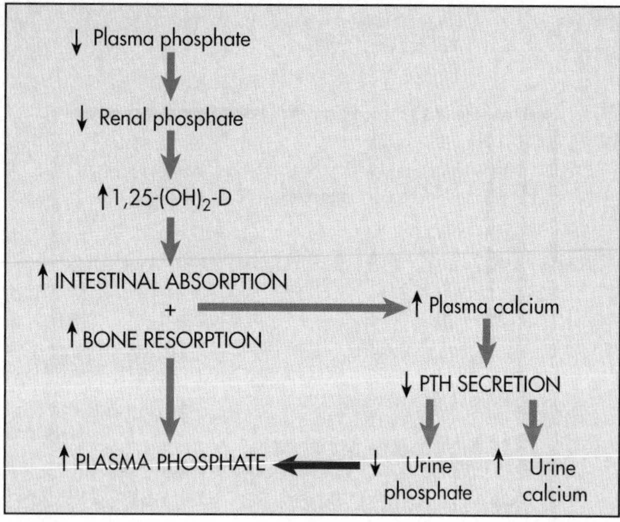

FIGURE 44–11. The compensatory response to a decrease in the plasma [Pi]. See text for explanation.

THIS COMBINED ARRANGEMENT OF DUAL HORMONE REGULATION AND DUAL HORMONE ACTION BY PTH AND VITAMIN D PERMITS A SELECTIVE DEFENSE OF EITHER THE PLASMA [Ca^{++}] OR THE PLASMA [Pi] WITHOUT CREATING A CIRCULATORY EXCESS OF THE OTHER. The same principles apply in reverse when excess loads of Ca^{++} or Pi are imposed on the body.

The renal responses to PTH provide the most rapid (within minutes) defense against sudden changes in Ca^{++} or Pi levels. The gastrointestinal responses to 1,25-(OH)$_2$-D occur over days. Bone responses to regulation by PTH and 1,25-(OH)$_2$-D are relatively slow when they are caused by osteoclastic resorption. However, the capacity for Ca^{++} and Pi uptake and release by the skeleton is enormous.

The compensatory responses of the kidney and the gut defend the total body and bone stores of Ca^{++} and Pi against erosion. In contrast, the skeletal mechanisms that defend the plasma [Ca^{++}] and [Pi] levels have the important disadvantage that they eventually sacrifice the chemical and structural integrity of the bone mass.

Summary

- ❖ Ca^{++} is critically involved in numerous functions, including neurotransmission, hormone secretion and action, enzyme activities, muscle contraction, and blood clotting. It is also the chief mineral that contributes to the structural integrity of the skeleton.
- ❖ Extracellular [Ca^{++}] is closely controlled, in part to help regulate the wide transient swings in intracellular concentration, which is 10,000-fold lower.
- ❖ Pi participates in the major enzymatic pathways of energy generation, substrate flux, and protein and other macromolecule synthesis. Pi is also the anion partner of Ca^{++} in bone structure.
- ❖ The Ca^{++} balance depends on dietary intake, gastrointestinal absorption, renal excretion, and internal transfers between extracellular Ca^{++} and the skeletal reservoir.
- ❖ The Pi balance reflects dietary intake, gastrointestinal absorption, renal excretion, and internal shifts among extracellular fluid, large soft tissue contents, and the skeletal reservoir.
- ❖ Bone is a complex organ with several cell types that are specifically devoted to a continuous process of remodeling. Mineralized bone is resorbed by osteoclasts (which release Ca^{++} and Pi), followed by osteoblasts reforming new bone (which reassimilates Ca^{++} and Pi). This coupled process is initiated by signals from osteocytes that possess mechanosensors. It is augmented during growth periods and slows with aging.
- ❖ Vitamin D is a steroid molecule that is both synthesized in the skin by UV light and absorbed from the diet. It undergoes successive hydroxylations in the liver and kidney to 1,25-(OH)$_2$-D, the active metabolite.
- ❖ 1,25-(OH)$_2$-D acts via its intestinal epithelial nuclear receptor to increase the absorption of ingested Ca^{++} (and Pi). The hormone is therefore critical for supplying Ca^{++} for bone formation and maintaining the normal plasma levels required for other Ca^{++}-dependent processes. Overall, 1,25-(OH)$_2$-D increases both plasma [Ca^{++}] and plasma [Pi].

- PTH is a straight-chain peptide synthesized as a preprohormone in four parathyroid glands. PTH and Ca^{++} form a classic negative-feedback pair. PTH is released in response to the decreased plasma Ca^{++} level perceived by a plasma membrane Ca^{++} receptor; PTH synthesis and secretion are suppressed by Ca^{++} and by 1,25-$(OH)_2$-D.
- PTH acts via a plasma membrane receptor and cAMP to increase osteoclastic bone resorption, to increase the renal tubular reabsorption of Ca^{++} and to decrease that of Pi, and to increase 1,25-$(OH)_2$-D synthesis in the kidney. Overall, PTH increases levels of plasma Ca^{++} and decreases levels of plasma Pi.
- Ca^{++} deficiency evokes a synergistic sequence that increases levels of PTH and 1,25-$(OH)_2$-D. Their combined actions restore plasma Ca^{++} levels to normal.
- Pi deprivation evokes a synergistic sequence that increases 1,25-$(OH)_2$-D secretion but decreases PTH secretion. The result is the restoration of plasma [Pi] to normal.
- CT is a peptide hormone synthesized in C cells within the thyroid gland. It is secreted in response to hypercalcemia and acts as a PTH antagonist that inhibits bone resorption and lowers the plasma [Ca^{++}].

Bibliography

Bodine PV, Komm BS: Tissue culture models for studies of hormone and vitamin action in bone cells, *Vitam Horm* 64:101, 2002.

Bouillon R: Vitamin D: from photosynthesis, metabolism, and action to clinical applications. In DeGroot LJ, Jameson JL, eds: *Endocrinology,* ed 4, Philadelphia, 2001, WB Saunders.

Brent GA et al: Relationship between the concentration and rate of change of calcium and serum intact parathyroid hormone levels in normal humans, *J Clin Endocrinol Metab* 67: 944,1988.

Bringhurst FR: Regulation of calcium and phosphate homeostasis. In DeGroot LJ, Jameson JL, eds: *Endocrinology,* ed 4, Philadelphia, 2001, WB Saunders.

Brown EM, MacLeod RJ: Extracellular calcium sensing and extracellular calcium signaling, *Physiol Rev* 81:240, 2001.

Coleman DT, Fitzpatrick LA, Bilezikian J: Biochemical mechanisms of parathyroid hormone action. In Bilezikian J, ed: *The parathyroids: basic and clinical concepts,* New York, 1994, Raven Press.

Dempster DW et al: Anabolic actions of parathyroid hormone on bone, *Endocr Rev* 14:690, 1993.

Gurlek A, Pittelkow MR, Kumar R: Modulation of growth factor/cytokine synthesis and signaling by 1α,25-dihydroxyvitamin D_3: implications in cell growth and differentiation, *Endocr Rev* 23:763, 2002.

Holick MF: Skin: site of the synthesis of vitamin D and a target tissue for the active form, 1,25-dihydroxyvitamin D_3, *Ann N Y Acad Sci* 548:14, 1988.

Jans DA, Thomas RJ, Gillespie MT: Parathyroid hormone–related protein (PTHrP): a nucleocytoplasmic shuttling protein with distinct paracrine and intracrine roles, *Vitam Horm* 66:345, 2003.

Jones G et al: Current understanding of the molecular actions of vitamin D, *Physiol Rev* 78:1193, 1998.

Manolagas SC: Birth and death of bone cells: basic regulatory mechanisms and implications for the pathogenesis and treatment of osteoporosis, *Endocr Rev* 21:115, 2000.

Martin TJ, Moseley JM: Parathyroid hormone–related protein. In DeGroot LJ, Jameson JL, eds: *Endocrinology,* ed 4, Philadelphia, 2001, WB Saunders.

Potts JT Jr et al: Parathyroid hormone: physiology, chemistry, biosynthesis, secretion, metabolism, and mode of action. In DeGroot LJ, Jameson JL, eds: *Endocrinology,* ed 4, Philadelphia, 2001, WB Saunders.

Roodman GD: Advances in bone biology: the osteoclast, *Endocr Rev* 17:308, 1996.

Schmid C: IGFs: function and clinical importance to the regulation of osteoblast function by hormones and cytokines with special reference to insulin-like growth factors and their binding proteins, *J Intern Med* 234:535, 1993.

Slatopolsky E et al: Phosphorus restriction prevents parathyroid gland growth: high phosphorus directly stimulates PTH secretion in vitro, *J Clin Invest* 97:2534, 1996.

Van der Eerden BCJ, Karperien M, Wit JM: Systemic and local regulation of the growth plate, *Endocr Rev* 24:782, 2003.

Whitfield JF, Morley P, Willick GE: Bone growth stimulators: new tools for treating bone loss and mending fractures, *Vitam Horm* 65:1, 2002.

Ylikomi T et al: Antiproliferative action of vitamin D, *Vitam Horm* 64:357, 2002.

Case Studies

Case 44–1

A 50-year-old overstressed businessman treats frequent "heartburn" with large daily doses of antacids containing aluminum hydroxide. This binds Pi in the gastrointestinal tract and causes the patient to have severe Pi deficiency.

1. **Which of the following would increase?**
   A. Plasma PTH levels
   B. Urine Pi levels
   C. Plasma 24,25-$(OH)_2$-D levels
   D. Plasma 1,25-$(OH)_2$-D levels
   E. Bone formation

2. **Which of the following would decrease?**
   A. Gastrointestinal absorption of Ca^{++}
   B. Plasma PTH levels
   C. Urine hydroxyproline levels
   D. Urine Ca^{++} levels
   E. Plasma CT levels

Case 44–2

A well-nourished, otherwise healthy 35-year-old woman who had three kidney stones in 18 months has an elevated plasma [Ca^{++}] of 13 mg/dL and is found to have hyperparathyroidism. Radiographs show bone resorption.

1. **Which of the following would be decreased?**
   A. Urine cAMP levels
   B. Urine [Pi]
   C. Number of osteoclasts
   D. Bone formation
   E. Plasma [Pi]

2. **After removal of a large parathyroid tumor, which of the following would increase rapidly?**
   A. Plasma [Pi]
   B. Nerve excitability
   C. Urine [Ca^{++}]
   D. Heart rate
   E. Plasma [Ca^{++}]

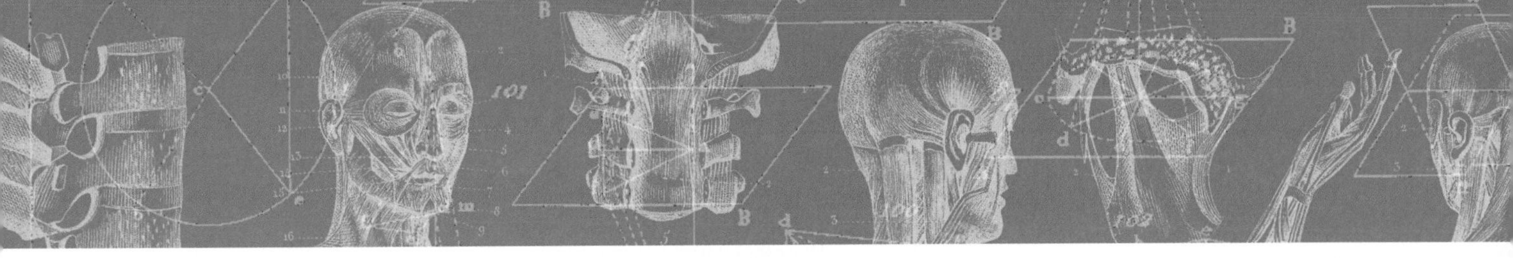

Chapter 45: Hypothalamus and Pituitary Gland

Objectives

- Describe the anatomical and functional relationships between the hypothalamus and the posterior and anterior pituitary gland.
- Explain the regulation of antidiuretic hormone and oxytocin (posterior pituitary hormones) secretion.
- Identify the actions of antidiuretic hormone and oxytocin on their target tissues.
- Explain the regulation of growth hormone and prolactin (anterior pituitary hormones) secretion.
- Identify the actions of growth hormone and prolactin on their target tissues.

The pituitary gland, once called the master gland, retains a preeminent position in endocrinology, even though it is now known to be under neural regulation by products from the hypothalamus and under feedback control by circulating products of its target glands and by other molecules arising in the periphery. The pituitary gland and hypothalamus, with their associated neural and vascular connections, form a complex functional unit that epitomizes the subtle interrelationship between the endocrine and nervous systems. THIS UNIT REGULATES WATER METABOLISM, MILK SECRETION, BODY GROWTH, REPRODUCTION, LACTATION, AND THE GROWTH AND SECRETORY ACTIVITIES OF THE THYROID, ADRENAL, AND REPRODUCTIVE GLANDS, THEREBY AFFECTING THE PHYSIOLOGICAL FUNCTIONING OF VIRTUALLY ALL OTHER ORGAN SYSTEMS IN THE BODY.

The neurons of the hypothalamus synthesize and secrete neurohormones **(Figure 45–1)**. Two of these neurohormones are transferred down the cell axons and are stored in secretory vesicles at the ends of the axons within the posterior pituitary gland, also known as the **neurohypophysis.** From there, they are released into the bloodstream and reach the general circulation to act on distant target cells (**neurocrine** function). Other hypothalamic neurohormones are transported down the cell axons to end in a neurovascular region known as the **median eminence,** which is situated just below the hypothalamus (Figure 45-1). From terminal secretory storage vesicles in the median eminence, these neurohormones are released into the bloodstream, and via local circulation, they reach the nearby anterior pituitary gland, also known as the **adenohypophysis.** There, they stimulate or inhibit endocrine target cells (again, neurocrine function). The endocrine cells in the adenohypophysis synthesize, store, and secrete a variety of peptide and protein hormones that are released into the bloodstream and reach the general circulation to act on distant peripheral target cells (**endocrine** function). In addition, the hormones of these closely intertwined endocrine cells may act on neighboring target cells within the adenohypophysis (**paracrine** function).

The Anatomy and Embryological Development of the Hypothalamus and Pituitary Gland Subserve Their Close Functional Relationship

The pituitary gland sits beneath the hypothalamus in a socket of bone **(sella turcica)** within the skull. The gland represents a fusion of two tissues. The

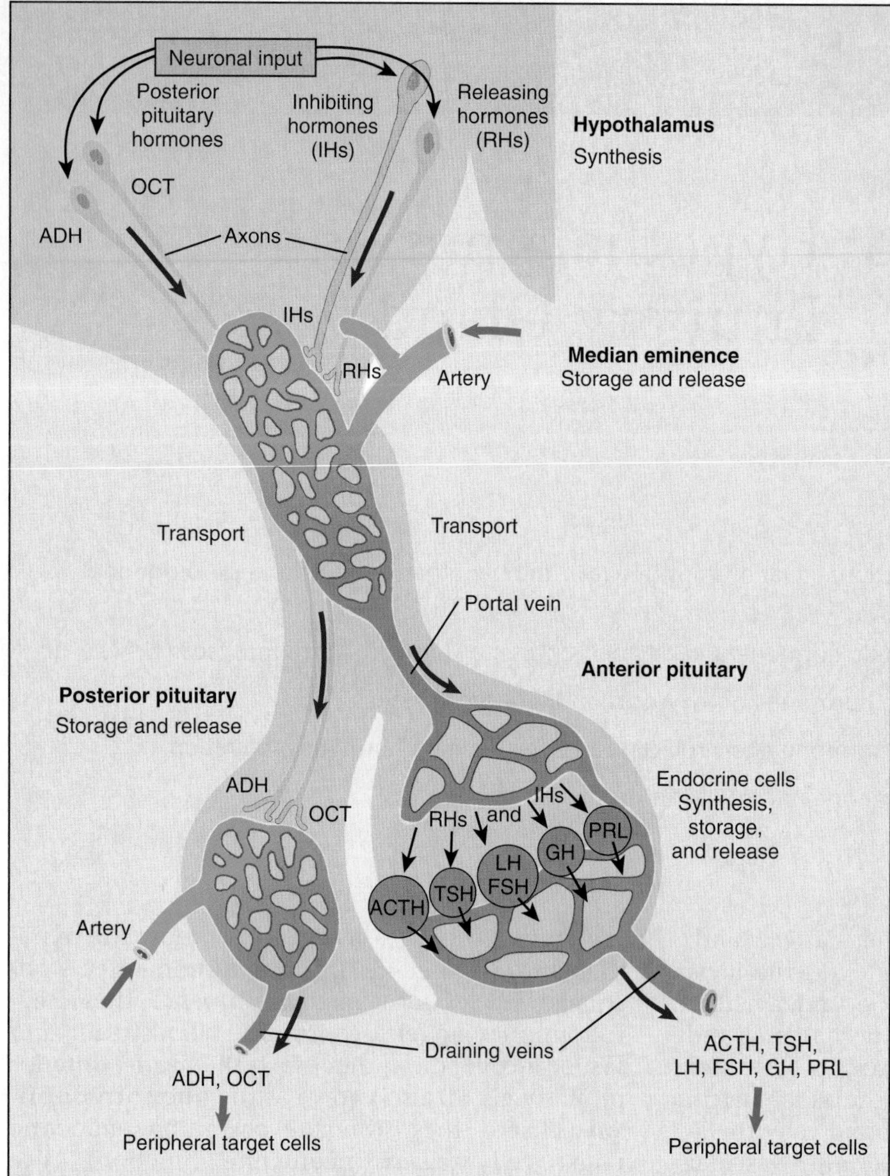

FIGURE 45–1. Anatomical and functional relationships between the hypothalamus and the pituitary gland. The posterior pituitary gland is an extension of neural tissue that stores neurohormones and has its own arterial blood supply. In contrast, the anterior pituitary gland is endocrine tissue with a blood supply derived largely from veins that first drain neural tissue in the median eminence. Because of this arrangement, the endocrine cells are exposed to high concentrations of neurohormones that originate in the hypothalamus and are stored in the median eminence. The hormones secreted by the posterior and anterior pituitary gland reach and act on peripheral target cells. ACTH, adrenocorticotropic hormone; ADH, antidiuretic hormone; FSH, follicle-stimulating hormone; GH, growth hormone; LH, luteinizing hormone; OCT, oxytocin; PRL, prolactin; TSH, thyroid-stimulating hormone.

posterior portion, or neurohypophysis, develops as a downward outpouching of neuroectoderm from brain tissue in the floor of the third ventricle. This differentiates into the neurons of the hypothalamus. The upper part of the neural stalk expands to form the median eminence. The lower part of the neural stalk grows downward to form the bulk of the posterior pituitary. Both the posterior pituitary and the median eminence consist largely of the terminals of various hypothalamic neurons. Both tissues are highly vascularized, and their capillaries contain fenestrations (intercellular windows) that allow the influx and efflux of protein molecules.

The posterior pituitary is supplied by the **inferior hypophyseal artery,** whose capillary plexus invests the terminal swellings of axons from the supraoptic and paraventricular areas of the hypothalamus. These terminals are the immediate source of the peptide neurohormones **antidiuretic hormone (ADH)** and **oxytocin (OCT);** ADH is also known as **arginine vasopressin.** These neurohormones are released into the capillary plexus, which carries them into the systemic circulation via draining veins (Figure 45–1).

The anterior pituitary develops from an upward outpouching of ectoderm from the floor of the oral cavity. After pinching off, the pouch becomes separated from the mouth by the sphenoid bone of the skull. At the junction of the anterior and posterior lobes of the pituitary gland is an intermediate zone, minuscule in humans but well developed in animals, from which another peptide hormone, **melanocyte-stimulating hormone,** is produced.

The median eminence is supplied mainly by the superior hypophyseal artery (and to a lesser extent by the inferior hypophyseal artery). Its capillary plexus invests terminal swellings of axons from a variety of hypothalamic neurons. These neurons are the source of hypothalamic **releasing** and **inhibiting hormones** that regulate anterior pituitary function. The capillary plexus of the median eminence forms a set of **portal veins** that descend into the anterior pituitary (Figure 45-1). These veins then give rise to a second fenestrated capillary plexus, which has a dual role. Hypothalamic releasing and inhibiting hormones, which are carried down from the median eminence, exit the second plexus and regulate secretion by the endocrine cells in the anterior pituitary. The protein hormone products of these cells then enter the same capillary plexus and are delivered via the circulation to distant target cells.

The anterior pituitary derives 90% of its blood supply from the portal veins and has little direct arterial input. Furthermore, its endocrine cells lie outside the blood-brain barrier. A reversal of flow upward in the portal veins may permit high concentrations of anterior pituitary hormones to reach the median eminence and even the hypothalamus, where they could feed back on neurons without impedance from the blood-brain barrier.

Just above the pituitary gland and sella turcica lies the crossing of the optic nerves as they course from the retina to the cerebral cortex. Any upward tumorous growth of the pituitary out of the sella turcica can compress the optic nerves and cause a characteristic loss of visual fields and visual acuity. This anatomy can be well visualized by magnetic resonance imaging **(Figure 45–2)**.

Hypothalamic Function Regulates Pituitary Gland Secretions to Coordinate with the Essential Needs of the Organism

A comprehensive discussion of the hypothalamus is provided in Chapter 10. From an endocrine standpoint, however, the hypothalamus may be viewed as a central relay station for collecting and integrating signals from diverse sources and funneling them to the pituitary gland **(Figure 45–3)**. The hypothalamus receives input from the thalamus, the reticular activating substance, the limbic system (amygdala, olfactory bulb, hippocampus, and habenula), the eyes, and remotely the neocortex. Through this input, PITUITARY FUNCTION CAN BE INFLUENCED BY SLEEP OR WAKEFULNESS, PAIN, EMOTION, FRIGHT, SMELL, LIGHT, AND POSSIBLY EVEN THOUGHT. It can be coordinated with other behavior, such as mating responses. INTERHYPOTHALAMIC AXONAL CONNECTIONS ALLOW THE OUTPUT OF PITUITARY HORMONES TO RESPOND TO CHANGES IN AUTONOMIC NERVOUS SYSTEM ACTIVITY AND TO THE NEEDS OF TEMPERATURE REGULATION, WATER BALANCE, AND ENERGY REQUIREMENTS.

The proximity of these various areas of the hypothalamus to one another has functional logic. For example, hormones of the thyroid gland increase energy expenditure, metabolic rate, and thermogenesis. The hypothalamic neurons that ultimately control thyroid gland output are located close to neurons that regulate temperature and energy intake via appetite control.

Separation of the hypothalamus into individual nuclei or distinct anatomical centers of endocrine function is relatively imprecise, with two exceptions. The supraoptic nucleus is a collection of large

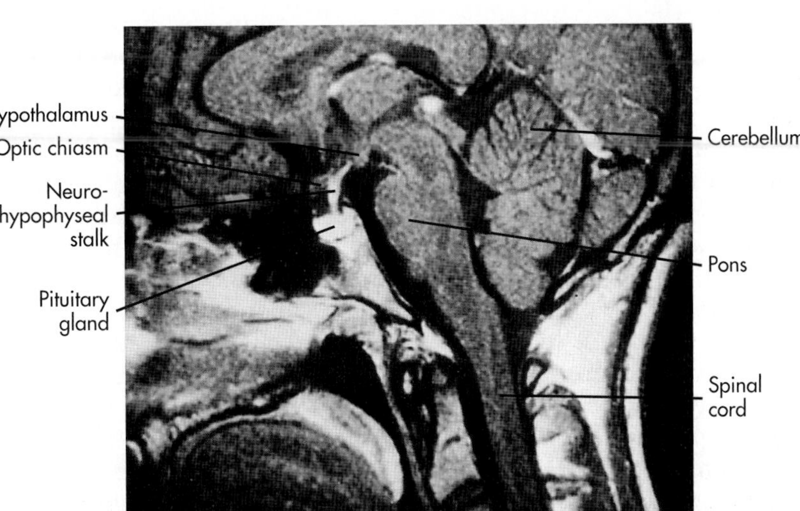

FIGURE 45–2. Magnetic resonance image of the brain showing the proximity of the hypothalamus and pituitary gland and their connection by a neurohypophyseal stalk. Also note the proximity of the optic chiasm (crossing of optic nerves) to the pituitary gland.

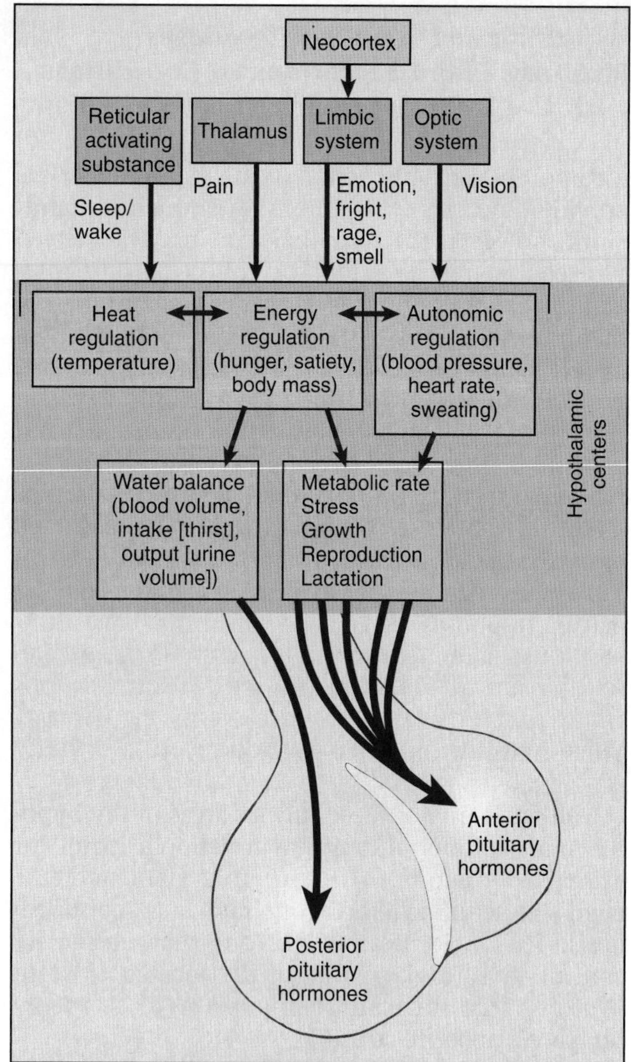

FIGURE 45–3. Interrelationships among various hypothalamic regulatory centers, their inputs from various parts of the brain, and their outputs to the pituitary gland. Note that sleep, pain, stressors, energy needs, temperature, and signals from the autonomic nervous system, as well as other factors, influence pituitary function.

neurons that secrete mainly ADH, and the paraventricular nucleus is a similar collection of neurons that secrete mainly OCT. These two neuronal pools overlap only slightly. In contrast, the small neurons that secrete the hypothalamic releasing and inhibiting hormones are more loosely aggregated in various areas, and they overlap more. As a general but not absolute rule, only one cell type secretes each neurohormone. In some hypothalamic neurons, neurotransmitters such as dopamine are also produced.

Each hypothalamic anterior pituitary releasing or inhibiting hormone can be assigned a primary target for which it has been named, such as **thyrotropin-releasing hormone** (a hormone that releases **thyrotropin,** an anterior pituitary hormone, which then stimulates the thyroid gland) or **somatostatin** (*soma,* "body growth"; *statin,* "halting of function"). However, some of these neuropeptides act on more than one anterior pituitary cell.

In addition to the hypothalamic neurons whose axons end in the posterior pituitary and median eminence, other neurons have axons that project to different parts of the brain. In these instances, the same hypothalamic peptides serve as neurotransmitters. Such neuropeptides have also been found in the spinal cord, sympathetic ganglia, sensory neurons, pancreatic islets, and neuroendocrine cells of the gastrointestinal tract.

Hypothalamic neurohormones are synthesized from preprohormones (see Chapter 41) and are typically secreted in pulses generated by an intrinsic neural oscillator **(Figure 45–4)**. This pulsatile pattern of signaling is necessary for optimal responses by target cells. Constant stimulation or inhibition of anterior pituitary cells by hypothalamic hormones down-regulates their receptors and leads to waning effects.

In women who are infertile because of hypothalamic dysfunction, ovulatory menstrual cycles can be restored only if the appropriate hypothalamic releasing hormone is administered in pulses of the correct size and frequency throughout the day. If the releasing hormone is administered continuously, the necessary anterior pituitary response is ultimately lost because of the down-regulation of the releasing hormone receptor. The same phenomenon is observed with regard to spermatogenesis in men.

Releasing and inhibiting hormones react with plasma membrane receptors in anterior pituitary cells; Ca^{++}, phosphatidylinositol products, and cAMP are generated as second messengers. The releasing hormones all stimulate the exocytosis of granules containing tropic hormones. In addition, they stimulate the transcription of tropic hormone genes and enhance hormone activity via posttranslational modification. Inhibiting hormones have the opposite effects.

Various neurotransmitters subserve hypothalamic function

Afferent impulses to hypothalamic neurons are transmitted via norepinephrine, serotonin, acetylcholine, the amino acid neurotransmitters (glutamate, aspartate, glycine, and γ-aminobutyric acid),

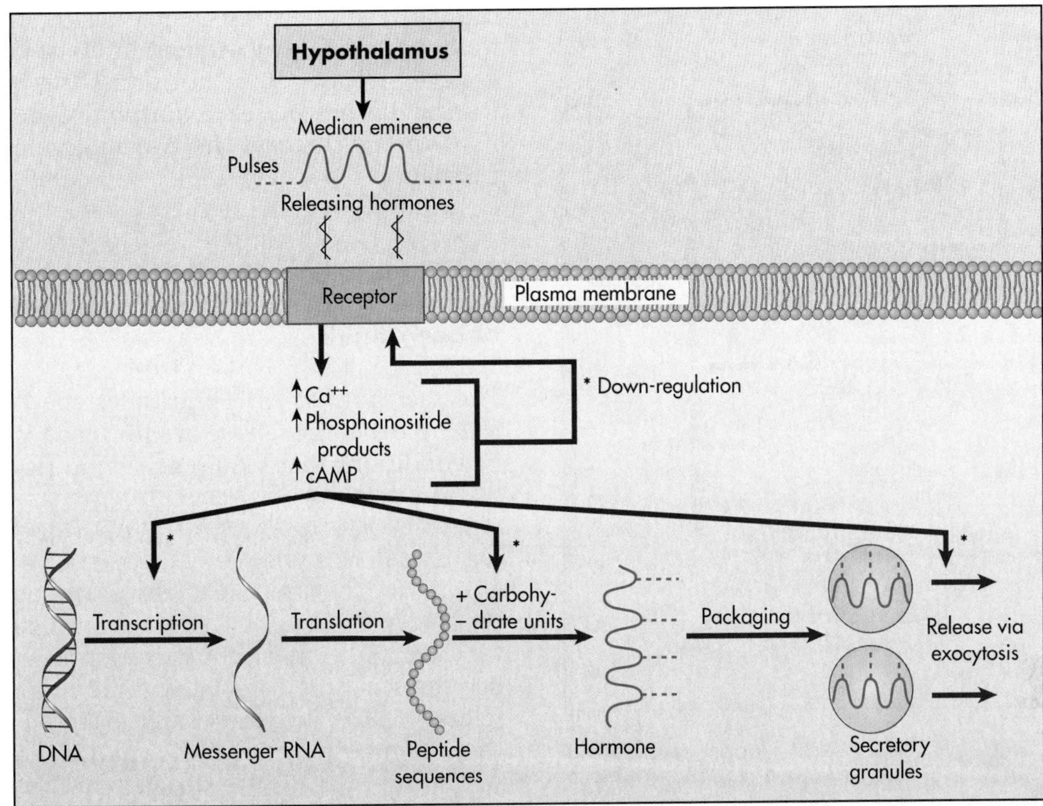

FIGURE 45–4. Action of hypothalamic releasing or inhibiting hormones on anterior pituitary cells. The neurohormones characteristically are released in pulses, bind to plasma membrane receptors, and act through Ca^{++} and other second messengers. They regulate gene expression, posttranslational processes, and secretion of anterior pituitary tropic hormones.

and numerous neuropeptides. From some hypothalamic neurons, dopamine and β-endorphin transmit signals to neighboring neurons via intrahypothalamic tracts and to the median eminence via efferent tracts. These signals directly or indirectly modulate the discharge of releasing and inhibiting hormones. In addition, neurotransmitters from the hypothalamus (e.g., dopamine) may themselves reach the portal vein blood and directly influence the output of anterior pituitary hormones.

The hypothalamus and pituitary gland respond to feedback control

The pituitary hypothalamic axis is under feedback control from its peripheral targets (**Figure 45–5**). Tropic hormones from the adenohypophysis regulate the concentrations of hormones secreted by the thyroid, adrenal, and reproductive glands; peripherally generated peptide products; and substrates such as glucose or free fatty acids. These in turn feed back to regulate the output of both the hypothalamus and the anterior pituitary. This is known as **long-loop feedback,** and it is usually negative, although it can transiently be positive. Negative feedback can also be exerted by the anterior pituitary hormones on the synthesis or discharge of the related hypothalamic releasing or inhibiting hormones. This is known as **short-loop feedback.** Because these hormones do not ordinarily cross the blood-brain barrier, short-loop feedback may occur either via fenestrated cells of the capillaries that bathe hypothalamic neurons or via retrograde flow through pituitary portal veins. Finally, a hypothalamic releasing hormone may even inhibit its own synthesis and discharge or the synthesis of a paired hypothalamic inhibiting hormone. This is called **ultrashort-loop feedback.**

The Posterior Pituitary Gland Regulates Water Metabolism and Breast Milk Secretion

ADH and OCT, two homologous peptides with nine amino acids and molecular weights of approximately 1000, are secreted by the posterior pituitary

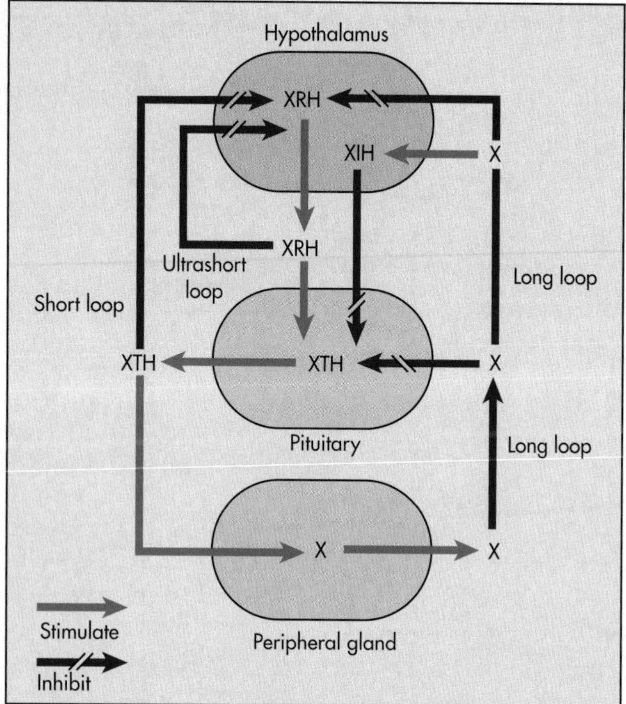

FIGURE 45–5. Negative-feedback loops regulating hormone secretion in a typical hypothalamus–pituitary–peripheral gland axis. Note that feedback from the periphery can regulate both hypothalamic and pituitary function. Ultrashort-loop feedback may be intrahypothalamic. X, peripheral gland hormone; XIH, hypothalamic inhibiting hormone; XRH, hypothalamic releasing hormone; XTH, pituitary tropic hormone.

gland. Each has two cysteines from which intramolecular disulfide rings are formed. THE PRIMARY ROLE OF ADH IS TO CONSERVE WATER AND REGULATE THE TONICITY OF BODY FLUIDS (see Chapter 38). A SECONDARY ROLE IS TO HELP MAINTAIN VASCULAR VOLUME. THE PRIMARY ROLE OF OCT IS TO EJECT MILK FROM THE LACTATING MAMMARY GLAND; AN ADDITIONAL ROLE IS TO STIMULATE CONTRACTION OF THE UTERUS. Although their main functions are different, both hormones are synthesized, stored, and secreted in similar fashion.

The similar genes that direct synthesis of the preprohormones for ADH and OCT probably have a common ancestor gene. In addition to the two neuropeptides, the gene products include distinctive small proteins known as **neurophysins.** Neurophysin 1 for OCT and neurophysin 2 for ADH are very similar. After processing, ADH and OCT are packaged with their respective neurophysins in neurosecretory granules. The neurophysins serve as carrier proteins during the transport of ADH and OCT down the axons to the posterior pituitary gland.

The release of ADH or OCT occurs when an electrical discharge is transmitted from the cell body in the hypothalamus down its axon, where it depolarizes the neurosecretory vesicle in the posterior pituitary. The subsequent influx of Ca^{++} into the vesicles releases the hormones via exocytosis. During this process, each hormone dissociates from its neurophysin, and the two molecules enter the circulation separately.

Antidiuretic hormone is secreted in response to changes in the osmolality of body fluids

The secretion of ADH illustrates the homeostatic principle that the release of a hormone is stimulated by conditions that require its action (**Figure 45–6**). WATER DEPRIVATION RAISES THE PLASMA OSMOLALITY, WHICH EVOKES THE RELEASE OF ADH. IN TURN, ADH CAUSES THE RETENTION OF FREE WATER BY THE KIDNEY AND AN INCREASE IN URINE OSMOLALITY, RESULTING IN A DECLINE OF PLASMA OSMOLALITY TO NORMAL (see Chapter 38). Conversely, ingestion of a water load decreases plasma osmolality. This suppresses ADH release, which increases water excretion and raises the plasma osmolality to normal. Thus, water and ADH form a negative-feedback loop that operates to defend total body water and osmolality.

A deficiency of ADH caused by disease or traumatic destruction of the ADH neurons, a condition known as **central diabetes insipidus,** has dramatic consequences. Urine volume can reach 500 to 1000 mL/hr, with osmolalities as low as 50 mOsm/kg. This forces frequent urination and requires the individual to drink equally large volumes of water to prevent collapse from volume depletion and hyperosmolality. Impairment of thirst or consciousness can therefore lead to death from dehydration. Treatment with ADH or longer acting synthetic analogues provides rapid relief.

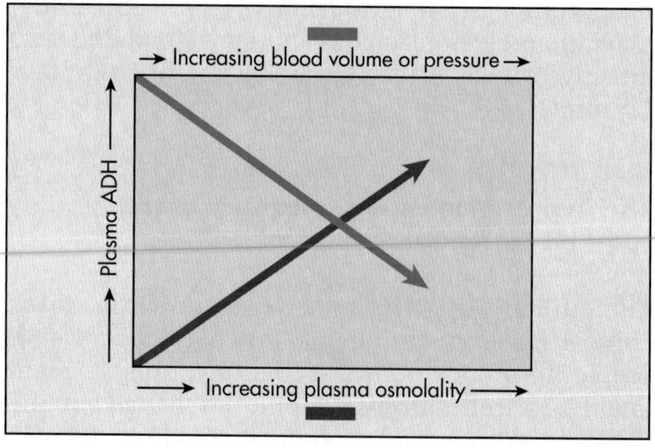

FIGURE 45–6. Positive correlation between the plasma ADH and increasing plasma osmolality. Negative correlation between plasma ADH and increasing blood volume or pressure.

The direct physiological stimulus of ADH release is an increase in the osmolality of fluids that bathe osmoreceptor neurons in the hypothalamus. This creates a gradient for water movement out of these neurons, and the consequent rise in intracellular osmolality causes them to fire and trigger the release of ADH from the ADH-producing neurons. Any administered solute that does not readily penetrate cell membranes (e.g., sodium) creates the same osmotic gradient and stimulates ADH secretion. In contrast, solutes that freely enter cells (e.g., urea) do not stimulate ADH release.

The hypothalamic osmoreceptors respond to changes in plasma osmolality of only 1% to 2%. The osmolar threshold for ADH release is approximately 280 mOsm/kg of body weight. Plasma ADH then increases 20% to 30% for each increase of 1 mOsm/kg in plasma osmolality. The generation of sufficient ADH to produce maximal retention of water and maximal urinary osmolality occurs when the plasma osmolality reaches 294 mOsm/kg. The osmolar threshold for the stimulation of thirst is close to or somewhat higher than that for ADH. Therefore, in defending normal body water content and tonicity, ADH secretion may precede the activation of thirst and is at least as important and more rapid.

ADH release is also stimulated by hypovolemia and hypotension (Figure 45-6). This is a much less sensitive response, requiring a 5% to 10% decrease in volume or blood pressure, that can be produced by hemorrhage, quiet standing, or positive-pressure breathing. The details of this pathway are given in Chapter 38. Severe hypovolemia and hypotension can override osmotic regulation and evoke large increases in plasma ADH, leading to water retention and a low plasma osmolality.

Pain, emotional stress, nausea and vomiting, heat, and a variety of drugs also stimulate ADH release. Ethanol, on the other hand, is a frequently encountered inhibitor that causes diuresis. Cortisol and thyroid hormone restrain ADH release; when they are deficient, ADH may be secreted even though the plasma osmolality is low.

A clinical syndrome of primary secretion of excess ADH in amounts inappropriate to the plasma osmolality occurs in a variety of settings. These include psychiatric or cerebral disease and pulmonary disease or tumor; it also occurs after major surgery and use of psychotropic drugs. Due to water retention, the plasma osmolality is low and can reach a point at which the patient becomes obtunded or has seizures. The restriction of water intake or the inhibition of ADH action is required to correct this situation, known as the **syndrome of inappropriate ADH secretion (SIADH).**

ADH circulates at basal concentrations of about 1 pg/mL (10^{-12} M). The plasma half-life is very short. Plasma levels of cosecreted neurophysin 2 also rise and fall in parallel with plasma levels of ADH.

Antidiuretic hormone acts on the kidney to conserve water

This action increases urine osmolality (**Figure 45–7**) to a maximum of about 1200 mOsm/kg at a plasma ADH level of 5 to 10 pg/mL. The details of ADH action via its plasma membrane V_2 receptor and cAMP as second messenger are given in Chapter 38.

Several factors can blunt the action of ADH on tubular cells. These include a mutant G protein, solute diuresis, chronic water loading (which reduces medullary hyperosmolality), K^+ deficiency, Ca^{++} excess, cortisol excess, and lithium administration. When any of these circumstances exist, the ineffectiveness of ADH leads to **nephrogenic diabetes insipidus.**

In addition to its major role in water metabolism, ADH subserves other functions. It contributes in a minor way to increasing vascular tone in response to hemorrhage. When ADH is administered systemically in large doses, it elevates the blood pressure and constricts the coronary and splanchnic beds. This action requires binding to a different V_1 receptor in vascular cells and is mediated by the phosphatidylinositol–protein kinase C second-

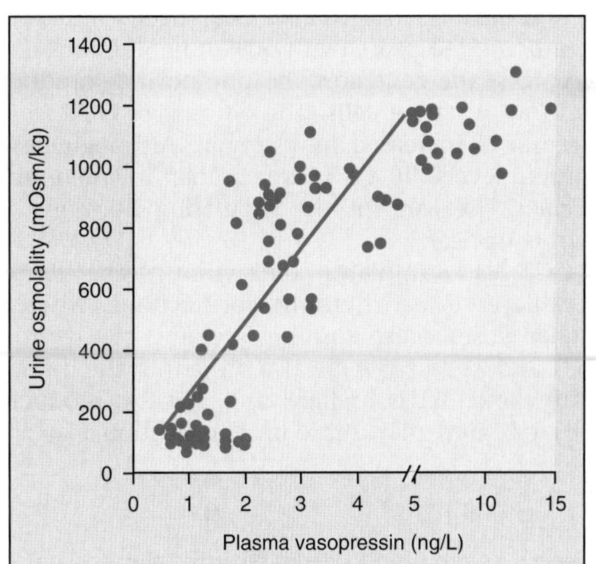

FIGURE 45–7. Relationship between urine osmolality and plasma ADH. Urine osmolality increases in proportion to plasma ADH until a maximum osmolality is reached at about 1200 mOsm/kg and an ADH level of 5 pg/mL. (Data from Berl T, Robertson G. In Brenner BM, ed: *The kidney,* ed 6, Philadelphia, 2000, WB Saunders.)

messenger system. ADH also functions as a hypothalamic releasing factor traveling down axons that project to the median eminence. Through another V_1 receptor, ADH stimulates the secretion of pituitary adrenocorticotropin, which in turn stimulates the secretion of adrenal cortisol.

Oxytocin is secreted in response to various reproductive needs

OCT is required for normal nursing. Known biologically as the milk let-down factor, it is secreted within seconds in response to suckling. Sensory receptors in the nipple generate afferent impulses that reach the hypothalamic paraventricular and supraoptic nuclei via various relays. A final cholinergic synapse causes the discharge of OCT and neurophysin 1 from the posterior pituitary in a manner similar to that of ADH. Continued suckling further stimulates the synthesis and transport of OCT to the posterior pituitary. In humans, there is little crossover secretion of ADH with suckling or of secretion of OCT with increased plasma osmolality. OCT secretion can also be stimulated by vaginal distention during sexual intercourse. The inhibition of OCT release by emotional distress can interfere with nursing.

Oxytocin acts on the breast and uterus

OCT causes the myoepithelial cells of the alveoli in the breast to contract. This forces the milk from the alveoli into the ducts and nipple, from which it is extracted by the infant. OCT acts via plasma membrane receptors (with 50% homology to ADH receptors) and generates phosphoinositide products and Ca^{++} in target cells. The binding of OCT to its receptor is increased by estrogen. Although basal plasma levels of OCT are similar in men and women, the role for the circulating hormone in men is unclear.

OCT also stimulates contraction of the uterus. Low doses cause rhythmic contractions, whereas higher doses cause sustained tetanic contraction. OCT and its receptor are also present in the human ovary and testis, where the locally produced hormone may play a role in reproduction.

There is controversial evidence regarding the function of maternal OCT in normal labor in humans, but the sustained contractions produced by OCT may be important in reducing blood loss from the uterus after the delivery of the conceptus. OCT in large doses is often used therapeutically to induce labor or to stop excessive postpartum bleeding.

The Anterior Pituitary Gland Secretes Numerous Hormones with Various Functions

The **anterior pituitary gland,** or **adenohypophysis,** makes up most of the 500 mg of pituitary tissue. It contains at least five types of endocrine cells, each being the source of a different hormone with a distinct function after which it is named. These cell types, their relative proportions in the pituitary, and their major secretory products are shown in **Figure 45–8**. Although the five types of functional cells aggregate in regions, they not only form unique enclaves but also are interspersed among one another. They vary somewhat in size and in the characteristics of their secretory granules, but they can be identified with certainty only by immunohistochemical staining of the hormones within. Cells that contain no known hormone are called **null cells.** They show evidence of protein hormone synthesis and contain a few secretory granules.

Each anterior pituitary cell is regulated by one or more hypothalamic neurohormones that reach it through the portal veins, as described previously. Three of the cell types produce hormones that regulate the function of the thyroid gland **(thyroid-stimulating hormone),** the adrenal glands **(adrenocorticotropic hormone),** and the gonads **(luteinizing hormone** and **follicle-stimulating hormone)**. The synthesis, secretion, and actions of these three tropic hormones are

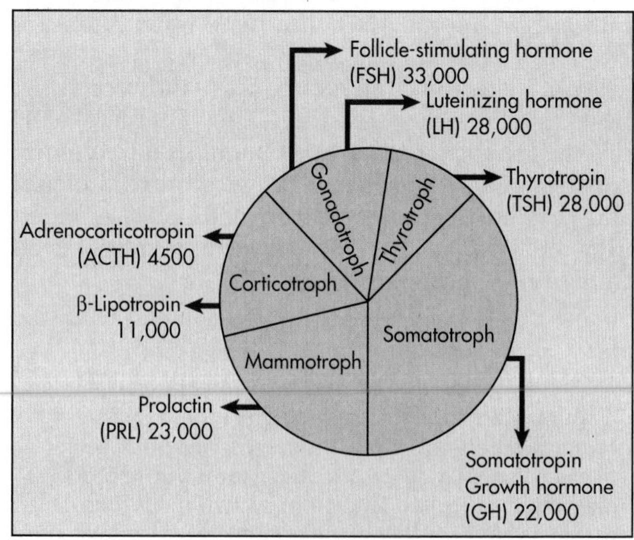

FIGURE 45–8. The relative proportions of cell types in the anterior pituitary gland, their major hormonal products, and the molecular weights of the products. Note the preponderance of cells secreting growth hormone and prolactin.

presented in conjunction with their peripheral target glands (see Chapters 46, 47, and 49). The differentiation of several types of anterior pituitary endocrine cells is stimulated by **Pit-1,** a transcription factor whose synthesis is increased by hypothalamic releasing hormones via cAMP as second messenger.

Mutations of Pit-1 cause hypoplasia of the anterior pituitary gland with deficient secretion of thyroid-stimulating hormone, growth hormone, and prolactin.

Growth hormone (somatotropin) stimulates growth and development

The major physiological effect of **growth hormone (GH)** is stimulation of postnatal somatic growth and development. Once childhood growth and puberty have been completed, GH continues to modulate the metabolism, body composition, and functional capabilities of adults.

GH is a hormone with profound anabolic action. In its absence, growth is stunted in humans. When the hormone is administered to unequivocally GH-deficient individuals, it causes prompt nitrogen retention and hypoaminoacidemia. Decreased urea production also results because the amino acids are diverted from oxidation to protein synthesis as growth ensues.

The synthesis and secretion of GH are stimulated and inhibited by hypothalamic factors and peripheral metabolic signals

Somatotrophs are the most numerous cells of the pituitary and are concentrated in its lateral wings (Figure 45-8). Their product, GH, is a single, large polypeptide chain with 191 amino acids and two disulfide bridges. Helical tertiary structures within the molecule are important in the binding of GH to its receptor. The human genome contains multiple genes that code for a family of molecules closely related to GH. Only one of these is expressed as normal pituitary GH. Messenger RNA directs the synthesis of a prehormone. After the removal of a signal peptide, the complete hormone is stored in granules. GH synthesis is increased by the specific hypothalamic peptide **growth hormone–releasing hormone (GHRH).** GHRH increases levels of cAMP, which with Pit-1 causes phosphorylation of a transcription factor for a cAMP response element on the GH gene. Thyroid hormone and cortisol also support GH synthesis.

GH secretion via exocytosis is stimulated by GHRH, which is a hypothalamic peptide with 44 amino acids. GHRH interacts with its plasma membrane receptor, after which Ca^{++}, phosphatidylinositol products, and cAMP are generated as second messengers.

Somatostatin, a hypothalamic peptide in either a 14- or a 28-amino acid form, is a powerful inhibitor of GH release. Somatostatin blocks GHRH stimulation noncompetitively. The inhibitor acts through its own plasma membrane receptor, in part by decreasing both the entry of Ca^{++} into the cells and the levels of cAMP. GH is secreted in pulses caused by the intermittent release of GHRH into portal pituitary vein blood. Somatostatin also diminishes the frequency and amplitude of GHRH pulses.

The secretion of GH is influenced by many factors (**Figure 45–9**). However, THE FINAL COMMON PATHWAY FOR MOST STIMULATORS OF GH IS AN INCREASE IN THE LEVELS OF GHRH, A DECREASE IN THE LEVELS OF SOMATOSTATIN, OR BOTH CHANGES. CONVERSELY, THE

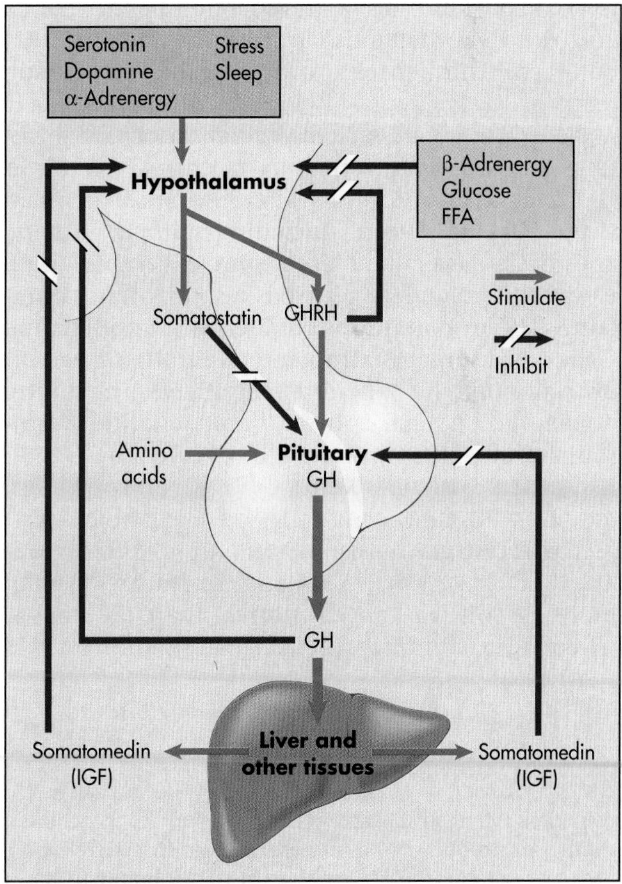

FIGURE 45–9. Regulation of GH secretion. Note that two hypothalamic peptides, one stimulatory (GHRH) and one inhibitory (somatostatin), regulate GH release. Negative feedback by insulin growth factor (IGF), the peripheral product, is exerted at the hypothalamic level by stimulating somatostatin release and at the pituitary level by directly suppressing responsiveness to GHRH. There is also complex regulation by substrates and neural influences. FFA, free fatty acid.

SUPPRESSORS OF GH DECREASE THE LEVELS OF GHRH, INCREASE THE LEVELS OF SOMATOSTATIN, OR CAUSE BOTH EFFECTS. Some agents can alter GH secretion via direct effects on the somatotroph.

The release of GH is regulated metabolically by the energy substrates glucose and free fatty acids and by amino acids. A sharp drop in the levels of either glucose or free fatty acid stimulates a large increase in the plasma levels of GH, whereas an elevation of the levels of either considerably reduces plasma GH levels. Protein ingestion or intravenous amino acid infusion stimulates GH release. Arginine is an especially effective amino acid. BOTH SHORT-TERM FASTING AND PROLONGED PROTEIN-CALORIE DEPRIVATION INCREASE GH SECRETION. IN CONTRAST, OBESITY REDUCES GH RESPONSES TO ALL STIMULI, INCLUDING GHRH.

A recently discovered endogenous stimulator of GH release is ghrelin, an acylated 28-amino acid peptide. Ghrelin, which also stimulates appetite (see Chapter 42), originates in both gastric glands and the hypothalamus. It synergizes with GHRH but acts through its own plasma membrane receptor.

Central nervous system regulation of GH secretion takes several forms. A nocturnal surge in GH occurs 1 to 2 hours after the onset of deep sleep. Various stresses, including trauma, surgery, anesthesia, fever, and even simple venipuncture, elevate plasma GH. Exercise is also a potent stimulant. These conditions influence hypothalamic GHRH and somatostatin neurons through a variety of monoamine neurotransmitters, including dopamine, norepinephrine, acetylcholine, serotonin, and γ-aminobutyric acid (Figure 45–9).

CHILDREN SECRETE MORE GH THAN ADULTS DO, ESPECIALLY DURING PUBERTY, WHEN ESTRADIOL AND TESTOSTERONE LEVELS RISE SHARPLY. IN AGED INDIVIDUALS, GH SECRETION DECLINES. Females are usually more responsive to GH stimuli than are males, reflecting a stimulatory effect of estradiol on GH synthesis.

Children who cannot secrete GH or respond to its actions grow at a reduced rate and are delayed in skeletal and sexual maturation. They are short in stature and modestly obese **(Figure 45–10)**. In some short children, deficiency is easily established because of the failure of plasma GH to rise acutely with any stimulus. In others, a fairly specific loss of nocturnal peaks or a diminution of total daily integrated secretion is used as evidence for a more subtle GH deficiency that justifies replacement therapy. GH secretion is reduced by a deficiency of thyroid hormone or by an excess of cortisol. In both conditions, the growth and maturation of children are also impaired.

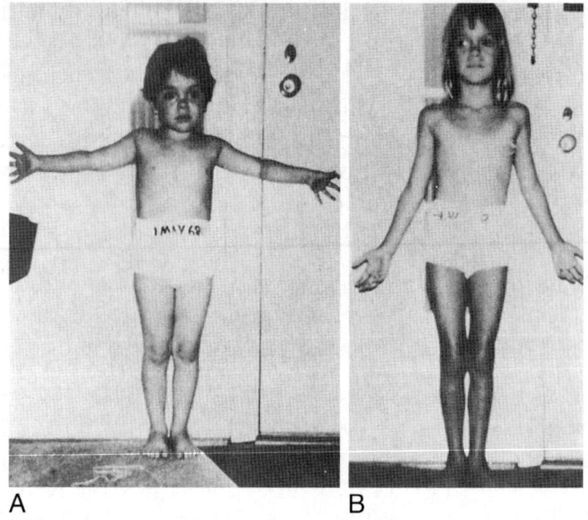

FIGURE 45–10. Effect of 15 months of GH replacement on a 6-year-old child with GH deficiency. Note that GH increases linear growth and decreases adiposity. (From Foster D, Wilson J, eds: *Williams textbook of endocrinology,* Philadelphia, 1985, WB Saunders.)

Resting basal plasma levels of GH are 1 to 5 ng/mL (10^{-10} M). The hormone circulates bound to a binding protein that is identical to the extracellular domain of plasma membrane GH receptors. Daily GH secretion is approximately 600 μg in prepubertal children, 1800 μg in individuals in late puberty, and 300 to 500 μg in adults.

Feedback regulation of GH secretion occurs at all levels (Figure 45–9). Long-loop negative feedback is exerted by **somatomedin,** which is a peripheral product of GH action (see the following section). Somatomedin inhibits the release of GHRH, inhibits the action of GHRH on the pituitary somatotroph, and stimulates somatostatin release. Short-loop negative feedback is exerted by GH itself via the stimulation of somatostatin release. Ultrashort-loop negative feedback is exerted by GHRH, possibly via synapses with somatostatin neurons.

Growth hormone acts through peripherally generated peptide mediators

GH interacts with several distinct plasma membrane receptors in target cells throughout the body. One GH molecule binds two neighboring receptor molecules. The intracellular tails of the receptors then "dock" and activate intracytoplasmic tyrosine kinases (see Chapter 5). The kinases phosphorylate transcription factor proteins, which mediate the effects of GH on gene expression. However, much of the growth-promoting effect of GH requires the peripheral generation of an entirely different family of peptides known as **somatomedins.** These peptides, which have a molecular weight of 7000, resemble proinsulin in structure (see Chapter 43). They were originally discovered in plasma and are commonly termed **insulin growth factors (IGFs).**

Two principal IGFs, their receptors, and the respective genes are well characterized. IGF-1 has 50% and IGF-2 has lesser amino acid homology with the A and B chains of insulin (see Chapter 43). IGFs are produced by many tissues in response to GH. However, circulating IGFs originate mainly in the liver, and the lag between the administration of GH and the subsequent increase in plasma IGF-1 and IGF-2 is about 12 hours. Both types of IGF circulate bound to a number of large insulin growth factor–binding proteins (IGFBPs) that regulate their availability to tissues. GH stimulates the production of some of these binding proteins, notably IGFBP-3, which is the most prevalent form, in the liver. The synthesis of IGFBP-1 is inhibited by insulin. The IGFBPs account for the relatively stable concentration and much longer half-lives of IGFs than that of GH itself. The IGFBPs are also synthesized in many tissues where they may modulate IGF actions. BOTH IGFs, BUT ESPECIALLY IGF-1, ARE GREATLY REDUCED IN THE PLASMA OF GH-DEFICIENT SUBJECTS.

Although IGFs can function as circulating hormones in classic endocrine fashion, they probably function mainly as locally produced hormones in paracrine and even autocrine fashion. GH induces the differentiation of precursor cells in target tissues—importantly, prechondrocytes in cartilage—into mature chondrocytes, which then express the IFG-1 gene under further GH stimulation. IGF-1 then acts through its own plasma membrane receptor, which has structural similarity to the insulin receptor and tyrosine kinase activity in the intracytoplasmic tail (see Chapter 43). (The IGF-2 receptor is dissimilar to both the IGF-1 and insulin receptors.) Pathways of mitogenic action downstream from the autophosphorylated IGF-1 receptor resemble those of insulin.

Insulin growth factors mediate the processes of growth

IGFs mediate the typical GH proliferative effects on cartilage, bone, muscle, adipose tissue, fibroblasts, and tumor cells in vitro. INDIVIDUALS WHO LACK THE ABILITY TO PRODUCE IGFs EXPERIENCE RETARDED GROWTH DESPITE HIGH GH LEVELS. Although fetal GH is not required for intrauterine growth, IGFs generated in the placenta or other fetal tissues may participate in regulating prenatal growth. A GH variant expressed in the placenta by a gene in the GH family probably stimulates the production of these growth factors. The IGF-2 gene and its receptor gene are expressed very early in fetal development.

During adolescence, plasma IGF-1 levels rise because of increases in GH secretion, with which they correlate. The progression of pubertal growth correlates with the increase in the levels of plasma IGF-1. Very tall people have a hyperresponsiveness to GHRH, which suggests that the GH secretory capacity is one determinant of final height.

In states of fasting and protein-calorie malnutrition, IGF levels in plasma are diminished; this finding correlates with the negative nitrogen balance in these conditions. Because GH levels are elevated in these catabolic states, factors other than GH must also regulate IGF production. In turn, the high GH levels most likely result from negative feedback caused by low IGF levels (Figure 45–9). IGF production is also diminished by cortisol and estrogens, hormones that antagonize GH action.

Insulin growth factors stimulate the processes of anabolism

GH, via IGFs, is a hormone with overall anabolic action (see Chapter 42). When it is administered to GH-deficient children or adults, it decreases plasma amino acid levels and urea production because the amino acids are shunted toward protein synthesis and away from oxidative degradation (see Chapter 42). The total body nitrogen balance, along with the related balances of the intracellular minerals K^+ and Pi, becomes positive. Lean body mass increases, whereas fat mass decreases. Bone formation is enhanced. The resting metabolic rate, exercise capacity, and sense of well-being all increase. These changes suggest that GH is essential to optimal health, even in adults. The decrease in GH with aging is likely to play a role in the changes of senescence, particularly in the declining lean body mass.

The multiplicity of GH targets and effects is indicated in **Figure 45–11**. The most striking and specific effect is the acceleration of linear growth (Figure 45–10) that results from GH action on the epiphyseal cartilage growth centers of long bones (see Chapter 44). All aspects of the metabolism of chondrocytes, the cartilage-forming cells, are stimulated. This includes the synthesis of collagen and the proteoglycan chondroitin, which together form the resilient extracellular matrix of cartilage. In addition, GH stimulates the synthesis and proliferation of proteins, RNA, and DNA in these cells. In support of the augmented protein synthesis, GH also stimulates the cellular uptake of amino acids.

Many tissues share in the anabolic response to GH. The width of bones increases, and in children, bone length increases. The visceral organs (i.e., liver, kidney, pancreas, intestines), endocrine glands (i.e., adrenals, parathyroids, pancreatic islets), skeletal muscle, heart, skin, and connective tissue all enlarge. This is also reflected in enhanced function of these organs.

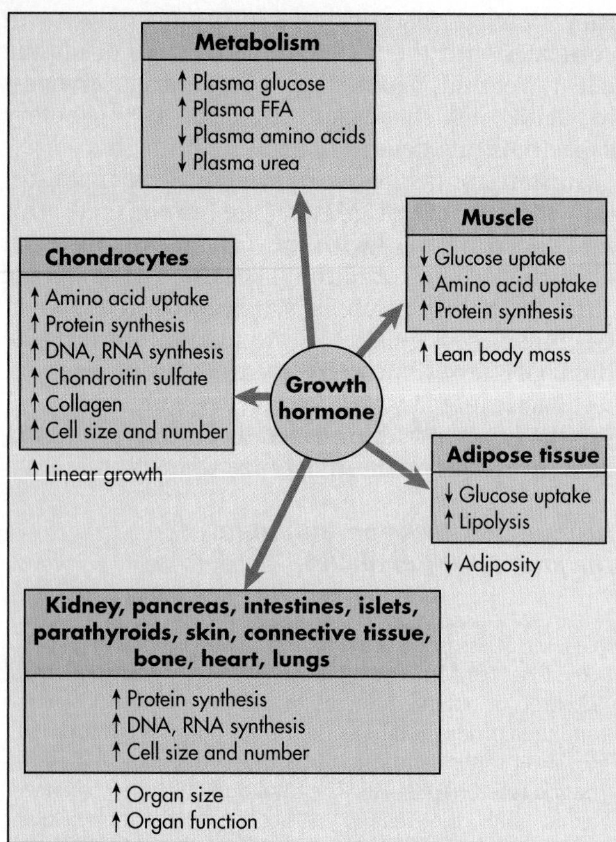

FIGURE 45–11. Overview of GH actions. FFA, free fatty acid.

Growth hormone opposes insulin actions

GH affects carbohydrate and lipid metabolism. It stimulates the expression of the insulin gene. HOWEVER, GH ALSO INDUCES RESISTANCE TO THE ACTION OF INSULIN. Glucose uptake by muscle and adipose cells is inhibited, and the plasma glucose concentration rises. Hyperinsulinemia results in compensation. In addition, GH enhances lipolysis and antagonizes insulin-stimulated lipogenesis. These actions increase plasma levels of free fatty acids and keto acids and decrease adipose tissue. Thus, GH is a diabetogenic hormone.

Sustained hypersecretion of GH from a slow-growing somatotroph tumor produces a unique syndrome called **acromegaly,** which reflects all these actions. In adults, the accumulation of excess soft tissue and the widening of bones lead to coarser features **(Figure 45–12)** and spadelike digits. Thick skin, enlarged muscles such as that in the tongue, and decreased subcutaneous fat are seen. Glomerular filtration and cardiac output are increased. Glucose intolerance or frank diabetes occurs in some individuals. Life expectancy is reduced via accelerated atherosclerosis. The diagnosis is confirmed by elevated plasma GH levels, which do not decrease when suppressive amounts of glucose are given, and by elevated IGF levels. If surgery is not curative, somatostatin analogues are effective treatment.

Growth hormone and insulin actions are also correlated

The secretion and actions of GH and insulin are metabolically coordinated:

- When protein and energy intake is ample, amino acids can be used for protein synthesis and growth. Thus, protein ingestion stimulates the secretion of both GH and insulin, and together, the hormones augment the production of IGFs. The IGFs in turn stimulate accretion of lean body mass. At the same time, the insulin-antagonistic effect of GH helps prevent hypoglycemia, which might otherwise result from the increased insulin secretion in the absence of ingested carbohydrate.
- When carbohydrate is ingested alone, insulin secretion is increased, but GH secretion is suppressed. In the absence of amino acids, the accelerated generation of IGFs is not advantageous. Insulin antagonism also is not necessary; on the contrary, unopposed expression of insulin action permits the efficient storage of excess carbohydrate calories.
- With fasting, insulin secretion falls, GH secretion rises, but IGF levels still decline. This combination seems appropriate in a situation in which protein catabolism is essential and protein synthesis must decline (see Chapter 42). However, the increase in GH is beneficial because it contributes to enhanced lipolysis and decreases peripheral tissue glucose use. This helps mobilize free fatty acids for oxidative purposes and helps provide glucose for central nervous system needs.

Prolactin is a protein hormone principally concerned with stimulating breast development and milk production in women

Prolactin (PRL) may play a role in reproductive function in both genders. The PRL-producing cells,

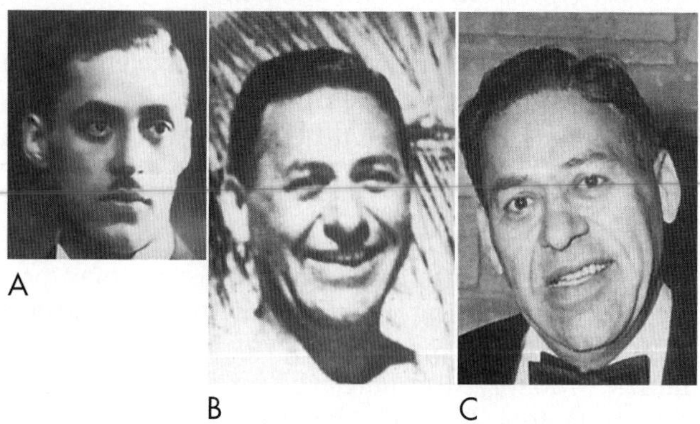

FIGURE 45–12. Coarsening of the face in a patient who developed GH hypersecretion (acromegaly). A, Age 24 years. B, Age 50 years. C, Age 58 years.

called **mammotrophs,** are the second most prevalent in the pituitary gland (Figure 45-8). They increase in number during pregnancy and lactation.

Pregnancy regulates the synthesis and secretion of prolactin

PRL is a single-chain protein with 198 amino acids and 3 disulfide bridges. It is structurally similar to GH, and the two genes are thought to have arisen from a common ancestor. The synthesis of PRL proceeds from a prehormone in the manner described for GH. Some molecules are also *N*-glycosylated and then secreted constitutively. A small number of pituitary cells called **mammosomatotrophs** secrete both PRL and GH. The transcription of the PRL gene is regulated by the same factors that regulate the secretion of the hormone.

THE MOST IMPORTANT INFLUENCE ON PRL SECRETION IS THE COMBINATION OF PREGNANCY, ELEVATED ESTROGEN LEVELS, AND NURSING (**Figure 45–13**). In preparation for lactation, PRL secretion increases steadily during pregnancy to a 20-fold plasma elevation. This is probably mediated by the high estrogen levels of pregnancy, which stimulates hyperplasia of the mammotrophs and transcription of the PRL gene. Although estrogen does not directly stimulate the release of PRL, it does enhance its release in response to other stimuli. If a new mother does not nurse her child, the plasma PRL level declines to the range that prevails in nonpregnant women by 6 weeks after delivery. Suckling, however, maintains elevated PRL levels for 8 to 12 weeks. PRL secretion rises at night and in conjunction with major stresses. The functional significance of such increases in PRL in these situations is unclear.

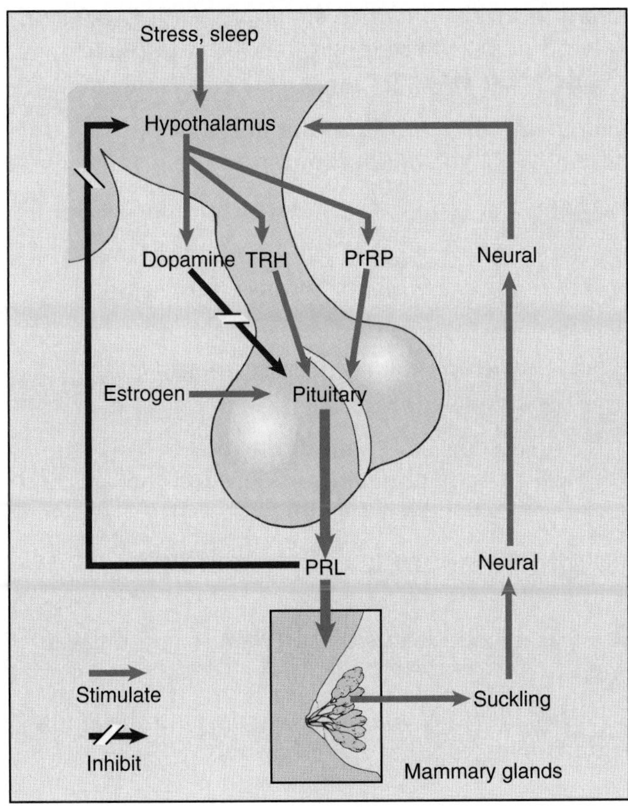

FIGURE 45–13. Regulation of PRL secretion. The predominant hypothalamic influence is normally inhibitory via dopamine. Pregnancy, high estrogen levels, and nursing (suckling) are the major physiological stimulators. TRH, thyrotropin-releasing hormone; PrRP, prolactin-releasing peptide. See text for details.

The hypothalamic regulation of prolactin secretion is both positive and negative

UNIQUE AMONG THE ANTERIOR PITUITARY HORMONES, THE SECRETION OF PRL IS PREDOMINANTLY UNDER INHIBITION BY HYPOTHALAMIC FACTORS (Figure 45–13). Disruption of pituitary connections to the hypothalamus leads to a great increase in PRL secretion, whereas the secretion rate of all other anterior pituitary hormones decreases. **Dopamine** released from the median eminence into the portal veins is the major hypothalamic inhibitory factor that suppresses the release and synthesis of PRL. Short-loop negative feedback also operates because PRL inhibits its own secretion by stimulating the synthesis and release of hypothalamic dopamine (Figure 45–13).

The hypothalamus is also the source of PRL-releasing factors. Thyrotropin-releasing hormone strongly stimulates the synthesis and release of PRL by acting through its receptors in mammotrophs. However, thyrotropin-releasing hormone probably does not primarily mediate the PRL response to nursing. A prolactin-releasing peptide homologous to vasoactive intestinal peptide has been found in hypothalamic neurons, whose axons also contact oxytocin neurons and project to the posterior pituitary. Given their physiological roles, some coordination between PRL and OCT is not unexpected.

Actions of prolactin

PRL PARTICIPATES IN STIMULATING THE ORIGINAL DIFFERENTIATION OF BREAST TISSUE AND ITS FURTHER EXPANSION DURING PREGNANCY. IT IS THE PRINCIPAL HORMONE RESPONSIBLE FOR LACTOGENESIS (MILK PRODUCTION). Together with estrogen, progesterone, cortisol, and GH, PRL stimulates the proliferation and branching of the breast ducts. During pregnancy, PRL, estrogen, and progesterone cause the development of glandular tissue (alveoli), within which milk production will occur. After parturition, milk synthesis and secretion require PRL along with cortisol and insulin.

PRL acts by combining with a plasma membrane receptor similar to that of GH and subsequently activating intracytoplasmic JAK-STAT tyrosine kinases. The result is a rapid transcription of RNAs for the milk proteins (casein, lactalbumin, and β-lactoglobulin) and enzymes such as galactosyltransferase—which is necessary for the synthesis of lactose, the major sugar in milk. These actions are antagonized by estrogen and progesterone.

A second area of PRL action may be on the reproductive axis. An excess of PRL blocks the synthesis and release of gonadotropin-releasing hormone and thus inhibits gonadotropin secretion. PRL also has immunomodulatory actions by suppressing proteins that enhance cytokine signaling.

Although the exact role of PRL in normal human reproduction is uncertain, an excess of PRL from a pituitary tumor has major consequences. Because the secretion of pituitary gonadotropins is suppressed, ovulation and menstruation are prevented in women, and spermatogenesis is blocked in men. Nonpregnant women secrete milk, and men may have breast enlargement. Surgical removal of the tumor and treatment with dopamine agonists reverse these effects.

Summary

- The hypothalamic-pituitary unit regulates water metabolism, growth, lactation, and the functions of the thyroid gland, adrenal glands, and gonads.
- Peptide hormones synthesized in some hypothalamic neurons pass down their axons to be stored in and released into the circulation from the posterior pituitary gland. Other hypothalamic peptides travel down axons to the median eminence, from which they are released into a portal venous circulation that carries them to the anterior pituitary gland. There, they stimulate or inhibit the release of target hormones.
- Hypothalamic releasing and inhibiting peptides are secreted in pulses and induce effects via Ca^{++}, cAMP, and phosphatidylinositol products as messengers. They stimulate or inhibit transcription, modulate translation, and stimulate or inhibit the secretion of target anterior pituitary hormones.
- ADH is a small peptide that is synthesized in the hypothalamus and secreted from the posterior pituitary in response to an increase in plasma osmolality or a decrease in plasma volume or blood pressure.
- ADH acts on renal tubule cells by use of cAMP as a second messenger to increase the reabsorption of free water and thus the final urine osmolality.
- OCT is structurally similar to ADH, but it acts specifically on the mammary gland to cause the release of milk. It is secreted in response to suckling.
- The anterior pituitary gland contains five functional cell types: thyrotrophs, adrenocorticotrophs, gonadotrophs, somatotrophs, and mammotrophs.
- GH is a protein hormone with anabolic effects. It stimulates cartilage development, bone growth, and the accretion of lean body mass, largely via a peptide mediator (IGF, or somatomedin) produced in the liver and many other target cells.
- GH secretion is stimulated by GHRH and inhibited by somatostatin. Glucose, free fatty acids, and the peripheral mediator IGF inhibit GH secretion.
- GH excess produces the disease acromegaly. GH deficiency in childhood leads to short stature and delayed maturation.
- PRL is structurally similar to GH, but it specifically stimulates the growth of mammary glands and the production of milk. Normally, PRL is tonically inhibited by dopamine from the hypothalamus.

Bibliography

Amato G et al: Body composition, bone metabolism, and heart structure and function in growth hormone (GH) deficient adults before and after GH replacement therapy at low doses, *J Clin Endocrinol Metab* 77:1671, 1993.

Asa SL, Horvath E, Kovacs KT: Functional pituitary anatomy and histology. In DeGroot LJ, Jameson JL, eds: *Endocrinology,* ed 4, Philadelphia, 2000, WB Saunders.

Berl T, Robertson GL: Pathophysiology of water metabolism. In Brenner BM, ed: *The kidney,* ed 6. Philadelphia, 2000, WB Saunders.

Cooke NE, Liebhaber SA: Molecular biology of the growth hormone–prolactin gene system, *Vitam Horm* 50:385, 1995.

Corpas E, Harman SM, Blackman MR: Human growth hormone and human aging, *Endocr Rev* 14:20, 1993.

Daughaday WH, Rotwein P: Insulin-like growth factors I and II: peptide, messenger ribonucleic acid and gene structures, serum, and tissue concentrations, *Endocr Rev* 10:68, 1989.

Freeman ME et al: Prolactin: structure, function, and regulation of secretion, *Physiol Rev* 80:1523, 2000.

Gimpl G, Fahrenholz F: The oxytocin receptor system: structure, function, and regulation, *Physiol Rev* 81:629, 2001.

Goffin V et al: Prolactin: the new biology of an old hormone, *Annu Rev Physiol* 64:47, 2002.

Horseman ND, Yu-Lee L-Y: Transcriptional regulation by the helix bundle peptide hormones: growth hormone, prolactin, and hematopoietic cytokines, *Endocr Rev* 15:627, 1994.

Kelly PA et al: The prolactin/growth hormone receptor family, *Endocr Rev* 12:235, 1991.

Kerrigan JR, Rogol AD: The impact of gonadal steroid hormone action on growth hormone secretion during childhood and adolescence, *Endocr Rev* 13:281, 1992.

Lee PD et al: Insulin-like growth factor binding protein-1: recent findings and new directions, *Proc Soc Exp Biol Med* 216:219, 1997.

Le Roith D et al: The somatomedin hypothesis, *Endocr Rev* 22:53, 2001.

Muller EE, Locatelli V, Cocchi D: Neuroendocrine control of growth hormone secretion, *Physiol Rev* 79:511, 1999.

Nielsen S et al: Aquaporins in the kidney: from molecules to medicine, *Physiol Rev* 82:205, 2002.

Patel YC: Neurotransmitters and neuromodulators in the control of anterior pituitary secretion. In DeGroot LJ, Jameson JL, eds: *Endocrinology,* ed 4, Philadelphia, 2000, WB Saunders.

Reichlin S: Neuroendocrinology. In Foster D et al, eds: *Williams textbook of endocrinology,* ed 9, Philadelphia, 1998, WB Saunders.

Rubinek T et al: Prolactin (PRL)–releasing peptide stimulates PRL secretion from human fetal pituitary cultures and growth hormone release from cultured pituitary adenomas, *J Clin Endocrinol Metab* 86:2826, 2001.

Theill LE, Karin M: Transcriptional control of growth hormone expression and anterior pituitary development, *Endocr Rev* 14:670, 1993.

Thissen JP, Ketelslegers JM, Underwood LE: Nutritional regulation of the insulin-like growth factors, *Endocr Rev* 15:80, 1994.

Thompson CJ, Selby P, Baylis PH: Reproducibility of osmotic and nonosmotic tests of vasopressin secretion in men, *Am J Physiol* 260:R533, 1991.

Thorner MO et al: The anterior pituitary. In Foster D et al, eds: *Williams textbook of endocrinology,* ed 9, Philadelphia, 1998, WB Saunders.

Case Studies

Case 45–1

A 49-year-old man complains of headache, sore feet from wearing the same shoes too many years ("Could my feet be growing?"), and a change in his facial appearance. His dentist has had to remake dental plates frequently. The patient's features appear coarse, and his hands are large and spade-like. Investigation for acromegaly reveals an elevated plasma GH level and a large pituitary tumor on magnetic resonance imaging.

1. **Which of the following genetic abnormalities could have produced this condition?**
   A. A mutant hyperactivating IGF gene
   B. A mutant hyperactivating IGF receptor gene
   C. A mutant inactivating IGF-1 gene
   D. A mutant hyperactivating GHRH receptor gene
   E. A mutant inactivating IGF-1 receptor gene

2. **Assuming the pituitary lesion is a monoclonal autonomous secreting GH-producing tumor, which of the following would you expect to find?**
   A. Increased GHRH release and increased IGF release
   B. Decreased GHRH release and decreased IGF release
   C. Decreased GHRH release and increased IGF release
   D. Increased GHRH release and decreased IGF release
   E. No change in GHRH or IGF release

3. **Which of the following metabolic changes from normal would be expected in the patient if he is maintained on a constant isocaloric and fixed-protein diet?**
   A. Decreased levels of IGF-1 binding protein
   B. Decreased levels of urea in urine
   C. Decreased plasma glucose levels after an oral glucose load

D. Decreased plasma insulin levels after an oral glucose load
E. Decreased plasma GH levels after an oral glucose load

Case 45–2

A 17-year-old girl sustains a severe head injury in a motorcycle accident and is virtually comatose for 3 days, requiring intravenous fluids (5% glucose in water) for maintenance. Beginning on the second day, she is noted to have a sharp increase in urine volume to 8 L/day. A quick check shows no glucose in her urine.

1. Which of the following would be expected?
A. Decreased serum osmolality
B. Decreased serum Na^+ levels
C. Decreased blood urea nitrogen levels
D. Increased plasma atrial natriuretic hormone levels
E. Decreased urine osmolality

2. The patient is treated with an intravenous infusion of ADH. This would result in which of the following?
A. Decreased cAMP levels in urine
B. Increased blood pressure
C. Increased serum osmolality
D. Decreased serum K^+ levels
E. Decreased plasma cortisol levels

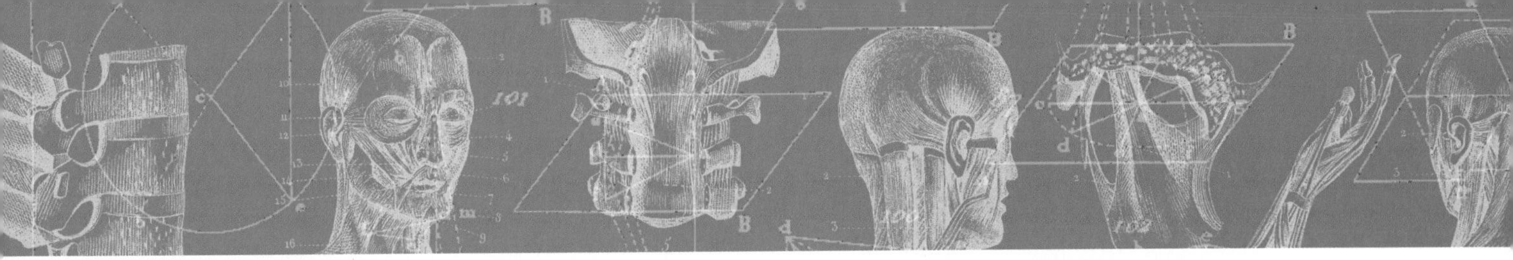

Chapter 46: Thyroid Gland

Objectives

- Explain the synthesis of thyroid hormones and the unique role of iodide therein.
- Explicate the regulation of thyroid hormone secretion by the hypothalamic–anterior pituitary axis and the reciprocal negative feedback of thyroid hormone on this axis.
- Describe how binding to serum proteins and the metabolism of thyroid hormone are important determinants of the hormone's effect on tissue.
- Describe the overriding effects of thyroid hormone on general metabolic processes.
- Explain the intracellular mechanism of thyroid hormone action.
- Delineate the profound effects of thyroid hormone on human physical and mental development.

The thyroid gland was the first endocrine gland to be recognized as such. Its absence or enlargement was correlated with altered biological findings at distant body sites, providing the clue that it produces a substance reaching tissue targets via the bloodstream. Extracts of the thyroid gland were subsequently shown to correct the striking disease state that resulted from its absence. The thyroid gland produces two hormones, **thyroxine (T_4)** and **triiodothyronine (T_3),** at a rather steady pace. THESE HORMONES INCREASE THE RATE OF BASAL O_2 USE AND METABOLISM AND THE CONSEQUENT RATE OF HEAT PRODUCTION SO THAT THYROID HORMONE LEVELS ARE ADJUSTED TO ALTERATIONS IN ENERGY NEED, CALORIE SUPPLY, AND ENVIRONMENTAL TEMPERATURE. Thyroid hormones concordantly modulate the delivery of substrates and O_2 by the cardiovascular and respiratory systems to sustain the metabolic rate in target tissues. The actions of thyroid hormone are critical for the normal growth and maturation of the fetus and the child. Virtually all other previously described organ systems in the body are affected by thyroid hormone.

Functional Anatomy

The thyroid gland develops from the endoderm of the pharyngeal gut. The gland descends to the anterior neck, where it lies adjacent to both sides of the trachea and can often be palpated **(Figure 46–1, *A*)**. It can also be visualized by several imaging techniques (e.g., nuclear scanning after administration of a radioactive iodine tracer, ultrasonography). By 12 weeks of human gestation, the gland synthesizes and secretes thyroid hormones under the stimulus of the fetal hypothalamus and pituitary gland. THIS ENTIRE AXIS IS REQUIRED FOR SUBSEQUENT NORMAL INTRAUTERINE DEVELOPMENT OF THE CENTRAL NERVOUS SYSTEM AND SKELETON because neither maternal thyroid hormone nor its pituitary-stimulating hormone can cross the placenta in sufficient quantities after the first trimester.

The thyroid gland in adults weighs approximately 20 g. The histological structure is shown schematically in Figure 46–1, *B*. The cuboidal endocrine cells are surrounded by a basement

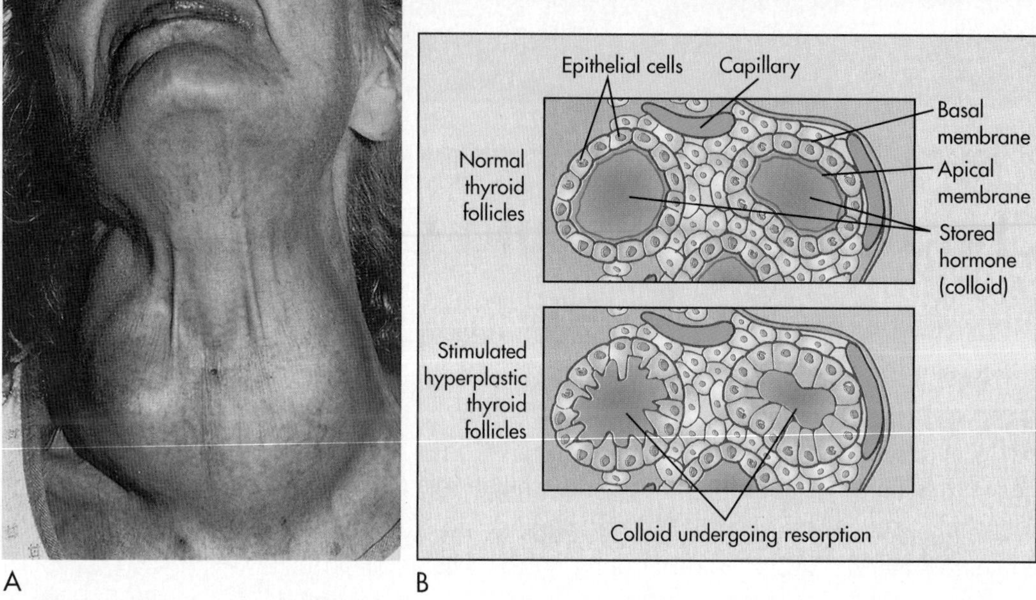

FIGURE 46–1. A, The anterior location of the thyroid gland permits visualization and palpation when it is enlarged and forms a goiter. B, Basic thyroid unit. A normal follicle consists of a central core of colloid material surrounded by a single layer of cuboidal cells. When stimulated by thyrotropin, the cells elongate, and the central core becomes scalloped because of resorption of the colloid.

membrane, and they form single-layered circular **follicles.** The lumens of the follicles contain thyroid hormones stored in the form of a **colloid** material. When they are stimulated, the endocrine cells enlarge and assume a columnar shape with the nuclei at their base. Because it is undergoing resorption, the colloid material in the lumen appears scalloped. Also scattered within the thyroid gland are the parafollicular cells, or C cells, which secrete calcitonin (see Chapter 44).

The synthesis of thyroid hormones is a stepwise process requiring iodine

Thyroid hormones are unique in that they incorporate an inorganic element, iodine, into an organic structure made up of two molecules of the amino acid tyrosine. The secretory products of the thyroid gland are known as **iodothyronines.** THE MAJOR PRODUCT IS **3,5,3′,5′-tetraiodothyronine,** KNOWN AS **THYROXINE** AND REFERRED TO AS **T_4.** This molecule functions largely as a circulating prohormone. Secreted in much less quantity is **3,5,3′-triiodothyronine,** known simply as **triiodothyronine** and referred to as **T_3.** This molecule, which provides almost all thyroid hormone activity in target cells, is produced mostly in various tissues from the circulating supply of the prohormone T_4. A trivial secretory product with no identified hormonal action is **3,3′,5′-triiodothyronine.** This is known as **reverse T_3 (rT_3)** because it differs from T_3 only in the location of one of the three iodine atoms. This inactive molecule is an alternative product of the prohormone T_4 and is produced when less thyroid hormone action is needed. The structures of T_4, T_3, and rT_3 are shown in **Figure 46–2.**

Three major steps are involved in the synthesis of thyroid hormones: (1) the uptake and concentration of iodide (I^-) within the gland, (2) the oxidation and incorporation of the I^- into the phenol ring of tyrosine, and (3) the coupling of two iodinated tyrosine molecules to form either T_4 or T_3 **(Figure 46–3).**

Before iodination and coupling, the tyrosine molecules must first be incorporated by standard peptide linkage into a protein known as **thyroglobulin.** Thyroglobulin is the substance actually iodinated on specific constituent tyrosines that are brought into proximity for coupling by the three-dimensional structure of the protein. The thyroid hormones formed remain in peptide linkage within thyroglobulin, and their release into the circulation requires proteolytic cleavage of the peptide bonds.

Step 1: Iodide metabolism is an intrinsic component of thyroid hormone synthesis

Iodide is an essential dietary element because of its thyroid role. The minimum daily I^- requirement for hormone synthesis is about 80 µg. In the United States, the average daily intake of I^- is 300 to 400 µg, and almost the same amount is excreted in the urine. About 80 µg, or 20% of the extrathyroidal I^- pool, is taken up daily by the gland. With I^-

3,5,3'5'-Tetraiodothyronine (thyroxine, or T_4)

3,5,3'-Triiodothyronine (T_3)

3,3',5'-Triiodothyronine (reverse T_3)

FIGURE 46–2. Structures of T_4, T_3, and rT_3. Note that T_3 and rT_3 differ only in the position from which an iodine atom was removed from T_4.

deficiency, the extrathyroidal pool of I^- shrinks; however, the gland can increase the daily percentage uptake to 80% to 90% and thereby still acquire sufficient I^- for hormone synthesis. A decrease in urinary excretion helps conserve I^-, as does the preferential synthesis of T_3 over T_4. Under steady-state conditions, about 80 μg of I^- is released from the gland daily, 90% in the form of T_4. The content of I^- within the thyroid gland is 100 times greater than the amount needed daily for hormone production. Because all this I^- is stored in the form of iodinated thyroglobulin, the human is protected for approximately 2 months from the effects of I^- deficiency.

I^- IS ACTIVELY TRANSPORTED INTO THE THYROID GLAND AGAINST CHEMICAL AND ELECTRICAL GRADIENTS BY A $2Na^+$-$1I^-$ COTRANSPORT SYSTEM LOCATED IN THE BASAL MEMBRANE OF THE CELLS (see Chapter 37). This $2Na^+$-$1I^-$ symporter (NIS), known as the **I^- trap,** maintains a high ratio of free [I^-] in the gland to the [I^-] in the plasma. One I^- atom is transported into the cell against an I^- gradient, while two Na^+ move down their gradient into the cell. This trapping mechanism requires energy generation via oxidative phosphorylation and is linked to a Na^+,K^+-ATPase in the plasma membrane. Various anions, such as thiocyanate (CNS^-), perchlorate (ClO_4^-), and

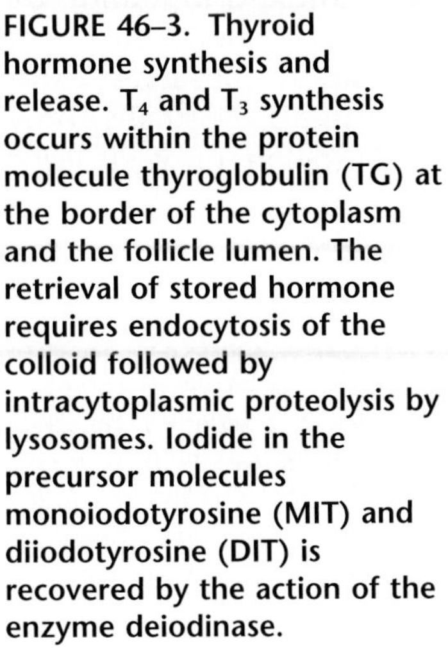

FIGURE 46–3. Thyroid hormone synthesis and release. T_4 and T_3 synthesis occurs within the protein molecule thyroglobulin (TG) at the border of the cytoplasm and the follicle lumen. The retrieval of stored hormone requires endocytosis of the colloid followed by intracytoplasmic proteolysis by lysosomes. Iodide in the precursor molecules monoiodotyrosine (MIT) and diiodotyrosine (DIT) is recovered by the action of the enzyme deiodinase.

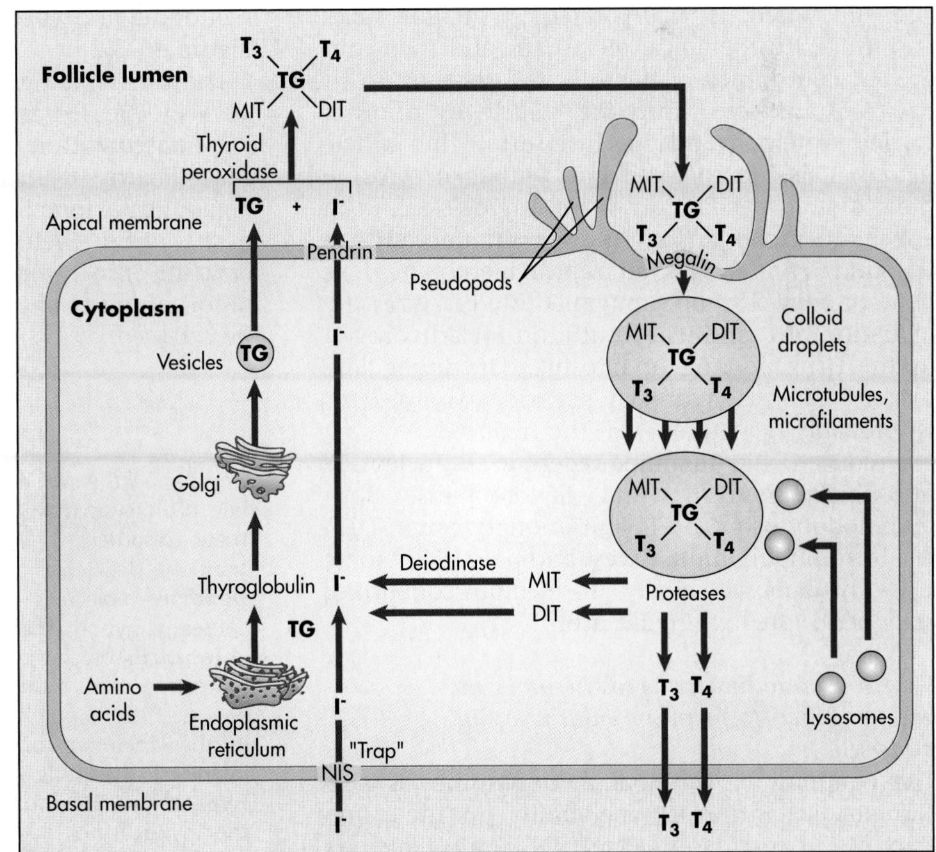

pertechnetate (TcO_4^-), act as competitive inhibitors of I^- transport.

Iodide is not plentiful in the environment, and deficiency of I^- is a major cause of **hypothyroidism** in such varied areas of the world as China and the Peruvian Andes. This tragic form of endemic **cretinism** (see later) can easily be prevented by public health programs that add I^- to table salt or that provide yearly injections of a slowly absorbed I^- preparation. The Environmental Protection Agency has also raised concerns about contamination of food or water with ClO_4^- and a potential hazard of hypothyroidism. The NIS gene is repressed by I^-. Mutations of NIS cause hypothyroidism and **goiter** (thyroid enlargement).

Small increases in dietary I^- intake lead to increases in the rate of thyroid hormone synthesis. However, as the daily dosage of I^- exceeds 2000 μg, the intraglandular concentration of free I^- or some iodinated product reaches a level that inhibits the I^- trap and the biosynthetic mechanism; thus, the hormone production declines back to normal.

Step 2: Tyrosine is iodinated within a storage protein called thyroglobulin

Thyroglobulin is a large glycoprotein that is synthesized as two separate peptide units. These combine and are then glycosylated in transit to the Golgi apparatus. The completed protein, which is also sulfonated, is incorporated in small vesicles and moves to the apical membrane and then into the adjacent lumen of the follicle (Figure 46–3).

I^- is transported into the follicle by another carrier protein, **pendrin.** Just inside the follicle lumen, I^- is incorporated into particular tyrosine molecules at specific sites within thyroglobulin. An enzyme complex known as **thyroid peroxidase** is bound to and traverses the apical membrane. This hemoprotein enzyme simultaneously catalyzes the oxidation of I^- and its substitution for a hydrogen in the benzene ring of tyrosine. The immediate oxidant of I^- is hydrogen peroxide (H_2O_2). This is probably generated via the reduction of O_2 by reduced nicotinamide adenine dinucleotide phosphate (NADPH) and flavoproteins. Both monoiodotyrosine (MIT) and diiodotyrosine (DIT) result from iodination. Excess and potentially toxic H_2O_2 is disposed of by a selenium-containing enzyme, thioredoxin reductase.

Step 3: Two iodinated tyrosine molecules are combined to form an iodothyronine molecule

The coupling of two iodinated tyrosines is also carried out within thyroglobulin by the same enzyme, peroxidase. One DIT molecule is juxtaposed either with another DIT molecule to form T_4 or with an MIT molecule to form T_3. The tertiary structure of thyroglobulin facilitates these juxtapositions. The usual ratio of T_4 to T_3 in the gland is 10:1. When I^- availability is restricted or when the thyroid gland is hyperstimulated, the formation of T_3 is favored; in this way, relatively more active hormone is provided.

Secretion of thyroid hormone requires its retrieval from storage in the follicle

Once thyroglobulin has been iodinated, it is stored within the follicle as **colloid.** The release of peptide-bonded T_4 and T_3 into the bloodstream first requires the retrieval of the thyroglobulin, which is transferred from the lumen of the follicle into the endocrine cell via **endocytosis** (Figure 46–3). In this process, facilitated by a receptor-like molecule called **megalin,** the cell membrane forms pseudopods, which engulf a pocket of colloid that is pinched off by the cell membrane and becomes a colloid droplet within the cytoplasm. The droplet moves in a basal direction, probably as a result of microtubule and microfilament function. At the same time, lysosomes move from the base toward the apex of the cell and fuse with the colloid droplets. Lysosomal proteases then release free T_4 and T_3, which leave the cell through the basal membrane and enter the adjacent capillary blood (Figure 46–3).

The uncoupled MIT and DIT molecules, which are also released from thyroglobulin, are rapidly deiodinated within the cell by the enzyme **deiodinase** (Figure 46–3). Because these compounds are metabolically inactive and, if secreted, would be lost in the urine, their deiodination conserves I^- for recycling into hormone synthesis. Normally, only minor amounts of intact thyroglobulin itself leave the cell.

Any step in the sequence from I^- trapping to thyroglobulin proteolysis may be defective in congenital biosynthetic disorders, and these defects result in thyroid hormone deficiency (hypothyroidism). Mutant NIS and **pendrin** molecules have already been identified as causes of hypothyroidism. A group of drugs known as **thiouracils** block the enzyme peroxidase and are useful in treating states of thyroid hyperfunction. A large excess of I^- itself, its competitive anion ClO_4^-, or Li^+ (widely used in the treatment of manic-depressive disorders) also inhibits T_4 synthesis. Iodide is sometimes used to treat **hyperthyroidism** for short periods until more definitive therapy takes hold.

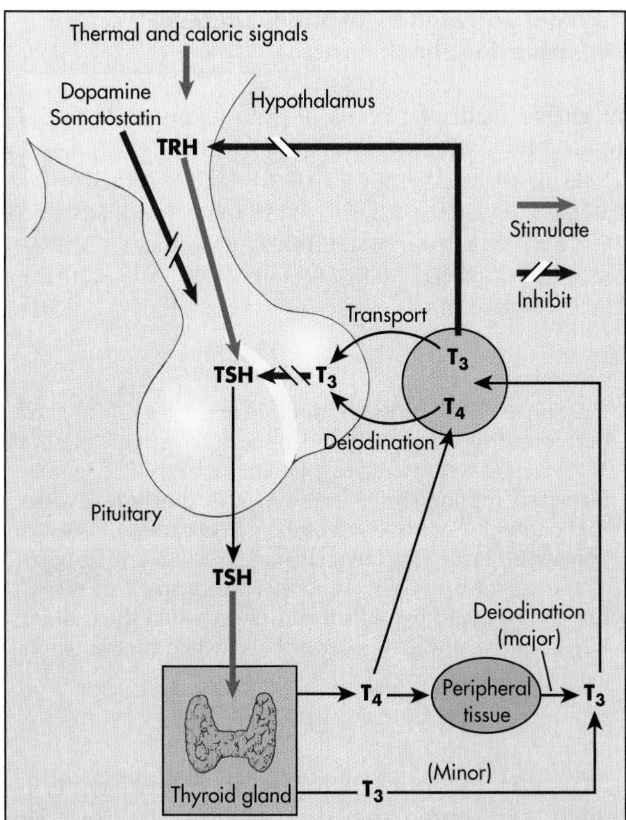

FIGURE 46–4. Hypothalamic-pituitary-thyroid axis. Thyrotropin-releasing hormone (TRH) stimulates the release of thyrotropin (TSH) from the pituitary gland. Thyrotropin stimulates T_4 secretion and to a minor degree T_3 secretion by the thyroid gland. T_3 arising from T_4 in peripheral tissues or within the pituitary gland itself blocks the effect of TRH and suppresses the release of thyrotropin via negative feedback. Dopamine and somatostatin also tonically inhibit thyrotropin release.

Thyroid Gland Activity Is Regulated by the Hypothalamus and Anterior Pituitary Gland

The thyroid gland is the effector component of a classic hypothalamic–anterior pituitary–peripheral gland axis (**Figure 46–4**; see Chapter 45). The major stimulator of thyroid hormone secretion is **thyrotropin,** or **thyroid-stimulating hormone (TSH),** which is secreted by the anterior pituitary gland. The direct stimulator of TSH secretion is **thyrotropin-releasing hormone (TRH)** from the hypothalamus. Via negative feedback, the thyroid hormones T_4 and T_3 inhibit the synthesis and release of TSH from the pituitary gland as well as TRH synthesis and release from the hypothalamus.

Thyrotropin-releasing hormone stimulates the synthesis and release of thyroid-stimulating hormone

TRH is a tripeptide, pyroglutamine-histidine-proline amide. The TRH gene codes for a large precursor molecule that contains the small tetrapeptide glutamine-histidine-proline-glycine. After translation, the glutamic acid undergoes cyclization, and the terminal glycine is replaced with an amino group. TRH is stored in the median eminence (see Chapter 45) and reaches its target cells via the pituitary portal vein. TRH binding to its plasma membrane receptor triggers increases in Ca^{++} and phosphatidylinositol product second messengers, which elicit TSH release via exocytosis. Prolonged stimulation with TRH also increases TSH synthesis and, via glycosylation, its bioactivity. TRH eventually down-regulates its own receptors and thereby diminishes its effectiveness.

Thyrotropin stimulates numerous processes involved in the growth and secretory activity of the thyroid gland

TSH is a glycoprotein hormone whose molecular weight is 28,000. It is composed of two peptide subunits that are encoded by separate genes on two different chromosomes. The α subunit is "nonspecific" because it is also part of two other pituitary tropic hormones (luteinizing and follicle-stimulating hormones) and chorionic gonadotropin from the placenta, all with reproductive function. In contrast, the β subunit of TSH is completely different and contains the specific biologically active sites of the hormone. Nonetheless, via noncovalent forces, the β subunit must be combined with the α subunit for TSH to stimulate thyroid cells. TSH is also sulfonated.

TSH circulates in concentrations of about 10^{-11} M. For technical reasons, these are usually reported in units of biological activity; the normal range is approximately 0.4 to 5.5 μU/mL. The α subunit also circulates.

TSH acts on the follicular cells of the thyroid gland to produce many effects, which are summarized in **Figure 46–5**. THE PROCESSES OF I^- TRAPPING (INCLUDING EXPRESSION OF THE NIS GENE) AND OF EACH STEP IN T_4 AND T_3 SYNTHESIS, AS WELL AS THE ENDOCYTOSIS OF COLLOID AND THE PROTEOLYTIC RELEASE OF T_4 AND T_3 FROM THE GLAND, ARE ALL RAPIDLY STIMULATED BY TSH. Sustained exposure to TSH leads to hyperplasia and hypertrophy of the follicular cells (Figure 46–1, *B*), which is manifested by increases in endoplasmic reticulum, ribosomes, size and complexity of the Golgi apparatus, and DNA synthesis. In the

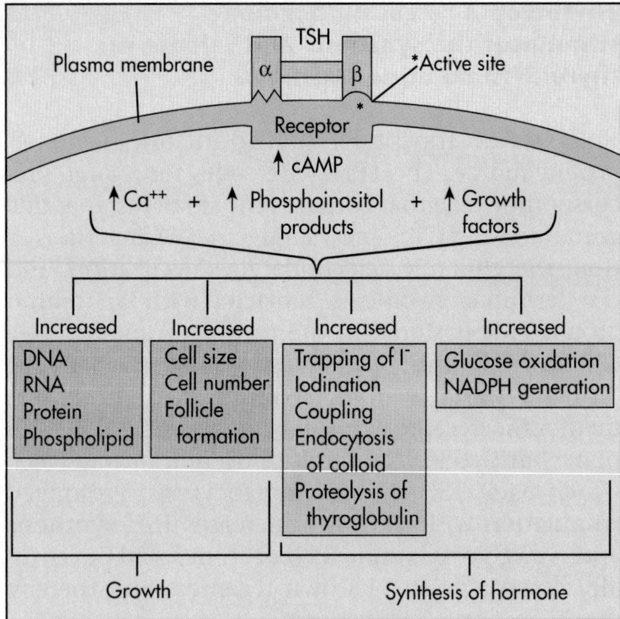

FIGURE 46–5. TSH actions on the thyroid cell. cAMP along with Ca^{++} and phosphoinositol products act as second messengers generated by TSH binding to its receptor. All steps in thyroid hormone production, as well as many aspects of thyroid cell metabolism and growth, are stimulated by TSH. α, α subunit; β, β subunit.

absence of TSH, the gland atrophies, although it still maintains a low basal level of thyroid hormone secretion. The trophic effects of TSH on the thyroid gland may be mediated by the local generation of growth factors such as insulin growth factors (IGF-1, IGF-2; see Chapter 45). TSH binding to its plasma membrane receptor activates adenylyl cyclase via a stimulatory G protein (see Chapter 5). cAMP then mediates the stimulation of I^- uptake by the cell. The phosphatidylinositol system may participate with cAMP in rapidly stimulating the peroxidase-catalyzed subsequent steps in thyroid hormone synthesis. Concurrently, TSH increases glucose oxidation, which may provide the NADPH needed for the peroxidase reaction. After several hours, TSH increases nucleic acid, protein, and phospholipid synthesis, actions that underlie the growth-promoting effects of TSH.

The trophic effects of TSH are commonly expressed pathophysiologically. A genetic biosynthetic defect, an acquired impairment of thyroid hormone synthesis caused by inflammation or drugs, and I^- deficiency all increase TSH secretion via negative feedback. Chronic stimulation of the thyroid gland by TSH hypersecretion may then produce a spectacular enlargement of the gland, known as a **goiter** (Figure 46–1, *A*).

Thyroid hormone output is under sensitive feedback control

Negative feedback keeps plasma levels of T_4 and T_3 relatively constant. INCREASES AND DECREASES IN THYROID HORMONE LEVELS OF ONLY 10% TO 30% ARE ENOUGH TO CHANGE TSH LEVELS (AND THEIR RESPONSE TO TRH) IN THE OPPOSITE DIRECTION. NEGATIVE FEEDBACK IS EXERTED PREDOMINANTLY AT THE PITUITARY LEVEL (Figure 46–4).

Individuals with long-standing deficiencies of thyroid hormone from thyroid gland disease have high plasma TSH levels as well as enlarged pituitary glands that contain increased numbers of thyrotroph cells and an elevated TSH content. Conversely, a pathological excess of thyroid hormone causes very low plasma TSH levels and atrophy of the thyrotroph cells. Abnormalities of the TSH receptor lead to hyperthyroidism and goiter when the mutant is hyperactive and to hypothyroidism when the mutant is inactive.

The effector molecule of negative feedback is T_3, which can enter the thyrotroph cell from the plasma. However, the T_3 generated within the pituitary gland by the deiodination of T_4 that is taken up from the plasma is more important (Figure 46–4). T_3 suppresses TSH release, represses transcription of the TSH gene, and down-regulates TRH receptors.

TSH secretion is also tonically inhibited by dopamine and somatostatin from the hypothalamus. Cortisol and growth hormone reduce TSH secretion as well, growth hormone probably by stimulating somatostatin release (see Chapter 45).

The operation of the hypothalamic-pituitary-thyroid axis results in a slightly pulsatile plasma TSH level and steady plasma T_4 and T_3 levels. This befits hormones whose actions on metabolism wax and wane slowly. Physiological conditions that alter TSH levels (and therefore T_4 and T_3 levels) are consonant with the action of thyroid hormones on energy use and thermogenesis. During total fasting, TSH responsiveness to TRH stimulation and possibly TRH release itself are diminished; T_3 levels also fall. This coincides with an advantageous decrease in the resting metabolic rate (see Chapter 42). In contrast, the ingestion of excess calories, especially carbohydrates, tends to increase T_3 availability. In animals, exposure to cold increases the secretion of TSH and thyroid hormone. In humans, this response is observed shortly after birth, when the change in temperature from the maternal to the external environment is accompanied by a sharp rise in plasma TSH and T_4 levels. The T_4 level remains above adult levels for some weeks.

The Metabolism of Thyroid Hormone Contributes to Its Actions

T_4 serves largely as a prohormone for T_3, but T_4 may provide some intrinsic intracellular action of its own. The average daily secretion of T_4 is 90 μg. The circulating storage function of plasma T_4 is reflected in its large pool size and long half-life (6 days). In contrast, the major portion of T_3 (35 μg/day) and virtually all rT_3 come from the deiodination of circulating T_4. T_3 has a much smaller pool size and a shorter half-life (1 day). Average plasma concentrations are T_4, 8 μg/dL; T_3, 0.12 μg/dL; and rT_3, 0.04 μg/dL.

The replacement of thyroid hormone in deficient individuals is almost always carried out with the prohormone, T_4, and not with the more active metabolite, T_3. This is done to mimic the physiological situation. The biochemical targets are a normal level of T_4 and a reduction to normal (via negative feedback) of TSH levels if they are elevated, as in primary hypothyroidism.

Protein binding of thyroid hormones determines their availability to tissues

T_4 and T_3 circulate almost entirely bound to proteins. The major binding protein is **thyroxine-binding globulin (TBG),** a glycoprotein that is synthesized in the liver. Each TBG molecule binds one molecule of T_4. About 70% of T_4 and T_3 is bound to TBG. The remainder is bound to **transthyretin** (thyroxine-binding prealbumin) and albumin. Transthyretin has a lower affinity for T_4 than TBG does and more readily transfers the hormone to target cells by dissociation. By creating a circulating reservoir of T_4, TBG and transthyretin buffer against acute changes in thyroid gland function. Even the sudden addition to the plasma of an entire day's thyroid gland output would cause only a 10% increase in the circulating T_4 concentration. After removal of the gland, it would take nearly 1 week for the plasma T_4 concentration to fall 50%.

Only 0.03% of total T_4 and 0.3% of total T_3 are in the free state. However, these are the critical biologically active fractions. Free T_4 and T_3 not only exert the thyroid hormone effects on target tissues but also are responsible for pituitary feedback. A chemical equilibrium between T_4 and TBG governs the distribution of the hormone between the free T_4 and bound $T_4 \cdot TBG$ fractions:

$$T_4 + TBG \leftrightarrow T_4 \cdot TBG \tag{46-1}$$

$$K_{eq} = \frac{[T_4 \cdot TBG]}{[T_4][TBG]} \tag{46-2}$$

$$\frac{\text{Free } T_4}{\text{Bound } T_4} = \frac{[T_4]}{[T_4 \cdot TBG]} = \frac{1}{K_{eq}[TBG]} \tag{46-3}$$

where K_{eq} is the equilibrium constant.

A temporary decrease in the plasma free T_4 level caused by a decrease in thyroid gland secretion can be rapidly reversed via a dissociation of bound T_4 (see Equation 46-1). Likewise, a temporary increase in free T_4 can be rapidly compensated for by the association of the excess T_4 with TBG, which has additional unoccupied binding sites. Sustained decreases or increases in the daily T_4 supply caused by thyroid disease, however, eventually lead to comparable sustained alterations in both the bound and free fractions.

A primary change in the TBG concentration itself disturbs the ratio of free to bound T_4 (see Equation 46-3). In this situation, the normal thyroid gland must increase or decrease its rate of hormone secretion until the new equilibrium state restores the absolute free T_4 level to normal. So long as thyroid gland function is normal, alterations in TBG do not cause disturbances in biological function.

Acute hepatic disease, pregnancy, or estrogen therapy raises serum TBG levels. In severe chronic hepatic disease (such as **cirrhosis**) or kidney disease (such as the **nephrotic syndrome**), serum TBG levels fall because of either reduced synthesis or loss of TBG in the urine. Any resultant changes in free T_4 levels are transient because negative feedback alters TSH secretion and thyroid gland secretion so that free T_4 levels can be restored to normal.

The metabolic fate of thyroid hormones determines their action

The liver, kidney, and skeletal muscle are the major sites of degradation of thyroid hormones. The rate of disposal of T_4 is proportional to the free T_4 concentration in plasma.

Because T_4 is only 25% as hormonally active as T_3, the initial step of converting it either to the active metabolite T_3 (by outer-ring deiodination; Figure 46–2) or to the inactive metabolite rT_3 (by inner-ring deiodination) is an important means of adjusting thyroid hormone action on tissues. Normally, the split between T_3 and rT_3 is equal. When it is physiologically desirable to have more thyroid hormone action, as in exposure to cold, more T_3 and less rT_3 are generated. The opposite, less T_3 and more rT_3, commonly occurs in critically ill persons and portends a poor outcome. There is one inner-ring **5 deiodinase** and two outer-ring **5′ deiodinases**. The 5′ deiodinases, which catalyze the conversion of T_4 to T_3, are important regulators of thyroid hormone activity. The 5 deiodinase converts T_4 to inactive rT_3. The rare trace element selenium, replacing the sulfur in cysteine, is necessary for the activity of these enzymes.

The Intracellular Actions of Thyroid Hormone Are Mediated by Nuclear Receptors and Changes in Gene Expression

T_4 and T_3 enter target cells via carrier-mediated, energy-dependent transport, after which most of the T_4 undergoes deiodination to T_3 **(Figure 46–6)**. Both T_4 and T_3 are transferred to the nucleus, where T_3 binds to a nuclear receptor with much greater affinity than T_4. Two main distinct forms of the T_3 receptor are expressed in a tissue-specific manner. The T_3-receptor complex interacts with DNA to stimulate or to inhibit the transcription of numerous messenger RNAs, which then direct the increased or decreased synthesis of many specific proteins in different tissues. The T_3 receptor often constitutively represses target genes. Binding of the T_3 ligand may relieve this repressive effect and in this way increase the transcription of the gene product. Examples of target genes include enzymes, growth hormone, myosin chains, osteocalcin (Chapter 44), TSH, and T_3 receptors.

The critical importance of the T_3 receptor is clinically illustrated by individuals whose hypothyroidism is caused by resistance to thyroid hormone. These patients have either mutant receptors that are unable to transduce the hormone signal efficiently or a single allele for a mutant receptor that blocks T_3 binding to the normal receptor. If the receptor dysfunction is generalized, the individual is hypothyroid. If the dysfunction is only in the hypothalamic-pituitary part of the axis and T_3 is not properly recognized, deficient negative feedback may lead to excessive TSH secretion and T_4 production with resultant hyperthyroidism.

The quantitative responses of tissues to T_3 correlate well with their nuclear receptor content and with the degree of receptor occupancy (see Chapter 41). Normally, about half the available receptor sites are occupied by T_3. Because T_3 acts largely through

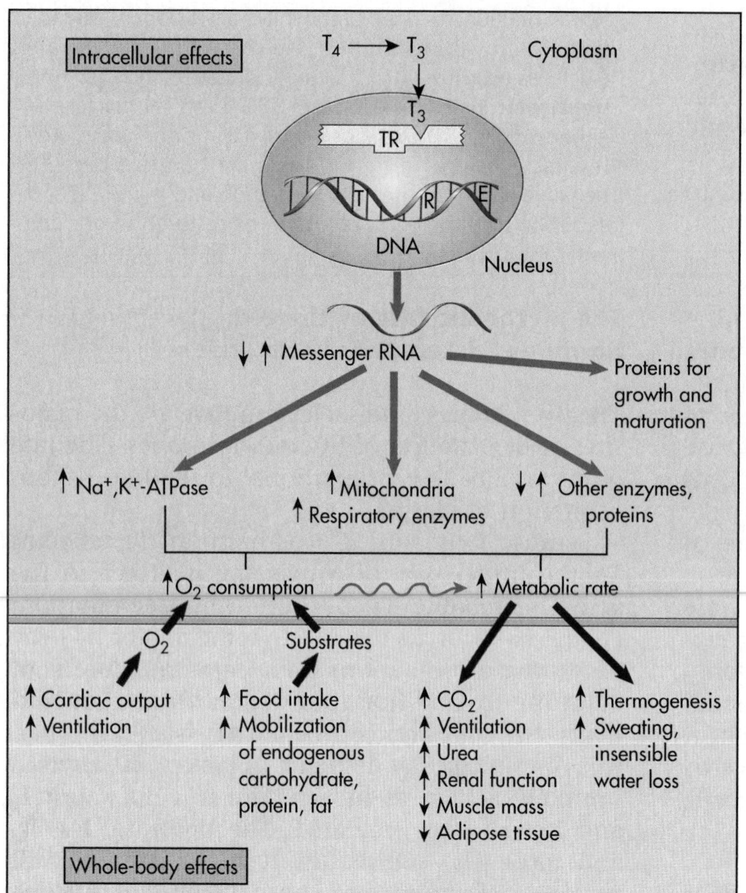

FIGURE 46–6. Thyroid hormone effects. ***Top,*** **Intracellular actions resulting from T_3 binding to its nuclear receptor (TR), which is linked to thyroid regulatory elements (TRE) in target DNA molecules.** ***Bottom,*** **All the various whole-body effects of thyroid hormone that sustain increased O_2 consumption and permit disposal of the excess CO_2, heat, and metabolic products.**

gene transcription, a 12- to 48-hour delay occurs before its effects become evident in vivo. Several weeks of hormone replacement are required before all the consequences of a deficiency state are corrected.

THE MOST OBVIOUS EFFECT OF THYROID HORMONE IS TO STIMULATE O_2 CONSUMPTION AND SUBSTRATE USE (Figure 46–6). A number of mechanisms are probably involved. T_3 increases the number, size, and membrane areas of mitochondria and increases the concentrations of certain key respiratory enzymes. T_3 also stimulates the activity of the Na^+,K^+-ATPase pump, which is responsible for membrane cation transport (see Chapter 1). Because large amounts of ATP are thereby consumed and much ADP is correspondingly generated by Na^+,K^+-ATPase, the extra ADP could be one "messenger" by which thyroid hormone stimulates mitochondrial O_2 use. Similarly, T_3 stimulates the Ca^{++}-ATPase of the sarcolemmal reticulum, requiring extra energy expenditure to resequester Ca^{++}. Another possibility is that thyroid hormone simultaneously stimulates the synthesis and oxidation of fatty acids and glucose, processes that create futile, wasteful cycles requiring energy input and heat generation. In brain tissue, O_2 consumption is not stimulated by T_3, but the hormone increases the synthesis of specific structural and functional proteins.

Most recently, the activity of brown adipose tissue has been shown to be T_3 sensitive. In cooperation with β-adrenergic stimulation (also potentiated by T_3 augmentation of β-adrenergic receptors), T_3 and cAMP induce expression of the UCP-1 (uncoupling) gene. UCP-1 increases facultative thermogenesis and energy-wasting heat production (Figure 46–6; see Chapter 42). Whether this accounts for energy wastage by human muscle and white adipose tissue is unproven.

The whole-body actions of thyroid hormone subserve an increase in O_2 use

In humans, O_2 use at rest is approximately 225 to 250 mL/min (see Chapter 42). It falls to about 150 mL/min in the absence of thyroid hormone and can increase to 400 mL/min with thyroid hormone excess. Of necessity, thermogenesis and body temperature increase or decrease concomitantly with O_2 use. Temperature changes, however, are moderated by thyroid hormone–induced increases or decreases in heat loss through appropriate changes in cutaneous blood flow, sweating, and ventilation.

Thyroid hormone could not stimulate O_2 use for long without augmenting O_2 supply to the tissues (Figure 46–6). Thus, thyroid hormone increases the resting rate of ventilation sufficiently to maintain a normal arterial O_2 pressure despite increased O_2 use and a normal CO_2 pressure in the face of increased CO_2 production. In addition, the O_2-carrying capacity of the blood is enhanced by a small increase in red cell mass.

ANOTHER IMPORTANT ACTION OF THYROID HORMONE IS TO INCREASE CARDIAC OUTPUT, WHICH ENSURES SUFFICIENT O_2 DELIVERY TO THE TISSUES. The resting heart rate and stroke volume are both increased, and the speed and force of myocardial contractions are enhanced (see Chapter 19). These effects are partly indirect, via adrenergic stimulation. However, thyroid hormone directly increases myocardial Ca^{++} uptake, adenylyl cyclase activity, and the active form of myosin-stimulated ATPase. The systolic blood pressure rises and diastolic blood pressure falls, reflecting the combined effects of the increased stroke volume with a substantial reduction in peripheral vascular resistance. The reduction in peripheral vascular resistance results from a direct effect of T_3 on resistance vessels and from blood vessel dilation produced by the increased tissue metabolism (see Chapter 23).

The stimulation of O_2 use also requires the provision of substrates for oxidation. Thyroid hormone potentiates the stimulatory effects of other hormones on glucose absorption from the gastrointestinal tract, on gluconeogenesis, on lipolysis, on ketogenesis, and on proteolysis of the labile protein pool. THE OVERALL METABOLIC EFFECT OF THYROID HORMONE HAS THEREFORE APTLY BEEN DESCRIBED AS ACCELERATING THE METABOLIC RESPONSE TO STARVATION.

Thyroid hormone also stimulates the biosynthesis of cholesterol and its oxidation, conversion to bile acids, and biliary secretion. The net effect is to decrease the body pool and plasma level of cholesterol. The rate of metabolic disposal of steroid hormones, B vitamins, and administered drugs is increased. Therefore, to maintain effective plasma levels of these substances in the presence of increased thyroid hormone, their endogenous production or their exogenous administration must be increased.

Thyroid hormone interacts with the sympathetic nervous system

A MAJOR INTERMEDIARY IN SOME THYROID HORMONE ACTIONS IS THE SYMPATHETIC NERVOUS SYSTEM. The sensitivity of tissues to the thermogenic, lipolytic, glycogenolytic, and gluconeogenic effects of epinephrine and norepinephrine is enhanced. Thyroid hormone may reinforce the cardiovascular responses to catecholamine hormones by increasing the number of β-adrenergic receptors, coupling them to adenylyl cyclase, and increasing cAMP levels. There are also reports that this increased sensitivity is accompanied by decreased plasma levels and urinary excretion of norepinephrine, the sympathetic neurotransmitter.

Hyperthyroidism presents a striking clinical picture because of the described effects. The increase in metabolic rate leads to weight loss, which is characteristically accompanied by an **increased** intake of food. The excessive generation of heat causes discomfort in warm environments, fever if the condition is severe, excessive sweating, thirst, and increased ventilation. Muscle weakness, atrophy, and even osteoporosis can result from increased protein degradation. The increase in β-adrenergic responsivity is manifested by tremor, nervousness, insomnia, and an anxious stare. The heart rate is rapid, atrial fibrillation may occur, and a high–cardiac output form of heart failure may develop in extreme cases. The use of β-adrenergic antagonists ameliorates the sympathetic nervous system manifestations.

Thyroid hormone modulates skeletal growth and central nervous system development

IN HUMANS, THYROID HORMONE STIMULATES THE LINEAR GROWTH, DEVELOPMENT, AND MATURATION OF BONE. A direct effect of T_3 on the activity of chondrocytes in the growth plate of bone may result from increases in insulin growth factor production and activity (see Chapter 45). T_3 also accelerates growth by stimulating the secretion of growth hormone. Although thyroid hormone is not required for linear bone growth until after birth, it is already essential for maturation of the growth centers in fetal bones.

Thyroid hormone also stimulates the remodeling of mineralized mature bone (see Chapter 44). T_3 stimulates bone resorption by increasing local release of resorptive cytokines, such as interleukins. T_3 receptors are present on osteoblasts and their precursors. Increased bone formation is evident from increases in osteocalcin and alkaline phosphatase levels; increased bone resorption is marked by increased hydroxyproline and pyridinium cross-link compounds (see Chapter 44). The regular progression of tooth development and eruption depends on thyroid hormone, as does the normal renewal cycle of the epidermis and hair follicles. Thyroid hormone accelerates shedding of the skin and hair. The synthesis of the mucopolysaccharides that form the intercellular ground substance is inhibited by thyroid hormone.

Normal skeletal muscle function also requires thyroid hormone. This may be related to the regulation of energy production and storage in this tissue. The muscle content of creatine Pi is reduced by an excess of thyroid hormone.

THYROID HORMONE HAS CRITICAL EFFECTS ON THE DEVELOPMENT OF THE CENTRAL NERVOUS SYSTEM. The T_3 receptor is expressed in the brain throughout fetal life. The activity of a 5′ deiodinase is augmented, ensuring efficient conversion of T_4 to T_3. Degradation of T_3 is diminished. Thus, during its development, the central nervous system is amply supplied with T_3 effects on gene expression. If thyroid hormone is deficient in utero, growth of the cerebral and cerebellar cortex, proliferation of axons and branching of dendrites, and myelinization are all impaired. Irreversible brain damage results when the deficiency of thyroid hormone is not recognized and treated immediately after birth. These anatomical defects are paralleled by biochemical abnormalities. Without thyroid hormone, RNA and protein content, protein synthesis, levels of enzymes necessary for DNA synthesis, protein and lipid content of myelin, neurotransmitter receptors, and neurotransmitter synthesis are decreased in various areas of the brain.

In children and adults, thyroid hormone enhances the speed and amplitude of reflexes, wakefulness, alertness, responsiveness to various stimuli, awareness of hunger, memory, and learning capacity. Normal emotional tone also depends on appropriate thyroid hormone levels.

The clinical effects of hypothyroidism **(Figure 46–7)** may be severe, especially in a newborn, in whom the condition is known as **cretinism.** The central nervous system manifestations can include mental retardation and delayed developmental milestones such as sitting, standing, and walking. Lethargy, growth retardation, skeletal immaturity, and poor school performance occur. In children and adults, the decreased metabolic rate causes intolerance of cold, decreased sweating, dry skin, low cardiac output, and weight gain. The weight gain results from both excess adipose tissue and edema fluid that accumulates in association with ground substance mucopolysaccharides **(Figure 46–8)**. All these abnormalities vanish with thyroid hormone replacement (except any signs resulting from irreversible central nervous system damage).

Thyroid hormone contributes to the regulation of reproductive function in both genders. The normal process of sperm production, the ovarian cycle of follicular development and maturation and ovulation, and the maintenance of a healthy pregnant state are all disrupted by significant deviations of thyroid hormone levels from normal. In part, these may be caused by alterations in the metabolism of sex steroid hormones.

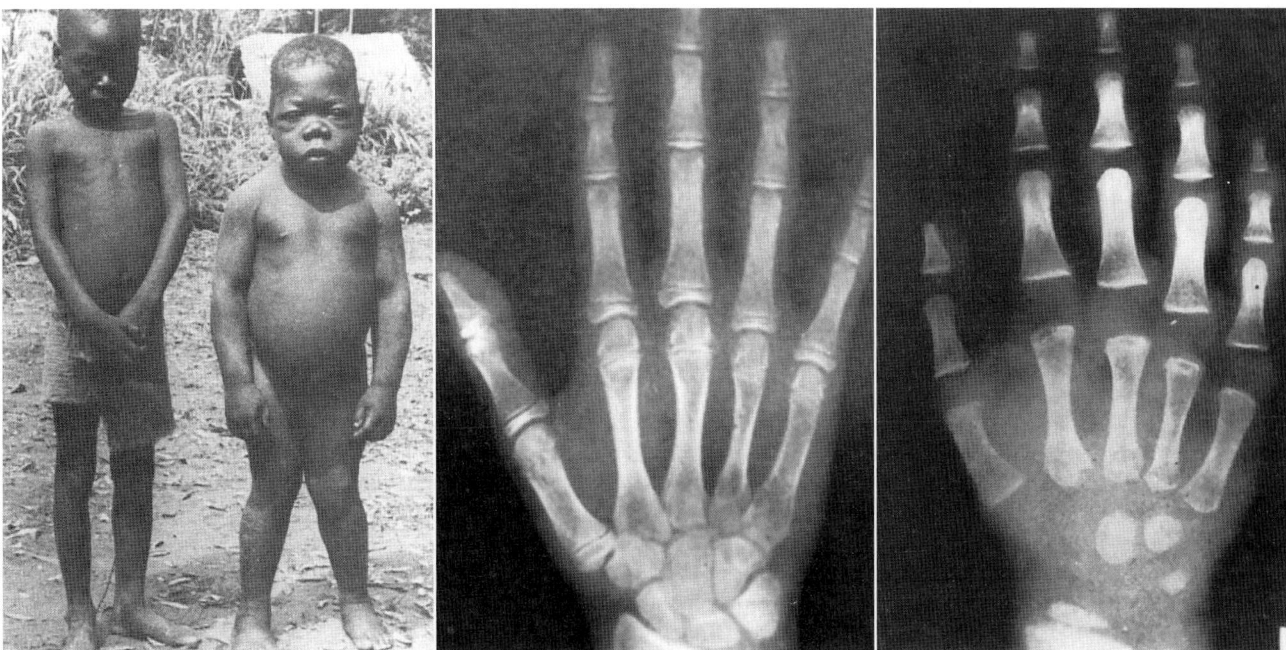

FIGURE 46–7. Normal 6-year-old child *(left)* and congenitally hypothyroid 17-year-old child *(right)* from the same village in an area of endemic cretinism **(A)**. Note especially the short stature, obesity, malformed legs, and dull expression of the mentally retarded hypothyroid child. Other features are a prominent abdomen; a flat, broad nose; a hypoplastic mandible; dry, scaly skin; delayed puberty; and muscle weakness. Hand radiographs of a 13-year-old normal child **(B)** and a 13-year-old hypothyroid child **(C)**. Note that the hypothyroid child has a marked delay in development of the small bones of the hands, in growth centers at either end of the fingers, and in the growth center of the distal end of the radius. (From Berne RM, Levy MN, Koeppen BM, Stanton BA: *Physiology,* ed 5, Philadelphia, 2004, Elsevier.)

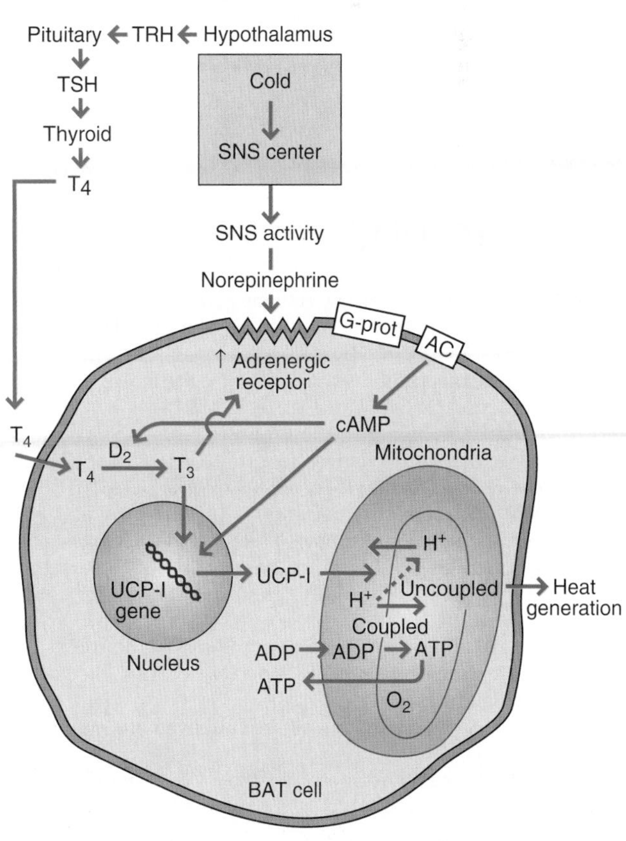

FIGURE 46–8. Interaction between thyroid hormones and the sympathetic nervous system (SNS) in regulating facultative thermogenesis in brown adipose tissue (BAT). In response to cold, T_4 is released and hypothalamic thermal sensors increase sympathetic outflow to adipose cells. Via β-adrenergic receptors, norepinephrine stimulates adenylyl cyclase (AC) activity and increased cAMP levels. T_4 enters the BAT cell, where it is converted to T_3, and T_3 increases the norepinephrine receptor. Together, T_3 and cAMP increase expression of the gene for uncoupling protein 1 (UCP-1). UCP-1 uncouples synthesis of ATP from O_2 utilization by creating *a leak* of protons back into the mitochondria. Thus, heat is generated. D_2, 5′-monodeiodinase 2.

Summary

- The basic endocrine unit of the thyroid gland is a follicle that consists of a single circular layer of epithelial cells surrounding a central lumen containing stored thyroid hormones (colloid). These hormones are tetraiodothyronine (thyroxine or T_4) and triiodothyronine (T_3).
- T_4 and T_3 are synthesized from tyrosine and I^- by the enzyme complex peroxidase. I^- is taken up by the gland via a $2Na^+$-$1I^-$ symporter. The tyrosine is incorporated in peptide links within the protein thyroglobulin. After iodination, two iodotyrosine molecules are coupled to yield the iodothyronines.
- The secretion of stored T_4 and T_3 requires the retrieval of thyroglobulin from the follicle lumen via endocytosis. To support hormone synthesis, I^- is actively concentrated by the gland.
- Thyrotropin (TSH) acts on the thyroid gland, largely via cAMP, to stimulate all steps in hormone production as well as growth of the epithelial cells. The secretion of TSH from the anterior pituitary is stimulated by thyrotropin-releasing hormone (TRH) from the hypothalamus and inhibited by T_4 and T_3.
- More than 99.5% of the T_4 and T_3 circulate bound to various proteins. Only the free fractions of T_4 and T_3 are biologically active.
- T_4 functions largely as a prohormone. Peripheral monodeiodination of the outer ring by a 5′ deiodinase yields most of the T_3, which is the principal active hormone.
- Thyroid hormone increases the basal metabolic rate. A nuclear T_3-receptor complex interacts with many target DNA molecules to induce or to suppress the synthesis of a variety of enzymes and other proteins. The result is to increase O_2 use and thermogenesis by numerous mechanisms.
- Additional important actions of thyroid hormone are to increase the heart rate, cardiac output, and ventilation and to decrease peripheral resistance. These subserve the increased tissue O_2 demand.
- Other effects of thyroid hormone on the central nervous system and skeleton are crucial to normal growth and development. In the absence of thyroid hormone, brain development is retarded, and cretinism results. Linear growth is restricted, and the bones fail to mature normally.

Bibliography

Bianco AC et al: Biochemistry, cellular and molecular biology, and physiological roles of the iodothyronine selenodeiodinases, *Endocr Rev* 23:38, 2002.

Brent GA: Mechanisms of disease: the molecular basis of thyroid hormone action, *N Engl J Med* 331:847, 1994.

Brown D et al: Amphibian metamorphosis: a complex program of gene expression changes controlled by the thyroid hormone, *Recent Prog Horm Res* 50:309, 1995.

Chin WW: Hormonal regulation of thyrotropin and gonadotropin gene expression, *Clin Res* 36:484, 1988.

Dohán O et al: The sodium/iodide symporter (NIS): characterization, regulation, and medical significance, *Endocr Rev* 24:48, 2003.

Dunn JT: Biosynthesis and secretion of thyroid hormone. In DeGroot LJ, Jameson JL, eds: *Endocrinology,* ed 4, Philadelphia, 2001, WB Saunders.

Klein I et al: Thyroid hormone and the cardiovascular system, *N Engl J Med* 344:501, 2001.

Kohn LD et al: The thyrotropin receptor, *Vitam Horm* 50:287, 1995.

Larsen PR, Silva JE, Kaplan MM: Relationships between circulating and intracellular thyroid hormones: physiological and clinical implications, *Endocr Rev* 2:87, 1981.

Lazar MA: Thyroid hormone receptors: multiple forms, multiple possibilities, *Endocr Rev* 14:184, 1993.

Lebon V et al: Effect of triiodothyronine on mitochondrial energy coupling in human skeletal muscle, *J Clin Invest* 108:733, 2001.

Mariotti S et al: The aging thyroid, *Endocr Rev* 16:686, 1995.

Oppenheimer JH, Schwartz HL, Strait KA: The molecular basis of thyroid hormone actions. In Braverman LE, Utiger RD, eds: *Werner and Ingbar's the thyroid,* ed 8, Philadelphia, 2000, Lippincott-Raven.

Porterfield SP, Hendrich CE: The role of thyroid hormones in prenatal and neonatal neurological development: current perspectives, *Endocr Rev* 14:94, 1993.

Robbins J: Thyroid hormone transport proteins and the physiology of hormone binding. In Braverman LE, Utiger RD, eds: *Werner and Ingbar's the thyroid,* ed 8, Philadelphia, 2000, Lippincott-Raven.

Scanlon MF, Toft AD: Regulation of thyrotropin secretion. In Braverman LE, Utiger RD, eds: *Werner and Ingbar's the thyroid,* ed 8, Philadelphia, 2000, Lippincott-Raven.

Silva JE: The multiple contributions of thyroid hormone to heat production, *J Clin Invest* 108:35, 2001.

Szkudlinski MW et al: Thyroid-stimulating hormone and thyroid-stimulating hormone receptor structure-function relationships, *Physiol Rev* 82:473, 2002.

Taurog A: Hormone synthesis: thyroid iodine metabolism. In Braverman LE, Utiger RD, eds: *Werner and Ingbar's the thyroid,* ed 8, Philadelphia, 2000, Lippincott-Raven.

Yen PM: Physiological and molecular basis of thyroid hormone action, *Physiol Rev* 81:1097, 2001.

Case Studies

Case 46–1

A 45-year-old recently divorced, obese male pharmacist complains of a rapid heart rate, a 20-pound weight loss in 2 months, and heat intolerance. His pulse rate is 110 beats/min at rest. The serum T_4 level is elevated, confirming the clinical impression of hyperthyroidism. On further questioning, the patient finally admits to taking large doses of exogenous T_4 tablets to help him lose weight so that he can more easily remarry.

1. **Which of the following would be decreased?**
   A. Serum T_3 levels
   B. Serum rT_3 levels
   C. Serum TSH levels
   D. Serum free T_4 levels
   E. Serum free T_3 levels

2. **Which one of the following cardiovascular factors would be increased?**
   A. Cardiac β-adrenergic receptors
   B. Muscle creatine Pi levels
   C. Plasma norepinephrine levels
   D. Systemic vascular resistance
   E. Diastolic blood pressure

3. **Which of the following might initially be increased in the thyroid gland?**
   A. I^- trap activity
   B. Content of colloid
   C. Peroxidase activity
   D. Height of thyroid epithelial cells
   E. Thyroglobulin synthesis

Case 46–2

A 16-month-old girl appears to be growing more slowly than normal. Her apathetic appearance alerts the pediatrician to the possibility of hypothyroidism. Her thyroid gland is greatly enlarged. Her serum T_4 level is low, and her serum TSH level is high.

1. **Which of the following could not be true?**
   A. Iodide deficiency caused her hypothyroidism.
   B. An inactive mutant peroxidase enzyme caused her hypothyroidism.
   C. She has the skeletal maturation of a 22-month-old child.
   D. She has excess body water.
   E. She has made no attempt to walk.

2. **As a result of T_4 therapy, which of the following would be expected?**
   A. Her heart rate would be reduced.
   B. Her systolic blood pressure would be reduced.
   C. Her height would be unchanged.
   D. Her weight would be unchanged.
   E. Her respiratory rate would be increased.

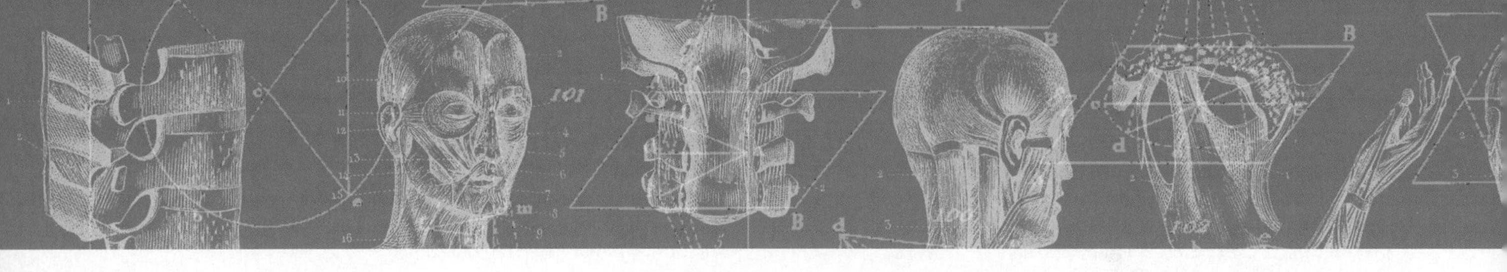

Chapter 47: Adrenal Cortex

Objectives

- ❖ Delineate the general biochemical pathway for the synthesis of all adrenal steroid hormones.
- ❖ Explain the complex regulation of adrenocortical function by the hypothalamic-pituitary-adrenal axis.
- ❖ Emphasize the extreme importance to life of the multiple effects of cortisol on body tissues.
- ❖ Describe the specific mechanisms of regulating aldosterone secretion in contrast to cortisol secretion.
- ❖ Explain how aldosterone affects kidney function and blood pressure.

Adrenal Hormones from Separate Anatomical Zones Regulate or Modulate Many Essential Physiological Processes

The adrenal glands are multifunctional endocrine organs that secrete a variety of hormones. Abundant experimental and clinical evidence has demonstrated that the adrenal glands are essential to life. THEIR SECRETIONS SUBSERVE A WIDE VARIETY OF PHYSIOLOGICAL FUNCTIONS, INCLUDING BLOOD GLUCOSE REGULATION; PROTEIN TURNOVER; FAT METABOLISM; Na^+, K^+, AND Ca^{++} BALANCE; MAINTENANCE OF CARDIOVASCULAR TONE; MODULATION OF TISSUE RESPONSE TO INJURY OR INFECTION; AND MOST IMPORTANT, SURVIVAL DURING SEVERE STRESS. These actions require modulation of the other organ systems whose functions are described elsewhere in this book.

Each adrenal gland is located just above the ipsilateral kidney (**Figure 47–1**), and their combined weight is 6 to 10 g. Each gland is a combination of two separate functional entities (**Figure 47–2**). The outer zone, or **cortex,** comprises 80% to 90% of the weight. It is derived from mesodermal tissue and is the source of **corticosteroid** hormones. The inner zone, or **medulla,** comprises the other 10% to 20%. It is derived from neuroectodermal cells of the sympathetic ganglia and is the source of **catecholamine** hormones. Paracrine actions between the inner cortical cells and the neighboring medullary cells are possible. The adrenal glands have one of the highest rates of blood flow per gram of tissue. Arterial blood enters the outer cortex and breaks up into capillaries; venous drainage is into the medulla. This exposes the inner cells of the cortex and the cells of the medulla to high concentrations of steroid hormones from the outer cortex.

The outermost **zona glomerulosa** of the adrenal cortex is only a few cells thick (Figure 47–2). The middle **zona fasciculata** is the widest layer and consists of long cords of columnar cells. The innermost **zona reticularis** contains networks of interconnecting cells. TYPICAL STEROID-SECRETING CELLS ARE RICH IN LIPID DROPLETS AND CONTAIN NUMEROUS LARGE MITOCHONDRIA WITH VESICLES IN THEIR MEMBRANES.

The major hormones of the cortex are the **glucocorticoid cortisol,** which has critical roles in carbohydrate and protein metabolism and in the adaptation to stress; the **mineralocorticoid aldosterone,** which is vital to maintaining normal extracellular fluid volume and K^+ levels; and **sex steroid precursors,** which contribute to maintaining secondary sexual characteristics.

The discovery and synthesis of cortisol were medical landmarks. Cortisol was lifesaving for patients whose adrenal glands were destroyed by disease, and it dramatically reversed their debilitation. Cortisol also has potent anti-inflammatory and antiimmune effects that are used to treat diseases in which autoimmunity plays an important pathogenetic role and to prevent rejection of organ transplants.

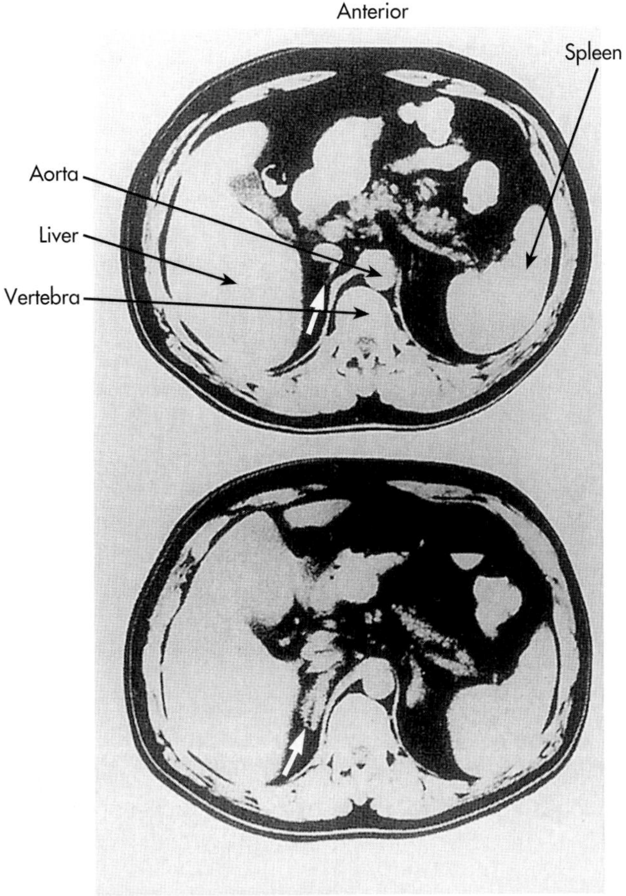

FIGURE 47–1. Computed tomographic scans of the abdomen. ***Top,*** **Small size of the left adrenal gland** ***(white arrow)*** **relative to other organs.** ***Bottom,*** **Marked hyperplasia of the left adrenal gland** ***(white arrow)*** **that occurred after 1 week of stimulation by an excess of endogenous adrenocorticotropic hormone. The right adrenal gland was less well seen on these images, but it also enlarged after excess amounts of this hormone. (From Mastorakos G et al:** ***J Clin Endocrinol Metab*** **77:1690, 1993.)**

The synthesis of corticosteroid hormones proceeds from cholesterol and is catalyzed by P-450 enzymes in the mitochondria and microsomes

THE PRECURSOR FOR ALL ADRENOCORTICAL HORMONES IS CHOLESTEROL, WHICH IS TAKEN UP FROM THE PLASMA VIA A SPECIFIC PLASMA MEMBRANE RECEPTOR FOR LOW-DENSITY LIPOPROTEINS (see Chapter 42). After transfer into the cell, the cholesterol is largely esterified and stored in vacuoles within the cytoplasm. Under basal conditions, cholesterol just taken up from plasma is immediately used for hormone synthesis. However, when hormone production is stimulated, stored cholesterol is rapidly mobilized and transferred to the mitochondria for the first synthetic step.

Most of the reactions in corticosteroid synthesis are catalyzed by **cytochrome P-450 enzymes** (**Figure 47–3**) located in the mitochondria and endoplasmic reticulum. The genes that direct their synthesis have considerable similarity. A single P-450 enzyme may catalyze more than one reaction, depending on its location in the adrenal cortex and on substrate availability. These enzymes catalyze hydroxylations of the steroid nucleus (Figure 47–3). The reactions require molecular O_2, reduced nicotinamide adenine dinucleotide phosphate (NADPH), a flavoprotein enzyme, and an iron-containing protein called **adrenoxin.** Molecular O_2 is split so that one O_2 atom is inserted between the carbon and one hydrogen at the reaction site. The other O_2 atom is reduced to H_2O.

Cortisol synthesis uniquely requires the addition of an 11-hydroxyl group to the steroid molecule

The synthesis of **cortisol,** the major glucocorticoid in humans (Figure 47–3), occurs largely in the zona fasciculata. The initial and rate-limiting reaction converts cholesterol to **pregnenolone** and is catalyzed by the mitochondrial side chain–cleaving enzyme complex P-450scc (also known as 20,22-desmolase). The pregnenolone is then converted to **progesterone,** after which hydroxyls are successively added at the 17 and 21 positions. These reactions take place within the endoplasmic reticulum. The resultant 11-deoxycortisol is transferred to the mitochondria and hydroxylated in the 11 position, the final and critical step in creating a glucocorticoid molecule.

NEITHER THE FINAL PRODUCT, CORTISOL, NOR ITS PRECURSORS ARE STORED IN THE ADRENOCORTICAL CELL. Thus, an acute need for increased cortisol secretion requires rapid activation of the initial controlling step: side chain cleavage of stored cholesterol.

Aldosterone synthesis uniquely requires oxidation of the 18 position on the steroid molecule

The synthesis of aldosterone, the major mineralocorticoid (Figure 47–3), is performed exclusively in the zona glomerulosa. The reactions from cholesterol to **corticosterone** (a glucocorticoid) occur as in the zona fasciculata. In the subsequent key step, the C-18 methyl group of corticosterone is oxidized to yield aldosterone (by the same or a similar mitochondrial enzyme that catalyzes 11-hydroxylation). **11-Deoxycorticosterone** and **18-hydroxydeoxycorticosterone** also have mineralocorticoid

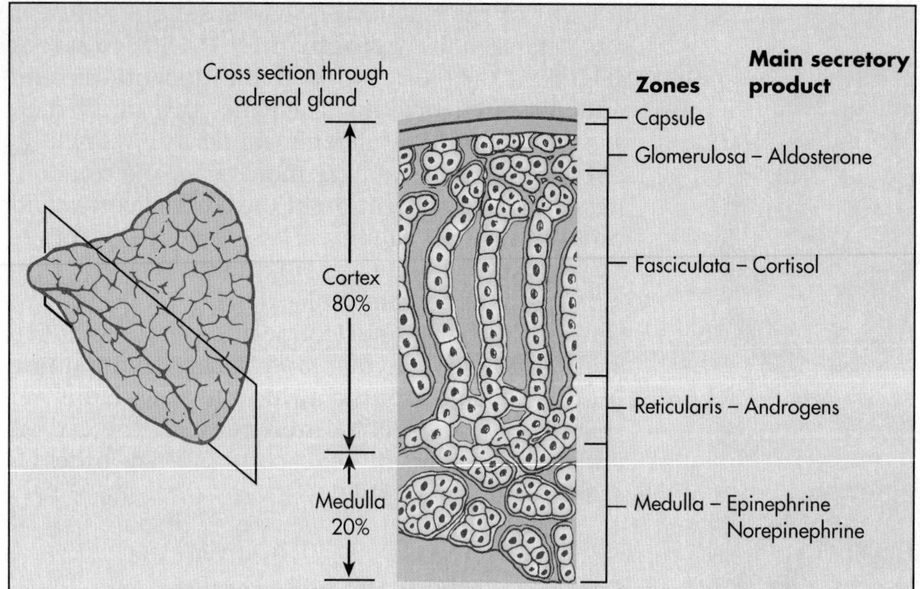

FIGURE 47–2. Structure and main secretory products of the adrenal gland.

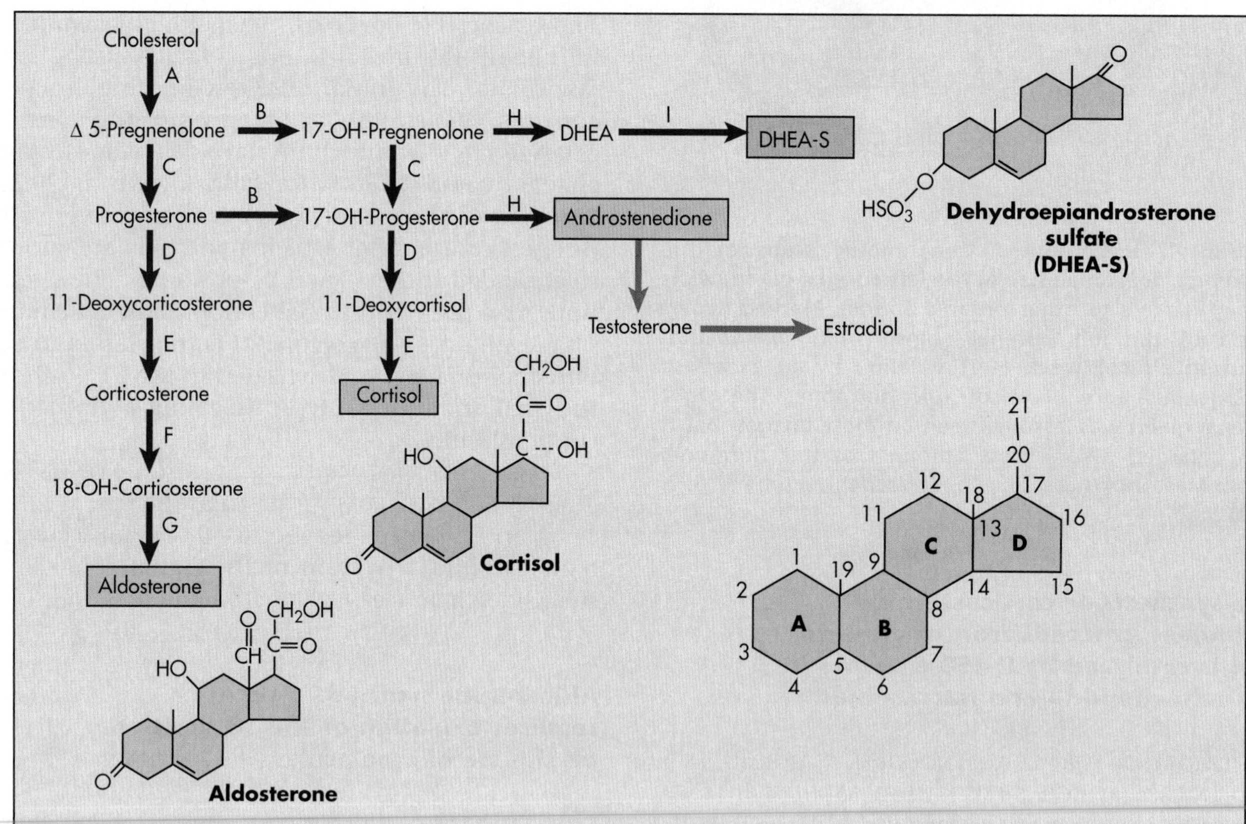

FIGURE 47–3. Sequence of reactions in the synthesis of adrenocorticosteroid hormones from the common precursor cholesterol. Step A is overall rate limiting. Step E is critical to glucocorticoid activity. Step G is critical to mineralocorticoid activity. Step B is essential to the formation of sex steroid precursors. DHEA, dehydroepiandrosterone; OH, hydroxy; *A,* 20,22-desmolase (P-450scc; CYP11A1); *B,* 17-hydroxylase (P-450c17; CYP17); *C,* 3β-ol-dehydrogenase, $\Delta^{4,5}$-isomerase; *D,* 21-hydroxylase (P-450c21; CYP21A2); *E,* 11-hydroxylase (P-450c11; CYP11B1); *F,* 18-hydroxylase; *G,* 18-OH-dehydrogenase; *H,* 17,20-desmolase (P-450c17; CYP17); *I,* sulfotransferase.

activity and are synthesized in small quantities in the zona fasciculata.

Androgen and estrogen precursors are 17-hydroxylated steroid molecules

The synthesis of sex steroids occurs largely in the zona reticularis. The potent androgen **testosterone** and the potent estrogen **estradiol** are normally secreted only in trace amounts by the adrenal cortex. However, substantial amounts of adrenal precursor steroids with weak androgenic activity are secreted and converted to testosterone and estradiol by peripheral tissues. These precursors—**androstenedione, dehydroepiandrosterone (DHEA),** and **dehydroepiandrosterone sulfate (DHEA-S)**—are synthesized from 17-hydroxyprogesterone and 17-hydroxypregnenolone, respectively, as shown in Figure 47–3 and in greater detail in Figure 49–1. In women, the adrenal precursors supply 50% of the androgenic hormone requirements. In men, they are ordinarily unimportant because the testes produce testosterone.

Genetic defects in cortisol biosynthesis have important and varied consequences for infants. A defect in either the 21- or 11-hydroxylase enzyme gene (see steps D and E in Figure 47–3) leads to overproduction of androgenic steroids from 17-hydroxyprogesterone and 17-hydroxypregnenolone, the accumulated precursors. This causes masculinization of female fetuses in utero and early secondary sexual changes in male infants and young boys. A severe deficiency of 21-hydroxylase activity may also cause manifestations of cortisol (glucocorticoid) and aldosterone (mineralocorticoid) deficiency. Deficiency of 11-hydroxylase leads to overproduction of the mineralocorticoid 11-deoxycorticosterone (Figure 47–3), which causes hypertension and hypokalemia.

Corticosteroid hormones are protein bound in serum and converted to metabolites excreted in urine

Basal plasma concentrations of cortisol in the morning are 5 to 20 μg/dL; by evening, they are often less than 5 μg/dL. The hormone circulates largely bound to a specific corticosteroid-binding globulin called **transcortin.** The concentrations of transcortin and total plasma cortisol are increased during pregnancy and estrogen administration. However, only free cortisol is biologically active, and the physiological effects of changes in transcortin levels are determined by principles similar to those discussed with regard to the effects of changes in thyroxine-binding globulin levels on T_4 and T_3 (see Chapter 46). Free cortisol is filtered by the kidney, and the small amount of daily urinary cortisol excretion (10 to 100 μg) is usually a valid index of cortisol secretion (see Chapter 41).

Cortisol is in equilibrium with its biologically inactive 11-keto analogue, **cortisone,** via type 1 and type 2 11β-hydroxydehydrogenase enzymes. The ubiquitous type 1 enzyme renders exogenous cortisone an effective source of cortisol activity by reducing cortisone to cortisol in cortisol target cells. The reverse conversion of cortisol to cortisone by the type 2 enzyme in the kidney is important in preventing cortisol from exerting excessive mineralocorticoid activity via aldosterone receptors, to which it binds (see later section). Almost all cortisol and cortisone is metabolized in the liver; the reduced metabolites are then conjugated and excreted in the urine as glucuronides. The measurement of these urinary metabolites, known generally as **17-hydroxycorticoids,** also provides a less specific index of cortisol secretion.

Aldosterone circulates bound to a specific aldosterone-binding globulin as well as to transcortin and albumin. Aldosterone and its liver-generated metabolites are excreted in the urine as glucuronide conjugates.

Adrenal androgen precursors are also metabolized in the liver and excreted in the urine in a fraction known as **17-ketosteroids.** However, these products are not specific for the adrenal gland because they also arise from gonadal androgens.

Cortisol Secretion by the Adrenal Cortex Is Basically Regulated Through Negative Feedback on the Hypothalamus and Pituitary Gland

The pattern of cortisol secretion is complex (**Figure 47–4**). The immediate stimulator of cortisol secretion is **adrenocorticotropin (ACTH)** from the anterior pituitary gland. The most important immediate stimulator of ACTH secretion is the neuropeptide **corticotropin-releasing hormone (CRH)** from the hypothalamus. Thus, a hypothalamic–anterior pituitary–adrenal cortex axis exists and forms a classic negative-feedback loop (Figure 47–4). Cortisol (or any synthetic glucocorticoid analogue, such as **dexamethasone** or **prednisone**)

1. feeds back (long loop) within minutes to inhibit the release of ACTH by blocking the stimulatory action of CRH on the corticotroph cells;

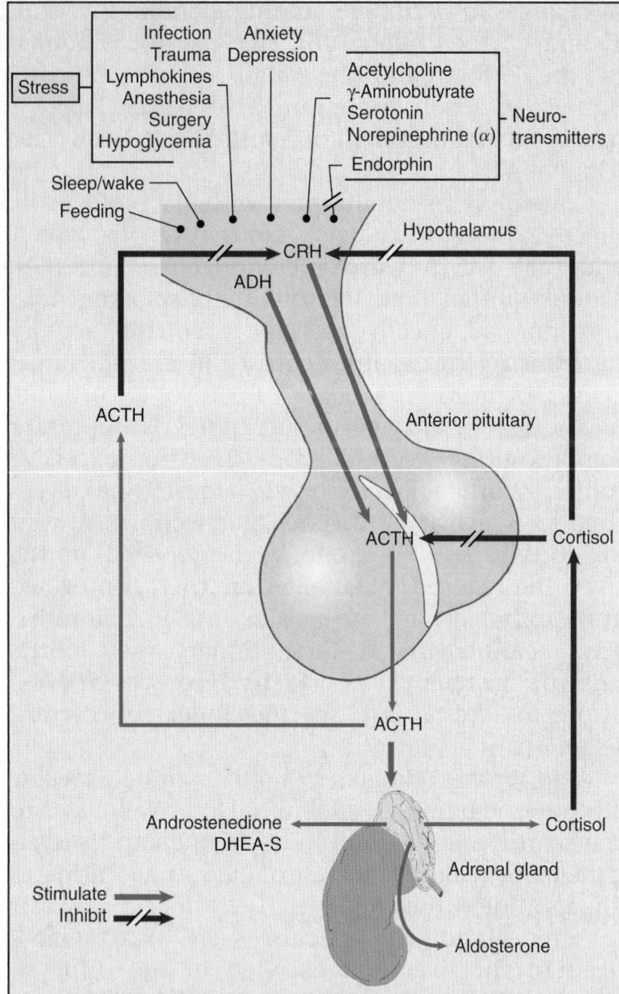

FIGURE 47–4. Regulation of cortisol secretion by the hypothalamic–anterior pituitary–adrenal cortex axis. A variety of stimuli to the hypothalamus activate the secretion of corticotropin-releasing hormone (CRH), which in turn increases the secretion of adrenocorticotropin (ACTH) and thence cortisol. Antidiuretic hormone (ADH) has an auxiliary stimulating effect on ACTH secretion, especially during stress. Cortisol exerts negative feedback at both the hypothalamic and the pituitary levels on CRH, ACTH, and ADH release.

2. feeds back more slowly (within hours) to inhibit ACTH synthesis by blocking the transcription of its gene; and
3. feeds back on the hypothalamus to block the release of CRH.

In short-loop feedback, ACTH inhibits the release of CRH (Figure 47–4). Antidiuretic hormone (ADH, arginine vasopressin; see Chapter 45) is another important stimulator of ACTH and therefore of cortisol secretion, especially in stressful situations, and cortisol feeds back to restrain ADH release.

Given in large doses for long periods, synthetic glucocorticoids profoundly suppress the function of the CRH neurons, the corticotroph cells, and consequently the cells of the zona fasciculata and zona reticularis. The ACTH-dependent adrenal cortex atrophies. After such therapy is withdrawn, full recovery of the inactivated hypothalamic–anterior pituitary–adrenal axis can take up to 1 year. During this time, patients must be protected against deficient responses to stress by receiving supplemental cortisol.

Corticotropin-releasing hormone stimulates adrenocorticotropin synthesis and release

CRH is a 41–amino acid peptide synthesized from a prepro-CRH in small cells of the paraventricular nucleus of the hypothalamus. CRH enters the pituitary portal veins and travels to the corticotroph cells (see Figure 45-1). After binding to a plasma membrane receptor, CRH stimulates the release of ACTH via Ca^{++} and cAMP as second messengers and also stimulates ACTH synthesis. CRH exhibits diverse other actions in the central nervous system. These include stimulating sympathetic nervous system activity and wakening, decreasing fever, suppressing food intake, suppressing reproductive function and sexual activity, suppressing growth hormone release, and altering behavior. CRH in immune cells stimulates cytokine release. Peripheral plasma levels of CRH are very low, but they mirror negative feedback because they are slightly increased by cortisol deficiency and decreased by glucocorticoid administration.

Adrenocorticotropin stimulates adrenocortical cell hyperplasia and corticosteroid hormone synthesis and release

ACTH is a 39–amino acid peptide that increases the synthesis and immediate release of cortisol, adrenal androgens, their precursors, and aldosterone. However, only cortisol feeds back negatively as previously described. ACTH is synthesized from a large precursor called **preproopiomelanocortin,** which gives rise to a number of cosecreted products, including **β-endorphin** and **melanocyte-stimulating hormone;** melanocyte-stimulating hormone increases skin pigmentation by dispersing melanin granules within melanocytes.

After binding to its adrenal plasma membrane receptor, ACTH stimulates the generation of cAMP, which is the major second messenger for its actions (**Figure 47–5**). The ultimate effects of ACTH are

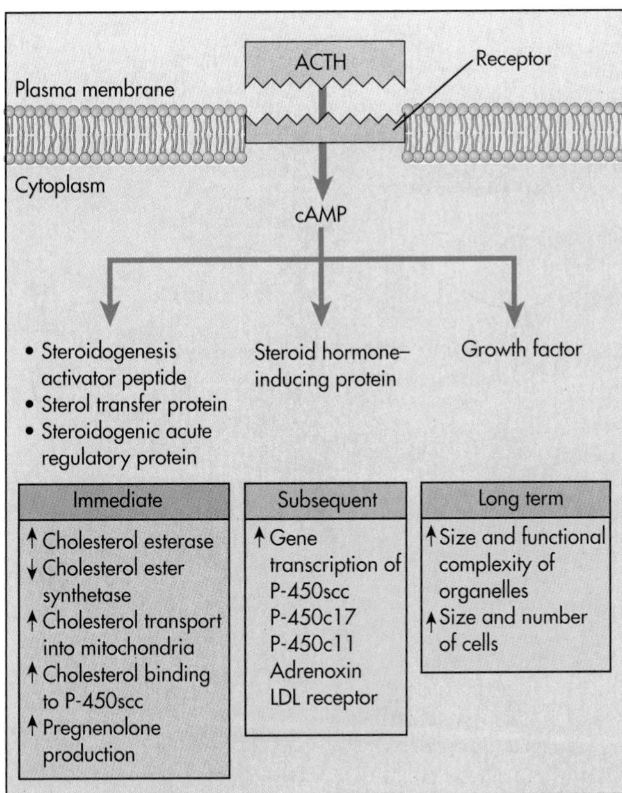

FIGURE 47–5. ACTH actions on target adrenocortical cells. Through cAMP as second messenger, ACTH activates and induces steroidogenic enzymes and stimulates adrenocortical cell growth. LDL, low-density lipoprotein. See text for details.

mediated by protein products that result from a cascade of enzyme phosphorylations catalyzed by protein kinases A and C. These products include enzyme activators, transcription factors, and growth factors. A **steroidogenesis activator protein** mediates hydrolysis of stored cholesterol esters, and a **sterol transfer protein** transports the cholesterol to the outer mitochondrial membrane. A phosphoprotein, **steroidogenic acute regulatory protein (StAR),** transfers cholesterol to the inner mitochondrial membrane, where the cholesterol is acted on by P-450scc. Later transcription factors, such as **steroidogenic factor 1 (SF-1),** stimulate expression of the synthetic enzyme genes and the genes for StAR, the LDL receptor, and adrenoxin. Thus, as with TSH and the thyroid, ACTH stimulates all the steps in corticosteroid hormone synthesis by the adrenal cortex. ACTH also alters the shape of the adrenocortical cell by affecting its cytoskeleton and by bringing the cholesterol vacuoles into contact with the mitochondria. Continuous stimulation with ACTH causes hyperplasia of the adrenal cortex (Figure 47–1) by stimulating synthesis of IGF-1 and other growth factors.

Cortisol secretion is pulsatile, diurnal, and stimulated by stresses

Bursts of cortisol secretion are induced by pulses of ACTH, which are caused by the pulsatile release of CRH in a diurnal pattern. Peak plasma ACTH and cortisol levels are achieved about 2 hours before awakening; the nadir of plasma ACTH and cortisol is reached just before a person falls asleep. The morning peak of cortisol constitutes 50% of its total daily secretion. The clock time of this peak can be altered by systematically shifting the sleep-wake cycle. THIS PHENOMENON IS OF OCCUPATIONAL SIGNIFICANCE, SUCH AS IN TRANSOCEANIC AIRLINE FLIGHTS. The circadian rhythm is intrinsic and generated within the hypothalamus by the suprachiasmatic nucleus. Negative feedback affects the setting of this center: exogenous glucocorticoid suppresses and prior cortisol deficiency accentuates the early morning ACTH peak. Loss of consciousness and constant exposure to either dark or light also blunt the circadian rhythm.

Cortisol is required for survival of the "stressed" organism. Severe pain and prolonged exercise also cause the release of cortisol, whereas the state of analgesia induced by endorphins (endogenous opiates) blocks the cortisol response. Stress can override the diurnal pattern of cortisol secretion as well as the suppressive effects of negative feedback. Several neurotransmitters mediate the stressful inputs that stimulate CRH (plus ADH) release (Figure 47–4). Low responders to one stress (e.g., exercise) tend to be low responders to another (e.g., psychological disturbance).

Extra cortisol is secreted in patients with serious medical illnesses (such as **sepsis**) or major fractures, those undergoing surgery or electroconvulsive therapy, and those experiencing hypoglycemia. In patients in intensive care units, plasma cortisol levels are elevated twofold to fivefold; there is an increased risk of mortality in patients with the highest levels.

Activation of cell-mediated immunity also increases ACTH and cortisol release. Lymphokines, such as interleukin-6, are secreted within the anterior pituitary, where they stimulate ACTH secretion (Figure 47–4). Some lymphocytes have ACTH receptors and can also secrete ACTH, so autocrine and even intracrine actions on lymphocytes may occur. Because infection and tissue trauma are accompanied by cell-mediated immune responses, and because cortisol is an important modulator of those responses (see following discussion), a significant feedback relationship exists between the immune and endocrine systems at several levels.

Cortisol (Glucocorticoids) Actions Permit Many Physiological Processes to Be Maintained at Normal Levels

CORTISOL IS REQUIRED TO SUSTAIN GLUCOSE PRODUCTION FROM PROTEIN AND TO SUPPORT VASCULAR RESPONSIVENESS. IN ADDITION, THIS HORMONE MODULATES CENTRAL NERVOUS SYSTEM FUNCTION, SKELETAL TURNOVER, HEMATOPOIESIS, MUSCLE FUNCTION, RENAL FUNCTION, AND IMMUNE RESPONSES. The term **permissive,** which has been used to describe cortisol's action, implies that the hormone may not directly initiate, so much as allow, critical processes to occur. For example, cortisol does not itself directly stimulate glycogenolysis. However, if cortisol is present, it enhances glycogenolysis stimulated by glucagon.

The intracellular mechanism of cortisol action is modulation of gene expression via a cytoplasmic-nuclear protein receptor

Almost all effects of cortisol are mediated via transcriptional mechanisms (see Figure 41–8). Cortisol enters target cells via facilitated diffusion and binds to either a type 1 or type 2 receptor that shuttles back and forth between the cytoplasm and nucleus. Binding of cortisol by the receptor displaces an inactivating protein from the receptor. The cortisol-receptor complex must undergo cytoplasmic activation by phosphorylation before it can move into the nucleus and bind to a target DNA molecule. The cortisol-liganded receptor activates acetylation of histones that bind chromatin to other nuclear constituents known as **nucleosomes.** This frees the genes for transcription. The final response is an increase in the gene transcription of specific messenger RNAs. Gene repression can also occur. Although other steroid hormones can bind to a cortisol receptor and other steroid receptors may bind to a similar regulatory element on the same DNA molecule, THE COMBINATION OF CORTISOL, ONE OF ITS RECEPTORS, AND A RESPONSIVE DNA MOLECULE IS REQUIRED TO ELICIT SPECIFIC CORTISOL ACTION. Nongenomic actions of cortisol may involve interactions with GABA and NMDA receptors (see Chapter 4) in the nervous system.

Cortisol affects metabolism

Cortisol causes the conversion of protein to glucose and a negative nitrogen balance

THE MOST IMPORTANT OVERALL EFFECT OF CORTISOL IS TO STIMULATE THE CONVERSION OF PROTEIN TO GLUCOSE AND THE STORAGE OF GLUCOSE AS GLYCOGEN, thus the term **glucocorticoid** (Figure 47–6). The type 2 receptor (also called the glucocorticoid receptor) mediates such actions. All phases of this process—mobilization of protein from muscle stores, entrance of the released amino acids into the hepatic gluconeogenetic pathway, conversion of pyruvate to glycogen, and disposition of the ammonia released from metabolism of the precursor amino acids—are augmented. Cortisol increases the activity of the enzymes involved in each of these steps. In some of these instances, the hormone "permits" substrate induction of its enzyme; in others, cortisol directly increases transcription of the target enzyme gene.

If the glucocorticoid effect is excessive and lengthy, the continuous drain on body protein produces serious deleterious effects because muscle, bone, connective tissue, and skin lose mass. This is

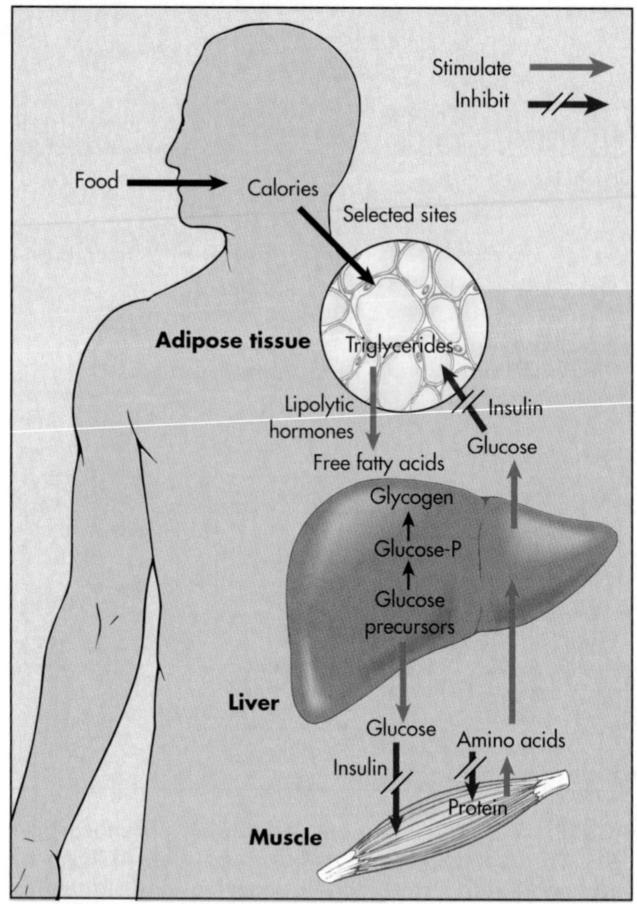

FIGURE 47–6. Effect of cortisol on the flow of fuels. Cortisol stimulates the mobilization of amino acids and their conversion to glucose. The glucose is preferentially but not exclusively stored as glycogen. Insulin-mediated glucose uptake by the peripheral tissues is inhibited. Cortisol facilitates the storage of fat in selected adipose tissue sites but also facilitates the release of free fatty acids.

exacerbated by the inhibitory effects of cortisol on the synthesis of constitutive proteins, such as collagen.

The clinical expression of the negative nitrogen balance that results from prolonged cortisol excess **(Cushing's syndrome)** is striking (**Figure 47–7**). Skin becomes so thin from loss of connective tissue that the capillaries show through, and because of fragile walls, they rupture spontaneously, causing bruises. Muscle weakness and atrophy are prominent. Osteoporosis results in atraumatic fractures and bone necrosis.

THE PRESENCE OF CORTISOL IS ESSENTIAL FOR THE MAINTENANCE OF PLASMA GLUCOSE LEVELS AND FOR SURVIVAL DURING PROLONGED FASTING. Without this hormone, death may occur from hypoglycemia once glycogen stores are gone. However, only a small increase in cortisol secretion occurs with fasting; the previous normal levels of the hormone help make possible the early mobilization of amino acids and gluconeogenesis. On the other hand, plasma cortisol levels increase sharply in response to acute hypoglycemia. In this situation, cortisol amplifies the glycogenolytic actions of glucagon and epinephrine, and it synergizes with them in rebuilding liver glycogen stores.

Cortisol opposes the key effects of insulin

Consonant with its role in preventing hypoglycemia, cortisol is a strong antagonist to insulin (Figure 47–6). Cortisol inhibits insulin-stimulated glucose uptake by muscle and adipose tissue and blocks the suppressive effect of insulin on hepatic glucose output. The interaction between cortisol and insulin is complex. Both hormones favor hepatic glycogen storage by increasing glycogen synthase activity (see Figure 42–3). However, they have opposite effects on the expression of genes for the gluconeogenetic enzyme phosphoenolpyruvate carboxykinase and the glucose-releasing enzyme glucose-6-phosphatase. Thus, cortisol induces expression of these genes, thereby stimulating glucose synthesis and output by the liver, whereas insulin inhibits both processes. The net result of cortisol excess is a rise in plasma glucose concentration and a compensatory increase in plasma insulin levels. WHEN THE INSULIN RESPONSE IS INSUFFICIENT, DIABETES MELLITUS CAN DEVELOP,

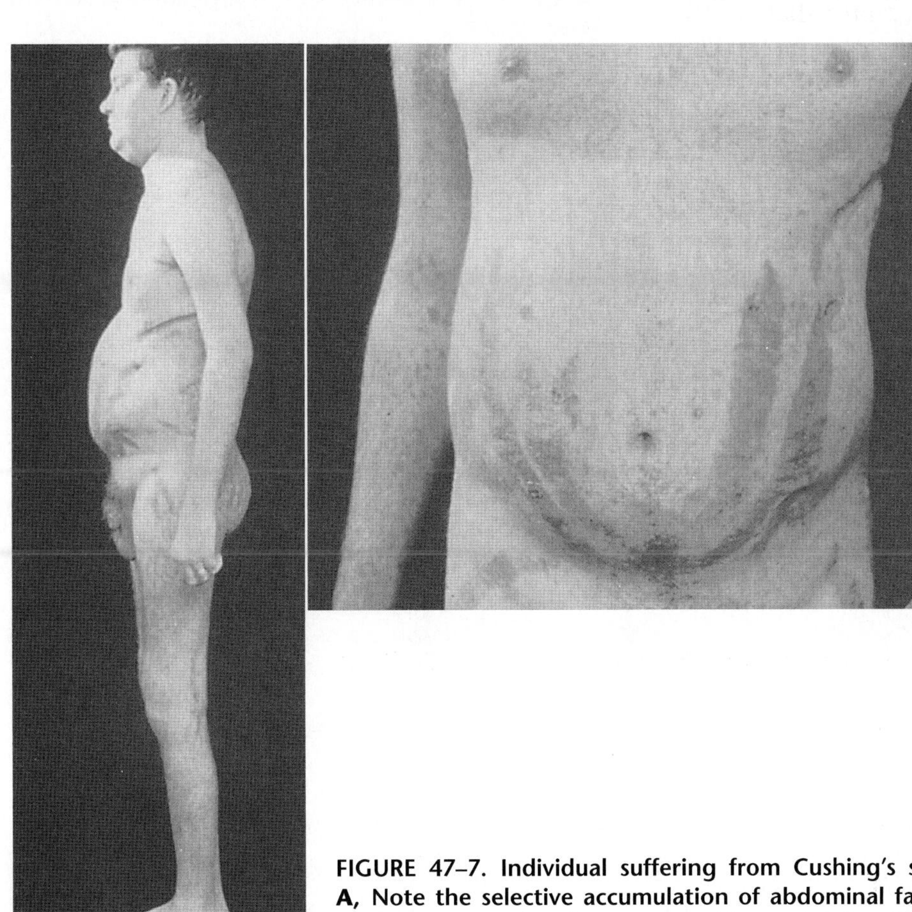

FIGURE 47–7. Individual suffering from Cushing's syndrome, an excess of cortisol. A, Note the selective accumulation of abdominal fat and the loss of musculature in the extremities. B, The extreme thinness of the skin reveals blood flowing through underlying blood vessels.

OR IF IT IS ALREADY PRESENT, IT CAN BE GREATLY WORSENED.

Cortisol also plays a complex role in fat metabolism (Figure 47–7). The presence of cortisol "permits" maximal stimulation of fat mobilization by growth hormone, epinephrine, and other lipolytic factors during fasting. However, the hormone also greatly increases appetite and stimulates lipogenesis in certain adipose tissue depots. THEREFORE, IN CUSHING'S SYNDROME, AN EXCESS OF CORTISOL ALSO RESULTS IN THE ACCUMULATION OF FAT, BUT THE OBESITY HAS A PECULIAR DISTRIBUTION, FAVORING THE FACE AND TRUNK BUT SPARING THE EXTREMITIES (Figure 47–7).

Thus, cortisol is a catabolic, antianabolic, and diabetogenic hormone. In stress situations, cortisol accentuates the hyperglycemia produced by other hormones and greatly accelerates the loss of body protein. These actions are amplified if insulin secretion is simultaneously deficient.

Cortisol affects diverse tissues and organs

Cortisol affects muscle, bone, the vascular system, the kidneys, and the central nervous system (**Figure 47–8**). It also affects the maturation of various systems and organs in the fetus.

Muscle

Basal levels of cortisol are required for the maintenance of normal contractility and for maximal performance of skeletal and cardiac muscle. In contrast, excess cortisol produces muscle atrophy and weakness through protein wastage (Figure 47–7).

Bone

The major effect of cortisol is to decrease bone formation. Less prominently, cortisol increases bone resorption. THE NET OUTCOME OF CORTISOL EXCESS CAN BE A PROFOUND REDUCTION IN BONE MASS AND, IN CHILDREN, A REDUCTION IN LINEAR GROWTH AS WELL. Several actions contribute to this outcome. Cortisol decreases the synthesis of 1,25-hydroxyvitamin D and blocks its action; therefore, Ca^{++} absorption from the gastrointestinal tract is defective (see Chapter 44). At the same time, urinary Ca^{++} excretion is increased. Thus, less Ca^{++} is available for the mineralization of bone. Cortisol also inhibits the differentiation of mesenchymal precursors into osteoblasts and the synthesis of collagen by these cells. In addition, apoptosis of osteoblasts and osteocytes is increased. Cortisol stimulates production of local inflammatory cytokines that cause bone resorption by activating osteoclasts.

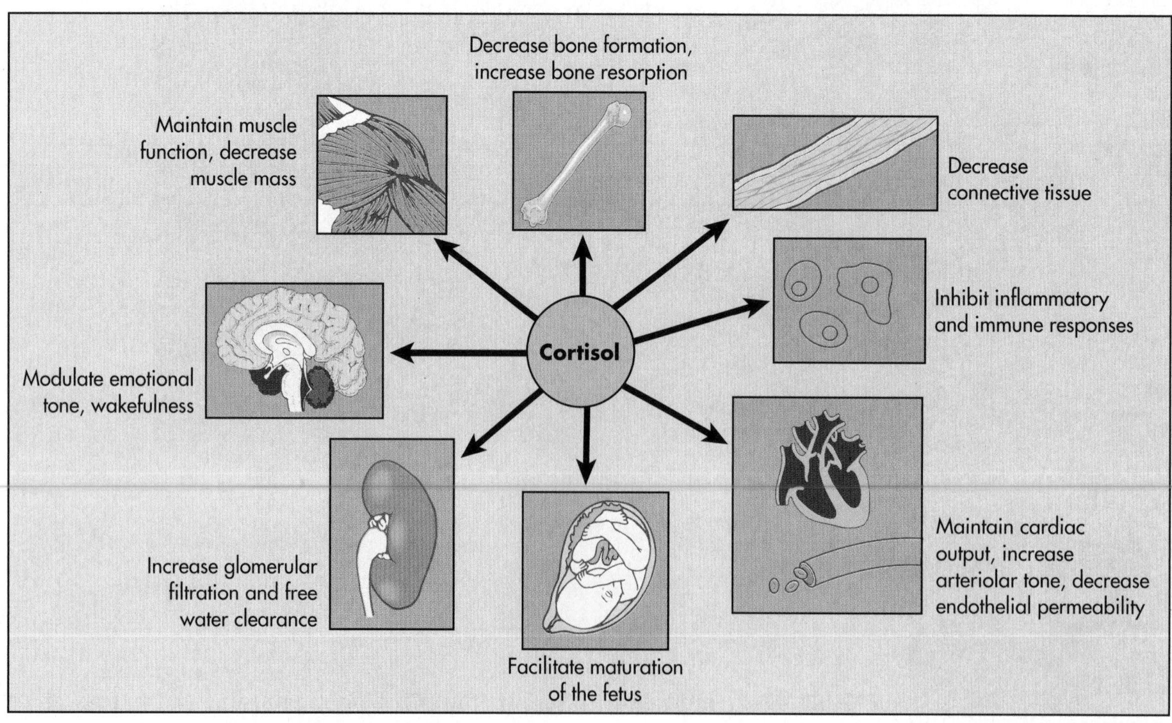

FIGURE 47–8. Effects of cortisol on various tissues and organs.

Vascular system

Cortisol is required for the maintenance of normal blood pressure. This hormone permits an enhanced responsiveness of arterioles to the constrictive action of adrenergic and angiotensin stimulation and also optimizes myocardial performance. Cortisol helps maintain blood volume by decreasing the permeability of the vascular endothelium. IN CUSHING'S SYNDROME, HYPERTENSION IS FREQUENTLY PRESENT.

Kidney

Cortisol increases the rate of glomerular filtration by decreasing preglomerular resistance and increasing flow of plasma into the glomerulus. It is also essential for the rapid excretion of a water load because it inhibits both the secretion of ADH and its action on the collecting duct tubules (see Chapter 45). CLINICALLY, THE ABSENCE OF CORTISOL MAY LEAD TO WATER RETENTION AND RESULTANT HYPONATREMIA.

Central nervous system

The type 1 receptor for cortisol (which is identical to the mineralocorticoid receptor) and the type 2 receptor are present in various areas of the brain. The type 1 receptor is concentrated in the hippocampus, reticular activating substance, and autonomic nuclei of the brainstem. Cortisol modulates perceptual and emotional functioning. In excess, cortisol causes insomnia and can strikingly elevate or depress the mood. A deficiency of cortisol accentuates auditory, olfactory, and gustatory acuity but may impair an organized response to external sensations. The increase in CRH pulses and cortisol levels just before awakening is important for normal arousal and initiation of daytime activity. CLINICALLY, AN EXCESS OF CORTISOL CAN CAUSE INSOMNIA AND EITHER EUPHORIA OR DEPRESSION.

Fetus

Cortisol facilitates in utero maturation of the lungs, gastrointestinal tract, central nervous system, retina, and skin. The development rate of the pulmonary alveoli, flattening of the lining cells, and thinning of the lung septa are increased. Most important, the synthesis of surfactant, a phospholipid vital for maintaining alveolar surface tension, is increased (see Chapter 27). These actions permit satisfactory breathing immediately after birth. Cortisol also facilitates the maturation of the enzyme capacity of the intestinal mucosa from a fetal to an adult pattern. This permits the newborn to digest the disaccharides in milk.

Cortisol inhibits inflammatory and immune responses

Cortisol has a profound influence on the complex set of reactions evoked by trauma, chemical irritants, foreign proteins, and infection. The overriding effect is to inhibit many important steps in the response to tissue injury.

Cortisol impedes the ability of tissues either to eliminate immediately noxious substances and invaders or to wall them off from the rest of the body. Thus, long-term treatment with pharmacological doses of any glucocorticoid increases a patient's susceptibility to opportunistic infections, allows their dissemination, and masks them. Normal wound healing after injury may also be prevented.

The mechanisms by which cortisol suppresses inflammatory responses are shown in **Figure 47–9**.

- Cortisol induces a phosphoprotein called **lipocortin** that inhibits the enzyme phospholipase A_2. This enzyme generates arachidonic acid. Because arachidonic acid serves as the precursor for the synthesis of prostaglandins and related compounds, the production of these mediators of inflammation is reduced. The production of **nitric oxide** and **platelet-activating factor** is also decreased, impairing vasodilation and leukocyte trapping at the site of an injury.
- Cortisol decreases the number of T lymphocytes and their production of **interleukin-1, interleukin-2, interleukin-6, interferon-**γ, and **tumor necrosis factor.** Initial presentation of antigens by macrophages is suppressed. This blocks the entire cascade of T cell–mediated immunity as well as the generation of fever. Antibody production stimulated by B cells may ultimately be affected.
- Cortisol stabilizes lysosomes and thereby reduces the release of enzymes capable of degrading foreign substances.
- Cortisol blocks the recruitment of neutrophils by inhibiting their ability to bind to chemotactic peptides and endothelial cell surface receptors. The production of stimulatory **leukotrienes** is inhibited in neutrophils, impairing their phagocytic and bactericidal capacity.
- Cortisol decreases the proliferation of fibroblasts and their ability to synthesize and deposit tissue fibrils and thus prevents the encapsulation of invaders.
- Many of cortisol's effects on cells are due to the hormone's effects on cell cycling, arresting the cycle in stages G_0 and G_1, and on apoptosis (programmed cell death).

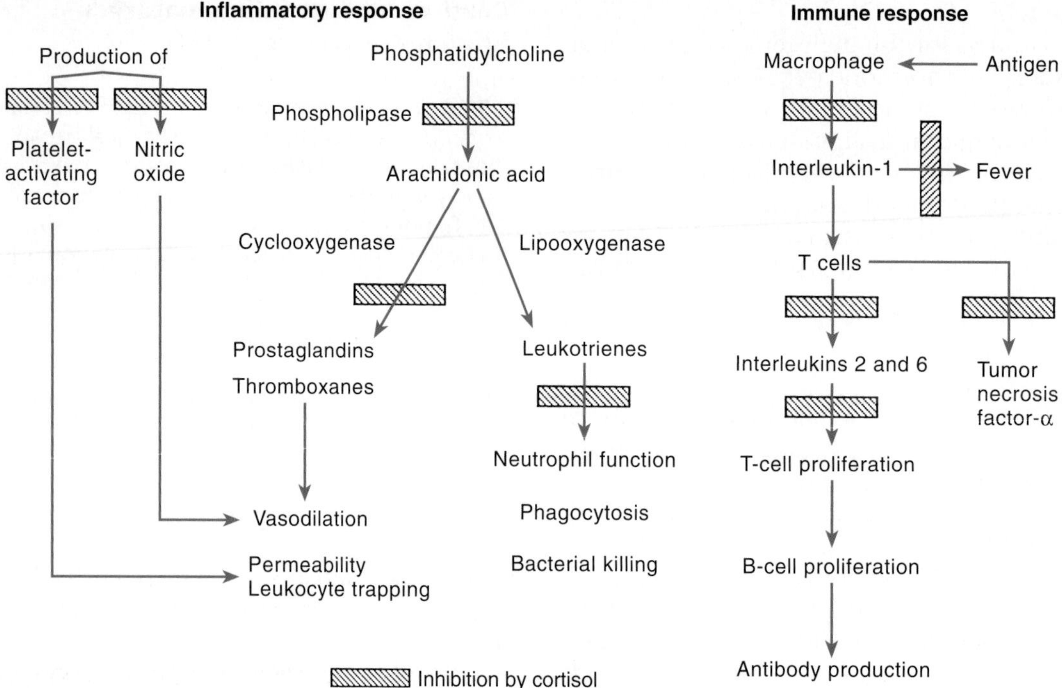

FIGURE 47–9. Mechanisms whereby cortisol inhibits many steps in the processes involved in inflammation and immune system responses. Inhibition of the enzymes phospholipase and cyclooxygenase and the synthesis of nitric oxide and platelet-activating factor impair the vascular component of inflammation. Inhibition of leukotriene actions impairs neutrophil phagocytosis and bactericidal abilities. Inhibition of antigen presentation and macrophage cytokine release impairs proliferation and cytokine release of T cells. Ultimately, B-cell function is reduced so that both cellular and humoral immunity are decreased.

The therapeutic use of glucocorticoids represents a two-edged sword. Glucocorticoids are dramatically beneficial when inflammatory reactions are so severe that they are functionally disabling or life-threatening (e.g., during a severe asthma attack) or when the rejection of transplanted organs, such as a kidney or heart, must be prevented. However, their adverse effects—vulnerability to serious infection, diabetes, osteoporosis, and psychiatric disorders—require physicians to PRESCRIBE GLUCOCORTICOIDS CAUTIOUSLY AND ONLY WHEN NO SAFER FORM OF TREATMENT EXISTS.

This injunction does not apply to the use of replacement doses of cortisol in patients who lack adrenocortical function **(Addison's disease).** Cortisol deficiency leads to anorexia, weight loss, fatigue, poor tolerance of stress, fever, hypoglycemia, and, in women, loss of sexual hair. The loss of negative feedback causes hypersecretion of ACTH and darkening of the skin through its melanocyte-stimulating activity. Suitable cortisol replacement therapy can reverse these findings without adverse effects.

Adrenal Sex Steroids Maintain the Skeletal System and Protect Against Osteoporosis

The recognized role for dehydroepiandrosterone (DHEA) and androstenedione in women is as substrates for extraadrenal and extragonadal testosterone and estradiol production. Both sex steroids help in maintenance of skeletal integrity and protection from osteoporosis. Testosterone stimulates pubic and axillary hair production.

DHEA-S may play a special role in childhood, puberty, and young adulthood. Plasma levels of DHEA-S increase at 6 to 8 years of age, reach a maximum at 20 to 30 years of age, and decline to 25% of the peak at the age of 70 years and to 5% of the peak at the age of 85 to 90 years. Whether a deficiency of DHEA-S contributes to the aging process in a pathological manner remains a moot point.

Aldosterone Secretion Is Regulated Primarily in Response to Changes in Na^+ Availability and Extracellular Fluid Volume

ALDOSTERONE, THE MAJOR PRODUCT OF THE ZONA GLOMERULOSA, HAS TWO PRINCIPAL FUNCTIONS: (1) SUSTAINING EXTRACELLULAR FLUID VOLUME BY CONSERVING BODY Na^+ AND (2) PREVENTING THE OVERLOAD OF K^+ BY ACCELERATING ITS EXCRETION (see Chapters 38 and

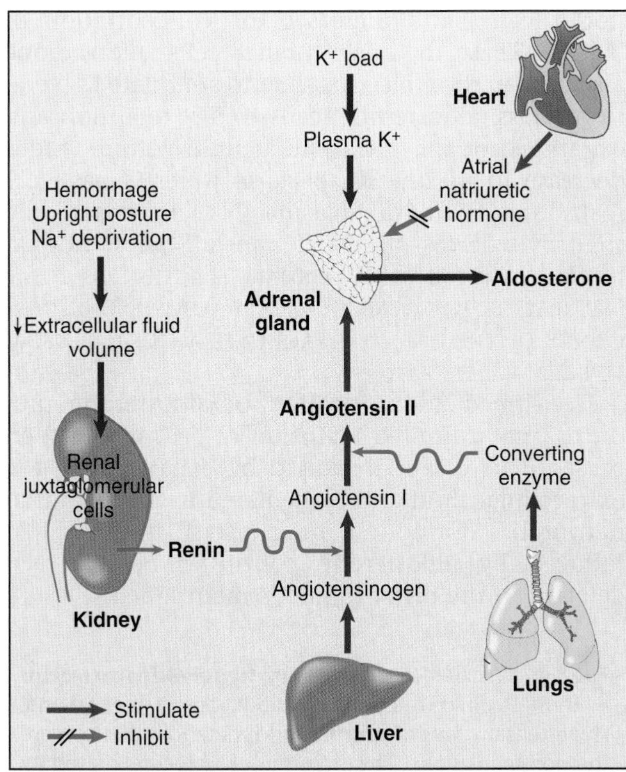

FIGURE 47–10. Regulation of aldosterone secretion. Activation of the renin-angiotensin system in response to hypovolemia is the predominant stimulus for aldosterone production. The kidney, liver, and lungs are required for the production of angiotensin II, the direct stimulator. An elevation of plasma K^+ levels is the other major stimulus of aldosterone secretion. Atrial natriuretic hormones inhibit aldosterone secretion. (See also Chapter 38.)

39). Thus, aldosterone is secreted largely in response to a reduced circulating fluid volume and an increased plasma [K^+] (**Figure 47–10**).

When the body Na^+ content is depleted, the fall in extracellular fluid and plasma volume causes a decrease in the arterial blood pressure and renal blood flow. The juxtaglomerular cells in the kidney respond by secreting the enzyme **renin** into the peripheral circulation (see Chapter 38). Renin acts on its substrate, **angiotensinogen,** to form **angiotensin I.** Angiotensin I is further cleaved by **angiotensin-converting enzyme** to the potent vasoconstrictors **angiotensin II** and **angiotensin III.** These bind to receptors in the zona glomerulosa and stimulate the key enzymatic steps in the synthesis (Figure 47–3) and release (Figure 47–10) of aldosterone. The Ca^{++} and the phosphatidylinositol messenger systems are mediators.

Basal plasma aldosterone levels range from 5 to 15 ng/dL. When hypovolemia is produced, either rapidly by hemorrhage or acute diuresis or slowly by chronic Na^+ deprivation, the aldosterone concentration increases markedly. Conversely, when excess Na^+ is ingested and the extracellular fluid volume expands, renin release and aldosterone secretion are suppressed. Thus, THE JUXTAGLOMERULAR CELLS AND ZONA GLOMERULOSA FORM A PHYSIOLOGICAL FEEDBACK SYSTEM TO DEFEND THE EXTRACELLULAR FLUID VOLUME (see Chapters 38 and 39).

The atrial natriuretic peptide (ANP) hormones, which are released by atrial myocytes in response to increased vascular volume, decrease aldosterone secretion directly by acting on the zona glomerulosa and indirectly by reducing the release of renin (see Chapter 38). The direct action is through ANP receptors, which then cause a decrease in cAMP and an increase in cGMP levels.

K^+ excess stimulates aldosterone secretion

Aldosterone also participates in a vital feedback relationship with K^+ (Figure 47–10). Aldosterone facilitates the clearance of K^+ from the extracellular fluid, and concordantly K^+ is an important stimulator of aldosterone secretion. In humans, raising the plasma [K^+] only 0.5 mEq/L immediately increases plasma aldosterone levels. Conversely, K^+ depletion lowers aldosterone secretion. K^+ acts by depolarizing the zona glomerulosa cell membrane, thereby allowing an influx of Ca^{++} and the activation of aldosterone biosynthesis. Therefore, Ca^{++} channel blockers decrease aldosterone secretion.

Other factors that influence renin release or angiotensin II formation secondarily affect aldosterone secretion. β-Adrenergic stimulation of the kidney in response to hypovolemia increases the output of renin and aldosterone. Certain prostaglandins produced within the kidney also increase renin release. Conversely, inhibitors of angiotensin-converting enzyme or blockers of angiotensin receptors decrease aldosterone secretion.

Therefore, β-adrenergic blocking agents (e.g., **propranolol**) used in the treatment of hypertension or angina, inhibitors of prostaglandin synthesis (e.g., **indomethacin**) used in the treatment of inflammatory conditions, and angiotensin-converting enzyme inhibitors (e.g., **captopril**) used in the treatment of hypertension or congestive heart failure can all depress aldosterone secretion and elevate plasma K^+ levels (see later section).

Aldosterone secretion is also stimulated by ACTH. However, this effect wanes after several days because as Na^+ is retained and extracellular fluid volume rises, renin and angiotensin levels decrease, whereas atrial natriuretic hormone levels increase. These

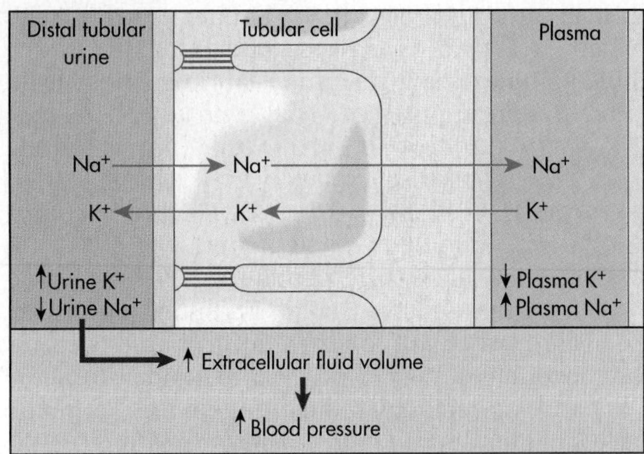

FIGURE 47–11. Action of aldosterone on the renal tubule. Na^+ reabsorption from tubular urine is stimulated. Simultaneously, K^+ secretion into the tubular urine is increased via responses to the electronegative gradient created by Na^+ movement. The net result is the expansion of extracellular fluid and kaliuresis.

responses return aldosterone secretion to basal levels. When ACTH is deficient, the aldosterone response to Na^+ depletion is modestly diminished.

Aldosterone (mineralocorticoids) causes Na^+ retention and K^+ excretion by the kidney

The kidney is the major site of mineralocorticoid action (**Figure 47–11**). As described in detail in Chapters 39 and 40, aldosterone acts on the thick ascending limb of Henle's loop, the distal convoluted tubule, and especially the collecting duct to increase Na^+ reabsorption. The combination of aldosterone and the mineralocorticoid receptor induces expression of Na^+ channel and Na^+-Cl^- symporter genes and increases the concentration of Na^+,K^+-ATPase in target tubular cells. Aldosterone also acts on the collecting duct to stimulate K^+ secretion. Thus, aldosterone leads to Na^+ retention and expansion of the extracellular fluid volume and a decrease in plasma K^+. Because water is passively reabsorbed with Na^+, plasma [Na^+] increases only slightly, whereas plasma K^+ can fall below normal levels. ALTHOUGH ONLY A SMALL FRACTION OF TOTAL Na^+ REABSORPTION IS REGULATED BY ALDOSTERONE, DEFICIENCY OF THE HORMONE PRODUCES A CRITICAL NEGATIVE Na^+ BALANCE.

Continued administration of aldosterone produces only a limited retention of Na^+, which then ceases. This escape is caused by expansion of the extracellular fluid and is mediated in part by atrial natriuretic hormones. In contrast, the K^+ loss induced by aldosterone continues because Na^+ delivery to the distal tubule is maintained.

The net clinical effect of **primary hyperaldosteronism** is modest fluid retention without detectable edema. Hypertension, **hypokalemia,** and metabolic alkalosis are the dominant signs. This situation can be ameliorated by the administration of aldosterone antagonists (e.g., **spironolactone**). In contrast, **aldosterone deficiency** leads to natriuresis, dehydration, hypotension, **hyperkalemia,** modest hyponatremia, and hyperchloremic acidosis. These findings are also present in **Addison's disease,** which is caused by adrenocortical destruction and loss of the zona glomerulosa.

Aldosterone significantly affects Na^+ and K^+ exchange across muscle cells. The net result is an increase in the K^+ content of the intracellular space, another effect that helps prevent hyperkalemia. Aldosterone also modestly stimulates Na^+ reabsorption from gastrointestinal fluids and enhances K^+ excretion in the feces.

Summary

- The adrenal cortex secretes three types of steroid hormones: cortisol, a glucocorticoid; aldosterone, a mineralocorticoid; and androgen precursors, largely dehydroepiandrosterone.
- The adrenal glands are richly vascularized and essential to survival because of the cortisol they produce.
- All adrenocorticosteroids are synthesized from cholesterol by sequential enzymatic steps consisting of side chain cleavage and hydroxylation of key sites in the steroid molecule. Cortisol specifically requires an 11-hydroxyl group; aldosterone, an 18-hydroxyl group; and androgens, a 17-hydroxyl group for their respective activities.
- Cortisol secretion and androgen secretion are stimulated by adrenocorticotropin (ACTH) from the pituitary gland. ACTH secretion is stimulated by CRH from the hypothalamus. Cortisol feeds back negatively to suppress the release of both ACTH and CRH.

- ACTH, via cAMP as second messenger, stimulates the cellular uptake of cholesterol, its movement from storage vacuoles into mitochondria, and all subsequent biosynthetic steps to cortisol.
- Cortisol acts via a nuclear receptor and modulates gene expression of numerous enzymes and proteins. Cortisol increases muscle proteolysis and hepatic conversion of the liberated amino acids into glucose and its storage as glycogen. Cortisol also inhibits insulin-stimulated glucose uptake by muscle.
- Cortisol stimulates calorie intake and favors the deposition of fat in selected sites. By inhibiting collagen synthesis, cortisol reduces bone formation and causes thinning of the skin and capillary walls.
- Cortisol strongly inhibits the entire process of inflammation, including the recruitment and function of neutrophils and the release of prostaglandin and leukotriene mediators. It also inhibits the immune system and prevents the proliferation of thymus-derived lymphocytes and the production of some lymphokines.
- Aldosterone is a major regulator of Na^+, K^+, and fluid balance. It acts on the renal tubule via a nuclear receptor. Na^+ reabsorption is increased, and there is concomitant expansion of extracellular fluid. Renal K^+ excretion is concurrently increased, and plasma $[K^+]$ is lowered.
- Aldosterone secretion is regulated primarily by the renin-angiotensin system.

Bibliography

Canalis E, Giustina A: Glucocorticoid-induced osteoporosis: summary of a workshop, *J Clin Endocrinol Metab* 86:5681, 2001.

Chrousos GP: The hypothalamic-pituitary-adrenal axis and immune-mediated inflammation, *N Engl J Med* 332:1351, 1995.

Chrousos GP, Gold PW: The concepts of stress and stress system disorders, *JAMA* 267:1244, 1992.

Horrocks PM et al: Patterns of ACTH and cortisol pulsatility over twenty-four hours in normal males and females, *Clin Endocrinol (Oxf)* 32:127, 1990.

Hunt PJ et al: Improvement in mood and fatigue after dehydroepiandrosterone replacement in Addison's disease in a randomized, double blind trial, *J Clin Endocrinol Metab* 85:4650, 2000.

Kim GH et al: The thiazide-sensitive Na-Cl cotransporter is an aldosterone-induced protein, *Proc Natl Acad Sci USA* 95:14552, 1998.

Masilamani S et al: Aldosterone-mediated regulation of ENaC α, β, and γ subunit proteins in rat kidney, *J Clin Invest* 104:R19, 1999.

Mastorakos G, Chrousos GP, Weber JS: Recombinant interleukin-6 activates the hypothalamic-pituitary-adrenal axis in humans, *J Clin Endocrinol Metab* 77:1690, 1993.

Meikle AW: Secretion and metabolism of the corticosteroids and adrenal function and testing. In DeGroot LJ, Jameson JL, eds: *Endocrinology,* ed 4, Philadelphia, 2001, WB Saunders.

Mortensen RM, Williams GH: Aldosterone action: physiology. In DeGroot LJ, Jameson JL, eds: *Endocrinology,* ed 4, Philadelphia, 2001, WB Saunders.

Munck A, Náray-Fejes-Tóth A: Glucocorticoid action: physiology. In DeGroot LJ, Jameson JL, eds: *Endocrinology,* ed 4, Philadelphia, 2001, WB Saunders.

Orth DN, Kovacs WJ, Debold CR: The adrenal cortex. In Wilson JD, Foster DW, eds: *Williams textbook of endocrinology,* ed 9, Philadelphia, 1998, WB Saunders.

Pearce D, Bhargava A, Cole TJ: Aldosterone: its receptor, target genes, and actions, *Vitam Horm* 66:29, 2003.

Pushkala K, Gupta PD: Steroid hormones regulate programmed cell death: a review, *Cytobios* 106:201, 2001.

Stewart PM, Krozowski ZS: 11β-Hydroxysteroid dehydrogenase, *Vitam Horm* 57:249, 1999.

Stocco DM: StAR protein and the regulation of steroid hormone biosynthesis, *Annu Rev Physiol* 63:193, 2001.

Takeda R et al: Aldosterone biosynthesis and action in vascular cells, *Steroids* 60:120, 1995.

Wallberg, AE, Wright A, Gustafsson JA: Chromatin-remodeling complexes involved in gene activation by the glucocorticoid receptor, *Vitam Horm* 60:75, 2000.

Wick G et al: Immunoendocrine communication via the hypothalamus-pituitary-adrenal axis in autoimmune diseases, *Endocr Rev* 14:539, 1993.

Case Studies

Case 47–1

A 56-year-old woman with a 40-year history of heavy tobacco use has recently begun coughing. She has gained 20 pounds in 6 months, mostly in the face and abdomen, and has noticed increasing facial hair. Her blood pressure is 160/108 mm Hg. She has bilateral edema of her legs. A chest radiograph shows a large mass in her right lung. Her physician suspects a lung cancer that is an ectopic source of ACTH production.

1. Which of the following would be increased?
- **A.** Serum [K^+] levels
- **B.** Skin pigmentation
- **C.** Pituitary ACTH secretion
- **D.** Hypothalamic CRH secretion
- **E.** Serum renin levels

2. The patient undergoes surgery to remove the tumor. On the first day after surgery, she develops a high fever, hypotension, profound anorexia, and hyponatremia. What is the diagnosis?
- **A.** She has acute cortisol deficiency resulting from atrophy of the adrenal zona fasciculata.
- **B.** She has acute ACTH deficiency resulting from atrophy of the adrenocorticotrophs.
- **C.** She has acute ADH deficiency.
- **D.** She has acute aldosterone deficiency resulting from atrophy of the adrenal zona glomerulosa.
- **E.** She has acute DHEA deficiency resulting from atrophy of the adrenal zona reticularis.

Case 47–2

A 65-year-old man with severe atherosclerosis abruptly develops hypertension. His blood pressure is 220/122 mm Hg. On auscultation, a harsh bruit (sound of blood flowing past an obstruction) is heard over the right kidney. The diagnosis of a partial occlusion of the renal artery is confirmed radiographically.

1. Which of the following would be decreased?
- **A.** Serum [K^+]
- **B.** Serum aldosterone levels
- **C.** Serum angiotensin levels
- **D.** Serum renin levels
- **E.** Serum atrial natriuretic hormone levels

2. Which of the following does not contribute to the patient's hypertension?
- **A.** Ca^{++}
- **B.** Angiotensin-converting enzyme
- **C.** Protein kinase C
- **D.** Na^+,K^+-ATPase
- **E.** cAMP

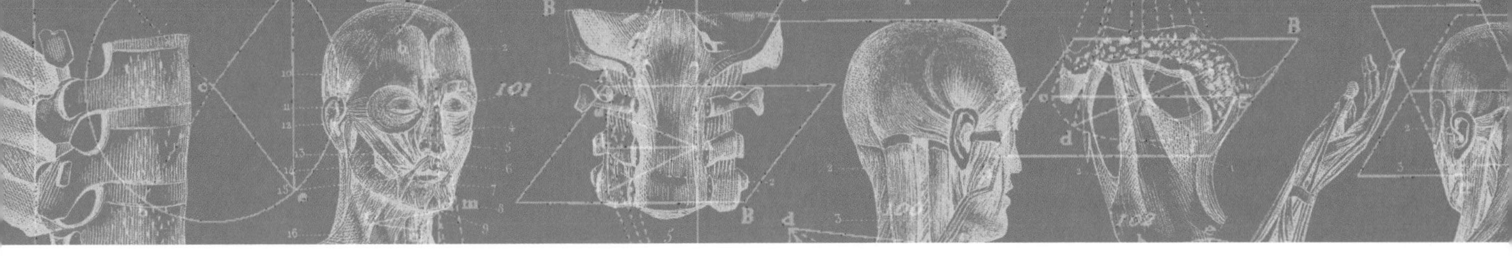

Chapter 48: Adrenal Medulla

Objectives

- ❖ Explain the relationship between the neural and endocrine functions of catecholamine hormones.
- ❖ Describe the biochemistry and intracellular sites of catecholamine hormone synthesis.
- ❖ Describe the factors that regulate epinephrine and norepinephrine secretion by the adrenal medulla.
- ❖ Examine the wide array of epinephrine and norepinephrine actions.
- ❖ Explain the concept of the stress reaction and the complex interplay of adrenocortical and medullary hormones in response to stress.

The Adrenal Medulla Functions Partly as a Sympathetic Nervous System Ganglion and Partly as an Endocrine Gland

The adrenal medulla forms the inner core of the adrenal gland (see Figure 47–2). It is the source of the circulating catecholamine hormone **epinephrine.** The medulla also secretes **norepinephrine,** primarily a neurotransmitter that can also function as a hormone. The catecholamine hormones are important mediators of rapid fuel mobilization; they increase the release of both glucose and free fatty acids, especially during acute stress. They also stimulate the cardiovascular system and cause contraction or relaxation of smooth muscles in the respiratory, gastrointestinal, and genitourinary tracts.

The adrenal medulla is essentially a specialized sympathetic ganglion (see Figure 10–2). However, the neuronal cells of the medulla do not have axons; instead, they discharge their products directly into the bloodstream, and thus they function in true endocrine fashion. The medulla is often activated along with the sympathetic portion of the autonomic nervous system and acts in concert with it in the fight-or-flight reaction. Some of the neurotransmitter actions of norepinephrine are duplicated and amplified by the hormone actions of epinephrine, which reaches similar targets via the circulation. However, epinephrine has other effects of its own, some of which modulate those of norepinephrine.

The adrenal medulla is formed in parallel with the peripheral sympathetic nervous system. At about 7 weeks of gestation, neuroectodermal cells invade the adrenal cortex, where they develop into the medulla. The development of this tissue and the induction of hormone synthesis are stimulated by nerve growth factor. The adrenal medulla begins to function during the gestational period.

The adult adrenal medulla weighs about 1 g and is composed of **chromaffin cells.** These are organized in cords in intimate relationship with venules that drain the adrenal cortex. THE CHROMAFFIN CELLS ARE INNERVATED BY CHOLINERGIC PREGANGLIONIC FIBERS OF THE SYMPATHETIC NERVOUS SYSTEM. Within these cells are numerous granules similar to those found in postganglionic sympathetic nerve terminals. These contain catecholamines, ATP, proopiomelanocortin products (see Chapter 47), **chromogranin,** and other neuropeptides. Approximately 85% of the chromaffin granules store epinephrine, and 15% store norepinephrine.

Catecholamine Hormones Are Synthesized in Sequential Steps Alternating Between the Cytoplasm and Storage Granules of the Adrenomedullary Cells

The catecholamines are synthesized by the series of reactions shown in **Figure 48–1**. The intermediates move back and forth in sequence between the cytoplasm and the storage granules. The first, rate-limiting step is the conversion of tyrosine to **dihydroxyphenylalanine (DOPA).** It occurs in the cytoplasm and requires molecular O_2, a tetrahydropteridine, and reduced nicotinamide adenine dinucleotide phosphate. The subsequent decarboxylation of DOPA to **dopamine** in the cytoplasm uses pyridoxal phosphate as a cofactor. The dopamine must then be taken up into the chromaffin granules, where the next enzyme in the sequence, dopamine β-hydroxylase, catalyzes the formation of norepinephrine from dopamine, molecular O_2, and a hydrogen donor. In a minority of granules, the sequence ends there, and the norepinephrine remains stored.

In most granules, norepinephrine reenters the cytoplasm, where it is *N*-methylated to epinephrine, with *S*-adenosylmethionine as the methyl donor. The epinephrine is then taken back up into the chromaffin granules for storage. Granule uptake of catecholamines and their storage at high concentrations require ATP. A total of 1 mole of the nucleotide complexes with 4 moles of catecholamine hormone and a protein known as chromogranin.

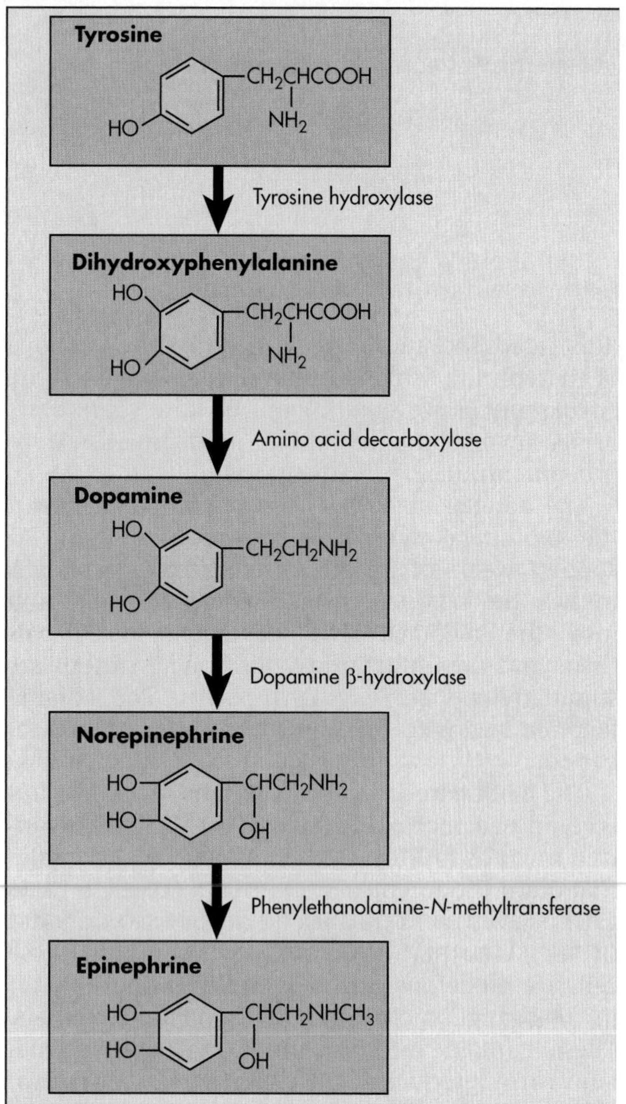

FIGURE 48–1. Pathway of catecholamine hormone synthesis in the adrenal medulla.

The synthesis and secretion of catecholamine hormones are regulated by sympathetic nerve impulses and cortisol

The synthesis of epinephrine and norepinephrine (Figure 48–1) is regulated by several factors. Acute sympathetic stimulation of the medulla activates the initial rate-limiting step. Chronic stimulation induces an increased concentration of tyrosine hydroxylase, and thereby catecholamine output is maintained in the face of continuous demand. cAMP mediates both of these effects. Cortisol specifically induces the last enzyme in the sequence, *N*-methyltransferase, and selectively stimulates epinephrine synthesis. The perfusion of the adrenal medulla with cortisol-enriched blood from the adrenal cortex facilitates this induction.

The effector pathway for the release of adrenal medullary hormones consists of **cholinergic** preganglionic fibers in the splanchnic nerves. On nerve stimulation, **acetylcholine,** which is released from the nerve terminals, depolarizes the chromaffin cell membrane by increasing its permeability to Na^+. This in turn induces an influx of Ca^{++}, which causes aggregation of the chromaffin granules. Exocytosis follows with the secretion of epinephrine, norepinephrine, ATP, dopamine β-hydroxylase, neuropeptides, and chromogranin. Although chromaffin cells contain about 30,000 granules each, a single stimulus–action potential releases less than 1 granule per cell. The major fibrinolytic enzyme **plasmin** is attracted to binding sites on the chromaffin cells and cleaves chromogranin as it is released from the cell. Peptide cleavage products of chromogranin in turn inhibit further release of catecholamines via exocytosis, forming an autocrine negative feedback regulatory arrangement.

In a complex set of reactions, catecholamine hormones are metabolized to products excreted in the urine

All the circulating epinephrine is derived from adrenal medullary secretion. Basal plasma epinephrine levels are 25 to 50 pg/mL. In contrast, almost all the circulating norepinephrine is derived from sympathetic nerve terminals and from the brain; this represents norepinephrine that escaped local reuptake from the synaptic clefts. Basal norepinephrine levels are 100 to 350 pg/mL. Both catecholamines have plasma half-lives of about 2 minutes, which allows rapid turnoff of their dramatic effects. Only 2% to 3% of catecholamines, the majority of which is norepinephrine, are excreted unchanged in the urine.

Epinephrine and norepinephrine are metabolized by *O*-methylation and oxidative deamination, predominantly in the liver and kidney. The major end products, **vanillylmandelic acid** and **metanephrines,** are excreted in the urine. They serve as indices of activity of the sympathetic nervous system or of pathological hypersecretion of the catecholamine hormones by tumors of the adrenal medulla called **pheochromocytomas.**

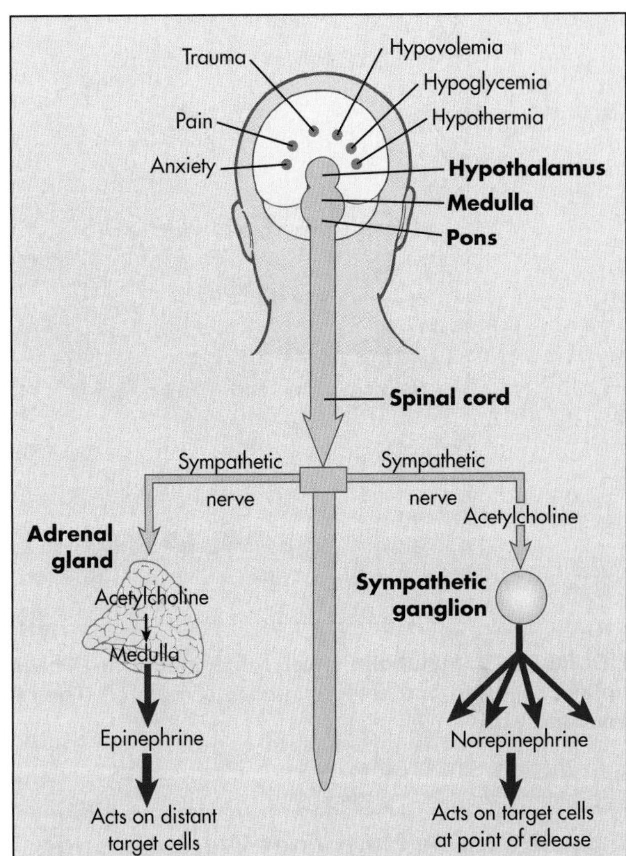

FIGURE 48–2. Activation of catecholamine effects via the sympathetic nervous system and the adrenal medulla. The adrenal medulla is homologous to a sympathetic ganglion, but the adrenal medulla releases its catecholamines into the bloodstream rather than into a synaptic cleft.

Adrenal medullary secretion is stimulated by many factors related to stress

Secretion from the adrenal medulla is part of the fight-or-flight reaction (**Figure 48–2**). Thus, THE PERCEPTION OR EVEN ANTICIPATION OF DANGER, FEAR, EXCITEMENT, TRAUMA, PAIN, HYPOVOLEMIA, HYPOTENSION, ANOXIA, HYPOTHERMIA, HYPOGLYCEMIA, AND INTENSE EXERCISE CAUSE THE RAPID RELEASE OF EPINEPHRINE AND NOREPINEPHRINE (see Chapter 26). These stimuli are sensed at various levels in the sympathetic nervous system, and responses are initiated in the hypothalamus and brainstem (see also Chapter 10). Epinephrine secretion may follow activation of the sympathetic nervous system by more intense stimuli. However, epinephrine secretion specifically increases in response to mild hypoglycemia, moderate hypoxia, and fasting even though sympathetic nervous system activity may remain constant or decrease.

Mild hypoglycemia causes a 5-fold to 10-fold increase in the plasma epinephrine concentration but little change in the norepinephrine concentration. The resulting epinephrine concentration can stimulate a compensatory increase in the plasma glucose level; the norepinephrine level cannot. The reduction in central venous pressure produced by a person assuming the upright position (see Chapter 24) increases both plasma epinephrine and norepinephrine concentrations 2-fold. However, only the epinephrine concentration is high enough to increase the heart rate and blood pressure. Thus, epinephrine functions as a true hormone in both situations, whereas norepinephrine does not. Norepinephrine, however, contributes as a neurotransmitter to the compensatory response to hypovolemia and to more severe hypoglycemia because the higher concentration necessary for its action is generated locally at the effector site (Figure 48–2). IN STATES OF MAJOR METABOLIC DECOMPENSATION, SUCH AS DIABETIC KETOACIDOSIS, THE CIRCULATING CONCENTRATIONS OF BOTH CATECHOLAMINES RISE HIGH ENOUGH TO EVOKE RESPONSES.

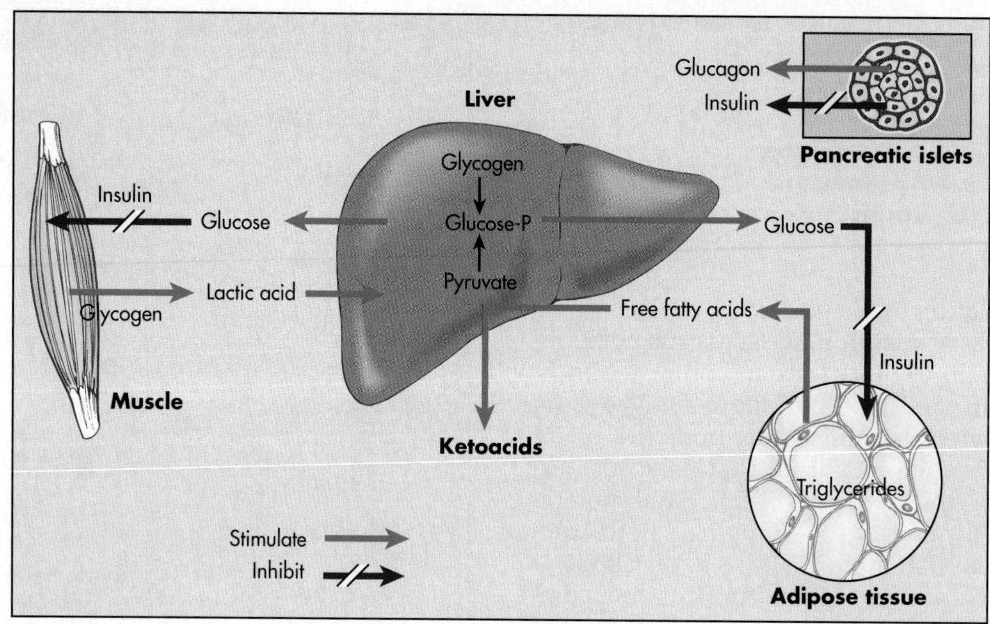

FIGURE 48–3. Metabolic effects of epinephrine. The hormone stimulates glucose production and inhibits glucose uptake. Lipolysis and ketogenesis are stimulated. The result is an increase in plasma levels of glucose, free fatty acids, and keto acids.

Catecholamine Hormones Work Through Several Plasma Membrane Receptors and Second Messengers

Epinephrine and norepinephrine exert their many effects via several plasma membrane receptors, designated β_1, β_2, β_3, α_1, and α_2. The β_1, β_2, and β_3 receptors are structurally similar glycoproteins. Each winds in and out of the plasma membrane so that more than one surface is presented extracellularly for hormone binding and intracellularly for signal generation (see Chapter 5). The β_1, β_2, and β_3 receptors are coupled to the stimulating G protein of adenylyl cyclase, and hormone binding increases cAMP levels. In contrast, the α_2 receptor is coupled to the inhibiting G protein of adenylyl cyclase, and hormone binding decreases cAMP levels. Catecholamine hormones therefore either trigger (β_1 or β_2) or suppress (α_2) a cascade of protein phosphorylations catalyzed by protein kinase A. The α_1 receptor is structurally different and is coupled to Ca^{++} and phosphatidylinositol products as second messengers.

Continuous exposure to catecholamines eventually down-regulates the number of receptors and induces partial refractoriness to hormone action. A distinctly different phenomenon—acute desensitization to successive doses of catecholamine hormones—is caused by hormone-induced activation of protein kinase A or C, which results in the phosphorylation of the receptor molecules themselves. This desensitization process constitutes a form of rapid intracellular negative feedback that almost immediately limits hormone actions.

Catecholamine hormones mobilize substrates for energy generation and increased energy expenditure

THE MAJOR METABOLIC EFFECT OF CATECHOLAMINES IS FUEL MOBILIZATION (**Figure 48–3**). Glycogenolysis in the liver is stimulated via the cAMP-mediated activation of phosphorylase, and glucose output increases. In the absence of glucagon, this epinephrine action is critical to recovery from insulin-induced hypoglycemia in type 1 diabetes (see Chapter 43). Glycogenolysis in muscle is similarly stimulated. This increases muscle glucose supply and glycolysis. Lactate is released and serves as a substrate for hepatic gluconeogenesis. In addition, gluconeogenesis is stimulated directly by catecholamines, through α_1 receptors in the liver. Plasma glucose levels also rise because catecholamines inhibit insulin secretion as well as insulin-stimulated glucose uptake by muscle tissue. The availability of free fatty acids is increased by activating the enzyme adipose tissue lipase. The enhanced lipolysis in turn leads to increased free fatty acid oxidation in the liver and ketogenesis.

The catecholamine hormones are diabetogenic. They contribute materially to the development of hyperglycemia and ketonemia in diabetic ketoacidosis, particularly when an intercurrent stress has provoked this metabolic emergency.

All of this sequence is an important response to exercise.

Catecholamines increase the basal metabolic rate by stimulating facultative, or nonshivering, thermogenesis (see Chapter 42). This action is an important part of the response to cold exposure. In adipose tissue, catecholamines stimulate energy expenditure and increase heat production by inducing transcription of the gene for an uncoupling protein (see Chapter 46). Catecholamines also increase diet-induced thermogenesis.

Sympathetic nervous system activity decreases during fasting and increases after feeding. In this way, norepinephrine adapts total energy use to energy availability and helps maintain balance between them. In contrast, epinephrine secretion increases slightly during prolonged fasting and also 4 to 5 hours after a meal, when the plasma glucose level is declining. This response serves a different purpose: sustaining glucose production for use by the central nervous system.

The activity of the sympathetic nervous system tends to be decreased in obese individuals. This characteristic favors storage of energy as fat when dietary calories are plentiful.

Epinephrine and norepinephrine activate the cardiovascular system

The cardiovascular and visceral effects of epinephrine are consonant with its metabolic actions (**Table 48–1**). For example, during exercise, epinephrine increases cardiac output by increasing the cardiac contractile force and heart rate (see Chapters 19 and 26). At the same time, muscle arterioles dilate (because of local metabolic factors), whereas renal, splanchnic, and cutaneous arterioles constrict because of increased epinephrine levels. Systolic blood pressure increases. The net effect is to shunt blood to exercising muscles and away from other tissues while essential coronary and cerebral blood flows are maintained (see Chapter 26). This guarantees the delivery of O_2 and substrate for energy production to the critical tissues in situations of danger or during whole-body exercise.

TABLE 48–1. ACTIONS OF CATECHOLAMINE HORMONES

β	α
Metabolic	
↑ Glycogenolysis	↑ Gluconeogenesis (α_1)
↑ Glucose use	
↑ Lipolysis and ketosis (β_1)	
↑ Calorigenesis (β_1)	
↑ Insulin secretion (β_2)	↓ Insulin secretion (α_2)
↑ Glucagon secretion (β_2)	
↑ Muscle K^+ uptake (β_2)	
Cardiovascular	
↑ Cardiac contractility (β_1)	
↑ Heart rate (β_1)	
↑ Conduction velocity (β_1)	
↑ Arteriolar dilation (β_2) (muscle)	↑ Arteriolar vasoconstriction (α_1) (splanchnic, renal, cutaneous, genital)
↓ Blood pressure	↑ Blood pressure
Visceral	
↑ Muscle relaxation (β_2)	↑ Sphincter contraction (α_1)
Gastrointestinal	Gastrointestinal
Urinary	Urinary
Bronchial	
Other	
—	Sweating (adrenergic)
	Dilation of pupils
	Platelet aggregation (α_2)

↑, increased; ↓, decreased.

In severe or prolonged states of shock, the compensatory hypersecretion of catecholamines can eventually contribute to fatal ischemic kidney and hepatic failure and to lactic acidosis (see Chapter 26). The catecholamine response to exercise may also be disadvantageous in patients who have coronary artery disease and who cannot adequately increase myocardial blood flow. β-Adrenergic antagonists are used to good therapeutic advantage in this situation; by decreasing heart rate, cardiac contractility, and systolic blood pressure, these drugs improve the balance between myocardial work and O_2 supply and prevent **angina pectoris** (chest pain).

Catecholamine hormones have effects that mimic those of the sympathetic nervous system

During exposure to cold, the constriction of cutaneous vessels helps conserve heat and reinforces epinephrine's thermogenic action. Other responses useful to the threatened individual are relaxation of the bronchioles, which improves alveolar gas exchange; dilation of the pupils, which permits better distant vision; and inhibition of temporarily unneeded gastrointestinal and genitourinary motor activity that could hinder escape from danger.

During acute asthma attacks, constriction of the bronchioles increases airway resistance (see Chapter 32) and causes wheezing and hypoxia. Synthetic β-adrenergic agonists of epinephrine, administered through inhalers, relax the bronchioles and provide critical relief to patients in respiratory distress.

The catecholamines also have significant actions on mineral metabolism. They increase Na^+ reabsorption by the kidney by stimulating renal tubular Na^+ transport and by stimulating renin release and consequently aldosterone secretion (see Chapter 38). They also stimulate the influx of K^+ into muscle cells via β_2 receptors and help prevent hyperkalemia (see Chapter 39).

Pathological hypersecretion of epinephrine and norepinephrine from a tumor of the chromaffin cells **(pheochromocytoma)** results in a distinct and dangerous syndrome. Bursts of catecholamine release can cause sudden tachycardia, extreme anxiety with a sense of impending death, cold perspiration, skin pallor resulting from vasoconstriction, blurred vision, headache, and chest pain. The blood pressure may rise greatly and cause stroke or heart failure. In addition to such episodes, chronic catecholamine excess may produce weight loss (as a result of the increased metabolic rate) and hyperglycemia. Prompt surgical removal of the tumor is mandatory.

Adrenomedullin, a small protein/large peptide containing 52 amino acids, is secreted by the adrenal medulla and endothelial and smooth muscle cells. Its most prominent action is to lower blood pressure by causing vasodilation through stimulating nitric oxide production, by decreasing aldosterone responses to K^+ and angiotensin, and by causing natriuresis. Excessive adrenomedullin release may contribute to the hypotensive state that often accompanies sepsis.

The Hypothalamic-Pituitary-Adrenocortical Axis, Adrenal Medulla, and Sympathetic Nervous System Together Integrate the Response to Stress

The adrenal medulla and adrenal cortex are both major participants in the adaptation to stress. Their intimate anatomical juxtaposition mirrors a fundamental functional relationship between the sympathetic nervous system and the corticotropin-releasing hormone–adrenocorticotropic hormone–cortisol axis (**Figure 48–4**). Stress is perceived by many areas of the brain, from the cortex down to the brainstem. Major stresses almost simultaneously activate corticotropin-releasing hormone (CRH) and ADH neurons and adrenergic neurons in the hypothalamus. The activation is mutually reinforcing because norepinephrine input increases CRH release and CRH increases adrenergic discharge (Figure 48–4). The release of CRH (and ADH) elevates plasma cortisol levels; adrenergic stimulation elevates plasma catecholamine levels. Together, these hormones increase glucose production and shift glucose use toward the central nervous system and away from peripheral tissues. Epinephrine also rapidly augments the supply of free fatty acid to the heart and to muscles, and cortisol facilitates this lipolytic response. Both hormones raise the blood pressure and cardiac output and improve the delivery of substrates to tissues critical to the immediate defense of the organism. If the stress involves tissue trauma or invasion by microorganisms, high cortisol levels eventually act to restrain the initial inflammatory and immune responses so that these responses do not themselves lead to irreparable damage.

Norepinephrine and CRH produce other adaptive responses to stress. A general state of arousal and vigilance, an activation of defensively useful behavior, and appropriate aggressiveness result from norepinephrine stimulation of pertinent brain centers. At the same time, CRH input to other hypothalamic neurons inhibits appetite, sexual activity, and growth hormone and gonadotropin release. This is reinforced by the excess of cortisol, which also suppresses growth and ovulation. Thus, the adaptation to stress represents a prime example of the integration between the nervous system and the endocrine system.

Although the description of the stress response appears unvarying and monolithic, there is evidence to suggest that individual stresses lead to specific patterns of response. Moreover, different persons may respond more or less strongly or in qualitatively different ways to the same stress.

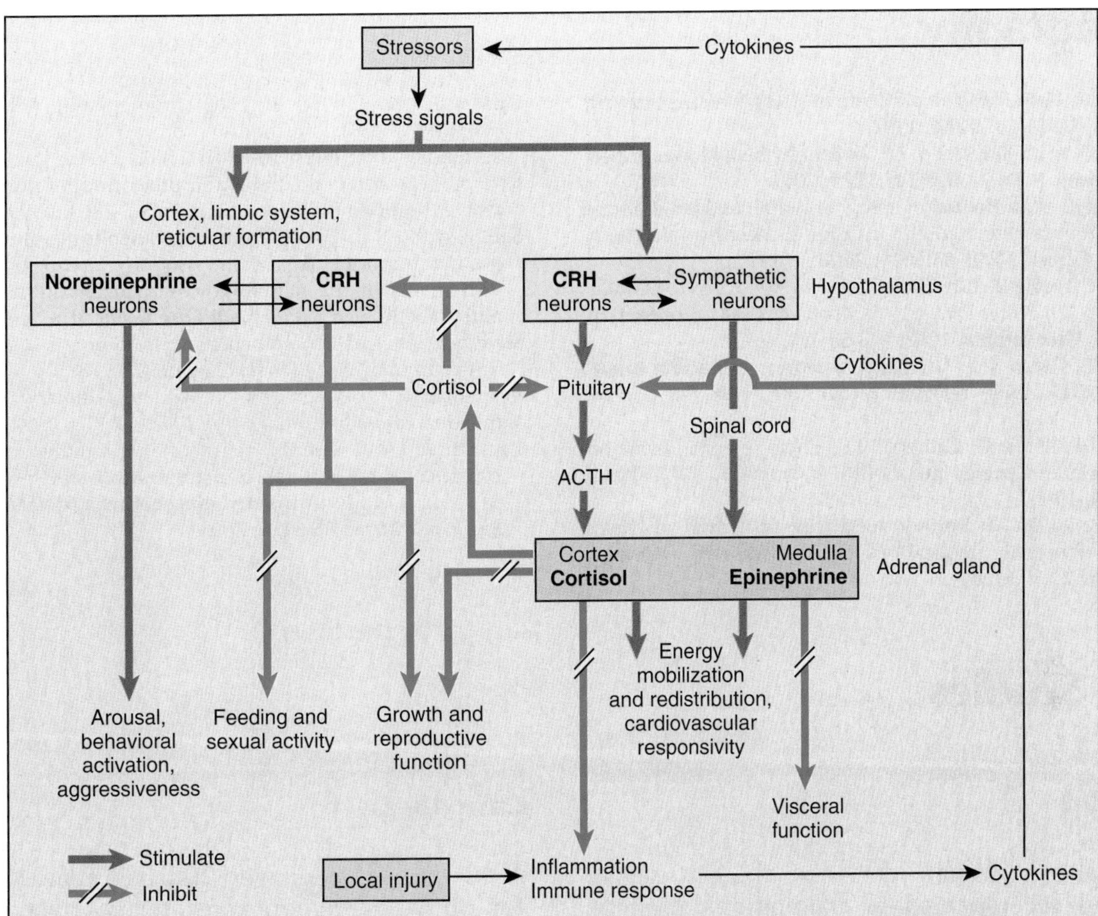

FIGURE 48–4. Integrated responses to stress mediated by the sympathetic nervous system and the hypothalamic-pituitary-adrenocortical axis. The responses are mutually reinforcing at both the central and peripheral levels. Inflammatory cytokines stimulate ACTH release, but negative feedback by cortisol also can limit an overresponse of inflammation that might be harmful to the individual.

Summary

- The adrenal medulla is an enlarged, specialized sympathetic ganglion that synthesizes epinephrine and norepinephrine from tyrosine and stores them in granules.
- Catecholamines are released from the medulla in response to activity in preganglionic cholinergic fibers of the sympathetic nervous system that are stimulated by hypoglycemia, hypovolemia, hypotension, exercise, or stress.
- Circulating epinephrine increases the concentrations of plasma glucose, free fatty acids, and keto acids by stimulating glycogenolysis and lipolysis and by inhibiting glucose uptake by muscle. The metabolic rate also rises. cAMP and Ca^{++} are second messengers.
- Cardiovascular actions include increases in heart rate and cardiac contractility and variable effects on different vascular beds.
- Circulating norepinephrine contributes to these effects, but more often the effects of epinephrine are reinforced by concurrent activation of the sympathetic nervous system, with norepinephrine as the neurotransmitter.

Bibliography

Chrousos GP, Gold PW: The concepts of stress and stress system disorders, *JAMA* 267:1244, 1992.

Herndon DN et al: Reversal of catabolism by beta-blockade after severe burns, *N Engl J Med* 345:1223, 2001.

Lainchbury JG et al: Hemodynamic, hormonal, and renal effects of short-term adrenomedullin infusion in healthy volunteers, *J Clin Endocrinol Metab* 85:1016, 2000.

Landsberg L, Young JB: Catecholamines and the adrenal medulla. In Wilson JD, Foster DW, eds: *Williams textbook of endocrinology,* ed 9, Philadelphia, 1998, WB Saunders.

Lefkowitz RJ, Caron MG: Adrenergic receptors: molecular mechanisms of clinically relevant recognition, *Clin Res* 33:395, 1985.

Matthews DE, Pesola G, Campbell RG: Effect of epinephrine on amino acid and energy metabolism in humans, *Am J Physiol* 258:E948, 1990.

Pacak K, Palkovits M: Stressor specificity of central neuroendocrine responses: implications for stress-related disorders, *Endocr Rev* 22:502, 2001.

Parmer RJ et al: Processing of chromogranin A by plasmin provides a novel mechanism for regulating catecholamine secretion, *J Clin Invest* 106:907, 2000.

Samson WK: Adrenomedullin and the control of fluid and electrolyte homeostasis, *Annu Rev Physiol* 61:363, 1999.

Santiago JV et al: Epinephrine, norepinephrine, glucagon, and growth hormone release in association with physiological decrements in the plasma glucose concentration in normal and diabetic man, *J Clin Endocrinol Metab* 51:877, 1980.

Silverberg A et al: Norepinephrine: hormone and neurotransmitter in man, *Am J Physiol* 234:E252, 1978.

Wortsman J, Frank S, Cryer PE: Adrenomedullary response to maximal stress in humans, *Am J Med* 77:779, 1984.

Zuckerman-Levin N et al: The importance of adrenocortical glucocorticoids for adrenomedullary and physiological response to stress: a study in isolated glucocorticoid deficiency, *J Clin Endocrinol Metab* 86:5920, 2001.

Case Studies

Case 48–1

A 25-year-old woman develops sudden, severe headaches accompanied by palpitations, anxiety, and clammy sweat. During one such episode, she is examined in an emergency department; her blood pressure is 260/140 mm Hg, her pulse is 56 beats/min, and her serum K^+ value is 3.4 mEq/L.

1. **An excess of which of the following hormones is the most likely cause?**
   A. Cortisol
   B. Epinephrine
   C. Norepinephrine
   D. Aldosterone
   E. 11-Deoxycorticosterone

2. **Which of the following drugs would quickly lower her dangerously high systolic and diastolic blood pressures?**
   A. An α_1-adrenergic blocker
   B. A β_1-adrenergic blocker
   C. A β_2-adrenergic blocker
   D. An α_2-adrenergic blocker
   E. An aldosterone antagonist

Case 48–2

A 40-year-old man who has had type 1 diabetes for 30 years demonstrates severe hyperglycemic damage to the peripheral parts of the sympathetic nervous system.

1. **Release of which of the following hormones is most likely impaired by this "neuropathy"?**
   A. C peptide
   B. Glucagon
   C. Epinephrine
   D. Cortisol
   E. Growth hormone

2. **If epinephrine cannot be released in response to hypoglycemia, which of the following hormones is most critical for promptly raising the blood glucose level?**
   A. Growth hormone
   B. Glucagon
   C. Cortisol
   D. Insulin
   E. Somatostatin

Chapter 49: Overview of Reproductive Function

Objectives

- ❖ Identify the synthetic pathway for androgens and estrogens, the gonadal steroid hormones.
- ❖ Identify the common elements of the hypothalamic-pituitary-gonadal axis in males and females.
- ❖ Describe the common hormonal components of puberty and senescence in males and females.
- ❖ Explain the differences between genetic sex, gonadal sex, and phenotypic (genital) sex.

The endocrine glands in general are essential to maintaining the life and well-being of the individual. In contrast, the endocrine function of the gonads is also concerned with the perpetuation and well-being of the species. Human reproduction requires highly complex patterns of hypothalamic-pituitary-gonadal function that ensure the development and maintenance of mature gametes, **ova** and **spermatozoa,** from primordial germ cells; their subsequent successful union **(fertilization);** and finally the growth and development of the conceptus within the body of the mother. Gonadal hormones also influence many other functions and structures described elsewhere in this book (e.g., hepatic function, skeletal structure). Although certain fundamental differences exist between male and female gonadal function, important conceptual similarities and operational homologies are also present. The gender differences are better appreciated if the common aspects of gonadal function are first understood.

The Gonads Contain Several Cell Types with Different Reproductive and Hormonal Functions

The gonad, whether ovary or testis, consists of two distinct anatomical and functional parts. One part encloses the developing germ cell line, with specialized membrane and cytoplasmic barriers that prevent its indiscriminate exposure to all constituents of plasma and interstitial fluid. In the ovary, the germ cell enclosure is the **follicle;** in the testis, it is the **spermatogenic (seminiferous) tubule.** The other part is composed of surrounding endocrine cells that secrete sex steroid hormones, protein hormones, and other products necessary for germ cell development. The most important sex steroids are **estradiol** and **progesterone** in the female and **testosterone** in the male. Protein hormones produced by the gonads include **inhibin, activin, follistatin, antimüllerian hormone, oocyte meiosis inhibitor**, **growth factors,** and **IGF-binding proteins** as well as various derivatives of proopiomelanocortin (see Chapter 47).

Acting locally in paracrine and autocrine fashion, the gonadal hormones stimulate the development of the respective germ cells into ova and spermatozoa. Acting systemically in endocrine fashion, these hormones stimulate the development and function of the secondary sex organs essential for the support and delivery of the ova and spermatozoa to the site of fertilization, regulate the secretion of hypothalamic-pituitary hormones essential to gonadal function, modify somatic shape and regulate certain physiological functions within each gender, and support the conceptus in the early phase of pregnancy in the female.

There are two principal types of endocrine cells in the gonads. Those immediately encompassing the germ cells are called **granulosa cells** in the ovary and **Sertoli cells** in the testis. Those more distant from the germ cells and separated from them by a basement membrane are called **theca** or **interstitial cells** in the ovary and **Leydig cells** in the testis. The homologous granulosa and Sertoli cells produce mainly estrogens, whereas the homologous theca and Leydig cells secrete mainly androgens. Only in females, progesterone is secreted in large amounts by transformed granulosa and theca cells known as **luteal cells.** The protein products come mostly from granulosa and Sertoli cells.

The Gonads Synthesize Androgens and Estrogens by the Same Biochemical Steps Used in the Adrenal Cortex

THE BIOSYNTHESIS OF GONADAL STEROID HORMONES FOLLOWS A COMMON PATHWAY IN BOTH GENDERS (**Figure 49–1**). THE ENZYMES, THEIR ORGANELLE LOCALIZATION, AND THEIR COFACTOR REQUIREMENTS ARE THE SAME AS THOSE DESCRIBED FOR THE ADRENAL CORTEX (see Chapter 47). Furthermore, the gonadal enzymes are identical to the adrenal enzymes, and the same genes direct their synthesis. Cholesterol, either synthesized in situ from acetyl coenzyme A or taken up from the low-density lipoproteins in plasma, is the starting compound. P-450scc (20,22-desmolase) catalyzes side chain cleavage of cholesterol and is the rate-limiting enzyme for the synthesis of progesterone, androgens, and estrogens. Within the testes, a small quantity of testosterone undergoes 5α-reduction to **dihydrotestosterone (DHT),** a potent androgen. However, a much larger and more important conversion of testosterone to DHT, catalyzed by the enzyme 5α-reductase, occurs in target tissues. Estradiol and estrone are synthesized from their respective obligate androgen precursors by the P-450 **aromatase** enzyme complex (Figure 49–1). This sequentially catalyzes the hydroxylation and

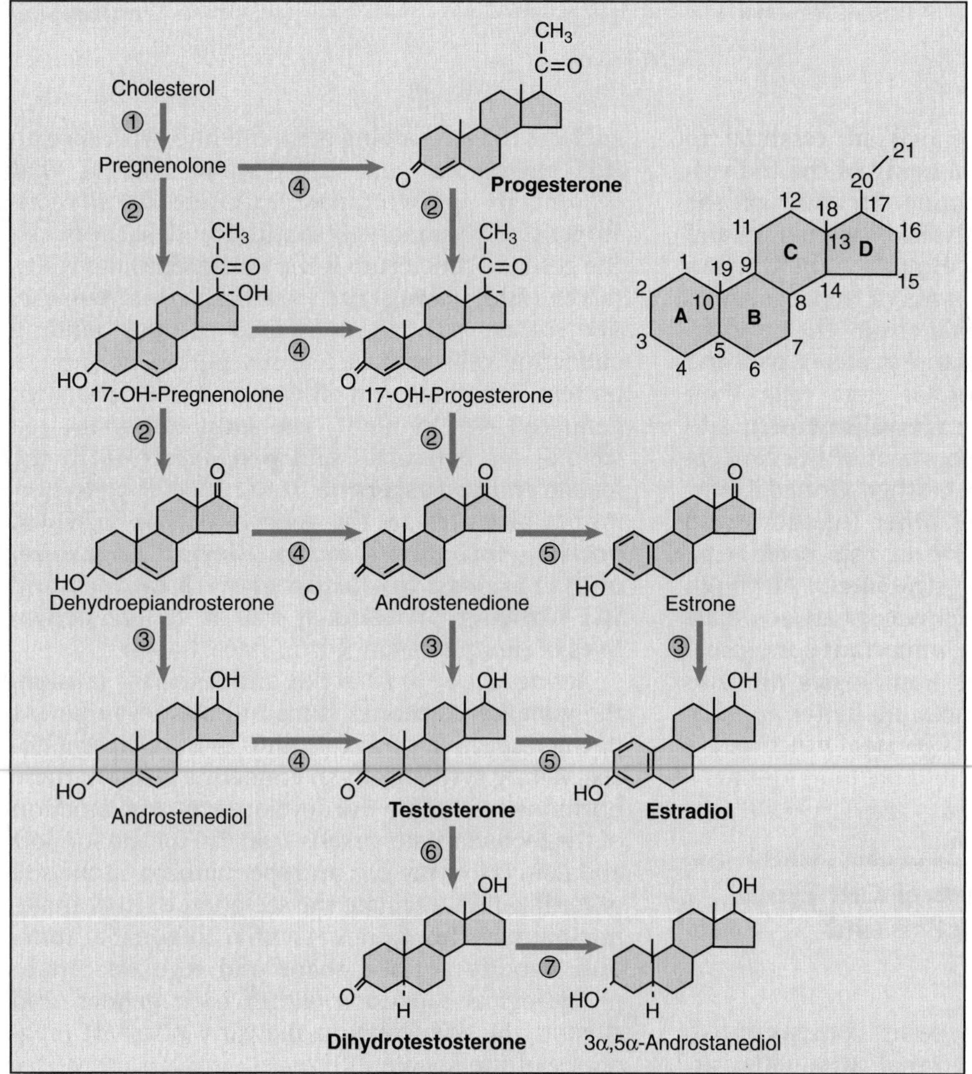

FIGURE 49–1. Pathways of synthesis of steroid hormones in the gonads. Testosterone is the major product of the testis. Estradiol and progesterone are the major products of the ovary. OH, hydroxy. The enzymes are 1: 20,22-desmolase (P-450scc; CYP11A1); 2: 17-hydroxylase/17,20-desmolase (P-450c17; CYP17); 3: 17β-hydroxysteroid dehydrogenase; 4: 3β-ol-dehydrogenase, $\Delta^{4,5}$-isomerase; 5: aromatase (P-450arom; CYP19); 6: 5α-reductase; 7: 3α-reductase.

oxidation of the 19-methyl group, the creation of a 1-2 double bond, the decarboxylation of position 19, and the formation of the characteristic benzene ring of estrogens.

Although the ratio of plasma testosterone to plasma estradiol is much greater in adult men than in women, the tissue levels may be much closer to each other. This is because of synthesis of both sex steroids from dehydroepiandrosterone sulfate (see Figure 49–1, steps 3, 4, and 5) in target cells. Moreover, their actions are not totally antagonist, and estradiol may even mediate some actions of testosterone.

Gonadal Steroid Hormone Secretion Is Regulated

A hypothalamic releasing hormone and two pituitary gonadotropins regulate the synthesis and secretion of sex hormones

A hypothalamic–anterior pituitary–gonadal axis, analogous to those involved in thyroid and adrenal function, is the basis for gonadal regulation (**Figure 49–2**). The components are **gonadotropin-releasing hormone (GnRH)** from hypothalamic neurons and two pituitary gonadotropins, designated **luteinizing hormone (LH)** and **follicle-stimulating hormone (FSH).** A single pituitary cell type, the gonadotroph, generally produces both LH and FSH, although occasional gonadotrophs contain only one or the other.

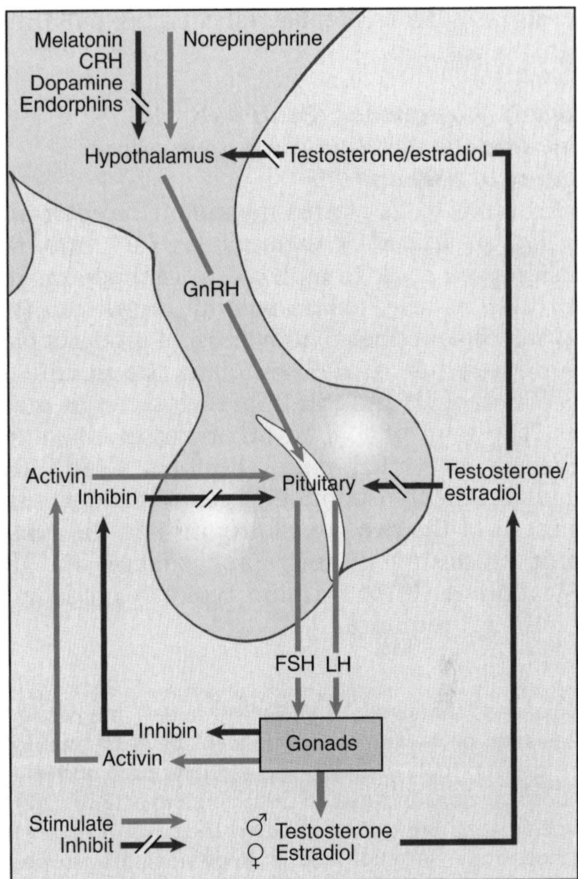

FIGURE 49–2. Hypothalamic–anterior pituitary–gonadal axis. The hypothalamic peptide gonadotropin-releasing hormone (GnRH) stimulates the release of two gonadotropins, luteinizing hormone (LH) and follicle-stimulating hormone (FSH), from the pituitary gland. The gonadotropins in turn stimulate gonadal secretion of primarily testosterone in males and primarily estradiol in females. These feed back negatively at both the pituitary and hypothalamic levels to inhibit the secretion of LH and FSH. In addition, FSH stimulates the gonadal release of inhibin, which feeds back negatively to preferentially block the release of FSH. In contrast, estradiol (in women) and the gonadal protein activin have positive-feedback effects on pituitary secretion. CRH, corticotropin-releasing hormone.

GnRH resides in the hypothalamus

GnRH, also known as **luteinizing hormone–releasing hormone,** stimulates both LH and FSH secretion but LH more so. GnRH, a decapeptide synthesized from a much larger preprohormone, is produced in two clusters of neurons in the arcuate and preoptic nuclei of the hypothalamus. These neurons originate in olfactory epithelium in an early embryonic stage and later migrate to the hypothalamus. From there, the hormone is transported axonally for storage in the median eminence. Input from other areas of the brain to the hypothalamus (see Chapter 45) permits reproduction to be influenced by light-dark cycles (probably via melatonin), by stress hormones such as corticotropin-releasing hormone, and by olfactory stimuli via airborne molecules known as **pheromones.** Pheromones react with specific receptors in the nose, distinct from those receptors that detect odors. The receptor neurons transmit signals via the olfactory bulb (Chapter 8) to GnRH neurons in the hypothalamus, whereby gonadal function and reproduction are responsive to the environment, including other individuals. Dopaminergic and endorphinergic tracts within the hypothalamus and the median eminence transmit important inhibitory influences on the release of GnRH (Figure 49–2). GnRH is released into the pituitary portal veins in pulses driven by a primary generator. Men have 8 to 10 pulses per day; in women, the frequency and periodicity of pulses vary with the menstrual cycle. In prepubertal children, pulsatility is greatly reduced.

Properly programmed GnRH pulses stimulate the secretion of an appropriate balance of FSH and LH

GnRH binds to its plasma membrane receptor and triggers an influx of extracellular Ca^{++} into the gonadotroph cells. Complexed to calmodulin, the Ca^{++} acts as the major second messenger (see Chapter 5), and phosphatidylinositol products play a subsidiary role. GnRH stimulates the simultaneous release of LH and FSH from their secretory granules. The ratio of FSH to LH increases when the frequency of GnRH pulses declines. GnRH also stimulates the transcription of genes that direct the synthesis of the two gonadotropins and the subsequent processing of their prohormones via glycosylation. A GnRH infusion typically produces a biphasic LH response.

Prolonged stimulation by GnRH causes the down-regulation of its receptor, consequent desensitization of the gonadotroph to GnRH, and resulting profound inhibition of gonadotropin secretion. Long-acting GnRH superagonists are commonly used therapeutically when gonadotropin secretion and androgen or estrogen production by the gonad must be suppressed. Such situations include **carcinoma of the prostate** in men and **endometriosis** in women. In participants of in vitro fertilization programs, it may be easier to produce ova at a specified time with an external program of FSH and LH administration (see Chapter 51) if endogenous secretion of these hormones is eliminated.

LH and FSH act via cAMP on different primary target cells in the gonads to stimulate the secretion of sex steroid hormones

LH and FSH are glycoproteins that resemble thyroid-stimulating hormone. The α subunits of all three hormones are identical, whereas their respective β subunits are different and are determined by unique genes. The α and β subunits in each gonadotropin are required for binding to its gonadal receptor, and proper carbohydrate components are necessary for full biological activity of the β subunits. Glycosylation and sialylation of FSH slow the metabolic clearance rate of FSH and decrease binding to its receptor.

LH MAINLY STIMULATES THE THECA CELLS OF THE FEMALE AND THE LEYDIG CELLS OF THE MALE TO SYNTHESIZE AND SECRETE ANDROGENS and, to a much lesser extent, estrogens. LH also stimulates granulosa cells, once LH receptors have been expressed by these cells during the female cycle. cAMP is the major second messenger for LH actions. Continuous stimulation by LH down-regulates its receptor and reduces responsivity to the hormone.

Analogous to adrenocorticotropic hormone, LH stimulates cholesterol transfer to the mitochondria and its conversion to pregnenolone. Subsequently, the concentrations of steroidogenic enzymes and adrenoxin are increased by stimulating transcription of their genes. Most important, LH INCREASES THE LEVELS OF 17-HYDROXYLASE/17,20-DESMOLASE, WHICH IS THE ESSENTIAL STEP IN ANDROGEN SYNTHESIS (Figure 49–1).

FSH stimulates **granulosa** and **Sertoli cells** to secrete estrogens. Acting via its plasma membrane receptor and cAMP as a second messenger, FSH INCREASES TRANSCRIPTION OF THE GENE FOR **AROMATASE**, THE ENZYME SPECIFIC TO ESTRADIOL SYNTHESIS. Another important effect of FSH is to increase the number of LH receptors in target cells and thereby to amplify their sensitivity to LH. FSH also stimulates the secretion of **inhibin** and other protein products of the granulosa and Sertoli cells (Figure 49–2).

Sex steroid hormones and protein products of the gonads feed back to regulate the release of GnRH and the secretion of pituitary gonadotropins

The regulation of gonadotropin secretion, sex steroid hormone production, and other aspects of gonadal function is complex, and those aspects distinctive to each gender are described in later sections. However, certain common principles exist (Figure 49–2). TESTOSTERONE, PRIMARILY IN MEN, AND ESTRADIOL, PRIMARILY IN WOMEN, INHIBIT THE SECRETION OF LH AND FSH. In this basic negative-feedback loop, the sex steroids act at the pituitary level by blocking the actions of GnRH on gonadotropin release and synthesis. They also act at the hypothalamic level by recruiting endorphin neurons to decrease GnRH levels. Both the frequency and the amplitude of LH and FSH pulses are diminished.

Negative feedback forms the basis for the use of current contraceptive drugs by women. Combinations of relatively small doses of estrogens and synthetic progestational agents, given orally, decrease the secretion of pituitary gonadotropins to levels below those needed to produce a mature ovum monthly. The cessation of oral contraceptives is generally followed by rapid reinstitution of fertility. Analogous administration of androgens for this purpose has not yet been successfully formulated for safe and effective use as a male contraceptive.

In women, an additional specific positive-feedback effect of estradiol on LH secretion is included in the basic framework (see Chapter 51). This effect depends on the dose, time, and duration of exposure to estradiol.

Another negative-feedback loop relates the protein **inhibin** from granulosa and Sertoli cells to FSH secretion. INHIBIN REDUCES GnRH RELEASE, FSH β SUBUNIT SYNTHESIS, AND THE STIMULATORY EFFECT OF GnRH ON FSH SECRETION. In contrast, from the same gonadal cells, **activin** exerts a positive-feedback effect to stimulate FSH secretion, whereas follistatin binds activin and thereby inhibits FSH (Figure 49–2). Thus, the output of LH and FSH from the pituitary gland can be exquisitely and differentially regulated by interactions among hypothalamic and gonadal products. At various times, the critical influence may be from either site. In this sense, the gonad can be viewed as much more self-regulatory than either the adrenal cortex or the thyroid. This is most apparent in women, as discussed later. Moreover, production of inhibin, activin, and follistatin within the pituitary gland adds a paracrine mode of regulation of FSH secretion.

The Secretion Pattern of Sex Steroid Hormones Varies Markedly at Different Stages of Life

The hypothalamic-pituitary-gonadal axis changes markedly throughout human life. Although the female and male patterns differ, certain common aspects bear emphasis (**Figure 49–3**).

Intrauterine and childhood patterns show GnRH present at various concentrations and at very low levels

In humans, GnRH is present in the hypothalamus by 4 weeks of gestation, and FSH and LH are present in the pituitary gland by 10 to 12 weeks of gestation. A peak of gonadotropin concentrations occurs in fetal plasma at midgestation. The concentrations drop to low levels before birth and then transiently increase (more prolonged in females), again at about 2 months of age. For the rest of childhood, FSH and LH are secreted at very low levels. These changes are mirrored by similar fluctuations of plasma testosterone in males and of plasma estradiol in females.

LH and FSH levels begin to increase during puberty

THE TRANSITION FROM A NONREPRODUCTIVE TO A REPRODUCTIVE STATE REQUIRES THE PUBERTAL MATURATION OF THE ENTIRE HYPOTHALAMIC-PITUITARY-GONADAL AXIS. Before a child reaches 10 years of age, plasma LH and FSH levels are low despite very low concentrations of gonadal hormones. Therefore, either the negative-feedback system is inoperative or

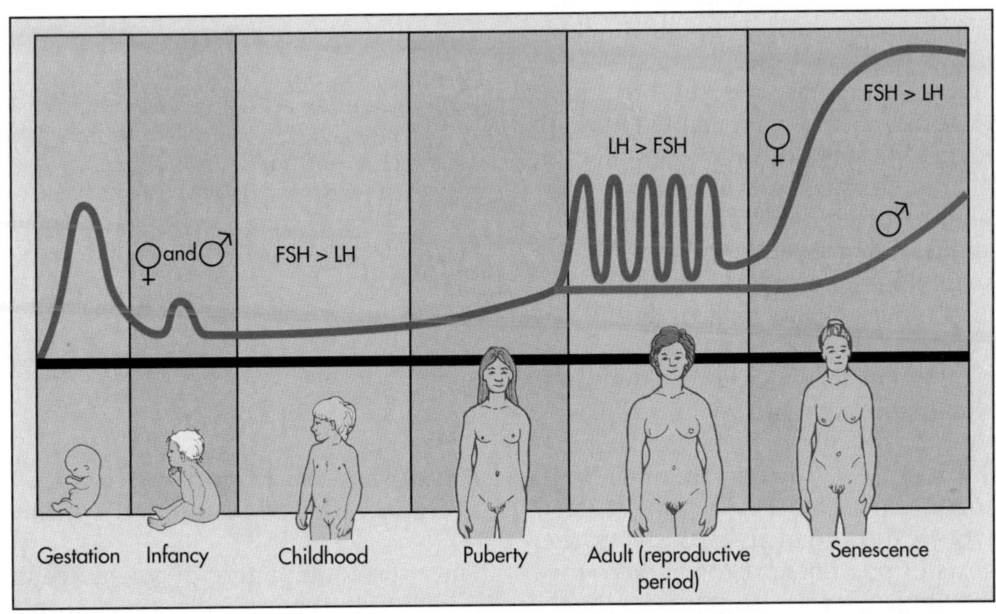

FIGURE 49–3. Pattern of gonadotropin secretion throughout life. Note the transient peaks during gestation and early infancy and low levels thereafter in childhood. Women subsequently develop monthly cyclic bursts, with LH concentrations exceeding FSH concentrations; men do not develop such a pattern. Both genders show increased gonadotropin production after 50 years of age, with FSH levels exceeding LH levels.

restrained by other central nervous system input to GnRH neurons (e.g., by melatonin, GABA, endorphin) or the hypothalamus and pituitary gland are exquisitely sensitive to testosterone, estradiol, and inhibin. One factor in puberty may thus be the gradual maturing of hypothalamic neurons, and this process leads to an increased synthesis and release of GnRH. Three factors that initiate this process may be (1) the maturation of the bones to a certain stage, (2) an increase in adipose tissue to a particular level, and (3) an increase in leptin stimulation of GnRH. A preceding increase in adrenal androgen secretion marked by increasing plasma levels of dehydroepiandrosterone sulfate may stimulate the required bone development.

The age at which this reproductive maturational process begins ranges from 9 to 17 years. It may also be preprogrammed because up to 80% of the variation is genetic and ethnic patterns are apparent. As puberty approaches, a pulsatile pattern of LH and FSH secretion becomes more evident. The ratio of plasma LH to FSH rises as the pulse frequency increases. Furthermore, during early and middle puberty but not usually thereafter, a distinct nocturnal peak in LH secretion is observed **(Figure 49–4)**. This coincides with but is not proved to be the result of a decrease in nocturnal melatonin secretion. These changes in GnRH and gonadotropins occur even in the absence of the gonads.

During early puberty, the responsiveness of the pituitary gland to GnRH changes so that LH exceeds FSH output. This may result from the increased synthesis and storage of LH in response to pulsatile GnRH secretion because pulses of GnRH allow better maintenance of GnRH receptors. Although the gonadal target cells can respond to LH in childhood, their responsiveness is augmented during puberty. Therefore, plasma levels of estradiol in females, testosterone in males, and inhibin in both genders increase sharply during these years. Early puberty and middle puberty can thus be viewed as a cascade of increasing maturation from the hypothalamic to the pituitary to the gonadal level.

The growth spurt during puberty is importantly contributed to by the increases in testosterone and estradiol, both acting in boys and girls. In addition to their endocrine effects, estradiol and testosterone are produced by bone cells, wherein they can have intracrine, autocrine, and paracrine actions. A later onset of puberty in boys than in girls allows the boys 2 extra years of prepubertal growth, accounting in part for their greater final height. The growth spurt averages 4 years in boys and 3 years in girls. On average, men have 10% greater height and 25% greater bone mass than women do because of these factors.

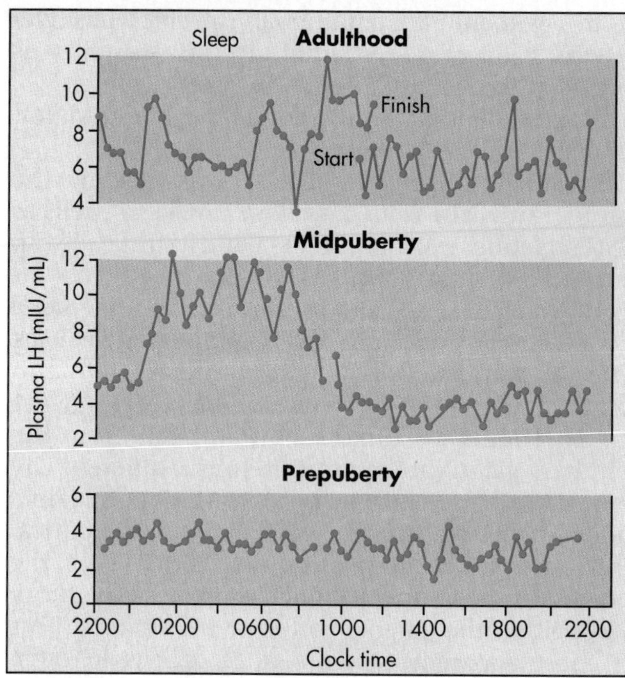

FIGURE 49–4. Changing pattern of diurnal LH secretion from childhood to adulthood. During puberty, LH secretion becomes much more pulsatile. In addition, a nocturnal peak appears early in puberty and then disappears when puberty is completed. Males and females both undergo these changes. Each day's sampling started and finished at approximately 10 AM. (Data from Boyar RM et al: *N Engl J Med* 287:582, 1972.)

Clinical endocrine testing often fails to distinguish between a late onset of normal puberty and a disorder of the hypothalamus that prevents the increased secretion of LH and FSH. Because failure to show physical signs of puberty by the age of 13 or 14 years (see Chapters 50 and 51) is psychologically distressing to the child, treatment with sufficient testosterone or estradiol to induce such changes and a growth spurt may be warranted. Such hormonal support can be withdrawn after an appropriate period to determine whether normal puberty has finally begun.

Adult patterns of gonadotropin secretion differ in men and women

Once the adult pattern of gonadotropin secretion is established, the basal plasma concentrations of LH and FSH (approximately 10^{-11} M) are similar in men and women. An important distinguishing feature between the genders is the additional establishment of a dramatic monthly gonadotropin cycle in women only (see Chapter 51); this is when the LH bursts greatly exceed the FSH bursts (Figure 49–3).

In both genders, a loss of gonadal responsiveness to gonadotropin stimulation develops around the fifth decade of life. In men, this is gradual, and some reproductive capacity usually persists even into the ninth decade. In women, reproductive capacity is eventually lost completely, and menopause occurs. In both genders, negative feedback leads to elevated plasma gonadotropin levels. The FSH level rises more than the LH level, and the increase in both gonadotropins is more distinct in women (Figure 49–3).

The Two Genders Are Normally Differentiated by Genetic, Gonadal, and Genital (Phenotypic) Factors

The most fundamental and obvious difference between the genders lies in the anatomy and consequent physiology of their reproductive tracts. During the first 5 weeks of gestation, however, the gonads of males and females are indistinguishable, and their genital tracts are unformed. From this stage of the "indifferent gonad" to that of the completed normal individual of either gender lies the process of sexual differentiation (**Figures 49–5 and 49–6**). The final maleness or femaleness is best characterized in terms of differences in genetic, gonadal, and genital (phenotypic) sex.

Maleness versus femaleness is determined positively and predominantly by the presence of the Y chromosome

The normal male has a chromosome complement of 44 autosomes and 2 sex chromosomes, XY. WITHOUT THE Y CHROMOSOME (OR IN RARE INSTANCES, CRITICAL DNA TRANSLOCATED FROM THE Y TO THE X CHROMOSOME), NEITHER TESTICULAR DEVELOPMENT NOR MASCULINIZATION OF THE GENITAL TRACTS AND EXTERNAL GENITALIA CAN OCCUR. The organization of the indifferent gonad into the characteristic spermatogenic tubules of the male is directed by a 14-kilobase segment known as the **sex-determining region of the Y chromosome (*SRY* gene),** which encodes a nuclear transcription factor known as the **testis-determining factor (TDF).** This gene is located on the short arm of the Y chromosome (Figures 49–5 and 49–6, *B*). The rest of this transcription factor family are known as SOX proteins and are products of autosomes. SOX-9 on chromosome 17 represses differentiation of the gonad into a testis and TDF relieves this repression, thereby stimulating formation of a testis steroidogenic factor 1 (SF-1), which on chromosome 9 induces the genes for gonadal steroidogenesis (see Chapter 47). Other loci on the Y chromosome are probably involved in guiding an orderly process of spermatogenesis. Even though it is essential, the Y chromosome by itself is not sufficient for maleness. Located on the X chromosome is the gene for the **androgen receptor,** which sensitizes the genital

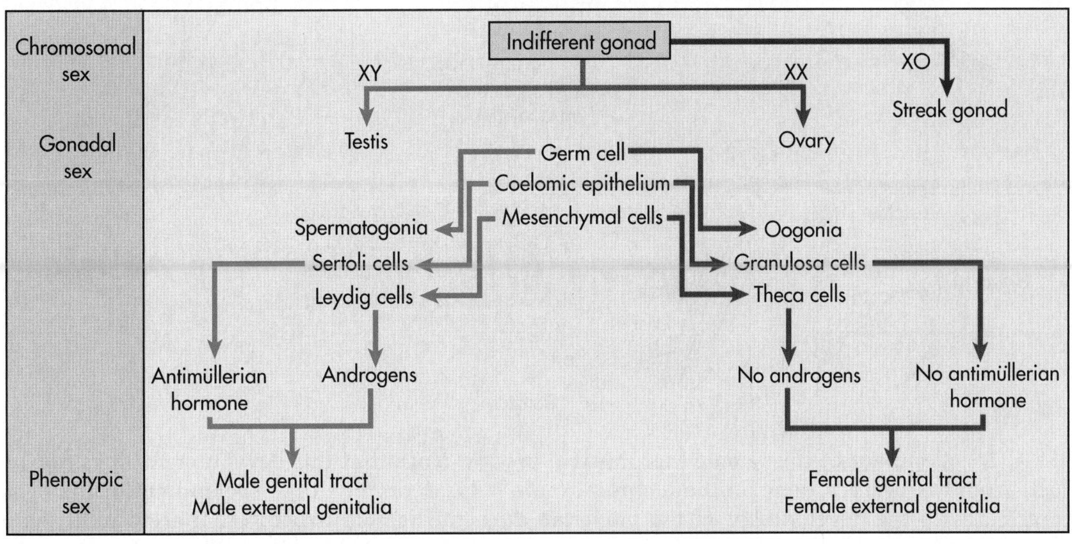

FIGURE 49–5. Overview of the development of the cells of the ovary and testis from the primitive indifferent gonad. Androgens and antimüllerian hormone from the normal testis induce the male pattern of differentiation of the genital tract and external genitalia. It is the lack of secretion of these products from the normal ovary at the critical times that determines differentiation of the genital tract and the external genitalia into the female pattern.

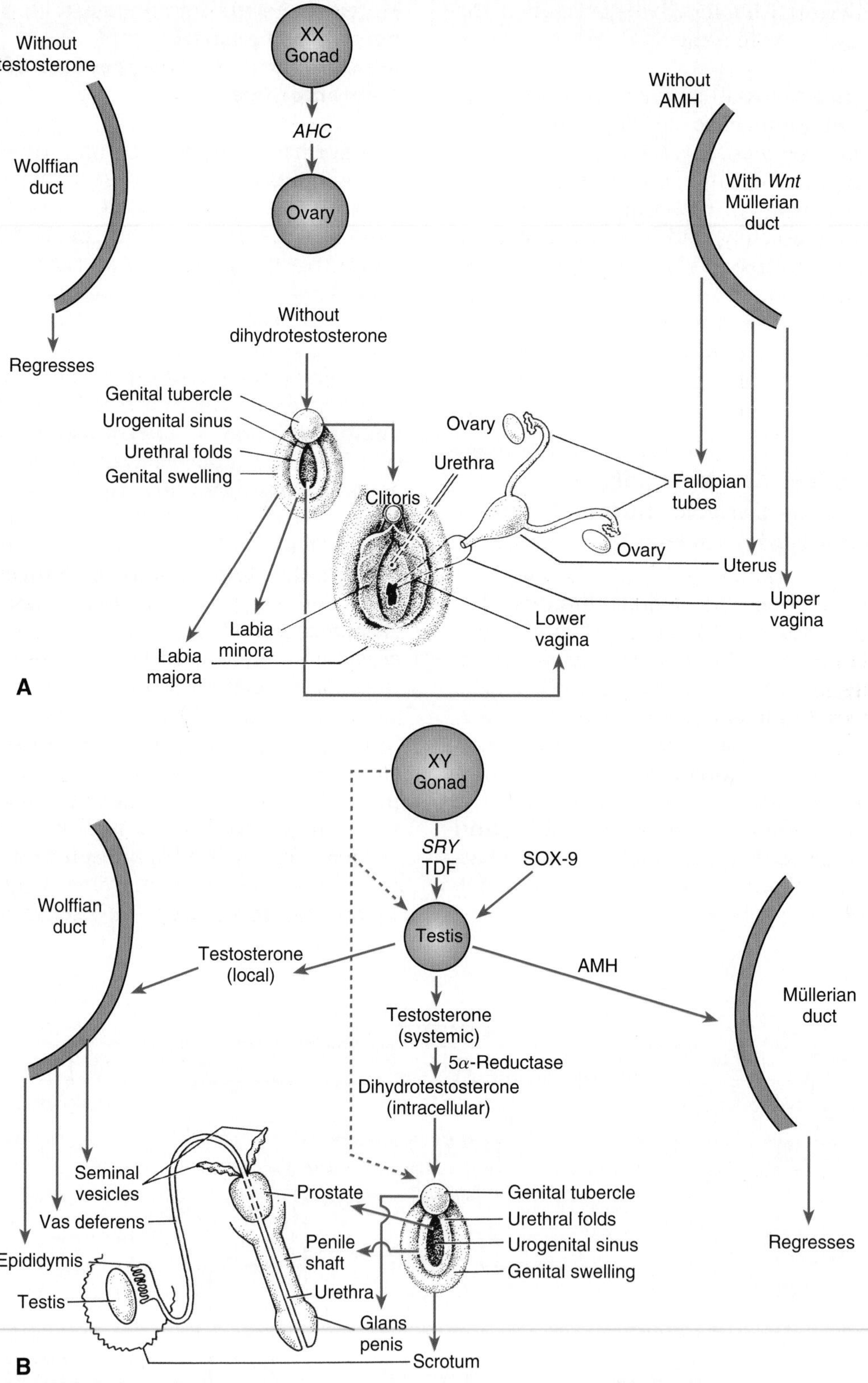

FIGURE 49–6. A, Development of the female reproductive organs. Note that this development does not require hormonal products from the ovary. A gene on the X chromosome helps determine the development of the ovary, and the *Wnt* gene contributes to the development of the müllerian duct into female structures. Therefore, in the absence of gonads, the female pattern results. *AHC*, adrenocortical hypoplasia (gene); AMH, antimüllerian hormone. B, Development of the male reproductive organs. Note that the complete male pattern requires the *SRY* gene product, TDF, as well as the secretion and local action of testosterone on the wolffian duct, the reduction of testosterone to DHT to provide androgen action in the anlage cells of the external genitalia, and the secretion of AMH to suppress development of the müllerian duct. (From Berne RM, Levy MN, Koeppen BM, Stanton BA: *Physiology,* ed 5, Philadelphia, 2004, Elsevier.)

ducts and the external genitalia to the masculinizing effects of testosterone and DHT.

In contrast, femaleness is determined positively by the presence of two X chromosomes but also negatively by the absence of a Y chromosome. The normal female chromosome complement is 44 autosomes and 2 sex chromosomes, XX. Both X chromosomes are active in germ cells and are essential for the genesis of a normal ovary (Figures 49–5 and 49–6, *A*). A gene located on the short arm of the X chromosome known as *AHC* (adrenocortical hypoplasia), formerly called *DAX1,* codes for a nuclear transcription factor that either positively stimulates ovarian development or negatively inhibits testicular development from the indifferent gonad. However, FEMALE DIFFERENTIATION OF THE GENITAL DUCTS AND EXTERNAL GENITALIA REQUIRES THAT ONLY A SINGLE X CHROMOSOME BE ACTIVE IN DIRECTING TRANSCRIPTION WITHIN THEIR CONSTITUENT CELLS. The second X chromosome of a normal XX female is randomly inactivated in all tissues outside the gonad. Both X alleles are equally affected. Thus, if an abnormality in **meiosis** or early **mitosis** produces an individual with only a single sex chromosome (an X), that individual will undergo normal female genital development even though her gonad is abnormal and without function (Figure 49–5).

The gonads of the two genders differentiate into organs with some functional homologies but important anatomical differences

Before the appearance of any gonad, primordial germ cells are identifiable in the 5-day-old blastocyst. The indifferent gonad of 5 weeks' gestation consists of a primordial mesonephric ridge with several components: coelomic epithelium, the precursor of granulosa and Sertoli cells; mesenchymal stromal cells, the precursors of theca and Leydig cells; and germ cells that have migrated there from the yolk sac endoderm (Figure 49–5). This neutral assembly lasts only 7 to 10 days and is organized as an outer cortex and an inner medulla.

In a normal male fetus, the spermatogenic tubules begin to form at 6 weeks, followed by differentiation of the Sertoli cells at 7 weeks under the influence of SOX-9 and the Leydig cells at 8 to 9 weeks. At this point, the testis is structurally recognizable, and testosterone secretion has begun. The germ cells have become enclosed within the medulla, whereas the cortex has regressed. No known hormonal influences are required for this differentiation of the indifferent gonad into a testis.

In a normal female fetus, differentiation of the indifferent gonad into an ovary does not start until 9 weeks' gestation. At this time, BOTH X CHROMOSOMES WITHIN THE GERM CELLS BECOME ACTIVE. The germ cells begin to undergo mitosis, giving rise to daughter cells called **oogonia,** which continue to proliferate. Shortly thereafter, meiosis is initiated in some oogonia, and each is surrounded by differentiating granulosa cells and precursor theca cells to form a **follicle.** The germ cells, now known as **primary oocytes,** remain in the first stage, or **prophase,** of meiosis until they are activated many years later. In contrast to the male arrangement of gonadal zones, the cortex, which contains the follicles, predominates in the developed ovary, whereas the medulla regresses. The primitive ovary begins to synthesize estrogenic hormones concurrent with these developments, and these hormones may contribute to later ovarian differentiation by blocking androgen actions.

Female internal and external genitalia are the neutral patterns that develop in the absence of androgen and protein products from the testes

Up to this point in fetal development, sexual differentiation is largely independent of known hormonal products. However, DIFFERENTIATION OF THE GENITAL DUCTS AND EXTERNAL GENITALIA REQUIRES SPECIFIC HORMONAL SIGNALS FROM THE NORMAL MALE GONAD TO PRODUCE THE MASCULINE FORMAT. WITHOUT SUCH INPUT, THE FEMININE FORMAT WILL RESULT.

During the sexually indifferent stage, from 3 to 7 weeks' gestation, two different genital ducts develop on each side. In the male, at about 9 to 10 weeks, the wolffian or mesonephric duct on each side begins to grow. Together, they give rise to the **epididymis, vas deferens, seminal vesicles,** and **ejaculatory duct** by 12 weeks (Figure 49–6, *B*). This constitutes the system for delivering sperm from the testis to the female. The growth and differentiation of each wolffian duct in the male are induced by testosterone, which is secreted by the **ipsilateral testis** and acts locally. Testosterone is not converted to the active metabolite DHT before acting on the wolffian duct cells, as it must be in other genital tissues. In the female, the wolffian ducts regress at 10 to 11 weeks because the ipsilateral ovary does not secrete testosterone.

Each müllerian duct arises parallel to the wolffian duct on its side. In the male, the müllerian ducts begin to regress at 7 to 8 weeks, about the same time that the Sertoli cells of the testis appear. These cells produce a glycoprotein, antimüllerian hormone (AMH), that causes atrophy of the müllerian ducts. AMH belongs to a superfamily of growth-regulating factors that are coded for by genes similar to each other and to the AMH gene; these include transforming growth factors (TGF-α, TGF-β), epidermal growth factor, and inhibin. AMH also initiates the descent of the testes into the inguinal area. The early critical secretion of AMH in the male may be initiated by a product of the *SRY* gene. Although the homologous granulosa cells of the ovary produce AMH, they do not do so until after the müllerian ducts have already developed to the point where AMH can no longer cause their regression. In addition, the Wnt gene product inhibits the action of AMH. Therefore, in the female, the net effect is that these ducts grow and differentiate into fallopian tubes at their upper ends and join at their lower ends to form a single uterus, cervix, and upper vagina (Figure 49–6, *A*).

The external genitalia of both genders begin to differentiate at 9 to 10 weeks. They are derived from the same primitive structures: the genital tubercle, genital swelling, urethral or genital folds, and urogenital sinus (Figure 49–6). FOR THE EXTERNAL GENITALIA TO DIFFERENTIATE INTO THE MASCULINE FORMAT, TESTOSTERONE MUST BE SECRETED INTO THE FETAL CIRCULATION AND MUST SUBSEQUENTLY BE CONVERTED TO DHT WITHIN THESE TISSUES. With DHT stimulation via the androgen receptor, the genital tubercle grows into the glans penis, the genital swellings fold and fuse into the scrotum, the urethral folds enlarge and enclose the penile urethra and corpora spongiosa, and the urogenital sinus gives rise to the prostate gland (Figure 49–6, *B*).

In the normal XX female, in an individual with an XO chromosome karyotype, or in an individual who has no gonads, the external genitalia develop into the clitoris, labia majora, labia minora, and lower vagina without significant positive androgenic influence (Figure 49–6, *A*). The critical importance of androgen molecules to the development of masculine external genitalia is emphasized by the presence of adequate androgen receptors in female urogenital tract cells. Estrogen molecules in the female may play a role by offsetting the possible virilizing actions of normal adrenal androgens in that gender.

A placental gonadotropin initially and a fetal pituitary gonadotropin later stimulate the androgen secretion involved in sexual differentiation

The initial androgen production necessary for male sexual differentiation does not depend on fetal pituitary gonadotropins. An LH-like hormone, **chorionic gonadotropin** from the placenta, stimulates early testosterone production by the Leydig cells of the testis. On the other hand, the continued growth of the male genitalia in the last 6 months of gestation requires fetal pituitary LH to support the necessary testicular androgen production. Similarly, the later molding of the female genitalia in utero may be modulated by ovarian estrogen production, which also depends on fetal pituitary gonadotropins.

Other aspects of phenotypic sexual differentiation are not evident until long after birth. These include differences between the unchanging daily pattern of gonadotropin secretion in the male and the monthly cyclic pattern in the female, the degree of breast development, and psychological identification with one gender. What factors imprint or regulate these traits in humans are not certain. Evidence from rodents suggests that circulating androgens program the fetal hypothalamus to set the ultimate noncycling pattern of gonadotropin secretion in the postpubertal male. (To do so, testosterone may paradoxically require conversion to estradiol within the target neurons.) Without androgens, the ultimate cyclic pattern of the female results. This would constitute another instance in which the female pattern is the "neutral pattern" but the male pattern requires an action derived from the Y chromosome.

Mammary gland development in the rodent embryo also is clearly regulated by androgens. In its absence, a normal female breast develops; in its presence, the elaborated ductal system is suppressed. In the human, however, male-female differences in breast tissue are not apparent until puberty. At that time, increased estrogen in the female induces the growth and differentiation of breast tissue; increased androgens in the male suppress these processes.

Psychological gender identity, and its expression as gender role behavior, is probably the result of a complex interaction of numerous factors. Genetic sex is not an absolute determinant: a Y chromosome does not guarantee male gender identity, nor does its absence guarantee a female gender identity. Sex assignment at birth almost always accords with the predominant anatomy of the external genitalia, which reflects early embryonic exposure to androgens, prenatal testosterone and DHT, and the essential mediation of the androgen receptor. Therefore, androgens can be said to influence gender identity. Parental rearing cues and social recognition in accord with sex assignment then establish and reinforce the initial gender identity. A possible later endocrine influence on gender identity is revealed by the natural history of individuals with defective synthesis of testosterone or DHT. Because of incomplete virilization at birth, these XY individuals are raised with female gender identities (or at least expectations). During puberty, compensatory

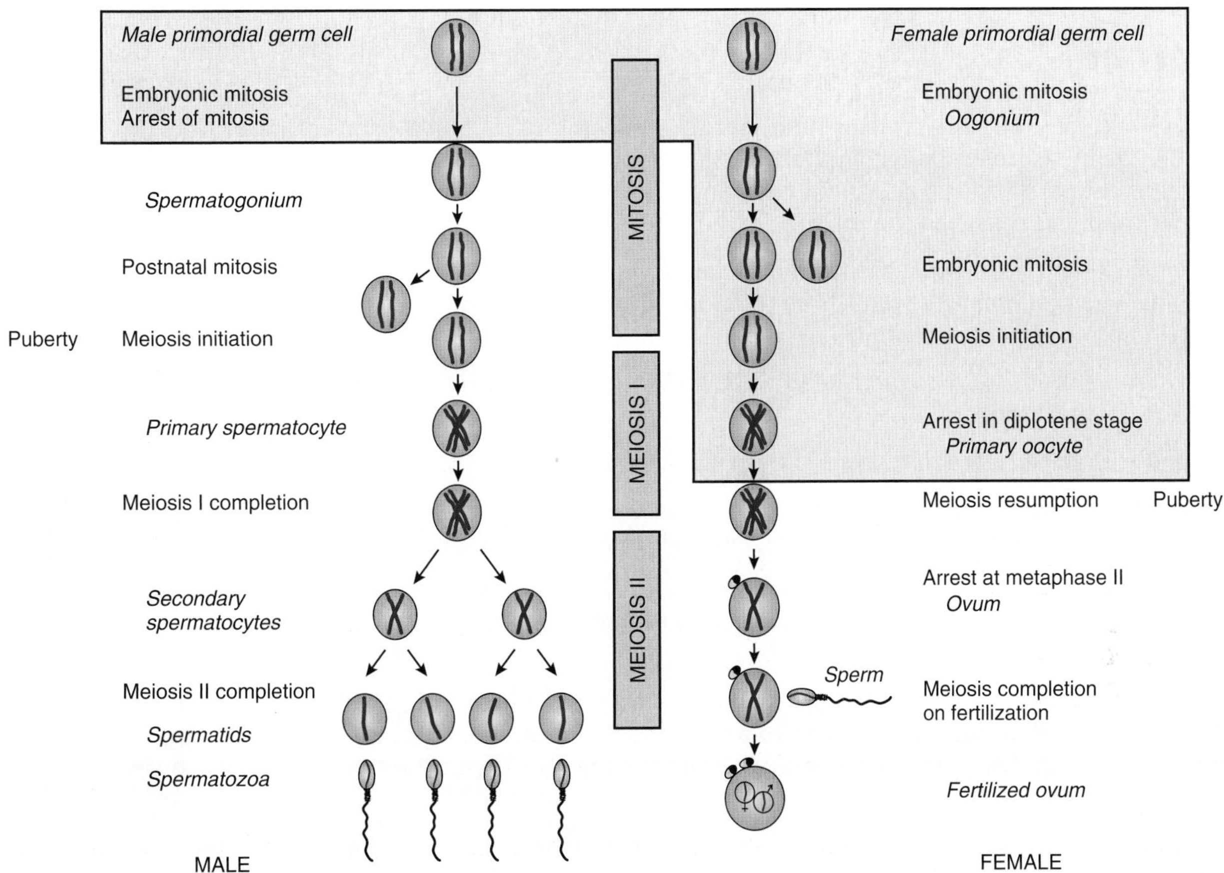

FIGURE 49–7. Comparison of male gamete and female gamete production from primitive germ cells. Whereas female germ cells enter meiosis in embryonic life and remain suspended in that state for many years before resuming development after puberty, male germ cells start into meiosis only after puberty. Each female germ cell yields a single ovum, whereas each male germ cell yields many sperm. Approximately 70 days elapse in each case, once meiosis is resumed or started, respectively, until an ovum or sperm is finally formed. (From Berne RM, Levy MN, Koeppen BM, Stanton BA: *Physiology,* ed 5, Philadelphia, 2004, Elsevier.)

mechanisms lead to normal testosterone or DHT production, growth of the penis, erections, and fertility. Most such individuals then change to male gender identity and male role behavior.

Germ Cell Development Is Determined by Gender

Before the gender-specific aspects of reproductive endocrine function are discussed, it is useful to examine the analogies and differences in male and female gamete production (**Figure 49–7**). In the embryonic state, primordial germ cells in the male undergo only mitosis to primitive spermatogonia, but development stops there. Meiosis (cell division with chromosomal reduction to the haploid state) does not begin until puberty, but once it does, the process continues through two meiotic divisions to the final emergence of spermatozoa within 2 months. In females in the embryonic state, not only do primordial germ cells undergo mitosis to oogonia, but also the oogonia already begin meiosis, which stops in the diplotene stage of prophase. The first meiosis does not resume until many years later, following puberty; but after its completion, the second meiosis again arrests in the metaphase II stage, with extrusion of one polar body. The second meiosis of the ovum is completed only after entry of a sperm, and then the second polar body is extruded. Finally, after fertilization, the two haploid pronuclei—one from the sperm and one from the ovum—begin DNA synthesis separately and then fuse into the final diploid nucleus of the zygote.

Summary

- ❖ Female and male gonadal structure and function have important homologous characteristics. In each gender, germ cells develop within sheltered and hormonally conditioned environments provided by granulosa cells (estrogens) and theca cells (androgens) in the female and by Sertoli cells (estrogens) and Leydig cells (androgens) in the male.
- ❖ Gonadal steroids are synthesized from cholesterol via the same enzymatic pathways that produce adrenal steroids. The predominant products are estradiol in the female and testosterone in the male. An important protein hormone product is inhibin.
- ❖ Testosterone production is stimulated by LH, and estradiol and inhibin production by FSH, from the anterior pituitary gonadotrophs.
- ❖ LH and FSH are secreted in response to a pulsatile hypothalamic release of GnRH.
- ❖ Estradiol and testosterone feed back negatively on the hypothalamus and pituitary to decrease LH and FSH release, and inhibin feeds back negatively on FSH release.
- ❖ Gonadotropin and sex steroid production have fetal peaks, are low during childhood, and rise to adult levels during puberty. Sex steroid levels decline during senescence, whereas gonadotropin levels increase because of negative feedback.
- ❖ Gender differences in reproductive function derive from the process of sexual differentiation. The Y chromosome is a positive determinant of the development of the indifferent gonad into a testis and of spermatogenesis. Two active X chromosomes are required for normal development of the ovary and for oogenesis.
- ❖ Regardless of karyotype, masculinization of the internal genital ducts and the external genitalia into a delivery system for sperm requires normal testosterone production and action. Suppression of the development of the female internal ducts requires AMH from the testis.
- ❖ In the absence of these testicular hormones, the internal ducts develop into organs for receiving sperm and housing a conceptus, and the external genitalia are feminized.

Bibliography

Achermann JC et al: Gonadal determination and adrenal development are regulated by the orphan nuclear receptor steroidogenic factor-1, in a dose-dependent manner, *J Clin Endocrinol Metab* 87:1829, 2002.

Brann DW et al: Leptin and reproduction, *Steroids* 67:95, 2002.

Brzezinski A: Mechanisms of disease: melatonin in humans, *N Engl J Med* 336:186, 1997.

Canning CA, Lovell-Badge R: Sry and sex determination: how lazy can it be? *Trends Genet* 18:111, 2002.

Delemarre-van de Waal HA: Regulation of puberty, *Clin Endocrinol Metab* 16:1, 2002.

Federman DD: Perspective: Three facets of sexual differentiation, *N Engl J Med* 350:323, 2004.

Friedman RC, Downey J: Neurobiology and sexual orientation: current relationships, *J Neuropsychiatry Clin Neurosci* 5:131, 1993.

Hawkins JR: The SRY gene, *Trends Endocrinol Metab* 4:328, 1993.

Hughes IA: Minireview: sex differentiation, *Endocrinology* 142:3281, 2001.

Josso N: Anatomy and endocrinology of fetal sex differentiation. In DeGroot LJ, Jameson JL, eds: *Endocrinology,* ed 4, Philadelphia, 2000, WB Saunders.

MacLaughlin DT, Donahoe PK: Sex determination and differentiation, *N Engl J Med* 350:367, 2004.

Odell WD: Endocrinology of sexual maturation. In DeGroot LJ, Jameson JL, eds: *Endocrinology,* ed 4, Philadelphia, 2000, WB Saunders.

Odell WD: Genetic basis of sexual differentiation. In DeGroot LJ, Jameson JL, eds: *Endocrinology,* ed 4, Philadelphia, 2000, WB Saunders.

Parent AS et al: The timing of normal puberty and the age limits of sexual precocity: variations around the world, secular trends, and changes after migration, *Endocr Rev* 24:668, 2003.

Reichlin S: Neuroendocrinology. In Foster D, Wilson J, eds: *Williams textbook of endocrinology,* ed 9, Philadelphia, 1998, WB Saunders.

Riggs BL, Khosla S, Melton LJ 3rd: Sex steroids and the construction and conservation of the adult skeleton, *Endocr Rev* 23:279, 2002.

Southworth MB et al: The importance of signal pattern in the transmission of endocrine information: pituitary gonadotropin responses to continuous and pulsatile gonadotropin-releasing hormone, *J Clin Endocrinol Metab* 72:1286, 1991.

Stern K, McClintock MK: Regulation of ovulation by human pheromones, *Nature* 392:177, 1998.

Wilson JD: Androgens, androgen receptors, and male gender role behavior, *Horm Behav* 40:358, 2001.

Wu FCW et al: Ontogeny of pulsatile gonadotropin releasing hormone secretion from midchildhood, through puberty, to adulthood in the human male: a study using deconvolution analysis and an ultrasensitive immunofluorometric assay, *J Clin Endocrinol Metab* 81:1798, 1996.

Yen SSC: Neuroendocrinology of reproduction. In Yen SSC, Jaffe RB, Barbieri RL, eds: *Reproductive endocrinology,* ed 4, Philadelphia, 1999, WB Saunders.

Case Studies

Case 49–1

A 22-year-old woman has never menstruated. Otherwise, she has been well. She is 5 feet 6 inches tall and weighs 130 pounds. Physical examination reveals well-developed, rather full breasts. There is no pubic or axillary hair. The external genitalia are feminine in pattern. The vagina is shortened and ends in a blind pouch without a recognizable cervix. No uterus or ovaries are felt or seen on an ultrasound examination. A small mass was felt in each inguinal area.

1. **The biological effects of which of the following hormones are missing?**
   A. Estrogen
   B. Androgen
   C. AMH
   D. FSH
   E. Insulin growth factor 1

2. **Measurement of plasma testosterone levels shows the value to be very high for a female. Which of the following is a likely finding?**
   A. Her chromosome karyotype is XX.
   B. The inguinal masses are ovaries.
   C. Her plasma LH level is low.
   D. She has an inactivating mutation of the androgen receptor.
   E. She has an inactivating mutation of the estrogen receptor.

Case 49–2

A 15-year-old boy delivered by a midwife in Appalachia develops inflammatory bowel disease, for which he is treated with high doses of glucocorticoids for 6 months. To his and his parents' consternation, he notes two episodes of bleeding from an orifice adjacent to his urethra for several days every month. On physical examination, he has a masculine adult voice, early beard growth, and a masculine format of pubic hair. Careful examination of the genitalia reveals incomplete fusion of the urethral folds around the shaft of what was thought to be a penis but is belatedly recognized to be an enlarged clitoris. The scrotum is also incompletely fused and deeply pigmented. A persistent urogenital sinus and a small orifice to an apparent vagina are noted. No testes are felt. The chromosome karyotype is XX.

1. **Which of the following structures might be absent?**
   A. Vas deferens (spermatic cord)
   B. Ovaries
   C. Uterus
   D. Fallopian tubes
   E. Adrenal zona reticularis

2. **What caused the pigmented "scrotum"?**
   A. Dehydroepiandrosterone
   B. Testosterone
   C. 17-Hydroxyprogesterone
   D. Luteinizing hormone
   E. Adrenocorticotropic hormone

Chapter 50: Male Reproduction

Objectives

- ❖ Describe the structural arrangement that subserves the reproductive function of the testis.
- ❖ Describe the biology of spermatogenesis and its hormonal regulation.
- ❖ Explain the pattern of secretion and metabolism of testosterone.
- ❖ Identify the various actions of androgenic hormones.

The testis is the site where male gametes, spermatozoa, are formed and mature in a specialized hormonal environment dominated by testosterone. This potent androgen also influences numerous processes described in other sections of the book, including skeletal development, hepatic protein synthesis, lipoprotein metabolism, red blood cell production, and renal tubular function.

The Anatomy of the Testis Creates Special Conditions Conducive to the Maturation of Germ Cells Under Endocrine, Paracrine, and Autocrine Regulation

The testes are situated in the scrotum, where they are maintained at 1°C to 2°C below the body core temperature, a situation that facilitates sperm production. Each adult testis weighs about 40 g and has a long diameter of 4.5 cm. A total of 80% of the testis is made up of the **spermatogenic** or **seminiferous tubules;** the remaining 20% is composed of connective tissue containing the **Leydig cells.** The spermatogenic tubules, a coiled mass of loops, empty into a ductal system that eventually drains into the **epididymis,** a maturation and storage site for spermatozoa. From there, spermatozoa are carried via the **vas deferens** and **ejaculatory duct** into the penis for emission.

The structure of the spermatogenic tubule is shown in **Figure 50–1**. Each tubule is bounded by a basement membrane that separates it from the Leydig cells, the **peritubular (myoid) cells,** and the adjacent capillaries. Beneath this membrane are **Sertoli cells** and immature germ cells, the **spermatogonia.** As the spermatogonia divide and develop around the circumference of the tubule, columns of maturing germ cells are formed below them. These columns reach from the basement membrane to the lumen and culminate in the spermatozoa. Each column of germ cells lies between the cytoplasms of two adjoining Sertoli cells, which extend all the way from the tubule's basement membrane to its lumen (Figure 50–1). SPECIAL PROCESSES OF THE CYTOPLASMS OF ADJACENT SERTOLI CELLS FUSE INTO TIGHT JUNCTIONS THAT CREATE TWO COMPARTMENTS OF INTERCELLULAR SPACE BETWEEN THE BASEMENT MEMBRANE AND THE LUMEN OF THE TUBULE. The spermatogonia lie within the proximal **basal** compartment, whereas their descendants that arise from subsequent stages in spermatozoon development lie in the distal **adluminal** compartment.

The compartmentalization of intercellular space between germ cells accomplishes two important functions

THE BASEMENT MEMBRANE, THE OVERLAPPING PERITUBULAR CELLS, AND THE SERTOLI CELL CYTOPLASM TOGETHER FORM A BLOOD-TESTIS BARRIER WITH IMPORTANT FUNCTIONS. First, this barrier can exclude harmful circulating substances from the intercellular fluid that

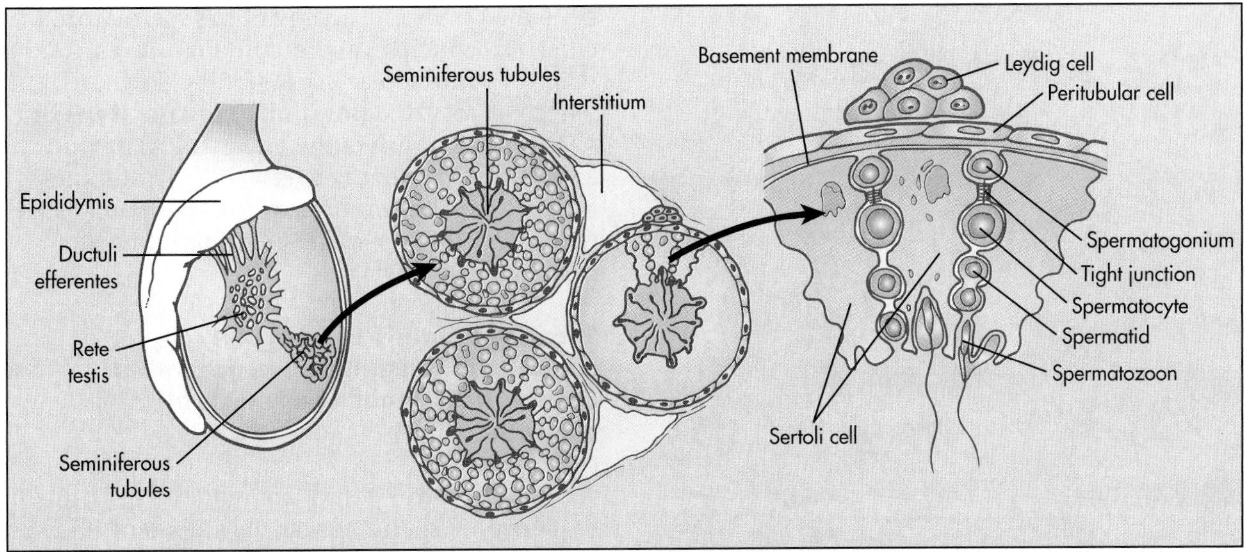

FIGURE 50–1. Architecture of the testis. The Leydig cells and peritubular cells are separated from the spermatogenic tubules. Within the tubules, the germ cell line is completely invested by the cytoplasm of the surrounding Sertoli cells. In addition, tight junctions between adjacent Sertoli cells separate the ancestral spermatogonia from their descendant spermatocytes, spermatids, and spermatozoa. Thus, a blood-testis barrier effectively filters plasma, permitting only selected substances to reach the developing germ cells from the cytoplasm of the Sertoli cells. (From Skinner MK: *Endocr Rev* 12:45, 1991.)

bathes the maturing germ cells and from the tubular fluid surrounding the spermatozoa. Second, products from the later stages of spermatogenesis are prevented from diffusing back into the bloodstream and producing antibodies. In addition, THE PROXIMITY OF THE LEYDIG CELLS PROVIDES GERM CELLS WITH HIGH LOCAL CONCENTRATIONS OF TESTOSTERONE. The proximity of the Sertoli cells provides protein and other products from the Sertoli cells in high concentrations that are essential for spermatogenesis.

Biology of Spermatogenesis

Spermatozoa are the products of a complex process of development from spermatogonia

Sperm production continues virtually throughout the normal male's life. At peak, 100 to 200 million sperm can be produced daily. To generate this large number, the spermatogonia must renew themselves continuously through cell division. This differs from the situation in the female, who at birth has a fixed number of germ cells that continually decrease throughout her life.

The descendants of the spermatogonia undergo an extraordinary metamorphosis to spermatozoa as they move from the basement membrane to the tubule. This process of differentiation depends on support from the abutting functional Sertoli cells. Within the basal compartment (Figure 50–1), a spermatogonium undergoes two mitotic divisions that give rise to three active cells and a single resting cell; the resting cell will be the "ancestor" of a later generation of spermatozoa. The active cells divide further to yield type B spermatogonia, which then generate a number of **primary spermatocytes** (**Figure 50–2**). These enter the prophase of meiosis, the first reduction division, in which they remain for about 20 days.

The complex process of chromosomal reduplication, synapsis, crossover, division, and separation completes meiosis. Within the adluminal compartment (Figure 50–1), the daughter cells, **secondary spermatocytes,** divide again. The products, called **spermatids** (Figure 50–2), then contain 22 autosomes and either an X or a Y chromosome. The spermatids lie near the lumen of the tubule and are attached to the abutting Sertoli cells by specialized junctions. They also remain connected to spermatocytes through intercellular bridges. The spermatids undergo nuclear condensation, shrinkage of cytoplasm, formation of an **acrosome,** and development of a tail, and then they emerge as flagellated spermatozoa (Figure 50–2). In the end, 64 spermatozoa arise from each spermatogonium. In the process of **spermiation,** the spermatozoa are then extruded into the tubular lumen, leaving behind most of their cytoplasm imbedded in Sertoli

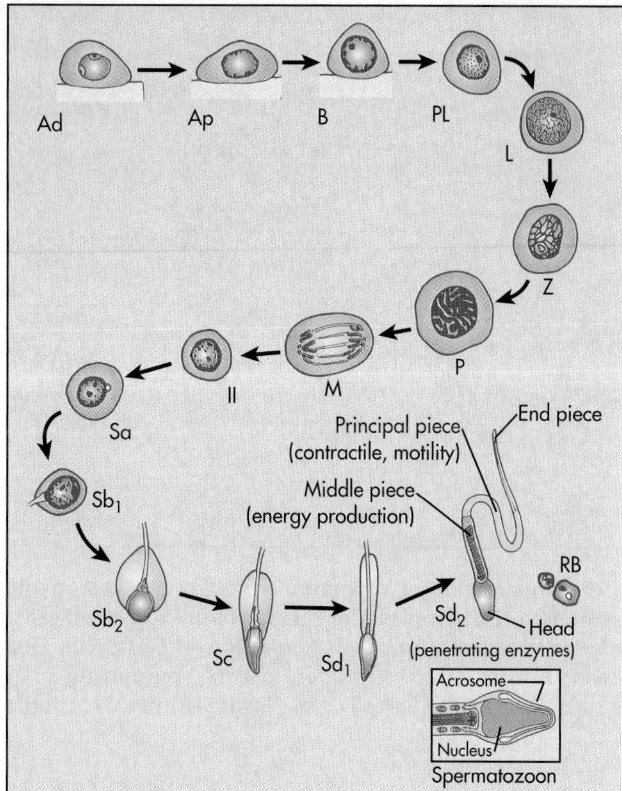

FIGURE 50–2. Development of spermatozoa from spermatogonia in the human. The final spermatozoon is almost devoid of cytoplasm. Ad, dark spermatogonium; Ap, pale spermatogonium; B, type B spermatogonium; PL, preleptotene primary spermatocyte; L, leptotene spermatocyte; Z, zygotene spermatocyte; P, pachytene spermatocyte; M, meiotic division; II, secondary spermatocyte; Sa, Sb, Sc, Sd, spermatids; RB, residual body. (From De Kretser DM et al. In DeGroot LJ, ed: *Endocrinology,* ed 3, Philadelphia, 1995, WB Saunders.)

cells, where it is phagocytosed and degraded. Movement of the spermatozoa into the epididymis is facilitated by fluid currents generated by the peritubular myoid cells and by fluid absorption of the **efferent ductules**, which connect the testis to the epididymis.

The components of spermatozoa are a head with penetrating power, a midportion with energy-generating capacity, and a tail with motile power

The mature spermatozoa are linear structures with several components (Figure 50–2). The head contains the nucleus and an acrosomal cap with concentrated hydrolytic and proteolytic enzymes that facilitate penetration of the ovum. The middle piece, or body, contains mitochondria, which generate the motile energy of the spermatozoa. The chief, or principal, piece contains stored ATP and pairs of contractile microtubules down its entire length. Cross-bridging arms contain **dynein,** an ATPase that transfers the energy of ATP bonds into a sliding movement between the microtubules. This imparts flagellar motion to the spermatozoa. Both Ca^{++} and cAMP promote sperm motility.

Spermatogenesis is an orderly, partially self-regulating process that occurs throughout the length of the tubule

A total of 60 to 70 days are required for the entire sequence of spermatozoal development. However, INDIVIDUAL RESTING SPERMATOGONIA DO NOT BEGIN THE PROCESS OF SPERMATOGENESIS RANDOMLY. There is a regular topographical association of particular stages of spermatogenesis in neighboring cycles around the circumference of the tubule. Groups of adjacent spermatogonia initiate a cycle of development about every 16 days, which constitutes one "generation." At about the same time that the primary spermatocytes of one cycle enter prophase, a second cycle of spermatogonia is activated. A third cycle begins about the time spermatids from the first cycle appear. When these spermatids have completed their transformation into spermatozoa, a fourth cycle of spermatogonia has begun. The individual descendants of any one type B spermatogonium that lie within the adluminal compartment of the tubule may not be totally separated. Continuity of cytoplasm and possibly cell-to-cell intercommunication may exist.

The whole sequence of spermatogenesis is under *intrinsic regulation* by a preprogrammed temporal pattern of germ cell expression that directs differentiation and morphogenesis. Some of the gene transcripts are unique to germ cells, and they are highly conserved in evolution, being shared among mammals, roundworms, fruit flies, and budding yeast. Some of these unique genes are expressed by germ cells only at certain stages of their development. Another form of regulation is *interactive;* that is, products from cells in one stage of spermatogenesis may influence cells in earlier or later stages. *Extrinsic* or hormonal regulation is engrafted on the intrinsic and interactive modes of regulation.

Changes in metabolism and structure occur during spermatogenesis. Glycolysis is ineffective in spermatids, whereas glucose utilization by sperm is an absolute requirement for fertilization to take place. In the last phase, nuclear histones are replaced by protamine, a basic molecule that allows packaging of the DNA into one-twentieth the volume that is required in somatic cells.

The spermatozoa traverse the epididymis in 2 to 4 weeks. During this time, they lose their remaining cytoplasm and become increasingly motile. The epididymis resembles renal tubules in that it is lined by specialized epithelial cells whose function includes progressive modulation of the chemical and osmotic environment in which the sperm advance. Proteins produced by these cells bind to sperm membranes and enhance their forward mobility and their ultimate ability to fertilize an ovum. After reaching the vas deferens, sperm may be stored viably for several months.

Delivery of Spermatozoa

Erectility of the penis and ejaculation of sperm are under autonomic nervous system control

The process of ejaculation delivers spermatozoa from the vas deferens out of the penile urethra and, for reproductive purposes, into the female genital tract. ERECTION OF THE PENIS RESULTS FROM AN EIGHT-FOLD INCREASE IN ITS BLOOD CONTENT CAUSED BY FILLING OF ITS CAVERNOSAL VENOUS SINUSES. THIS IS ACCOMPLISHED THROUGH SIMULTANEOUS DILATION OF ARTERIOLES AND COMPRESSION OF DRAINING VEINS BY THE ENGORGED SINUSES AND IS UNDER PARASYMPATHETIC CONTROL. NITRIC OXIDE, cGMP, AND PROSTAGLANDIN E MEDIATE THE CHANGES IN VESSEL TONE THAT RESULT IN PENILE ENGORGEMENT. EJACULATION IS THEN EFFECTED BY SYMPATHETIC ACTIVATION.

Inability to ejaculate, or impotence, is a common problem. It may be caused by structural and functional disorders, including neuropathies and spinal cord lesions, or by psychogenic complications. Direct self-injection of α-adrenergic antagonists or appropriate prostaglandins into the cavernosa at the base of the penis generates erections that last 1 to 3 hours. Drugs that inhibit cGMP phosphodiesterase increase cGMP and facilitate erection under conditions of sexual stimulation.

Just before ejaculation, successive fluids are added to the contents of the vas deferens. The initial alkaline secretions from the **prostate** gland help neutralize the acid pH of the female genital secretions. The terminal portion of the ejaculate is composed of secretions from the **seminal vesicles.** These contain fructose, another important oxidative substrate for the spermatozoa, and prostaglandins. Seminal fluid also contains Ca^{++}, Zn^{++}, luteinizing hormone (LH), follicle-stimulating hormone (FSH), prolactin, testosterone, estradiol, inhibin, oxytocin, endorphins, and a variety of enzymes. Their exact source within the genital tract and the role of each in fertilization remain to be determined.

A typical seminal emission contains 200 to 400 million spermatozoa in a volume of 3 to 4 mL. Once they are within the vagina and aided by contractions of the smooth muscle, the spermatozoa rapidly move inward. Their life span in the female genital tract is approximately 2 days. The transport of sperm to the ovum requires mechanical assistance by smooth muscle contractions of the other female reproductive organs.

THE FERTILIZING ABILITY OF SPERMATOZOA NORMALLY REQUIRES EXPOSURE TO FEMALE GENITAL SECRETIONS. In vivo, human sperm cannot fertilize an ovum until they have been in contact with the female reproductive tract for several hours; the process is termed **capacitation.** In vitro, however, fertilization can occur after the ejaculated sperm have been washed free of seminal fluid. Penetration requires the **acrosomal reaction,** in which the acrosomal membrane and the outer sperm membrane fuse to create pores through which the enclosed proteolytic enzymes can escape and degrade the protective wall of the ovum.

Capacitation has proved to be a regulated process. A fertilization-promoting peptide (FPP) originates in the prostate gland and in other male reproductive tissues. FPP is a tripeptide, pGlu-Glu-Pro-NH_2, that is similar to thyrotropin-releasing hormone (see Chapter 46). FPP interacts with its receptor to increase cAMP in uncapacitated sperm, and cAMP stimulates capacitation. In the course of capacitation, cholesterol is withdrawn from the sperm membrane, and the surface proteins of the membrane redistribute. In addition, Ca^{++} influx occurs, and motility becomes more whiplike. This increases the forward velocity of sperm and enhances its ability to penetrate the ovum. Most important, capacitation permits the acrosomal reaction, also stimulated by cAMP. In this reaction, the acrosomal membrane fuses with the outer sperm membrane (Figure 50–2). Pores are created through which the acrosomal hydrolytic and proteolytic enzymes can escape. These enzymes then create a path though the protective membranes of the ovum for penetration of the sperm. Activation of guanylyl cyclase and production of cGMP play important roles in many of these sperm functions.

During Puberty, Males Develop Adult Levels of Androgenic Hormones and Full Reproductive Function

Puberty begins at an average age of 10 to 11 years and ends at about 15 to 17 years. Activation of the testes results in adult size and function of the accessory organs of reproduction, complete secondary sexual characteristics, and adult musculature. Boys undergo a linear growth spurt, and the epiphyseal growth centers (see Chapter 44) close when adult height is attained. A composite picture of the sequence is shown in **Figure 50–3.**

Enlargement of the testes is the first physical sign of puberty. This principally represents an increase in the volume of the spermatogenic tubules, and it is preceded by small increases of plasma FSH. Leydig cells appear, and testosterone secretion rises secondary to increases of the plasma LH level. The plasma testosterone level climbs rapidly during a 2-year period, when pubic and axillary hair appear, the penis enlarges, muscle mass increases, and the peak velocity of linear growth is achieved (Figure 50–3). Growth ceases 1 to 2 years after adult testosterone levels are reached. In about one third of boys, a transient stimulation of breast growth occurs, probably reflecting increased production of estradiol. As testosterone levels become dominant, the breast tissue regresses.

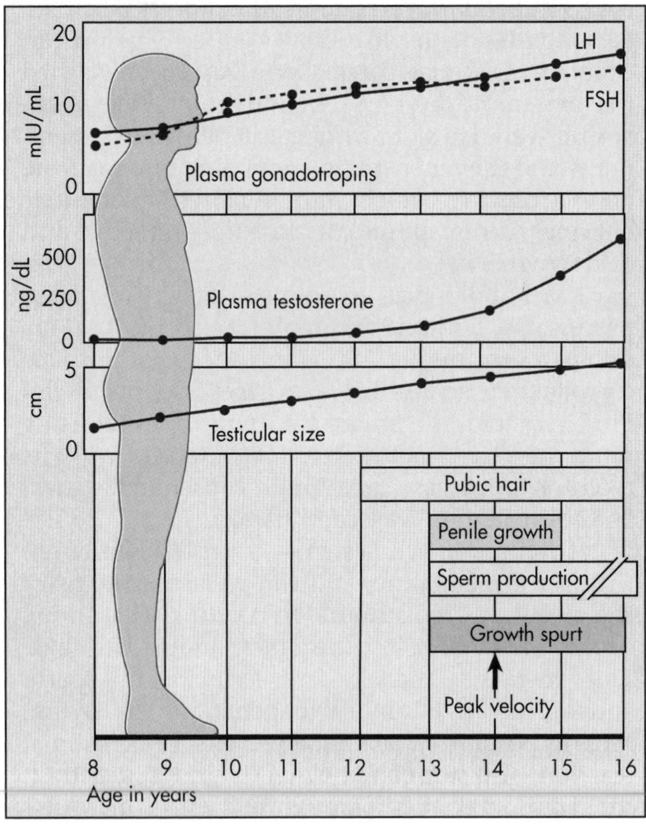

FIGURE 50–3. Average chronological sequence of hormonal and biological events in normal male puberty. The secretion of FSH and LH initiates testicular enlargement and testosterone secretion, respectively. Testosterone then stimulates somatic growth and skeletal development as well as maturation of the organs of reproduction. (Data from Marshall WA, Tanner JM: *Arch Dis Child* 45:13, 1970; and Winter JSD et al: *Pediatr Res* 6:126, 1972.)

When the boy is about 13 years of age, sperm production begins. The spermatogonia initiate meiosis, and the sequence described earlier ensues.

Hormonal Regulation of Spermatogenesis

For various reasons, the hormonal regulation of spermatogenesis is more difficult to elucidate and less completely understood than that of oogenesis. Numerous hormones and hormonal products are involved, and circumstances exist for paracrine and autocrine interactions among Leydig, peritubular, Sertoli, and germ cells. Given that spermatogenesis is genetically programmed, the role of the endocrine system is to optimize the rate of sperm production, the total quantity produced, and the ability of the sperm to reach and fertilize the ovum.

For normal sperm production, the adult gonadotropin-releasing hormone, luteinizing hormone, follicle-stimulating hormone, and testosterone axis must function normally

THE PULSATILITY OF GONADOTROPIN-RELEASING HORMONE (GnRH) RELEASE AND OF FSH/LH ACTIONS ON THEIR TARGET CELLS AND THE PRODUCTION OF HIGH INTRATESTICULAR CONCENTRATIONS OF TESTOSTERONE ARE ESSENTIAL COMPONENTS IN SPERMATOGENESIS. In normal adults, experimental induction of transient FSH and LH deficiency via total suppression of the pituitary gonadotrophs almost completely halts sperm production. Selective replacement of either FSH or LH then reinitiates sperm production but not to normal levels, which can be achieved only by restoring FSH and LH together. Adult men who lack GnRH neurons can be made fertile by properly programmed multiple pulses of GnRH delivered daily. A suitable period of pubertal exposure to FSH is essential to spermatogenesis; however, after that, sperm production can sometimes be maintained adequately by LH or high levels of testosterone alone in adults with hypopituitarism.

FSH, LH, and testosterone may also coordinate with dihydrotestosterone (DHT) and estradiol, derived locally from testosterone, other sterols, inhibin, and activin, as well as pituitary-secreted prolactin and growth hormone in the regulation of spermatogenesis. For example, growth hormone deficiency delays the onset of reproductive function, probably because of a resulting lack of local production of insulin-like growth factors (somatomedins) (see Chapter 45).

The prepubertal testis contains only resting spermatogonia and quiescent Sertoli cells that do not exhibit cyclic alterations in structure or in biochemical functioning. Neither Leydig cells nor peritubular cells of the adult myoid character are present (Figure 50–1). Pubertal activation of gonadotropin secretion leads to dramatic and complex changes. The proximity of several stimulated endocrine cell types (with multiple secretory products) to each other and to the germinal cell line creates many possible paracrine effects. These effects are in addition to central feedback actions.

During fetal life, the transient midgestation surge of FSH, LH, and testosterone release may stimulate the transformation of some primordial germ cells into resting spermatogonia. Reduction in fetal gonadotropins then leaves the spermatogonia in suspended development throughout childhood. Shortly after FSH and LH secretion begins to rise at the onset of puberty, the spermatogonia are activated. The maximum rate of sperm production may be set by the number of Ap spermatogonia present at the end of puberty.

Although FSH alone cannot initiate and complete spermatogenesis, the process is arrested in its absence. Men with inactivating mutations of the FSH β subunit gene have had azoospermia (complete absence of sperm from the ejaculate). Men with inactivating mutations of the FSH receptor have quantitatively and qualitatively abnormal spermatogenesis. FSH may promote transformation of Ap to more mature type B spermatogonia, rather than to Ad spermatogonia. Downstream, FSH appears to facilitate the normal structural changes during spermiogenesis and ultimately to ensure adequate acrosomal activity and motility of sperm. Most important, FSH stimulates the Sertoli cells, whose functions are required for initial germ cell mitotic and early meiotic activity.

LH stimulates the Leydig cells to secrete testosterone, which presumably diffuses across the basement membrane and enters Sertoli cells. The Sertoli cells contain a high density of androgen receptors. The high local concentration of testosterone (50- to 100-fold greater than in plasma) is essential for completion of the later stages of spermatogenesis. Testosterone prevents premature separation of the next to last stage spermatids from the Sertoli cell, thus promoting normal separation of the last stage of spermatids at the proper time (spermiation). This effect of testosterone may be explained by stimulation of Sertoli cell secretion of adhesion molecules, such as N-cadherins. In men who lack LH, testosterone administration to attain normal systemic plasma levels, even if it is given with FSH, cannot sustain spermatogenesis. It is possible that DHT may also enter and act within the germ cells. Conversion of small amounts of testosterone to estradiol within the Leydig and Sertoli cells makes this estrogen available as another local spermatogenesis modulator. Men with inactivating mutations of either estrogen receptors or the aromatase enzyme (necessary for estradiol synthesis) have diminished fertility and abnormal spermatogenesis.

Once regular spermatogenesis has been established during puberty, it can continue to a small extent in adults who have very low levels of FSH and LH, provided testosterone is present in high amounts. Under these circumstances, type B spermatogonia are decreased 80% to 90%, spermiation is impaired, and the number of sperm is markedly reduced, but the sperm are normal in appearance. Selective restoration of either FSH alone or LH alone can increase sperm numbers, but both are required for normal levels to be reached.

Other pituitary hormones are also involved in spermatogenesis. Prolactin increases the number of LH receptors and synergizes with LH to stimulate androgen production. Growth hormone is essential for the normally timed onset of reproductive function. Growth hormone stimulates growth of the wolffian duct structures, penis, and prostate gland and increases the Leydig cell response to LH (i.e., it raises testosterone levels). Insulin growth factor also enhances testosterone synthesis.

Sertoli Cell Function and Its Regulation

The Sertoli cells and their responses to FSH and testosterone are crucial to spermatogenesis. Sertoli cells proliferate during the infancy peak of FSH secretion (see Figure 49–3) and again during puberty. Thereafter, the Sertoli cells do not undergo further cell divisions. Each cell remains in contact with up to five other Sertoli cells and with many more germ cells in different stages of development. Because each Sertoli cell can support only a limited number of germ cells, the number of functioning Sertoli cells is a major determinant of the maximum rate of sperm production. Ectoplasmic processes from Sertoli and germ cells invaginate into each other's plasma membranes. In close association with the cycle of spermatogenesis, Sertoli cells undergo regular changes in the activity and shape of the nucleus; the size, shape, and branching of the cytoplasmic processes; the concentrations of lipid and glycogen; mitochondrial function; and enzyme content. These changes relate to the processing of the germ cells in an intimate and regular manner, which suggests that the Sertoli cells are responding in part to signals from the germ cells. One candidate germ cell signal is the cytokine **tumor necrosis factor-α (TNF-α),** which is secreted by spermatids. Sertoli and Leydig cells have TNF-α receptors, and Sertoli cells secrete inhibin in response to TNF-α.

The cytoplasm of the Sertoli cells extends from the basement membrane to the lumen of the seminiferous tubule. The investing cytoplasm acts as conduits, between which the germ cells move in their developmental passage to the lumen (Figure 50–1). As spermatocytes mature, new tight junctions between the investing Sertoli cells develop behind them while the old tight junctions ahead of them "unzip." In this way, spermatocytes pass from the basal to the adluminal compartment without breaking the integrity of the blood-testis barrier that is formed by Sertoli cell cytoplasm.

More than 100 proteins are synthesized and secreted by the Sertoli cells in response to FSH. Some of these secretions are directed into the lumen of the seminiferous tubule. FSH induces the enzyme aromatase, which makes estradiol locally available from testosterone. FSH up-regulates the androgen receptor and makes the Sertoli cell more responsive to testosterone. In response to FSH and testosterone, which act synergistically, an **androgen-binding glycoprotein (ABP),** with an amino acid sequence identical to that of the circulating sex steroid–binding globulin (see later), is synthesized. ABP binds testosterone, DHT, and estradiol with high affinity. Germ cells lack androgen receptors, but ABP may make testosterone (and other steroids) available to germ cells by endocytosis of testosterone complexed to ABP. ABP is also secreted into epididymal fluid, where it prevents reabsorption of sex steroids and ensures their continued presence for sperm needs.

Inhibin B, activins, and various growth factors are also synthesized under the influence of FSH and testosterone. *Destruction or spontaneous loss of the spermatogenic cells suppresses inhibin secretion, thereby increasing FSH secretion.* This influence suggests that a signal from spermatogenic cells stimulates the synthesis of inhibin by the Sertoli cells (**Figure 50–4**). FSH promotes the availability of iron, copper, vitamin A, and crucial sphingolipids to the germ cells by stimulating synthesis of their binding proteins. Binding proteins then extract their respective ligands from plasma and transfer them to the germ cells. FSH-stimulated proteases and plasminogen activator are probably involved in the process of spermiation.

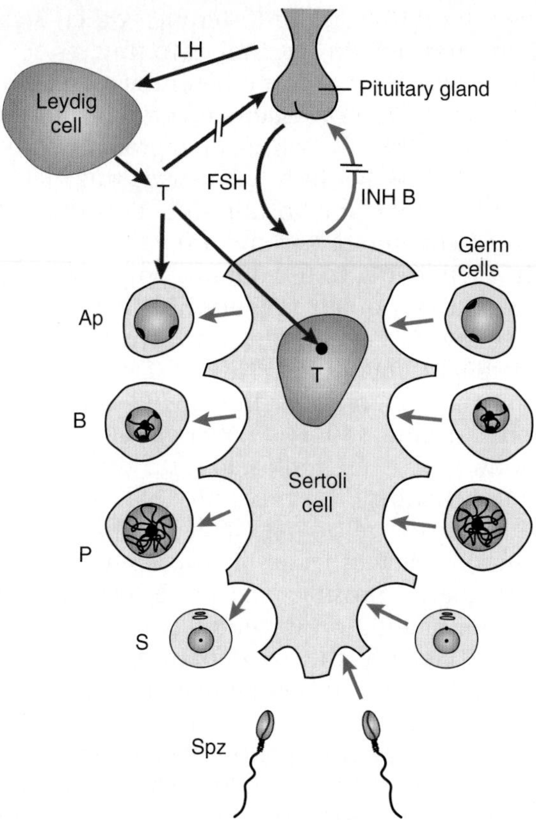

FIGURE 50–4. Endocrine and paracrine regulation of spermatogenesis. The preprogrammed development of sperm from spermatogonia is facilitated and maintained at a basal rate by T (testosterone) effects on the Sertoli cell and possibly directly on the germ cells themselves. The Sertoli cells receive signals from various stages of the germ cell progression and also send signals to the germ cells. FSH augments the rate of spermatogenesis by stimulating Sertoli cells. The Sertoli cells feed back on the pituitary negatively via inhibin. When the rate of spermatogenesis is too low, signals from the germ cells (Ap and B, spermatogonium; P, primary spermatocyte; S, spermatid; Spz, spermatozoa) reduce inhibin secretion from the Sertoli cell, thereby causing an increase in FSH and a consequent increase in sperm production. Sperm count and FSH levels demonstrate a negative feedback relationship. Support of the necessary T concentration is effected by a separate negative feedback relationship with LH. (From Berne RM, Levy MN, Koeppen BM, Stanton BA: *Physiology,* ed 5, Philadelphia, 2004, Elsevier.)

One conceptual way to summarize and integrate the relationship between spermatogenesis and its major hormonal regulators is illustrated in Figure 50–4. Spermatogenesis proceeds at a preprogrammed rate that the germ cells themselves can increase or decrease by **eliciting** the appropriate hormonal regulators. When sperm production is too great, germ cells signal Sertoli cells to **increase** secretion of inhibin. Inhibin then suppresses FSH release from the pituitary gland. The lower FSH levels lead to a reduction in spermatogenesis. Conversely, when the rate of sperm production is inadequate, the germ cells signal Sertoli cells to repress inhibin synthesis. This allows pituitary FSH secretion to increase, and the higher FSH levels restore spermatogenesis to the desired rate. Thus, sperm count and plasma FSH have an inverse relationship, much like that of plasma testosterone and LH (Figure 50–4), a relationship that acts to maintain the appropriate local concentration of testosterone for optimal spermatogenesis.

Approximately 10% of otherwise normal males are completely or relatively infertile, often because of inadequate spermatogenesis, for which no current therapy is reliably effective. The ejaculate may contain no sperm **(azoospermia),** an inadequate number (<10,000,000/mL) of sperm **(oligospermia),** a high percentage of sperm with reduced mobility, or a high percentage of sperm with immature or abnormal morphological characteristics. With azoospermia, the serum FSH level is elevated secondary to loss of negative feedback by inhibin, which is deficient. However, in other situations, routine measurements of plasma gonadotropin and testosterone levels may be normal, yet testicular biopsy specimens may show spermatogenic arrest at various stages from spermatogonia to spermatids, with few normal-appearing spermatozoa, or failure of Sertoli cells to form properly functioning junctional complexes with germ cells. It is not clear whether the timing, frequency, or amplitude of FSH/LH pulses may still be abnormal, whether paracrine hormonal effects may be defective, or whether the Y chromosome genes that program spermatogenesis are ineffective mutants.

Testosterone, an Androgen, Is in Part Only a Circulating Prohormone

Testosterone, the major androgenic hormone, is synthesized as described in Chapter 49. In adults, plasma testosterone levels show small pulses throughout the day that correspond to pulses of LH. Much of androgen action is supplied by the reduction of testosterone to DHT and **5α-androstenediol** in target tissues. The key enzyme, 5α-reductase, exists in two types. Type 2 is present in genital tissues, and it is essential to differentiation of these tissues in the male pattern in utero. This enzyme isotype is greatly down-regulated at puberty, and the type 1 5α-reductase is responsible for DHT and androstenediol production thereafter in target tissues, such as the prostate gland. Circulating testosterone is the major source of systemic estradiol in men, produced by aromatization in such sites as adipose tissue and the liver. In certain instances, estradiol may be the mediator of an apparent testosterone action.

Only 1% to 2% of plasma testosterone is in a free form. Testosterone and DHT circulate mostly bound to a sex steroid–binding globulin (SSBG), which is identical in amino acid sequence to ABP of Sertoli cell origin. The remaining testosterone is bound to albumin. Thus, SSBG-bound fractions serve as circulating androgen reservoirs, similar to those of thyroid hormone and cortisol. In general, only the free and the loosely bound albumin fractions of testosterone diffuse into cells and are biologically active. The concentration of SSBG is increased by estrogens and decreased by androgens.

Most testosterone is metabolized to products oxidized at the 17 position (see Figure 49–1) and excreted in the urine; these products constitute 30% of the 17-ketosteroid fraction (see Chapter 47). Of the average normal production of testosterone (7 mg daily), about 1% is excreted in the urine as a glucuronide.

Plasma testosterone levels vary throughout life. As shown in **Figure 50–5**, the plasma testosterone level rises to adult values in the fetus at the same time as plasma gonadotropins (see Figure 49–3) and when the external genitalia are undergoing differentiation. By birth, however, the testosterone levels have declined greatly. After a brief postnatal surge, plasma testosterone (and LH) levels fall to low values throughout childhood, and Leydig cells cannot even be identified in the testis. At the age of about 11 years, Leydig cells reappear, and plasma

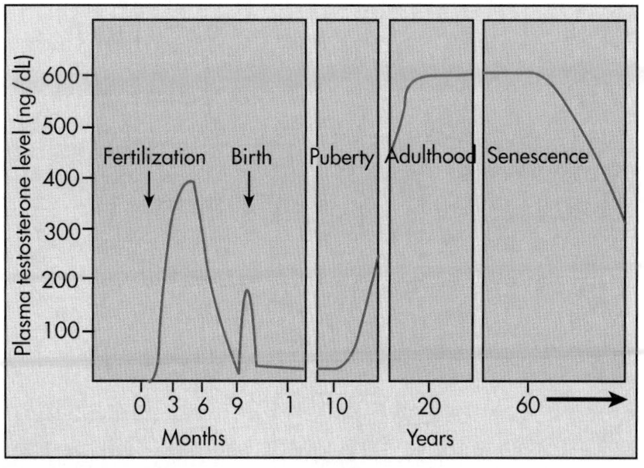

FIGURE 50–5. Plasma testosterone profile during the life span of a normal male. The intrauterine surge corresponds with completion of masculinization of the external genitalia in the fetus. The adult plateau is achieved rapidly during puberty. The senescent decline is relatively modest, and there is slight if any loss of androgen effects. (Data from Griffin JE et al. In Bondy PK, Rosenberg LE: *Metabolic control and disease,* Philadelphia, 1980, WB Saunders; and Winter JSD et al: *J Clin Endocrinol Metab* 42:679, 1976.)

testosterone concentration begins a steep rise to approximately 600 ng/dL at about the age of 17 years (Figure 50–5). This plateau is sustained until the third decade of life when total and free testosterone levels begin to decrease 0.5% to 1.0% per year. This occurs because there is a reduction in GnRH release and the Leydig cells lose their responsiveness to LH stimulation. Because of negative feedback, plasma LH levels rise slowly (as do FSH levels from reduction in inhibin). Although there may be a decline in sperm production, spermatogenesis still occurs in most octogenarians. However, in the senescent era, there is a decline in libido, a decrease in bone and muscle mass, and an increased risk of fractures and falls.

Outside the Testis, Androgens Act on Reproductive Organs, Produce Secondary Sexual Characteristics, Stimulate Somatic Growth and Maturation, and Influence Metabolism

The extratesticular effects of testosterone and related androgens can be divided into two major categories: (1) effects that pertain specifically to reproductive function and to secondary sexual characteristics and (2) effects that pertain more generally to stimulation of nonreproductive tissue growth and maturation (**Figure 50–6**). Similar intracellular mechanisms are involved in both categories of effects. In general, the model for steroid hormone effects is applicable (see Figure 41–8).

Testosterone diffuses freely into cells. In many but not all target cells, it rapidly undergoes reduction to DHT and, in some cells, to 5α-androstenediol (see Figure 49–1). DHT is much more potent than testosterone in some biological actions, and it has a threefold greater affinity for the androgen receptor.

The androgen receptor is a member of the steroid receptor superfamily. The DNA-binding domain is 56% homologous with that of the estrogen receptor. The androgen hormone–receptor complex is phosphorylated, disassociates from a chaperone heat shock protein, dimerizes, and then interacts with target DNA molecules. It is sometimes assisted by other nuclear transcription factors. As a result, RNA polymerase, various messenger RNAs, and the synthesis of proteins are stimulated. In addition, the activities of enzymes, such as thymidine kinase

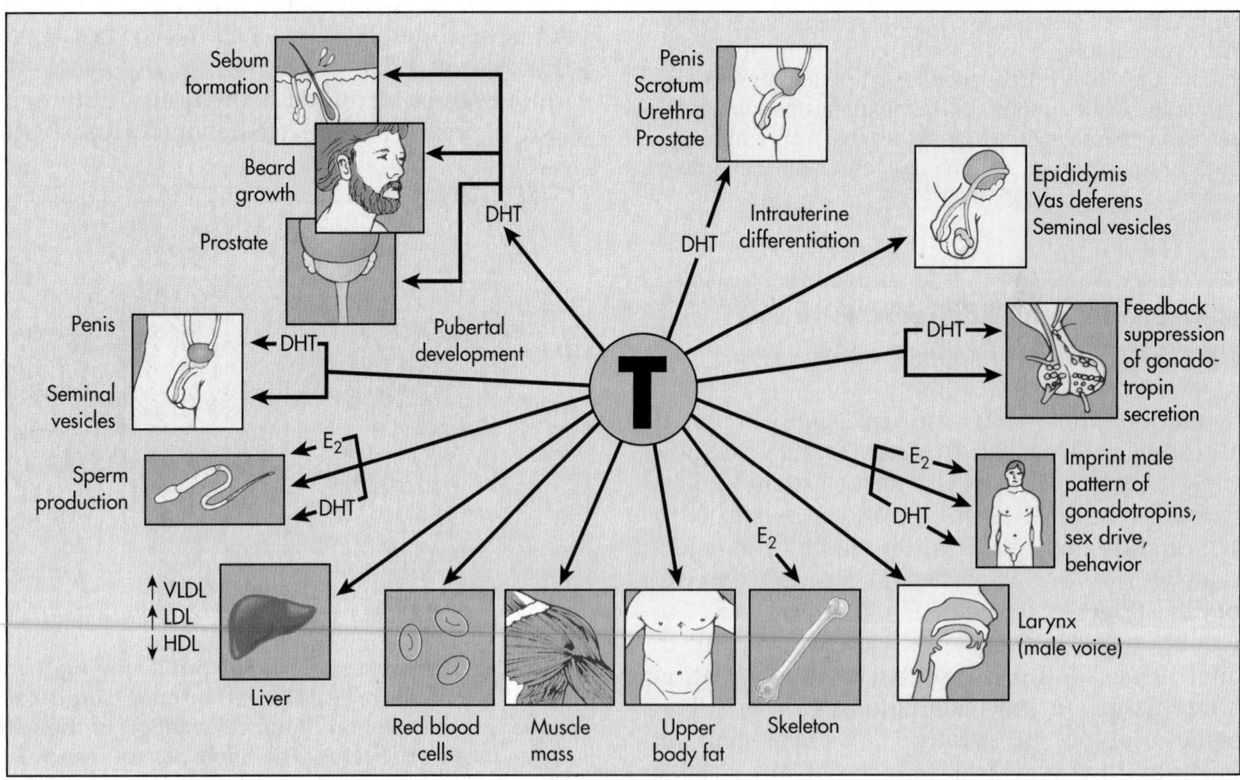

FIGURE 50–6. Spectrum of androgen effects. The final or most important effector molecule is not known with certainty in all cases. Some effects, such as increases in muscle mass, result from the action of testosterone (T) itself. Other effects, such as prostate growth and development, are definitely mediated by DHT. The role of estradiol (E_2) produced from testosterone in the testis itself is uncertain, but estradiol does mediate skeletal actions. HDL, high-density lipoprotein; LDL, low-density lipoprotein; VLDL, very-low-density lipoprotein.

and DNA polymerase, that play roles in DNA synthesis are increased.

In the prostate gland and seminal vesicles, spermine and putrescine synthesis is stimulated by testosterone, and these compounds in turn increase RNA synthesis. Androgens also stimulate the remarkable growth of these accessory organs of reproduction. This growth is characterized by hypertrophy and hyperplasia of the epithelial cells, stromal components, and blood vessels. In the prostate gland, a prostate-specific antigen is induced. The DHT-liganded androgen receptor causes prostate mesenchymal cells to secrete positive growth regulators of epithelial cells, such as keratinocyte growth factor and fibroblast growth factor; on the other hand, TGF-β, a repressor of prostate growth, is down-regulated by DHT. In the absence of androgen action, apoptosis of prostate cells is accelerated.

The mitogenic effects of androgens (and specifically of DHT) on the prostate gland are of great clinical importance. The conditions known as **benign prostatic hypertrophy** and **prostate cancer** are common after the age of 50 years. Benign prostatic hypertrophy interferes with bladder function, and it can even cause renal failure by obstruction. The presence of prostate cancer is suggested by an elevated serum level of prostate-specific antigen. Growth of prostate cancer is at least partly androgen dependent, and removal of androgen action is a mainstay of treatment. Methods include excision of the testes, markedly reducing LH and hence testosterone secretion with long-acting GnRH agonists that down-regulate their receptors, and inhibiting testosterone and DHT actions with a receptor blocker or with estrogens.

The spectrum of androgen effects is shown in Figure 50–6. DHT is specifically required in the fetus for differentiation of the genital tubercle, genital swellings, genital folds, and urogenital sinus into the penis, scrotum, penile urethra, and prostate, respectively. During puberty, DHT is required again for growth of the scrotum and prostate and for stimulation of prostatic secretions.

DHT or 5α-androstenediol stimulates the hair follicles and produces the typical male pattern of hair growth characterized by beard growth, diamond-shaped pubic escutcheon, relatively large amounts of body hair, and recession of the temporal hairline. In some men, this last response culminates in baldness. DHT or 5α-androstenediol is also responsible for increased production of sebum by the sebaceous glands and the consequent development of acne, especially during puberty.

Testosterone, on the other hand, specifically stimulates the differentiation of the wolffian ducts into the epididymis, vas deferens, and seminal vesicles. During puberty, testosterone, with or without DHT, causes enlargement of the penis and the seminal vesicles. It also causes enlargement of the larynx and thickening of the vocal cords, which result in a deeper voice.

Testosterone itself first stimulates the pubertal growth spurt. It then terminates linear growth by closing the epiphyseal growth centers. Androgen receptors in osteoblasts transduce testosterone-stimulated increases in collagen synthesis and in the levels of transforming growth factors. Estradiol is an essential partner of testosterone and a mediator of testosterone's action on bone maturation in males. Estradiol also mediates effects of testosterone in the hypothalamus and reproductive tract.

In the male reproductive tract, estradiol regulates the reabsorption of luminal fluid by cells of the efferent ductules (Figure 50–1). These cells contain Na^+,K^+-ATPase, Cl^- channels, and aquaporin. Normally, 90% of the fluid in the rete testes is reabsorbed. This process concentrates the sperm in the final ejaculate and improves their maturation and survival. Without estradiol action, fluid reabsorption is defective and infertility results.

Testosterone causes enlargement of the muscle mass in boys during puberty. In subsequent adult life, administration of testosterone to either sex causes nitrogen retention, which reflects protein anabolism. Androgen suppression of gonadotropin secretion by negative feedback is largely a function of testosterone since the hypothalamus lacks significant 5α-reductase activity. However, aromatase is present, and estradiol mediates this testosterone effect.

Testosterone has important actions on lipid metabolism. It increases levels of circulating low-density lipoprotein cholesterol and decreases levels of circulating high-density lipoprotein cholesterol (see Chapter 42). It also favors accumulation of upper body, abdominal, and visceral fat. These effects are associated with a greater risk of cardiovascular disease in men than in premenopausal women.

Certain other diverse androgenic actions can be ascribed to testosterone. These include stimulation of erythropoietin synthesis and maturation of erythroid precursors, which help maintain a normal red blood cell mass; stimulation of renal Na^+ reabsorption; suppression of hepatic synthesis of SSBG, cortisol-binding globulin, and thyroxine-binding globulin; suppression of mammary gland growth; initiation of sexual drive (libido) and the ability to achieve a physiologically complete erection (potency); and stimulation of aggressive behavior.

Summary

- The anatomical arrangement of the testis permits spermatogenesis to occur in a protective and conditioned environment within the spermatogenic tubules behind a blood-testis barrier, formed largely by cytoplasm of flanking Sertoli cells.
- Spermatogenesis is a process preprogrammed by genes, but the rate of production of sperm is regulated by hormone action.
- Sertoli cells are stimulated by FSH to provide ABP, growth factors, inhibin, mineral- and vitamin-binding proteins, and enzymes required for the development, sustenance, maturation, and transit of spermatozoa.
- Leydig cells in the interstitium of the testis are stimulated by LH to secrete testosterone, which in high local concentrations is essential for spermatogenesis.
- Testosterone and its active, more potent product, DHT, are required for pubertal masculinization to occur.
- Testosterone also increases muscle mass and linear body growth but ultimately halts any further increase in height by closing the epiphyseal growth centers of bones.
- Estradiol mediates some testosterone actions.

Bibliography

Andersson K-E, Wagner G: Physiology of penile erection, *Physiol Rev* 75:191, 1995.

Cheng CY, Mruk DD: Cell junction dynamics in the testis: Sertoli-germ cell interactions and male contraceptive development, *Physiol Rev* 82:825, 2002.

De Kretser DM, Risbridger GP, Kerr JB: Male reproduction: functional morphology. In DeGroot LJ, Jameson JL, eds: *Endocrinology,* ed 4, Philadelphia, 2001, WB Saunders.

De Kretser DM et al: Spermatogenesis, *Hum Reprod* 13:1, 1998.

Eddy EM: Male germ cell gene expression, *Recent Prog Horm Res* 57:103, 2002.

Fawcett DW: Ultrastructure and function of the Sertoli cell. In Hamilton DW, Greep RO, eds: *Handbook of physiology, section 7, Male reproductive system, vol 5,* Bethesda, Md, 1975, American Physiological Society.

Fraser LR, Adeoya-Osiguwa SA: Fertilization promoting peptide: a possible regulator of sperm function in vivo, *Vitam Horm* 63:2, 2001.

Heckert L, Griswold MD: The expression of the follicle-stimulating hormone receptor in spermatogenesis, *Recent Prog Horm Res* 59:129, 2002.

Hull KL, Harvey S: GH as a co-gonadotropin: the relevance of correlative changes in GH secretion and reproductive state, *J Endocrinol* 172:1, 2002.

Jensen TK et al: Inhibin B as a serum marker of spermatogenesis: correlation to differences in sperm concentration and follicle-stimulating hormone levels: a study of 349 Danish men, *J Clin Endocrinol Metab* 82:4059, 1997.

Kierszenbaum AL: Mammalian spermatogenesis in vivo and in vitro: a partnership of spermatogenic and somatic cell lineages, *Endocr Rev* 15:116, 1994.

Lindzey J et al: Molecular mechanisms of androgen action, *Vitam Horm* 49:383, 1994.

McLachlan RI et al: Identification of specific sites of hormonal regulation in spermatogenesis in rats, monkeys, and man, *Recent Prog Horm Res* 57:149, 2002.

McLachlan RI et al: The endocrine regulation of spermatogenesis: independent roles for testosterone and FSH, *J Endocrinol* 148:1, 1996.

Plant TM, Marshall GR: The functional significance of FSH in spermatogenesis and the control of its secretion in male primates, *Endocr Rev* 22:764, 2001.

Revelli A et al: Guanylate cyclase activity and sperm function, *Endocr Rev* 23:484, 2002.

Rhoden EL, Morgentaler A: Risks of testosterone-replacement therapy and recommendations for monitoring, *N Engl J Med* 350:482, 2004.

Saez JM: Leydig cells: endocrine, paracrine, and autocrine regulation, *Endocr Rev* 15:574, 1994.

Skinner MK: Cell-cell interactions in the testis, *Endocr Rev* 12:45, 1991.

Spiteri-Grech J, Nieschlag E: The role of growth hormone and insulin-like growth factor I in the regulation of male reproductive function, *Horm Res* 38(suppl 1):22, 1992.

Steinberger E, Steinberger A: Hormonal control of spermatogenesis. In DeGroot LJ, Jameson JL, eds: *Endocrinology,* ed 4, Philadelphia, 2001, WB Saunders.

Tapanainen JS, Aittomädaki K, Huhtaniemi IT: New insights into the role of follicle-stimulating hormone in reproduction, *Ann Med* 29:265, 1997.

Veldhuis JD: Male hypothalamic-pituitary-testicular axis. In Yen SSC, Jaffe RB, Barbieri RL, eds: *Reproductive endocrinology,* ed 4, Philadelphia, 1999, WB Saunders.

Wilson JD: Androgens, androgen receptors, and male gender role behavior, *Horm Behav* 40:358, 2001.

Yamamoto M, Turner TT: Epididymis, sperm maturation, and capacitation. In Lipshultz LI, Howards SS, eds: *Infertility in the male,* St. Louis, 1991, Mosby.

Case Studies

Case 50–1

A 32-year-old XY male has a congenital deficiency of GnRH caused by the intrauterine failure of GnRH neurons to send their axons to the median eminence.

1. **Which of the following abnormalities would be expected?**
   A. Relatively short arms and legs
   B. Female external genitalia
   C. Prostatic hypertrophy
   D. Small testes
   E. Arrest of spermatogenesis at the spermatid stage

2. **Which would be the optimal treatment to make this man fertile?**
   A. Testosterone injections
   B. FSH injections
   C. LH injections
   D. A long-acting GnRH agonist injected daily
   E. GnRH injected by a pump programmed to deliver multiple pulses daily

Case 50–2

A 46-year-old man with multiple autoimmune diseases developed an autoantibody to the FSH receptor that blocked FSH activity.

1. **Which of the following plasma levels would be higher than normal?**
   A. Inhibin
   B. Antimüllerian hormone
   C. LH
   D. FSH
   E. Testosterone

2. **Which of the following would be lower than normal?**
   A. Plasma testosterone level
   B. Plasma low-density lipoprotein level
   C. Sperm count
   D. Red blood cell count
   E. Bone density

Chapter 51: Female Reproduction

Objectives

- ❖ Describe the complex developmental sequence of ovarian follicles.
- ❖ Explain the hormonal regulation of oogenesis.
- ❖ Delineate the critical actions of estradiol on reproductive and other tissues.
- ❖ Identify the many functions of the placenta.
- ❖ Describe the changes in maternal metabolism caused by pregnancy.
- ❖ Explain the concepts of parturition.

The ovary is the site where the female gametes, the ova, develop and mature in a sheltering and supportive environment. In addition, the ovaries secrete estrogens, hormones that act on numerous peripheral tissues and organs described earlier in this book. Estrogens affect the cardiovascular system, renal function, skeletal structure, and hepatic protein synthesis.

The ovaries, along with the fallopian tubes and uterus, are situated in the pelvis. In adults, each ovary weighs approximately 15 g and consists of three zones. The dominant zone is the **cortex,** which is lined by **germinal epithelium** and contains all the **oocytes,** the germ cells, each enclosed in a **follicle.** Follicles in various stages of development and regression are present throughout the cortex (**Figure 51–1**). The surrounding stroma is composed of connective tissue elements and **interstitial cells.** The other two zones of the ovary, the **medulla** and the **hilum,** contain scattered steroid-producing cells whose function is unknown. The ovaries and follicle development can be visualized by ultrasonography and computed tomography.

The **granulosa** and **theca cells** of the ovary produce hormones and other substances that act locally to modulate the development of the ovum and its extrusion from the follicle. The hormones are also secreted into the blood and act on the fallopian tubes, uterus, vagina, breasts, hypothalamus, pituitary gland, adipose tissue, liver, kidney, bones, and vasculature. Many of these endocrine effects also subserve the process of reproduction. THE FUNDAMENTAL REPRODUCTIVE UNIT IN THE OVARY IS THE FOLLICLE, WHICH CONSISTS OF ONE OOCYTE SURROUNDED BY A CLUSTER OF ENDOCRINE GRANULOSA AND THECA CELLS. When it is fully developed and functional, the follicle maintains, nurtures, and matures the oocyte and releases it at the proper time; prepares the female genital tract to facilitate fertilization of the ovum and implantation of the zygote in the uterus; and provides hormonal support for the fetus until the placenta can assume this function.

Biology of Oogenesis

Germ cells initially differentiate into oocytes suspended in the prophase of meiosis

Oogonia arise from primordial germ cells that migrate to the genital ridge at 5 to 6 weeks of gestation. In the developing ovary, they undergo mitosis until 20 to 24 weeks have elapsed, when the total number of oogonia has reached a maximum of 7 million. Beginning at 8 to 9 weeks and continuing until 6 months after birth, oogonia start

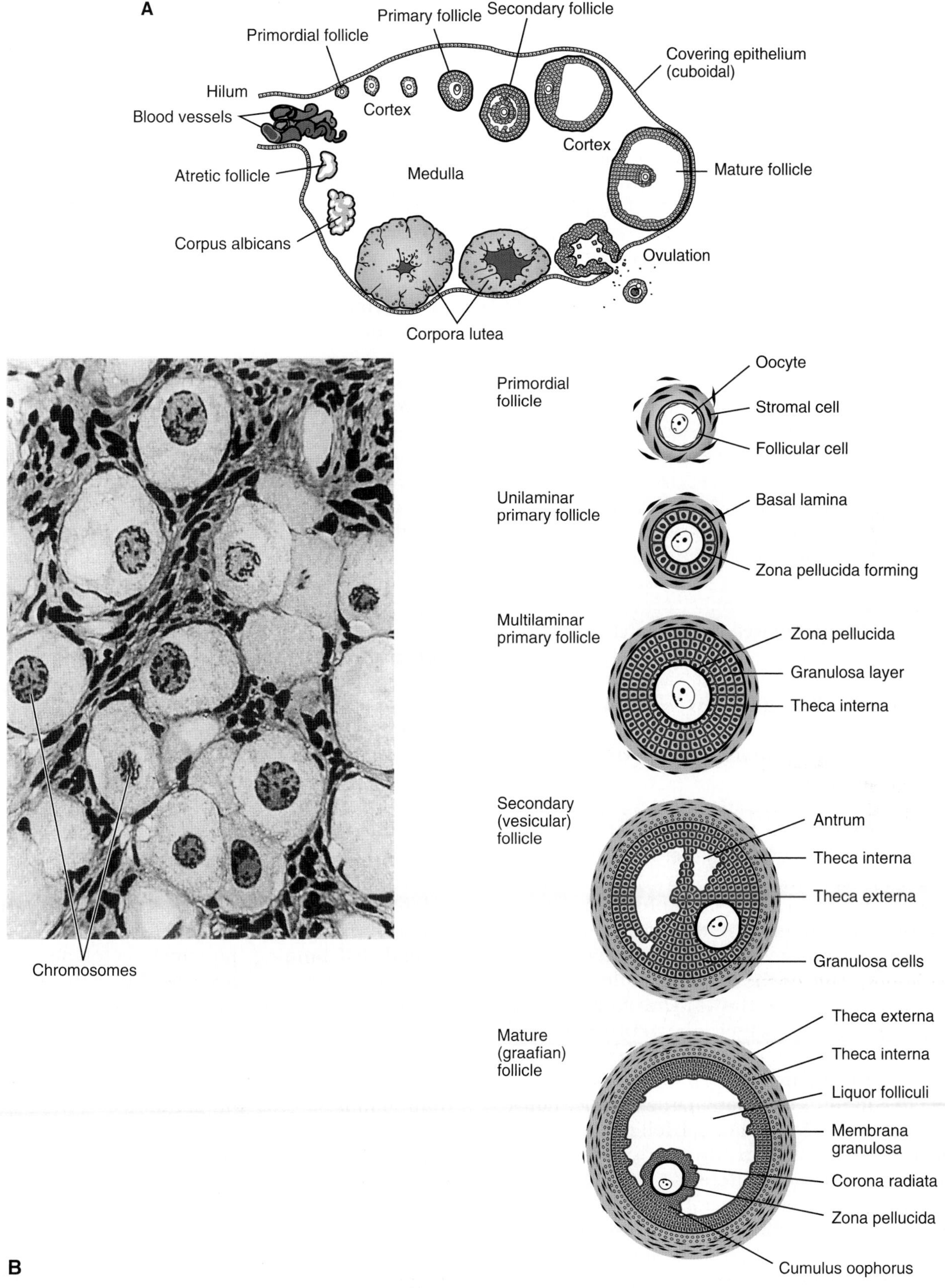

FIGURE 51–1. **A,** Schematic representation (not to scale) of the structure of the ovary showing the various stages in the development of the follicle and its successor structure, the corpus luteum. **B,** Details of each stage showing how the oocyte draws successive layers of nutritive, supportive, and protective cells around it as it reaches its maximum size in the secondary follicle. Note the chromosomes that are visible in the photomicrograph because the oocytes are suspended in meiosis. Hormones and other constituents in the follicular fluid regulate this process. (From Berne RM, Levy MN, Koeppen BM, Stanton BA: *Physiology,* ed 5, Philadelphia, 2004, Elsevier.)

into the prophase of meiosis and become primary oocytes. The primary oocytes grow from 10 to 25 µm in diameter when meiosis begins and reach 50 to 120 µm at maturity. The process of meiosis is kept suspended in prophase by inhibitory hormones, at least until sexual maturation of the individual and, in some primary oocytes, until menopause. The first meiotic division is not completed until the time of **ovulation** (release of the ovum). Thus, primary oocytes have life spans of up to 50 years, and both X chromosomes are required for their survival.

Oocytes undergo attrition

From the start of oogenesis, a process of oocyte attrition by apoptosis occurs simultaneously so that only 2 million primary oocytes exist by birth and only 400,000 remain by the onset of puberty. THIS CONSTITUTES THE ENTIRE SUPPLY OF POTENTIAL OVA FOR THE WOMAN'S REPRODUCTIVE LIFE BECAUSE NO NEW OOGONIA CAN BE FORMED. With continuing attrition, few oocytes are left when menopause begins and reproductive capacity ends. This contrasts sharply with the male, in whom the supply of spermatogonia is continually being renewed (see Chapter 50).

The ovarian follicle develops in stages

Oocytes induce a surrounding supportive and protective follicle

The follicle develops in distinct stages (Figure 51–1). The first stage parallels the prophase of the oocyte and occurs slowly. It begins in utero and ends at any time during reproductive life. As an oocyte enters meiosis, it induces a single layer of spindle-shaped cells from the stroma to surround it completely. They form cytoplasmic processes that attach to the plasma membrane of the oocyte. Simultaneously, a membrane called the **basal lamina** forms outside the spindle cells. This delimits the **primordial follicle,** which has a diameter of 25 µm, from the surrounding stroma (Figure 51–1).

At 5 to 6 months of gestation, the spindle-shaped cells in some of the primordial follicles are transformed into cuboidal **granulosa cells,** thereby forming a **primary follicle.** As these granulosa cells divide and create several layers around the oocyte, the complex becomes a **secondary follicle.** The granulosa cells secrete mucopolysaccharides, which form a protective halo, the **zona pellucida,** around the oocyte (Figure 51–1). However, the cytoplasmic processes of the granulosa cells continue to penetrate the zona pellucida and provide nutrients and hormonal signals to the enclosed maturing primary oocytes. The cytoplasm of the granulosa cells also forms a filter through which plasma substances must pass before reaching the germ cell (compare with Sertoli cells and spermatocytes in Figure 50–1).

The secondary follicle grows to a diameter of about 150 µm. At this point, the oocyte has reached its maximum diameter of 80 µm. Concurrently, a new layer of cells from the stroma is "recruited" outside the basal lamina and forms the **theca interna.** The granulosa cells then begin to extrude small collections of fluid around and among them. This completes the first, or preantral, stage and is the maximal degree of follicular development ordinarily found in the prepubertal ovary.

A small number of follicles enlarge and develop further functional capability after menarche

The second stage of follicular development ordinarily begins only after the onset of menstrual cycling. This stage may require up to 70 to 85 days, and it spans parts of three menstrual cycles until completion. Past the midpoint of each cycle, a small number of secondary follicles are recruited for further development. The small collections of follicular fluid coalesce into a single area called the **antrum** (Figure 51–1). The fluid of the antral follicle contains a complex of substances, some secreted by the granulosa and theca cells and some transferred from the plasma through the granulosa cell cytoplasm. Included are mucopolysaccharides, plasma proteins, electrolytes, enzymes of steroid synthesis, steroid hormones, follicle-stimulating hormone (FSH), luteinizing hormone (LH), inhibin, activin, follistatin, oxytocin, arginine vasopressin, corticotropin-releasing hormone (CRH), and proopiomelanocortin derivatives. In addition, antral fluid contains growth factors (including IGF-1, IGF-2, and IGF-binding proteins), cytokines (interleukin-1 and tumor necrosis factor-α), and the components of the renin-angiotensin system. All of these presumably play some role in particular events of follicle development or ovulation. The steroid hormones reach the antrum via secretion from granulosa cells and via diffusion from theca cells. A nonsteroidal substance capable of inhibiting oocyte meiosis, possibly inhibin or antimüllerian hormone, is also present in the antrum.

As the granulosa cells proliferate, they form a syncytium with electrical and chemical intercommunication. The oocyte is displaced into an eccentric position on a stalk, where it is surrounded by a distinctive layer, the **cumulus oophorus,** which is two to three cells thick (Figure 51–1). The cells of the theca interna also proliferate and are transformed into cuboidal steroid-secreting cells. Additional layers of spindle cells from the stroma form an outer vascularized layer called the **theca externa.** The new blood vessels carry blood-borne substances such as LH and FSH to the follicle. At the end of this stage, the entire complex, which is called an **antral** or **graafian follicle** (Figure 51–1), has reached an average diameter of 2 to 5 mm.

The selection of a dominant follicle precedes and is essential for ovulation

In the final stage of follicular development, one of the graafian follicles is "selected" by day 5 to 7 of a menstrual cycle, and it dominates the other second-stage follicles. This **dominant follicle** now undergoes further rapid expansion via cellular growth and augmented production of antral fluid. The colloid osmotic pressure of this fluid increases because of depolymerization of the mucopolysaccharides. However, the total pressure remains unchanged at 16 to 20 mm Hg. The granulosa cells spread apart, the cumulus oophorus loosens, and the vascularity of the theca layers increases greatly. With exponential growth, the total size of the dominant follicle reaches up to 20 mm during the last 48 hours before the midpoint of the cycle, when ovulation occurs. At a critical point, the basal lamina adjacent to the surface of the ovary undergoes proteolysis. The follicle gently ruptures, releasing the oocyte with its adherent cumulus oophorus into the peritoneal cavity. At this time, the initial meiotic division of the oocyte is completed. The resulting **secondary oocyte** is drawn into the closely approximated fallopian tube. The other daughter cell receives very little cytoplasm. It is called the first **polar body** and is discarded. In the fallopian tube, sperm penetration completes the second meiotic division, resulting in a haploid (23-chromosome) **ovum** and a second polar body. The remaining nondominant and unsuccessful follicles from that cycle undergo **atresia** (see later section) within the ovary (Figure 51–1).

Corpus luteum forms from the ruptured follicle and supports a zygote resulting from fertilization of the ovum

The residual elements of the ruptured dominant follicle next form a new endocrine unit, the **corpus luteum** (Figure 51–1). THE CORPUS LUTEUM PROVIDES THE NECESSARY STEROID HORMONE BALANCE THAT OPTIMIZES CONDITIONS FOR IMPLANTATION OF A FERTILIZED OVUM AND FOR SUBSEQUENT MAINTENANCE OF THE ZYGOTE UNTIL THE PLACENTA IS ABLE TO DO SO. The corpus luteum is 80% made up of granulosa cells. These hypertrophy in rows and take on characteristics of cells secreting steroid hormones at a high rate. They have active-appearing mitochondria with dense matrices and tubular cristae, proliferating endoplasmic reticulum, and numerous lipid droplets within their cytoplasm. This process, which is called **luteinization,** begins just before ovulation and is greatly accelerated by the exit of the oocyte from the ruptured follicle. The rest of the corpus luteum consists of somewhat luteinized theca cells arranged in folds along its outer surface. In the next important step, the basal lamina disappears, allowing ingrowth of more blood vessels that supply the granulosa cells directly. Vascular endothelial growth factor drives the rapid vascularization process.

If conception does not follow ovulation, the corpus luteum regresses after a 14-day life span. During regression, known as **luteolysis,** the granulosa and theca cells undergo necrosis, and after the structure is invaded by leukocytes, macrophages, and fibroblasts, the corpus luteum degenerates to an avascular scar (Figure 51–1).

The fate of unsuccessful follicles is programmed cell death (atresia)

During an average woman's reproductive life span, only 400 to 500 oocytes (usually only one per month) undergo the complete sequence that culminates in ovulation. The remaining millions of oocytes disappear in a process called **atresia,** which begins almost with the appearance of the initial primordial follicles. Atresia is caused by **apoptosis,** or programmed cell death. In first-stage follicles, the oocyte simply becomes necrotic, and the granulosa cells degenerate. This accounts for almost all of the oocytes. In second-stage follicles (Figure 51–1), necrosis of the granulosa cells farthest from the oocyte may precipitate a resumption of meiosis in the oocyte to the point of extrusion of the first polar body. However, the granulosa cells in the cumulus oophorus also eventually die, the unsupported oocyte degenerates, and everything inside the basal lamina collapses into a scar. The theca cells dedifferentiate and return to the stroma.

Hormonal patterns vary during the menstrual cycle

The menstrual cycle is divided physiologically into three phases (**Figure 51–2**) that correspond with the dominant events in the monthly development of each ovum. The **follicular phase** begins with the onset of menstrual bleeding and averages 15 days

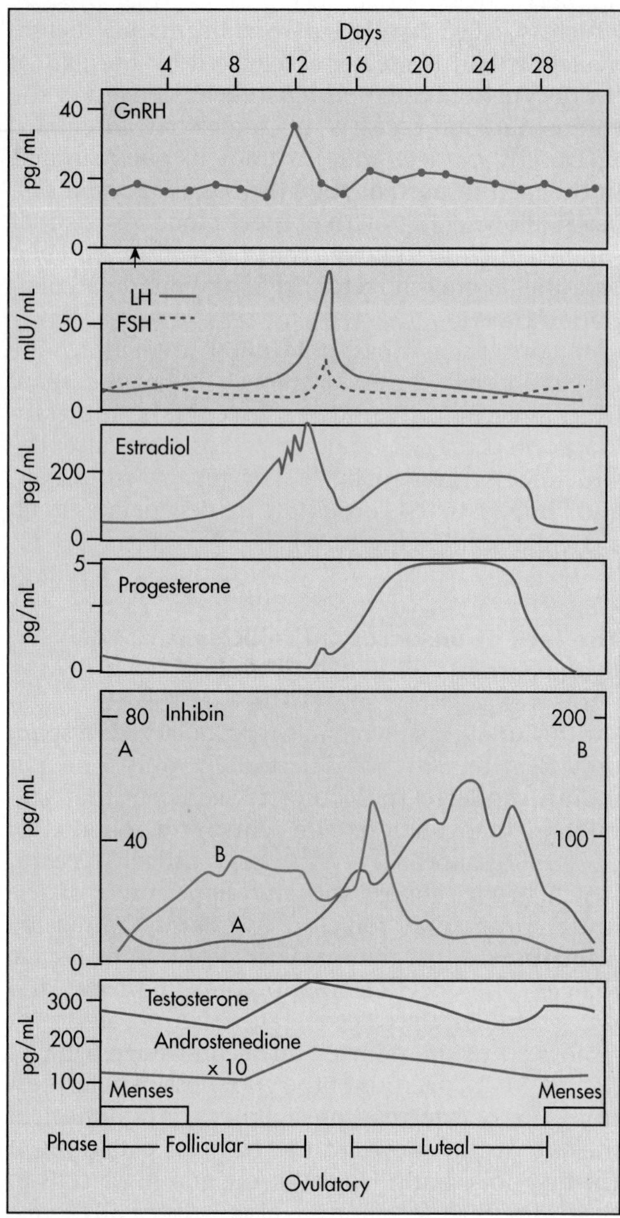

FIGURE 51–2. Profile of plasma hormone levels throughout the menstrual cycle. The dominant follicle is the source of the rising estradiol level in the later part of the follicular phase. The ovulatory surges of LH and FSH are preceded by increases in the levels of estradiol and gonadotropin-releasing hormone (GnRH). The broad peaks of progesterone and estradiol in the luteal phase result from secretion by the corpus luteum. The earlier inhibin B peak results from follicle production; the later inhibin A peak originates from corpus luteum production.

(range, 9 to 23 days). The succeeding **ovulatory phase** lasts only 1 to 3 days. The final **luteal phase** lasts 13 to 14 days and ends with the onset of menstrual bleeding. A normal menstrual cycle may range from 21 to 35 days, depending mainly on the length of the follicular phase.

Levels of pituitary gonadotropins and ovarian steroids fluctuate in a regular, interrelated pattern throughout the cycle

Normal reproductive function is characterized by cyclic changes in ovarian steroid hormone and inhibin production that are consequent to cyclic changes in LH and FSH secretion resulting from greater sensitivity of the pituitary gonadotrophs to hypothalamic gonadotropin-releasing hormone (GnRH) and to increased GnRH pulses. Both negative- and positive-feedback loops are involved in creating this complex pattern.

The critical regulators of the ovarian cycle are FSH and LH. Just before the start of the follicular phase, plasma FSH and LH concentrations are at their lowest (Figure 51–2), and the LH/FSH ratio is slightly greater than 1. The FSH level begins to rise gradually 1 day before menses begins, and it continues to do so through the first half of the follicular phase. The level of LH rises later.

During the second half of the follicular phase, the FSH level falls slightly, whereas the LH level continues to rise so that the LH/FSH ratio reaches about 2. Stimulated by the early rise in FSH levels, the plasma estradiol concentration also increases gradually during the critical first 6 to 8 days of the cycle. Later in the follicular phase, the plasma estradiol level increases much more sharply and reaches a peak just before the ovulatory phase (Figure 51–2). THIS ESTRADIOL IS SECRETED BY THE GRANULOSA CELLS OF THE DOMINANT FOLLICLE. The higher estradiol level, along with increased granulosa cell secretion of inhibin B (Figure 51–2), then feeds back to decrease the plasma FSH concentration during the second half of the follicular phase. LH levels continue to rise slowly, as do androgens produced by theca cells. Progesterone levels remain low.

The succeeding ovulatory phase is uniquely characterized by a large but transient spike in the plasma LH level, with a lesser spike in the FSH level; the LH/FSH ratio increases to 5. This surge in gonadotropin is preceded first by the "sawtooth" estradiol peak of the late follicular phase and then by an increase in GnRH pulses (Figure 51–2). At the same time, the plasma progesterone level rises slightly. Together these changes suggest that both the ovary and the hypothalamus contribute to the ovulatory surge of LH and FSH. The surge takes 14 hours to peak and remains at its peak for another 14 hours. The downside of the surge takes 20 hours.

Plasma estradiol levels begin to plummet during the upswing of FSH and LH.

Corpus luteum function determines the hormone pattern in the postovulatory second half of the cycle

After ovulation, negative feedback from the corpus luteum causes LH and FSH levels to decline further during the luteal phase and to reach their nadirs toward its end (Figure 51–2). The pulse frequency of gonadotropin secretion is also diminished. The most distinctive feature of the luteal phase is a 10-fold increase in plasma levels of progesterone, secreted by the corpus luteum. Levels of estradiol, which is also secreted by the corpus luteum, increase again, and there is a large rise in inhibin A concentrations. If pregnancy does not occur and the corpus luteum degenerates, progesterone, estradiol, and inhibin A levels decrease dramatically to their lowest at the end of the luteal phase, FSH secretion increases, and menstrual bleeding starts.

Hormonal Regulation Is Part of Oogenesis

The first stage of follicle formation is not absolutely hormonally dependent

The initial growth of the primordial follicle appears to be a local phenomenon that is independent of gonadotropins and one in which factors from the oocyte stimulate granulosa cell development. Genes coding for zona pellucida proteins appear to be essential to development of the follicle. Granulosa cell products initiate formation of the theca and then stop maturation of the oocyte once it reaches about 80 μm in diameter. Other gene products protect germ cells by inhibiting their apoptosis. This first stage, from primordial to primary follicle, continues to occur until menopause, apparently independent of the state of reproductive cycling. However, the transient surge of FSH and LH in midgestation and even the low levels of gonadotropins secreted during childhood appear to be necessary for an adequate rate of follicular growth throughout the rest of life. Females with inactivating mutations of the FSH β subunit gene or of the FSH receptor gene are infertile.

The exact mechanism by which a particular group of resting primordial follicles is recruited to descend from the cortex into the interstitium toward the medulla and to initiate development into primary follicles is unknown. However, the most "selectable" follicles are those whose theca interna begins to develop during the periovulatory phase of that cycle, when the surge of gonadotropin release increases the vascularity of the follicles and helps protect them from atresia.

In follicular development, a high level of estradiol production is essential to a follicle's "success"

The second stage of follicular development begins in the early luteal phase of one cycle and continues gradually until the late luteal phase two cycles later. A small number of follicles that have acquired FSH and LH receptors are recruited, and they grow slowly during this period (**Figure 51–3**). From each group of approximately 20 follicles of 2 to 4 mm, a single dominant follicle is "selected" by the fifth to seventh day of the ensuing follicular phase, usually in only one ovary each month. The early rise in FSH

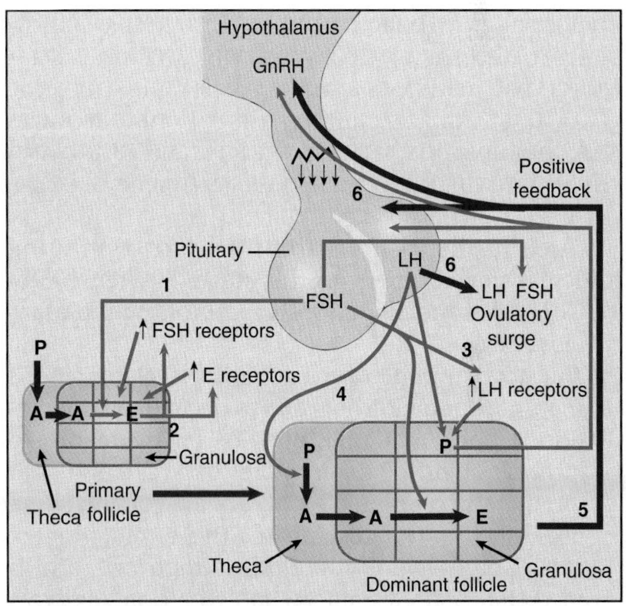

FIGURE 51–3. Hormonal regulation of follicular development. 1, FSH stimulates granulosa cell growth and estradiol (E) synthesis in a small cohort of primary follicles. 2, The local estradiol increases its own receptors and FSH receptors, amplifying the effects of both hormones. Thus, a self-propelling mechanism is set into motion. 3, FSH later increases LH receptors, initiating granulosa responsiveness to LH. 4, LH stimulates theca cell growth and androgen (A) production. Androgen is then converted to estradiol in the granulosa cells. LH also stimulates progesterone (P) production in the granulosa cells and adds to the effects of FSH by increasing cAMP levels. 5, As a result of theca and granulosa cell synergism, the dominant follicle emerges as an efficient secretor of estradiol. 6, Rising estradiol levels, with late potentiation by progesterone, feed back positively on the pituitary gland and hypothalamus to evoke the preovulatory surge of LH and FSH.

levels during the follicular phase stimulates mitosis and proliferation of the granulosa cells in the selected follicle to a 600-fold increase in cell number. FSH acts by inducing gene expression and production of cyclin D_2, one of the regulators of the cell cycle clock apparatus during the G_1 phase. FSH ALSO INDUCES THE GENE AND STIMULATES ACTIVITY OF THE KEY ENZYME AROMATASE, CAUSING ESTRADIOL SYNTHESIS FROM ANDROGENS TO BE MARKEDLY ENHANCED IN THE DOMINANT FOLLICLE (Figure 51–3). Steroidogenic factor 1 (SF-1) and cAMP liganded to its binding protein assist in induction of aromatase at separate DNA sites. The high local estradiol concentration then increases its own receptors as well as FSH receptors. This further sensitizes the granulosa cells to both hormones, and even more estradiol is produced, which with locally produced activin accelerates the process. In addition, granulosa cell hypertrophy and hyperplasia are enhanced by local generation of insulin-like growth factors (IGF-1 and IGF-2) as well as transforming growth factor and epidermal growth factor. ONCE IT IS STARTED, SECOND-STAGE FOLLICULAR DEVELOPMENT THUS BECOMES A SELF-PROPELLING MECHANISM THAT COMBINES ENDOCRINE, AUTOCRINE, AND PARACRINE EFFECTS AND THAT REQUIRES FINE COORDINATION BETWEEN THE PITUITARY GLAND AND THE OVARY. THE OUTCOME IS EXPONENTIAL FOLLICULAR GROWTH.

Three further actions contribute to continuing follicular development in this stage (Figure 51–3):

1. FSH and estradiol induce LH receptors on the granulosa cells.
2. The slowly rising plasma estradiol level conditions the GnRH-gonadotropin axis to decrease FSH secretion slightly but still permits LH secretion to increase slightly. Pituitary stores of LH are also built up, thereby creating a supply for the coming surge of LH in the ovulatory phase. This estradiol effect occurs partly within the gonadotroph cells and is mediated partly via interaction with dopaminergic and endorphinergic neurons that inhibit GnRH release.
3. Estradiol increases LH receptors on theca cells, making them able to maximize production of androgen substrates that aromatase will convert to estradiol.

Theca and granulosa cells cooperate to boost estradiol synthesis and to induce the ovulatory surge of luteinizing hormone

THE UNIQUE ROLE OF LH IN THE SECOND HALF OF THE FOLLICULAR PHASE IS TO STIMULATE THECA CELLS TO PRODUCE INCREASING AMOUNTS OF ANDROSTENEDIONE AND TESTOSTERONE. These androgens diffuse across the basal lamina into the granulosa cells, where they serve as essential precursors to estradiol (see Figure 49–1). LH acts through increases in P-450scc and StAR (Chapter 47). In addition, LH stimulates more granulosa cell production of progesterone.

The maturation of the dominant follicle depends on a complex set of interactions between its component theca and granulosa layers (Figure 51–3). These interactions underlie the critical goal: a high enough output of estradiol to trigger ovulation. The FSH-specific granulosa cells are greatly dependent on the LH-specific thecal cells for a sufficient supply of androgens to be converted to estrogens. This reaction is catalyzed by the action of aromatase, which is up-regulated by FSH-stimulated cAMP levels. The FSH-induced recruitment of LH receptors on granulosa cells also allows LH to augment cAMP levels in those cells and thus to directly contribute to estradiol production. Another granulosa cell product induced by FSH (namely, inhibin B) stimulates androgen production by the theca cells. In turn, androgens stimulate inhibin production by granulosa cells. This local positive-feedback loop, as well as paracrine effects of locally produced IGF-1 and its binding proteins, contributes to the striking synthetic momentum of the dominant follicle and its production of estradiol. The entire process is also stimulated by insulin and growth hormone as well as by **locally produced** growth hormone–releasing hormone (GHRH), somatostatin, and possibly GnRH itself.

FSH also stimulates enhanced granulosa cell production of trace metal– and vitamin-binding proteins and substrates for energy generation in the oocytes, as Sertoli cells do for spermatocytes. Levels of molecules involved in the mechanism of ovulation (such as plasminogen activator and cytokines) are also increased by FSH during the preovulatory period.

Both ovaries presumably receive similar amounts of FSH and LH. Therefore, THE EMERGENCE OF ONE DOMINANT FOLLICLE IN EACH CYCLE MAY RESULT FROM ITS POSSESSING MORE FSH RECEPTORS AND GREATER AROMATASE ACTIVITY AT THE OUTSET. Such characteristics would permit this particular follicle to exceed the others in early estradiol production. Conversely, the other second-stage follicles undergoing atresia have relatively low ratios of estradiol to androgen in the antral fluid. This probably reflects declining FSH availability as FSH secretion is reduced by estradiol and by inhibin B released from the dominant follicle.

Whatever the mechanism for achieving dominance, this follicle secretes sufficient estradiol to inhibit growth of its sister follicles, to prime the GnRH-LH/FSH part of the axis to generate the LH ovulatory surge, and to prepare the genital tract to receive and accept a conceptus.

Ovulation is dependent on hormonal activity

The ovulatory surge of LH and FSH is triggered by a positive-feedback effect of estradiol

A critical plasma estradiol level of at least 200 pg/mL, sustained for at least 2 preceding days, is required to trigger ovulation (Figures 51–2 and 51–3). The proportionally smaller preovulatory increase in plasma progesterone synergizes with estradiol to amplify and prolong the gonadotropin surge. This positive-feedback effect takes place at both pituitary and hypothalamic levels. Estradiol and progesterone augment the flow of GnRH pulses from the hypothalamus to the pituitary gland, partly by decreasing inhibitory activity of dopaminergic and endorphinergic neurons on GnRH neurons. The pituitary gland, appropriately primed by the preceding pattern of ovarian steroid exposure, now responds to these repetitive GnRH pulses in exaggerated fashion. Furthermore, the sialic acid content of the secreted LH molecules, modified by estradiol, makes the LH more biologically active.

A hormonally stimulated pseudoinflammatory response ruptures the follicle and releases the ovum

The hypothalamic-pituitary unit is conditioned by ovarian steroids to provide a sudden increase in gonadotropin (mainly LH) stimulation of the dominant follicle. This triggers ovulation 12 hours later via a multicomponent mechanism:

- LH neutralizes the action of a peptide oocyte maturation inhibitor. A sterol (4,4-dimethylzymosterol) in follicular fluid also activates meiosis. These effects allow the completion of meiosis. At the same time, further replication of granulosa cells is halted.
- LH stimulates progesterone synthesis; the increased progesterone augments proteolytic enzyme activity, which loosens the wall and increases the distensibility of the follicle.
- A pseudoinflammatory response ensues; this response is characterized by local synthesis of prostaglandins, leukotrienes, and thromboxanes, some of which are required for follicular rupture. The LH surge induces the key enzyme **prostaglandin endoperoxide synthase** to stimulate production of these inflammatory factors.
- FSH stimulates the production of glycosaminoglycans, which mucify the environment and disperse the cumulus oophorus. FSH also induces proteolytic enzymes and plasminogen activator, which catalyze the final breakdown of the follicular wall.
- Immediately after ovulation, there is a rapid fall in estradiol production, which also contributes to the loss of integrity of the follicle.
- Establishment of the corpus luteum from the disrupted follicle is subsequently favored by suppressing the inflammatory response with extra cortisol generated locally from cortisone by an increase in the ratio of type 1 to type 2 11-hydroxysteroid dehydrogenase (see Chapter 47).

The development and functioning of the corpus luteum are under hormonal control

The ovulatory LH surge stimulates the luteinization of granulosa cells. Subsequent lower frequency, higher amplitude luteal phase pulses of LH can then maintain a high rate of progesterone production by the corpus luteum as well as a substantial rate of estradiol production (Figure 51–2). Exposure to proper amounts of FSH in the preceding follicular phase ensures the presence of sufficient corpus luteum receptors for LH action. Vascular ingrowth into the corpus luteum, stimulated by vascular endothelial growth factor, is also important for delivery of the LH and cholesterol necessary to sustain progesterone secretion. The lower levels of FSH and LH during the luteal phase withdraw support from the other follicles of this cohort and hasten their atresia.

When pregnancy occurs, an early placental hormone saves the corpus luteum from atresia

If pregnancy is initiated, the earliest placental cells rapidly begin secreting **human chorionic gonadotropin (hCG)** with LH bioactivity. If pregnancy does not ensue and the declining LH levels of the late luteal phase are not replaced by the equivalent hCG, the corpus luteum begins to regress after the eighth postovulatory day, and its secretion of progesterone and estradiol ceases completely by the fourteenth day. By then, corpus luteum secretion has fallen low enough to release the pituitary gland from feedback inhibition of FSH by estradiol and inhibin A and to allow the FSH rise of the next cycle to begin. The apoptosis of luteal cells is partly mediated by prostaglandins and by interactions between oncogenic and tumor suppressor gene products.

Extraordinary coordination between the various elements of the female hypothalamic-pituitary-ovarian axis is required for ovulation and conception. This creates numerous possibilities for failure, and infertility arising from dysfunction of this system is common. Disease or conditions that disrupt GnRH release or impair the gonadotrophic responsiveness prevent the necessary initial FSH pattern to recruit a dominant follicle, and they may result in complete loss of menses **(amenorrhea).** A dominant follicle may produce enough estrogen for uterine bleeding to occur (see later section) but not enough to induce a midcycle peak of LH; this causes **anovulatory cycles.** On the other hand, an elevated ratio of LH to FSH in the follicular phase is associated with excessive theca cell production of androgens and the formation of numerous atretic and cystic follicles; this constitutes the **polycystic ovary syndrome.** Even if ovulation occurs, an **inadequate luteal phase,** either too short or substandard in progesterone production, may lead to poor preparation of the reproductive tract for either fertilization or implantation.

Various manipulative medical therapies are available for female infertility, in contrast to the situation in men. For example, the drug **clomiphene** is an estrogen antagonist that blocks the estrogen receptor in the hypothalamus. By simulating estrogen deficiency and the absence of negative feedback, clomiphene produces an increase in GnRH and gonadotropin secretion in women with a hypothalamic origin of infertility. Alternatively, endogenous pituitary function can be suppressed with a long-acting GnRH superagonist, and ovulation can be induced by carefully timed doses of exogenous FSH and LH or by pulses of native GnRH.

The menstrual cycle originates in the ovary

Substantial evidence supports the thesis that in humans, THE MONTHLY CYCLE OF THE LH/FSH SURGE AND CONSEQUENT OVULATION IS MAINLY A RHYTHM INDUCED BY THE OVARY ITSELF RATHER THAN THE RESULT OF AN INHERENT RHYTHM GENERATED WITHIN THE CENTRAL NERVOUS SYSTEM. No cycle of LH/FSH release is observed in the absence of functional ovaries. The gonadotropin surge occurs only when the dominant follicle has reached the receptive preovulatory stage of development irrespective of the number of days required for this to occur. Estradiol itself, administered in a proper fashion, can induce an LH surge. Finally, in primates, if the pituitary gland is experimentally severed from the hypothalamus and GnRH pulses of appropriate frequency and amplitude are provided externally to the pituitary gland in a proper but fixed pattern, a preovulatory surge of LH and ovulation occur without abruptly altering the profile of the GnRH input.

Undoubtedly, a GnRH pulse generator in the central nervous system is required to initiate and sustain follicular development. However, it is the subsequent developing pattern of ovarian events and secretions, most critically in the dominant follicle, that conditions this pulse generator and the pituitary gonadotrophs to respond later with an ovulatory LH/FSH surge. Perhaps no other phenomenon so clearly illustrates the intricate nature of the interactions among endocrine, paracrine, autocrine, and neural mechanisms of regulation.

The close coordination between the emergence of a single dominant follicle and the ovulatory signal it recruits makes multiple pregnancies unlikely in humans. For example, the natural rate of occurrence of **dizygotic twins** is less than 1% of live births. This is further emphasized by the much higher rate (15%) of multiple ova produced during cycles in which follicular development and ovulation are produced artificially "from above" by superimposed profiles of stimulation with exogenous FSH and LH. Multiple pregnancies are also more common (5%) when endogenous FSH and LH are released in response to clomiphene administered on the fifth day of the cycle to infertile women.

The ovarian signals that induce ovulation can be overridden by other influences. Loss of cyclic gonadotropin secretion can result from calorie deprivation, loss of adipose tissue mass, habitual strenuous exercise, stress, emotional disturbances such as depression, physical translocation, change of climate, and chronic inflammatory disease. The inhibitory influences on GnRH or LH and FSH secretion may be mediated by endorphins, dopamine, or CRH and in some instances by changing the levels of cortisol, androgens, or thyroid hormone.

Well-known examples of anovulation or even complete loss of menses occur in women with **anorexia** nervosa, in ballet dancers, and in marathon runners. The ovarian dysfunction can be so serious that it causes profound estrogen deficiency with consequent **osteoporosis.**

Seasonal variation in reproduction activity suggests modulation by melatonin because human conception rates are lowest in the winter months (when darkness is most prevalent, and the secretion of inhibitory melatonin is highest). It has also been observed that women who live close to one another can adopt a common timing of their menstrual cycles, possibly because of chemical signals **(pheromones)** emitted by one individual that affect a nearby individual. In humans, little evidence exists that ovulation is directly stimulated by sexual behavior, as it is in other animals. However, female-initiated sexual activity is reportedly increased around the time of ovulation.

The Cyclic Changes in Ovarian Hormone Secretion Affect All the Reproductive Tract Tissues Involved in Conception

Fertilization normally occurs in the fallopian tubes, a circumstance associated with the highest rate of pregnancy

Each fallopian tube ends in fingerlike projections called **fimbriae** that lie close to the adjacent ovary. The tubes consist of a muscle layer enclosing an epithelial lining containing secretory and ciliated cells that beat toward the uterus. During the follicular phase of the cycle, estradiol increases the number of cilia and their rate of beating. At ovulation, the fimbriae undulate to draw the shed ovum into the tube, and tubal contractions move the ovum toward incoming sperm. During the luteal phase, progesterone maximizes this ciliary beat, thereby facilitating movement of any fertilized ovum toward the uterus. Estradiol stimulates secretion of mucus, which facilitates upward movement against the current created by the cilia. Estradiol and progesterone also regulate the tubal secretion of ions and substrates that facilitate movement of the ovum and sperm and help sustain a zygote.

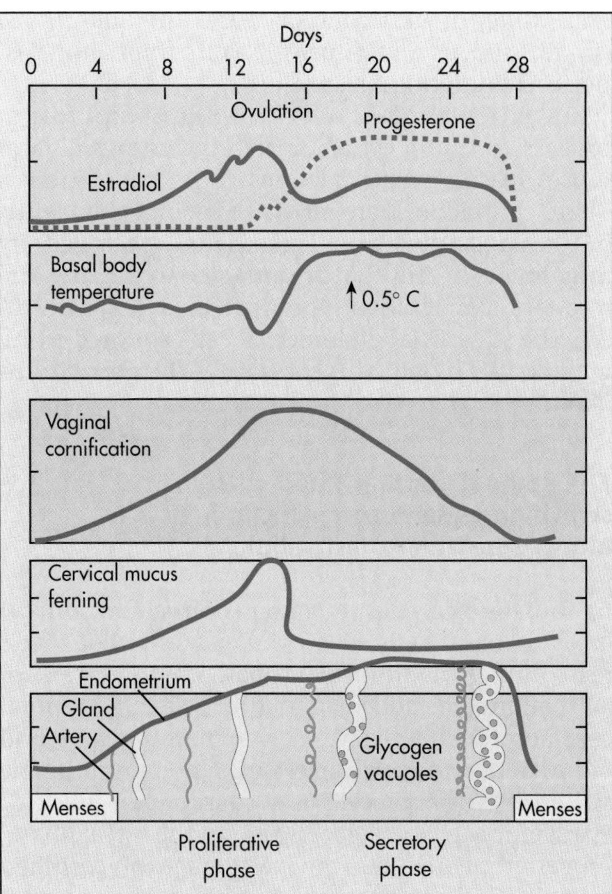

FIGURE 51–4. Correlation of changes in body temperature, vaginal cytology, and endometrial structure and function with the profiles of plasma estradiol and progesterone concentrations. (Data from Odell WD. In DeGroot LJ, ed: *Endocrinology,* ed 2, Philadelphia, 1989, WB Saunders.)

The uterus houses and nurtures the developing conceptus and ultimately evacuates the mature fetus

This muscular organ encloses a cavity lined with a mucous membrane called the **endometrium** and stromal cells. At the start of each menstrual cycle, the endometrium is thin, and its glands are sparse and straight, with a narrow lumen (**Figure 51–4**); it exhibits few mitoses and is incapable of receiving a conceptus. After menstruation has ceased, the rise in plasma estradiol concentration during the follicular phase increases endometrial thickness threefold to fivefold to a maximum of 8 to 10 mm. Mitoses appear in the glands and stroma, the glands become tortuous, and the spiral arteries that supply the endometrium elongate. This is the characteristic appearance of the **proliferative phase** of the endometrium. During this phase, estradiol induces high levels of the enzyme telomerase, which repairs the shortened ends of chromosomes and thereby prevents apoptosis. Estradiol also changes the mucus elaborated by the cervix (the opening to the uterus) from a scant, viscous material to a copious, more watery but more elastic substance. This mucus can be stretched into a long, fine thread, and it produces a characteristic fernlike pattern when it is dried. Such cervical mucus creates channels that facilitate the entrance of the sperm into the uterine cavity.

Shortly after a woman ovulates, the rise in the plasma concentration of progesterone greatly alters the endometrium and produces the characteristic appearance of the **secretory phase** (Figure 51–4). The rapid growth and mitotic activity of the endometrium are inhibited as progesterone suppresses telomerase, telomeres are lost, and apoptosis is increased. The glands become much more tortuous and accumulate glycogen. As the luteal phase of the cycle progresses, the glycogen vacuoles move from the base toward the lumen, and the glands greatly increase mucus secretion. The stroma of the endometrium becomes edematous; the spiral arteries elongate further and coil. Glycoproteins, glycolipids, and glycogen in the progesterone-stimulated secretions enable the endometrium to accept, implant, and nourish a conceptus. At the same time, progesterone decreases the quantity of cervical mucus and returns it to its thick, nonelastic, and nonferning state.

If conception does not occur, the abrupt loss of progesterone and estradiol from the corpus luteum causes spasmodic contractions of the spiral arteries. These contractions are mediated by increased levels of prostaglandins and leukotrienes, provided by inflammatory cells that are attracted to the site. The resultant loss of blood supply produces tissue death, and the superficial endometrial cells are shed along with clotted blood. This constitutes the **menstrual flow.**

The vaginal canal is lined with a stratified squamous epithelium that is highly sensitive to estradiol

In the absence of a squamous epithelium, only a layer of basal cells is present. As estradiol levels rise during the follicular phase, more layers of epithelium are added, and the maturing vaginal cells accumulate glycogen. They become large and **cornified,** and their nuclei shrink or disappear. The percentage of such cells is a quantitative index of estrogenic activity (Figure 51–4). In the luteal phase, progesterone reduces the percentage of cornified cells. Vaginal secretions that enhance the prospect for fertilization are also increased by estradiol.

Reproductive sexual functioning involves several processes

Several processes combine to accomplish the acceptance and inward transmission of sperm. In some women, the desire for sexual activity is increased just before ovulation by the midcycle rise in plasma androgens (Figure 51–2). With sexual stimulation, vascular erectile tissue beneath the clitoris is activated by parasympathetic impulses. During heterosexual intercourse, this causes the vagina to be tightened around the penis. Simultaneously, the glands beneath the labia and in the vaginal entrance secrete copious amounts of mucus. The secretions lubricate the vagina and help it produce a massaging effect on the penis. These glands are maintained by estradiol action. Orgasm results from spinal cord reflexes that are similar to those involved in male ejaculation. Orgasm consists of involuntary contractions of the skeletal muscle of the perineum; musculature of the vagina, uterus, and fallopian tubes; and rectal sphincter.

Many spermatozoa are trapped and within a few hours are destroyed in the vagina. The remainder reach the cervix, where they dwell in storage crypts formed by the estrogen-stimulated convoluted mucosa and its mucus. From this reservoir, capacitated spermatozoa migrate into the uterine cavity and fallopian tubes during 24 to 48 hours. Of these, as few as 50 to 100 spermatozoa (1 in 100,000) eventually reach an ovum, but they are sufficient for fertilization.

The mammary glands consist of lobular ducts lined by an epithelium capable of secreting milk

These ducts empty into larger milk-conveying ducts that converge at the nipple. The glandular structures are embedded in supporting adipose and connective tissue. Before puberty, the breasts grow only in proportion to the rest of the body. The development of adult breasts depends on estradiol, but progesterone, insulin, growth hormone, IGF-1, cortisol, epidermal growth factor, and prolactin have synergistic effects. After puberty, estradiol stimulates the growth of lobular ducts in the area around the nipple. Estradiol also selectively increases the adipose tissue, giving the breast its distinctive female shape. Local production of estradiol from circulating androgens and effects of the estrogen on stromal cells are important components in breast development. Progesterone stimulates outpouching of the lobular ducts to form numerous alveoli capable of milk secretion. Cyclic changes in the breast occur in conjunction with the fluctuations in estradiol and progesterone levels during the menstrual cycle.

Ovarian steroid effects on other tissue are important to sexual development

During puberty, estradiol is to the female what testosterone is to the male. Estradiol causes almost all the somatic changes that result in the female adult appearance. In addition to stimulating growth of the internal reproductive organs and breasts, estrogens cause pubertal enlargement of the labia majora and labia minora. Linear body growth is accelerated by estradiol; however, because the epiphyseal growth centers are more sensitive to estradiol than to testosterone, they close sooner. This is another reason that the average height of women is less than that of men. The hips enlarge, and the pelvic inlet widens, facilitating future accommodation of pregnancy. The predominance of estradiol over testosterone is responsible for women's total weight of adipose tissue being twice as great as that of men, whereas muscle and bone mass are only two thirds that of men.

The skeleton, the kidney, the liver, and the vasculature are also important target tissues of estrogens. Estradiol restrains bone turnover in adults and keeps bone formation equal to bone resorption. Osteoclast formation and activity are decreased, and osteoclast apoptosis is increased. Osteoclast recruitment is reduced by estradiol's inhibition of the production of interleukin-1, tumor necrosis factor-α, and granulocyte-macrophage colony-stimulating factor, all of which are lymphokines that stimulate proliferation of osteoclasts (Chapter 44). Estradiol may also increase the formation, differentiation, and activity of osteoblasts. These skeletal effects are achieved through estrogen receptors in cortical bone different from those in trabecular bone. Loss of estrogen action after the menopause shifts the balance markedly toward bone resorption.

Estradiol increases hepatic synthesis of binding proteins for thyroid and steroid hormones, of the renin substrate angiotensinogen, of clotting factors, and of very-low-density lipoproteins. The last actions can lead to hypertension, venous thrombosis, and hyperlipidemia in estrogen-treated women.

The effects of estradiol on the vasculature are vasodilatory and antivasoconstrictive. It increases the local release of vasodilators such as nitric oxide, prostaglandin E_2, and prostacyclin, and it decreases the production or activity of endothelin-1, a potent local vasoconstrictor. The marked fall in estradiol secretion at the end of the luteal phase alters the endometrial balance from vasodilator to vasoconstrictor and helps initiate the ischemic necrosis of the endometrium. The vasodilatory effect of estradiol may offer some women protection from coronary thrombosis and myocardial infarction before menopause.

The presence of estrogen receptors in areas of the brain outside the hypothalamus supports the existence of significant estrogen effects on central nervous system functioning. Estrogens interact with *N*-methyl-D-aspartate receptors in the hippocampus to induce formation of new synapses between axons and dendrites. Estradiol improves memory and learning in rats. Estradiol deficiency in women is associated with deficits in declarative memory and with subtle motor incoordination.

Progesterone produces the 0.5°C rise in body temperature that occurs shortly after ovulation (Figure 51–4). Central nervous system actions of progesterone include an increase in appetite, a decrease in wakefulness, and a heightened sensitivity of the respiratory center to CO_2.

Estrogens and Progesterone Modulate Gene Expression

Estradiol, estrone, other estrogens, and progesterone all enter cells freely and bind to cytoplasmic receptors of the steroid, thyroid, and vitamin D superfamily (see Figure 41–8). Two distinct estrogen receptors exist, coded for by different genes located on separate chromosomes. They are termed ERα and ERβ. Although the DNA-binding domains are similar, the ligand-binding domains of the ERα and ERβ are only 55% homologous in amino acid sequence. Although they have equal affinity for estradiol, their affinities for estrone and numerous synthetic agonists and antagonists vary widely. The tissue distributions of ERα and ERβ overlap somewhat, but distinct localizations have been noted. Uterine endometrium contains mostly ERα, whereas granulosa cells and osteoblasts contain ERβ. After ligand binding by the receptor, heat shock proteins are displaced and phosphorylation and dimerization occur. After transfer to the nucleus, the hormone-receptor complex binds to variant estrogen response elements on DNA molecules. Estrogen receptors can also be activated by various kinases in the absence of ligand. Numerous coactivators and corepressors of the activated liganded estrogen receptor have also been discovered. Moreover, estradiol-ERα complexes activate transcription, whereas estradiol-ERβ complexes repress transcription at estrogen response element sites.

The importance of understanding the estrogen receptors has been greatly heightened by the discovery of **selective estrogen receptor modulators,** such as raloxifene and tamoxifen. These pharmaceutically produced nonsteroidal estrogen receptor ligands have varied estrogen receptor profiles. Tamoxifen antagonizes the action of estrogens on the breast but mimics the action of estrogens on the uterine endometrium. It is an excellent chemotherapeutic agent for breast cancer, but it can rarely also produce endometrial cancer of the uterus. Raloxifene has beneficial agonist effects on bone and serum lipids but not on breast or endometrium. It is therefore safe for treatment of osteoporosis, but its antagonist effects on the brain produce, as a side effect, the hot flashes associated with estrogen deficiency.

Nongenomic actions of estradiol that are evident within minutes also occur. These are mediated by estrogen receptors contained in plasma membrane invaginations known as **caveolae**. These liganded receptors are linked to MAP kinases, which phosphorylate other proteins that yield such rapid effects of estradiol as dilation of coronary arteries.

Some other relatively early and rapid target cell responses to estrogen are likely to be due to protooncogenes, such as c-*jun* and c-*fos*, whose expression is induced by liganded estrogen receptors. These transcription factors may then facilitate later actions of the estrogen receptor via its estrogen response elements within more specific target DNA molecules. Numerous genes are regulated by estrogen receptors in various tissues. Examples include ovalbumin, ovomucoid, growth factors, the LDL receptor, and type I collagen.

The **progesterone receptor** interacts with progesterone and progesterone regulatory elements on DNA molecules similarly to the glucocorticoid receptor–cortisol format. Indeed, these interactions overlap in such a manner that a progesterone inhibitor that binds to a progesterone receptor (mifepristone, an abortifacient drug) also inhibits the binding of cortisol to its receptor. Thus, mifepristone is used to treat endogenous hypercortisolism.

One of estradiol's important actions is to increase the synthesis of estrogen receptor and progesterone receptor. In this way, estradiol amplifies its own effects on growth of the follicle and on proliferation of the endometrium. This action also prepares target tissues for subsequent, efficient progesterone action. Conversely, progesterone decreases the synthesis of estrogen receptor. This action accounts for the inhibition by progesterone of further endometrial proliferation during the luteal phase.

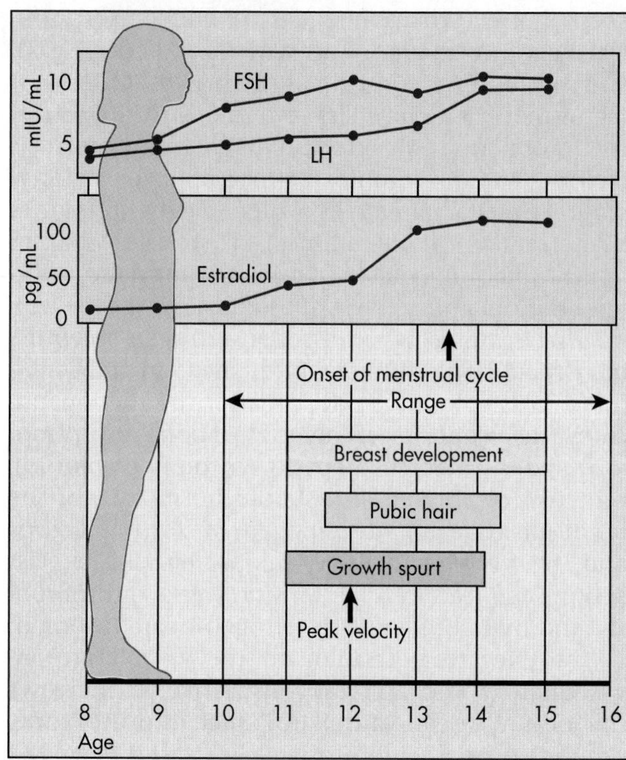

FIGURE 51–5. Average chronological sequence of hormonal and biological events in female puberty. The growth spurt starts earlier and is shorter than in males. (Data from Lee PA et al: *J Clin Endocrinol Metab* 43:775, 1976; and Marshall WA, Tanner JM: *Arch Dis Child* 45:13, 1970.)

Estradiol and Progesterone Circulate Bound to Protein

Estradiol and estrone bind to sex steroid–binding globulin, but their affinities are lower than that of testosterone. They also circulate bound to albumin, and this fraction, along with the free steroids, is biologically active. In women who menstruate, most of the circulating estrogen is estradiol from the ovaries; in postmenopausal women, it is largely produced in extraovarian tissues where it also acts, such as in bone and adipose tissue cells. In preadipocytes, the key enzyme of estradiol synthesis, aromatase, is induced by cytokines and inhibited by peroxisome proliferator–activated receptor δ (see Chapter 42). In this way, estradiol may mediate some of the effects of these regulators of differentiation of preadipocytes to adipocytes. Estrogens are excreted in the urine as sulfate and glucuronate conjugates, and hydroxylation of the aromatic ring produces **catechol estrogens** that may have antiestrogen effects in the brain. Progesterone circulates bound largely to albumin. It is reduced to pregnanediol, which is then excreted in the urine.

Female Puberty Begins with the Increase of Gonadotropin Secretion

The general process of the initiation of puberty is described in Chapter 49. Reproductive function begins after gonadotropin secretion increases from the low levels of childhood (**Figure 51–5**). Budding of the breasts is the first physical sign of puberty, and it coincides with the initial increase in plasma estradiol concentration. The onset of menses occurs approximately 2 years later, at 11 to 15 years of age, after LH levels have risen more sharply.

The positive-feedback effect of estradiol on gonadotropin secretion is the last step in the maturation of the hypothalamic-pituitary-ovarian axis; thus, ovulation usually does not occur in the first few menstrual cycles. These cycles are irregular in length because the bleeding is induced by the withdrawal of estrogen secretion from graafian follicles undergoing atresia.

The growth spurt and peak velocity of growth are characteristically attained earlier in girls than in boys. Height increase usually stops 1 to 2 years after the onset of menses. The development of pubic hair precedes menses and correlates best with rising levels of adrenal dehydroepiandrosterone sulfate (DHEA-S). The time at onset of female puberty is influenced by race and individual heredity, and it occurs earlier in tropical zones. Menarche can be delayed by undernutrition or regular strenuous exercise but is accelerated by obesity and blindness.

Estrogen Deficiency Characterizes Menopause

The reproductive capacity of women usually wanes in the fifth decade of life, and menses terminate at an average age of 50 years. For several years before, the frequency of ovulation decreases. Menses occur at variable intervals, and the decreased menstrual flow is caused by irregular peaks of estradiol secretion and inadequate secretion of progesterone in the luteal phase. With the disappearance of almost all follicles, ovarian secretion of estradiol virtually ceases, and estrone produced from theca cell and adrenal androgens becomes the predominant circulating estrogen.

As menopause approaches, follicular sensitivity to gonadotropin stimulation diminishes, and plasma FSH and LH levels gradually increase. Once menopause occurs, loss of negative feedback from estradiol and inhibin increase plasma gonadotropins to levels four to ten times those characteristic of the follicular phase, and FSH levels exceed LH levels (see Figure 49–3). Although the cycle of gonadotropin secretion is lost, pulsatility persists.

The manifestations of ovarian insufficiency, most particularly estradiol deficiency, depend on the stage of female life. **Intrauterine estradiol deficiency**—even caused by complete absence of the ovaries—does not prevent expression of the basic feminine phenotype (see Chapter 49), although the external genitalia may appear somewhat undersized. During puberty, estrogen deficiency causes a lack of breast development and menses. The uterus and ovaries remain infantile in size. In an **XX individual,** instead of a growth spurt, there is slow but prolonged growth until the epiphyses close late.

In women whose reproductive function is terminated early by disease and in postmenopausal women, estrogen deficiency causes thinning of the vaginal epithelium, loss of its secretions, and discomfort during intercourse. A decrease in breast mass and thinning of the skin also occur. Vascular flushing and emotional lability are disturbing symptoms. Of great importance is a sharp increase in the incidence of **coronary artery disease.** In women with relatively low bone mass caused by other factors, such as poor intake of calcium earlier in life, accelerated further bone loss from estrogen deficiency causes **osteoporosis,** with fractures of the wrist, spine, and hips. Hip fractures become a common and major source of morbidity after the age of 80 years. Short-term estrogen replacement can be safely provided to alleviate symptoms such as hot flashes. The benefit (prevent osteoporosis) to risk (breast cancer) ratio of long-term estrogen replacement and the effect on cardiovascular outcomes are still being debated.

The Endocrine Aspects of Pregnancy Are Many and Varied

Fertilization of an ovum by a single sperm depends on a complex set of interactions

Sexual encounters during the 6 days before ovulation are most likely to result in fertilization. After the ovum enters the widened proximal end of the fallopian tube (ampulla), it is transported down to the junction with the isthmus. There, the ovum must encounter sperm within 12 to 24 hours for fertilization to occur. The sperm in turn must reach the ovum within 48 hours after entering the vagina. Nitric oxide produced by the female genital tissues increases sperm motility. Contact between the sperm and ovum is facilitated by a mixing motion of the fallopian tube. Contact is also promoted by chemotaxis, which may be mediated in part by atrial natriuretic peptide (ANP) elaborated by the follicle and ANP receptors present on the sperm.

When sperm come very close to an ovum, they undergo the **acrosomal reaction,** which may also be triggered by ANP. Access of the sperm to the ovum then begins with dispersal of the granulosa cells of the cumulus oophorus (Figure 51–1). Dispersal is achieved through the action of **hyaluronidase,** a **corona-dispersing enzyme,** a neuraminidase, and a trypsin-like enzyme, all of which are contained in the acrosomal cap of the sperm (see Figure 50–2). The underlying zona pellucida of the ovum (Figure 51–1) contains species-specific receptors for sperm. The single fertilizing sperm penetrates this barrier by releasing **acrosin,** a proteolytic enzyme. Penetration is followed by Ca^{++} uptake into the ovum, which then releases ovum materials contained in granules. These substances along with **glycodelin,** a glycosylated, sialylated protein secreted by decidual cells stimulated by progesterone, block the entrance of other sperm. This prevents **polyploidy,** which is the production of an individual with more than two sets of homologous chromosomes. The polar body resulting from the second reduction division is then ejected from the ovum, leaving a haploid female pronucleus with 23 chromosomes. After fusion of their respective membranes, the DNA of the sperm head is engulfed by the ovum and forms the male pronucleus with 23 chromosomes. The two pronuclei then generate a spindle on which the chromosomes are arranged, and a zygote with 46 chromosomes is created. The sperm mitochondria are essentially eliminated so that only maternal mitochondrial DNA is inherited by offspring.

Implantation of a zygote within the uterine endometrium requires complex interactions

The zygote develops by mitosis into a **blastocyst,** which traverses the fallopian tube in about 3 days. Within another 2 or 3 days, implantation in the uterus begins. This is successful only if it occurs in the "receptive window" of the uterus during days 20 to 24 of the cycle. IMPLANTATION CONSISTS OF THREE CONSECUTIVE PROCESSES: ADHESION, PENETRATION, AND INVASION. The blastocyst must find a suitable area of the endometrium to adhere to. The requisite dissolution of the zona pellucida is initiated by alternate contraction and expansion of the blastocyst as well as by the action of lytic substances in the uterine secretions. Epidermal growth factor and its receptors in the blastocyst are critical to implantation, as are endogenous cannabinoids and their receptors. These and other maternal factors necessary for implantation depend on adequate maternal levels of progesterone and estradiol and early paracrine signals such as GnRH from the zygote. Attachment of the embryo to the endometrium is brought about by binding of cell surface receptors called **integrins** to the extracellular matrix and by bridging molecules secreted by the receptive endometrium.

From the initial solid mass of cells, a layer of **trophoblasts** separates. Microvilli of these cells interdigitate with those of endometrial cells, and junctional complexes form between the cell membranes. Adhesion is aided by a variety of endometrially produced molecules, such as **laminin** and **fibronectin.** Once they are firmly attached, trophoblasts penetrate between and beneath endometrial cells by lysing the intercellular matrix with a variety of enzymes and by phagocytosing and digesting dead endometrial cells.

The depth of penetration by the trophoblasts is limited by changes in the endometrium. Late in the luteal phase, uterine stromal cells, stimulated by progesterone, enlarge and accumulate glycogen and lipid. Now called **decidual cells,** they disappear unless pregnancy supervenes and the corpus luteum is maintained. In that case, continuing progesterone and estrogen stimulation rapidly changes the entire stroma into a sheet of decidual cells. This **decidua** functions initially as a source of nutrients for the embryo, until trophoblastic invasion establishes vascular connections between the fetus and the mother. Thereafter, the decidua provides a mechanical and an immunological (via glycodelin) barrier to further invasion of the uterine wall. The decidua also secretes prolactin, relaxin, prostaglandins, and other molecules with paracrine effects on the uterine muscle and on the fetal membranes (**chorion** and **amnion**).

Implantation is even more susceptible to mishap than conception is. Approximately 70% of all conceptions result in **miscarriage.** The majority occur within 14 days and are unrecognized by the woman, who may only have a slightly delayed menstrual period. Miscarriages later in the first trimester may still reflect suboptimal maternal-fetal attachment but are also caused by fetal anomalies.

The placenta is an endocrine organ whose products affect both the mother and the fetus

Pregnancy is marked by the development of a unique organ, the **placenta,** which has a limited life span. This organ serves as the fetal gut, supplying nutrients; as the fetal lung, exchanging O_2 and CO_2; and as the fetal kidney, regulating fluid volumes and disposing of waste metabolites. In addition, the placenta is an extraordinarily versatile endocrine gland capable of synthesizing and secreting numerous protein and steroid hormones that affect maternal and fetal metabolism. These hormones can be found in fetal plasma and amniotic fluid, and they exhibit characteristic concentration profiles in maternal plasma (**Figure 51–6**).

Trophoblasts differentiate into an inner layer of **cytotrophoblasts** and an outer layer of **syncytiocytotrophoblasts,** which are fused. The inner cytotrophoblasts secrete hypothalamic-like stimulatory and inhibitory peptides, such as CRH, that may regulate in paracrine manner the secretion of pituitary-like peptides, such as adrenocorticotropic hormone (ACTH), by the outer syncytiocytotrophoblasts. The outer syncytiocytotrophoblasts also secrete increasingly large amounts of sex steroid hormones as pregnancy progresses.

Human chorionic gonadotropin replaces luteinizing hormone as the hormone that sustains corpus luteum function

hCG is the first key hormone of pregnancy. PLACENTAL SYNCYTIOCYTOTROPHOBLAST CELLS STIMULATED BY GnRH FROM ADJACENT CYTOTROPHOBLASTS SECRETE hCG. THIS GONADOTROPIN CAN BE DETECTED IN MATERNAL PLASMA AND URINE WITHIN 9 DAYS OF CONCEPTION, AND IT SERVES AS A RELIABLE PREGNANCY TEST. hCG is a glycoprotein with two subunits. The α subunit is identical to that of thyroid-stimulating hormone (TSH), FSH, and LH. The β subunit is closely homol-

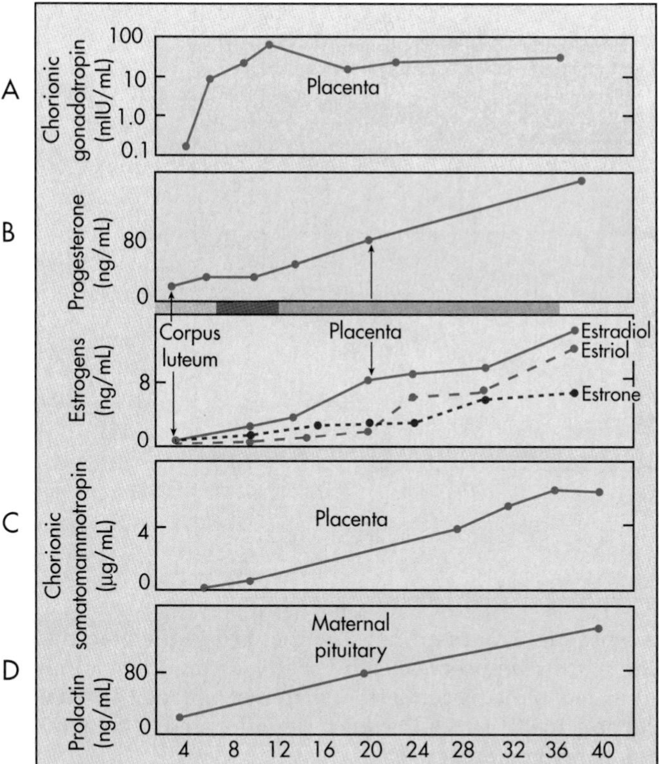

FIGURE 51–6. Profile of maternal plasma hormone changes in human pregnancy. A, Note the logarithmic scale for hCG. B, Between 6 and 12 weeks, the source of estrogens and progesterone shifts from the corpus luteum to the placenta. C, The placenta also secretes large amounts of chorionic somatomammotropin. D, The maternal pituitary contributes the excess prolactin. (Data from Goldstein DP et al: *Am J Obstet Gynecol* 102:110, 1968; Rigg LA et al: *Am J Obstet Gynecol* 129:454, 1977; Selenkow HA et al. In Pecile A, Frinzi C: *The foetoplacental unit,* Amsterdam, 1969, Excerpta Medica; Tulchinski D et al: *Am J Obstet Gynecol* 112:1095, 1972.)

ogous to that of LH, and the two hormones have indistinguishable biological actions. Maternal plasma hCG concentrations increase at an exponential rate, reach a peak at 9 to 12 weeks of gestation, and then decline to a stable plateau for the remainder of pregnancy (Figure 51–6).

hCG maintains the function of the corpus luteum, which would otherwise degenerate in the absence of pregnancy. It stimulates the corpus luteum to secrete progesterone and estradiol via mechanisms identical to those of LH. Later, when the placenta itself synthesizes these steroids in adequate amounts, hCG secretion declines, and the corpus luteum regresses. hCG also stimulates essential DHEA-S production by the fetal zone of the adrenal gland (see later section). In males, hCG stimulates the early secretion of testosterone by the Leydig cells, an action that is critical to masculine genital tract differentiation (see Chapter 49). The very high hCG levels also have enough homology with TSH to stimulate increased maternal thyroid activity early in pregnancy.

Progesterone is essential for successful implantation, initial sustenance, and long-term maintenance of the fetus

Progesterone stimulates the endometrial glands to secrete nutrients on which the early zygote depends. Thereafter, progesterone maintains the decidual lining of the uterus, where it induces prolactin synthesis. Prolactin helps inhibit maternal immune responses to fetal antigens of male parent origin, and thus it helps prevent rejection of the fetus. Progesterone transferred to the fetus is the substrate for the synthesis of cortisol and aldosterone by the fetal adrenal cortex (**Figure 51–7**). The fetal adrenal cortex cannot itself synthesize progesterone from pregnenolone because it lacks 3β-ol-dehydrogenase, $\Delta^{4,5}$-isomerase activity (see Figures 47–3 and 49–1).

Progesterone quiets uterine muscle activity by inhibiting prostaglandin production and responsivity to oxytocin (see Chapter 45). This prevents premature expulsion of the fetus. Also, it stimulates mammary gland development and greatly enhances the eventual capacity to secrete milk. Finally, progesterone increases the rate of maternal ventilation, which is needed for removal of the increased load of CO_2 created by metabolism in the pregnant state.

The placenta begins to synthesize progesterone at about 6 weeks, and by 12 weeks, it produces enough to replace the corpus luteum source (Figure 51–6). Cholesterol extracted from maternal plasma serves as the major precursor for placental progesterone. The synthetic pathway is identical to that of the adrenal gland and ovary. By the end of pregnancy, placental progesterone production reaches a level that is 10-fold greater than peak production by the corpus luteum during the menstrual luteal phase.

Estrogens prepare maternal tissues for labor, delivery, lactation, and nursing

Progressive increases in **estradiol, estrone,** and **estriol** occur throughout pregnancy. These estrogens stimulate continuous growth of the uterine muscles necessary for labor. They foster relaxation and softening of the pelvic ligaments and junction of the pelvic bones; this allows better accommodation of the expanding uterus. In addition, estrogens

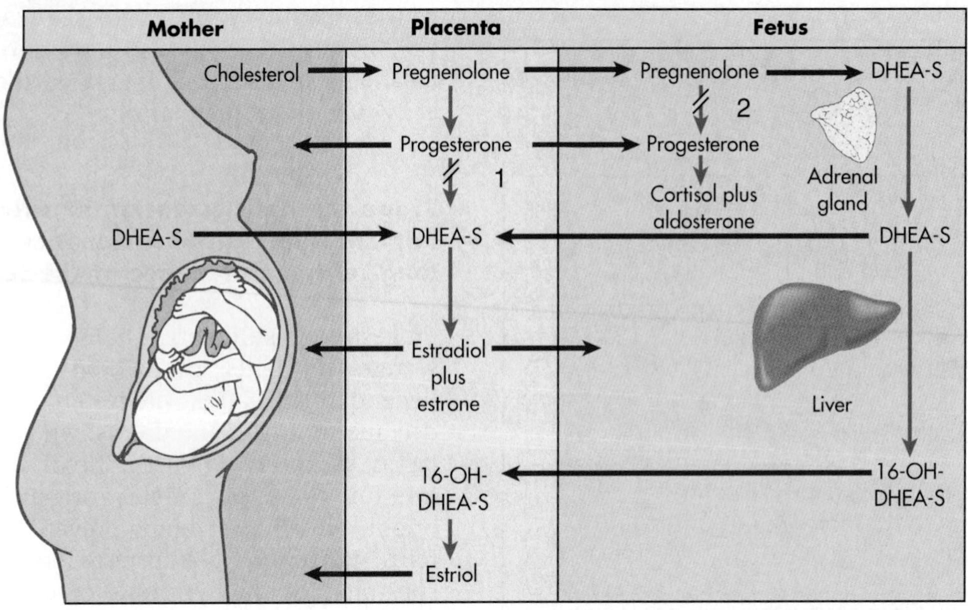

FIGURE 51–7. Maternal-fetal-placental unit in steroid hormone synthesis. Progesterone is synthesized in the placenta from maternal cholesterol. In turn, this progesterone acts on the mother and serves as the precursor to fetal adrenal cortisol and aldosterone synthesis. Estradiol and estrone are synthesized in the placenta from maternal and fetal adrenal DHEA-S and estriol from 16α-hydroxydehydroepiandrosterone sulfate (16-OH-DHEA-S), which is synthesized in the fetal liver. 1, 17-hydroxylase/17,20-desmolase; 2, 3β-ol-dehydrogenase, $\Delta^{4,5}$-isomerase.

augment growth of the ductal system of the breast to prepare it for lactation. Within the placenta, estradiol augments progesterone synthesis.

Estrogens are initially produced by the corpus luteum. The placenta subsequently assumes this role, but because it lacks 17-hydroxylase/17,20-desmolase activity, it cannot produce the necessary androgen precursors (see Figure 49–1). Therefore, the placenta requires androgen substrates from the maternal and fetal compartments (Figure 51–7). This exemplifies coordinated maternal-placental-fetal function. Thus, the placenta extracts DHEA-S derived from the maternal and fetal adrenal glands, removes the sulfate, and aromatizes the androgen to estradiol and estrone (Figure 51–7). In the case of **estriol,** the fetal liver must first 16-hydroxylate DHEA-S before the placenta can act on this precursor androgen (Figure 51–7). Estriol in the form of conjugates accounts for 90% of the estrogens in maternal urine.

Human chorionic somatomammotropin

A protein hormone unique to pregnancy is **human chorionic somatomammotropin (hCS),** also called **human placental lactogen.** Its structure is determined by a gene in the growth hormone (GH) family.

hCS synthesis by placental trophoblasts is regulated by GHRH and somatostatin from other trophoblasts and occurs within 4 weeks; maternal plasma hCS concentration rises steadily throughout pregnancy. The peak hCS production rate far exceeds that of any other human protein hormone. Although its growth-promoting activity is only a small fraction of that of GH, the high maternal plasma concentration of hCS makes it capable of contributing to anabolism in the mother. hCS stimulates lipolysis and is an insulin antagonist. Thus, hCS raises maternal free fatty acid and glucose levels. As discussed later, a major function of hCS is to direct maternal metabolism to shunt these substrates to the fetus. hCS may also contribute to fetal growth by stimulating synthesis of IGF-2 in the placenta (see Chapter 45).

Other placental hormones

The placenta produces hypothalamic- or pituitary-like peptides, including GnRH, TRH, CRH, GHRH, somatostatin, ACTH, and TSH. CRH levels, in particular, become very high in maternal plasma and peak during labor. In addition, a unique placental GH variant is synthesized and becomes the dominant GH in maternal plasma. Placental ACTH and TSH may augment maternal adrenal and thyroid gland activity, and placental GH acts on maternal target tissues. The placenta also synthesizes 1,25-dihydroxyvitamin D, which helps regulate Ca^{++} homeostasis and skeletal formation in the fetus (see Chapter 44). Maternal plasma inhibin levels reach an early peak within 7 days of conception. This source of inhibin A is mostly fetal trophoblasts, with some contribution from the corpus luteum in response to stimulation by hCG. A later steady rise in the inhibin A level to a peak at term represents placental production. In contrast, inhibin B levels remain low throughout pregnancy. The increased inhibin A level may suppress the mother's FSH secretion and unneeded ovarian follicle formation.

Both activin A and follistatin levels also increase steadily in maternal plasma. These hormones are derived from placental, decidual, and fetal membrane sources. Activin stimulates hCG and progesterone synthesis by the placenta, whereas follistatin interferes with this effect. The outcome of these interactions may depend on the time at which they occur and on countervailing influences from both mother and fetus.

Prolactin and relaxin are hormones of maternal origin

Prolactin maintains breast milk production and suppresses ovulation in the nursing mother

Prolactin secretion from the maternal pituitary gland increases greatly (Figure 51–6) in response to high maternal estrogen levels. The prolactin is in the nonglycosylated active form, and it specifically stimulates the lactogenic apparatus of the breast (see Chapter 45). During pregnancy, however, lactation itself is largely suppressed by the great excess of estrogen and progesterone. After delivery of the fetus, true milk synthesis is initiated by the precipitous drop in steroid hormone levels. Thereafter, milk synthesis is maintained in a nursing mother by prolactin and is facilitated by insulin and cortisol. Although basal prolactin concentrations gradually decline by 8 weeks after delivery, they are transiently elevated during each period of suckling. This helps sustain milk secretion.

Prolactin also suppresses reproductive function in the nursing mother. During the first 7 to 10 days after delivery, plasma FSH and LH levels remain low. FSH levels then rise, but LH levels do not; this pattern simulates that in early puberty. In the nursing mother, this pattern persists because of the inhibitory effects of prolactin on GnRH secretion. A decrease in circulating prolactin that follows the cessation of nursing triggers LH release and initiates a resumption of menstrual cycling.

Relaxin is a peptide hormone that is structurally similar to proinsulin

Relaxin is produced by the corpus luteum, decidua, and placenta under hCG stimulation. Maternal plasma relaxin levels rise to a peak in the first trimester and then decline somewhat. This hormone relaxes the mother's pelvic outlet and softens the cervix by increasing collagenase activity and decreasing tissue collagen content. Relaxin also decreases uterine muscle contractility by reducing the activity of myosin kinase. Thus, relaxin acts initially to maintain uterine quiescence and to prevent early abortion, but later it facilitates easier passage of the fetus into the birth canal once labor has begun.

The pregnant state induces changes in the function of all maternal endocrine glands

After the third month of pregnancy, maternal insulin secretion increases in response to glucose challenge or meals. It peaks during the last trimester and acts to compensate for the insulin resistance caused by hCS, placental GH, and cortisol.

Aldosterone secretion increases throughout pregnancy because of estrogen-induced augmentation of renin and angiotensinogen levels. The higher levels of angiotensin II stimulate the adrenal zona glomerulosa to increase aldosterone secretion (see Chapter 47). This induces a positive Na^+ balance, which is needed to support a high maternal plasma volume and to build the extracellular fluid of the fetus. Another mineralocorticoid, deoxycorticosterone (see Chapter 47), is synthesized by maternal kidneys during pregnancy, and it also contributes to Na^+ retention.

Total plasma thyroxine and cortisol levels are elevated because of estrogen-induced increases in their respective binding globulins. Levels of free thyroxine and triiodothyronine may be increased in the first trimester, and these necessary hormones may be transferred to the fetus and serve before the fetal thyroid begins to function. The level of plasma free cortisol also rises modestly, and this may contribute to maternal adipose tissue gain and to mammary gland development. The ultimate cause of maternal hypercortisolism is production by the placenta of high CRH levels that stimulate ACTH secretion from the maternal pituitary.

Parathyroid hormone secretion also increases. This hormone augments maternal plasma levels of 1,25-hydroxyvitamin D, which with 1,25-dihydroxyvitamin D, also produced by the placenta, in turn increases dietary Ca^{++} absorption, enhancing the maternal supply of Ca^{++} for the growing fetal skeleton (see Chapter 44).

Maternal FSH and LH secretion is suppressed by high concentrations of estrogen, progesterone, and prolactin and by inhibin A from the corpus luteum and placenta. Similarly, maternal pituitary GH secretion is decreased through negative feedback resulting from the actions of hCS and placental variant GH actions.

Maternal Metabolism Is Adapted to the Changing Needs of the Mother and Fetus

During pregnancy, the average gain in maternal weight is 11 kg. Approximately half of this can be attributed to changes in maternal tissues and half to the fetus and placenta. The mother must ingest approximately 300 extra kilocalories and 30 extra grams of protein daily to support fetal development and energy needs, to enlarge maternal energy stores, and to sustain growth of certain maternal tissues.

DURING THE FIRST HALF OF PREGNANCY, THE MOTHER IS IN AN ANABOLIC STATE, and the conceptus represents an insignificant nutritional drain. This phase is characterized by normal or even increased maternal sensitivity to insulin. Maternal plasma levels of glucose, free fatty acids, glycerol, and amino acids are normal or slightly decreased. Dietary carbohydrate and protein loads are rapidly used. Maternal lipogenesis is favored, glycogen stores are expanded, and protein synthesis is enhanced. These actions support the early growth of the breasts and uterus and prepare the mother to withstand the later metabolic demands of the enlarging fetus during maternal fasting periods.

DURING THE SECOND HALF OF PREGNANCY, THE MOTHER SHIFTS INTO A CATABOLIC STATE APTLY DESCRIBED AS "ACCELERATED STARVATION" (see Chapter 42). INSULIN SENSITIVITY IS REPLACED BY INSULIN RESISTANCE. This resistance causes elevation of postprandial plasma levels of glucose and amino acids as the uptake of dietary carbohydrate, protein, and fat by maternal tissues is reduced. Consequently, the diffusion of glucose and the facilitated transport of amino acids across the placenta into the fetus are accelerated. During maternal fasting intervals, plasma glucose and amino acid levels fall more rapidly than in nonpregnant women because the fetus continues to siphon off these substances. Maternal lipolysis is excessively stimulated, ensuring alternative oxidative fuels for the mother and even for the fetus, to whom keto acids and free fatty acids can be transferred across the placenta. hCS is a key hormone responsible for maternal insulin resistance and for lipid mobilization during fasting in this later stage of pregnancy. Elevated estrogen, progesterone, and cortisol levels also antagonize insulin action in the mother. Estrogens also stimulate hepatic production of very-low-density lipoproteins (see Chapter 42). The extra triglycerides are stored in breast tissue to be used later for milk production.

The insulin resistance of pregnancy, when it is added to an underlying vulnerability to diabetes, produces **gestational diabetes** in 4% of pregnancies. Hyperglycemia appears around week 24 to 28 of gestation, and this occurrence may have serious consequences for the fetus. Maternal hyperglycemia is transmitted to the fetus and stimulates fetal hyperinsulinemia; this causes heavier babies that are more difficult to deliver and a tendency toward hypoglycemia in the newborn infant. Immature lungs that lack surfactant can cause respiratory distress, and sudden death caused by heart muscle abnormalities may occur in utero, even near term.

Just as the Maintenance of the Pregnant State Depends on a Unique Hormonal Milieu, Its Termination Probably also Depends on Specific Hormonal Changes

In humans, the exact mechanism by which parturition, or the process of giving birth, is initiated remains uncertain. Cortisol, estrogen, progesterone, CRH, prostaglandins, oxytocin, catecholamines, and inflammatory cytokines may all participate in complex interrelationships that result in the initiation and maintenance of labor and in the final uterine evacuation. Because species variations exist, it is difficult to extrapolate data from animal studies directly to humans. **Figure 51–8** illustrates current concepts of the endocrine regulation of parturition.

Throughout pregnancy, the uterine myometrium exhibits long episodes of low-amplitude contractions referred to as **contractures.** These are perceived by the mother beginning at least 1 month before the end of gestation and are called **Braxton Hicks** contractions. They are uncoordinated and ineffective. Progesterone helps maintain this myometrial state of functional quiescence.

The onset of true labor has a circadian rhythm, with a peak between midnight and 5 AM, during which period the sensitivity of the myometrium to stimulation by prostaglandins and oxytocin is heightened and the secretion of maternal oxytocin peaks. Some signal from the fetus probably initiates labor contractions. In sheep, fetal cortisol has been strongly implicated as the signal. Although gestation is prolonged in women when the fetus lacks an intact hypothalamic-pituitary-adrenal unit, the evidence for a surge of fetal cortisol secretion immediately preceding human parturition is weak. However, a marked late gestational increase in fetal

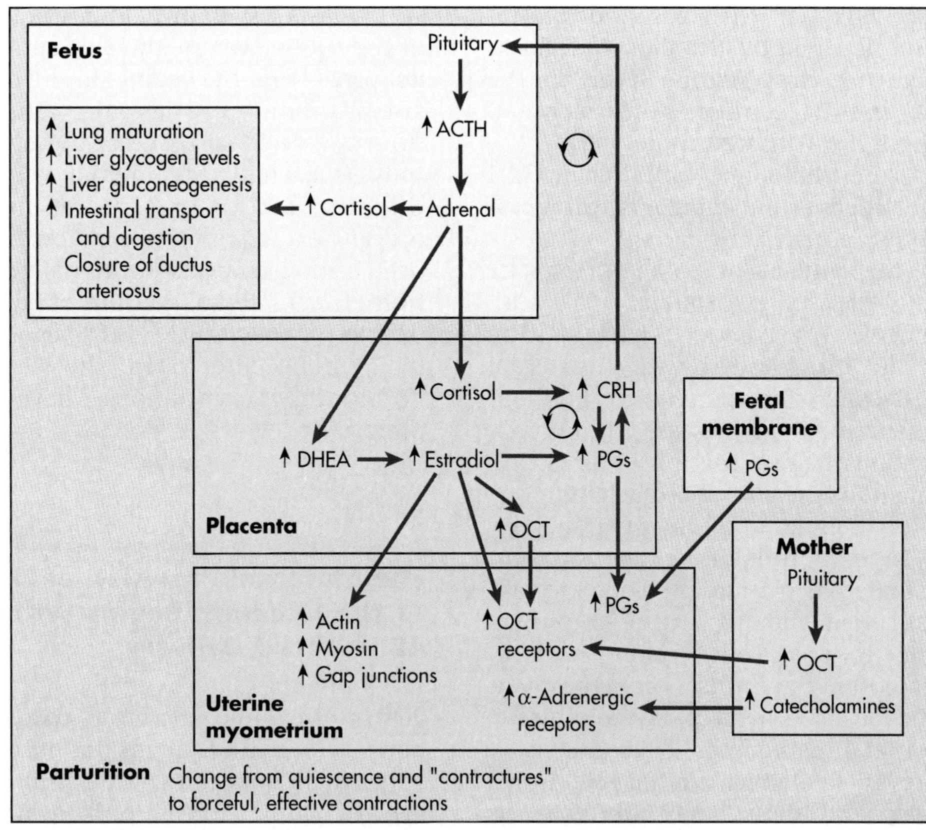

FIGURE 51–8. Endocrine regulation of parturition. A positive-feedback loop between cortisol and placental CRH production appears to initiate parturition. A rising fetal adrenal supply of dehydroepiandrosterone (DHEA) augments estradiol production. This leads to increased prostaglandin (PGs) levels, which are the main stimuli of uterine labor contractions. Oxytocin (OCT) produced locally in the placenta and decidua and a small maternal component coupled with increased myometrial oxytocin receptors may contribute to labor but are not essential. However, oxytocin sustains uterine contractions after expulsion of the fetus to minimize maternal loss of blood. Maternal catecholamines may add to the hormonal cascade stimulating contractions. Cortisol also prepares the fetus to maintain its own supply of O_2 and substrates after birth.

cortisol secretion is important to survival of the newborn (Figure 51–8).

CRH produced by the placenta stimulates the fetal pituitary to secrete ACTH, which in turn increases fetal cortisol and dehydroepiandrosterone (DHEA) production. The extra DHEA substrate fuels placental estradiol production (Figure 51–7), which is also increased by cortisol stimulation. In an unusual positive-feedback effect, the fetal cortisol also amplifies (rather than inhibits, as expected) placental CRH synthesis (see Chapter 47). This phenomenon generates a powerful momentum to increase both factors exponentially. The late rapid rise in CRH production is reflected by escalating levels of maternal plasma CRH.

A central and determinant role for CRH in the initiation of labor is supported by several other observations. CRH receptors are present in the myometrium, and CRH potentiates the contractile responses to both oxytocin and prostaglandins. In another positive-feedback loop, CRH and prostaglandins stimulate each other's production. Finally, an inverse correlation exists between maternal plasma CRH levels early in pregnancy and the absolute length of the gestational period. Higher CRH levels predict shorter gestational periods. Thus, a placental clock based on the inherent ability of the placenta to produce CRH may be set early in pregnancy; cortisol from the fetus may trigger a CRH "alarm" to start labor once the hormone reaches a high enough level in the uterus. Increased fetal cortisol levels also stimulate lung maturation, increase stores of liver glycogen, induce intestinal transport systems and digestive enzymes, and promote closure of the ductus arteriosus, all of which prepare the fetus for the abrupt transition to extrauterine life (Figure 51–8).

Late in pregnancy, increases in the secretion of estradiol by the placenta prepare the myometrium to contract in a forceful and coordinated manner by increasing the concentrations of contractile proteins, myosin and actin, as well as the gap junctions between fibers. Oxytocin receptors and prostaglandins are also increased by estradiol. A decrease in local effective free progesterone levels in the uterus may be an essential component to the overall process. Progesterone withdrawal augments the effects of increased estradiol and would favor CRH production. The progesterone antagonist **mifepristone** (RU-486) is a potent abortifacient.

A LARGE INCREASE IN THE LOCAL CONCENTRATION OF PROSTAGLANDINS INCREASES MYOMETRIAL CELL Ca^{++} LEVELS AND TRIGGERS UTERINE CONTRACTIONS. The prostaglandins are produced by the maternal uterine tissues (decidua) and the fetal chorion and amnion as evidenced by an increase in amniotic fluid prostaglandins before the onset of labor. Certain prostaglandins are also abortifacients.

Another major stimulator of myometrial contractions is **oxytocin.** Although the concentration of oxytocin in maternal plasma does not increase consistently just before labor, the frequency of oxytocin pulses does increase. Furthermore, myometrial oxytocin receptor content rises dramatically at term, as does the local synthesis of oxytocin by the decidua and the fetal membranes. Thus, maternal, placental, and even fetal oxytocin may reinforce labor contractions, and immediately after delivery, oxytocin probably maximizes the contractions that minimize maternal blood loss from the placental vessels. Uterine contractions can also be modulated by catecholamines; α adrenergy is stimulatory, and β adrenergy is inhibitory. Both estradiol and prostaglandins increase myometrial α-adrenergic receptors.

In addition to uterine contractions, the rapid changes that occur in placental and cervical tissue are also important components of labor. Progesterone maintains rigidity of the cervix by inhibiting the enzyme matrix metalloproteinase. At term, the decrease in progesterone action allows the enzyme to lyse the matrix and soften the cervix, making it more pliable. The concentrations of inflammatory cytokines, such as interleukin-6 and interleukin-8, rise sharply in amniotic fluid. These cytokines are produced by maternal decidua and fetal membranes, probably under hormonal paracrine stimulation. They attract neutrophils, which then release collagenase. This enzyme loosens the attachments between the maternal and fetal tissue planes and further decreases the cervical resistance to pressure from the fetal head.

Once labor has begun, it proceeds in three clinically recognized stages. In the first stage, which lasts several hours, the uterine contractions, which originate at the fundus and sweep downward, force the head of the fetus against the cervix. Under this pressure, the cervix progressively widens and thins the opening to the vaginal canal. In the second stage, which lasts less than 1 hour, the fetus is forced out of the uterine cavity and through the cervix and is delivered from the vagina. In the third stage, which lasts 10 minutes or less, the placenta is separated from the decidual tissue of the uterus and is forcefully evacuated. Myometrial contractions during this stage act to constrict the uterine vessels and prevent excessive bleeding. Once the placenta has been removed, all its hormonal products disappear from the maternal plasma at a rate determined by their characteristic half-lives. In general, by 48 to 72 hours after birth, the steroid and protein hormone concentrations have reached non-pregnancy levels.

The Maternal Provision of Nutrients to the Newborn Begins Within 48 Hours of Delivery

First, a thin fluid known as **colostrum** that contains lactose and proteins but little fat is secreted in very small quantities. True milk delivery follows shortly. Human breast milk contains 1% protein, largely as casein, lactalbumin, and lactoglobulin. In addition, it contains 7% lactose and 3.5% fat, equivalent to about 70 kcal/100 mL. By 1 week, 550 mL/day is produced; later, maximum amounts of up to 2000 mL/day may occur. Large quantities of Ca^{++} and Pi are also needed by and provided to the infant. Milk also contains immunoglobulins, which protect against infection. There are more than 160 other constituents, including many peptide hormones and growth factors, that are synthesized in the breast or actively transported from maternal plasma into the milk. In addition to supporting breast tissue and milk formation (cortisol and insulin, in particular), these may act directly on the infant's gastrointestinal tract or even be absorbed to act systemically. Typically, infants nurse for 6 to 12 months.

Mammary cells package proteins, lactose, Ca^{++}, and Pi in secretory vesicles and fat in droplets. Prolactin is essential to these processes (see Chapter 45). Immunoglobulins, combined with membrane receptors in vesicles, enter the cells. All these products are then secreted into the alveoli. Suckling and even anticipatory signals, such as the infant's cry, stimulate oxytocin release via neural sensory pathways and the central **nucleus tractus solitarius.** Oxytocin causes contraction of myoepithelial cells around the alveoli and smooth muscle cells in the duct walls. This "lets the milk down" into the areolar area, where the infant obtains it through holes in the nipple.

Summary

- In the ovary, oocytes that are suspended in the prophase of meiosis are secluded in primordial follicles. These follicles undergo slow, hormonally independent development to primary follicles, which are composed of nurturing, surrounding granulosa cells.
- Monthly cohorts of follicles are stimulated sequentially by FSH and LH to progress in development. From each cohort, a single dominant follicle emerges each month and grows exponentially.
- The dominant follicle produces enough estradiol and inhibin to inhibit its cohort follicles, to prepare reproductive organs for fertilization, and to condition the hypothalamus and pituitary gland to provide a timed surge of LH and FSH to cause ovulation.
- Estradiol production by the follicular granulosa cells depends on androgen substrate, which is provided by neighboring theca cells.
- The monthly cyclicity of ovulation is determined mainly by the ovary. A surge of LH and FSH secretion occurs when the dominant follicle secretes sufficient estradiol in an appropriate temporal pattern.
- After ovulation, the granulosa and theca cells form a corpus luteum. This endocrine structure secretes sufficient progesterone and estradiol to condition the reproductive organs so that they can receive and implant a zygote.
- Estradiol and progesterone in sequence and together induce cyclic changes in the structure and secretory function of the vagina, endometrium of the uterus, and fallopian tubes.
- Estrogens also have important actions on bone remodeling, the hepatic synthesis of proteins, and other systemic target tissues.
- After implantation of a conceptus, the placenta is formed from fetal trophoblasts, which initially secrete hCG that sustains the corpus luteum. Eventually, the placenta itself produces the important hormones of pregnancy, such as estrogens, progesterone, and a variety of proteins and peptides that resemble hypothalamic and pituitary hormones.
- Early in pregnancy, the mother is in a metabolic state that facilitates the growth of reproductive tissues and energy stores. Later, she becomes insulin resistant, which allows her to shunt substrates to the growing fetus.
- The endocrine mechanism of parturition is not yet completely defined. An increased ratio of estradiol to progesterone in uterine tissue augments the production of prostaglandins, which are the main stimulators of uterine contractions. Corticotropin-releasing hormone, as an initiator of labor, and oxytocin, as a stimulator of contractions during and immediately after labor ceases, also play important roles.

Bibliography

Apter D et al: Gonadotropin-releasing hormone pulse generator activity during pubertal transition in girls: pulsatile and diurnal patterns of circulating gonadotropins, *J Clin Endocrinol Metab* 76:940, 1993.

Dey SK et al: Molecular cues to implantation, *Endocr Rev* 25:341, 2004.

Erickson GF: Folliculogenesis, ovulation, and luteogenesis. In DeGroot LJ, Jameson JL, eds: *Endocrinology,* ed 4, Philadelphia, 2001, WB Saunders.

Gougeon A: Regulation of ovarian follicular development in primates: facts and hypotheses, *Endocr Rev* 17:121, 1996.

Gruber CJ et al: Production and actions of estrogens, *N Engl J Med* 346:340, 2002.

Hillier SG: Gonadotropic control of ovarian follicular growth and development, *Mol Cell Endocrinol* 179:39, 2001.

Hillier SG: Current concepts of the roles of follicle stimulating hormone and luteinizing hormone in folliculogenesis, *Hum Reprod* 9:188, 1994.

Hillier SG, Whitelaw PF, Smyth CD: Follicular oestrogen synthesis: the "two-cell, two-gonadotrophin" model revisited, *Mol Cell Endocrinol* 100:51, 1994.

Hsueh AJW, Billig H, Tsafriri A: Ovarian follicle atresia: a hormonally controlled apoptotic process, *Endocr Rev* 15:707, 1994.

Junquiera LC, Carneiro J, Kelley RO: The female reproductive system. In *Basic histology,* ed 9, Norwalk, Conn, 1999, Appleton & Lange.

Kelly RW: Pregnancy maintenance and parturition: the role of prostaglandin in manipulating the immune and inflammatory response, *Endocr Rev* 15:684, 1994.

Klein NA et al: Ovarian follicular concentrations of activin, follistatin, inhibin, insulin-like growth factor I (IGF-I), IGF-II, IGF-binding protein-2 (IGFBP-2), IGFBP-3, and vascular endothelial growth factor in spontaneous menstrual cycles of normal women of advanced reproductive age, *J Clin Endocrinol Metab* 85:4520, 2000.

Lessey BA, Arnold JT: Paracrine signaling in the endometrium: integrins and the establishment of uterine receptivity, *J Reprod Immun* 39:105, 1998.

Lorenzo J: A new hypothesis for how sex steroid hormones regulate bone mass, *J Clin Invest* 111:1641, 2003.

Marshall JC: Hormonal regulation of the menstrual cycle and mechanisms of ovulation. In DeGroot LJ, Jameson JL, eds: *Endocrinology,* ed 4, Philadelphia, 2001, WB Saunders.

McLean M et al: A placental clock controlling the length of human pregnancy, *Nat Med* 1:460, 1995.

Neville MC, Morton J: Physiology and endocrine changes underlying human lactogenesis II, *J Nutr* 131:3005S, 2001.

Nilson S et al: Mechanisms of estrogen action, *Physiol Rev* 81:1535, 2001.

Olson DM, Mijovic JE, Sadowsky DW: Control of human parturition, *Semin Perinatol* 19:52, 1995.

Richards JS et al: Ovulation: new dimensions and new regulators of the inflammatory-like response, *Annu Rev Physiol* 64:69, 2002.

Seppälä M et al: Glycodelin: a major lipocalin protein of the reproductive axis with diverse actions in cell recognition and differentiation, *Endocr Rev* 23:401, 2002.

Simpson ER et al: Aromatase—a brief overview, *Annu Rev Physiol* 64:93, 2002.

Stern K, McClintock MK: Regulation of ovulation by human pheromones, *Nature* 392:177, 1998.

Weiss G: Clinical review 118: endocrinology of parturition, *J Clin Endocrinol Metab* 85:4421, 2000.

White MM et al: Estrogen, progesterone, and vascular reactivity: potential cellular mechanisms, *Endocr Rev* 16:739, 1995.

Yeh J, Adashi EY: The ovarian life cycle. In Yen SSC, Jaffe RB, Barbieri RL, eds: *Reproductive endocrinology,* ed 4, Philadelphia, 1999, WB Saunders.

Yen SSC: The human menstrual cycle: neuroendocrine regulation. In Yen SSC, Jaffe RB, Barbieri RL, eds: *Reproductive endocrinology,* ed 4, Philadelphia, 1999, WB Saunders.

Case Studies

Case 51–1

A 28-year-old healthy woman with regular menstrual cycles since the age of 12 years was a passenger on a bus that overturned and submerged in a lake. She was uninjured but was one of only four passengers who escaped death by drowning. Her menses ceased completely in the ensuing year, during which she had frequent recurring nightmares about the accident.

1. **Which of the following most likely mediates her amenorrhea?**
   A. Increased CRH secretion
   B. Decreased prolactin secretion
   C. Decreased dopamine secretion
   D. Decreased endorphin secretion
   E. Increased norepinephrine levels

2. **Which of the following findings would be expected in this estrogen-deficient patient?**
   A. Hyperplasia of the endometrium
   B. Cornification of the vaginal epithelium
   C. Profuse secretion of an elastic cervical mucus
   D. Decreased libido
   E. Decreased breast mass

Case 51–2

A 30-year-old married woman consults her physician for infertility. She has regular menstrual cycles. Daily home urine LH measurement shows a midcycle surge in LH secretion, and intercourse has been appropriately timed thereby. Her husband's sperm count and analysis are normal. Findings of her physical examination are entirely normal.

1. **Which of the following is the most likely cause of her infertility?**
   A. Progesterone excess
   B. Inhibin A excess
   C. Failure to form an adequately functioning corpus luteum
   D. Failure to develop a dominant follicle
   E. Estradiol deficiency

2. **Which of the following findings would confirm the diagnosis?**
   A. Low plasma estradiol on day 28 of her cycle
   B. Low plasma estrone on day 1 of her cycle
   C. High plasma prolactin on day 14 of her cycle
   D. Low plasma progesterone on day 21 of her cycle
   E. Low plasma progesterone on day 7 of her cycle

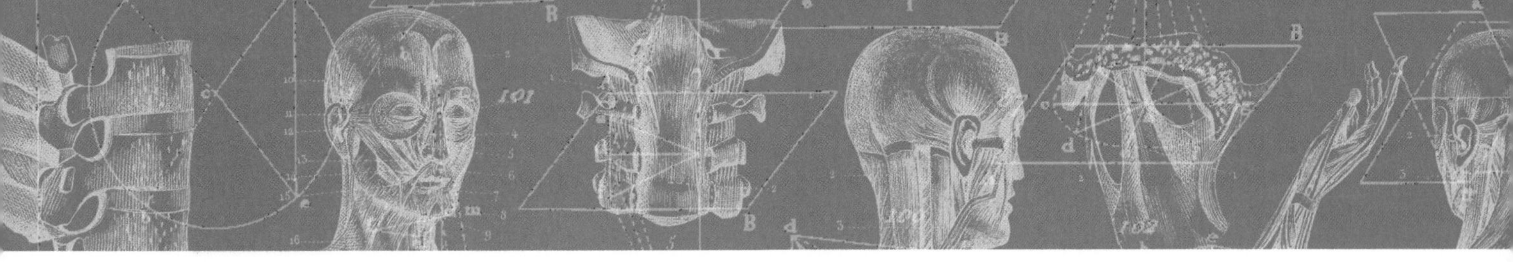

Answers to Case Studies

Self-Assessment 1

1. A is incorrect because the rate of diffusion is directly proportional to the diffusion coefficient.
   B *is correct because the time required for the average molecule to diffuse a given distance is proportional to the square of distance.*
   C is incorrect because diffusion is rapid on a scale of micrometers or smaller.
   D is incorrect because many cells are small enough for diffusion to suffice for intracellular transport.
2. A is incorrect because the smaller the molecular weight (MW) of X, the faster its diffusion.
   B *is correct because molecules that are soluble in nonpolar (hydrophobic) solvents, due to greater solubility in membrane lipids, diffuse more rapidly across membranes.*
   C is incorrect because the diffusion of water across membranes is relatively rapid.
   D is incorrect because membranes are relatively impermeable to water-soluble molecules with MW = 400.
3. A is incorrect because an ideal semipermeable membrane is impermeable to all solutes.
   B *is correct because water does flow from where osmotic pressure is lower to where osmotic pressure is higher.*
   C is incorrect because the more concentrated the solution, the less accurate is van't Hoff's law.
   D is incorrect because the osmotic pressure of a solution is proportional to its boiling point elevation.
4. A is incorrect because transport via a transporter is faster than by diffusion.
   B *is correct because transport proteins do have chemical specificity.*
   C is incorrect because ion channels, but not transporters, spontaneously alternate between rapidly and slowly transporting states.
   D is incorrect because for transporters, the transport rate saturates at high concentrations of the transport substrate.
5. A *is correct because the Na^+,K^+-ATPase derives its energy directly from ATP.*
   B is incorrect because the Na^+-glucose symporter is a secondary active transporter.
   C is incorrect because the Na^+-H^+ antiporter is a secondary active transporter.
   D is incorrect because the $3Na^+$-$1Ca^{++}$ antiporter is a secondary active transporter.

Self-Assessment 2

1. A is incorrect because both the concentration and the electrical forces tend to make Cl^- flow from A to B.
   B is incorrect because K^+ would be in equilibrium only when the membrane potential (A minus B) is equal to –60 mV.
   C *is correct because the electrical force moving K^+ from B to A is larger than the concentration force tending to make K^+ flow from A to B.*
   D is incorrect because K^+ tends to flow from B to A as explained in answer C.
2. A is incorrect because the impermeant ion has negative charge, so that the [Li^+] in the cell

will be greater than that in the extracellular fluid.

B is incorrect. Since the impermeant ion has negative charge, the [Cl^-] in the extracellular fluid will be greater than that in the cell.

C *is correct because the sum of [Li^+] and [Cl^-] is greater in the cell than in the extracellular fluid. This is a property of Gibbs-Donnan equilibria.*

D is incorrect. Since these ions are in Gibbs-Donnan equilibrium, the product of [Li^+] and [Cl^-] in the cell is equal to that in the extracellular fluid.

3. **A** is incorrect because the membrane is impermeable to K^+.

B *is correct because the equilibrium potential for Cl^- is +60 mV.*

C is incorrect because an infinitesimal amount of Cl^- will flow from A to B.

D is incorrect because only the permeant ion, Cl^-, will attain equilibrium.

4. **A** *is correct because the membrane potential causing Cl^- to leave the cell is smaller in magnitude than E_{Cl}.*

B is incorrect because the membrane potential tending to hold K^+ in the cell is smaller in magnitude than E_K.

C is incorrect since both forces on Na^+ tend to make it flow into the cell.

D is incorrect since Cl^- is the ion closest to equilibrium.

5. **A** is incorrect because if the conductances (g's) for Na^+, K^+, and Cl^- are equal, the membrane potential would be equal to the average of E_{Na}, E_K, and E_{Cl} (about –40 mV).

B *is correct because if the only ion with significant conductance is K^+, then $E_m = E_K =$ –92.6 mV.*

C is incorrect because if Na^+ is the only permeant ion, then $E_m = E_{Na} = +64.8$ mV.

D is incorrect because if g_{Cl} is 0 and $g_{Na} = g_K$, then E_m will be the average of E_{Na} and E_K (–13.9 mV).

Self-Assessment 3

1. **A** is incorrect because the rising phase of the action potential is due to a rapid increase in the Na^+ conductance.

B is incorrect because the peak of the action potential never reaches the equilibrium potential for Na^+.

C is incorrect because the repolarizing phase is due to closing of Na^+ channels and the delayed opening of K^+ channels.

D *is correct because the hyperpolarizing afterpotential is due to the prolonged increased conductance to K^+.*

2. **A** *is correct because voltage-gated Na^+ channels first activate but then inactivate in response to depolarization of the membrane.*

B is incorrect because K^+ channels in neurons open more slowly than do Na^+ channels after a depolarization.

C is incorrect because the plateau phase of the cardiac action potential is due predominantly to Ca^{++} channels that open and close slowly.

D is incorrect because ion channels open and close randomly.

3. **A** is incorrect because the absolute refractory period is due primarily to voltage inactivation of Na^+ channels.

B *is correct because if a neuron is depolarized very slowly, it may reach threshold without firing an action potential.*

C is incorrect because early in the relative refractory period, the cell can fire an action potential in response to a stronger than normal stimulus.

D is incorrect because during the early part of the relative refractory period, elevated conductance to K^+ and inactivation of Na^+ channels both contribute to refractoriness.

4. **A** is incorrect because a subthreshold depolarization will not elicit an action potential.

B *is correct because action potentials are conducted by electrotonic conduction.*

C is incorrect because the length constant is the length over which an electrotonically conducted signal loses 63% of its strength.

D is incorrect because decreasing the membrane resistance will decrease the length constant.

5. **A** is incorrect because myelination greatly increases membrane resistance.

B is incorrect. By confining membrane potential generation to the nodes, saltatory conduction results in greatly decreased use of energy.

C *is correct. Due to myelination and the concentration of ion channels at the nodes of Ranvier, only the nodal membrane can initiate an action potential.*

D is incorrect because the length constant of a myelinated fiber is much greater than that of an unmyelinated fiber of the same diameter.

Self-Assessment 4

1. A is incorrect because opening of voltage-gated Ca^{++} channels (not Mg^{++} channels) in the nerve terminal triggers exocytotic release of ACh.
   B is incorrect because ACh does not bind appreciably to membrane lipids.
   C is incorrect because the action potential is generated by the voltage-gated Na^+ and K^+ channels of the nonjunctional muscle membrane.
   D *is correct because reuptake of about 50% of the choline released into the junctional cleft is mediated by a secondary active transporter in the nerve terminal.*
2. A *is correct because the channel opened by ACh is roughly equally conductive to Na^+ and K^+.*
   B is incorrect because in the presence of an inhibitor of cholinesterase, the EPP will be larger in amplitude than in the absence of the inhibitor.
   C is incorrect because in health, the EPP always elicits an action potential in the muscle cell.
   D is incorrect. Because of lower numbers of ACh receptors in myasthenia gravis, EPPs may be smaller in amplitude.
3. A is incorrect because ACh is bound to the α subunit of AChR.
   B is incorrect because AChR is gated by ACh.
   C *is correct because AChR are much more concentrated in the postjunctional membrane than in the rest of the muscle cell plasma membrane.*
   D is incorrect because AChR are reduced in number, but not absent, in myasthenia gravis.
4. A is incorrect because an IPSP is a transient hyperpolarization of a postsynaptic cell.
   B *is correct. This phenomenon is called facilitation.*
   C is incorrect because most IPSPs are caused by increased Cl^- conductance of the postsynaptic cell.
   D is incorrect because EPSPs are caused by increased Na^+ and K^+ conductance of the postsynaptic cell.
5. A is incorrect because nitric oxide is unstable and persists only for seconds.
   B is incorrect because GABA is the most common inhibitory transmitter in the brain.
   C is incorrect because glutamate is an important excitatory transmitter.
   D *is correct because many neuropeptides are present in the brain and in the gastrointestinal system, which contains a great many neurons.*

Self-Assessment 5

1. A is incorrect because activation involves binding GTP.
   B is incorrect because interaction with an agonist-bearing receptor promotes activation of a G protein.
   C is incorrect because activation occurs when GTP is bound.
   D *is correct because, on activation, the α subunit tends to separate from βγ.*
2. A *is correct because activation of G_q increases the activity of phospholipase Cβ.*
   B is incorrect because cleavage of phosphatidylinositol bisphosphate produces InsP3 and diacylglycerol.
   C is incorrect because protein kinase C is stimulated at the plasma membrane by diacylglycerol.
   D is incorrect because InsP3 causes release of Ca^{++} from the endoplasmic reticulum.
3. A is incorrect because acetylcholine binding to muscarinic receptors leads to opening of K^+ channels.
   B *is correct because the action of acetylcholine on K^+ channels is mediated by βγ subunits.*
   C is incorrect because cGMP-gated Na^+ channels in rod cells are closed by light.
   D is incorrect because cAMP-activated Na^+ channels in olfactory cells are opened by odorants.
4. A is incorrect because protein kinase A is activated when regulatory subunits are released.
   B is incorrect because calmodulin-dependent protein kinases are activated by calmodulin with bound Ca^{++}.
   C is incorrect because no isoforms of protein kinase C are activated by cholesterol.
   D *is correct because phosphorylation of a myosin light chain by myosin light-chain kinase promotes contraction of smooth muscle.*
5. A is not correct because protein-tyrosine kinases have single transmembrane α helices.
   B is incorrect because protein kinases couple binding of growth factors to cellular responses.
   C *is correct because the MAP kinase cascade is involved in numerous pathways initiated by receptor protein-tyrosine kinases.*

D is incorrect because mutated forms of Ras promote uncontrolled growth of cells.

Case 6–1

1. A is incorrect because the motor deficit is uncharacteristic for this disease.
   B is incorrect because a brain tumor was not revealed in the magnetic resonance imaging study and microorganisms were found in the CSF.
   C is incorrect because encephalitis would not generally be associated with markedly dilated ventricles, and it would have a more acute course.
   D *is correct because the hydrocephalus is due to obstruction of the ventricles as a result of cryptococcal meningitis.*
   E is incorrect because the results of the blood chemistry tests were normal.
2. A is incorrect because the magnetic resonance image would show distention of the subarachnoid space, and cryptococcal meningitis is more likely to affect the base of the brain.
   B is incorrect because if the cerebral aqueduct were occluded, only the lateral and third ventricles would be dilated.
   C is incorrect because if one interventricular foramen were blocked, only one lateral ventricle would be distended.
   D *is correct because the roof of the fourth ventricle can be occluded by meningitis at the base of the brain.*
   E is incorrect because obstruction of the third ventricle would result in distention of only the lateral ventricles and the interventricular foramina.

Case 6–2

1. A is incorrect because astrocytes affect nerve impulse activity only indirectly.
   B is incorrect because the patient has disruption of sensation (vision, hearing) as well as motor difficulties, and the motor disorders included interruption of the voluntary motor pathways; for example, the stretch reflexes were increased on one side, whereas diseases of motor neurons result in reduced stretch reflexes.
   C *is correct because oligodendroglia provide myelin sheaths for CNS axons, and demyelinating diseases that affect these cells disrupt function by slowing or interrupting nerve impulse conduction.*
   D is incorrect because the function of these neurons on one side was temporarily affected secondarily to the disorder of oligodendroglial cells that provided the myelin sheaths for pyramidal cell axons.
   E is incorrect because Schwann cells myelinate axons in the PNS, whereas the disorder in this patient affected the CNS.
2. A is incorrect because there are no known diseases that cause localized and changeable disorders of axonal transport.
   B *is correct because the disorder, multiple sclerosis, affects localized groups of oligodendroglial cells, resulting in demyelination of axons of neurons in a particular location and therefore having a particular function. Remissions often occur as the oligodendroglial cells recover and remyelinate axons.*
   C is incorrect because chromatolysis results from transection of axons, which could not occur in a disease in which symptoms recover in as short a time as a few weeks; the interruption of axons in the CNS usually results in a permanent impairment because of the limited capability of CNS axons to regenerate.
   D is incorrect because no disorders are known that result in localized and migratory failures of synaptic transmission in different neural systems.
   E is incorrect for the same reasons that are discussed in answer C.

Case 7–1

1. A is incorrect because such a lesion might interrupt the medial lemniscus and pyramid, causing some of the symptoms, but the spinothalamic tract would be unaffected, and chronic pain would not be expected.
   B is incorrect because it would be unlikely for a cortical lesion to involve both the arm and the leg, since these are supplied by different cerebral arteries.
   C is incorrect because peripheral polyneuropathies are symmetrical and would not be restricted to one side.
   D *is correct because the somatosensory loss can result from a lesion affecting the VPL nucleus.*

The motor deficit could be caused by extension of the lesion into the internal capsule. A thalamic pain syndrome can result from a lesion of the VPL nucleus.

E is incorrect because a hemisection of the spinal cord above C5 on the right would result in a loss of fine tactile discrimination on the right and of pain and temperature sensation on the left.

2. A is incorrect because if these ascending projections of the reticular formation were interrupted, the patient would be comatose.

B is incorrect because the pain in patients who have the thalamic syndrome is very real and can lead to suicide.

C *is correct because the spinothalamic input to the VPL nucleus is largely interrupted, but plastic changes are known to occur in denervated cortical circuits.*

D is incorrect because mechanoreceptors do not convert to nociceptors, although their activation can trigger discharges in wide-dynamic-range nociceptive neurons in the CNS.

E is incorrect because nociceptive neurons would not stop responding to pinprick, although they might well develop more spontaneous activity and discharge more vigorously to tactile stimuli after injury to the nervous system.

Case 7–2

1. A is incorrect because morphine is unlikely to reach the periaqueductal gray.

B *is correct because there are opiate receptors in the spinal cord dorsal horn, and their activation will reduce nociceptive transmission.*

C is incorrect because there is no evidence that morphine would act on cancer cells in the pelvic region, preventing these cells from inducing pain.

D is incorrect because nociceptors in the meninges are unlikely to be responsible for the pain, unless metastases have reached the spinal cord; even in this case, morphine would not act like a local anesthetic to block their activity.

E is incorrect because when morphine reaches the spinal cord, it will diminish the release of substance P from the terminals of nociceptors in the dorsal horn.

2. A is incorrect because morphine could cause respiratory depression if it reached the medulla.

B is incorrect because the local infusion of morphine may cause itching sensations.

C is incorrect because tolerance to morphine may develop.

D is incorrect because morphine will block only some types of pain.

E *is correct because morphine will block only pain, whereas a local anesthetic will block all types of somatosensory sensations.*

Case 8–1

1. A is incorrect because this visual field defect involves a loss of vision in the temporal half of the visual field in each eye.

B is incorrect because a scotoma implies an area of visual loss that corresponds to an area within the visual field of one eye.

C *is correct because homonymous means that the visual field loss is in the corresponding region in both eyes (e.g., on the left or on the right in both eyes). Hemianopia means "half-blindness," so the loss is in half of each visual field. Macular sparing means that vision in the central parts of the visual fields is relatively spared.*

D is incorrect because this visual field defect is a loss of vision in the lower quadrants in the two eyes. Homonymous means that the loss is in the corresponding quadrants (e.g., both left or right quadrants).

E is incorrect because the loss is in the upper right or upper left quadrant in both eyes.

2. A is incorrect because this artery supplies the medial parts of the frontal and parietal lobes and has nothing to do with vision.

B is incorrect because although it does supply the optic tract, a lesion of the optic tract would probably produce homonymous hemianopia without macular sparing. In addition, this artery supplies structures belonging to the motor system that are not impaired in this patient.

C is incorrect because one of the branches of the internal carotid is the ophthalmic artery, which supplies the retina. Occlusion of the blood flow in the ophthalmic artery would cause blindness in one eye.

D is incorrect because interruption of the middle cerebral artery on the left side might produce a homonymous hemianopia without macular sparing by interrupting the optic radiation, but it would also cause motor and somatosensory impairments and a language disorder.

E *is correct because it supplies the striate cortex. Macular sparing can result if there is enough collateral circulation (e.g., from the middle cerebral artery).*

3. A is incorrect because destruction of a lateral geniculate nucleus would produce a homonymous hemianopia without macular sparing.

   B *is correct. Macular sparing can occur because of the large representation of the macula in the cortex near the occipital pole and the possibility of collateral circulation from branches of the middle cerebral artery.*

   C is incorrect because a lesion of the optic chiasm would produce a bitemporal hemianopia. This would happen only if the crossing fibers from the nasal hemiretina were interrupted. This is unlikely with a vascular lesion but can occur in cases of pituitary tumor.

   D is incorrect because a lesion of the optic tract is likely to result in homonymous hemianopia without macular sparing.

   E is incorrect because a lesion within the retina would cause a scotoma.

Case 8–2

1. A is incorrect because with a conduction deficit, the Rinne tests would be expected to show that bone conduction is better than air conduction.

   B is incorrect because the boy can hear, although his hearing is impaired.

   C is incorrect because in this case, the sound should have been localized to the impaired side in Weber's test, and bone conduction should have been better than air conduction on that side.

   D *is correct. Weber's test is inconclusive because the hearing loss is symmetrical. The Rinne tests show the normal relationship of air to bone conduction. Audiometry shows a severe hearing loss that includes part of the region important in understanding spoken language.*

   E is incorrect because in this case, sound should have been localized to the left side in Weber's test.

2. A is incorrect because deafness is generally not associated with a cortical lesion, although problems with language are.

   B is incorrect because although damage to both cochlear nerves would result in a similar pattern of sensorineural deafness, the history of listening to loud music suggests another cause.

   C *is correct because the loud music has evidently resulted in damage to hair cells as a result of excessive deflections of the basilar membrane in the region corresponding to the range of hearing loss detected by audiometry.*

   D is incorrect because such a disruption would result in a conduction deficit.

   E is incorrect because a problem with the tympanic membrane would also cause conduction deafness.

Case 9–1

1. A is incorrect because disorders of the basal ganglia do not produce weakness or hyperactive stretch reflexes.

   B is incorrect because cerebellar disorders are likely to reduce muscle tone and stretch reflexes.

   C *is correct because the corticospinal, corticobulbar, and corticoreticulospinal pathways as well as the thalamocortical projections from the somatosensory thalamus could all be interrupted by a lesion of the internal capsule.*

   D is incorrect because the face, arm, and leg areas of the precentral and postcentral gyri would probably not all be damaged in a stroke that left the patient able to function relatively well. The cerebral arterial blood supply of the leg area differs from that of the arm and face areas.

   E is incorrect because although a high cervical lesion of the spinal cord could cause spastic paralysis of the arm and leg and interrupt transmission of somatic sensations in the dorsal column, no paralysis or sensory loss would occur in the head.

2. A is incorrect because Babinski's sign indicates that the lateral corticospinal tract has been interrupted; however, this sign can be elicited whether or not the paralysis is of the spastic type.

   B *is correct because spasticity is characterized by hyperactive stretch reflexes.*

   C is incorrect because sensory loss is independent of the presence or absence of spasticity.

   D is incorrect because the tongue can be weak from either interruption of the corticobulbar tract or a lesion of the hypoglossal nucleus or nerve.

E is incorrect because weakness can be present without spasticity.

Case 9–2

1. A *is correct because individuals with Parkinson's disease have lost many of the dopaminergic neurons in the substantia nigra, and so dopamine levels in the striatum are reduced. The result is a motor disorder with the characteristics seen in the case.*
   B is incorrect because damage to the corticoreticulospinal inhibitory pathway contributes to spasticity.
   C is incorrect because a lesion of these nuclei will result in cerebellar signs, such as ataxia.
   D is incorrect because a lesion in the primary motor cortex will cause weakness and also Babinski's sign if the leg area is affected.
   E is incorrect because a lesion in the supplementary motor cortex may interfere with motor performance, but it will not produce Parkinson's disease.
2. A *is correct because the main problem is the reduction in the number of dopaminergic neurons in the substantia nigra. Replacement of the dopamine by L-dopa can be an effective therapy, at least in the early stages of Parkinson's disease, because it can cross the blood-brain barrier before it is used for dopamine synthesis.*
   B is incorrect because epinephrine will not cross the blood-brain barrier, nor would it react effectively with dopamine receptors if it did enter the basal ganglia.
   C is incorrect because this inhibitory neurotransmitter will not cross the blood-brain barrier.
   D is incorrect. Glutamate is used in many excitatory synapses in the brain, including in the basal ganglia. If it crossed the blood-brain barrier, it would have generalized effects.
   E is incorrect because substance P would be broken down in the blood by peptidases.

Case 10–1

1. A is incorrect because the ascending pathways from the spinal cord are interrupted, as is the hypothalamospinal tract.
   B is incorrect because the bladder may become excessively distended in the spinal shock phase of spinal cord injury, but it becomes spastic in the chronic phase. No pain can be felt in either phase.
   C is incorrect because the main concern with bacterial infection is hypotension and shock if bacterial products reach the systemic circulation.
   D is incorrect because the target organs of sympathetic postganglionic neurons have not been denervated, so there should be no change in postsynaptic receptors in the target organs.
   E *is correct because both autonomic and somatic reflexes become exaggerated after spinal cord transection.*
2. A *is correct because the hypothalamus is disconnected from the spinal cord autonomic centers.*
   B is incorrect. Although relatively vasodilated because of loss of central autonomic drive, the patient will not be able to lose heat via increased vasodilation and sweating in response to a hot environment.
   C is incorrect because the patient would not be able to shiver effectively.
   D is incorrect because the thermoreceptors would presumably react to thermal stimuli in a normal fashion, but in any event, the hypothalamic signals that mediate thermoregulation are impaired.
   E is incorrect because hypothalamic regulation in either direction is prevented by the spinal cord transection.

Case 11–1

1. A is incorrect because interruption of the corpus callosum will produce problems other than a language disorder.
   B *is correct because Broca's area has been damaged, which leads to an expressive aphasia.*
   C is incorrect because in most people, Broca's area is in the left hemisphere.
   D is incorrect because this region of the superior temporal gyrus is part of Wernicke's area, and damage here would result in a receptive aphasia.
   E is incorrect because damage to this region does not result in expressive aphasia.
2. A *is correct because language functions of all types, not just speech, would be impaired.*
   B is incorrect because this type of tremor would be expected from a cerebellar lesion.
   C is incorrect because this would involve the right hemisphere.

D is incorrect because unilateral deafness is usually due to a conduction deficit or to a sensorineural deficit involving the cochlea, cochlear nerve, or cochlear nuclei, not a brainstem or cortical lesion.

E is incorrect because the motor deficit would be on the right; the patient could have Babinski's sign on the right if projections from the leg representation are interrupted in the internal capsule.

Case 12–1

1. A is incorrect because many conditions besides muscular dystrophy can cause necrosis of skeletal muscle and hence the release of skeletal muscle proteins into the serum. Injury of skeletal muscle could also release these proteins into the serum.
   B *is correct since injury or necrosis of skeletal muscle usually results in disruption of the sarcolemma of the skeletal muscle cell and hence the release of intracellular (soluble) skeletal muscle proteins into the serum.*
   C is incorrect. Skeletal muscle proteins are usually not secreted into the serum.
   D is incorrect. Exercise does not usually result in injury of skeletal muscle cells.
   E is incorrect because atrophy indicates a decrease in size of the muscle cell and does not involve a disruption of the sarcolemma.
2. A *is correct because the defective gene is X-linked and recessive. That is, for a female to develop Duchenne's muscular dystrophy, both parents must contain the defective gene; but given the severe muscle wasting by the age of 12 years and lethality in adolescence and early adulthood, few adult men with Duchenne's muscular dystrophy procreate. Consequently, the disease is typically passed down generations by heterozygous females mating with normal males, resulting in some male children who have the defective gene and thus develop Duchenne's muscular dystrophy and some females who are heterozygous for the mutant gene (but do not show evidence of the disease).*
   B is incorrect.
   C is incorrect. Dystrophin appears to contribute to the cytoskeleton within skeletal muscles and may be important for intracellular signaling cascades, independent of gender.
   D is incorrect. Dystrophin deficiency usually becomes manifest in childhood.
   E is incorrect.
3. A is incorrect. Muscle wasting associated with Duchenne's muscular dystrophy occurs in childhood, at a time when there is little if any skeletal muscle proliferation.
   B is incorrect. Muscle wasting associated with Duchenne's muscular dystrophy involves necrosis and death of muscle cells, which is distinct from the reversible changes in muscle size due to hypertrophy or atrophy.
   C *is correct. Dystrophin is located on the cytoplasmic surface of the sarcolemma and contributes to the structural integrity of the cell. Deficiencies in dystrophin increase the likelihood of rupture of the sarcolemma and hence death of the muscle cell.*
   D is incorrect. Although inadequate O_2 supply could lead to muscle weakness, cramping, and in extreme cases necrosis, the muscle wasting associated with Duchenne's muscular dystrophy is linked to a deficiency of the structural protein dystrophin (not tissue oxygenation).
   E is incorrect.

Case 12–2

1. A is incorrect. This is not pertinent to malignant hyperthermia but represents a viable means of promoting contraction (e.g., with tetanus toxin).
   B is incorrect. This is also not pertinent to malignant hyperthermia but represents another mechanism of promoting contraction (e.g., with some nerve gases).
   C is incorrect since contraction of skeletal muscle does not require Ca^{++} influx through the sarcolemma.
   D *is correct. Malignant hyperthermia is a genetic disorder characterized by mutations within the skeletal muscle SR* Ca^{++} *channel that increase SR* Ca^{++} *release (particularly in the presence of muscle relaxants and volatile anesthetics). In this case study, the muscle relaxants facilitated opening of the SR* Ca^{++} *channel, resulting in an increased cytosolic* $[Ca^{++}]$ *and thereby promoting massive contractions.*
   E is incorrect. An increase in Ca^{++} sensitivity of the thin filaments could promote or increase contraction but is not pertinent to malignant hyperthermia.
2. A *is correct. The heat produced by ATP hydrolysis during muscle contraction is significant.*
   B is incorrect. The heat produced by ATP hydrolysis during SR Ca^{++} reaccumulation is small.

C is incorrect. The overall efficiency of energy transfer to ATP by glycolysis/oxidative phosphorylation is approximately 65%, indicating that only a third of the energy is lost (as heat) during the synthesis of ATP.

D is incorrect because heat dissipation did not decrease.

E is incorrect. Ca^{++} influx through the sarcolemma is minimal in skeletal muscle and follows an electrochemical gradient. Consequently, any small amount of Ca^{++} influx would occur by diffusion and thus not require ATP.

Case 13–1

1. A is incorrect because training does not alter the organization of the sarcomere.

   B is incorrect. Changes in ATP production by mitochondria do not alter sarcomeric structure. Moreover, one would expect an athlete to have a high oxidative capacity, not decreased ATP production.

   C is incorrect.

   D is incorrect since a myocardial infarction results in the death of cells, and the development of scar tissue, rather than a reorganization of the sarcomere.

   E *is correct and refers to a special form of cardiac hypertrophy induced by a mutant muscle protein (e.g., myosin). Specifically, transgenic studies have shown that expression of only a small amount of mutant myosin in heart muscle can induce hypertrophy of cardiac muscle cells, with a concomitant disarray of the sarcomere, and abnormal electrophysiological characteristics. This phenomenon, termed the poison peptide hypothesis, has been implicated in the development of familial cardiac hypertrophy. Note that this form of hypertrophy is pathological, whereas more physiological forms of hypertrophy (such as after a training regimen) do not involve an alteration of sarcomere structure.*

Case 13–2

1. A is incorrect. Patients with exertional angina usually exhibit normal regulation of intracellular Ca^{++}.

   B is incorrect. Regulation of actin-myosin interactions also appears to be normal in patients with exertional angina.

   C is incorrect because depletion of ATP would result in death of the cardiac muscle cells.

   D *is correct. Partially clogged coronary vessels, for example, may provide sufficient* O_2 *to the heart at rest but fail to meet the energy needs of the heart muscle during periods of exercise, resulting in exertional angina.*

   E is incorrect. Regulation of sarcolemmal Ca^{++} channels also appears normal in patients with exertional angina.

2. A is incorrect. Phospholamban is an inhibitor of SERCA, but given the high endogenous level of phospholamban in the heart, it is unlikely that the DNA transfer technology would further reduce SERCA activity. Furthermore, inhibition of SERCA could be detrimental (as indicated in B).

   B is incorrect. Inhibition of SERCA would decrease the force of contraction and slow the rate of relaxation, resulting in weak, prolonged contractions that could significantly decrease cardiac output, compromise perfusion of the heart, and severely limit exercise capacity.

   C is incorrect. Creatine supplements are thought to increase anaerobic capacity of skeletal muscle by slightly increasing creatine phosphate stores but would be of limited use to the heart, which is highly aerobic.

   D is incorrect and would be expected to exasperate the situation, facilitating the onset of exertional angina by increasing heart rate.

   E *is correct because vasodilators can increase* O_2 *supply to the cardiac muscle cells by dilating coronary vessels. As the response to vasodilators such as nitroglycerin decreases with prolonged exposure to the agonist, nitroglycerin is typically reserved for the reversal of angina during an attack (rather than as a preventive measure).*

Case 14–1

1. A is incorrect. Constriction of the airways is causing the difficulty in breathing and hence low oxygenation of the blood. The low oxygenation of blood and labored breathing then promote a feeling of severe fatigue.

   B is incorrect. Narrowing of the airways by edema would not have been easily reversed by a β_2-adrenergic agonist.

   C *is correct, as indicated by the action of the* β_2*-adrenergic agonist. Specifically, the* β_2*-adrenergic* *agonist inhibited contraction of bronchial smooth muscle, thereby improving her breathing.*

D is incorrect.

2. A is incorrect because the heart contains few β_2-adrenergic receptors and thus would exhibit minimal phosphorylation of phospholamban. Instead, phosphorylation of cardiac phospholamban typically follows β_1-adrenergic stimulation. Also note that β_1-adrenergic stimulation of the heart under this condition would exasperate the situation, increasing O_2 demand of the heart at a time when breathing is compromised.

   B is incorrect since β_2-adrenergic agonists do not increase cGMP level.

   C *is correct. β_2-Adrenergic agonists increase the cAMP level in the smooth muscle, resulting in cAMP-dependent phosphorylation of myosin light-chain kinase (MLCK) and hence an inhibition of MLCK. Decreased activity of MLCK results in a lower level of phosphorylated myosin, thereby relaxing the smooth muscle.*

   D is incorrect for the reason given in B.

   E is incorrect since smooth muscle does not contain troponin.

Case 14–2

1. A is incorrect. The oxygenation of the blood is normal in Raynaud's, with the paleness resulting from local vasoconstriction.

   B is incorrect for the reason given in A.

   C *is correct and represents a localized cold-induced vasospasm.*

   D is incorrect.

   E is incorrect.

2. A *is correct and represents a return of the oxygenated blood supply as the vasospasm subsides.*

   B is incorrect because further vasoconstriction would produce more blanching and cyanosis.

   C is incorrect. CO_2 decreases O_2 binding to hemoglobin, which would decrease the redness of the blood (as in venous blood).

   D is incorrect.

   E is incorrect.

Case 15–1

1. A is incorrect because the wide pulse pressure produces a pulsatile flow in the nail bed.

   B *is correct. The circulation time will be shortened because some blood passes through the shunt (short circuit).*

   C is incorrect because the pulse pressure is increased secondary to reduced peripheral resistance.

   D is incorrect because the velocity of blood flow is still greatest in the aorta, where the cross-sectional area of the vasculature is smallest.

   E is incorrect because the right atrial pressure is less than vena caval pressure; otherwise, blood would not be able to return to the heart.

2. A is incorrect because autonomic reflexes will compensate to maintain circulation to the heart.

   B is incorrect because the autonomic reflexes will also compensate to maintain cerebral circulation.

   C *is correct because the artery and vein involved are muscular in nature.*

   D is incorrect because circulation beyond the region of the shunt will diminish and therefore decrease capillary flow in the affected leg.

   E is incorrect because the shunt will deliver blood at a higher than normal pressure to the iliac vein.

Case 15–2

1. A is incorrect because chronic blood loss results in red cells with considerable size variation, typical of microcytic anemia.

   B is incorrect because the hematocrit would be greatly reduced below a normal of 45%.

   C is incorrect because the red cell count would be below the normal level of 5 million cells/mm^3.

   D *is correct because the normal blood hemoglobin level is 15 g/dL. A value of 6 g/dL indicates severe anemia.*

   E is incorrect because the hemoglobin/red cell ratio would be reduced. Each red cell would contain less than the normal amount of hemoglobin.

2. A is incorrect because the stool sample would show red blood.

   B is incorrect because bleeding from a renal artery would not reveal a guaiac-positive stool sample.

   C is incorrect because there would be no sign of blood in the stool.

D *is correct because the epigastric pain relieved by food, milk, or antacid tablets indicates the presence of a bleeding gastric ulcer.*
E is incorrect because this would cause accumulation of blood and swelling in leg tissues.

Case 16–1

1. A is incorrect because a less negative transmembrane potential (V_m) inactivates fast Na^+ channels, and this decreases propagation velocity.
   B is incorrect because ventricular myocardial cells are fast-response fibers, and such fibers do not display post-repolarization refractoriness.
   C *is correct because when the extracellular [K^+] increases, the Nernst equation indicates that the transmembrane potential will become less negative.*
   D is incorrect because ordinary myocardial cells do not possess the property of automaticity.
   E is incorrect because reentry is more likely to occur when propagation is retarded.
2. A is incorrect because the slope of the automatic cell upstroke does not appreciably affect the firing frequency.
   B *is correct because when the slope of the slow diastolic depolarization is increased, the firing threshold of the automatic cells is reached more quickly.*
   C is incorrect because increasing the firing threshold would actually decrease the firing frequency of the automatic cells.
   D is incorrect because increasing the maximum negativity would prolong the time required for V_m to reach threshold.
   E is incorrect because changes in the amplitude of the action potential upstroke of an automatic cell do not appreciably affect the firing frequency of that cell.
3. A is incorrect because if a bypass tract had been present, the ventricle would contract at the same frequency (90 beats/min) as did the atria.
   B is incorrect because ordinary ventricular myocytes can become automatic only under unusual conditions.
   C is incorrect because if such ventricular cells did exist, they would fire at the prevailing frequency (90 firings/min) of the SA node cells.
   D *is correct because the Purkinje fibers are automatic, and they generate action potentials at a low frequency when they are not depolarized (overdrive suppression) by action potentials originating in higher frequency pacemaker sites.*
   E is incorrect because myoneural junctions (between nerve and muscle cells), such as those in skeletal muscle, do not exist in cardiac muscle.
4. A *is correct because pacing cardiac tissue at a frequency substantially greater than the natural firing frequency of the intrinsic ventricular pacemakers (Purkinje cells) causes an excessive influx of Na^+ into the cardiac cells, including the automatic cells, and this leads to overdrive suppression.*
   B is incorrect because overdrive suppression is readily induced in isolated cardiac tissues that have been completely denervated.
   C is incorrect because overdrive suppression is readily induced in isolated cardiac tissues that have been completely denervated.
   D is incorrect because overdrive suppression is a characteristic of automatic, not of ordinary, myocardial cells.
   E is incorrect because overdrive suppression is readily induced in isolated cardiac tissues that have been completely denervated.

Case 17–1

1. A is incorrect because SA node rhythm is determined from the P-P interval.
   B is incorrect because bundle branch conduction is not measured by the PR interval.
   C *is correct because the PR interval indicates that the time for conduction from atria through the AV node and ventricular conducting system to the ventricle is normal.*
   D is incorrect because atrial excitation is indicated by P waves.
   E is incorrect because the electrocardiogram does not report on the contractile state of the heart.
2. A is incorrect because the interval between SA node impulses is measured by the P-P interval.
   B is incorrect because atrial impulses are indicated by P waves.
   C is incorrect because the PR interval measures conduction time from atrium to ventricle.

D is incorrect because the ventricular conducting system is shown by His bundle electrograms.
E *is correct because the QT interval measures the duration of the average ventricular action potential.*

3. A *is correct because the heart rate can be taken from either the R-R or P-P intervals when conduction is normal.*
B is incorrect because the PR interval measures conduction time from atrium to ventricle.
C is incorrect because QRS duration indicates conduction through the ventricles.
D is incorrect because P waves indicate atrial excitation.
E is incorrect because R wave amplitude indicates mass of ventricular tissue.

4. A is incorrect because greater closing of repolarizing K^+ channels would reduce the QT interval.
B is incorrect because the QT interval is increased.
C is incorrect because greater inactivation of Na^+ channels would reduce the QT interval.
D *is correct because greater activation of repolarizing K^+ channels would reduce the QT interval.*
E is incorrect because the increase of the QT interval arises from either greater inward or diminished outward cation currents.

Case 18–1

1. A is incorrect because the patient's murmur is diastolic, not systolic.
B is incorrect for the same reason as for A.
C is incorrect because the characterizations of this murmur (soft, high pitched) and its location are compatible with aortic regurgitation, not mitral stenosis.
D *is correct because the murmur is characteristic of mitral stenosis.*
E is incorrect for the same reason as for A.

2. A is incorrect because cardiac rhythm is irregular in atrial fibrillation.
B is incorrect because some weak beats are not palpable at the wrist but are heard over the precordium.
C *is correct because the pulse is totally irregular.*
D is incorrect because beats after inadequate ventricular filling are felt as weaker than those after adequate ventricular filling.
E is incorrect because P waves are replaced by F waves in the electrocardiogram.

3. A is incorrect because a pacemaker cannot take over the rhythm in atrial fibrillation.
B *is correct because a phlebotomy would relieve the excessive preload and allow the ventricles to contract more efficiently.*
C is incorrect because a saline infusion would add to the high preload and aggravate the congestive failure.
D is incorrect because adenosine will have no effect on atrial fibrillation.
E is incorrect because the heart needs more intracellular Ca^{++}, not less.

4. A is incorrect because the serum albumin level would not be elevated. It might even be reduced.
B *is correct because the elevated left atrial pressure would be transmitted back to the wedged catheter (wedge pressure).*
C is incorrect because Na^+ excretion would be reduced in a patient in congestive heart failure.
D is incorrect because peripheral resistance would be increased in a patient with heart failure and a low cardiac output.
E is incorrect because the pulse pressure would be either normal or reduced in a patient with a low cardiac output.

5. A is incorrect because dicumarol would prevent clot formation in the fibrillating atria and thereby prevent the release of emboli from the atria.
B is incorrect because digoxin strengthens the cardiac contractions by raising intracellular Ca^{++} levels.
C is incorrect because procainamide can sometimes stop atrial fibrillation.
D is incorrect because the diuretic hydrochlorothiazide enhances the renal excretion of NaCl and water, thereby reducing blood volume and cardiac preload.
E *is correct because nitroglycerin is prescribed for angina pectoris caused by myocardial ischemia and is not prescribed for congestive heart failure.*

6. A is incorrect.
B is incorrect.
C *is correct because*

$$300 / (0.18 - 0.08) = 300 / 0.10 = 3000 \text{ mL/min} = 3 \text{ L/min}$$

D is incorrect.
E is incorrect.

Case 19–1

1. A is incorrect because a decrease in the arterial pressure would reflexly increase sympathetic activity and decrease vagal activity, both of which would increase myocardial contractility.
   B is incorrect because a decrease in the arterial pressure would reflexly increase sympathetic activity and decrease vagal activity, both of which would shorten the cardiac cycle.
   C is incorrect because a decrease in the arterial pressure would reflexly increase sympathetic activity and decrease vagal activity, both of which would enhance AV conduction.
   D *is correct because a decrease in the arterial pressure would reflexly increase sympathetic activity and thereby increase the neuronal release of norepinephrine.*
   E is incorrect because a decrease in the arterial pressure would increase the neuronal release of norepinephrine and thereby increase Ca^{++} conductance.
2. A is incorrect because the acetylcholine (ACh) released by the vagal fibers markedly shortens the atrial action potentials, which curtails the influx of Ca^{++} into the myocytes and thus weakens their contractions.
   B is incorrect because the ACh released from vagal endings inhibits the release of norepinephrine from nearby sympathetic nerve endings.
   C is incorrect because the distribution of vagal nerve fibers and of muscarinic cholinergic receptors is sparse in these tissues.
   D *is correct. The ACh released from vagal fibers acts on muscarinic receptors on SA node automatic cells, and these receptors interact quickly with specific K^+ channels because no second messenger intervenes.*
   E is incorrect because the neurally released ACh hyperpolarizes the conduction fibers and thereby retards conduction.
3. A *is correct because the cardiac responses to vagal stimulation develop and decay rapidly, but the responses to sympathetic stimulation develop and decay slowly. Hence, respiratory arrhythmia is mediated almost entirely by the vagus nerves, and this arrhythmia would be abolished by a potent muscarinic antagonist.*
   B is incorrect because vagally released ACh weakens the contractions of atrial myocytes; a muscarinic antagonist would prevent this effect.
   C is incorrect because vagally released ACh retards AV conduction; a muscarinic antagonist would prevent this effect.
   D is incorrect because vagally released ACh decreases the action potential duration of atrial myocytes; a muscarinic antagonist would prevent this effect.
   E is incorrect because vagally released ACh hyperpolarizes the atrial myocytes during phase 4; a muscarinic antagonist would prevent this effect.
4. A *is correct because the heart rate increases during inspiration in this arrhythmia; this increase is mediated mainly by a reduction in vagal activity.*
   B is incorrect because decreased sympathetic activity would tend to decrease the heart rate during inspiration.
   C is incorrect because a decreased rate of slow diastolic depolarization would decrease the heart rate during inspiration.
   D is incorrect because hemorrhage decreases vagal activity and would thereby attenuate the arrhythmia.
   E is incorrect because propranolol attenuates the sympathetic effects on the heart; such effects have little influence on the respiratory arrhythmia.
5. A is incorrect because if the cardiac automatic cells became more responsive, the heart rate response would decay less rapidly.
   B is incorrect because ACh is removed from the cardiac interstitium by hydrolysis, not by uptake by the vagus nerve endings.
   C is incorrect because ACh is removed from the cardiac interstitium by hydrolysis, not by uptake by the cardiac myocytes.
   D is incorrect because the synthetic mechanisms in the nerve endings can usually produce new ACh at a rate equal to its release rate.
   E *is correct because acetylcholinesterase is abundant in atrial tissues, especially the SA and AV nodes.*

Case 20–1

1. A is incorrect.
   B *is correct because*
   $P_a - P_v / Q = [(100 - 80) + (80 - 10)] / 300$
   $= 0.3$ mm Hg/mL/min
   C is incorrect.
   D is incorrect.
   E is incorrect.

2. A is incorrect.
   B is incorrect.
   C is incorrect.
   D *is correct because the left [(100 – 10)/500] and right [(100 – 10)/300] vascular resistances were 0.18 and 0.30 mm Hg/mL/min, respectively, and the reciprocals of those resistances were 5.56 and 3.33 mL/min/mm Hg, respectively. Hence, the reciprocal of the sum (8.89 mL/min/mm Hg) of these reciprocals equals 0.11 mm Hg/mL/min.*
   E is incorrect.
3. A *is correct because*
   Resistance to flow =
   Pressure difference across the plaque/
   Flow past the plaque =
   100 – 80 mm Hg / 300 mL/min =
   0.066 mm Hg/mL/min
   B is incorrect.
   C is incorrect.
   D is incorrect.
   E is incorrect.

Case 21–1

1. A *is correct because the mean arterial pressure in the systemic and pulmonary vascular beds depends on the outputs of the left and right ventricles and the systemic vascular resistances. Over any substantial time interval, the outputs of the two ventricles are equal, but the systemic vascular resistance far exceeds the pulmonary vascular resistance.*
   B is incorrect because the mean arterial pressure is not affected by the arterial compliance.
   C is incorrect because over any substantial time interval, the outputs of the right and left ventricles must equal each other.
   D is incorrect because the total cross-sectional area of the systemic capillary bed is much greater than the total cross-sectional area of the pulmonary capillary bed.
   E is incorrect because the durations of the rapid ejection phases of the right and left ventricles are virtually equal.
2. A is incorrect because the systemic vascular resistance increases considerably in patients with essential hypertension.
   B is incorrect because the duration of the reduced ejection phase of the left ventricle has only a negligible effect on the arterial pulse pressure.
   C *is correct because when the arterial pressure rises, the arteries become less compliant (as does a balloon); also, the arterial compliance decreases with age.*
   D is incorrect because the total cross-sectional area of the systemic capillary bed does not change substantially in hypertensive subjects.
   E is incorrect because if the aortic compliance increased, the arterial pulse pressure would tend to decrease.

Case 22–1

1. A is incorrect.
   B is incorrect.
   C is incorrect.
   D *is correct because* (44 + 2) – (23 + 8) = 15.
   E is incorrect.
2. A is incorrect because dialysis would be of no value. It is used in cases of kidney failure to remove waste products normally eliminated by the kidneys.
   B is incorrect because a high-fat diet is contraindicated since it would put an added burden on the cirrhotic liver.
   C *is correct because portal-caval shunt (portal vein to inferior vena cava) could reduce the high venous pressure in the mesentery by allowing mesenteric blood to bypass the high vascular resistance in the liver. This would aid in eliminating the ascites.*
   D is incorrect because cholecystectomy would be of no value.
   E is incorrect because erythromycin is an antibiotic and would not be indicated in alcoholic cirrhosis, which is not an infectious disease.
3. A is incorrect because Na^+, NaCl, and K^+ are equally distributed across the capillary membrane and hence do not exert an osmotic force between intravascular and extracellular spaces.
   B *is correct because albumin is small enough (low molecular weight) to exert the main osmotic force of plasma and large enough to remain within the vascular compartment.*
   C is incorrect because Na^+, NaCl, and K^+ are equally distributed across the capillary membrane and hence do not exert an osmotic force between intravascular and extracellular spaces.
   D is incorrect because globulin is a large protein (high molecular weight) and hence exerts only a small osmotic force.
   E is incorrect because Na^+, NaCl, and K^+ are equally distributed across the capillary

membrane and hence do not exert an osmotic force between intravascular and extracellular spaces.

E is incorrect because capillaries do not constrict. They are passive in response to intravascular pressure changes.

Case 22–2

1. A is incorrect because although saline can help restore blood volume, it would be rapidly lost from the burned surfaces.
   B is incorrect because although whole blood can restore blood volume, it would not be the most effective treatment. The patient has a high hematocrit, which indicates a concentration of red cells in his circulation. Therefore, red cells are not needed, and whole blood would not correct the hemoconcentration.
   C is incorrect because isotonic glucose would only temporarily restore blood volume, and as with saline, the water would be lost from the burned surfaces.
   D is incorrect because although dextran can help restore blood volume and the oncotic pressure, it would not restore albumin levels to normal.
   E *is correct because the albumin concentration in the patient's blood is low due to loss of albumin from the burned tissues. This results in a decreased plasma oncotic pressure; this plus the loss of fluid from the damaged microvessels leads to a decreased blood volume and an increased red cell concentration. Therefore, a plasma transfusion, which supplies albumin plus saline without red cells, is the most effective treatment.*
2. A is incorrect because a reflex constriction of arterioles in the feet would not occur as a consequence of standing erect.
   B is incorrect because tissue pressure is normally close to atmospheric pressure, and it could reach high levels only if severe subcutaneous edema occurred. Even then, the pressure would not equal intracapillary pressure in the feet in the standing position.
   C is incorrect because the total capillary cross-sectional area is not involved. The pressure would be high and equal in all of the capillaries of the feet.
   D *is correct because the small diameter (or radius) of the capillaries is responsible for the low wall tension, according to the law of Laplace: T (wall tension) = P (pressure) × r (radius of capillary). The low wall tension protects against capillary rupture.*

Case 23–1

1. A is incorrect because the intravascular pressure in the arterioles is decreased, not increased, and because the arterioles are maximally dilated by the local release of metabolites.
   B *is correct because the arterioles are maximally dilated secondary to the inadequate blood flow that causes the local release of vasodilator metabolites.*
   C is incorrect because maximally dilated vessels do not autoregulate.
   D is incorrect because local metabolites override a myogenic response.
   E is incorrect because this would occur only with the washout of metabolites, not with their presence.
2. A *is correct because use of tobacco is believed to be a contributing factor to the cause and exacerbation of thromboangiitis obliterans.*
   B is incorrect because a vasodilator drug would be valueless. The resistance vessels are already maximally dilated.
   C is incorrect because the arterioles cannot be dilated further by interrupting their nerve supply.
   D is incorrect because heat would increase the metabolic rate of the ischemic tissue and would thereby aggravate the problem.
   E is incorrect because a vasoconstrictor drug would reduce blood flow to the lower leg and exacerbate his symptoms.

Case 23–2

1. A is incorrect because a hypersensitive carotid sinus can produce fainting, especially with tight collars.
   B is incorrect because episodes of heart block can produce fainting (Stokes-Adams syndrome) when the ventricular rate falls to very low levels and blood pressure falls.
   C is incorrect because some individuals experience severe hypotension when they change from the horizontal to the vertical position, a condition usually observed in astronauts when they return to earth.

D is incorrect because severe tachycardia can interfere with ventricular filling, which can result in low blood pressure and syncope.

E *is correct because diabetic coma is not characterized by repeated brief bouts of unconsciousness.*

2. A is incorrect because adenosine as a bolus injection is the drug of choice in the treatment of supraventricular tachycardia (SVT).

B is incorrect because the Valsalva maneuver can terminate SVT by depressing atrial ventricular conduction via enhanced cardiac vagal activity.

C *is correct because digitalis is not prescribed for SVT unless there is also impaired myocardial function.*

D is incorrect because carotid sinus massage can terminate SVT by the same mechanism as with Valsalva's maneuver.

E is incorrect because in severe and prolonged cases of SVT, the ectopic focus is located with a cardiac catheter tip and ablated with an electric current.

Case 24–1

1. A is incorrect because the blood loss would decrease the central venous pressure, but this reduction in cardiac preload would decrease the cardiac output.

B is incorrect because the blood loss would decrease the central venous pressure.

C *is correct because the blood loss would decrease the central venous pressure; this reduction in cardiac preload would decrease the cardiac output.*

D is incorrect because the reduced cardiac preload would decrease the cardiac output and thus would decrease the mean arterial pressure.

E is incorrect because the decrease in the central venous pressure (preload) would decrease the stroke volume and thus the aortic pulse pressure.

2. A *is correct because a drug that improves cardiac contractility would increase cardiac output, which would tend to increase the arterial blood volume. Hence, if the total blood volume remains constant, the venous blood volume would decrease. Consequently, the central venous pressure would decline.*

B is incorrect because a drug that improves cardiac contractility would increase cardiac output. Consequently, mean arterial pressure would increase.

C is incorrect because a drug that improves cardiac contractility would increase cardiac output. Consequently, the increased cardiac output would redistribute the blood volume such that the arterial volume would increase and the venous volume would decrease. Hence, central venous pressure would decrease.

D is incorrect because a drug that improves cardiac contractility would, by definition, enhance the efficacy of the cardiac contractile proteins and thereby increase cardiac output.

E is incorrect because a drug that improves cardiac contractility would increase cardiac output and would therefore decrease central venous pressure.

3. A is incorrect because gravity acts to pool blood in the compliant, dependent veins. Hence, the volume of blood in the central veins diminishes, and central venous pressure falls.

B is incorrect because gravity acts to pool blood in the compliant, dependent veins, and hence pressure increases in the foot veins.

C is incorrect because gravity acts to pool blood in the compliant, dependent veins; hence, the central venous volume and pressure diminish. The consequent reduction in preload reduces the cardiac output and therefore the mean arterial pressure.

D is incorrect because gravity acts to pool blood in the compliant, dependent veins, and hence the pressure in the foot veins will increase.

E *is correct because gravity acts to pool blood in the compliant, dependent veins; hence, the pressure in the foot veins will increase. The redistribution of the venous blood volume will cause the central venous volume and pressure to diminish. The consequent reduction in preload decreases the cardiac output.*

4. A is incorrect because when the heart rate is abnormally high (250 beats/min), the cardiac output declines substantially, and hence mean arterial pressure is diminished.

B *is correct because when the heart rate is abnormally high, cardiac filling is inadequate; therefore, stroke volume and cardiac output are decreased.*

C is incorrect because cardiac filling is inadequate; therefore, stroke volume is decreased.

D is incorrect because cardiac filling is inadequate; therefore, cardiac output is decreased.
E is incorrect because cardiac filling is inadequate; therefore, stroke volume is decreased. The reduction in stroke volume causes the arterial pulse pressure to decrease.

Case 25–1

1. A is incorrect because in severe bradycardia, blood pressure and hence coronary perfusion pressure are low, and the reduced transmural pressure might elicit a myogenic dilation but not a constriction.
   B is incorrect because myocardial metabolic activity is reduced and would produce vasoconstriction.
   C is incorrect because local factors predominate over neural factors. Also, there is no reason to invoke a reflex response.
   D *is correct because two factors operate in bradycardia. At the slower rate, more time is spent in diastole, which decreases coronary resistance (less extravascular compression). However, at the slower rate, the heart uses less O_2 and fewer vasodilator metabolites are present, which permits greater expression of basal tone (coronary constriction). The result is the algebraic sum of these two opposing actors.*
   E is incorrect because the epicardial-endocardial blood flow rate is not significantly affected in bradycardia.
2. A *is correct because the coronary vessels are maximally dilated as a result of the accumulation of vasodilator metabolites consequent to an inadequate O_2 supply to the myocardial cells. If any vasoconstriction occurred, it would be transient.*
   B is incorrect because both the atrial and ventricular rates would increase.
   C is incorrect because both the atrial and ventricular rates would increase.
   D is incorrect because the coronary resistance vessels are already maximally dilated.
   E is incorrect because the accumulated vasodilator metabolites would override a neural vasoconstrictor response.
3. A is incorrect because nitroglycerin is a vasodilator.
   B *is correct because endothelin is a powerful vasoconstrictor.*
   C is incorrect because prostacyclin is a vasodilator.
   D is incorrect because adenosine is a vasodilator.
   E is incorrect because acetylcholine is a vasodilator.
4. A is incorrect because a transplanted heart is denervated.
   B is incorrect because a transplanted heart is denervated.
   C is incorrect because a transplanted heart is denervated and the respiratory effect on heart rate is mediated by the cardiac nerves.
   D is incorrect because a transplanted heart is denervated and the respiratory effect on heart rate is mediated by the cardiac nerves.
   E *is correct because with exercise, a denervated heart increases the stroke volume more than the heart rate to meet the required cardiac output. Any increase in heart rate must come from release of epinephrine and norepinephrine from the adrenal medulla.*

Case 25–2

1. A *is correct because hepatic fibrosis increases the hepatic vascular resistance; therefore, the pressure in the vessels downstream to the liver is elevated. Consequently, the balance of Starling forces in the splanchnic capillaries favors the movement of fluid out of the capillaries and into the abdominal cavity.*
   B is incorrect because the hepatic artery pressure would be equal to the aortic pressure, which is not appreciably affected by cirrhosis.
   C is incorrect because the resistance vessels between the portal and hepatic vessels cause a pressure drop as blood flows from the portal to the hepatic veins.
   D is incorrect because the pressure in the splenic vein virtually equals that in the portal vein, since the splenic vein is a tributary of the portal vein. Hence, the resistance vessels between the splenic and hepatic veins cause a pressure drop, as explained in C.
   E is incorrect because the hepatic vascular resistance was increased.

Case 26–1

1. A is incorrect because the active muscles were capable of using more O_2 if it were provided by the circulation.

B is incorrect because the arterial blood was fully saturated with O_2 even at a high rate of blood flow through the lungs.

C is incorrect because there is no reason to suspect that the splanchnic vessels and those in the inactive muscle were not constricted.

D *is correct because his heart became unable to pump enough blood per unit time as a result of a decrease in stroke volume and hence in cardiac output.*

E is incorrect because the arteriovenous O_2 difference was at maximum.

2. A *is correct because his body temperature reached an alarmingly high level as a result of inadequate heat loss via the skin (vasoconstriction secondary to decrease in blood pressure) in the face of the great heat production in the active muscles.*

B is incorrect because the heart rate reached a maximum level before his collapse.

C is incorrect because his skin blood vessels constricted in response to a fall in blood pressure.

D is incorrect because his blood pH decrease was caused by the release of lactic acid from the active muscles.

E is incorrect because his blood pressure fell as a result of the reduction of stroke volume.

Case 26–2

1. A is incorrect because there are very few parasympathetic nerves to the skin and because the released acetylcholine would dilate, not constrict, the cutaneous vessels.

B is incorrect because there are very few parasympathetic nerves to the skin; the released vasoactive intestinal peptide would dilate, not constrict, the cutaneous vessels.

C is incorrect because there are very few parasympathetic nerves to the skin; they do not release neuropeptide Y.

D is incorrect because the sympathetic nerves to the skin do not release much nitric oxide; the nitric oxide would dilate, not constrict, the cutaneous vessels.

E *is correct because the hypotension would act via the arterial baroreceptors to activate the sympathetic nerves to the skin. The consequent release of norepinephrine would constrict the cutaneous arterioles, and the skin temperature would drop.*

2. A *is correct because the abnormally low mean arterial pressure (≈72 mm Hg) would signify an abnormally small cardiac output. The low mean arterial pressure could not have been caused by arteriolar vasodilation because the baroreceptor reflex response to such a low pressure would be vasoconstriction, not vasodilation. The low pulse pressure (20 mm Hg) would signify an abnormally small stroke volume.*

B is incorrect because over any substantial time, the outputs of the two ventricles must be equal.

C is incorrect because the small pulse pressure (20 mm Hg) denotes a small stroke volume (and there is no reason to believe that the arterial compliance is abnormally great).

D is incorrect because blood loss would lead to reflex vasoconstriction. A normal cardiac output would lead to a higher than normal mean arterial pressure if generalized vasoconstriction prevailed.

E is incorrect because over any substantial time, the output of the two ventricles must be equal.

3. A is incorrect because any acute change in red cell volume would most likely be produced by a change in the osmolarity of the plasma; blood loss does not acutely alter the osmolarity of the extracellular fluid (or blood plasma) substantially.

B *is correct because the decrease in capillary hydrostatic pressure draws interstitial fluid into the plasma compartment and thereby dilutes the red cell component of whole blood.*

C is incorrect because hemorrhage would have no direct effect on the leukocytes, but the dilution effect of the influx of interstitial fluid into the plasma compartment would tend to dilute the leukocyte component of whole blood.

D is incorrect because the dilution effect of the influx of interstitial fluid into the plasma compartment would tend to diminish the concentration of albumin in the plasma.

E is incorrect because the dilution effect of the influx of interstitial fluid into the plasma compartment would tend to diminish the concentration of globulin in the plasma.

Case 27–1

1. A is incorrect because a history of fever accompanied by left-sided chest pain and decreased breath sounds is highly suggestive

of a pneumonia, which would most likely be illustrated as an abnormal finding on the chest film.

B is incorrect because both the pain and decreased breath sounds have been associated with the left side.

C *is correct because the topographical location of the left lower lobe is along the lower edge of the left rib cage.*

D is incorrect because the superior segment of the left lower lobe does not correlate with the topographical location of the physical findings.

E is incorrect because the location of the lingula does not correlate with the topographical location of the physical findings.

Case 27–2

1. A is incorrect because this patient's history is highly suggestive of an obstructive disease, such as bronchitis, which would be manifested by ventilation abnormalities, not perfusion abnormalities.

B is incorrect because perfusion is usually not affected by obstructive lung diseases associated with increased mucus production until the condition becomes severe with cardiac complications.

C *is correct because the increased mucus production will obstruct this man's airways to varying degrees. As a result, ventilation will be affected. This man's history is most compatible with chronic bronchitis.*

D is incorrect because the increased mucus production will obstruct this man's airways to varying degrees. As a result, ventilation will be affected.

E is incorrect because perfusion is usually not affected by obstructive lung diseases associated with increased mucus production until the condition becomes severe with cardiac complications.

Case 27–3

1. A is incorrect because the most common causes of emphysema are cigarette smoking and a genetic abnormality, α_1-antitrypsin deficiency. This individual does not have a history of either of these diseases.

B *is correct because this man has immotile cilia syndrome, in which all ciliated structures in the body are abnormal. As a result, he will experience abnormalities in mucociliary transport due to failure of the cilia located on the airway epithelium to beat. Mucus will be retained in the lung, and secondary infection will develop. The abnormality affects all cilia in the lung, and so the disease will affect all areas of the lung.*

C is incorrect because a major defense system in the lung, the mucociliary transport system, is abnormal in structure and function. In addition to poor particulate removal from the lung, he will accumulate large amounts of mucus, which is also conducive to increased bacterial growth.

D is incorrect because the problem is throughout the lung, not in a localized area; thus, all areas of the lung will be affected.

Case 27–4

1. A is incorrect because surfactant therapy has become a standard of care for premature infants, especially at the level of development of this infant.

B is incorrect because the anti-stick properties of surfactant contribute significantly to inhibiting atelectasis, and thus, in its absence as in premature infants, atelectasis is a prominent feature.

C is incorrect because ventilation will certainly be decreased as a result of surfactant deficiency and atelectasis.

D *is correct because this infant is significantly premature and will most likely experience respiratory distress syndrome. If he is not treated with surfactant, this infant will experience airway closure (atelectasis) with decreased ventilation and abnormalities in gas exchange.*

Case 28–1

1. A is incorrect. Asthma gets better and worse on its own, irrespective of therapy. It would also be unusual for asthma to cause a barrel chest or distant breath sounds.

B is incorrect. This man does not have chronic bronchitis because he has a reduced DLCO.

C *is correct because the man's history of cigarette smoking puts him at risk for obstructive pulmonary disease, which is confirmed by the changes in pulmonary function that demonstrate decreased expiratory flow rates and air trapping (increased RV/TLC). But is it chronic bronchitis or emphysema? The answer lies in the decreased surface area for gas exchange (decreased DLCO) and the increase in lung compliance. This man has emphysema.*

D is incorrect. Pulmonary fibrosis would cause a restrictive pattern on pulmonary function testing.

E is incorrect. This is a disease of newborn infants due to a lack of surfactant.

2. A is incorrect. The diaphragm would be flattened (hyperinflated lungs), and the lung fields would not appear normal.

B is incorrect. The diaphragm would be flattened, and the lung fields would not have increased markings as you might see in someone with chronic bronchitis.

C *is correct because on the chest radiograph, there should be evidence of air trapping with a flattened diaphragm and a decrease in lung markings. Because of tissue destruction in emphysema, there is enlargement of the air spaces (decreased surface area for gas exchange) and bullae formation. Many of these bullae form in the apices of the lung.*

D is incorrect. The diaphragm would be flattened, but the lung markings would be decreased, not increased.

E is incorrect. The lung markings would be most decreased in the lung apices where bullae are most commonly formed.

Case 28–2

1. A is incorrect.

B is incorrect.

C is incorrect.

D *is correct because compliance is the measurement of how much pressure is required to overcome the elastic forces of a structure (in this case, the lungs and chest wall together). It is important that this measurement be made in a patient who is not exerting effort and at the point of no airflow so that airway resistance will not affect the pressure being measured. The compliance of the respiratory system in this patient is*

$$\frac{1000 \text{ mL}}{25 \text{ cm } H_2O - 0 \text{ cm } H_2O} = 40 \text{ mL/cm } H_2O$$

E is incorrect.

2. A is incorrect.

B is incorrect.

C is incorrect.

D *is correct because airway resistance is equal to the change in pressure divided by airflow. The pressure difference in this situation is the difference between the pressure at the mouth (P_{ao}) and the alveolar pressure (P_{alv}). In an intubated patient, the peak airway pressure during airflow is P_{ao}, and pressure during occlusion (i.e., air is not flowing) is equal to P_{alv}. Therefore:*

$$\text{Airway resistance (Raw)} = \frac{P_{ao} - P_{alv}}{\text{Flow}}$$

$$= \frac{35 \text{ cm } H_2O - 25 \text{ cm } H_2O}{1 \text{ L/sec}}$$

$$= 10 \text{ cm } H_2O/\text{L/sec}$$

E is incorrect.

Case 28–3

1. A is incorrect because the nodular tumor would result in obstruction of the airways, not a loss of elastic recoil.

B *is correct because this patient has a tumor that is obstructing her airway. The tumor narrows the size of the airway and results in an increase in airway resistance.*

C is incorrect because this woman has obstructive pulmonary disease.

D is incorrect because there is no evidence that this woman has muscle weakness that would cause restrictive lung disease.

E is incorrect because of the nodular tumor in her airway on bronchoscopy.

2. A is incorrect.

B is incorrect.

C *is correct because compliance is defined as the change in volume per change in pressure. In this example, the change in volume is 1 L and the change in pressure is 5 cm H_2O. Thus, the compliance of the lung at this volume is 0.2 L/cm H_2O.*

D is incorrect.

Case 28–4

1. A *is correct because this individual demonstrates a decrease in the $FEF_{25\text{-}75}$, which significantly improves after inhalation of albuterol. By history, he most likely has asthma.*

B is incorrect because there is a significant increase in FEV_1 and $FEF_{25\text{-}75}$ after the bronchodilator, demonstrating reversibility.
C is incorrect because this patient has evidence of obstructive pulmonary disease (decreased $FEF_{25\text{-}75}$).
D is incorrect because this patient has evidence of obstructive pulmonary disease (decreased $FEF_{25\text{-}75}$).
E is incorrect because pulmonary function is usually normal in pulmonary vascular disease.

Case 28–5

1. A *is correct because this woman is experiencing an asthma attack, a type of obstructive pulmonary disease. There will be air trapping and decreases in expiratory flow rates and in the FEV_1. In addition, with moderate to severe asthma attacks, the vital capacity will be decreased.*
   B is incorrect because in obstructive pulmonary disease, the FEV_1/FVC is decreased.
   C is incorrect because during an asthma attack, there is airway obstruction that results in a decrease in FEV_1, in the FEV_1/FVC, and in the expiratory flow rates.
   D is incorrect because during an asthma attack, there are abnormalities in pulmonary function.
   E is incorrect because in obstructive pulmonary disease, the FEV_1/FVC is decreased.

Case 28–6

1. A is incorrect because this man has a major risk factor for pulmonary disease (smoking) but has no respiratory symptoms or physical signs of disease.
   B *is correct because in individuals who have smoked less than 20 pack-years, a chest radiograph is frequently normal, the DLCO may be normal, and the sputum shows no signs of infection. He is a young man, and a positive exercise stress test is likely to be normal. The earliest indicator of pulmonary disease secondary to smoking is a change in pulmonary function. This change will occur in the absence of all symptoms. If this man were to stop smoking now, most if not all of these changes could be reversed.*
   C is incorrect because at this point in the spectrum of smoking-induced lung disease, he has no symptoms or signs of lung disease.
   D is incorrect because he has no signs or symptoms of infection or lung disease.
   E is incorrect because he is a young man and the likelihood of coronary artery syndrome at 35 years of age in the absence of a family history of early, sudden death would be unusual.

Case 29–1

1. A is incorrect.
   B *is correct because by the alveolar gas equation, his alveolar O_2 at Pikes Peak is*
   $(445 \text{ mg Hg} - 47 \text{ mm Hg}) \times 0.21 - 40/0.8 =$
   34 mm Hg
   C is incorrect.
   D is incorrect.
   E is incorrect.

Case 29–2

1. A is incorrect because $\dot{V}/\dot{Q}$mismatch is a cause of hypoxemia and a component of emphysema.
   B *is correct because in emphysema, there is a loss of the surface area for gas exchange with destruction of the capillary bed and the alveoli. There is also premature closure of the airways due to loss of elastic recoil, resulting in bronchial obstruction and changes in the distribution of ventilation. The man's low blood pressure and poor capillary refill are indicators of a reduced cardiac output. Not a feature of emphysema is a right-to-left shunt in the lung, which is also known as a pulmonary arteriovenous malformation, a type of lung-derived anatomical shunt.*
   C is incorrect because there is destruction of the capillary bed that results in a diffusion to gas transfer in individuals with emphysema.
   D is incorrect because low cardiac output is the only nonpulmonary factor that can cause hypoxemia.
   E is incorrect because with pneumonia, there is edema and mucus in the airways, resulting in obstruction.
2. A is incorrect because there is usually no difference between alveolar and arterial CO_2.

B is incorrect because the Aa gradient for O_2 in the normal lung is usually less than 15 mm Hg.
C is incorrect because in hypoventilation, the Aa gradient is normal; in $\dot{V}/\dot{Q}$ mismatch, the Aa gradient is increased.
D *is correct because CO freely diffuses across the alveolar-capillary interface, and therefore there is no gradient. This is the basis for the DLCO. A reduction in DLCO is indicative of a loss of surface area for gas diffusion.*
E is incorrect because the alveolar air equation that is used to calculate the alveolar O_2 requires knowledge of the barometric pressure.

3. A is incorrect.
B is incorrect.
C is incorrect.
D *is correct because*
$PAO_2 = (760 \text{ mm Hg} - 47 \text{ mm Hg}) \times 0.21 - 67/0.8 = 87 \text{ mm Hg}$
The Aa gradient is therefore 87 mm Hg – 48 mm Hg = 39 mm Hg.
E is incorrect.

Case 29–3

1. A is incorrect.
B *is correct because*
$PAO_2 = (760 \text{ mm Hg} - 47 \text{ mm Hg}) \times 0.21 - 54/0.8 = 82 \text{ mm Hg}$
The Aa gradient = 82 mm Hg – 70 mm Hg = 12 mm Hg.
C is incorrect.
D is incorrect.
E is incorrect.

2. A is incorrect because this man has muscle weakness. Muscle weakness will cause hypoventilation, a cause of hypoxemia.
B is incorrect because there is no history suggestive of an anatomical shunt. Rather, the history suggests ventilatory muscle weakness.
C is incorrect because this man has muscle weakness that puts him at risk for hypoventilation.
D *is correct because of all the causes of hypoxemia, only one is associated with a normal Aa gradient, and that is hypoventilation.*
E is incorrect because this man has muscle weakness that puts him at risk for hypoventilation.

Case 30–1

1. A *is correct. Since carbon monoxide has about 200 times greater affinity for Hgb than O_2 does, it competes for the Hgb sites and thus directly prevents O_2 binding. The presence of carbon monoxide increases the affinity of Hgb for O_2, which has the effect of inhibiting its release from Hgb at tissue sites (shifts the dissociation curve to the left).*
B is incorrect. Although CO prevents O_2 binding to Hgb and increases the affinity of O_2 for Hgb, it inhibits the release of O_2 from Hgb and thus shifts the dissociation curve to the left, not the right.
C is incorrect. CO does not decrease the affinity of O_2 for Hgb.
D is incorrect. CO does not decrease the affinity of O_2 for Hgb, nor does it shift the dissociation curve to the right.
E is incorrect. CO does not enhance the binding of O_2 to Hgb.

2. A is incorrect. Blood pressure would be increased, not decreased, in an attempt to compensate for the poor tissue delivery of O_2.
B is incorrect. Although the blood pressure and heart rate would be increased in attempts to compensate for poor tissue delivery of O_2, it is unlikely that the respiratory rate would be increased until the acidosis becomes severe.
C is incorrect. The blood pressure would be increased, not decreased, to compensate for the poor tissue delivery of O_2.
D is incorrect. The blood pressure would be increased, not decreased, to compensate for the poor tissue delivery of O_2.
E *is correct. Blood pressure and heart rate will be increased in attempts to compensate for the poor tissue O_2 delivery due to the limited amount of O_2 bound to Hgb and the lowered ability of O_2 to dissociate from Hgb. The respiratory rate can be increased, but this would occur only in severe cases when acidosis has resulted.*

Case 30–2

1. A is incorrect. At 10 months of age, it would be expected that some adult HgbS should be present in addition to fetal HgbF.

B is incorrect. Although the 10-month-old infant should have adult Hgb, it would be the abnormal HgbS, not HgbA.
C is incorrect. At 10 months of age, there still should be some HgbF remaining, and the adult Hgb would be the abnormal HgbS.
D *is correct. HgbF is the predominant Hgb at birth and is slowly replaced by HgbA by the end of the first year of life. Since this infant has HgbS and not HgbA at 8 months of age, this child most likely has both HgbF and HgbS. The symptoms are beginning to occur now because the protection provided by HgbF during the first few months after birth is now disappearing as it is replaced by the adult HgbS.*
E is incorrect. At 10 months of age, there still should be some HgbF remaining.

2. A is incorrect. Although the liver can be damaged by infarction, it is unlikely to lead to immunosuppression since the liver is not a major lymphoid organ.
B *is correct. The spleen is the major site for normal red blood cell filtration and destruction and is a common site for infarction due to red blood cell sickling. This results in recurrent tissue destruction in the spleen, which is a major immune system organ, and thus an immunocompromised state manifested by recurrent infections. The splenic damage becomes more pronounced later in life after multiple recurrent infarctions.*
C is incorrect. Although the thymus is a major lymphoid organ, its lack of development in sickle cell disease is not a common feature.
D is incorrect. Although the kidney can be damaged by infarction, it is unlikely to lead to immunosuppression since the kidney is not a major lymphoid organ.
E is incorrect. Although undernourishment can lead to immunosuppression, it is not the primary cause of immunosuppression in individuals with sickle cell disease.

Case 31–1

1. A is incorrect because injury to the pons will result in apneustic breathing.
B is incorrect because injury to the medulla would result in apnea.
C is incorrect because injury to the DRG would result in apnea.
D is incorrect because injury to the VRG would result in a prolonged inspiratory breathhold.
E *is correct because the phrenic nerve has been severed and the diaphragm has been paralyzed. Ventilation is now achieved by the (unopposed) contraction of the intercostal muscles.*

2. A *is correct because in the absence of diaphragmatic motion, there will be a reduced vital capacity and hypoventilation. The hypoventilation will result in a mild increase in* Pa_{CO_2} *and a mild decrease in* Pa_{O_2} *(with a normal Aa gradient). Maximal inspiratory pressure depends on normal muscle activity and will be decreased.*
B is incorrect because injury to the phrenic nerve is associated with a decrease in the vital capacity and muscle weakness that would result in a decrease in the maximal inspiratory pressure.
C is incorrect because in the presence of a reduced vital capacity, the P_{CO_2} would increase and the P_{O_2} would decrease. Absence of diaphragmatic muscle activity would also result in a decrease in the maximal inspiratory capacity.
D is incorrect because control of respiration is normal in this condition, and thus periods of apnea are unlikely to occur.
E is incorrect because the pons was not injured. Apneustic breathing is a sign of injury to the pons.

Case 31–2

1. A is incorrect because the snoring episodes with arousal that are reported are suggestive of obstructive sleep apnea, and the hypoxemia suggests that the process is severe.
B is incorrect because by history, this man has severe obstructive sleep apnea. Brief episodes would be compatible with mild obstructive sleep apnea.
C is incorrect because this man has obstructive sleep apnea, not the central sleep apnea associated with no attempt to breathe.
D *is correct because this individual has severe obstructive sleep apnea with the complications of cor pulmonale (right-sided cardiac failure) and polycythemia secondary to hypoxemia.*
E is incorrect because this man has severe obstructive sleep apnea with evidence of hypoxemia and hypercapnia.

Case 31–3

1. A *is correct because this woman has severe obstructive pulmonary disease with chronic hypercapnia. Her breathing is driven by hypoxemia. When her PaO_2 increases and the hypoxia is relieved, her minute ventilation decreases and her $PaCO_2$ begins to rise; 1 L of O_2 sufficiently relieves her hypoxemia without causing dangerous respiratory suppression.*
   B is incorrect because as this woman's PaO_2 rises, so does her $PaCO_2$. This demonstrates that her ventilatory drive is on a hypoxic and not a hypercapnic basis.
   C is incorrect because the respiratory rate decreases with an increase in O_2, suggesting that her rapid respiratory rate on room air is hypoxemia driven.
   D is incorrect because should this young woman go to sleep on 2 L O_2, the hypoventilation that normally accompanies sleep with a further increase in the $PaCO_2$ could result in marked acidosis with effects on the heart and sudden death.
   E is incorrect because this woman has a 15 mm Hg increase in PCO_2 on room air (55 mm Hg – 40 mm Hg). If this were an acute change, her pH would have fallen 0.12 (0.08 change in pH per 10 mm Hg change in PCO_2). Her pH is borderline normal, however. This could only have occurred had the CO_2 retention and respiratory acidosis been chronic and allowed renal compensation (retention of HCO_3^-).

Case 32–1

1. A is incorrect. Although the FVC and FEV_1 are reduced, the FEV_1/FVC is normal; thus, the subject does not have an obstructive disease. Also, the subject does not have a history of smoking.
   B is incorrect. Although the FVC and FEV_1 are reduced, the FEV_1/FVC is normal; thus, the subject does not have an obstructive disease. Also, the subject does not have a history of smoking.
   C is incorrect. Although the decreased FVC and FEV_1 with a normal ratio are suggestive of a restrictive disease, there are no indications of infection, such as a fever or increased white blood cell count.
   D *is correct. The patient does not have an obstructive disease because of the normal FEV_1/FVC. Her decreased FVC and FEV_1 would suggest a restrictive disease. She is at high risk for restrictive disease from silica exposure at her work.*
   E is incorrect. Although the FVC and FEV_1 are reduced, their ratio is normal; thus, the subject does not have an obstructive disease.
2. A is incorrect. Although interstitial hemorrhage, edema fluid, and a neutrophil infiltrate can be common features of specific types of restrictive disease, these are not characteristic of this type of occupational exposure.
   B *is correct. The alveolar macrophages can phagocytose the silica but cannot destroy it, resulting in a chronic progressive interstitial disease with characteristic granulomatous-like lesions and interstitial fibrosis.*
   C is incorrect. Although a predominant macrophage infiltrate is common in this type of occupational exposure, the interstitial hemorrhage and edema fluid are not.
   D is incorrect. Silica exposure is characterized predominantly by the large foamy macrophages, not a neutrophil infiltrate, although it can occur.
   E is incorrect. Silica exposure is characterized by a granulomatous response. The appearance of "bullae" is more characteristic of an emphysematous lung.
3. A is incorrect. The DLCO and lung volume will usually be decreased in an individual with restrictive lung disease.
   B is incorrect. The DLCO and lung volume will usually be decreased in an individual with restrictive lung disease.
   C *is correct. The DLCO and lung volume will usually be decreased in an individual with restrictive lung disease.*
   D is incorrect. The DLCO will usually be decreased in an individual with restrictive lung disease.
   E is incorrect. The lung volume will usually be decreased in an individual with restrictive lung disease.

Case 32–2

1. A is incorrect. The individual will have an obstructive disease due to poor mucociliary clearance and should have an abnormal FEV_1/FVC.
   B is incorrect. The FEV_1/FVC should be decreased with a normal DLCO.
   C *is correct. This patient would have a problem with mucociliary clearance because of dysfunctional cilia and will have an obstructive disease with a decreased FEV_1/FVC and a*

normal DLCO demonstrating normal surface area for gas diffusion.

D is incorrect. The DLCO would most likely be normal.

E is incorrect. The FEV_1/FVC should be decreased.

2. A *is correct. In obstructive lung diseases, the chest x-ray can appear quite normal except in the late stages, when the heart appears enlarged. Because this is a young man, the heart most likely will be of normal size.*

B is incorrect. In most instances, the chest x-ray appears normal in individuals with obstructive lung disease, although the heart can be enlarged in severe disease and after many years of being overworked. Also, it is common for individuals with obstructive lung disease to have concomitant viral or bacterial pneumonia (acute exacerbations), which may appear as infiltrates on chest x-ray. During episodes of acute exacerbation, the observed lung infiltrates are a result of the pneumonia and not the obstructive lung disease.

C is incorrect (see answer B).

D is incorrect (see answer B).

E is incorrect (see answer B).

Case 33–1

1. A is incorrect because the normal resting pressure in the lower esophageal sphincter is about 30 mm Hg. In this patient, the value measured is 60 mm Hg.

B *is correct because the elevated pressure in the lower esophageal sphincter at rest and after a swallow contributes to the dilation of the lower esophagus during a barium swallow.*

C is incorrect because decreased resting pressure in the upper esophageal sphincter would not account for the dilation of the lower esophagus seen on the barium swallow examination.

D is incorrect because increased pressure of the upper esophageal sphincter would cause difficulty of material entering the esophagus, whereas in this patient, the problem is the slow rate of material leaving the esophagus.

E is incorrect because reverse peristalsis would not cause dilation of the lower esophagus.

2. A is incorrect because the pressure in the lower esophageal sphincter is abnormally high both before and after a swallow.

B is incorrect because the high pressure in the lower esophageal sphincter is likely to have a neural component.

C *is correct because increased pressure in the lower esophageal sphincter is often associated with hypertrophy of the lower esophageal sphincter.*

D is incorrect because diffuse esophageal spasm is not consistent with the radiographic finding during a barium swallow, that is, dilation of the lower esophagus.

E is incorrect because there is no apparent malfunction of the upper esophageal sphincter.

3. A is incorrect because the improvement caused by dilation of the lower esophageal sphincter is often temporary.

B is incorrect because drugs that relax the lower esophageal sphincter might well alleviate the patient's swallowing difficulties.

C *is correct because surgical weakening of the lower esophageal sphincter may cause long-term improvement of the patient's swallowing.*

D is incorrect because another dilation of the lower esophageal sphincter would probably alleviate the symptoms again, but only temporarily.

E is incorrect because resolution of the patient's swallowing difficulties is unlikely to occur spontaneously.

Case 33–2

1. A is incorrect because the normal reflex relaxation of the internal anal sphincter is absent in a significant number of normal infants.

B is incorrect because the next step should be a suction biopsy of the mucosa since this does not require general anesthesia.

C is incorrect because the absence of ganglion cells in the submucosal plexus and the presence of enlarged nerve trunks in the mucosa would help confirm the diagnosis.

D *is correct because enlarged nerve trunks in the mucosa are characteristic of Hirschsprung's disease.*

E is incorrect because fasting should not cause improvement.

2. A is incorrect because eating solid food will not affect the underlying problem of lack of enteric nervous system in the terminal part of the colon.

B is incorrect because the disorder rarely improves with age.

C is incorrect because there is currently no effective drug therapy for Hirschsprung's disease.

D *is correct because surgical removal of the affected section of colon is frequently an effective therapy.*
E is incorrect because balloon dilation of the colon will not affect the underlying problems of the enteric nervous system.

3. A is incorrect because this might result in subsequent rupture of this part of the colon.
B is incorrect because only the aganglionic part of the colon need be removed.
C is incorrect because in most cases, an anastomosis of the unaffected part of the colon to the rectum proximal to the anal canal is effective.
D *is correct because there is no reason to remove the normal part of the colon and because of the effectiveness of the procedure described for C.*
E is incorrect because of the reasons stated for B and C.

Case 34–1

1. A is incorrect because HCl and gastrin are both effective secretagogues for pepsinogens.
B is incorrect because the duodenal mucosa is poorly protected against acid and pepsin.
C *is correct because pancreatic lipase is inactivated at a low pH, leading to steatorrhea.*
D is incorrect because the actions of gastrin, both on parietal cells and on ECL cells, are potentiated by acetylcholine.

2. A is incorrect because hyposecretors of HCl also have elevated gastrin levels due to lack of feedback inhibition of H^+ on gastrin secretion.
B is incorrect because if the diagnosis is correct, the patient has an ectopic gastrin-secreting tumor that will not respond to amino acids and peptides in the stomach and duodenum.
C *is correct because gastrin is trophic and increases the number of oxyntic glands and the number of parietal cells in the glands.*
D is incorrect because high rates of HCl secretion are rarely associated with gastric ulcers.

3. A is incorrect because treatment with an antagonist of somatostatin would still further augment HCl secretion.
B is incorrect because H_2 receptor blockers will reduce HCl secretion, but to a lesser extent than in a normal individual.
C is incorrect because sectioning these vagal branches would substantially diminish HCl secretion.
D *is correct because omeprazole directly inhibits H^+,K^+-ATPase; it will strongly suppress HCl secretion, even in the presence of elevated gastrin levels.*

Case 34–2

1. A *is correct because when cholesterol secretion into bile is high relative to the amounts of bile acids and phospholipids in bile, cholesterol gallstones tend to form.*
B is incorrect because hypomotility of the gallbladder frequently contributes to gallstone formation.
C is incorrect because mucus secretion enhances gallstone formation.
D is incorrect because nonsteroidal antiinflammatory drugs depress mucus secretion by the gallbladder and thereby decrease the likelihood of gallstone formation.

2. A *is correct because 70% of gallstones in the United States are cholesterol stones.*
B is incorrect because when gallstones contain Ca^{++} salts, they are radiopaque.
C is incorrect because ultrasonography is effective at detecting gallstones.
D is incorrect because the data do not rule out bile pigment gallstones.

3. A is incorrect because treatment with the bile acids would tend to dissolve cholesterol gallstones, but it would take many months or even years of treatment to dissolve stones 5 to 10 mm in diameter.
B is incorrect because this patient is a good candidate for lithotripsy based on the size of the gallstones and their lack of calcification.
C *is correct because treatment with an inhibitor of cholesterol synthesis would diminish the rate of cholesterol secretion into bile; in combination with other therapies, this would be useful.*
D is incorrect because gallstones recur in about 50% of patients who have previously had them.

Case 35–1

1. A is incorrect because the absorption of neutral amino acids from dipeptides and tripeptides is usually adequate to maintain good nutrition.
B *is correct because even though dietary niacin is above the minimum daily requirement, the patient is missing some of the large fraction of niacin that is synthesized from tryptophan.*

Since 60 mg of tryptophan is required to produce 1 mg of niacin, the patient will require doses of niacin much greater than the minimum daily requirement.

C is incorrect because with the absorption of neutral amino acids in dipeptides and tripeptides, plasma levels of the neutral amino acids will not be markedly reduced.

D is incorrect because high urinary levels of most neutral amino acids are the hallmark of Hartnup disease.

2. A *is correct because a diet richer in protein would improve the patient's protein nutrition and, by providing him more tryptophan, help remedy his niacin deficiency.*

B is incorrect because the intestinal transporter that is responsible for absorbing most of the neutral amino acids in the jejunum is defective in Hartnup disease.

C is incorrect because the disorder is recessive, so that both parents are most likely carriers and each of his siblings probably has 25% probability of having Hartnup disease.

D is incorrect because pellagra is, strictly speaking, due to a dietary deficiency of niacin. The patient is deficient in niacin but has a niacin intake in excess of the minimum daily requirement.

3. A is incorrect because the amino acid transporter that transports these amino acids across the brush border membrane of jejunum is deficient.

B is incorrect because glycine, methionine, and cystine are reabsorbed from the renal proximal tubule by other transporters that are not defective in Hartnup disease.

C *is correct because Hartnup disease is quite rare. It is highly likely that both parents are carriers since this is a recessive disorder.*

D is incorrect because the patient's ability to absorb dipeptides and tripeptides is not deficient.

Case 35–2

1. A is incorrect because pancreatic insufficiency is common in cystic fibrosis.

B is incorrect because cystic fibrosis is the most common autosomal recessive disorder, occurring in about 1 in 2000 live births.

C *is correct. Because of destruction of the pancreas in utero, the baby is likely to be deficient in pancreatic proteases and in pancreatic lipases.*

D is incorrect because a low-fat diet would exacerbate the baby's malnutrition.

2. A *is correct because the enzymes will improve digestion of fats, carbohydrates, and proteins.*

B is incorrect because decreased gastric acid secretion will decrease acid inactivation of pancreatic enzymes.

C is incorrect because absorption of fat-soluble vitamins is likely to be deficient.

D is incorrect because medium-chain triglycerides will be more completely digested and absorbed than long-chain triglycerides.

3. A is incorrect. Because of destruction and fibrosis of pancreatic tissue, as the child develops, there is an increased likelihood that islets of Langerhans will be destroyed and diabetes mellitus will ensue.

B is incorrect because there is no deficiency of brush border enzymes associated with cystic fibrosis.

C *is correct because ongoing destruction of acinar cells will release trypsinogen. In later life, when the exocrine pancreas is essentially gone, serum trypsinogen levels may be below normal.*

D is incorrect. Because of protein malnutrition, the baby may have decreased levels of plasma proteins.

Case 36–1

1. A is incorrect because the serum creatinine concentration is not normally dependent on changes in RBF.

B is incorrect because the serum creatinine concentration does not normally depend on urine output or volume, as this is determined by the need to maintain water balance. Only if renal failure were to occur, which is not the case in this woman, would a decrease in urine output be expected to increase the serum creatinine concentration.

C is incorrect because creatinine metabolism rarely changes other than in exceptional circumstances, such as loss of muscle mass or damage to muscles, neither of which occurred in this woman.

D *is correct because the serum creatinine concentration is inversely related to GFR.*

E is incorrect. The blood volume in this woman is increased because the ECF volume is increased. This would tend to decrease rather than to increase the serum creatinine concentration.

2. A is incorrect because prostaglandin causes vasodilation and thereby increases RBF. Therefore, inhibition of prostaglandin

production by nonsteroidal antiinflammatory pain relievers will allow sympathetic input to the kidney to go unopposed, induce renal vasoconstriction, and decrease RBF.

B *is correct because decreased prostaglandin levels would cause constriction of the glomerular arterioles, which would reduce GFR.*

C is incorrect because decreased prostaglandin levels would decrease GFR, which in turn could lead to a decrease in urine output.

D is incorrect because prostaglandins do not affect protein excretion, since they do not have an effect on the amount of protein in the glomerular ultrafiltrate or the reabsorption of filtered protein by the proximal tubule.

E is incorrect because even though prostaglandins can affect creatinine excretion by their effect on GFR, the decrease in prostaglandin levels seen with nonsteroidal antiinflammatory pain reliever use would tend to decrease, not increase, creatinine excretion.

Case 36–2

1. A is incorrect because the filtration rate of Na^+ is not affected by the integrity of the filtration barrier (i.e., Na^+ is filtered freely), and the amount of Na^+ in the urine is determined by its rates of reabsorption along the nephron.

   B is incorrect because the filtration rate of K^+ is not affected by the integrity of the filtration barrier (i.e., K^+ is filtered freely), and the amount of K^+ in the urine is determined by the rates of K^+ secretion and reabsorption along the nephron.

   C *is correct because serum albumin is not normally found in the urine. However, when the glomerular filtration barrier is damaged, the amount of albumin filtered increases and overwhelms the ability of the proximal tubule to reabsorb albumin. Thus, albumin appears in the urine.*

   D is incorrect because the filtration rate of creatinine is not affected by the integrity of the filtration barrier (i.e., creatinine is filtered freely).

   E is incorrect because the filtration rate of urea is not affected by the integrity of the filtration barrier (i.e., urea is filtered freely), and the amount of urea in the urine is determined by the rates of urea secretion and reabsorption along the nephron.

Case 37–1

1. A is incorrect because damage to the glomerulus would not increase the excretion of organic molecules (except protein). Glucose and amino acids are normally filtered freely and reabsorbed by the nephron.

   B *is correct because the proximal tubule is the portion of the nephron responsible for reabsorbing the organic molecules entering the tubular fluid via glomerular filtration.*

   C is incorrect because damage to the thick ascending limb of the loop of Henle would not result in the increased excretion of organic molecules, since they are reabsorbed by the proximal tubule.

   D is incorrect because damage to the distal tubule would not result in the increased excretion of organic molecules, since they are reabsorbed by the proximal tubule.

   E is incorrect because damage to the collecting duct would not result in the increased excretion of organic molecules, since they are reabsorbed by the proximal tubule.

2. A *is correct because a decrease in extracellular fluid volume will activate the renin-angiotensin-aldosterone system (see Chapter 38). Aldosterone will act on the collecting duct to increase the reabsorption of Na^+, the appropriate adaptive response (e.g., increase renal Na^+ reabsorption).*

   B is incorrect because ANP is secreted in response to an increase in the extracellular fluid volume. Also, ANP inhibits Na^+ reabsorption by the collecting duct.

   C is incorrect because urodilatin is produced by the kidneys in response to an increase in the extracellular fluid volume. Also, urodilatin inhibits Na^+ reabsorption by the collecting duct.

   D is incorrect because dopamine is released in response to an increase in the extracellular fluid volume. Also, dopamine inhibits Na^+ reabsorption by the proximal tubule.

   E is incorrect because hydrostatic pressure in the peritubular capillaries (P_c) will be decreased in the setting of reduced extracellular fluid volume.

Case 37–2

1. A is incorrect because the glomerulus is not a site of action of diuretics. Diuretics inhibit

specific membrane transport proteins along the nephron.

B is incorrect because the increase in fractional excretion of Na^+ observed does not reflect the fraction of the filtered load of Na^+ that is normally reabsorbed by the proximal tubule. In addition, if the diuretic were acting on the proximal tubule, it would be expected that the excretion of organic molecules and other ions reabsorbed by the proximal tubule (e.g., HCO_3^-, Pi, and K^+) would also increase.

C *is correct because the magnitude of the increase in Na^+ excretion is exactly what is expected for a diuretic acting on the thick ascending limb of Henle's loop.*

D is incorrect because diuretics that act on the distal tubule will not cause the degree of natriuresis seen with this agent. The distal tubule normally reabsorbs less than 10% of the filtered load of Na^+.

E is incorrect because diuretics that act on the collecting duct will not cause the degree of natriuresis seen with this agent. The collecting duct normally reabsorbs only a small percentage of the filtered load of Na^+.

2. A is incorrect because the Na^+-glucose symporter is found in the proximal tubule and because no glucose was found in the urine.

B is incorrect because inhibition of the Na^+-H^+ antiporter would likely be seen with diuretics affecting the proximal tubule. Also, inhibition of this transporter would result in the excretion of large amounts of HCO_3^- (see Chapter 40).

C *is correct because the $1Na^+,1K^+,2Cl^-$ symporter is responsible for NaCl reabsorption by the thick ascending limb of the loop of Henle, this diuretic's site of action.*

D is incorrect because the Na^+-Cl^- symporter is localized to the distal tubule.

E is incorrect because the Na^+ channel is localized to the collecting duct.

Case 38–1

1. A is incorrect because changes in Na^+ balance (e.g., decreased NaCl ingestion) usually lead to alterations in the volume of the ECF, not the serum [Na^+]. Hyponatremia most often indicates a disorder of water balance, not Na^+ balance.

B is incorrect because as noted, this man has a problem with water balance, not a problem with Na^+ balance.

C *is correct because hyponatremia indicates a problem with water balance. In this case, the amount of water excreted by the kidneys is less than the amount ingested. Also, this man's kidneys are producing concentrated urine, a finding that indicates ADH levels are elevated. This, in turn, prevents the kidneys from excreting water. The elevated level of ADH is unexpected because his body fluid osmolality is reduced ($2 \times [Na^+] = 260$ mOsm/kg H_2O), and his ECF volume appears to be normal. Therefore, he must have inappropriate secretion of ADH, probably caused by the infection in his lungs.*

D is incorrect even though a shift of water from the ICF to the ECF would cause the serum [Na^+] to decrease. However, this man has developed hyponatremia as a result of positive water balance. Therefore, the ECF becomes diluted, which causes water to move from the ECF to the ICF.

E is incorrect because the distribution of Na^+ between the ICF and ECF is maintained by the Na^+,K^+-ATPase. Because the activity of this transporter is not altered in this case, a shift of Na^+ from the ECF into the ICF is not expected.

2. A is incorrect because this man's ADH level is already elevated and causes reduced excretion of water. Administration of ADH would only make this situation worse.

B *is correct because this is a case of positive water balance, in which the ability of the kidneys to excrete water is impaired by inappropriately elevated levels of ADH. To reestablish water balance, water intake must be reduced.*

C is incorrect because as noted, water intake needs to be restricted. Increased water intake would make the hyponatremia worse.

D is incorrect because the man is in Na^+ balance. Therefore, altering NaCl intake would not correct the problem of water balance.

E is incorrect because as noted, the man is in Na^+ balance. Therefore, altering NaCl intake would not correct the problem of water balance.

Case 38–2

1. A is incorrect because the woman is in both positive water balance and Na^+ balance.

Water intake and NaCl intake must be restricted and not increased.

B is incorrect. Although restriction of NaCl intake would be beneficial in treating her ECF volume expansion, increasing water intake will intensify her hyponatremia.

C is incorrect. Although restriction of water intake would be beneficial in treating her hyponatremia, increasing NaCl intake would further increase the volume of her ECF and make the edema worse.

D *is correct. This woman is in positive Na^+ balance (presence of edema) and positive water balance (presence of hyponatremia) because the ability of her kidneys to excrete NaCl and water is impaired. Her heart failure has impaired tissue perfusion. As a result, her volume sensors are sending signals to the kidneys to reduce both NaCl and water excretion. To bring her back into balance, both water and NaCl intake should be restricted.*

E is incorrect because as noted, this woman is in positive Na^+ and water balance due to reduced excretion of NaCl and water by her kidneys. For balance to be reestablished, her current levels of NaCl and water ingestion must be reduced.

2. **A** is incorrect.

B is incorrect.

C is incorrect.

D *is correct because the ACE inhibitor blocks the conversion of angiotensin I to angiotensin II. As a result, angiotensin II levels decrease. Because angiotensin II inhibits renin secretion (negative feedback), renin levels increase after administration of the ACE inhibitor. Also, angiotensin-converting enzyme breaks down bradykinin, a potent vasodilator. After administration of the ACE inhibitor, bradykinin levels increase.*

E is incorrect.

Case 39–1

1. **A** is incorrect because frequent urination (i.e., an increase in urine flow rate) would tend to increase urinary K^+ excretion and cause hypokalemia.

B is incorrect because ketoacidosis would have no effect on plasma $[K^+]$. Organic acids such as the keto acids do not cause K^+ to shift out of cells.

C *is correct because increased plasma glucose levels would increase plasma osmolality. An increase in plasma osmolality causes K^+ to leave cells and thereby increase plasma $[K^+]$.*

D is incorrect because the presence of glucose and ketones in the urine produces an osmotic diuresis that would be expected to increase urinary K^+ excretion and cause hypokalemia.

E is incorrect because the patient does not have a metabolic alkalosis.

2. **A** *is correct because insulin promotes K^+ uptake into cells.*

B is incorrect. Although insulin corrects the ketoacidosis, K^+ will not enter the cells in exchange for H^+ as the ketoacidosis is corrected. Keto acids are organic acids, and they do not cause K^+ to be exchanged for H^+ across cell membranes.

C is incorrect because as insulin reduces the levels of glucose and keto acids in the plasma, their excretion by the kidneys will decrease. This will stop the osmotic diuresis, and as a result, excretion of K^+ by the kidneys will decrease. Thus, this would tend to increase, not decrease, the plasma $[K^+]$.

D is incorrect because stimulation of glucose uptake by cells will decrease, not increase, the plasma osmolality.

E is incorrect because insulin does not inhibit but rather stimulates the Na^+,K^+-ATPase.

Case 39–2

1. **A** *is correct because you would expect to see an increase in the serum $[Ca^{++}]$ and a decrease in the serum [Pi] as a result of an elevation of PTH levels.*

B is incorrect.

C is incorrect.

D is incorrect.

E is incorrect.

2. **A** is incorrect.

B is incorrect.

C is incorrect.

D *is correct because PTH stimulates Ca^{++} reabsorption only in the distal tubule.*

E is incorrect.

3. **A** is incorrect.

B *is correct because PTH decreases Pi reabsorption only in the proximal tubule.*

C is incorrect.

D is incorrect.

E is incorrect.

Case 40–1

1. A *is correct because this is a case of diabetic ketoacidosis due to the lack of insulin. The blood gas analysis shows that he has a metabolic acidosis with appropriate respiratory compensation, which is secondary to the generation and accumulation of keto acids that occurs when insulin levels are not adequate.*
   B is incorrect because the man is acidotic, not alkalotic.
   C is incorrect because with respiratory acidosis, the P_{CO_2} is increased. The laboratory data show a decreased P_{CO_2} consistent with respiratory compensation for a metabolic acidosis.
   D is incorrect because the man is acidotic, not alkalotic.
   E is incorrect. Although a mixed disorder composed of a metabolic acidosis and respiratory alkalosis would have decreased $[HCO_3^-]$ and P_{CO_2}, the history and laboratory values are more consistent with a simple metabolic acidosis with appropriate respiratory compensation.
2. A is incorrect because an increase in ventilation will decrease, not increase, his P_{CO_2}.
   B is incorrect because although hypoxemia stimulates ventilation, the man has a normal P_{O_2}.
   C *is correct because the normal respiratory response to a metabolic acidosis is to increase the ventilation rate (i.e., rapid and deep breathing) to reduce the P_{CO_2}. This respiratory compensation is mediated by the respiratory center's response to the acidosis.*
   D is incorrect because although this man reports "having the flu," there is no evidence that he has a lung infection. If he did have an infection that impaired gas exchange, he would probably have hypoxemia.
   E is incorrect because although aspirin can stimulate the respiratory centers, it does so only at doses exceeding the two tablets that he reported he took for his headache. Moreover, an aspirin overdose would more likely present as a mixed acid-base disorder.
3. A is incorrect because the decrease in plasma $[HCO_3^-]$ caused by the ketoacidosis decreases the filtered load of HCO_3^- in this man.
   B is incorrect because the activity and expression of proximal tubule H^+ secretory transporters are increased, not decreased, in this situation as a result of the systemic acidosis.
   C *is correct because the renal compensatory response to a metabolic acidosis is to increase the excretion of net acid. This occurs primarily through the production and excretion of NH_4^+. Moreover, expression and activity of the proximal tubule enzymes responsible for glutamine metabolism are increased by acidosis.*
   D is incorrect because collecting duct H^+ secretion is increased, not decreased, in this situation as a result of the systemic acidosis.
   E is incorrect because collecting duct HCO_3^- secretion is stimulated in alkalosis, not acidosis.

Case 40–2

1. A is incorrect because the woman is alkalotic, not acidotic.
   B *is correct because the loss of gastric contents from vomiting and the nasogastric suction has resulted in the development of a metabolic alkalosis. The arterial blood gas values also confirm the presence of a metabolic alkalosis.*
   C is incorrect because the woman is alkalotic, not acidotic.
   D is incorrect because with respiratory alkalosis, the P_{CO_2} is decreased. The laboratory data show an increased P_{CO_2} consistent with respiratory compensation for a metabolic alkalosis.
   E is incorrect. Although a mixed disorder composed of a metabolic alkalosis and respiratory acidosis would have increased $[HCO_3^-]$ and P_{CO_2}, the history and laboratory values are more consistent with a simple metabolic alkalosis with appropriate respiratory compensation.
2. A *is correct because the loss of gastric fluid has resulted in volume depletion. As a result, the kidneys are conserving Na^+. An important mediator of this response is the renin-angiotensin-aldosterone system (see Chapter 38). Because Na^+ reabsorption in the proximal tubule is coupled to the secretion of H^+, and Na^+ reabsorption is enhanced, all of the filtered load of HCO_3^- is reabsorbed. The elevated levels of aldosterone stimulate not only collecting duct Na^+ reabsorption but also intercalated cell H^+ secretion. As a result, HCO_3^- excretion is reduced, collecting duct H^+ secretion is*

stimulated, and urine pH is acidic. This occurs despite the presence of a metabolic alkalosis.

B is incorrect because as just described, proximal tubule H^+ secretion is enhanced secondary to the need for this nephron segment to increase its reabsorption of Na^+.

C is incorrect because although the plasma $[HCO_3^-]$ is increased, the glomerular filtration rate is reduced by the volume depletion. Therefore, the filtered load of HCO_3^- is probably decreased, not increased. Moreover, an increase in the filtered load of HCO_3^- would result in an alkaline urine, not the acidic urine seen in this woman.

D is incorrect because NH_4^+ production and excretion would be reduced secondary to the metabolic alkalosis.

E is incorrect because the most abundant urinary buffer is phosphate. Because phosphate is reabsorbed in the proximal tubule with Na^+ (see Chapter 39), less will be excreted in the setting of volume depletion.

Case 41–1

1. **A** is incorrect. A mutant receptor with a reduced affinity for hormone X or a decreased concentration of receptors for the hormone could be overcome by increasing the concentration of the hormone, as was the case in this patient. [XR], which initially determines the biological effect, can be increased by increasing [X] to overcome a decrease either in K or in [R] (see Equation 41–5).

   B is incorrect for the same reasons as in A.

   C is incorrect because an excess of a competitive antagonist (A), such as another hormone that cross-reacts with the same receptor to bind to the receptor but not generate a signal, can be overcome by increasing the concentration of hormone X. This would lead to more [HR] and less inactive [AR].

   D *is correct. If the patient's problem were inability to transduce the primary signal of hormone X because its second messenger could not be generated as a result of a severe lack of the necessary enzyme, then no amount of hormone X could be expected to elicit a normal response. The patient would be resistant to the hormone with a decrease in maximal responsiveness.*

   E is incorrect because if a mutant hormone X were altered in structure so that it could bind to the receptor but not generate a signal, then it would act like a competitive antagonist as in C.

   NOTE: In A through C and E, the patient would be resistant because of decreased sensitivity to hormone X. In all the answers, the lack of normal hormone effect would generate negative feedback on the gland of origin and thus increase the secretion and plasma levels of hormone X (as measured by immunoassay).

2. **A** is incorrect because the patient would need all the hormone X that he or she could possibly secrete to bind to a mutant receptor with decreased affinity for the hormone, so an inhibitor of secretion would be counterproductive.

   B is incorrect because when there is a deficiency of the receptor, a higher hormone concentration would increase the concentration of the hormone-receptor complex.

   C is incorrect because the effect of a competitive antagonist could be overcome by more hormone.

   D is incorrect because less hormone would only magnify the problem of generating too little second messenger.

   E *is correct because reduction of the level of mutant hormone X would allow greater access of genuine hormone X to its receptor binding sites and thus decrease the dose of hormone X that would be needed for therapy.*

Case 42–1

1. **A** *is correct because the avid hepatic uptake and conversion to glucose of this important gluconeogenic amino acid would exceed its release from protein stores.*

   B is incorrect because urine nitrogen levels would increase in the first 2 or 3 days, reflecting an increased protein breakdown. However, after another 10 to 12 days, metabolic adaptation to prolonged fasting would decrease protein breakdown to conserve body structure and function, and urine nitrogen would decline to a constant low level.

   C is incorrect because markedly increased lipolysis of stored triglycerides would raise plasma free fatty acid levels.

   D is incorrect because markedly increased beta oxidation of free fatty acids would raise plasma keto acid levels.

E is incorrect because plasma glucose level would be decreased. This would occur because the brain continues to use glucose despite the lack of exogenous carbohydrate and because the increase in hepatic production of glucose does not initially quite keep up with the substrate's use.

2. A is incorrect because 2550 g would require that he had expended a normal total of 2300 calories/day; however, he cannot move, so this is highly unlikely.
   B is incorrect because 1550 g would require that his basal metabolic rate had remained at a constant 1400 calories/day for the whole time.
   C *is correct because in a resting state, the metabolic rate would be about 20 cal/kg body weight, or 1400 calories/day. After about 3 days of fasting and a lower body temperature, the BMR would decline. Assuming a decrease in the BMR of about 10% to 1260 calories,* $(3 \times 1400) + (7 \times 1260) = 13{,}020$ *calories expended in the 10 days of fasting. At 9 calories/g, this would be provided by 1450 g of fat.*
   D is incorrect because the caloric value of 4 calories/g for carbohydrate was used in the final step of the calculation performed in C.
   E is incorrect because both the caloric value of 4 calories/g was used in the final step in the calculation and the value of 2300 calories/day was used as in A.

Case 42–2

1. A is incorrect because neuropeptide Y stimulates eating. An inactive mutant would cause decreased appetite, not obesity.
   B *is correct because an inactive mutant β-adrenergic receptor would prevent normal sympathetic nervous stimulation of obligatory thermogenesis in adipose tissue, thus preventing increased energy expenditure when even occasional ingestion of excess calories occurred. This could lead to obesity.*
   C is incorrect because an overactive leptin receptor would falsely report the presence of an excess of adipose tissue. This would stimulate downstream mechanisms to reduce adipose tissue, not increase it.
   D is incorrect because overactivity of UCP would increase thermogenesis and decrease adipose tissue mass.
   E is incorrect because lipoprotein lipase is required to transfer free fatty acid from circulating triglycerides into adipose tissue for reesterification with glycerol and storage. An inactive form of the enzyme would decrease fat storage.

2. A is incorrect. Theoretically, a single abnormal set point for appetite would have made weight loss more difficult, and such an abnormality could have been compensated for at least partially by an increase in energy expenditure for thermogenesis.
   B is incorrect because leptin secretion stimulated by a lower than normal adipose mass should cause lower than normal body weight, not obesity.
   C is incorrect because theoretically, a single abnormal set point for energy expenditure could have been compensated for at least partially by a decrease in appetite.
   D is incorrect because if UCP production was stimulated at a lower than normal adipose mass, this should cause a lower than normal body weight, not obesity.
   E *is correct because her return after weight loss to about her original weight suggests an abnormal set point for energy stores (i.e., adipose tissue mass).*

Case 43–1

1. A is incorrect because although her dietary protein intake is reduced, her endogenous protein breakdown is excessive as a result of the lack of insulin's inhibitory action on proteolysis. The carbon skeletons of the excess amino acids are used for accelerated gluconeogenesis, and the amino groups are incorporated into urea and excreted in urine.
   B is incorrect because plasma glucagon levels will be high in the absence of insulin's inhibitory action on glucagon secretion.
   C is incorrect because both free fatty acid and acetoacetate levels will be high as a result of the loss of insulin's inhibitory action on lipolysis and ketogenesis and as a result of elevated glucagon levels.
   D *is correct because the patient is almost certainly in diabetic ketoacidosis caused by insulin deficiency. To compensate for this metabolic acidosis, she is hyperventilating to excrete the extra* CO_2 *generated from* $NaHCO_3$*, which is used to buffer the large amounts of strong keto acids produced by the liver. Therefore, the* P_{CO_2} *will be reduced.*
   E is incorrect (see C).

2. A is incorrect because lipoprotein lipase activity will decrease, enhancing clearance of VLDL triglycerides from the plasma.
   B is incorrect because insulin will cause K^+ to move back into cells.
   C *is correct because lipoprotein lipase activity is stimulated by insulin. Therefore, plasma triglyceride levels will decrease, making A incorrect.*
   D is incorrect because the restoration of insulin will decrease adipose tissue lipase activity, in part by decreasing cAMP levels in that tissue.
   E is incorrect because insulin promotes phosphate uptake by cells. It also promotes glucose uptake.

Case 43–2

1. A is incorrect because this insulin/glucagon state will not promote lipolysis in adipose tissue and gluconeogenesis in the liver as efficiently as the state in D.
   B is incorrect for the same reason as in A.
   C is incorrect for the same reason as in A.
   D *is correct because to support prolonged aerobic exercise, this woman needed to mobilize endogenous substrates (i.e., free fatty acids, glucose) at maximum rates. This required a decrease in insulin levels and an increase in glucagon concentrations to promote lipolysis in adipose tissue and gluconeogenesis in the liver, respectively.*
   E is incorrect for the same reason as in A.
2. A is incorrect because the formation of fructose 6-phosphate (gluconeogenesis) would be favored over that of fructose 1,6-bisphosphate (glycolysis).
   B is incorrect because the activity of this key enzyme of gluconeogenesis would be increased.
   C *is correct because when insulin levels are deficient and glucagon levels excessive, the formation of fructose 2,6-bisphosphate is decreased. This favors the activity of fructose-1,6-bisphosphatase over that of 6-phosphofructokinase so that gluconeogenesis predominates over glycolysis.*
   D is incorrect because glucose-6-phosphatase activity would be high to catalyze release of glucose from the liver.
   E is incorrect because phosphorylase activity would be high to favor glycogenolysis over glycogen synthesis and prevent storage of glucose when glucose needs to be exported to the exercising muscles.

Case 44–1

1. A is incorrect because increased 1,25-$(OH)_2$-D would slightly increase plasma Ca^{++} levels. Both would then decrease PTH levels via negative feedback.
   B is incorrect because a decrease in PTH levels would lead to increased renal tubular Pi reabsorption and hence decreased urine Pi levels.
   C is incorrect because increased 1,25-$(OH)_2$-D and Ca^{++} levels would decrease 1,24-$(OH)_2$-D formation.
   D *is correct because Pi deficiency would decrease plasma and renal cortical Pi levels. This would increase 1,25-$(OH)_2$-D synthesis.*
   E is incorrect because bone formation would decrease as a result of lack of Pi for mineralization.
2. A is incorrect because the 1,25-$(OH)_2$-D increase would enhance the gastrointestinal absorption of Ca^{++}.
   B *is correct because 1,25-$(OH)_2$-D levels would increase secondary to Pi deficiency. This would tend to raise plasma [Ca^{++}], which with the rise in 1,25-$(OH)_2$-D values would decrease PTH levels.*
   C is incorrect because to the extent that the increased amount of 1,25-$(OH)_2$-D could increase bone resorption, this action would increase hydroxyproline excretion.
   D is incorrect because urine Ca^{++} excretion would increase, partly as a result of the decrease in PTH levels.
   E is incorrect because an increase in plasma Ca^{++} levels would increase calcitonin secretion.

Case 44–2

1. A is incorrect because urine cAMP levels would be increased by excess PTH action on renal tubular cells.
   B is incorrect because urine Pi levels would be increased by excess PTH action on renal tubular cells.
   C is incorrect because excess PTH would increase the differentiation of osteoclast precursors into active osteoclasts and increase their number.

D is incorrect because although excess PTH secretion stimulates bone resorption, the principle of coupling suggests that bone formation would secondarily increase.

E *is correct because excess PTH action on the kidney would decrease plasma Pi levels.*

2. A is incorrect because the sudden cessation of excess PTH-stimulated bone resorption would shift the balance to the coupled excess of bone formation. This action would "pull" phosphate out of the plasma into bone, and plasma Pi levels would decrease.

   B *is correct because nerve excitability had previously been suppressed by hypercalcemia and would increase rapidly. Plasma Ca^{++} levels might well drop below normal for reasons stated in C through E, and the patient might develop tetany.*

   C is incorrect because unopposed bone formation would also "pull" Ca^{++} out of the plasma, plasma Ca^{++} levels would decrease, the renal filtered load of Ca^{++} would decrease, and urine Ca^{++} concentrations would decrease (despite a decrease in the tubular reabsorption of Ca^{++}).

   D is incorrect because neither PTH nor Ca^{++} primarily affects the heart rate.

   E is incorrect because the loss of PTH would lower plasma Ca^{++} levels. Moreover, PTH does not directly affect the equilibrium between ionized and protein-bound Ca^{++} levels. However, withdrawal of the excess PTH would remove the hormone's inhibition of renal tubular HCO_3^- reabsorption. This would tend to increase the pH of plasma, which in turn would decrease the ionized Ca^{++} fraction.

Case 45–1

1. A is incorrect because IGF inhibits GH secretion.

   B is incorrect because IGF action inhibits GH secretion.

   C is incorrect because the combination of IGF-1 with its receptor mediates many of the actions on tissue growth of GH. E might also lead to a compensatory increase in IGF-1 levels, which would inhibit GH secretion via negative feedback.

   D *is correct because increased GHRH receptor activity would generate excess cAMP in the pituitary somatotroph, causing hyperplasia of somatotroph cells, excess GH secretion, and consequent tissue overgrowth.*

   E is incorrect (see C).

2. A is incorrect because GHRH release would be decreased through negative feedback.

   B is incorrect because IGF release would be increased by the action of excess GH.

   C *is correct because high levels of GH and its peripheral product IGF-1 would feed back negatively on GHRH neurons to decrease their activity and would feed back to increase the secretion of the GH inhibitor somatostatin. Both actions would have the effect of trying to decrease the excess secretion of GH.*

   D is incorrect (see A and B).

   E is incorrect because it does not take into account the regulatory pathways stimulated by GH.

3. A is incorrect because GH stimulates the production of some IGF-1–binding proteins.

   B *is correct because high GH levels stimulate protein synthesis, putting the patient in positive nitrogen balance. Hence, the amount of urea produced and excreted would be less than expected.*

   C is incorrect because GH is an antagonist to insulin action. Therefore, plasma glucose levels would be higher, not lower.

   D is incorrect because GH is an antagonist to insulin action. Therefore, compensatory plasma insulin levels would be higher, not lower.

   E is incorrect because although glucose normally suppresses GH secretion, it would fail to do so when GH is secreted autonomously by a tumor. Plasma GH levels may even rise paradoxically after a glucose load.

Case 45–2

1. A is incorrect because the loss of water would increase the serum concentrations of Na^+.

   B is incorrect because the loss of water would increase the serum concentrations of Na^+ and hence osmolality.

   C is incorrect because a water deficit of large magnitude would lead to a decrease in circulating blood volume and hence glomerular filtration rate, so blood urea concentrations would rise.

   D is incorrect because a low circulating blood volume would distend the cardiac atria less and decrease atrial natriuretic peptide production.

   E *is correct because the sudden onset of such severe polyuria strongly suggests traumatic hypothalamic damage resulting in ADH deficiency. In the absence of ADH, the kidney cannot conserve water, and the urine is very dilute (i.e., hypoosmolar).*

2. A is incorrect because cAMP is the second messenger for ADH action on the renal tubules, and its levels would increase in the urine.
   B *is correct because ADH has a vasoconstrictive effect through its V_1 receptor.*
   C is incorrect because water retention caused by ADH would decrease serum osmolality.
   D is incorrect because ADH has no significant effect on the metabolism of K^+.
   E is incorrect because ADH stimulates adrenocorticotropin and hence cortisol secretion.

Case 46–1

1. A is incorrect because it is a product of T_4, which is present in excessive amounts. There may be relatively less excess T_3 than rT_3 to compensate for the increased effects of the active T_3 metabolite on tissues.
   B is incorrect because it is a product of T_4, which is present in excessive amounts.
   C *is correct because exogenous T_4 will feed back negatively on the hypothalamus-pituitary axis to decrease TRH and TSH secretion.*
   D is incorrect because high levels of total T_4 will also increase levels of free T_4 unless thyroxine-binding globulin is also increased. If anything, this globulin may actually be slightly decreased.
   E is incorrect because high levels of total T_3 will also increase levels of free T_3 unless thyroxine-binding globulin is also increased.
2. A *is correct and largely accounts for the rapid heart rate.*
   B is incorrect because hyperthyroidism causes defects in generating ATP and leads to reduced stores of creatine phosphate.
   C is incorrect because the activity of the sympathetic nervous system is diminished by excess thyroid hormone, and this is reflected in lower levels of plasma norepinephrine.
   D is incorrect because thyroid hormone increases tissue use of O_2 and production of CO_2, which causes vasodilation and lowers systemic vascular resistance.
   E is incorrect because the vasodilation noted in D decreases the diastolic blood pressure.
3. A is incorrect because a low TSH level (see previous question) would decrease I^- trap activity.
   B *is correct because the low TSH stimulation (see previous question) would decrease the proteolysis of thyroglobulin and the release of T_4, so some colloid might initially accumulate.*
   C is incorrect because it is dependent on the action of TSH, so peroxidase activity, the height of thyroid epithelial cells, and thyroglobulin synthesis would all decrease eventually, since TSH levels remain low.
   D is incorrect for the same reasons as in C.
   E is incorrect for the same reasons as in C.

Case 46–2

1. A is incorrect because iodide deficiency could cause hypothyroidism and thyroid enlargement secondary to the elevated TSH. The patient's thyroid gland uptake of a radioactive iodide isotope would be increased.
   B is incorrect because loss of peroxidase activity could cause hypothyroidism and thyroid enlargement secondary to the elevated TSH. Thyroid uptake would be decreased because iodide could not be incorporated into tyrosine.
   C *is correct because the patient's skeletal maturation would be retarded, not accelerated, by thyroxine deficiency.*
   D is incorrect because water does accumulate in the tissues held by increased ground substance.
   E is incorrect because central nervous system development would be retarded in hypothyroidism.
2. A is incorrect because sensitivity to adrenergic stimulation would increase and so would heart rate, contractile force of cardiac muscle, and systolic blood pressure.
   B is incorrect for the same reasons as in A.
   C is incorrect because linear growth at the epiphyseal centers of long bones and consequently height would increase.
   D is incorrect because diuresis of excess interstitial water would occur, and enhanced lipolysis would decrease adipose tissue; both effects would contribute to an initial weight loss.
   E *is correct because O_2 use and CO_2 production would increase, necessitating increased ventilation.*

Case 47–1

1. A is incorrect because the high cortisol levels will bind to the type 1 glucocorticoid (mineralocorticoid) receptor in the renal tubules and stimulate K^+ excretion. As a result, serum K^+ levels would be decreased.
   B *is correct because ACTH is cosecreted with molecules that have melanocyte stimulating activity from a common precursor, proopiomelanocortin. Therefore, high levels of expression of the ACTH gene cause increased skin pigmentation.*
   C is incorrect because ACTH from the tumor is stimulating the adrenal cortex to secrete excessive amounts of cortisol. The cortisol suppresses both hypothalamic CRH and pituitary ACTH secretions via negative feedback.
   D is incorrect for the same reasons as in C.
   E is incorrect because the mineralocorticoid effect of cortisol expands extracellular fluid volume, and this effect would suppress renin.
2. A is incorrect because the zona fasciculata will be hyperplastic, not atrophied, from stimulation by tumor ACTH.
   B *is correct. Excessive amounts of cortisol from tumor ACTH have blocked the effects of CRH on the pituitary adrenocorticotrophs, causing suppression of their ACTH release and loss of CRH's trophic effect on these cells; hence, they atrophy and cannot immediately provide sufficient ACTH to meet the major stress of lung surgery. The patient's hypotension, fever, and anorexia reflect the resultant acute cortisol deficiency, as does the hyponatremia, which results from the retention of water given as intravenous infusions.*
   C is incorrect because ADH deficiency would cause hypernatremia, not hyponatremia, and it would not cause fever and anorexia.
   D is incorrect because the zona glomerulosa will be maintained via stimulation by tumor ACTH. However, renin and angiotensin levels will be decreased because of the expanded extracellular fluid volume.
   E is incorrect because the zona reticularis will also be hyperplastic from tumor ACTH stimulation. Dehydroepiandrosterone secretion may be excessive; because this steroid is largely an androgen precursor, it is likely to be the cause of the excessive hair growth.

Case 47–2

1. A *is correct because this patient probably has hyperaldosteronism secondary to reduced blood flow in the right renal artery. This would increase renin secretion from the juxtaglomerular apparatus of the right kidney, in turn increasing angiotensin levels and aldosterone secretion. The latter would increase renal K^+ excretion and lower serum K^+.*
   B is incorrect because it would be increased for the reasons stated in A. The elevated angiotensin level is causing the acute rise in blood pressure.
   C is incorrect because it would be increased for the reasons stated in A.
   D is incorrect because it would be increased for the reasons stated in A.
   E is incorrect because high aldosterone levels would cause Na^+ retention and elevated extracellular fluid volume. The increased pressure on the atrial myocytes would increase the secretion of atrial natriuretic peptide.
2. A is incorrect because Ca^{++} is involved in generating the effects of the increased angiotensin level on the zona glomerulosa and causing hyperaldosteronism.
   B is incorrect for the same reasons as in A.
   C is incorrect for the same reasons as in A.
   D is incorrect for the same reasons as in A.
   E *is correct because angiotensin does not work through cAMP as second messenger.*

Case 48–1

1. A is incorrect because cortisol acts via gene transcription, and this mechanism is unlikely to cause abrupt hypertension.
   B is incorrect because the bradycardia would be an uncharacteristic effect of epinephrine, which typically causes tachycardia.
   C *is correct because paroxysmal hypertensive episodes of such severity suggest sudden secretion of a catecholamine hormone. Norepinephrine causes extreme vasoconstriction, and the resultant hypertension activates baroreceptors and produces a reflex bradycardia. Stimulation of K^+ uptake into muscle cells would explain the slight hypokalemia.*
   D is incorrect for the same reason as in A.
   E is incorrect for the same reason as in A.
   NOTE: All three of the steroid hormones (those in A, D, and E) could produce the

hypokalemia by stimulating the excretion of renal K^+.

2. A *is correct because it would rapidly relieve vasoconstriction in the renal, splanchnic, and cutaneous vascular beds and lower the blood pressure.*
   B is incorrect because reduced cardiac contractility would not decrease the diastolic blood pressure, which prevails during two thirds of the cardiac cycle.
   C is incorrect because blocking the β_2 action could further decrease an already slow heart rate and might raise the blood pressure by leaving α_1 effects unopposed by the vasodilator action of the β_2 receptors.
   D is incorrect because α_2 receptors are primarily located not in blood vessels but in platelets and gastrointestinal cells.
   E is incorrect because the hypertension is not caused by an excessive amount of aldosterone; even if it were, the response to an aldosterone antagonist would be much too slow.

Case 48–2

1. A is incorrect because C peptide is released with insulin in response to hyperglycemia, not hypoglycemia. In addition, there would be no functioning β cells left after 40 years of type 1 diabetes.
   B is incorrect because although α cells of the pancreatic islets are innervated by the sympathetic nervous system, these cells can also respond directly to a low ambient glucose level by releasing glucagon.
   C *is correct because epinephrine release by the adrenal medulla requires stimulation by the sympathetic splanchnic nerve with acetylcholine as the preganglionic mediator.*
   D is incorrect because cortisol release depends on ACTH, not sympathetic nerve stimulation.
   E is incorrect because growth hormone release is modulated both negatively (β adrenergy) and positively (α adrenergy) by the sympathetic nervous system at the hypothalamic, not the peripheral, level. Hypoglycemia triggers growth hormone release by decreasing the release of somatostatin, an inhibitor of growth hormone secretion.
2. A is incorrect because growth hormone does not directly stimulate glycogenolysis.
   B *is correct because glucagon immediately stimulates glycogenolysis in the liver as well as the rapid release of glucose.*
   C is incorrect because cortisol does not directly stimulate glycogenolysis. Cortisol does increase gluconeogenesis, which would be necessary for a sustained increase in glucose.
   D is incorrect because insulin lowers blood glucose levels.
   E is incorrect because somatostatin would have counterproductive effects on the response to hypoglycemia by inhibiting glucagon and growth hormone release.

Case 49–1

1. A is incorrect because the patient has excellent breast development, which requires estrogen.
   B *is correct because the external genitalia are not masculinized and there is no pubic or axillary hair—all effects that require androgen action.*
   C is incorrect because the patient lacks a uterus and upper vagina. That is, antimüllerian hormone has been present to suppress development of the müllerian ducts into female internal genitalia.
   D is incorrect because FSH has no known direct effect on differentiation of the genitalia. In addition, the biological action of estrogen on the breast suggests FSH stimulation of either ovarian granulosa cells or analogous testicular cells.
   E is incorrect because there is no known effect of IGF-1 on genital patterning. In addition, the patient is of normal height, implying normal growth hormone and IGF-1 action.
2. A is incorrect because the patient would be very unlikely to have a high testosterone level and evidence of antimüllerian hormone without a Y chromosome.
   B is incorrect because a Y chromosome would direct formation of the testes, not the ovaries.
   C is incorrect because LH levels would be elevated as a result of lack of negative feedback caused by inactive androgen receptors in the pituitary.
   D *is correct because this explains the absence of androgen effects despite a high testosterone level. The high testosterone level has resulted from the lack of negative feedback by*

testosterone on pituitary gonadotrophs that are also missing a competent androgen receptor.

E is incorrect because the patient's well-developed breasts show the presence of estrogen receptors.

Case 49–2

1. A *is correct because although androgen stimulates the wolffian duct to develop into the vas deferens, it is local testosterone from the ipsilateral testis that is responsible. However, the patient has two X chromosomes, and no testes should be present. The patient probably has 21-hydroxylase deficiency (congenital adrenal hyperplasia), which was inadvertently treated for the first time with glucocorticoids at the age of 15 years. These suppressed the greatly elevated ACTH levels and reduced the high adrenal androgen levels, which had been suppressing LH and FSH secretion. Removal of these androgens permitted expression of her hypothalamic-pituitary-ovarian axis and menstrual bleeding.*

   B is incorrect because in an individual with two X chromosomes, ovaries will develop. Without testes, antimüllerian hormone will be lacking, and the müllerian duct will develop into a uterus and fallopian tubes.

   C is incorrect for the same reasons as in B.

   D is incorrect for the same reasons as in B.

   E is incorrect because this individual with two X chromosomes has had enough masculinization of her external genitalia since birth to have led to assignment of the male gender and to rearing as a male. Because there are no testes, the requisite androgen derives from the adrenal zona reticularis (see A).

2. A is incorrect because no steroid hormone directly causes skin to darken.

   B is incorrect for the same reason as in A.

   C is incorrect for the same reason as in A.

   D is incorrect because LH has no melanocyte-stimulating hormone activity.

   E *is correct because ACTH has melanocyte-stimulating hormone activity.*

Case 50–1

1. A is incorrect because the lack of the pubertal increase in testosterone level, stimulated by GnRH and LH secretion, leads to failure of the epiphyses (growth centers) to close. Hence, the long bones continue to grow slowly for years after the normal closure time of 15 to 18 years, leading to long arms and legs relative to height.

   B is incorrect because sexual differentiation occurs before the Leydig cells of the testes become dependent on fetal pituitary LH secretion stimulated by fetal GnRH. The testosterone necessary for the male pattern of external genitalia is secreted by the fetal testis in response to chorionic gonadotropin secreted by fetal placental cells.

   C is incorrect because the lack of pubertal testosterone and its product DHT would not allow the prostate to develop to even a normal size.

   D *is correct because lack of FSH to initiate spermatogenesis would lead to its absence and to small testes, since 80% of testicular volume is accounted for by the seminiferous (spermatogenic) tubules.*

   E is incorrect because without FSH, the spermatid stage of spermatogenesis is unlikely to be reached.

2. A is incorrect because testosterone produced in high concentrations by LH stimulation within the testis must synergize with FSH to initiate and maintain spermatogenesis.

   B is incorrect because neither it nor LH alone can sustain spermatogenesis. However, some men with this problem produce sperm if both gonadotropins are injected in proper doses with proper timing.

   C is incorrect because neither it nor FSH alone can sustain spermatogenesis. However, some men with this problem produce sperm if both gonadotropins are injected in proper doses with proper timing.

   D is incorrect because constant GnRH stimulation of the pituitary gonadotrophs down-regulates GnRH receptors and leads to LH and FSH deficiency.

   E *is correct because pulsatile stimulation of the pituitary will generate pulses of gonadotropins to the testis, which will result in the optimum intratesticular hormonal environment to initiate and support spermatogenesis.*

Case 50–2

1. A is incorrect because inhibin is a product of FSH action.

B is incorrect because there is presently no known relationship between FSH action and antimüllerian hormone secretion.
C is incorrect because inhibin has less of a negative-feedback effect on LH secretion than on FSH secretion.
D *is correct because FSH action on Sertoli cells would be lacking. This would lead to low inhibin levels. The lack of negative feedback of inhibin on the pituitary gonadotrophs would then result in elevated FSH levels.*
E is incorrect because FSH action on the testis has no direct effect on testosterone secretion.

2. A is incorrect because testosterone levels would remain normal with selective loss of FSH action but retention of LH action.
B is incorrect because LDL is increased by testosterone and both would remain normal, as in A.
C *is correct because without FSH, spermatogenesis would be reduced; hence, sperm count would decrease below normal.*
D is incorrect because red blood cell production is increased by testosterone, which is not deficient in this case.
E is incorrect because testosterone increases bone density, but testosterone is not deficient here.

Case 51–1

1. A *is correct because this is classic, stress-induced amenorrhea with increased CRH secretion suppressing GnRH release.*
B is incorrect because prolactin inhibits GnRH release.
C is incorrect because dopamine inhibits GnRH release.
D is incorrect because endorphin inhibits GnRH release.
E is incorrect because α-adrenergic pathways stimulate GnRH release.

2. A is incorrect because estrogen increases endometrial hyperplasia.
B is incorrect because estrogen increases vaginal epithelial cornification.
C is incorrect because estrogen increases secretion of an elastic cervical mucus.
D is incorrect because insofar as is known, there is no direct effect of estrogens on libido. Androgens are stimulatory. However, prolonged CRH excess might decrease the patient's libido.
E *is correct because the estrogen-sensitive ductal tissue of the breast would partly atrophy.*

Case 51–2

1. A is incorrect because progesterone helps elicit the LH surge and is required to support a conceptus.
B is incorrect because inhibin A is a product of the corpus luteum and is probably deficient in this woman.
C *is correct because the LH surge suggests that the patient probably ovulates, but after the ovum is fertilized, the zygote probably fails to implant. This suggests inadequate progesterone secretion from the corpus luteum. This causes poor preparation of the endometrium to support a conceptus adequately.*
D is incorrect because without a well-functioning dominant follicle, no LH surge would occur.
E is incorrect because a late rise in estradiol during the follicular phase is essential for an LH surge to occur.

2. A is incorrect because this is a normal finding on day 28, when corpus luteum functioning has normally just ceased and no dominant follicle has yet formed.
B is incorrect because this is a normal finding on day 1, when corpus luteum functioning has normally just ceased and no dominant follicle has yet formed.
C is incorrect because there is no notable variation in prolactin secretion during the menstrual cycle. Moreover, prolactin helps increase LH receptors, which would enhance corpus luteum function.
D *is correct because with a normally functioning corpus luteum, plasma progesterone levels would be greatly elevated on day 21.*
E is incorrect because plasma progesterone levels are at a relatively low point normally on day 7.

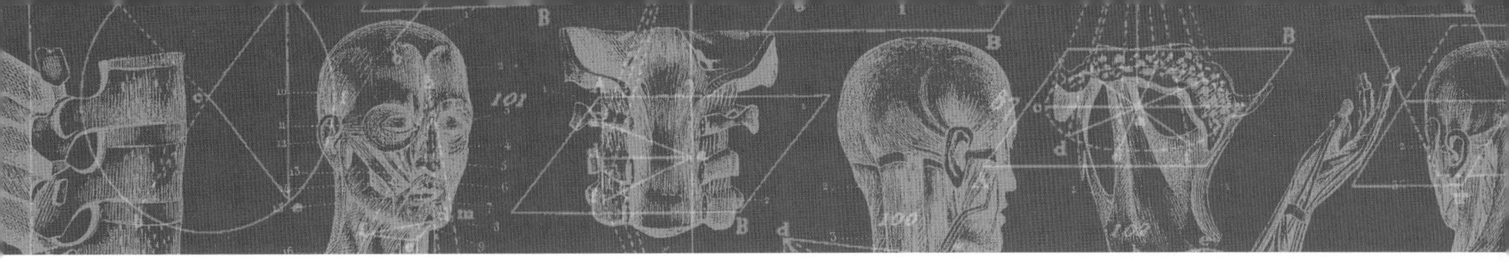

Index

Note: Page numbers followed by the letter f refer to figures, those followed by t refer to tables, and those followed by b refer to boxed material.

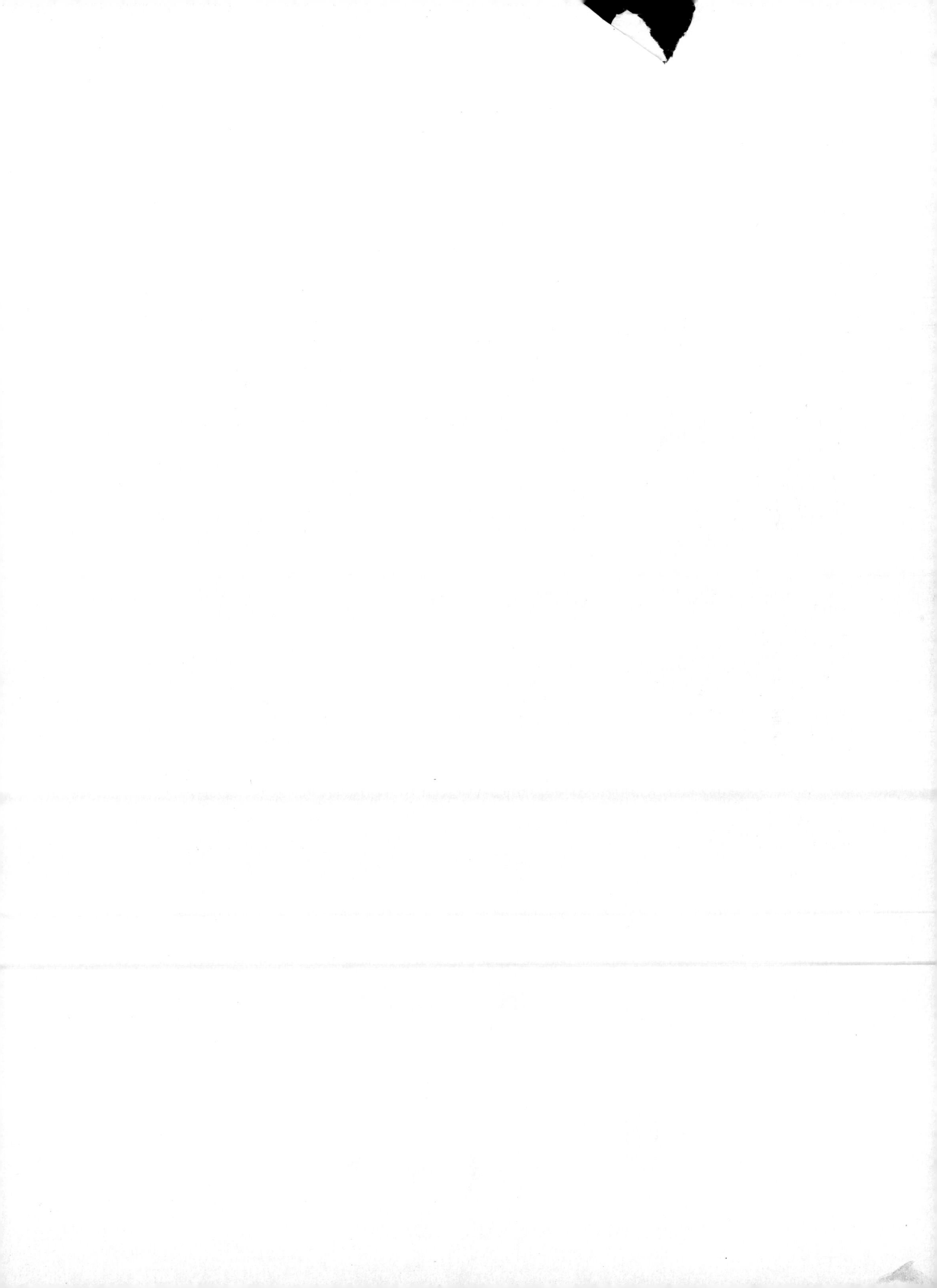